Second Edition

INFERTILITY

A Comprehensive Text

Prentice Hall International (UK) Limited, *London*
Prentice Hall of Australia Pty. Limited, *Sydney*
Prentice Hall Canada, Inc., *Toronto*
Prentice Hall Hispanoamericana, S.A., *Mexico*
Prentice Hall of India Private Limited, *New Delhi*
Prentice Hall of Japan, Inc., *Tokyo*
Simon & Schuster Asia Pte. Ltd., *Singapore*
Editora Prentice Hall do Brasil Ltda., *Rio de Janeiro*
Prentice Hall, *Upper Saddle River, New Jersey*

Library of Congress Cataloging-in-Publication Data

Infertility : a comprehensive text / [edited by] Machelle M. Seibel.
 — 2nd ed.
     p.   cm.
   Includes bibliographical references.
   ISBN 0-8385-4258-1 (Case : alk. paper)
   1. Infertility.   I. Seibel, Machelle M.
   [DNLM: 1. Infertility.   WP 570 I4305 1996]
 RC889.I556   1996
 616.6'92—dc20
 DNLM/DLC
 for Library of Congress   96-17607

Senior Managing Editor, Development: Kathleen McCullough
Production Service: Spectrum Publisher Services
Designer: Janice Barsevich Bielawa

Printed in the United States of America

ISBN: 0-8385-4258-1

9 780838 542 3

90000

This book is dedicated to my children, Amy Nicole, Sherry Renee, and Alexander Nathan who, by allowing me to experience being a parent, provided me with a clearer understanding of why infertile patients are so motivated to succeed, and to Bette McNamee, my administrative secretary for 16 years, who typed the first edition and most of the second edition of this book, and whose experience as a mother of five helped shape and mold a beautiful capacity to deal with people and with life.

CONTRIBUTORS

Reuwen Achiron, MD
Head of Ultrasound Unit
Department of Obstetrics and Gynecology
Sheba Medical Center
Senior Lecturer, Department of Obstetrics and Gynecology
Sackler School of Medicine, Tel-Aviv University
Tel Hashomer, Israel

Eli Y. Adashi, MD
Director, Division of Reproductive Endocrinology
University of Maryland Medical System
Professor, Departments of Obstetrics and Gynecology
  and Physiology
University of Maryland School of Medicine
Baltimore, Maryland

Lori B. Andrews, JD
Professor of Law
Chicago-Kent College of Law
Chicago, Illinois

Diane D. Aronson
Executive Director
RESOLVE
Somerville, Massachusetts

Mary Lou Ballweg
President and Executive Director
Endometriosis Association
Milwaukee, Wisconsin

Shalom Bar-Ami, PhD
Director of Embryology Research
Faulkner Hospital
Instructor
Harvard Medical School
Boston, Massachusetts

G. William Bates, MD
Principal Care Incorporated
Clinical Professor Obstetrics and Gynecology
Vanderbilt University
Brentwood, Tennessee

Joel H. Batzofin, MD
Director
Huntington Reproductive Center
Pasadena, California

Michael W. Berns, PhD
Beckman Lasar Institute and Medical Clinic
The Arnold and Mabel Beckman Professor
Professor of Surgery, Department of Surgery
University of California at Irvine
Irvine, California

Charla M. Blacker, MD
Director, In Vitro Fertilization-Embryo Transfer
Hutzel Hospital
Assistant Professor, Department of Obstetrics and Gynecology
Wayne State University
Detroit, Michigan

Richard E. Blackwell, PhD, MD
Professor, Department of Obstetrics and Gynecology
University of Alabama at Birmingham
Birmingham, Alabama

Richard A. Bronson, MD
Director of Andrology
Health Science Center
Associate Professor, Departments of Obstetrics and
  Gynecology and Physiology
State University of New York
Stony Brook, New York

Ivo A. Brosens, MD
Professor of Medicine and Gynecology
University Hospital Gasthuisberg
Belgium

William J. Butler, MD
Director
Section of Reproductive Endocrinology
Department of Obstetrics and Gynecology
Associate Professor
Medical University of South Carolina
Charleston, South Carolina

Diran Chamoun, MD
Fellow, Division of Reproductive Endocrinology
University of Maryland Medical System
Instructor, Department of Obstetrics and Gynecology
University of Maryland School of Medicine
Baltimore, Maryland

John A. Collins, MD
McMaster University Medical Centre
Professor
McMaster University
Hamilton, Ontario, Canada

Carolyn B. Coulam, MD
Director, Division of Reproductive Immunology
Center for Human Reproduction
Chicago, Illinois

F. Czyglic
Laboratoire d'Histologie-Embryologie
CECOS
Centre Hospitalier Kremlin Bicetre
France

Mark A. Damario, MD
Assistant Attending
Department of Obstetrics and Gynecology
New York Hospital–Cornell Medical Center
Instructor of Obstetrics and Gynecology
Center for Reproductive Medicine and Infertility
Cornell University Medical College
New York Hospital–Cornell Medical Center
New York, New York

Alan H. DeCherney, MD
Chairman and Professor, Department of Obstetrics
 and Gynecology
University of California at Los Angeles
Los Angeles, California

Paul Devroey
Clinical Director
Centre for Reproductive Medicine
Academisch Ziekenhuis
Vrije University Brussels
Brussels, Belgium

Michael P. Diamond, MD
Department of Obstetrics and Gynecology
Hutzel Hospital
Detroit, Michigan

Alexander M. Dlugi, MD
Director, Center for Reproductive Endocrinology
Atlantic Health System
Morristown, New Jersey

Alice D. Domar, PhD
Staff Psychologist, Division of Behavioral Medicine
New England Deaconess Hospital
Assistant Professor of Medicine
Harvard Medical School
Boston, Massachusetts

Professor R. G. Edwards, FRCOG, FRS
Emeritus Professor
Cambridge University
Cambridge, England

Asgerally T. Fazleabas, PhD
Professor
Department of Obstetrics and Gynecology
University of Illinois at Chicago
Chicago, Illinois

Rene Frydman, MD
Laboratoire d'Histologie-Embryologie
CECOS
Centre Hospitalier Kremlin Bicetre
France

Jeffrey Garber, MD
Chief, Endocrinology Health Center Division
Harvard Pilgrim Health Care
Beth Israel Hospital
Instructor in Medicine
Harvard Medical School
Brookline, Massachusetts

Isaac Z. Glatstein, MD
Reproductive Science Center of Boston
Deaconess-Waltham Hospital
Waltham, Massachusetts

Victor Gomel, MD
Department of Obstetrics and Gynecology
Vancouver Hospital Health Sciences Center
Vancouver, British Columbia, Canada

David S. Guzick, MD, PhD
Professor and Chairman
University of Rochester Medical Center
Rochester, New York

Karen R. Hammond, MSN, CRNP
Nurse Practitioner and Nurse Coordinator
Division of Reproductive Biology and Endocrinology
Department of Obstetrics and Gynecology
University of Alabama at Birmingham
Birmingham, Alabama

Mary G. Hammond, MD
North Carolina Center for Reproductive Medicine
Pittsboro, North Carolina

Andrew G. Herzog, MD
Director, Neuroendocrine Unit
Beth Israel Hospital
Associate Professor, Department of Neurology
Harvard Medical School
Boston, Massachusetts

Robert B. Hunt, MD
Clinical Instructor, Department of Obstetrics and Gynecology
Harvard Medical School
Boston, Massachusetts

Arye Hurwitz, MD
Senior Obstetrician and Gynecologist and Senior Lecturer
Hadassah University Hospital, Mount Scopus
Jerusalem, Israel

Scot M. Hutchison, MD
Department of Obstetrics and Gynecology
Johns Hopkins Hospital
Baltimore, Maryland

Howard S. Jacobs, MD, FRCP, FRCOG
Professor of Reproductive Endocrinology
University College, London Medical School
Middlesex Hospital
London, England

Ami S. Jaeger, JD
Attorney and Consultant
National Center for Genome Resources
Santa Fe, New Mexico

Sharon Heim Jette, RNC, MS, MPH
Nurse Practitioner
Private Practice
Andover, Massachusetts

Pierre Jouannet, MD
Groupe Hospitalier Cochin
Paris, France

Eric S. Knochenhauer, MD
Assistant Professor of Reproductive Endocrinology
  and Infertility
Assistant Professor of Obstetrics and Gynecology
University of Alabama at Birmingham
Birmingham, Alabama

Neri Laufer, MD
Chairman and Professor
Department of Obstetrics and Gynecology
Hadassah Mount Scopus University Hospital
Jerusalem, Israel

Gad Lavy, MD
Director
New England Fertility Institute
Stamford, Connecticut

Ingeborg Liebaers
Centre for Medical Genetics
University Hospital and Medical School
Vrije Universiteit Brussels
Laarbeeklaan, Brussels

Larry I. Lipshultz, MD
Professor, Scott Department of Urology
Baylor College of Medicine
Houston, Texas

Bruno Lunenfeld, MD
Professor Emeritus Endocrinology
Bar Ilan University
Tel-Aviv, Israel

Eitan Lunenfeld, MD
Professor of Endocrinology
Bar Ilan University
Tel-Aviv, Israel

Mary B. Mahowald, PhD
Assistant Director, Center for Clinical Medical Ethics
Professor, Department of Obstetrics and Gynecology
University of Chicago Hospitals
Chicago, Illinois

George B. Maroulis, MD, PhD
Professor and Director, Department of Obstetrics
 and Gynecology
Division of Reproductive Endocrinology
University of South Florida
Tampa, Florida

Colin R. McArdle, MD
Director of Obstetric and Gynecologic Ultrasound
Beth Israel Hospital
Associate Professor, Department of Radiology
Harvard Medical School
Boston, Massachusetts

Howard D. McClamrock, MD
Director, In Vitro Fertilization Program
Universitiy of Maryland Medical System
Associate Professor, Department of Obstetrics
 and Gynecology
University of Maryland School of Medicine
Baltimore, Maryland

Paul G. McDonough, MD
Department of Obstetrics and Gynecology
Medical College of Georgia
Atlanta, Georgia

Michael S. Mersol-Barg, MD
Director, Division of Reproductive Endocrinology
 and Infertility
Henry Ford Medical Center
Henry Ford Somerset Center for Reproductive Medicine
Assistant Professor, Department of Obstetrics
 and Gynecology
Case Western Reserve University
Troy, Michigan

Clarke F. Millette, PhD
Professor, Department of Cell Biology
 and Neuroscience
University of South Carolina School of Medicine
Columbia, South Carolina

Gilles R. G. Monif, MD
Professor, Department of Obstetrics and Gynecology
Creighton University School of Medicine
Omaha, Nebraska

David Morris, MA, MRCP
Division of Endocrinology
Royal Victoria Hospital
Associate Professor of Medicine
McGill University
Montreal, Quebec
Canada

Steven T. Nakajima, MD
Assistant Professor, Department of Obstetrics
 and Gynecology
Division of Reproductive Biology and Medicine
University of California at Davis
Davis, California

Camran Nezhat, MD
Director, Stanford Endoscopy Center For Training
 and Technology, Stanford, California
Director, Center for Special Pelvic Surgery
Atlanta, Georgia
Clinical Professor of Gynecology and Obstetrics
 and of Surgery
Stanford University School of Medicine
Stanford, California
Clinical Professor of Gynecology and Obstetrics
Mercer University School of Medicine
Macon, Georgia

Ceana H. Nezhat, MD
Director, Center for Special Pelvic Surgery
Atlanta, Georgia
Codirector, Stanford Endoscopy Center for Training
  and Technology, Stanford, California
Clinical Assistant Professor, Department of Obstetrics
  and Gynecology
Stanford University School of Medicine
Stanford, California
Clinical Associate Professor, Department of Obstetrics
  and Gynecology
Mercer University School of Medicine
Macon, Georgia

Farr Nezhat, MD
Director, Center for Special Pelvic Surgery
Atlanta, Georgia
Codirector, Stanford Endoscopy Center for Training
  and Technology, Stanford, California
Clinical Professor of Obstetrics and Gynecology
Stanford University School of Medicine
Stanford, California
Clinical Professor, Department of Obstetrics and
  Gynecology, Mercer University School of Medicine
Macon, Georgia

John Thomas Queenan, Jr, MD
Medical Director
Southeastern Fertility Center
Assistant Professor
Medical University of South Carolina
Mount Pleasant, South Carolina

Patrick Quinn, PhD, HCLD
IVF Laboratory
Alvarado Hospital Medical Center
San Diego, California

Zev Rosenwaks, MD
Attending Obstetrician-Gynecologist
The New York Hospital–Cornell Medical Center
Revlon Distinguished Professor of Reproductive Medicine
  in Obstetrics and Gynecology
Professor, Department of Obstetrics and Gynecology
Cornell University Medical College
New York, New York

Susan A. Rothmann, MD, PhD
Fertility Solutions Incorporated
Cleveland, Ohio

Joseph G. Schenker, MD
Director and Chairman, Department of Obstetrics
  and Gynecology
Hadassah University Medical Center
Professor, Department of Obstetrics and Gynecology
Hebner University of Jerusalem
Jerusalem, Israel

Eric K. Seaman, MD
Scott Department of Urology
Baylor College of Medicine
Houston, Texas

Machelle M. Seibel, MD
Medical Director, Faulkner Centre for Reproductive Medicine
Associate Clinical Professor of Surgery (Gynecology)
Harvard Medical School
Boston, Massachusetts

Daniel S. Seidman, MD
Department of Obstetrics and Gynecology
Sheba Medical Center
Tel-Aviv University
Tel-Aviv, Israel

Sherman J. Silber, MD
Director
Infertility Center of St. Louis
St. Luke's Hospital
St. Louis, Missouri

Alex Simon, MD
In Vitro Fertilization Unit
Hadassah University, Mount Scopus
Senior Lecturer of Obstetrics and Gynecology
Hebrew University School of Medicine
Jerusalem, Israel

Michael R. Soules, MD
Department of Obstetrics and Gynecology
University of California School of Medicine
Sacramento, California

Yona Tadir, MD
Beckman Lasar Institute and Medical Clinic
Professor, Obstetrics and Gynecology
Department of Surgery
University of California at Irvine
Irvine, California

Luther M. Talbert, MD
North Carolina Center for Reproductive Medicine
Cary, North Carolina

Seang Lin Tan, MBBS, FRCOG, FRCS(C), MMed(O&G)
Obstetrician and Gynecologist-in-Chief
Royal Victoria Hospital
James Edmund Dodds Professor and Chairman
McGill University
Montreal, Quebec, Canada

Patrick J. Taylor, MD
Department of Obstetrics and Gynecology
Saint Paul's Hospital
Vancouver, British Columbia
Canada

Togas Tulandi, MD, FRCS(C), FACOG
Director, Division of Reproductive Endocrinology
  and Infertility
Royal Hospital
Jewish General Hospital
Professor, Department of Obstetrics and Gynecology
Director, Division of Reproductive Endocrinology
  and Infertility
McGill University
Montreal, Quebec, Canada

Judith L. Vaitukaitis, MD
Division of Resources
National Institutes of Health
Bethesda, Maryland

E. Van den Abbeel
Academic Hospital VUB
Brussels, Belgium

André C. Van Steirteghem, MD, PhD
Scientific Director
Centre for Reproductive Medicine
Academic Ziekenhuis-Vrije Universiteit Brussels
Full Professor
Dutch-Speaking Brussels University
Brussels, Belgium

Ariel Weissman, MD
Senior Physician, In Vitro Fertilization Unit
Department of Obstetrics and Gynecology
Kaplan Hospital
Rehovat, Israel

Stephen J. Winters, MD
University of Pittsburgh Medical Center
Professor of Medicine
University of Pittsburgh School of Medicine
Pittsburgh, Pennsylvania

J. P. Wolf
Laboratoire d'Histologie-Embryologie
CECOS
Centre Hospitalier Kremlin Bicetre
France

Howard A. Zacur, MD, PhD
Theodore and Ingrid Baramski Professor
Johns Hopkins University School of Medicine
Director
Division of Reproductive Endocrinology
Department of Obstetrics and Gynecology
Johns Hopkins Hospital
Baltimore, Maryland

Moshe Zilberstein, MD
Faulkner Centre for Reproductive Medicine
Clinical Instructor, Department of Gynecology (Surgery)
Harvard Deaconess Surgical Program
Boston, Massachusetts

CONTENTS

Preface xv
Foreword xvii

PART I. EVALUATION OF INFERTILITY 1

1. Diagnostic Evaluation of an Infertile Couple 3
   Machelle M. Seibel

2. Emotional Aspects of Infertility 29
   Alice D. Domar, Machelle M. Seibel

3. Semen Analyis: A Practical Guide to Performance
   and Interpretation 45
   Susan A. Rothmann

4. Endocrine Testing in Infertility 59
   Shalom Bar-Ami

PART II. ENDOCRINOLOGY OF FEMALE INFERTILITY 79

5. Oocyte Development and Meiosis in Humans 81
   Shalom Bar-Ami, Machelle M. Seibel

6. Anovulation and Amenorrhea 111
   Judith L. Vaitukaitis

7. Polycystic Ovary Syndrome 121
   Howard S. Jacobs

8. Luteal-Phase Inadequacy .135
   Steven T. Nakajima, Michael R. Soules

9. Prolactin Disorders in Infertility 155
   Richard E. Blackwell, Karen R. Hammond,
   Eric S. Knochenhauer

10. Thyroid Disorders and Reproduction 171
    Jeffrey Garber

PART III. ENDOMETRIOSIS 187

11. Pathophysiology and Medical Treatment
    of Endometriosis-Associated Infertility 189
    Ivo A. Brosens

12. Endometriosis: Surgical Treatment 203
    Camran Nezhat, Farr Nezhat, Ceana H. Nezhat,
    Daniel S. Seidman

PART IV. MALE INFERTILITY 219

13. Reproductive Physiology of Men 221
    Clarke F. Millette

14. Relationship of Abnormal Semen Values
    to Male-Factor Infertility .253
    Sherman J. Silber

15. Pathogenesis and Medical Management
    of Male Infertility 261
    Stephen J. Winters

16. Surgical Management of Male-Factor
    Infertility 277
    Sherman J. Silber

17. Assisted Reproductive Treatments
    of Oligospermia 297
    Joel H. Batzofin, Eric K. Seaman, Larry I. Lipshultz

18. Therapeutic Insemination 309
    Mary G. Hammond, Luther M. Talbert

PART V. SPECIFIC CATEGORIES OF INFERTILITY 321

19. Unexplained Infertility 323
    John A. Collins

20. Immunology 341
    Richard A. Bronson

21. Infections 359
    Gilles R. G. Monif

22. Molecular Genetics and Infertility 371
    William J. Butler, Paul G. McDonough

23. Genetic Issues in Reproduction 387
    Moshe Zilberstein, Machelle M. Seibel

24. Neurologic Considerations 397
    Andrew G. Herzog

25. Body Weight and Reproduction 409
    G. William Bates

26. Recurrent Pregnancy Loss 417
    Carolyn B. Coulam

27. Aging and Reproduction 435
    George B. Maroulis

PART VI. ULTRASOUND 445

28. Ultrasound in Infertility 447
    Ariel Weissman, Colin R. McArdle, Reuwen Achiron

PART VII. HORMONAL TREATMENT
         OF INFERTILITY OF WOMEN 493

29. Ovulation Initiation with Clomiphene Citrate 495
    *Diran Chamoun, Howard D. McClamrock,
    Eli Y. Adashi*

30. Ovulation Induction with Human
    Menopausal Gonadotropin 507
    Bruno Lunenfeld, Eitan Lunenfeld

31. Ovulation Induction with
    Follicle-Stimulating Hormone 525
    Machelle M. Seibel

32. The Role of Gonadotropin-Releasing Hormone
    and Its Agonists in Infertility 537
    Seang Lin Tan, David Morris, Togas Tulandi

33. Treatment of Infertility with Dopamine Agonists 557
    Scot M. Hutchison, Howard A. Zacur

PART VIII. SURGICAL TREATMENT
          OF FEMALE-FACTOR INFERTILITY 571

34. Diagnostic and Operative Hysteroscopy 573
    Patrick J. Taylor, Victor Gomel

35. Operative Laparoscopy 591
    Robert B. Hunt

36. Technical Aspects of Tubal Surgery by Means
    of Laparotomy 611
    Robert B. Hunt

37. Laser Physics and Applications
    in Reproductive Medicine 629
    Yona Tadir, Michael W. Berns

38. Diagnosis and Management
    of Ectopic Pregnancy 643
    Michael P. Diamond, Gad Lavy, Alan H. DeCherney

39. Pelvic Adhesions and Infertility 655
    Charla M. Blacker, Michael P. Diamond

PART IX. REPRODUCTIVE TECHNOLOGY 669

40. Embryo-Uterine Interactions
    During Implantation 671
    *John Thomas Queenan, Jr.,
    Asgerally T. Fazleabas*

41. Gamete Intrafallopian Transfer 687
    *Alexander M. Dlugi, Michael S. Mersol-Barg,
    Machelle M. Seibel*

42. In Vitro Fertilization 703
    *Neri Laufer, Alex Simon, Arye Hurwitz,
    Isaac Z. Glatstein*

43. Assisted Fertilization Techniques 751
    *André C. Van Steirteghem, Ingeborg Liebaers,
    Paul Devroey*

44. Preimplantation Genetics and
    Preimplantation Diagnosis 761
    Moshe Zilberstein, Machelle M. Seibel

45. Ovum Donation 773
    Mark A. Damario, Zev Rosenwaks

46. Cryopreservation and Infertility 793
    *Patrick Quinn, Pierre Jouannet, Rene Frydman,
    André C. Van Steirteghem, J. P. Wolf, F. Czyglik,
    E. Van den Abbeel*

47. Legal Aspects of Infertility 807
    Lori B. Andrews, Ami S. Jaeger

48. Ethical Considerations in Infertility 823
    Mary B. Mahowald

49. Religious Aspects of Reproduction 829
    Joseph G. Schenker

PART X. ADOPTION 843

50. The Adoption Alternative 845
    Sharon Heim Jette

PART XI. PATIENT PERSPECTIVES 851

51. RESOLVE: Patient Support for the
    Infertility Experience 853
    Diane D. Aronson

52. Endometriosis and Infertility:
    The Patient Perspective 859
    Mary Lou Ballweg

PART XII. STATISTICS 873

53. Statistical Analysis of Infertility Data 875
    David S. Guzick

Index 887

PREFACE

As we approach the second millennium, infertility diagnosis and treatment stands out as one of the most rapidly evolving areas in medicine. Recombinant technology has changed the way gonadotropins are manufactured, micromanipulation has altered our approach to male-factor infertility, molecular genetics has transformed infertility techniques into preventive measures for inherited diseases, and egg donation has blurred the limits of the reproductive lifespan. It is no wonder that all of these advances have simultaneously evoked enormous emotional, ethical, and legal considerations.

Although many excellent reproductive endocrinology textbooks relegate infertility to a single chapter or section, my goal in this second edition of *Infertility: A Comprehensive Text* was to utilize reproductive physiology and endocrinology as a vehicle for understanding infertility and its treatments. As in the first edition, I have incorporated both endocrine and surgical aspects of male and female infertility and have provided individual chapters on each of the ovulatory-inducing drugs. To address the enormous expansion in molecular biology, I have expanded the one chapter on genetics and molecular biology into three separate chapters on genetic counseling, preimplantation genetic diagnosis, and a basic discussion of molecular biology. Chapters on the importance of weight, religion, and aging on infertility have also been added along with updated chapters on immunology, ultrasound, infections, neurologic considerations, the emotional, legal, and ethical aspects of infertility,

adoption, and statistical analysis of infertility data. The surgical section has been expanded to include a chapter on adhesion prevention. A chapter has also been added on both andrology and endocrine laboratory testing to explain and better understand the methodology and significance of ordered tests. I have also invited two important consumer groups, RESOLVE and the Endometriosis Association, to define their services and roles for patients experiencing infertility.

I am proud of and grateful to each of my contributors. Many of their names are synonymous with the topics they wrote about. Each one conveyed their knowledge and experience clearly. Their ability to convey current thinking and insights is superb.

As in the first edition of this book, a decision tree was used at the beginning of each chapter where applicable. Illustrations and tables were used throughout to clarify key points. Descriptive chapters, such as those explaining surgical techniques and the chapter on ultrasound, made particularly abundant use of illustrations.

The end result of our efforts is a current, authoritative, and comprehensive textbook written for the medical student, resident, fellow, or practicing clinician in numerous specialties caring for infertile patients. It is my express hope that, as with the first edition, readers will find this resource useful and stimulating.

Machelle M. Seibel, MD

FOREWORD

Everyone is aware that there are now many single-authored and multiauthored books on assisted human conception. The plethora of such books is no handicap to editors, authors, or readers, because this field of study has virtually exploded since the first child was born as a result of in vitro fertilization in 1978. Where there once were queues of patients attending the few available infertility clinics, often returning time and time again for simple and frequently ineffective treatments, there are now numerous clinics worldwide offering the most advanced techniques. This revolution in the treatment of infertility has come about through a series of novel discoveries in many aspects of the field and through the introduction of new methods or the elaboration of existing methods. Consequently, a rapidly expanding and comprehensive system of infertility treatments is now available to patients suffering from their own individual problems. The result of this vast expansion of infertility services is the need for practitioners in the field to have readily available a constant stream of new books for training purposes and to update their knowledge.

This textbook is therefore most welcome. It gives numerous experts in the field of infertility management the opportunity to expound their most recent medical and surgical concepts within a largely clinical framework. The text provides both theoretical and practical advice about a whole variety of conditions associated with infertility in both men and women. The chapter authors are highly distinguished in their areas of expertise, and each of them has considerable experience in the field of assisted human conception and has made his or her own special contribution to it. This book will be welcome internationally both in countries where in vitro fertilization has been practiced over many years and in developing nations where the number of clinics treating infertility continues to expand. The text presents current, tried, and tested treatments of infertility along with new and rapidly advancing concepts. All the subdisciplines involved in assisted human conception are represented fairly, so that a comprehensive approach to the alleviation of infertility is provided. Some of the newer disciplines, such as the preimplantation diagnosis of genetic disease in human embryos and the application of laser physics to reproductive medicine, make their own distinctive mark on the book.

This is the second edition of *Infertility: A Comprehensive Text*. The first edition was just published in 1990. The ongoing, extremely rapid advances in the field of reproductive medicine, and the incursion of molecular genetics into it, will doubtless soon create the need for a third edition. This headlong pace is likely to continue for many years to come since, in one sense, reproductive medicine is entering new domains. In effect, the years since 1981 have involved a period of catching up on a preexisting science. Many currently used clinical and laboratory methods can be identified in scientific studies in the field of reproductive medicine published as long ago as 1986 or even 1976. Two such examples are studies on micromanipulative techniques in mammalian fertilization and the preimplantation diagnosis of genetic disease, which were published in the 1960s and 1970s by investigators working with laboratory or domestic species. Earlier investigators would not have had much difficulty coming to terms with many modern forms of ovarian stimulation, at least until recently.

This situation, however, does not hold true today. Many clinical studies in humans now are further advanced than scientific studies in animals. The pace of change has accelerated, being sustained by the urgent need of clinicians to bring the newest, best, and safest treatments to their patients. Clinical studies have become highly sophisticated since 1976 and clinicians now work side-by-side with scientists in most hospitals and units to the benefit of both. The introduction of gonadotropin-releasing hormone agonists and antagonists, for example, is transforming the concepts of ovarian stimulation and the new recombinant hormones could well demand a revolution in our thinking. The astounding clinical success of Intracytoplasmic sperm injection (ICSI) could not have been foreseen by our teachers, even if the details of the technique itself would not have occasioned much surprise among them. New scientific advances are now rapidly translated into both applied and clinical work, unlike the older days.

We live today in a world where fundamental knowledge is essential in many clinical assisted human reproduction situations. Consequently, new interdisciplinary books are needed for new interdisciplinary people. The second edition of *Infer-*

tility: A Comprehensive Text is therefore most timely and, as its title states, comprehensive. It will appeal to the in vitro scientist as much as to the clinician who is treating patients. I wish it well.

Professor R. G. Edwards, FRCOG, FRS

Second Edition

INFERTILITY

A Comprehensive Text

PART I

Evaluation of Infertility

CHAPTER 1

Diagnostic Evaluation of an Infertile Couple

MACHELLE M. SEIBEL

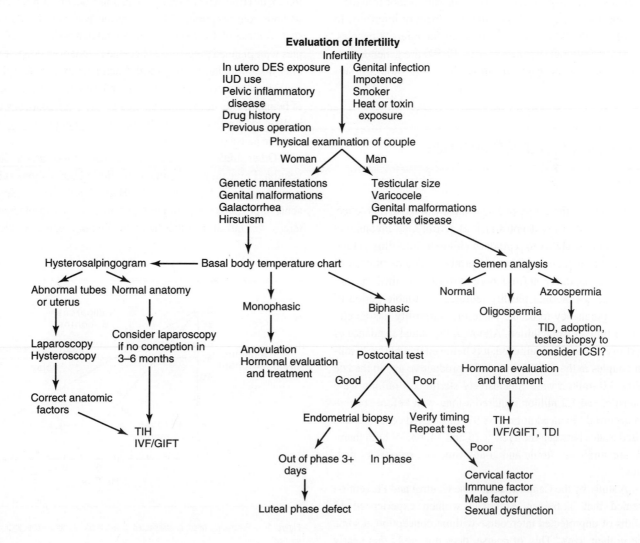

Evaluation of Infertility

Infertility

In utero DES exposure / Genital infection
IUD use / Impotence
Pelvic inflammatory / Smoker
 disease / Heat or toxin
Drug history / exposure
Previous operation

Physical examination of couple

Woman / Man

Genetic manifestations / Testicular size
Genital malformations / Varicocele
Galactorrhea / Genital malformations
Hirsutism / Prostate disease

Hysterosalpingogram ← Basal body temperature chart / Semen analysis

Abnormal tubes / Normal anatomy / Monophasic / Biphasic / Normal / Oligospermia / Azoospermia
or uterus

Laparoscopy / Consider laparoscopy / Anovulation / Postcoital test / TID, adoption,
Hysteroscopy / if no conception in / Hormonal evaluation / testes biopsy to
 / 3–6 months / and treatment / Good / Poor / Hormonal evaluation / consider ICSI?
 / and treatment

Correct anatomic / Endometrial biopsy / Verify timing / TIH
factors / Repeat test / IVF/GIFT, TDI

TIH / Out of phase 3+ / In phase / Poor
IVF/GIFT / days

Luteal phase defect / Cervical factor
 / Immune factor
 / Male factor
 / Sexual dysfunction

3

The desire to reproduce is an intensely motivating human force. After all, it is through our children that we attain a measure of immortality. Because of its personal nature, couples may also experience strong religious, cultural, and societal pressures to conceive. Therefore, it is understandable that people experiencing infertility often perceive it as a serious life crisis.

This central role of reproduction in the human experience has contributed greatly to the desire of couples to overcome infertility. To some extent, it has led to the rapid evolution of technologic advances in reproductive biology. Few, if any, other specialty fields have given rise to so many emotional, ethical, and legal considerations. Advances in diagnosis and treatment have led many physicians to believe that all infertility must be treated by a subspecialist. This notion is compounded by the fact that experts themselves disagree on the best management. The literature also has produced confusion; results of similar trials often are inconsistent, and controls are not always included. Nevertheless, if an obstetrician-gynecologist, family practitioner, or urologist has a clear understanding of the basic principles, there is no reason why he or she cannot provide a large portion of diagnosis and initial treatment of infertility. In fact, of the 45,600 physicians who care for infertile couples, 20,000 are obstetrician-gynecologists, 12,500 are generalists or family practitioners, 6100 are urologists, and 1400 are surgeons.[1]

GENERAL PRINCIPLES OF INFERTILITY CARE

Definition

Fertility denotes the ability of a man and a woman to reproduce. Conversely, infertility denotes lack of fertility, an involuntary reduction in the ability to reproduce children. Infertility is relative; sterility is total inability to reproduce. The definitions of these words are different from those of most other medical conditions because normal fertility requires a variable period of time for pregnancy to occur. Therefore, infertility has an element of time in its definition. Although the actual incidence of infertility can only be estimated, it is believed that of the 28 million couples in the United States of reproductive age in the late 1980s, 3.0 million were conclusively sterile, 2.8 million were subfertile, and 1.2 million required a long wait before conception occurred.[2] In an additional 38.9% of married couples in the United States between the ages of 15 and 44, one or both members are surgically sterile and at any time can reconsider their status.[1]

A study by the Centers for Disease Control and Prevention revealed that 32.6% of American women experienced 12 months of unprotected intercourse without conception at some time in their lives.[3] This, of course, does not imply that nearly one third of U.S. couples are infertile. The same study revealed that 20.6% of women experienced at some time 2 years of unprotected intercourse without conception. However, only 12.5% stated that they had tried to conceive for 2 years, and only 9.6% sought medical attention about the condition. Studies such as this one illustrate the need to ask specific questions about motivation and use of health services when defining and measuring infertility. They also demonstrate that the prevalence of infertility has not increased since 1965. Infertility rates in that year, adjusted to exclude both surgically sterilized women and those who had a hysterectomy, revealed the prevalence to be 13.3% compared with 13.9% in 1982 and 13.7% in 1988. That the absolute number of 500,000 women with primary infertility in 1965 doubled to 1 million in 1988 appears in large part caused by the baby-boom generation's reaching childbearing age or choosing to start their families after voluntary delays.[4]

The widely accepted definition proposed by the American Fertility Society states that "a marriage is to be considered barren or infertile when pregnancy has not occurred after coitus without contraception." This definition was based on studies such as those of Tietze et al,[5] who found that 90% of 1727 couples with planned pregnancies became pregnant in the first year after discontinuing birth control. Such a study suggests that a couple not achieving pregnancy after 1 year has a 90% chance of being outside the norm. Examination of these couples would be likely to uncover a clinically significant and potentially correctable cause of the infertility.

Other studies caution physicians against too early an intervention. Pregnancy rates among unselected populations follow a predictable pattern (Fig 1–1). Half of nulliparous patients achieve pregnancy within the first 5 months of unprotected intercourse. Half of the other half who are not pregnant at the be-

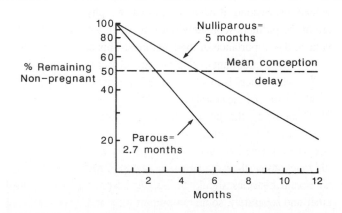

Figure 1–1. Pregnancy rates in unselected populations of nulliparous and parous women.

ginning of each subsequent 5 months will remain nonpregnant.[6] Therefore, among 1000 unselected nulliparous women, 500 will remain nongravid after 5 months, 250 after 10 months, and 125 after 15 months. Women who have already completed one or more pregnancies follow a similar, more rapid and predictable pattern. From these figures it follows that if patients were considered to have an infertility problem after only 5 or even 10 months, a large cure rate could be obtained without treatment. It is imperative to share this information with couples at their initial interview. It also underscores the need for necessary controls in all treatment of infertility. Finally, it implies that at least 5 months are required for any treatment regimen to be considered having been given a reasonable trial toward correcting a problem contributing to infertility. This concept is important because the number of annual office visits for infertility in the United States has risen from 600,000 in 1968 to 2 million in the 1990s. Couples with primary infertility are about twice as likely to seek medical attention as those with secondary infertility (51.2% versus 22.4%).

The Couple as a Unit

To evaluate adequately the potential of a couple to achieve pregnancy, the physician must from the outset view the couple as a unit. Individuals are often neither "fertile" nor "infertile," but for a number of reasons their fertility may be reduced to varying degrees. For example, a man with a somewhat low fertility potential whose partner is very fertile may never need medical attention. In contrast, that same man, if his partner has a somewhat low fertility potential, may have an infertility problem. Similarly, a woman who has oligoovulation but whose partner is very fertile may not be aware of her condition. Indeed, as a couple these partners are not infertile.

The concept of the couple as a unit may affect patient care in several other ways. First, it establishes the need for examining both partners, a practice that is not always used in infertility evaluations. Second, it necessitates that two physicians taking care of the partners separately must maintain a close liaison to evaluate the importance of their findings. This communication is particularly important during therapy so that the relative fertility of the partners is increased simultaneously, enhancing the overall fertility of the couple.

Even when the partners are being treated by separate physicians, they should be interviewed together at the initial visit. The information obtained from talking with both partners tells much about their dynamics as a couple. Medical, marital, and sexual histories should be obtained from the couple together and separately, so that important facts or events that one partner may not wish to reveal to the other may be elicited. The physician may also ascertain whether one partner is more motivated or saddened by the infertility or whether one is indifferent

or resistant to participating in the evaluation. Finally, one can determine the degree of stress the couple is experiencing as a result of infertility. It is imperative to be aware that since fertility may be due to problems experienced by one partner, he or she may feel guilty or at fault. In this way infertility may devastate the person's self-esteem.[7] Working with the pair as a team can help sustain them through what may be a long battery of inconvenient and painful tests and treatment. Even if they do not conceive, if the partners work together, they may more readily accept that they have tried their utmost and in active cooperation with their physician have been offered the best of medical science and compassionate understanding.

Multiplicity of Factors

Reduced fertility in many cases is brought about by a number of factors alone not important enough to prevent pregnancy but added together sufficient to cause reproductive failure. Therefore, a rational approach is that each partner undergoes a basic minimum evaluation. This generally uncovers most of the contributing factors. Simultaneous treatment of both the man and woman may be initiated, reducing the percentage of patients who ultimately require complicated and extensive testing or who unnecessarily are referred for assisted reproduction techniques. Furthermore, testing for and managing one factor at a time while others are ignored can be avoided.

APPROACH TO THE INITIAL INFERTILITY INVESTIGATION

The initial evaluation is often perceived as a stressful experience. Couples may have waited many months for their appointment and have hoped that somehow pregnancy would occur before the visit. The couple is seen together. It is helpful and saves time to have a questionnaire for them to fill out on arrival. The questionnaire includes a menstrual history, documentation of previous pregnancies, birth control history, tests and operations previously performed and results, and general medical information. The age of the couple, how long they have been married or living together, whether they had previous partners, and how long they have been trying to conceive are ascertained. This information helps determine the degree of urgency they are experiencing. It also provides an opportunity to point out the statistical probability that pregnancy may occur without intervention if the infertility has been of relatively short duration. The questionnaire is not intended to replace the history; it provides a basis for review and additional questioning.

Careful questioning concerning ethanol and drug consumption must be obtained because of the frequency with which these substances are abused and the potential deleterious effects they may have on reproduction.[8] Exposure to environ-

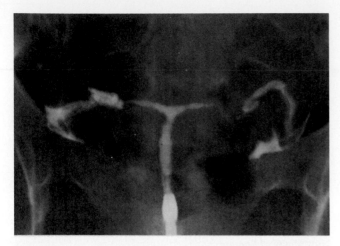

A

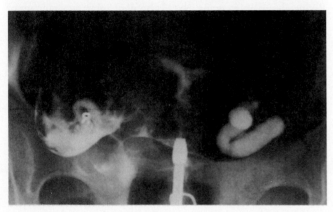

B

Figure 1–2. Hysterosalpingograms of two women (**A** and **B**) prenatally exposed to diethylstilbestrol. Note the characteristic T shape of the uteri. **B.** Patient (**B**) also has a left hydrosalpinx. She delivered a 5-lb, 6-oz daughter at 36 weeks' gestation despite the small uterine size.

mental toxins such as estrogens (through diet, steroids, or environmental chemicals), ethylene glycol ether solvents (semiconductor manufacturing), or nitrous oxide (dental assistants, anesthetists) should be explored.[9–12] A history of abortion, venereal disease, impregnating a previous partner, and discord between the partners must be sought. Frequently, more accurate information is obtained if these questions are asked separately during the individual examinations. A pedigree of both patients should also be obtained to identify potential genetic diseases. After the answers are obtained, a more directed history is elicited.

Ovulatory Factors

Ovulatory factors account for approximately 25% of infertility. Ovulation can be affected by means of a multitude of factors. The three most common ones are (1) excessive weight loss or weight gain, (2) excessive exercise, and (3) extreme emotional stress. Twenty percent above or below ideal body weight may affect ovulation. Furthermore, it must be remembered that obese people may be protein deficient and thin people may be eating quite well. A dietary history is essential. People who are more than 20% above or below their ideal body weight may experience ovulatory dysfunction. The relationship between excess body fat and ovulatory disturbances appears stronger for early-onset obesity (see Chapter 25).

Although an exercise history is easily obtained, factors affecting stress often are not apparent. For example, many people hold several jobs to improve their lifestyle. The stress inherent in such a schedule is compounded by the need to leave work frequently for infertility testing. The death of a parent or other loved one might have precipitated the desire to conceive; many couples relocate and have no support base in their new homes. Any of these factors may result in sufficient stress to impair fertility.

Other important information to request of the woman includes age of menarche, menstrual history, and if and when menstrual cyclicity changed. Questioning the patient regarding preference for hot or cold weather, changes in mood and energy, hair loss, and changes in bowel habits may help uncover subtle thyroid disease. She must always be asked directly about excessive hair growth. Hirsute women may spend hours daily removing unwanted hair and thus appear not to have a problem. Acne and oily skin are other clues of androgen excess. Information concerning galactorrhea must be obtained because of its frequent association with ovulatory dysfunction.[13] Diverse causes of infertility such as seizure disorders may also greatly affect ovulatory function.[14]

Peritoneal Factors

Peritoneal factors are uncovered in approximately 25% of infertility evaluations. Pertinent history includes a history of ap-

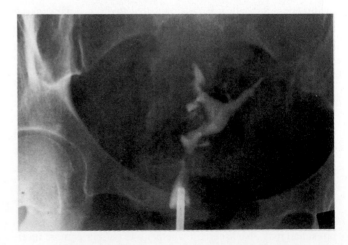

Figure 1–3. Intrauterine synechiae typical of Asherman's syndrome.

pendicitis, particularly if the appendix ruptured,[15] and abdominal or pelvic operations. The patient must be asked if she has ever been treated for pelvic inflammatory disease (PID) as an inpatient or an outpatient.[16] Approximately 267,000 hospitalizations for PID occur annually in the United States. Many more patients go untreated or the disease is not recognized. As many as 30% of women with pelvic adhesions and who are seropositive for chlamydial infection have a history negative for PID. For this reason, testing for evidence of chlamydial infection is an important component of an infertility evaluation. A seropositive test for chlamydial heat shock protein with a molecular weight of 60 kD is strongly correlated with tubal disease.[17] Previous use of an intrauterine device (IUD) is associated with as much as a fourfold increased risk for pelvic adhesions and an increased rate of PID.[18] Premenstrual spotting, dysmenorrhea, and dyspareunia are associated with endometriosis.[19]

Cervical Factors

Cervical factors are present in less than 5% of women with infertility. Because the cervix is a necessary passage for sperm, however, a careful evaluation is important. Factors that reduce either the quantity or quality of cervical mucus may reduce sperm viability and, ultimately, fertility. Previous operations on the cervix, particularly an overzealous cryosurgical procedure, cauterization (LEEP), or cone biopsy, may cause cervical stenosis or destruction of cervical glands with resultant scant mucus. Postpartum dilation and curettage (D&C) or previous abortion could result in either cervical stenosis or incompetence and ha-

bitual abortion. A history of prenatal exposure to diethylstilbestrol (DES) must be elicited because of associated stenosis and other cervical abnormalities.[20]

A chronic vaginal discharge or spotting suggests chronic cervicitis. Infection may destroy cervical glands or contaminate the mucus with leukocytes. Additional information regarding douching and use of vaginal lubricants must be obtained because both practices are associated with potential spermicidal effects.

Uterine Factors

Uterine factors are revealed in approximately 5% of infertility evaluations. They are commonly associated with a history of prenatal exposure to DES,[21] which causes a T-shaped uterus (Fig 1–2). Other pertinent historical information includes a previous D&C or therapeutic abortion, which can cause intrauterine synechiae (Fig 1–3). Patients with this problem may complain of reduced quantity of menstrual flow. Spontaneous abortion, particularly if it is recurrent, could signify uterine fibroids (Fig 1–4) or congenital abnormality of the uterus (Fig 1–5). Both uterine fibroids and polyps (Fig 1–6) are commonly associated with increased menstrual bleeding.

Smoking and Reproduction

Despite increasing realization of the many potentially harmful effects of smoking, almost one third of men and women of reproductive age in the United States smoke, and the percentage of adolescents and teenage girls who smoke is increasing. Cig-

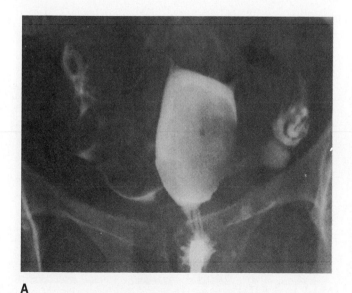

A

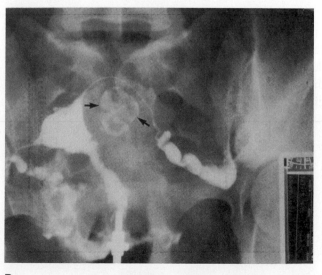

B

Figure 1–4. A. Uterine cavity markedly distorted by fibroid. **B.** Arrows point to an intraligamentous fibroid, which changes the course of the left fallopian tube and deviates the uterine fundus to the right. (*continued*)

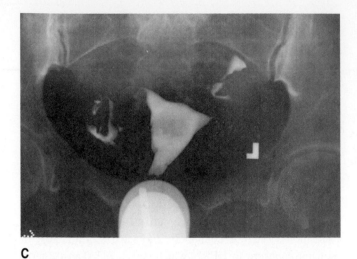

C

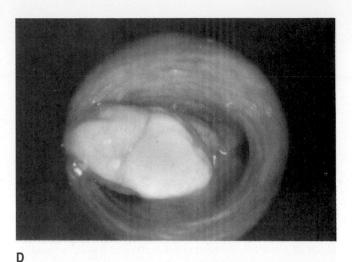

D

Figure 1–4. (*cont.*) C. Hysterosalpingogram shows fibroid within the uterine cavity. **D.** Same fibroid as in **C** at hysteroscopy.

arette smoke is known to contain hundreds of toxic substances, including nicotine, carbon monoxide, and the recognized carcinogens and mutagens radioactive polonium, benzo-(α)-pyrine, dimethylbenz-(α)-anthracene, dimethylnitrosamine, naphthalene, and methylnaphthalene.[22] It has been estimated that an average of 5.5 minutes of life are lost for each cigarette smoked, on the basis of an average reduction in life expectancy for cigarette smokers of 5 to 8 years.[23]

The impact of smoking on reproduction has been less emphasized. Epidemiologic studies have demonstrated a con-

sistent and highly significant trend of decreased fertility with increasing numbers of cigarettes per day, especially among women who smoke more than 16 cigarettes a day.[24] A trend toward a dose-response effect of heavier smoking on fecundity has been observed.[25] Fertility among light smokers (up to 20 cigarettes per day) was 75% of that of nonsmokers, and fertility among heavy smokers (more than 20 cigarettes per day) fell to 57% of that of nonsmokers. Infertility has been reported in as many as 46% more smokers than nonsmokers.[26]

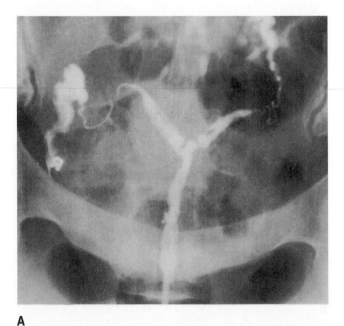

A

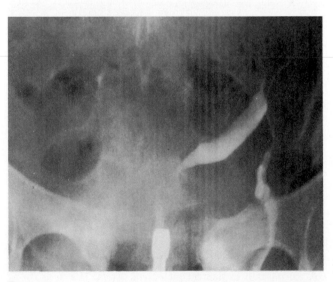

B

Figure 1–5. Hysterosalpingograms demonstrate (**A**) bicornuate uterus (note Asherman's syndrome), (**B**) unicornuate uterus. (*continued*)

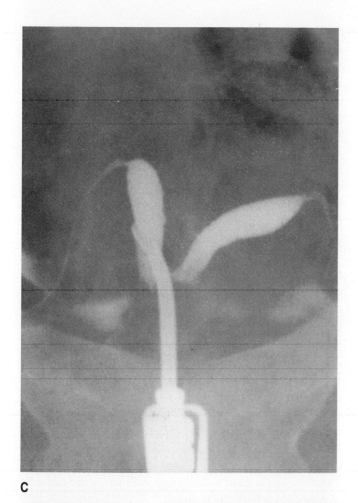

C

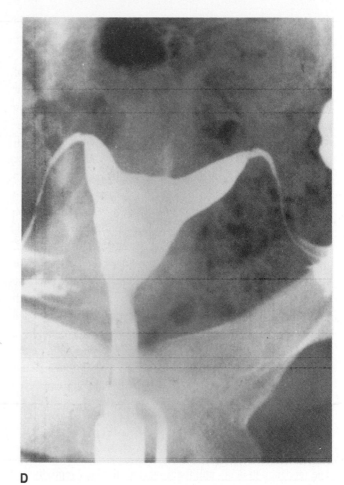

D

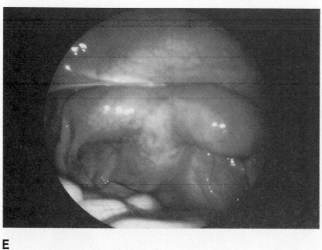

E

Figure 1–5. (*cont.*) Hysterosalpingograms demonstrate (**C**) septate uterus appearing bicornuate before metroplasty and (**D**) normal appearing uterus after metroplasty. **E.** Anatomic appearance of a bicornuate uterus.

Smoking affects reproduction in many and varied ways. Cigarette smoke has been shown to increase uterotubal wave amplitude and tonus, probably because of the effects of nicotine.[27] This can partially explain the increase in ectopic gestation among smokers compared with controls[28] and the finding that women with both cervical-factor infertility and tubal disease are likely to have been smokers.[29] Nicotine also has been demonstrated to impair decidualization in pseudopregnant rats and to cause delays in conceptus cleavage from two-cell to four-cell stage, impair entrance of the conceptus into the uterus, and impair blastocyst formation, shedding of the zona pellucida, implantation and in vitro fertilization (IVF) outcomes.[30–32] The effects are probably amplified; nicotine is ten times more concentrated in the uterine fluid than it is in plasma. This may explain the reputed associations between smoking and spontaneous abortion.[33]

Smokers have been shown to have a high frequency of amenorrhea and menstrual abnormalities. The findings appear to be dose related; they are most common among women who smoke 20 or more cigarettes a day.[34] These effects may be centrally mediated by nicotine through enhancement of vasopressin, which can diminish levels of luteinizing hormone (LH),[35] or peripheral effects due to the reduction of aromatase in granulosa cells.[36] Cigarette smoking also may have an adverse effect on male reproduction. Sperm density is reduced an average of 22% among smokers, and sperm motility and morphology are less consistently affected. Cigarette smoke, nicotine, and polycyclic aromatic hydrocarbons have produced testicular atrophy, block spermatogenesis, and alter sperm morphologic features in experimental animals.[37] Furthermore, smokers with testicular varicoceles have a frequency of oligospermia ten times greater than that of men who smoke but who do not have a testicular varicocele.[38] Therefore, for couples with unexplained infertility who smoke or for men whose semen values are marginal, the importance of stopping smoking cannot be overemphasized.

Influence of Age on Reproduction

The tendency to delay childbearing until the later reproductive years has increased since the 1950s. Factors such as easily available contraception, particularly with oral contraceptives, increasing numbers of women with occupations besides home-

making, changing sexual mores, and the social acceptability of delayed marriage contribute to this phenomenon. The result is that many couples are faced with a relatively shorter period of time in which to conceive.[39] This fact is enhanced by general and medical publications that emphasize reduced fecundity among persons older than 35 years. One of the earlier of these studies reported that among 2193 women who underwent therapeutic insemination with donor sperm (TDI) whose husbands were azoospermic, the probability of success of TDI in 12 cycles was 74% for those younger than 31 years, 61% for women 31 to 35 years of age, and 54% for women older than 35 years.[40] Similar data have been found among patients treated with donor insemination at my institution (Fig 1–7).[41]

One study evaluated the effect of age and ovarian reserve status on cumulative pregnancy rates by having 1200 women undergo a clomiphene citrate challenge test in the first few months of the initial infertility evaluation. The patients had a serum sample collected on cycle day 3 for measurement of follicle-stimulating hormone (FSH), received clomiphene citrate (100 mg) on cycle days 5 through 9, and had serum again collected for FSH measurement on cycle day 10. Cycles were considered abnormal if either the day 3 or the day 10 FSH concentration exceeded 10 IU/l.[42] Women with evidence of diminished ovarian reserve had uniformly poor pregnancy rates. Patients with normal ovarian reserve had much higher pregnancy rates, but a statistically significant age-related decline in pregnancy rate was clearly identified. Therefore, age remains a clearly important prognostic factor for women seeking infertility treatment.

Reduction in fecundity with increasing age is not limited to women. Only one third of males older than 40 years impreg-

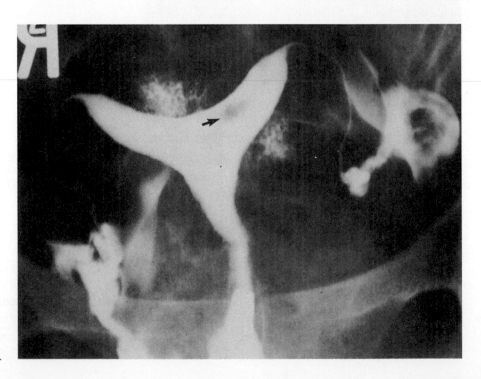

Figure 1–6. Intrauterine polyp.

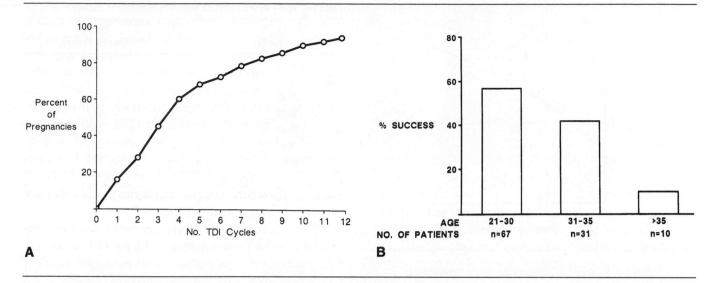

Figure 1-7. Pregnancy rates for patients receiving donor insemination (**A**) regardless of age and (**B**) according to age. (**A** *from Yeh J, Seibel MM: Artificial insemination with donor sperm: A review of 108 patients. Obstet Gynecol 70:313, 1987.*)

nate their partners within 6 months compared with men younger than 25 years (Fig 1-8). The graph in Figure 1-8 does not correct for the age of the woman; therefore it is possible that the reduction in conception rate is in part due to the compound effect of paternal and maternal age. These data also do not correct for frequency of intercourse. It was argued that fecundity declines linearly from age 20 through age 40 almost entirely because of the progressive decline in the frequency of intercourse.[43] Although frequency of coitus in all probability is not totally accountable for decreased fertility, it is clear that less frequent intercourse substantially reduces the percentage of conceptions within a 6-month period (Fig 1-9).[44] A sexual history is of particular importance in interviews of infertile couples, particularly among patients of advanced reproductive age.

Changes in the endocrinologic function of reproductively older women contribute to reduced fertility. When levels of estradiol, progesterone, LH, and FSH were measured in regularly cycling women 40 and 41 years of age, the hormonal profiles did not differ from those of women 18 to 30 years of age. Women older than 45 years with regular menses did have altered endocrine function.[45] Follicular-phase, midcycle, and luteal-phase estradiol levels were lower in the women older than 45 years; early follicular-phase FSH levels were substantially elevated compared with those of younger women. These data are reflected in the increasingly irregular cycle length with advancing age (Table 1-1)[45] and the resultant reduction in ovulatory frequency. Such changes are in part due to aging of the ovaries and the hypothalamus-pituitary axis and to altered neurotransmitters.[46] That the uterus itself is also affected by advancing age is reflected by increasing risk for spontaneous abortion (Table 1-2).[47] The effect of age on the uterus was also suggested by the demonstration of higher pregnancy rates

among younger than among older oocyte recipients who share oocytes during an egg donation cycle.[48]

The risk for congenital abnormalities among older women is well established (Table 1-3).[49] In addition, the absolute frequency of autosomal dominant disease due to new mutations among offspring of fathers 40 years or older is at least 0.3% to 0.5%.[50] This risk is many times greater than that among children of young fathers and is similar in magnitude to the risk for Down syndrome among the offspring of mothers 35 to 45 years of age. For these reasons, amniocentesis or chorionic villus biopsy must be discussed with respect to a potential pregnancy

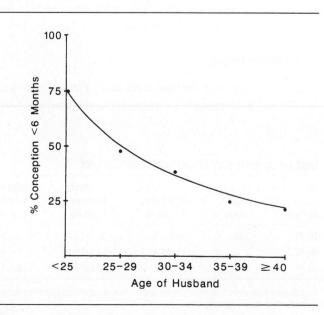

Figure 1-8. Relationship of paternal age to conception rate.

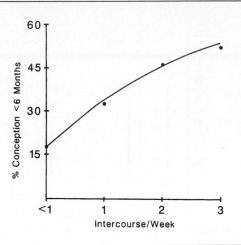

Figure 1–9. Relationship of intercourse frequency to conception rate.

TABLE 1–2. RISK FOR SPONTANEOUS ABORTION WITH INCREASED AGE

Maternal Age (yr)	Risk for Spontaneous Abortion (%)
15–19	9.9
20–24	9.5
25–29	10.0
30–34	11.7
35–39	17.7
40–44	33.8
≥45	53.2

From Warburton D, et al: Cytogenic abnormalities in spontaneous abortions of recognized conceptions. In: Porter IH, Willey A (eds), Perinatal Genetics: Diagnosis and Treatment. New York: Academic Press, 1986:133.

when either partner is biologically older, and genetic counseling should be offered.

Men also demonstrate endocrinologic and anatomic changes with advancing age. Involution of testicular function, deceased levels of free and total testosterone, decreased sperm production and quality, and maturation arrest of spermatogenesis have been reported.[51] These changes underscore the need to view the couple as a unit.

Despite all these concerns, a report on women older than 40 years demonstrated that they could expect a good pregnancy outcome.[52] This was particularly true for women whose weight was less than 67.5 kg and those who were of low parity. Nevertheless, when either partner is reproductively older, the infertile couple deserves an expedited and complete evaluation. This should include testing the woman's overall general health, since the stress of pregnancy places considerable stress on both the cardiovascular and the endocrine system.[53]

Male-Factor Infertility

A careful history from the man is essential. Prenatal exposure to DES has been associated with anatomic abnormalities such as epididymal cysts, microphallus, and hypertrophy of the prostatic utricle. Reproductive dysfunction, including altered semen analysis, is also well documented although recent reports questioned the validity of this association.[54,55] A history of childhood diseases or undescended testes is important. The overall semen quality of men born with either unilateral or bilateral undescended testes is lower than that of other men regardless of time of orchiopexy.[56] In the presence of a unilateral undescended testis, spermatogenesis is impaired in the descended as well as undescended gonad. A history of prepubertal mumps does not appear harmful. After the onset of puberty, however, mumps causes unilateral orchitis in 30% and bilateral orchitis in 10% of affected men. Such men often have markedly atrophic gonads.

A history of operations on the bladder neck or prostate must be sought, particularly for men with reduced seminal volume and azoospermia or oligospermia. A history of testicular cancer must be explored. Return of sperm production after radiation therapy or chemotherapy may require 4 to 5 years; when sperm is produced, it is generally reduced in quantity.[57] Decreased ejaculatory volume may be a clue to diabetes mellitus. If the disease is associated with peripheral neuropathy, a lack of emission or retrograde ejaculation may occur. Delayed sexual maturation may be a clue to hypogonadotropic hypogonadism (Kallmann's syndrome).

Special care must be taken to enquire about ethanol ingestion, smoking, and drug use.[8] Environmental toxins such as pesticides and occupational exposure to toxins such as Agent Orange, may reduce semen values.[55] Removal of these toxins may reverse the adverse effects. Medication such as sulfasalazine,[58] cimetidine, and nitrofurantoin may be gonadotoxic. Androgenic steroids are occasionally administered to improve gonadal function, and young athletes more and more com-

TABLE 1–1. CHANGES IN CYCLE LENGTH WITH INCREASED AGE

Age (yr)	No. of Patients	Total Cycle Length (d)	Length of Follicular Phase (d)	Length of Luteal Phase (d)
18–30	10	30.0±3.6	16.9±1.8	12.9±1.8
40–45	7	25.4±2.3	10.4±2.9	15.0±0.9
46–56	8	23.2±2.9	8.2±2.8	15.9±1.3

From Sherman B, Korenman S: Hormonal characteristics of the human menstrual cycle throughout reproductive life. J Clin Invest 55:699, 1975.

TABLE 1–3. RISK OF CHROMOSOMAL ABNORMALITY BY MATERNAL AGE

Maternal Age (yr)	Risk for Down Syndrome	Total Risk for Chromosomal Abnormalities
20	1/1667	1/526
21	1/1667	1/526
22	1/1429	1/500
23	1/1429	1/500
24	1/1250	1/476
25	1/1250	1/476
26	1/1176	1/476
27	1/1111	1/455
28	1/1053	1/435
29	1/1000	1/417
30	1/952	1/385
31	1/909	1/385
32	1/769	1/322
33	1/602	1/286
34	1/485	1/238
35	1/378	1/192
36	1/289	1/156
37	1/224	1/127
38	1/173	1/102
39	1/136	1/83
40	1/106	1/66
41	1/82	1/53
42	1/63	1/42
43	1/49	1/33
44	1/38	1/26
45	1/30	1/21
46	1/23	1/16
47	1/18	1/13
48	1/14	1/10
49	1/11	1/8

From Antenatal diagnosis of genetic disorders. ACOG Technical Bulletin, no 108, Sept 1987.

monly are taking anabolic steroids. Use of these substances should be stopped, because they inhibit gonadotropin secretion and interfere with normal spermatogenesis.

Finally, the physician must ask the man if he has difficulty achieving or maintaining an erection or in ejaculating. Problems of this nature are often embarrassing, and questions may be best asked of both partners separately.

PHYSICAL EXAMINATION

After the infertility history is complete, a careful physical examination of both partners is performed. The woman's head should be examined for temporal balding, acne, or hirsutism, all of which are signs of androgen excess. Large amounts of facial hair at the angle of the jaw, chin, or upper lip should be noted. Care is taken to evaluate the size of the thyroid. Galactorrhea is evaluated by attempting to express discharge from the nipples. Presternal hair or acne, hair or acne on the back, an increase in suprapubic hair, and a male escutcheon are additional clues to androgen excess. The presence of clitoromegaly should be determined.

Visualization of the cervix includes inspection of the cervical mucus. Copious amounts suggest either impending ovulation or estrogen associated with conditions such as polycystic ovary syndrome. In the presence of cervical mucus, a postcoital test should be performed if intercourse has occurred within the last 3 days. Occasionally abundant sperm is found at this initial visit, and further testing of the cervix can be eliminated. Attention must be paid to the position of the uterus and whether it is fixed or mobile. The size and mobility of the ovaries should be determined. A rectovaginal examination must be done to determine the presence of uterosacral nodularity or tenderness suggestive of endometriosis.[19]

Examination of the man includes emphasis on the genitalia. General body habitus and limb length are evaluated to determine the presence of genetic conditions such as Klinefelter's syndrome. Limited body hair, gynecomastia, and eunuchoid proportions may suggest inadequate virilization. The location of the urethral meatus is determined to evaluate placement of the ejaculate in the vagina. The scrotal contents are carefully palpated with the patient standing to determine testicular consistency and size to the nearest millimeter. The volume of the testes also can be estimated with an orchidometer. The long measurement should be at least 4 cm and the volume at least 20 mL.[56] A small testicular size is often associated with impaired spermatogenesis. The epididymis is palpated for induration or cystic changes, and the vas deferens is palpated for nodularity. The presence of a varicocele, vascular engorgement of the pampiniform plexus, can easily be established by asking the patient to perform a Valsalva maneuver while standing.

In addition to the physical information obtained, these individual examinations provide the opportunity for brief separate interviews, which are often invaluable in treating and understanding the couple as a unit. On completion of these examinations, the couple is asked to return to the consultation room, where an evaluation plan is described.

BASIC INFERTILITY TESTS

The basic evaluation outlined by the American Society for Reproductive Medicine (formerly the American Fertility Society) and followed by most specialists consists of history and examination of the female partner with evaluation of insemination (postcoital test), hormonal (endometrial biopsy), and tubal factors (hysterosalpingography [HSG]) and history and examination of the male partner and two semen analyses 4 to

6 weeks apart. The use of hysteroscopy is gaining wider acceptance, especially in association with unexplained infertility or a history of IUD use, D&C, or abortion. Incomplete evaluations, such as only one or two tests, or immediately performing laparoscopy, often do not explain the cause of infertility. Typically the basic minimum evaluation can be completed in 2 to 3 months.

After the tests that are to be performed have been explained, the couple is asked to speak with the fertility nurse, who gives the man a semen-collection container with printed instructions and explains to the woman how to take and record her basal body temperature (BBT). The woman is asked to call the nurse at the start of her next menstrual flow (or on Monday if her period begins on a weekend) and to begin keeping a BBT at that time. She is then given appointments for HSG and an endometrial biopsy. The woman is asked to bring a semen sample from her partner during one of these appointments to avoid their both having to miss work. The woman mails her temperature chart at the onset of her next menstrual period and at that time makes appointments for a postcoital test and another consultation. The postcoital test is optimally done in a cycle separate from the endometrial biopsy to reduce the risk that the biopsy will interrupt a pregnancy. The couple brings the second semen sample on the day of the consultation appointment.

The Cervical Factor

The importance of sperm survival in the cervix after coitus was first described by J. Marian Sims in 1888.[59] His findings were expanded by Huhner in 1913.[60] Since that time, the Sims-Huhner postcoital test has been widely accepted as an important tool in infertility diagnosis.

During most of the menstrual cycle, the cervical mucus is thick and tenacious. Under the influence of rising levels of estrogen in the preovulatory period, however, it becomes thin and watery with the consistency of egg white. This midcycle mucus is rich in mucin, glycoproteins, and salts and is relatively free of endocervical cells. It develops increased elasticity, called *spinnbarkeit*. The drying of mucus at this time results in the development of arborization, or ferning (Fig 1–10). The external ostium of the uterus and probably the endocervical canal become dilated. At this stage in the cycle the cervical mucus serves as a passageway for spermatozoa. It also acts as a filter to remove abnormal sperm and as a reservoir for sperm, which continuously make their way to the distal end of the fallopian tubes during the periovulatory period.[53,54]

Postcoital Test

Timing in the Cycle

Except during the preovulatory period, sperm routinely do not live well in the cervical canal. In the 1 to 2 days before ovulation, however, they have the capability of living for many hours, if not days, in the cervical mucus. For that reason, in a 28-day cycle, the best time to perform the postcoital test is cycle day 12 to cycle day 14, which should correspond with or precede by a day or two the low point in the temperature chart. For women with irregular cycles, it may be necessary to repeat the test at 2-day intervals. For women with extremely irregular cycles, it may be necessary to prescribe an ovulatory agent such as clomiphene citrate to regulate the cycle to prevent the need for repeated office visits. Although over-the-counter LH kits have been advocated by some gynecologists for timing a postcoital test, in my opinion this should not be necessary.

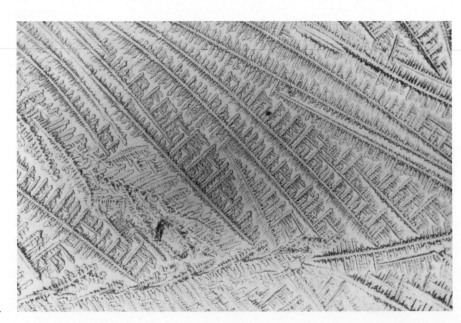

Figure 1–10. Ferning pattern of cervical mucus.

Timing After Coitus

There is considerable confusion about when after coitus the postcoital test should be performed.[61] Many authors state that 2 hours after intercourse is the optimum time; however, this recommendation does not take into consideration the function of the cervix as a reservoir. To ensure a high rate of fertilization, active spermatozoa must be, and normally are, available for 24 hours. Therefore the postcoital test should be performed approximately 12 hours after intercourse. This serves two functions. First, it allows the physician to ascertain whether the sperm are living for an extended period after intercourse; this answers the question whether the cervical mucus functions as an adequate reservoir. Second, it allows the couple to have sexual relations in preparation for the test under relatively natural circumstances and with less time pressure.[62]

Procedure

With the patient in the lithotomy position, a bivalve speculum, lubricated only with warm water, is placed into the vagina. A large dressing forceps and a cotton ball are used to remove vaginal secretions from the exocervix. The closed forceps is then inserted about 1 cm into the cervical canal, opened, rotated 180°, closed tightly, and withdrawn. The mucus is placed on a microscopic slide.

The amount of mucus is classified as scant, moderate, or profuse. The degree of clarity is noted. One tests the sample for *spinnbarkeit* by placing a glass coverslip on the mucus, slowly drawing it from the slide, and recording the number of centimeters the mucus stretches; 6 to 10 cm suggests impending ovulation. Using a metal dressing forceps instead of a glass coverslip to determine the number of centimeters of *spinnbarkeit* gives a falsely low reading.

Under the microscope the degree of cellularity is observed, and the sperm are counted. It is best first to scan the slide under low microscopic power until a representative field is found. One can then switch to high power and count the number of active, sluggishly motile, and nonmotile sperm per high-power field (hpf). Although one would assume that the more sperm present, the better the chance of pregnancy, this relationship has not been proved. Only two numbers are important in the postcoital test—more than 20 sperm/hpf, which has been positively correlated with pregnancy; and 0, which suggests faulty sperm production in the man, poor coital technique, or the presence of antibodies that are destroying the sperm in situ (Fig 1–11). Sperm found shaking in place but not moving progressively are also associated with immunologic infertility. After the slide is read, it is dried with an alcohol lamp and evaluated for fern formation. The person performing the postcoital test must recognize the importance of the results to patients, who often feel a poor outcome suggests that they have "failed their love-making test" or that they are "allergic" to each other.

Special Tests

Fractional postcoital tests have been described in which samples are taken at three levels of the endocervical canal by means of a special polyethylene catheter. Although a correlation has been noted between sperm at various levels, no correlation with conception has been found. Other studies have shown that sperm distribution is uniform throughout the cervical canal.[63] Therefore, fractional tests do not appear to be a more reliable method than the Sims-Huhner test.

In vitro sperm migration tests are recommended when the semen analysis is normal but results of the postcoital test are poor. The physician must first make absolutely certain that the postcoital test was performed at the appropriate time and that the mucus was preovulatory. This is best done by reviewing the temperature chart from the cycle in which the test was performed. If the timing was appropriate, a sperm penetration test should be performed. The first penetration test was described in 1928 by Kurzrok and Miller. One performed the test by placing a small drop of cervical mucus on a slide with a coverslip over it. The corners of the coverslip are supported by small pillars of petrolatum jelly. Semen is applied to the edge of the coverslip and allowed to flow around the cervical mucus. The slide is then placed in a moist chamber at room temperature and read after 3 to 4 hours as follows: degree 0, sperm found only in peripheral parts of the mucus; degree 1, most of the sperm have invaded the periphery and some are present in the center of the mucus; degree 2, semen are equally distributed throughout the mucus.

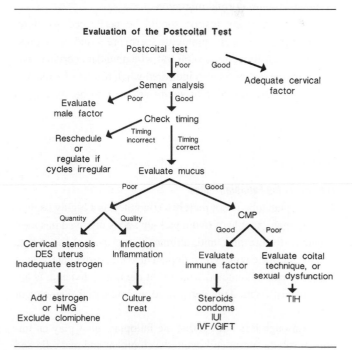

Figure 1–11. Decision tree for evaluation of a poor postcoital test. CMP, cervical mucus penetration.

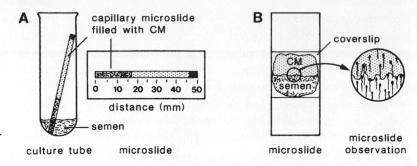

Figure 1–12. A. Cervical mucus penetration test. **B.** Microslide penetration test. CM, cervical mucus.

The capillary tube mucus penetration test described by Kremer is a more widely used in vitro test.[64] Mucus is taken from the cervix as for the postcoital text. It is placed on a microscopic slide and, with a flat capillary tube, suctioned with negative pressure by mouth. The mucus is drawn into the capillary tube, care being taken to ensure that no air bubbles are present. The capillary tube is then placed vertically into a test tube containing 1 mL of the male partner's sperm, and this tube is placed in a rack for 1 hour. At the end of that time, the distance the spermatozoa have traveled is measured (Fig 1–12). It is important to compare sperm penetration of the patient's mucus with that of donor mucus. This test is made simple by the commercial availability of bovine cervical mucus already drawn in flat capillary tubes. In general, failure to penetrate the mucus implies an immune factor, as does the presence of immotile sperm. Motile sperm seen throughout the 30-mm column of mucus implies normal migration.

Sperm antibody testing should be performed when no sperm or predominately nonmotile sperm are found in the presence of a well-timed postcoital test with abundant cervical mucus. Immune testing is also indicated when results of a mucus-penetration test are poor or sperm are seen to be shaking in place on the postcoital test.

Tubal Factor

Function of the Fallopian Tubes

The fallopian tube is not merely a conduit. It is a highly sophisticated organ capable of ovum pick-up and is involved in sperm transport, fertilization, and, ultimately, transport of the zygote into the uterine cavity. The fallopian tube is approximately 9 cm long. Its widest diameter, which is at the fimbriated end, is approximately 2 cm. This narrows to an interstitial diameter of 0.5 mm.

Although it is known that the fallopian tubes play an important role in sperm and ovum development and that cilia and muscular activity are important elements in ova, diagnostic evaluation is limited to determination of tubal patency or lack of patency. Three nonsurgical methods are available for this purpose: tubal insufflation with carbon dioxide, hysterosalpingography, and hysterosonography.

Tubal Insufflation with Carbon Dioxide

Tubal insufflation with carbon dioxide was originally described by Rubin in 1920.[65] This test should always be performed in the preovulatory phase so as not to interfere with a newly fertilized ovum. The position of the uterus is ascertained, a tenaculum is placed on the anterior lip of the cervix, and a hollow cannula with an acorn tip is placed into the cervix. An instrument for recording the speed and pressure of flow of the carbon dioxide is required. This recording instrument can produce either a permanent record on a graph or temporary marks on a screen to be visualized by the operator. The insufflation is carried out slowly, 25 to 35 mL/minute. The flow is maintained for 1 minute, after which the cannula is removed and reinserted twice more. The patient is asked to sit up. If she feels shoulder pain due to phrenic irritation, the carbon dioxide has passed through the fallopian tubes and into the peritoneal cavity.

Although this test has been performed for more than 50 years as a screening procedure to rule out complete blockage, it is seldom used now because it gives no information about unilateral or bilateral patency. In addition, comparison of Rubin test results with findings of direct visualization of the tubes at laparoscopy has shown that the Rubin test is negative when tubes are patent approximately 25% of the time. Nevertheless, it is rare for tubal insufflation to suggest patency when the fallopian tubes are closed, so the procedure can be used as an initial screening tool for patients with no history of tubal disease. The procedure is described herein because of its limited expense at this time of cost consciousness.

Hysterosalpingography

HSG is an integral part of an infertility evaluation. It is performed in the first half of the menstrual cycle after bleeding has stopped and before ovulation. This timing is designed to prevent reflux of endometrial tissue and thus eliminate a potential source of endometriosis. In addition, it precludes the possibility that the test will interfere with conception in the uterus or cause

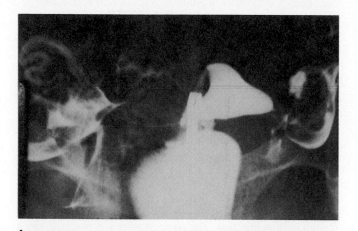

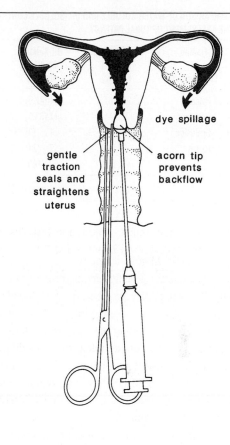

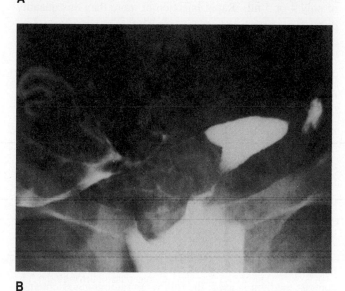

A

B

C

Figure 1–13. Retroverted uterus (**A**) before and (**B**) after traction is applied to cervix. **C**. Schematic depicts technical points.

an ectopic pregnancy by pushing a conceptus from the fallopian tube into the peritoneal cavity.

Any history of PID warrants determination of the patient's sedimentation rate. If the rate is elevated, it is good practice to have the patient take prophylactic antibiotics beginning on the day of HSG and for 2 or 3 days afterward. In general, doxycycline, 100 mg twice a day for 5 days, is adequate. If tenderness or a pelvic mass is found at the pelvic examination before HSG, the procedure should be cancelled.

The procedure is performed in a radiologic setting, but it is helpful to have a gynecologist perform the instrumentation. Having her own physician present may decrease the patient's anxiety, and gynecologists are usually more adept than other physicians at instrumentation of the uterus.

The patient is placed in the dorsal lithotomy position, and a plastic speculum is introduced into the vagina. It is important that the speculum be plastic; a metal speculum precludes

radiologic visualization of the cervix. If a metal speculum is used, it should be removed before the radiograph is obtained. Several methods may be used for instrumentation of the uterus, which follows cleaning of the vaginal cavity with an aseptic substance such as benzalkonium chloride (Zephiran) or povidone-iodine (Betadine). A paracervical block placed on the anterior lip of the cervix at the 4 o'clock and 8 o'clock positions is helpful in diminishing discomfort. Taking a prostaglandin inhibitor 1 to 2 hours before the procedure has been found effective in reducing discomfort. A Jarco cannula in association with a tenaculum on the anterior lip of the cervix or special suction devices that grasp the cervix through negative pressure may be used. A Foley catheter often interferes with visualization of the endometrial cavity and does not allow adequate traction (Fig 1–13).

Both water-soluble and oil-soluble contrast materials can be used for HSG; each has its advantages and disadvantages (Ta-

TABLE 1–4. COMPARISON OF WATER-SOLUBLE AND OIL-SOLUBLE CONTRAST MEDIUM IN THE ASSESSMENT OF TUBAL PATENCY

Finding at HSG	Finding at Laparoscopy	Water-Soluble Medium No. (%)	Oil-Soluble Medium No. (%)	Combined No. (%)
Patent	Patent	27 (61)	14 (42.5)	41 (53)
Occlusion	Occlusion	5 (11)	11 (33.5)	16 (21)
Patent	Occlusion	3 (7)	1 (3)	4 (5)
Occlusion	Patent	9 (21)	7 (21)	16 (21)
Totals		44 (100)	33 (100)	77 (100)

From Loy RA, Weinstein FG, Seibel MM: Hysterosalpingography in perspective: The predictive value of oil and water soluble contrast media. Fertil Steril 51:170, 1989.

bles 1–4 and 1–5).[66] Oil-soluble material is associated with a slightly increased risk for granulomatous formations in the peritoneal cavity. It is also poorly absorbed from occluded tubes and thus may remain there until surgical intervention, although the exact importance of this finding has not been determined. The positive aspect of use of an oil-soluble contrast medium is that it is associated with an increased pregnancy rate. Under no circumstance, however, should HSG be considered a therapeutic study. It is a diagnostic study that has a slight short-term association with improved outcome.

A more serious concern with use of oil-soluble contrast medium is emolization, which was reported in 1% of patients in

TABLE 1–5. CHOOSING THE BEST TREATMENT FOR INFERTILE COUPLES

Clinical Situation	Surgical Treatment	IVF	GIFT
Tubal implantation	No	Yes	No
Tubocornual anastomosis	Yes	No	No
Tubal reanastomosis (≥3.5 cm tubal length)	Yes	No	No
Tubal reanastomosis (<3.5 cm tubal length)	No	Yes	No
Previous fimbriectomy	No	Yes	No
Salpingostomy	No	Yes	No
Repeated tubal operations	No	Yes	No
Pelvic adhesions (mild)	Yes	Yes	Yes
Pelvic adhesions (severe)	No	Yes	No
Previous ectopic pregnancy	Yes	Yes	No
Endometriosis			
Stages I–IIa	No	No	No
Stages III–IV	Yes	Yes	No
Age >35 yr, surgical option	No	Yes	Yes
Unexplained infertility <3 yr duration	No	No	No
Unexplained infertility ≥3 yr duration	No	Yes	Yes

GIFT, gamete intrafallopian transfer.
[a]Other treatment options and adequate observation recommended first.

one series.[67] Intravasation produces a spiderweb appearance adjacent to the uterus with opacified streaks that extend toward the pelvic side wall (Fig 1–14). The reported causes of lymphatic or venous intravasation include excessive pressure during instillation, direct trauma to the uterine mucosa, surgically altered cervix or endometrium, and organic or congenital anomalies of the uterine cavity. If the spiderweb pattern is seen, HSG should be stopped at once to prevent emolization.

Water-soluble contrast medium is slightly more irritating than oil-soluble medium. It is reabsorbed quickly, however, and does not appear to be associated with adhesion formation in the peritoneal cavity.

Regardless of which medium is used, the most important feature is slow injection. The uterine cavity is a potential space of only 4 or 5 mL. Rapid injection of more than this quantity distends the uterus and causes cramping and pain. If pain does occur, a temporary pause in the procedure often proves helpful.

A fluoroscope with an image intensifier is the recommended radiologic equipment. If fluoroscopy is not possible, no more than three or four radiographs should be obtained. A preliminary radiograph is obtained before the contrast agent is injected. A second radiograph after injection of 1 mL of contrast medium outlines uterine contour and defines intrauterine abnormalities such as polyps. Air bubbles are occasionally mistaken for intrauterine polyps or fibroids; they are differentiated by asking the patient to shift positions, which causes the bubbles to rise to a new location (Fig 1–15). A third radiograph obtained after injection of 5 mL of medium should determine tubal patency.

A final follow-up radiograph should be obtained to depict the spread of dye through the peritoneal cavity. If oil-soluble contrast medium is used, the follow-up radiograph is obtained in 24 hours; if water-soluable medium is used, the follow-up radiograph may be obtained in 10 minutes. Accumulation of contrast medium in the pelvis indicates that peritubal adhesions have been trapped in the contrast medium. When proximal tubal occlusion is encountered, selective fallopian tube catheterization performed by means of insertion of a 5F catheter directly into the ostium of the fallopian tube and injection of contrast medium overcomes pseudo-obstruction due to spasm or debris.[68] True obstruction may be recanalized by means of coaxial advancement of a fine, floppy, 0.015-inch (0.038-cm) angiographic guide wire through a 3F catheter (Fig 1–16).

Hysterosonography

Doppler ultrasound has been used to observe the insufflation of saline solution into the uterine cavity in an attempt to access flow through the fallopian tubes. A 3-mm catheter is inflated inside the uterus to occlude the cervix and 10 cc of saline is injected. Preliminary results with this technique as a screening tool are

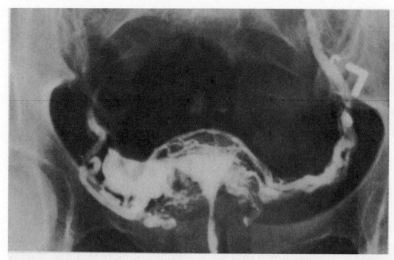

A

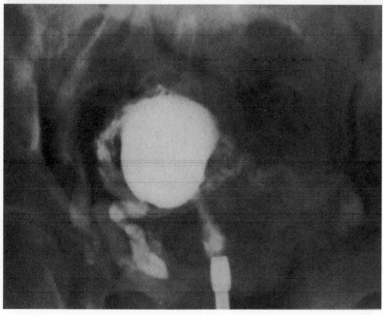

B

Figure 1–14. A. Spiderweb appearance of intravasation into uterine lymphatics. **B.** Venous drainage looks like fallopian tubes.

encouraging. However, the ultimate role in the evaluation of the female reproductive tract is yet to be determined.

The Ovulatory Factor

The presence or absence of ovulation and the quality of corpus luteum function, both important factors in infertility, may be evaluated in three ways: (1) determination of BBT; (2) performance of endometrial biopsy; and (3) measurement of progesterone levels in the blood. These approaches yield only presumptive evidence of ovulation, all dependent on the secretion of progesterone by the corpus luteum. Occasionally, a luteinized unruptured follicle (LUF) secretes progesterone, imitating ovulation.

Basal Body Temperature Chart

The BBT chart, first described in 1904, is the simplest and most inexpensive method of assessment of the presence or absence of ovulation. A biphasic chart, characterized by a sustained rise of at least 0.4°F (0.2°C) for 12 to 15 days, is typical of ovulation and an adequate luteal phase. It is generally accepted that ovulation occurs on the day of the lowest temperature and is followed by a sustained rise in temperature. This may actually

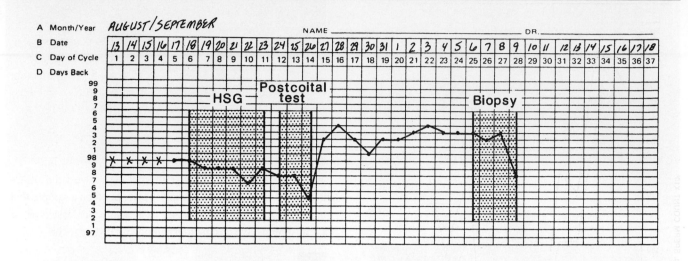

A	Month/Year	AUGUST/SEPTEMBER

Figure 1–17. Basal body temperature chart demonstrates schedule for testing.

nmol/L) 1 week after ovulation. Because progesterone levels vary considerably and no sharp demarcation exists between what is normal and what is abnormal on any given day, this assessment is not as useful as endometrial biopsy.

The Male Factor: Semen Analysis

Because the man may have a factor causing infertility in as many as one third of couples, it is imperative that he not be neglected during the evaluation. If the couple lives near a urologist who is interested in infertility, it is appropriate for the man

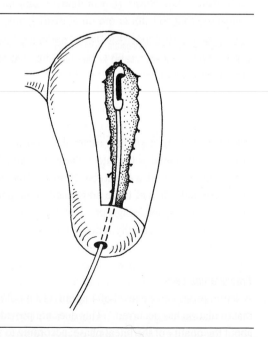

Figure 1–18. Endometrial biopsy.

to be examined by that physician. Usually, however, it is the gynecologist who first examines the woman and thus has the responsibility of ensuring that the man is properly examined and treated. A postcoital test alone is not sufficient. It is necessary to obtain a history and perform a physical examination of the man and to perform two semen analyses. One must bear in mind that there is a circannual rhythm in human sperm counts. The trend is toward highest values in February and March and the lowest in September (Fig 1–19).[72]

The semen should be collected in a small, clean, widemouthed, 1- to 2-ounce (30- to 60-mL) glass jar. Use of a larger jar often allows the specimen to dry along the sides while it is being transported to the office or laboratory. The preferred method of sperm collection is masturbation. If this is objectionable, coitus withdrawal may be used, but a portion of the semen is lost. Latex condoms without spermicidal agents can be used, but one must be sure that the patients are not allergic to latex. Condoms that contain a spermicidal agent should never be used.

The man should abstain from sexual relations for approximately 48 hours before collecting the specimen. The specimen should reach the laboratory within 2 to 3 hours; it is not necessary that the sperm be examined immediately after collection. During transportation the specimen should be kept as near to room temperature as possible. In cold weather it can be held close to the body. After delivery to the laboratory, the specimen is evaluated for viscosity and volume. Semen normally is ejaculated as a coagulum, but it liquefies in 5 to 20 minutes, after which it flows easily and freely. Continuation of the viscous state is abnormal and may reduce fertility.

Volume between 2.5 and 8.0 mL is considered normal. Less than 2.5 mL often results in poor cervical insemination. If

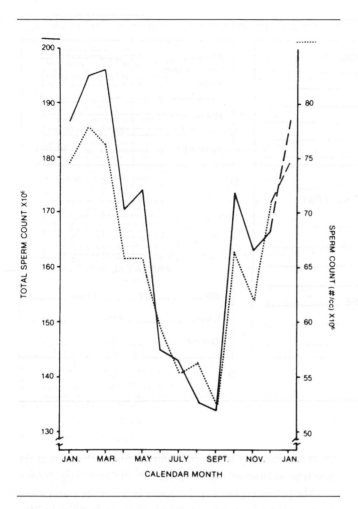

Figure 1–19. Circannual rhythm in human total sperm count and concentration.

the small ejaculatory volume is oligospermic or azoospermic and is alkaline, a postejaculation urine sample should be examined to exclude retrograde ejaculation. This condition is particularly likely among men who are diabetic or who have undergone prostate or bladder operations. A volume greater than 8 mL is usually accompanied by diminished sperm density. This finding is an indication for the use of homologous insemination with a split ejaculate.

After thorough mixing, a drop of semen is placed on a microscopic slide, and the number of leukocytes and the presence of agglutination are assessed. One determines the percentage of motile sperm by dividing the mean of the number of active forms by the number of inactive forms in four or five high-power fields. Because sperm longevity may be another important factor in conception, a second evaluation of motility should be performed 5 to 6 hours after ejaculation. Well-mixed semen is drawn up to the 0.5 mark on a pipette used to count white blood cells. The pipette is then filled with tap water and thoroughly shaken. The cells are counted in the red blood cell field of a hemocytometer or other chamber designed for semen. All

the cells lying within five blocks of the 16 cells are counted. The total number of sperm cells counted gives the count in millions per milliliter. If the count is low, the semen should be brought to the 1.0 mark of the pipette (1:10 dilution) and the number of cells doubled to give the count in millions. This reduces the counting error in severe cases of oligospermia. A chamber has been developed in which direct counting is made from an undiluted sample. Counting the number of sperm heads in 10 squares of the grid immediately provides concentration in millions per milliliter.

Sperm morphology is evaluated as a routine part of the semen analysis; new criteria for morphology have been established.[73] Morphologic evaluation is performed on a sample that represents the sperm population as a whole. At least 60% of sperm should have normal morphology according to the old criteria and 14% according to the new criteria. A high percentage of tapering forms has been associated with varicocele. It has been reported that abnormal forms are twice as frequent in non-motile sperm as they are in motile sperm.[74]

Although there is no absolute standard of fertility, guidelines for semen analysis have been established. Semen is considered fertile if the count is greater than 40 million/mL, the percentage of motility at 6 hours is greater than 50%, and morphology of more than 60% of sperm is normal (14% by new criteria). An infertile specimen is one with a count less than 20 million/mL, motility at 6 hours less than 35%, and less than 60% normal forms (5% by new criteria). Patients with counts and motility percentages between these two levels (20 and 40 million, 35% and 50%) have a state of relative infertility and deserve to be treated. These values are not absolute; sometimes men achieve conception even when their semen morphology approaches zero.[75] Computerized sperm analyzers provide precise quantification of sperm motility, speed, and motion patterns. Although they may be useful in the future, they do not appear to provide more useful data for improving pregnancy outcome than an experienced technician.[73]

FINAL STEPS OF THE BASIC EVALUATION

Consultation

After the minimum evaluation is completed, the couple meets with the physician to discuss the test results and to determine how best to proceed. This consultation is extremely important. The results of all previous tests are reviewed with verification that they were obtained at the correct time in the cycle. This task is made simpler with the use of a summary sheet. Use of rubber stamps for each procedure to highlight the test results of the evaluation also helps in the review of the data (Fig 1–20). Problem areas are explained and discussed, and a treatment plan is outlined.

CHAPTER 2

Emotional Aspects of Infertility

ALICE D. DOMAR · MACHELLE M. SEIBEL

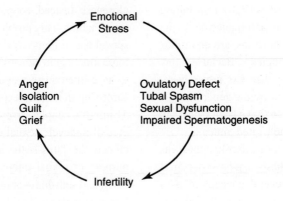

Infertility
The simple union of man and wife
in love creates a brand new life.
A child to cherish, play with, and be
their link with immortality.

What bliss and joy they anticipate!
Unless infertility becomes their fate
and buries dreams which die within
as they mourn their child who might have been.
M. M. Seibel, 1988

Conception, pregnancy, and childbirth are among the most deeply meaningful parts of our lives and arouse the strongest of feelings. So it is not surprising that these areas, so highly charged with emotion, are themselves sensitive to the effects of stress.[1]

The link between emotions and fertility has been appreciated since biblical times. Consider the story of Hannah, from the first chapter of the first book of Samuel.

A man named Elkanah had two wives: Peninah, who had many children, and Hannah, who was ridiculed by Peninah for her inability to conceive. Eventually, Hannah became so distressed she would not eat. She prayed and wept bitterly; her lips moved, but she was unable to utter a sound.

A priest saw her in this state and accused her of drunkenness. But when Hannah explained the reason for her sorrow, the priest said to her, "Go in peace. May the God of Israel grant your petition." Comforted and calmed, Hannah returned home, began to eat, and shortly thereafter conceived a son, Samuel.

It is estimated that infertility affects 15% of the childbearing-age population in the United States, or approximately 10 million couples. Numerous factors, including postponement of childbearing and the rising frequency of sexually transmitted disease, use of contraceptive tools such as an intrauterine device (IUD), and the number of therapeutic abortions, are contributing to increased numbers of infertile couples.[1,2] Because infertility results in the loss of something that has never been, however, its impact often goes unnoticed by the general population.[3] For these reasons, infertile couples have been called the most neglected and silent minority in the United States.[4]

The study of the emotional aspects of infertility must incorporate three important shifts in emphasis that have occurred during the past 15 years. First, the general concept of psychogenic infertility has been reversed so that, with few exceptions, distress is now seen as the result, not the cause, of infertility.[5] Nevertheless, psychologic, physiologic, and neuroendocrine factors are interactive and interdependent.[6] Second, the evaluation and management of infertility have evolved from being viewed exclusively as a woman's problem; physiologic male factors are being studied extensively. The emotional impact of infertility on men is considered, but less intensively.[7] Finally, the emphasis on managing infertility as an individual matter has changed to treating a couple as a unit. Both partners are viewed as enduring a personal and a family crisis.[6,8]

Infertility may be experienced as an emotional loss in many ways. For some, it is similar to the amputation of a limb or the diagnosis of a chronic illness. For all, the diagnosis represents being denied the choice of having a biologic child. Although as recently as the late 1960s, 50% of infertility cases were classified as emotionally determined, improved methods in diagnosing defects in reproductive endocrinologic processes and infertility rule out emotional causes in all but 5% of cases. Nonetheless, the physical and mental consequences of the in-

fertility evaluation, treatment, and lack of success may cause or contribute to a psychologic problem. Thus physicians who treat infertile couples must be aware of the enormous stresses that infertility places on both partners and must understand the psychologic interventions that are effective in alleviating some of these stresses.

THE EVALUATION

For many couples, infertility has come to be viewed as a physical disease awaiting appropriate medical or surgical therapy. The evaluation becomes a consuming, long-term preoccupation. It also can be psychologically, socially, physically, and financially devastating. The relation between the amount of treatment failure and distress is independent of age, years infertile, or years in treatment.[9] The timing of certain tests and sexual relations is so critical that other aspects of living become subordinate.[1] Coitus is no longer an expression of affection or closeness. Instead, couples stop making love and start trying to make babies. This problem has been exacerbated by the widespread use of home ovulation-detection kits. Couples purchase these kits to gain control over their cycles, only to feel required to have intercourse when the indicator dot turns blue. It is not surprising that many express personal distress. In one study of 51 infertile couples, five couples (10%) demonstrated some degree of midcycle sexual dysfunction.[10] Contributing factors included the "this-is-the-night" syndrome, the change in the purpose of sexual intercourse, the stress of testing by a third party, and self-doubt about the adequacy of future performance. Some patients cope with their anxiety by avoiding medical examinations, as suggested by repeated cancellations of the postcoital test.

During the initial evaluation, the requisite sexual review may be seen by some patients as embarrassing, intrusive, inappropriate, and demeaning. Questions that focus on sexual habits and patterns may themselves cause sexual dysfunction, further contributing to infertility.[11] The simplest manner in which psychologic factors can be thought of as causing infertility is through their effect on sexual performance: Reduced frequency can contribute to infertility.[12] The pressures of having sex during ovulation may have considerable negative impact on desire; sex for pleasure fades away into the job of procreation.[13]

Therapy for infertility can continue for more than a decade. Many couples marshal all their strength and stamina in the belief that the infertility can be corrected. As long as they are receiving active therapy, couples usually put aside crucial decisions about career, life plans, and adoption and delay confronting childlessness.[2] Despite such outward appearances of stalwart determination, however, living with infertility means working through complex emotional reactions, often with little outside assistance.[11,13]

THE PSYCHOLOGIC IMPACT ON WOMEN

Some women consider the infertility investigation to be the worst experience of their lives. Infertility becomes the all-encompassing focus of their existence, affecting nearly every aspect of their lives. Many feel controlled by the drive to achieve conception and find it difficult to concentrate on long-term goals when taking medications, recovering from operations, dealing with their emotional reactions, and living with the daily hope that "it" will end soon.[14] Job security and advancement are often affected; women may decline promotions that require relocation, because they are invested with their physician, and avoid career changes that might interfere with the freedom to continue treatment. Taking time off from work for doctor's appointments, blood tests, operations, and other procedures may endanger job security.

In addition to the many practical stresses, a woman's desire to have a child is so powerful that the emotional toll of infertility is enormous. When questioned why they wanted to have a child, the most common answer given by a group of women was, "It is just a feeling." Conception is frequently viewed as the ultimate expression of love between a man and a woman.[15] Furthermore, because of the emphasis society places on parenthood, many infertile women feel unfeminine. This is particularly true for those with conditions such as polycystic ovary disease, in which hirsutism and excess of male hormones add to the problem.[16]

Infertile women may feel guilty for upsetting their partner and disappointing their families. The guilt may focus on sexual behaviors such as early promiscuity, premarital or extramarital sex, past abortion, homosexual experiences, masturbation, prior contraceptive use, or even taking pleasure in sex.[17] For some, continued painful or stressful treatments may represent atonement for past behaviors.[17] In addition, women with the pelvic pain often associated with infertility-causing conditions such as endometriosis often experience high levels of depression and anxiety.[18] One must also be mindful that women with chronic pelvic pain are more likely to have been physically and sexually abused in their past,[19] a circumstance that could add to the distress caused by infertility. Anger is connected to a sense of unfairness and may be stimulated by seeing pregnant women or babies, resulting in envy or jealousy. Sadness can be pervasive, and is associated with helplessness, lack of control, despair, and grief.[6]

Continued pressures can eliminate self-confidence, a sense of competence, and a sense of control. These losses can lead to a decreased feeling of security, compromised health, and inter-ference with close relationships, and they can destroy hopes and goals for the future.[14]

Infertility can take a substantial psychologic toll. Infertile women have statistically significantly higher levels of depressive symptoms than fertile women and twice the prevalence of depressive symptoms.[20] In a 1992 study that compared infertile women and fertile women undergoing routine gynecologic care, 11.0% of the infertile women, compared with 3.6% of the fertile women, met the criteria for a current major depressive episode.[21] In another study of 449 infertile women at their first clinic visit, the scores on depression, anxiety, cognitive difficulties, and hostility were statistically significantly higher than the scores for a large normative sample on the Index of Psychiatric Symptomatology.[22]

The psychologic impact of infertility may be equivalent to the impact of life-threatening illness. When infertile women were compared with women with cancer, hypertension, aftermath of myocardial infarction or bypass operation, chronic pain, or human immunodeficiency virus (HIV)–positive status, the infertile women had depression and anxiety scores on the Symptom Checklist 90R (SCL-90R) equivalent to those of all other patients except for the patients with chronic pain.[23] This study dramatically demonstrates the extreme psychologic impact of the infertility experience.

THE PSYCHOLOGIC IMPACT ON MEN

The emphasis in the literature on the psychologic impact of infertility has been on women. A review of 121 articles published between 1948 and 1985 revealed that only 18% emphasized the male partner, and most of these were written since the late 1960s.[24] Before 1970, knowledge of male responses to infertility was virtually nonexistent; physiology, not psychology, was emphasized.[25] The main problem in assessing the emotional response to infertility has been men's lack of availability and willingness to undergo evaluations. Many associate the inability to impregnate a woman with reduced masculinity and virility, and they appear threatened when psychologic factors are discussed.[17] One report noted that when a psychiatrist was introduced to investigate the psychogenic components of infertility, husbands dropped out of the program rapidly.[26] Many men who willingly undergo semen analysis and elaborate physical examinations consider the discussion of psychogenic impotence to be humiliating and devastating.

The infertility evaluation can be extremely stressful to men because of performance appraisal and expectation. The post-coital test seems to increase anxiety markedly. Men are unaccustomed to being told exactly when they have to make love; the knowledge that their performance is to be assessed by a third party and given a grade results in many men finding it difficult or impossible to perform. Sexual dysfunction and impotence can occur as a direct result of the infertility evaluation.

The popular concept of male responsibilities during the infertility assessment focuses on giving support to the partner.[27] The man is viewed as the stable, calm partner who tries his best to help the woman through painful and stressful treatments. When it is he being treated, however, his responses may be very different. He must cope with his own physical pain, frequent medical appointments, attitudes of others, and his own and his partner's emotional responses. In addition to shouldering his own complex feelings, a man may feel responsible for denying his partner the opportunity to have a child.[14] Therefore, infertile men must deal with many of the same emotions as infertile women.

The desire to have a child may not be less in men than in women, although it may be expressed differently. When questioned why they wanted to have a child, the most frequent response given by infertile men was, "To make life worth living."[15] That most men shun the suggestion of psychologic intervention does not mean that the psychologic impact is any less severe among men. Research findings support the concept that women report more infertility-specific distress than men.[28]

It may be that the experience of infertility is different for men and women. Research has shown that when compared with men, women feel it is more important to have a natural child, experience more discomfort when reminded of others' fertility such as at baby showers, and assume more personal responsibility for the fertility problem than do men.[29]

The impact of infertility on men apparently is determined by the presence or absence of male-factor infertility. In a study of 36 infertile couples undergoing treatment, the men reported emotional distress levels similar to that of their wives if the infertility was attributed to a male factor, but distress levels among men who did not have male-factor infertility were considerably less than among their wives.[30]

THE COUPLE

Although the psychologic burden of infertility may not be experienced equally by both partners, it is certainly experienced together. Most of the literature focuses on the individual rather than on the couple as a unit despite the fact that psychologic issues are important to both.[6]

Infertile couples face a number of issues that affect their relationship. One of the most difficult with which to deal is their individual perceptions of infertility. Women are often more emotionally expressive than men. They often cope by discussing their anxiety and depression with their partners, who may feel powerless to help. Men may feel a need to contain their emotions, not only to maintain the stoicism expected of them but also out of a sense of responsibility to be the stable one in the relationship. A woman may interpret silence as lack of concern and may escalate her complaints, causing the man to retreat further. This can lead to the woman's feeling abandoned, the man's feeling overwhelmed, and both feeling resentment. At a time when the two individuals most need support from each other, they may instead grow apart.[14,17,22]

Guilt and blame may strain a couple's relationship. If an organic factor is identified in one partner, that person may feel guilty at depriving the other of parenthood. Conversely, the unaffected member may feel anger toward the other at the same time feeling guilty at being impatient with the partner's depression. As the investigation continues, the man may grow to resent the continued scheduling of sexual activity. Tests such as the zona-free hamster egg–penetration test can be particularly significant. The man may feel that in addition to being unable to impregnate his partner, he is unable even to impregnate an animal egg. These feelings may lead to the man's unwillingness either to continue with the investigation or to comply with intercourse at the prescribed time. These stresses often lead to anger, which may account for reports of atypical sexual behavior during the infertility evaluations.[23]

Most infertile couples experience marked isolation. The social unacceptability of childlessness may result in real or perceived stress from family, friends, acquaintances, and even strangers, which results in reluctance to reveal the infertility. Because others may consider that the couple has experienced no tangible loss and find it difficult to empathize, the couple concludes that no one truly understands. In addition, couples may isolate themselves because of a self-protective impulse as outsiders in a fertile world. In a series of interviews with infertile couples, all expressed feelings of abnormality, rejection, abandonment, and being outcasts and unlovable.[5,14,31] Finally, infertile couples may isolate themselves because social contact is seen as an extra demand. The couple's time and energy are drained by procedures and physical regimens to such an extent that social interaction is not worth the effort it entails.

THE CRISIS OF INFERTILITY

Although many patients who are treated for infertility do eventually become pregnant, almost half must come to terms with the fact that they will never be the parents of a biologic child. The subsequent psychologic impact has been described as the crisis of infertility.[4] Patients typically evolve through a series of stages, including surprise, denial, anger, isolation, guilt, grief, and resolution. The crisis is biopsychosocial; it affects all areas of life, including psychologic, moral, and religious aspects and may exacerbate existing biologic, emotional, and social problems.[11]

One of the most important aspects of the infertility crisis is the sense of losing control. In our society, increasing numbers of individuals rely on birth control until their individual circumstances are optimal for childbearing. Thus, they have a sense of control over their bodies and over procreation. When faced with the loss of the choice of having a baby, the sense of order in their world is disturbed.[13]

Only a few formal investigations have assessed the reaction to infertility. In one study, 48 women were interviewed in an unstructured manner during their infertility treatment.[32] In addition to loss of control, the most common themes were ambiguity centering on the reason for the infertility and toward the physician, floundering in the pursuit of life goals, uncertainty about the efficacy and safety of treatment, and suspicion about future fertility. Another theme centered on the need for a time frame for everything, including sexual relations, basal body temperature, and all treatments. The women also acknowledged a sense of otherness, feeling unfairly singled out, left out, defective, and not being understood by others. Private-practice patients reported more distress than clinic patients.

A second study surveyed 500 infertile couples.[4] Most reported sexual dissatisfaction or dysfunction; however, actual sexual dysfunction was not more common than among fertile patients. The female partners felt less need to achieve orgasm; they were more concerned with becoming pregnant than in enhancing pleasure. In a third study, 24 infertile couples were interviewed 1 month before and 2 years after reconstructive tubal operations.[33] Over the 2-year period after the operation, there was a nonsignificant trend for the relationship to deteriorate as partners' feelings became more negative. Women had considerably more emotional effects than men, but over the 2 years the men's feelings of grief and depression increased. Women reported avoiding children, whereas the men reported increasing contact. None of the individuals had been offered professional help before the study, whereas at the end, half the women reported that they had needed help in solving problems with their partner, sexual relations, crisis reactions, or anxiety.

In one study of 16 couples who had recently been informed of the man's sterility, five of the men reported a period of impotence lasting 1 to 3 months after learning the diagnosis.[34] Five men suffered insomnia and depressed mood, and one had exacerbation of peptic ulcer symptoms. Only 3 of the 16 men reported no change in sexual patterns or mood. None of the women reported decreases in sexual desire, although 6 of the 16 women felt anger toward their partner. The author recommended that all men who receive the diagnosis of azoospermia receive therapy to assure them that impotence is common and typically resolves over the ensuing months.

THE PHYSICIAN'S ROLE

The physician's role in the treatment of infertile couples is extremely complex and challenging. He or she must simultaneously provide state-of-the-art medical and surgical management while never losing sight of the need for empathy and compassionate listening and understanding. By the time a couple first requests an infertility evaluation, the partners are already emotionally charged. The deep desire to have a child makes them depend on the physician. The resulting relationship may become characterized by a high degree of affection for and confidence in the physician with willingness to be helped. Alternatively, the physician may become a convenient target for frustration and anger that evolve to overdependence or noncompliance.[35]

The physician must be aware of the psychologic and social repercussions of the infertility evaluation in order to reduce or modify the couple's stress and to facilitate adaptation. It is important to consider the additional tensions produced by tests and treatment.[9,29] For example, the temperature chart may serve as a constant daily reminder of infertility. Not only can it be viewed as a sexual report card, but also it often results in the couple's having sex on schedule, which can lead to decreased sexual desire, impotence, or ejaculatory failure. Therefore, physicians must emphasize that the purpose of the temperature chart is to evaluate the timing of tests, not of intercourse. Some experts believe that with the exception of the basic evaluation or during ovulation induction, it is a mistake to ask patients to take their temperature daily for extended periods of time. With each patient, the medical information must be weighed in relation to the stress that results from a daily reminder of infertility.

There are a number of ways in which the physician can help the couple cope. The first is to treat the infertility as a problem of both partners. This is established by requesting that both partners attend the initial interview. In addition, the plan of tests and treatments should be developed with the couple as active participants; rationales, explanations, goals, and time frames should be shared. To increase the couple's sense of control, the physician should provide as many treatment choices as possible, encouraging the partners to share responsibility in making decisions.[17]

Starting with the initial interview, the physician should make an effort to provide specific medical information to reduce anxiety. Anxious patients cannot hear or understand subsequent information. In relaying the information, however, the physician should choose medical terms carefully. Terms such as *hostile mucus, habitual aborter, blighted ovum,* and *pregnancy wastage* should be avoided, since they may be misunderstood and contribute to feelings of inadequacy, guilt, and worthlessness.[26]

An open atmosphere must be established for asking questions. For example, many patients may secretly fear that performing sex incorrectly is the cause for their infertility; the opportunity to discuss these fears must be provided. Such questions allow the physician to recognize feelings of inadequacy, hopelessness, and depression. Some patients may hide their feelings, because they are self-conscious, afraid of being criticized, or thought of as being crazy. The physician must be alert for changes in personality, alterations in appetite or sleep patterns, loss of friends, sexual difficulties, excessive crying, or serious employment problems.[14] Optimistic assessments should not be substituted for direct confrontations of such emotional difficulties. It must be appreciated that infertility is a process rather than a series of independent emotional events. Data suggest that the distress experienced during infertility is a necessary part of the evolution toward acceptance of the infertility.[9]

Although not all patients need psychiatric help, the physician must provide emotional support and education and offer adequate time for expression of feelings. If a psychiatric referral is indicated, it should be made carefully so as not to give the patient the impression that she or he is crazy, or worse, is being abandoned.[36]

THE EFFECT OF EMOTIONS ON INFERTILITY

Psychoneuroendocrinology of Infertility

In the past, indirect evidence associated infertility with the secretion of biogenic amines and hypothalamic gonadotropin-releasing hormone (GnRH). Medications that interfered with catecholamine synthesis, metabolism, reuptake, or receptor binding were found to disturb gonadotropin release and subsequently result in anovulation. Common examples include reserpine, a catechol-depleting antihypertensive medication; d-methyl-p-tyrosine, an antihypertensive medication that inhibits tyrosine hydroxylase and depletes dopamine and norepinephrine; and phenothiazine, a dopamine receptor blocker that frequently causes amenorrhea or chronic anovulation.

Norepinephrine has been measured in human plasma during the periovulatory period, and its level been found to rise sharply either immediately before or simultaneously with the luteinizing hormone (LH) surge.[37] In rats, the depletion of norepinephrine during diestrus prevents the growth of ovarian follicles and the release of LH expected during proestrus and estrus.[38]

Large accumulations of catecholamines in the mammalian brain have been localized in the median eminence with cell bodies arising outside the basal hypothalamus. In the rhesus monkey, this part of the brain has been shown to be the nec-

essary nucleus in the pulsatile gonadotropin center and the predominant location of GnRH.[39] Neurons that carry catecholamines are distinct from those that carry GnRH. In monkeys subjected to ovariectomy, adrenergic-blocking agents immediately inhibited the pulsatile pattern of gonadotropin release.

Both norepinephrine and epinephrine are present in axons and nerve terminals in the arcuate nucleus, preoptic area, and other regions of the hypothalamus.[40] The arcuate-median eminence regions of the hypothalamus also contain the highest concentration of β-endorphins (endogenous opioids) in the human brain.[41] Furthermore, estradiol and dihydrotestosterone are concentrated in the nuclei of catecholaminergic neurons in the medial basal hypothalamus, and the target neurons of those two steroids are surrounded by catecholaminergic terminals.

Midcycle levels of sex steroids administered to women in the early to midfollicular phase appear able to elicit a midcycle follicle-stimulating hormone (FSH) but not LH surge to levels typically seen at midcycle.[42] These data suggest factors other than estrogen and progesterone are required to generate a normal midcycle LH surge.[42] Other workers localized axo-axonic interaction between dopamine and GnRH nerve terminals in the rat median eminence. This information is supported by the finding of a transient depression in circulatory LH after the administration of L-dopa, a precursor of dopamine. In addition, opiate receptors exist on dopamine neurons, and the naloxone-induced release of LH is abolished by dopamine.[43]

The mammalian pineal gland is innervated by the superior cervical ganglia. Activation of this network by the sympathetic nervous system may excite the pineal gland to secrete melatonin, which inhibits LH and stimulates prolactin. The mode and site of action of melatonin are still incompletely understood, but most studies suggest that melatonin suppresses pituitary function either by suppressing the pituitary response to GnRH or by inhibiting the frequency and amplitude of GnRH pulses. Basal LH levels in menopausal women can be suppressed with melatonin.[44] In ovulating women, however, melatonin has been shown to enhance the amplitude of spontaneous LH peaks and mean LH levels during the follicular but not the luteal phase of the menstrual[45] cycle and to enhance the LH and FSH response to GnRH in the follicular but not the luteal phase of the menstrual cycle.[46] We showed that the preovulatory LH surge occurs when serum melatonin levels are rapidly falling, which suggests that the early-morning onset of the LH surge may be related to the concurrent decline in melatonin secretion, as is the case in lower animals.[47] We also identified higher melatonin levels in preovulatory follicular fluid compared with plasma.[48] Subsequent studies have identified melatonin receptors on human granulosa cell membranes, which strongly suggests that melatonin in follicular fluid may have a physiologic role.[49]

Serotonin, from which melatonin arises, also stimulates prolactin in laboratory rodents. Serotonin may counteract the actions of the catecholamines by inhibiting GnRH. It has also been shown to stimulate prolactin in humans. Melatonin in human beings has been shown to be present at its highest levels 12 days before ovulation and at its lowest levels at the time of ovulation.[50,51] Norepinephrine has been shown to stimulate the pineal gland of some animals to secrete melatonin. In one report, ovulation was induced in a group of formerly anovulatory women after procaine blockade of their superior cervical ganglia. Therefore, strong evidence exists that gonadotropin secretion is intimately associated with biogenic amines.[52]

Mental depression has been found to be related to disorders of turnover or metabolism of central biogenic amines.[53] Some authors have postulated that an alteration in central catecholamine function may be causative in the development of acyclicity in patients with stress-induced, hypothalamic, chronic anovulation.[54] Normogonadotropic patients with amenorrhea and discernible psychologic disturbances were evaluated. Basal pituitary and ovarian hormone levels and the diurnal rhythm of cortisol were within normal limits. The pituitary-ovarian system was fully operational in those patients. They responded normally to GnRH, and spontaneous reversal of amenorrhea occurred after appropriate counseling. Subsequent studies showed that impairment of GnRH secretion is the likely underlying cause, since, in general, the frequency and amplitude of LH pulses are diminished.[55]

There is evidence of increased dopaminergic and opioid activity in patients with hypothalamic hypogonadotropic amenorrhea.[56] The study was based on the knowledge that opioid substances inhibit LH and augment prolactin secretion by the hypothalamic-pituitary system and that naloxone, an opioid receptor antagonist, could competitively inhibit these effects. These data tied in with those in previous reports showing that endogenous opioids increase pituitary prolactin levels through their interaction with opiate receptors located on dopamine nerve terminals in the median eminence.[57] A statistically significant elevation in circulating LH levels occurred in response to both a dopamine receptor antagonist (metoclopramide) and an opiate receptor antagonist (naloxone). These findings suggest that LH inhibition is due to increased hypothalamic opiate or dopamine activity. Because these patients responded normally to exogenous GnRH, it is reasonable to assume that this effect of endogenous opiates is on GnRH rather than on the pituitary gland directly.

Several other studies showed strong indirect evidence that psychologic trauma can lead to alterations in levels of catecholamines and endorphins that result in anovulation. Endorphins have been shown to decrease appetite. It may be that they are responsible for the low basal gonadotropin levels in persons with anorexia nervosa. Neuropharmacologic data suggest that excess dopamine and possibly norepinephrine are responsible for the clinical aspects of anorexia nervosa: (1) dopamine induces anorexia and weight loss; (2) amphetamine, a drug that increases brain catecholamines by inhibiting the reuptake of dopamine and epinephrine and affecting their release, causes anorexia and weight loss in habitual users; (3) apomorphine, a dopamine agonist, produces similar effects; (4) apomorphine and amphetamine both cause hypothermia; and (5) central catecholamine changes may cause amenorrhea.

Hormonal studies provide a different theory about how emotional factors affect infertility. Stress has been shown to stimulate the adrenal cortex to produce hirsutism and acne in some women. In addition, whereas exercise induces a response of the sympathetic nervous system, psychologic stress has been shown to induce a primarily adrenal response.[58] Some authors have suggested that the most important neuroendocrine response to stress is that of the adrenocorticotropic hormone (ACTH)–adrenal axis with the subsequent release of glucocorticoids and catecholamines.[59,60] In addition to releasing ACTH, corticotropin-releasing factor (CRF), together with vasopressin and oxytocin, modulates mood, behavior, and learning. It stimulates central noradrenergic activity, which activates peripheral norepinephrine release and adrenomedullary secretion of epinephrine. When CRF reaches the portal circulation, it stimulates the anterior pituitary gland to release ACTH and β-endorphin. The resulting release of cortisol can affect metabolism, the immune system, and mood. Corticotropin-releasing factor also affects reproductive function. Castrated rats exposed to noxious stimulation demonstrated both an inhibited pulsatile pattern of LH release and markedly lower plasma concentrations of LH. The central administration of a CRF antagonist reversed the inhibitory action of stress. Neither peripheral nor intraventricular injection of an inactive CRF analog was effective.[61] The CRF secreted by the brain during stress also inhibits GnRH secretion into the hypophyseal portal circulation. It has been shown that a high proportion of patients with hypothalamic chronic anovulation had psychosexual problems and socioenvironmental trauma before or around the time of puberty.[61] It is therefore possible that chronic and recurrent tension, or even the normal stress of adolescence, might affect adrenal steroidogenesis. The resultant excess of androgens could upset the balance of LH and FSH secretion, resulting in chronic anovulation and polycystic ovaries.

Another aspect of stress and amenorrhea can be found in the relation between stress and hyperprolactinemia. Follicular prolactin concentrations greater than 25 ng/mL were shown to suppress the normal follicular steroidogenic response to gonadotropins.[62] Women with hypothalamic amenorrhea may have increased levels of dopaminergic hormones. Patients with hyperprolactinemic amenorrhea also are believed to have increased dopamine activity. In addition, increased prolactin levels have been shown to suppress gonadotropins. This finding could provide an additional mechanism whereby stress could inhibit ovulation and ultimately lead to amenorrhea. Further evidence of the role of prolactin is gained by the fact that women with hyperprolactinemic amenorrhea treated with bromocriptine, a dopamine receptor agonist, resume normal gonadal function as long as prolactin levels are reduced. This finding adds support to the concept that prolactin inhibits gonadotropin release, and that dopamine plays an important role in the hypothalamic-pituitary control of ovulation.

Autonomic Control of the Reproductive Tract

The rich autonomic innervation of the pelvic viscera helps explain mechanisms through which emotional stress might affect ovulation, uterotubal function, or pregnancy maintenance (Fig 2–1).[63] Sympathetic centers in the lower thoracic segments of the spinal cord (T-10 to T-11) supply the ovary and part of the oviduct. The rest of the oviduct, the uterus, and the vagina are supplied by spinal nerves T-12 to L-2. The uterine cervix in humans is innervated from three plexuses of the pelvic autonomic nervous system—the superior, middle, and inferior hypogastric plexuses. Norepinephrine is the principal sympathetic neurotransmitter, although dopamine, epinephrine, acetylcholine, and prostaglandins are also involved. Two types of receptors, α and β, exist for the catecholamines. α-Receptors are most responsive to epinephrine and are usually excitatory, causing uterine contractions. Conversely, β-receptors are inhibitory and usually relax the uterus. It is by means of this mechanism that β-mimetic drugs such as ritodrine and terbutaline suppress uterine contractility in premature labor. The parasympathetic fibers arise from spinal nerves S-2 to S-4. The principal neurotransmitter is acetylcholine.

The ovary itself contains a few nerve bundles and small nonmyelinated adrenergic fibers in the parenchyma. These nerves transmit impulses to vascular smooth muscles within the ovary and could influence the hemodynamic state of blood vessels around the follicle. In this manner, the relative amount of hormones reaching the follicle could be affected and alter ovulation. In addition, distributed throughout the stroma are adrenergic and cholinergic fibers that terminate in neuromuscular connections in the theca interna.[64] Stress-related circumstances could modulate steroid production directly in this way.

Other fibers are located around follicles in all stages of growth, particularly graafian follicles, which contain smooth muscle cells in the theca interna. This allows the follicles to display spontaneous motor activity both in vivo and in vitro. Contractions are mediated both by α-adrenergic receptors and by muscarinic cholinergic receptors. Relaxation is mediated by

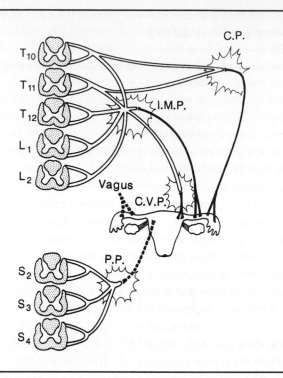

Figure 2–1. Autonomic control of the female reproductive tract. Preganglionic fibers are shown in white, sympathetic postganglionic fibers in solid black, and parasympathetic postganglionic fibers in broken lines. CP, celiac plexus; IMP, inferior mesenteric plexus; CVP, cervicovaginal plexus; PP, pelvic plexus (parasympathetic). *(From Pauerstein CJ: Anatomy. In: The Fallopian Tube: A Reappraisal. Philadelphia, Lea & Febiger, p. 18, 1974.)*

β-receptors. The nerve supply does not cross the basement membrane of the follicles. The proximity of adrenergic and cholinergic nerve fibers with smooth muscle fibers located throughout the stroma and theca interior resembles a neuromuscular system. This anatomic relation controlled by normal stimuli might be responsible for ovulation. Both norepinephrine and acetylcholine have induced contractions in follicular walls and increased intrafollicular pressure; dibenzyline, an α-adrenergic blocker, has been shown to inhibit ovulation in rabbits. Despite the interesting conjecture, sufficient evidence to the contrary has been reported to cast doubt on ovarian contractility as the sole mechanism of ovulation. One might theorize, however, that an excess of catecholamines resulting from stress might affect ovulation.

Stress-related catecholamine excess might affect oviductal activity. In humans, the ampulloisthmic junction and the uterotubal junction are richly endowed with adrenergic nerves.[65] Both α- and β-receptors have been found in the circular muscle of the isthmus and ampulloisthmic junction. In rabbits, excitatory α-receptors that are stimulated by norepinephrine have been identified in both circular and longitudinal muscles. Inhibitory β-receptors are located in the circular muscle, whereas longitudinal muscle possesses inhibitory α-receptors.

Steroids have been shown to influence receptor properties. Estrogen enhances and progesterone reduces the activity of excitatory receptors in the oviducts of rabbits, and the inhibitory action of β-receptors is stronger in the luteal phase. During the luteal phase in humans, norepinephrine similarly causes inhibitory responses in the oviduct. This change in sensitivity of α-adrenergic receptors has led some workers to speculate that high levels of preovulatory estrogen cause the isthmus to function as a sphincter at midcycle. As progesterone level rises over the next few days, β-adrenergic receptors are stimulated, and the isthmic sphincter relaxes. This mechanism may be very important in ovum transport. Further evidence supporting the isthmus as a factor in egg transport comes from recordings of pressure differences on either side of the ampulloisthmic junction. These differences are understandable, since the isthmus is richly innervated in contrast to the sparse innervation of the ampulla. In addition, the isthmus is more sensitive than the ampulla to norepinephrine. Owing to the rich innervation of the uterus, the tubes, and the ovaries by the autonomic nervous system, there is a sound neurologic basis for the effect of stress-related excess catecholamine secretion on ovulation, ovum transport, and implantation.

These comments are not intended to be all inclusive. They only provide an overview of the enormous interplay between the psychologic and the physiologic factors involved in infertility.

It has been known since ancient times that a relation exists between the menstrual cycle and the psyche.[1] The study of the emotional aspects of infertility is rapidly moving from consideration of psychologic presets, psychic trauma, and developmental influences to investigation of the production, reception, and effects of transmitter amines in brain centers associated with emotions and reproduction. The best-known brain transmitters are dopamine and norepinephrine (which are catecholamines), serotonin, and indolamine. The most notable direct effects of emotional stress on infertility involve these biogenic amines.

Other Psychogenic Factors

Psychogenic infertility has been documented in males.[66] Decreased libido and impotence are sequelae of psychologic problems.[67] Evidence shows that stress may result in retrograde and sham ejaculation due to malfunction in the sympathetic nervous system. Possible explanations include closure of the posterior sphincter of the urethra during orgasm, abnormal response to sympathetic stimuli in seminal vesicles and the ampullary part of the vasa deferentia, and a spastic permanent contraction of the ejaculatory duct. Stress may also result in a need for greater tactile stimulation because of alterations in tactile thresholds for touch and vibratory stimuli in men.[68] There is also evidence that psychologic stress can lead to abnormal spermatogenesis

through aberrant regulation of the hypothalamic-hypophysial axis.

Despite solid biochemical evidence of the effects of stress on the reproductive system, the question remains of underlying psychopathology as the root of infertility. Experts in analytic psychology propose that an unconscious psychologic defense mechanism defends the ego against the physiologic process of motherhood, which is basically feared. However, the most reports in the literature do not support a psychopathologic basis for infertility. A review of 235 papers written between 1935 and 1963 revealed no conclusive evidence that specific psychologic factors alter fertility.[69] Other work continues to support this hypothesis.[70] All these studies and theories fail to take into account the stress that infertility itself places on a couple. It is quite possible that infertility results in emotional problems, rather than the opposite.[71]

Conception After Adoption

It is commonly assumed, especially among the general public, that infertile couples frequently conceive after adoption. This concept was studied by several investigators, who had conflicting results. One investigator reported that in couples whose organic factors were adequately managed and who had continuing emotional tensions, adoption facilitated conception.[72] He reported evidence that adoption relieves emotional stress and thus results in conception. Several other groups of investigators have refuted these claims. A study of 100 adopting couples determined that adoption was responsible for conception among only four couples.[73]

In many studies, the diagnosis of definite infertility was not adequately controlled. Among 388 couples who adopted children, less than 12 subsequent pregnancies (3%) could be attributed to adoption.[74] A comparison of 249 adoptive infertile parents and 113 nonadoptive infertile couples revealed no evidence that adoption increased the tendency to conceive.[75] Thus, the statistical evidence documents that adoption itself does not appear to increase the likelihood of conception beyond that expected over time. Alternatively, pregnancies that did occur could possibly be explained by a reduction in stress that altered the neuroendocrinologic characteristics of the couple.[1]

PSYCHOLOGIC TREATMENT OF AN INFERTILE COUPLE

It is probably true that all persons who experience the stress of infertility could benefit from counseling. There are three times when such intervention is particularly beneficial: (1) the start of an infertility evaluation, (2) when a psychiatric indication is present, and (3) the termination of unsuccessful treatment. Evidence suggests that previously infertile couples who experience a successful pregnancy may also benefit from psychologic assistance during their transition to parenthood.[76] Previously infertile women who have a child experience higher levels of anxiety, avoidance behavior, and lack of preparation for taking home a newborn.

Few clinics and private practitioners routinely require contact with a counselor before or concurrent with commencement of an infertility evaluation. Even fewer consider the special needs of women who become pregnant after infertility. At the minimum, however, the impact of the diagnostic and therapeutic procedures should be addressed. An initial interview with a mental health professional should focus on identifying and explaining possible sources of anxiety, preparing the couple for future tests and treatments, and exploring sexual and marital problems, concerns, and unrealistic beliefs.[77] Ideally, the couple should be seen both together and individually, preferably with a counselor of the same sex. It must be remembered, however, that despite the degree of emotional stress experienced by couples at the initial visit, they are usually quite resistant to therapy at this point because of their optimism that at long last their problem will soon be solved.

Many patients become overwhelmed by the anxiety and stress that accompany infertility therapy.[78,79] This is particularly true if treatment has been prolonged. At this point, therapy can help the couple increase the feeling of control over their lives and lessen the impact of the medical and surgical interventions.

A psychiatric referral must be made when patients express an inability to cope with their emotions, or if they display depressive or suicidal symptoms, exacerbated alcohol or drug use, signs of unresolved grief, or sexual disorders.[80] It is critical to explain to patients that a referral to a mental health professional does not mean the termination of medical care; the reasons for referral should be clarified.[13] Patients are often resistant, however, because of the additional appointments for which they must miss work, the added costs, or the added perceived loss of control over their minds as well as their bodies.

The termination of unsuccessful treatment represents a crisis for most couples and is an appropriate time for short-term counseling. This is a critical period in which self-image, sexuality, and life plans must be reassessed. Patients must close an important chapter in their lives. Those who are told that they cannot bear children may require help mourning that loss. The most effective therapy is education to modify the emotional conflicts. Couples should be assisted with recognizing that because they are infertile does not imply that they are defective as human beings. They require help to maintain feelings of self-worth, self-esteem, and equanimity. Again, most couples resist therapy based on the feeling that they can "handle it themselves." The more likely reason, however, is the desire of one or both partners not to give up, because the reality is too painful to accept.

Most patients who receive a mental health referral either do not follow through to obtain services or delay calling the therapist for months or even years. In one study of 212 infertile couples who had been offered counseling services, only 62 attended any sessions.[81] At the end of the therapy, all 62 couples received a questionnaire concerning the frequency of psychologic symptoms and the response to counseling. The 31 couples (50%) who responded reported that counseling enhanced the quality of life; the women were more overtly affected than the men, but both benefited. Long-term counseling appeared to be more beneficial than short-term counseling. Because only half the couples responded, the results could represent self-selection of patients. However, because those who did respond reported therapy to be beneficial, at least half, if not more, of the couples who accepted counseling benefited.

Group therapy is valuable for infertile patients, because so many of them report that they feel alone in the world. Groups demonstrate that the members are not alone and that they can share thoughts, problems, experiences, and concerns with others in similar circumstances. In addition, participants can give support, which is often beneficial and rewarding. Group therapy can lead to improved communication with physicians as patients become aware of special needs and learn to express their frustrations about medical interventions. Group therapy is cost effective, and good results can be obtained without expensive, intensive individual psychotherapy.[82]

In one report, a group of five infertile women met with a registered nurse.[83] All women reported initial dissatisfaction with medical treatment and took their anxiety out on their husbands. At the outset of group therapy, the overwhelming impressions were a great amount of pressure and a marked sense of personal failure. At the end of the group work, all patients reported that the main value of the counseling sessions was a release of pressure and frustration, deeper insight into their own situation, and a general increased sense of well-being and security. Three years after undergoing group therapy, two of the patients had had a livebirth, one had had a miscarriage, one had declined tubal reconstructive surgery, and one was not available for follow-up data collection.

In another group for infertile patients, the emphasis was on attempts to internalize the patients' locus of control. The participants shared feelings, did role playing, explored free associations, used sentence completions, and searched for alternative patterns of behavior. In addition, they discussed societal pressure, blame and guilt, fears of medical testing and treatment, anger, feelings of family incompletion, sexual dysfunction, and alternatives to biologic parenting. These sessions led to marked decreases in fear, anxiety, isolation, and depression and resolution of feelings of blame and guilt.

Another study of infertile couples required both partners to complete a battery of psychologic tests before starting a six-session group counseling program.[36] The discussions covered denial, guilt, anger, depression, and self-concept in large and small groups and included role playing. The women experienced decreases in grief, depression, and anger and increases in self-concept. In another study, similar benefits were often informally reported by patients simultaneously going through ovulation induction or in vitro fertilization (IVF) as a result of meeting daily in the ultrasound or phlebotomy waiting areas.[84]

There is a lack of systematic appraisal of the impact of psychotherapy on infertile patients. Most of the conclusions in the literature are based on clinical assertions rather than precise evaluations of the problems experienced by couples or the methods used to resolve the problems. It is clear that infertility is stressful, and emotional support is beneficial but patients are resistant to receiving psychologic care.

The application of behavioral techniques such as relaxation training, stress management, and nutritional and exercise counseling to a wide variety of medical and psychiatric symptoms has met with widespread success, both in research and clinical settings. The first group clinical program to apply these techniques to infertile women was started in 1987 by these authors.[85] Participants learn numerous ways to elicit the relaxation response, "mini" relaxation techniques, cognitive restructuring, nutrition and exercise counseling, and methods for dealing with negative emotions, such as keeping a journal. Patients in the program must have documented infertility and be under a physician's care.

Patients completed a battery of psychologic questionnaires before beginning the program and again after completion. Participants demonstrated statistically significant reductions in every factor measured, including anxiety, depression, and anger.[86] In addition to the documented and subjective improvement in psychologic and physical symptoms, 34% of the participants conceived within 6 months of completion of the program. Within this group, 37% of the participants who attempted in vitro fertilization conceived on their first attempt.

Although the relation between stress and conception is still somewhat murky, the data support the efficacy of a behavioral approach in reducing psychologic distress. Because most patients with infertility report high levels of psychologic distress, a referral to a mental health professional with a specialization in relaxation training and stress management should be made with the goal of reducing distress, not solely for the purpose of conception enhancement.

IDIOPATHIC INFERTILITY

In the 1960s, it was estimated that 30% of all infertile patients suffered idiopathic infertility. By the 1980s, that number had been reduced to 5% or less. As biomedical knowledge increases, it is possible that anatomic, neuroendocrinologic, or pathophysiologic causes may eventually be found to explain virtually all infertility. Because evidence increasingly supports a biochemical connection between stress and the neuroendocrine system, a psychosomatic mechanism may operate in mediating some cases of infertility. When two partners are apparently healthy but infertile, there are two possible explanations: (1) the sophistication of modern testing is inadequate and undiagnosed organic abnormalities exist, or (2) alternatively but not exclusively, psychologic factors are operating. There may be a feedback loop mechanism to incorporate both hypotheses; delayed conception for an unknown reason leads to anxiety, and this leads to physiologic changes that delay conception even more. Stress can be both the cause and the effect of infertility (see the algorithm at the beginning of this chapter).

A woman is assumed to be psychogenically infertile if all known organic reasons have been excluded.[87] In a study that compared 22 couples with unexplained infertility with 10 fertile couples who acted as controls, the former had higher mean anxiety scores for all emotional factors.[88] In another study, 19 women with unexplained infertility were compared with 19 fertile women. No statistically significant differences occurred in assessment of traditional sex roles. The infertile patients had significantly more guilt than the controls, but there were no other statistically significant differences in attitudes toward sexuality. It is not known which comes first in these patients. It would seem logical that unexplained infertility could cause anxiety and guilt about the inability to become pregnant rather than the psychologic factors causing the infertility. A review of the claims that psychologic factors cause nonorganic female infertility concluded that the available data do not support the hypothesis.[89]

Despite the lack of evidence supporting the impact of psychologic factors on idiopathic infertility, numerous studies have documented increased conception rates after various psychologic interventions. One group followed 16 patients with unexplained infertility and depressive illness for 3 years.[90] The length of infertility ranged from 2 to 11 years. Seven patients had depressive symptoms of long duration, and nine reported such symptoms only after becoming aware of their infertility. Nine patients consented to undergo psychiatric treatment. Of the five patients with long-standing depression who underwent therapy, three became pregnant. None of the other patients became pregnant over the next 3 years. In another study, women who had unexplained infertility for a minimum of 3 years met in group sessions for 4 to 6 weeks.[91] Discussions included marriage, sex, infertility tests, husbands, childlessness, and clarification of medical questions. In addition to marked improvement in psychologic variables, attitudes toward medical treatment, and sexual functioning, 21.0% became pregnant within the first 3 months, and 26.5%

had become pregnant by the end of 6 months. In another group therapy study, five patients with unexplained infertility participated in a discussion group.[83] They acknowledged guilt, inadequacy, and problems with the marital relationship. All expressed benefits from the group sessions and felt they had achieved deeper insight into their own situation. Three of the five patients became pregnant, with two of these pregnancies resulting in livebirths.

One drug-intervention study supported the role of anxiety reduction in conception among 452 women with unexplained infertility.[92] Three hundred ten women were given 5 mg of thioridazine, a mild anxiolytic at that dosage, 1 hour after dinner from days 8 to 18 of their menstrual cycles; 142 women took a placebo (lactobacillus). All women were followed for 1 year. Ninety-four (30.3%) of the women who took the drug conceived, compared with 22 (15.5%) of the controls, a statistically significant difference. There were no significant differences between the two groups in miscarriages, malformations, or perinatal mortality.

A two-part study further documented the effects of stress in infertility. Forty-two women with unexplained infertility completed a psychologic battery before intensive medical treatment. During the follow-up period, 12 became pregnant. All 12 women showed statistically significant decreases in measured anxiety before pregnancy. Thus, anxiety seemed to predict pregnancy. The predictor was not anxiety as a general trait, however, but anxiety as it related to infertility. In the second part of the study, 14 of the women who had not become pregnant were randomly assigned to a behavioral treatment group or to a waiting-list control group. The 16 weekly behavioral sessions included relaxation training, cognitive restructuring, modeling of positive self-verbalizations, stress-inoculation training, anxiety management training, and self-instructional management. Patients were asked to perform progressive relaxation daily. Of the seven women who underwent behavioral treatment, four became pregnant within 3 months. None of the seven control patients became pregnant. The author concluded that situation anxiety may be an important antecedent variable contributing to unexplained infertility. In addition, it is apparent that behavioral therapy may be highly effective.

Although few data document that psychologic factors cause idiopathic infertility, four studies that examined the effects of psychologic interventions revealed subsequent pregnancy rates ranging from 26.5% to 60%. In most of these studies, the patients had long-standing histories of documented unexplained infertility. Three of the four interventions involved group treatment. It appears that group therapy provides effective treatment of patients suffering from unexplained infertility; it not only apparently provides important psychologic benefits but also may serve to increase the likelihood of conception.

ASSISTED REPRODUCTION: A PSYCHOLOGIC CHALLENGE

The new era of assisted reproductive technology has offered couples new hope and opportunity for conceiving a family. Women with blocked or missing fallopian tubes can bypass their anatomic problem by means of in vitro fertilization. Men with low sperm counts can fertilize their partner's eggs with intracytoplasmic single-sperm injection (ICSI). Women who no longer have eggs capable of being fertilized can receive an egg from another woman. Those without a uterus can designate another woman to carry the pregnancy for them.[93] As a result of preimplantation genetic testing, couples can also anticipate a higher likelihood of having a child without congenital anomalies. Despite the enormous advances these new technologies represent, they also cause psychologic concerns. Knowing when to stop treatment has become increasingly complex, as has knowing what options represent acceptable treatment to a particular couple, knowing whom to tell about a particular treatment option, and how to minimize the potential legal, ethical, and psychosocial complications that could arise.[94]

Many fears and anxieties are associated with participating in an IVF program, such as the time spent waiting to begin, the expense that is often not covered by insurance, and the possibility of failure at each stage of the cycle, including ovulation induction, oocyte retrieval, fertilization and cleavage, and embryo transfer. Many patients find the most anxious time to be between embryo transfer and pregnancy confirmation. This can be caused by a perceived lack of support from the IVF team, since there is no daily contact as during the first half of the cycle, and the unrelenting fear that the transferred embryos will be lost.[84] Patients also realize that the outcome beyond this point not only is out of their control but also is out of the control of the physician.

Emphasis in IVF often is on technology, and the human aspects are frequently ignored. An IVF team may unintentionally focus on monitoring the physiologic aspects of the cycle, leaving patients caught between trying to understand the importance of daily hormone levels and ultrasound examinations and simultaneously experiencing the tremendous emotional turmoil caused by the process. Failures during the cycle may be interpreted differently by the couple. For example, failure to ovulate or to produce sufficient sperm may result in self-blame, which can be devastating when superimposed on the emotional, physical, and financial expense of the process.

The impact of IVF failure can be profound. In a study of women undergoing IVF, 34% were found to have depressive symptoms before starting a cycle; of the women who did not conceive, 64% had depressive symptoms.[95]

The high prevalence of depressive symptoms among women who do not conceive during IVF may have an adverse impact on the success of future cycles. In a study of 330 women who completed psychologic questionnaires as they were preparing to undergo IVF, there was a statistically significant association between depression and conception among women who had already experienced an unsuccessful IVF cycle.[96] There was a 29% conception rate among women who were not depressed before treatment compared with a 13% conception rate among the women who reported depressive symptoms before treatment.

Psychologic interventions for patients undergoing IVF should be at two levels: (1) psychosocial assessment before entering the program and (2) counseling and support during and after each cycle. The initial psychologic evaluation should address ambivalence, anxiety, and unrealistic expectations, and it should assess abilities to tolerate stress and the potential for disappointment. During this initial session, enough time is needed to establish a relationship, provide information, and set appropriate goals. Counseling should be continued throughout each cycle to aid patients in dealing with the emotional roller coaster that accompanies IVF.[97]

When counseling is offered on a voluntary basis, few patients choose to participate. Thus, contact with a mental health professional is mandatory at many IVF centers. One reason this support is needed is that many couples become so distressed during the process that they drop out of the program, often at great personal and financial cost. In a survey of women who had dropped out of an IVF program, the reason most cited was cost, followed by anxiety and depression.[98] It appears obvious that patients need advice on how to deal with the stress before or simultaneously with being admitted to the program. Even patients who achieve pregnancy after in vitro fertilization experience higher levels of anxiety, avoidance behavior, and lack of preparation for taking home a newborn.[76] Practice guidelines must be developed to meet the special needs of women pregnant after infertility.

The use of behavioral medicine techniques by patients undergoing IVF can be accomplished in a group, and there is preliminary evidence that 2 to 4 hours of training may lead to increased conception rates in IVF patients. Fourteen of 63 women scheduled to begin IVF treatment self-selected to attend a two-session IVF preparation program.[99] The sessions included training in focused breathing to reduce pain, emotion-focused coping techniques, instruction in deep muscle relaxation, and information about what to expect during a treatment cycle. The women who attended the sessions had statistically significantly higher conception rates on their first IVF cycle than the women who did not attend. The women who attended the behavioral sessions were more likely to continue trying if the first attempt was unsuccessful, so they also achieved more subsequent pregnancies than the women who did not attend the sessions.

Infertile women have psychologic distress scores equivalent to those of women facing terminal illness. Infertility treatment is painful, expensive, and often unsuccessful. Psychologic interventions, especially group behavioral interventions and other forms of stress reduction, are underutilized and underappreciated. Infertile persons do not need to suffer as much as they do.

Additional psychologic attention should be provided for individuals and couples when undergoing less conventional forms of family building. Issues of being a single parent,[100] conceiving after menopause,[101] and introducing a third party into the reproductive process[102,103] all require and deserve special psychologic attention. In so doing, we are providing the necessary psychologic support our patients require as they experience the new reproductive technologies.

ACKNOWLEDGMENTS

The authors thank Herbert Benson, MD, for his support. Supported in part by grant MH50024 from the National Institute of Mental Health, Washington, DC.

REFERENCES

1. Seibel MM, McCarthy JA: Infertility, pregnancy, and the emotions. In: Goleman D, Gurin J (eds), *Mind Body Medicine*. Yonkers, NY, 1993:207
2. Domar AD, Seibel MM: Emotional aspects of infertility. In: Seibel MM (ed), *Infertility: A Comprehensive Text*, ed 1. Norwalk, CT, Appleton & Lange, 1990:23
3. Koropanick S, Daniluk J, Pattiuson HA: Infertility: A non-event transition. *Fertil Steril* 59:163, 1993
4. Menning B: The emotional needs of infertile couples. *Fertil Steril* 34:313, 1980
5. Berg BJ, Wilson JF: Psychological functioning across stages of treatment for infertility. *J Behav Med* 14:11, 1991
6. Seibel MM, Taymor ML: Emotional aspects of infertility. *Fertil Steril* 37:137, 1982
7. Collins A, Freeman EW, Boxer AS, Jureck R: Perceptions of infertility and treatment stress in females as compared with males entering in vitro fertilization treatment. *Fertil Steril* 57:350, 1992
8. Wright J, Duchesne C, Sabourin S, et al: Psychosocial distress and infertility: Men and women respond differently. *Fertil Steril* 55:100, 1991
9. Boivin J, Takefman JE, Tulandi T, Brender W: Reactions to infertility based on extent of treatment failure. *Fertil Steril* 63:801, 1995
10. Drake T, Grunert G: A cyclic pattern of sexual dysfunction in the infertility investigation. *Fertil Steril* 32:542, 1979
11. Cook E: Characteristics of the biopsychosocial crisis of infertility. *J Counseling Dev* 65:465, 1987
12. Berger D: The role of the psychiatrist in a reproductive biology clinic. *Fertil Steril* 28:141, 1977
13. Honea-Fleming P: Psychosocial components on obstetric/gyneco-

logic conditions with a special consideration of infertility. *Ala J Med Sci* 23:27, 1986

14. Mahlstedt P: The psychological component of infertility. *Fertil Steril* 43:335, 1985

15. Lalos A, Jacobsson L, Lalos O, von Schoultz B: The wish to have a child: A pilot study of infertile couples. *Acta Psychiatr Scand* 72:476, 1985

16. Jeffcoate W: The treatment of women with hirsutism. *Clin Endocrinol (Oxf)* 39:143, 1993

17. Spencer L: Male infertility: Psychological correlates. *Postgrad Med* 81:223, 1987

18. Waller KG, Shaw RW: Endometriosis, pelvic pain, and psychological functioning. *Fertil Steril* 63:796, 1995

19. Rapkin AJ, Kames LD, Darke LL, Stampler FM, Naliboff BD: History of physical and sexual abuse in women with chronic pelvic pain. *Obstet Gynecol* 76:92, 1990

20. Domar AD, Broome A, Zuttermeister PC, Seibel MM, Friedman R: The prevalence and predictability of depression in infertile women. *Fertil Steril* 58:1158, 1992

21. Downey J, McKinney M: The psychiatric status of women presenting for infertility evaluation. *Am J Orthopsychiatry* 62:196, 1992

22. Wright J, Duchesne C, Sabourin S, Bissonette F, Benoit J, Girard Y: Psychosocial distress and infertility: Men and women respond differently. *Fertil Steril* 55:100, 1991

23. Domar AD, Zuttermeister PC, Friedman R: The psychological impact of infertility: Comparison with patients with other medical conditions. *J Psychosom Obstet Gynecol* 14:45, 1993

24. Bents H: Psychology of male infertility: A literature survey. *Int J Androl* 8:325, 1985

25. Pantesco V: Nonorganic infertility: Some research and treatment problems. *Psychol Rep* 58:731, 1986

26. Farrer-Meschan R: Importance of marriage counseling to infertility investigation. *Obstet Gynecol* 38:316, 1971

27. MacNab RT: Male infertility: The psychological issues. In: Seibel MM, Kiessling AA, Bernstein J, Levin S (eds), *Technology and Infertility.* New York, Springer-Verlag, 1993:297

28. Stanton A, Tennen H, Affleck G, Mendola R: Cognitive appraisal and adjustment to infertility. *Women Health* 17:1, 1991

29. Berg B, Wilson J, Weingartner P: Psychological sequelae of infertility treatment: The role of gender and sex-role identification. *Soc Sci Med* 9:1071, 1991

30. Connolly K, Edelmann R, Cooke I, Robson J: The impact of infertility on psychological functioning. *J Psychosom Res* 36:459, 1992

31. Daniels K, Gunby J, Legge M, Williams T, Wynn-Williams D: Issues and problems for the infertile couple. *N Z Med J* 97:185, 1984

32. Sandelowski M, Pollock C: Women's experiences of infertility. *Image* 18:140, 1986

33. Lalos A, Lalos O, Jacobsson L, von Schoultz B: The psychosocial impact of infertility two years after completed surgical treatment. *Acta Obstet Gynecol Scand* 64:599, 1985

34. Berger D: Impotence following the discovery of azoospermia. *Fertil Steril* 34:154, 1980

35. Frick-Bruder C, Braendle W, Bettendorf G: Doctor-patient relationship during treatment of infertility. In: Insler V, Bettendorf G (eds), *Advances in Diagnosis and Treatment of Infertility.* Amsterdam, Elsevier North-Holland, 1981

36. Rosenfeld D, Mitchell E: Treating the emotional aspects of infertility: Counseling services in an infertility clinic. *Am J Obstet Gynecol* 135:177, 1979

37. Rosner J, Nagle C, deLaborde N, et al: Plasma levels of norepinephrine (NE) during the periovulatory period and after LH-RH stimulation in women. *Am J Obstet Gynecol* 124:567, 1976

38. Maeda K-I, Cagampang FRA, Coen CW, Tsukamura H: Involvement of the catecholaminergic input to the paraventricular nucleus, and of corticotropin-releasing hormone in the fasting-induced suppression of luteinizing hormone release in female rats. *Endocrinology* 134:1718, 1994

39. Kaufman J-M, Kesner JS, Wilson RC, Knobil E: Electrophysiologic manifestation of the LH-RH pulse generator activity in the rhesus monkey: Influence of α-adrenergic and dopaminergic blocking agents. *Endocrinology* 116:1327, 1985

40. Jarry H, Leonhardt S, Wuttke W: α-Aminobutyric acid neurons in the preoptic anterior hypothalamic area synchronize the phasic activity of the gonadotropin-releasing hormone pulse generator in ovariectomized rats. *Neuroendocrinology* 53:261, 1991

41. Brann DW, Zamorano PL, Putman-Robers CD, Mahesh UB: α-Aminobutyric acid–opioid interactions in the regulation of gonadotropin secretion in the immature female rat. *Neuroendocrinology* 56:445, 1992

42. Taylor AE, Whitney H, Hall JE, Martin K, Crowley WF: Midcycle levels of sex steroids are sufficient to recreate the follicle-stimulating hormone but not the luteinizing hormone midcycle surge: Evidence for the contribution of other ovarian factors to the surge in normal women. *J Clin Endocrinol Metab* 80:1541, 1995

43. Matera C, Freda PU, Ferin M, Wardlaw SL: Effect of chronic opioid antagonism on the hypothalamic-pituitary-ovarian axis in hyperprolactinemic women. *J Clin Endocrinol Metab* 80:540, 1995

44. Aleem FA, Wertzman ED, Weinberg V: Suppression of basal luteinizing hormone concentrations by melatonin in postmenopausal women. *Fertil Steril* 49:923, 1985

45. Cagnacci A, Soldani R, Yen SSC: Exogenous melatonin enhances luteinizing hormone levels of women in the follicular but not in the luteal menstrual phase. *Fertil Steril* 1995

46. Cagnacci A, Paoletti AM, Soldani R, Orru M, Maschio E, Melis GB: Melatonin enhances the luteinizing hormone and follicle-stimulating hormone responses to gonadotropin-releasing hormone in the follicular, but not in the luteal menstrual cycle. *J Clin Endocrinol Metab* 80:1095, 1995

47. Brzezinski A, Lynch H, Wurtman R, Seibel M: Possible contribution of melatonin to the timing of the luteinizing hormone surge. *N Engl J Med* 316:1550, 1987

48. Brzezinski A, Seibel MM, Lynch HJ, Deng MH, Wurtman RF: Melatonin in human preovulatory follicular fluid. *J Clin Endocrinol Metab* 64:865, 1987

49. Yie S-M, Niles LP, Younglai EV: Melatonin receptors on human granulosa cell membranes. *J Clin Endocrinol Metab* 80:1747, 1995

50. Webley G, Leidenberger F: The circadian pattern of melatonin and

its positive relationship with progesterone in women. *J Clin Endocrinol Metab* 63:323, 1986

51. Berga SL, Yen SSC: The human circadian pattern of plasma melatonin during four menstrual cycle phases. *Neuroendocrinology* 51:606, 1990

52. Novak E, Woodruff J: *Gynecologic and Obstetric Pathology with Clinical and Endocrine Relations.* Philadelphia, WB Saunders, 1974

53. Schidkrant J: Biogenic amines and affective disorders. *Annu Rev Med* 25:333, 1974

54. Reference unavailable

55. Crowley W, Felicori M, Spratt D, Santoro N: The physiology of gonadotropin-releasing hormone (GnRH) secretion in men and women. *Recent Prog Horm Res* 41:473, 1985

56. Quigley M, Sheehan K, Casper R, Yen S: Evidence for increased dopaminergic and opioid activity in patients with hypothalamic hypogonadotropic amenorrhea. *J Clin Endocrinol Metab* 50:949, 1980

57. Rasmussen DD: The interaction between mediobasohypothalamic dopaminergic and endorphinergic neuronal systems as a key regulator of reproduction: An hypothesis. *J Endocrinol Invest* 14:323, 1991

58. Dimsdale J, Moss J: Plasma catecholamines in stress and exercise. *JAMA* 243:340, 1980

59. Axelrod J, Reisine T: Stress hormones: Their interactions and regulation. *Science* 224:452, 1984

60. Biller BMK, Federoff HJ, Koenig JI, Klibanski A: Abnormal cortisol secretion and responses to corticotropin-releasing hormone in women with hypothalamic amenorrhea. *J Clin Endocrinol Metab* 70:311, 1990

61. Rivier C, Rivier J, Vale W: Stress-induced inhibition of reproductive function: Role of endogenous corticotropin-releasing factor. *Science* 231:607, 1986

62. McNatty K, Sawers R, McNeilly A: A possible role for prolactin control of steroid secretion by the human graafian follicle. *Nature* 250:653, 1974

63. Pauerstein CJ: Anatomy. In: Powerstein CJ, *The Fallopian Tube: A Reappraisal.* Philadelphia, Lea & Febiger, 1974

64. Amsterdam A, Lindner H, Groschel-Stewart U: Localization of actin and myosin in the rat oocyte and follicle wall by immunofluorescence. *Anat Rec* 187:311, 1977

65. Edward R: The adult ovary. In: Edwards R (ed), *Conception in the Human Female.* London, Academic Press, 1980

66. Abbey A, Andrews FM, Holman LJ: Gender's role in responses to infertility. *Psychol Women Q* 15:295, 1991

67. Greil AL, Porter KL, Leitko TA: Sex and intimacy among infertile couples. *J Psychol Hum Sex* 2:117, 1989

68. Rowland DL, Greenleaf, Mas M, et al: Penile and finger sensory thresholds in young, aging and diabetic males. *Arch Sex Behav* 18:1, 1989

69. Noyes R, Chapnick E: Literature on psychology and infertility: A critical analysis. *Fertil Steril* 15:543, 1964

70. Brand H: Psychological stress and infertility. II. Psychometric test data. *Br J Med Psychol* 55:385, 1982

71. Greenfield DA: Psychological issues in infertility. *Infertil Reprod Med Clin North Am* 4:3, 1993

72. Sandler B: Conception after adoption: A comparison of conception rates. *Fertil Steril* 16:313, 1965

73. Tyler E, Bonapart J, Grant J: Occurrence of pregnancy following adoption. *Fertil Steril* 11:581, 1960

74. Aronson H, Glienke C: A study of the incidence of pregnancy following adoption. *Fertil Steril* 14:547, 1963

75. Rock J, Tietze C, McLaughlin H: Effect of adoption on infertility. *Fertil Steril* 16:305, 1965

76. Bernstein J, Lewis J, Seibel MM: Effect of previous infertility on maternal-fetal attachment, coping styles, and self-concept during pregnancy. *J Wom Health* 3:125, 1994

77. Abbey A, Halman LJ, Andrews FM: Psychosocial treatment and demographic predictors of the stress associated with infertility. *Fertil Steril* 57:122, 1992

78. Andrews FM, Abbey A, Halman LJ: Is fertility problem stress different? The dynamics of stress in fertile and infertile couples. *Fertil Steril* 57:1247, 1992

79. Hirsch AM, Hirsch SM: The effect of infertility on marriage and self-concept. *J Obstet Gynecol Neonatal Nurs* 19:13, 1989

80. Bernstein J, Potts N, Mattox J: Assessment of psychological dysfunction associated with infertility. *J Obstet Gynecol Neonatal Nurs* 14:635, 1985

81. Bresnick E, Taymor ML: The role of counseling in infertility. *Fertil Steril* 32:154, 1979

82. Lukse M: The effect of group counseling on the frequency of grief reported by infertile couples. *J Obstet Gynecol Neonatal Nurs* 67S, 1985

83. Wilchins S, Park R: Use of group "rap sessions" in the adjunctive treatment of five infertile females. *J Med Soc N J* 1:951, 1974

84. Seibel MM, Levin S: A new era in reproductive technologies: The emotional stages of in vitro fertilization. *J IVF/ET* 4:135, 1987

85. Domar AD, Seibel MM, Benson H: The mind/body program for infertility: A new behavioral treatment approach for women with infertility. *Fertil Steril* 53:246, 1990

86. Domar AD, Zuttermeister PC, Seibel MM, Benson H: Psychological improvement in infertile women following behavioral treatment: A replication. *Fertil Steril* 58:144, 1992

87. Downey J, Yingling S, McKinney M: Mood disorders, psychiatric symptoms and distress in women presenting for infertility evaluation. *Fertil Steril* 52:425, 1989

88. Harrison R, O'Moore A, O'Moore R, McSweeny J: Stress profiles in normal infertile couples: Pharmacological and psychological approaches to therapy. In: Insler V, Betteadorf G (eds), *Advances in Diagnosis and Treatment of Infertility.* Amsterdam, Elsevier North-Holland, 1981:

89. Denber H: Psychiatric aspects of infertility. *J Reprod Med* 20:23, 1978

90. Ellenberg J, Koren Z: Infertility and depression. *Int J Infertil* 27:219, 1982

91. Arbanel A, Bach G: Group psychotherapy for the infertile couple. *Int J Infertil* 4:151, 1959

92. Sharma J, Sharma S: Role of thioridazine in unexplained infertility. *Int J Gynecol Obstet* 37:37, 1992

93. Seibel MM: A new era in reproductive technology: In vitro fertil-

ization, gamete intrafallopian transfer, and donated gametes and embryos. *N Engl J Med* 318:828, 1988

94. Seibel MM, Kiessling AA, Berskin J, Levin S: *Technology and Infertility: Clinical, Psychological, Legal and Ethical Aspects.* New York, Springer-Verlag, 1993

95. Garner C, Aronold E, Gray H: The psychological impact of in vitro fertilization. *Fertil Steril* 41:28, 1984

96. Thiering P, Beaurepaire J, Jones M, et al: Mood state as predictor of treatment outcome after in vitro fertilization/embryo transfer technology (IVF/ET). *J Psychosom Res* 37:481, 1993

97. Mahlstedt P, MacDuff S, Bernstein J: Emotional factors and the in vitro fertilization embryo transfer process. *J IVT/ET* 4:232, 1987

98. Mao K, Wood C: Barriers to treatment of infertility by in vitro fertilization and embryo transfer. *Med J Aust* 140:1532, 1984

99. Farrar D, Holbert L, Drabman R: Can behavioral-based preparation counseling increase pregnancy after in vitro fertilization? Presented at the Meeting of In Vitro Fertilization Psychologists, July 1990; Melbourne, Australia

100. Williams LS, Power PW: The emotional impact of infertility in single women: Some implications for counseling. *J Am Med Wom Assoc* 32:327, 1977

101. Hutchinson KA: Psychological aspects of menopause. *Infertil Reprod Med Clin North Am* 4:503, 1993

102. Mechanick-Braverman A, Corson SL: Characteristics of participants in a gestational carrier program. *J Asst Reprod Genetics* 9:4, 1992

103. Bolton V, Golombok S, Cook R, et al: A comparative study of attitudes toward donor insemination and egg donation in recipients, potential donors and the public. *J Psychosom Obstet Gynecol* (in press)

CHAPTER 3

Semen Analysis

A Practical Guide to Performance and Interpretation

SUSAN A. ROTHMANN

Semen Specimen Collection
Instructions
Laboratory accession
Macroscopic Analysis
Liquefaction
Color
Volume
Consistency (viscosity)
pH
Microscopic Analysis
General conditions
General analysis

Sperm concentration
Sperm motility
Sperm morphology
Sperm classification—World Health Organization
Sperm classification—strict criteria
Nonsperm morphology
How to Recognize a Quality Semen Analysis Laboratory
Limitations of Semen Analysis

Semen analysis includes examination of the spermatozoa and the seminal fluid delivered at the time of ejaculation. Because the reproductive potential of a man is suggested by the quality and number of spermatozoa delivered to the genital tract of a woman, semen analysis serves as the primary assessment of male fertility.[1] In this role, semen analysis indirectly provides the clinician with a global view of the entire male reproductive system. Without proper function of the pituitary gland, the testis, the accessory glands, and spermatogenesis itself, one or more factors of the semen analysis will be abnormal. This perspective allows the semen analysis to serve as an ideal test for male reproductive toxicity studies.[2] Sperm analysis provides a critical quality control in fertility programs.[3] It is often used as a quality indicator of sperm freezing and sperm processing protocols and can be used to determine quality of culture media and contact materials. Semen analysis can be divided into several

components: sample collection, macroscopic examination, and microscopic analysis (Table 3–1). Good laboratory practice and quality control form the essential framework for an analysis (Table 3–2).

SEMEN SPECIMEN COLLECTION

Semen values generally are quite stable in most men over time.[4-6] Three samples should be analyzed to establish a reliable baseline profile of an individual man's semen measures.[6,7] An important source of variation and misleading results is improper or incomplete semen specimen collection. Patients need clear and thorough instructions and need to understand the importance of compliance. Because many men are embarrassed about undergoing a semen analysis, they often do not want to discuss

TABLE 3–1. COMPONENTS OF SEMEN ANALYSIS

Macroscopic	Microscopic
Liquefaction	Agglutination
Consistency	Concentration
General appearance	Percentage motile
Color	Kinematics
Volume	Sperm morphology
pH	Semen cytology
	Sperm viability

the collection requirements. Written instructions should be provided at the time the test is ordered. Compliance is usually enhanced if reasons for the instructions are included and the patient understands that results will be accurate only if the sample is collected properly. The following instruction items are essential.

Instructions

Ejaculatory Abstinence Time

The usual recommendation for time of ejaculatory abstinence before specimen collection is 48 to 72 hours. The patient needs to understand that all types of ejaculatory activity should be avoided prior to collection. The accessory sex glands replenish secretions within 2 to 3 days of ejaculation.[8] Shorter times may yield a low semen volume, and longer times may be associated with the presence of aged, immotile sperm in the ejaculate because of stasis.[9]

Collection Container

Semen should be collected into a disposable tissue-culture grade polypropylene wide-mouthed container with a securely fitting cap, ideally provided by the laboratory after the lot has been tested for toxicity. A 130-mL sterile urine specimen container is commonly used. Use of jars and containers from home should be discouraged, because they may contain residual detergent or contents that may alter sperm motility or viability.

Collection Method

Ideally semen should be collected by masturbation. Before collection, the patient should carefully wash and rinse his hands

TABLE 3–2. ESSENTIAL ROUTINE LABORATORY QUALITY PROCEDURES

Verification of equipment function
Daily quality control for all procedures (minimum of two levels required)
Regular internal proficiency testing (recommended once a month)
External proficiency testing (minimum of twice a year required)
Routine personnel training

and penis. Patients who need additional stimulation or who have objections to masturbation should use a silicone condom. Lubricants should not be used, because virtually all such agents contain preservatives that immobilize sperm.[10]

Transport Conditions

Semen sample temperature should be maintained close to body temperature (carried in an inside shirt pocket). Extremes of temperature should be avoided but reported.

Transport Interval

Semen samples should reach the laboratory within 30 to 45 minutes of collection.

Sample Labeling

The patient should label the sample with his name, date, time of collection, and any unique laboratory identifier. If the female partner has a different last name, it is helpful to include her name.

Authorizing Requisition

All laboratory tests must be accompanied by a written request. Oral orders can be accepted but must be followed with a written request.

Laboratory Accession

The laboratory should obtain the aforementioned data and ascertain whether any deviations from the recommended collection conditions occurred. The sample should receive a unique accession number. The time of collection and receipt should be noted. Because the semen analysis often is ordered by the female partner's physician, adding the partner's name to the report can help the physician link the report with the appropriate patient.

MACROSCOPIC ANALYSIS

Liquefaction

Liquefaction and consistency (viscosity) are completely separate characteristics that often are confused by testing laboratories and physicians.[9,11] A brief review of semen composition should help differentiate the two phenomena. Most of the seminal fluid is contributed by the seminal vesicles and contains fructose and gel-forming proteins.[12] At initial ejaculation, a small volume of epididymal fluid containing a high sperm concentration is emitted with secretions of the prostate gland, about 30% of total volume, which is followed by emission and mixing of seminal vesicle secretions, about 70% of volume.[13] As the fluids combine, a thick gel forms immediately. Normally the gel liquefies in 15 to 30 minutes as prostatic enzymes cleave the gel-forming proteins into fragments.[13]

Failure of semen gelation appears to be a rare pathologic condition. However, the condition may go undetected because it can only be evaluated when a sample is collected at the laboratory and examined immediately after collection. Gelation failure occurs in cases of ejaculatory duct obstruction or when seminal vesicles are absent or function abnormally.[14] Delayed or incomplete liquefaction is more common and easier to detect than gelation failure. At macroscopic examination the semen should be a homogeneous fluid that one can examine grossly by holding the specimen container against a bright light. The presence of mucus-like streaks or jelly-like grains indicates incomplete liquefaction. Samples should be evaluated at 20- to 30-minute intervals and should display complete liquefaction by 1 hour after ejaculation. Incubation at 37°C can be useful.

Abnormal liquefaction is an indicator of prostatic dysfunction. However, abnormalities have not been clearly associated with specific fertility impairment. Microscopic observation often reveals that sperm appear trapped between gel streams or clot-like structures, which can mechanically reduce their access to the female reproductive tract. Biochemical studies have shown that men with oligoasthenozoospermia have markedly reduced protein- and zinc-containing prostatic secretions, which are involved with liquefaction.[15]

Color

Normal semen is opalescent and grayish white in color. Color deviations are important, because unless they are of exogenous pharmaceutical origin, they may indicate a serious pathologic condition.[16] A reddish tinge indicates erythrocyte contamination and suggests collection difficulties, accessory gland (usually prostate) disease, or a genital tract tumor. Yellow is associated with infection or urine contamination causing decreased motility or viability.

Volume

The suffix -spermia is used to refer to semen volume. *Normospermia* is 1.5 to 5 mL of semen per ejaculation. Volume should be measured after the sample has liquefied. A convenient measurement technique is to use a 5-mL serologic pipette graduated in 0.1-mL increments to transfer the specimen from the collection container to a test tube.

Deviations from the normal range can be useful in identifying a number of common nonpathologic situations and pathologic ones. *Hypospermia* may indicate semen loss during collection or a very short sexual abstinence time. Discussion with the patient may clarify the possibilities; however, patients often are too embarrassed to admit collection difficulties. It is useful to request this information in a questionnaire that the patient can complete at the time the sample is submitted. Ejaculate loss during semen collection is fairly common, occurring in 10 percent of collections, usually with loss of the first fraction.[17] Loss of the initial epididymal and prostatic portion of the ejaculate results in a low sperm count and basic pH. Loss of the last part of the ejaculate, which contains the seminal vesicle secretions results in a normal to high sperm count but low fructose concentration.

If collection errors are ruled out, a low ejaculate volume suggests a clinically significant pathologic condition that can affect fertility. If no sperm are present, a centrifuged urine sample should be examined immediately after orgasm to detect retrograde ejaculation. Caused by incomplete closure of the bladder neck at the time of emission, retrograde ejaculation can follow a wide range of clinical situations, including bladder reconstruction, retroperitoneal operation, and diabetes.[7] It also can be experienced by men who use inadequate stimulation during masturbation although they have normal postcoital tests. Retrograde ejaculation may respond to pharmacologic treatment with α-adrenergic receptor stimulators, such as pseudoephedrine and phenylpropanolamine.[18] If no sperm are present in the urine and fructose is not detected in the semen, the patient probably has a serious anatomic anomaly, such as total obstruction of the ejaculatory ducts or congenital absence of the vas deferens and seminal vesicles.

Hyperspermia sometimes occurs in men who are undergoing an infertility evaluation, but its relevance to the couple's fertility problem is questionable. It is possible that a dilutional effect of hyperspermia could reduce fertility, but evidence for this is lacking.[9]

Consistency (Viscosity)

At the same time that volume is measured, consistency can be determined. Normally, semen can be released from a narrow-bore pipette in discrete drops. As consistency increases, the semen becomes more difficult to pipette. Although scales have been described to differentiate degrees of consistency,[11] the utility of these scales is unclear because no definite association of infertility with hyperconsistency exists beyond mechanical slowing of sperm motility. The seminal plasma consistency may not resemble the consistency in ovulatory cervical mucus.[9]

Hyperconsistency is more important to the laboratory than to the clinician, because it makes mixing and pipetting of samples difficult and can cause misleading volume, count, and motility results. Sperm processing for artificial insemination also is difficult with very thick samples. For this reason, consistency should be noted as normal or high with disclaimers about analytic accuracy with high consistency. Techniques to reduce consistency include mechanical disruption by passage through an 18-gauge syringe needle,[11] addition of mucolytic agents,[72] or aspiration of the mucus plug from the semen sample before preparation.[20] The use of enzymatic disruption with chymotrypsin/galactose treatment also reduces consistency and improves sperm separation before intrauterine insemination.[21]

pH

Semen pH is normally slightly alkaline, in the range of 7.2 to 8.0.[22] Routine measurement of pH adds little useful information.[9] When the volume abnormalities described earlier are encountered, one can measure pH by spreading a drop onto quantitative litmus paper in a range from 6.5 to 9.0.[23,24] The accuracy of the pH paper should be verified with known standards.

MICROSCOPIC ANALYSIS

General Conditions

Semen should be evaluated with phase contrast optics. The microscope must be calibrated properly with a centered light source and phase annulus rings. Sperm motility is altered by changes in temperature, thus the laboratory temperature at the time analysis begins should be noted. The optimal temperature for motility studies is 37°C, but this requires a heat block and temperature-regulated microscope stage. For this reason, most semen analyses are performed at room temperature, which is acceptable as long as the temperature is controlled and noted on the semen analysis report.

General Analysis

When the volume has been measured, the sample should be thoroughly mixed and examined with a microscope. Many authors describe this step of the semen analysis as a wet preparation and recommend making a coverslipped droplet for examination. At my laboratory, the examination is performed on a sperm-analysis chamber just before the sample aliquot is counted. For some specimens a dilution must be made and the sample replated, but for many specimens our procedure can save an analytic step.

The examination should include a subjective estimate of sperm count and motility to determine if dilution should be performed. The presence of non–sperm cells, such as epithelial cells, bacteria, and round cells, which may be leukocytes or immature germ cells, should be recorded. Immature sperm cells should be positively identified from a stained semen smear (see Sperm Morphology). Any evidence of agglutination (sperm cells adhering to sperm cells) or aggregation (sperm cells adhering to debris or other cells) should be reported. Agglutination is most commonly associated with antisperm antibodies,

and investigation of this possibility should be recommended in the report.

Sperm Concentration

Numerous articles and monographs[11,23,25] and the World Health Organization (WHO) manual[22] describe techniques for manual determination of sperm concentration. A variety of chambers are available for semen analysis, including several disposable types. Each has advantages and limitations that are well characterized and must be weighed before one is selected for a particular laboratory.

No matter what chamber is used, several procedural operations are essential. The sample must be well mixed before aliquoting. Several 3-second vortex pulses at medium setting usually provide sufficient mixing without damaging the sperm. The chamber should be loaded with a volume specified by the manufacturer, and care should be taken not to overload the chamber. The sample should be analyzed at a concentration known to provide acceptable precision. As concentration increases, precision decreases. The laboratory should establish its range of reliability.

The accuracy of sperm counting can be increased by immobilizing the sperm prior to analysis.[11] If the sample has a concentration of less than 60 million per milliliter the sample can be placed in a 56°C water bath for 5 to 10 minutes to immobilize. If the concentration is greater, the sperm may clump during heat treatment and should be diluted in an immobilizing diluent such as buffered formalin.[23] When dilution must be made, the sample should be diluted in duplicate and each duplicate counted.

Several kinds of quality-control materials can be used for sperm counting ranging from latex heads to cryopreserved sperm. The most appropriate controls resemble the substance being analyzed, are reproducible, and are cost effective. At my laboratory we use stabilized sperm. Repetitive counts are used to construct control charts, which are posted at the workbench. Before patient samples are analyzed, two levels of control are counted and plotted. The visual display gives immediate feedback about accuracy and serves as permanent documentation (Fig 3–1). The control material or a retained patient specimen can be counted later in the day to establish testing precision.

The suffix -zoospermia is used to describe sperm. Normozoospermic values are derived from large population studies that established a statistically low likelihood of conception when sperm concentration is less than 20 million per milliliter.[70,71] Average sperm concentration is 70 to 80 million per milliliter.[7] When oligozoospermia is observed and collection errors are ruled out, an evaluation should be performed for endocrine dysfunction or exposure to toxic agents. If the analysis reveals complete azoospermia, the specimen should be concen-

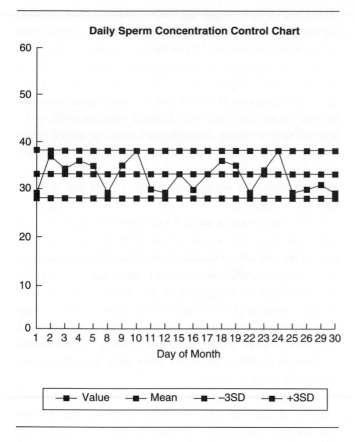

Daily Sperm Concentration Control Chart

—■— Value   —■— Mean   —■— –3SD   —■— +3SD

Figure 3–1. A statistical process control chart for sperm concentration. Upper and lower limits were calculated from 20 replicate counts of the stabilized sperm control sample.

trated by means of centrifugation and the pellet examined for sperm. The seminal plasma should be reserved for fructose evaluation if indicated. If no sperm are found and the sample has abnormally low volume, a postejaculatory urine specimen should be examined to rule out retrograde ejaculation. If sperm are not present, the reserved seminal plasma should be tested for the presence of fructose. If fructose is detected, spermatogenic failure should be suspected and serum follicle-stimulating hormone (FSH) levels measured. If fructose is not detected, congenital bilateral absence of the vas deferens and seminal vesicles is likely. This anatomic defect has been associated with mutations of the cystic fibrosis transmembrane-conductance regulator gene, which can be confirmed by means of genetic analysis.[27] Polyzoospermia is not clearly associated with fertility problems unless other abnormalities are present.[11]

Sperm Motility

Many laboratories use a subjective determination of motility by estimating the number of moving sperm in a wet-mount preparation. This technique should be discouraged because it is difficult to reproduce and motility is often substantially overesti-

mated in specimens with a moderate to high percentage of motility or rapid velocity.[28]

Strategies for reducing variability include careful counting,[29] but the simplest and easiest method is that described by Keel.[11] First, the nonmoving sperm in the sample are counted (count A). An aliquot of the specimen is treated to immobilize the moving sperm in one of two ways: (1) if the sample concentration is low to moderate (sperm widely distributed and easy to count), an aliquot is incubated in a 56°C waterbath for 5 to 10 minutes; (2) if the sample concentration is high, an aliquot is diluted 1:1 with buffered 10% formalin.[23] A count of all the sperm in the immobilized sample is performed (count B). Each step should be counted in duplicate to increase accuracy. Percentage motility is calculated as:

$$\frac{\text{Count B} - \text{Count A}}{\text{Count B}} \times 100$$

This method has the added advantage of using the same quality-control preparation as sperm-counting methods. Motility quality controls such as videotapes are awkward to use except with automated sperm analyzers, and cryopreserved sperm are difficult to prepare and are expensive to obtain and store.

Decreased percentage motility, termed *asthenozoospermia,* can be caused by varicocele, prolonged ejaculatory abstinence, ultrastructural or biochemical abnormalities of the flagellar apparatus or sperm differentiation, epididymal transport, or antisperm antibodies.[30] It is also associated with infection and inflammation, possibly due to leukocyte production of oxygen radical species[31–33] or nitric oxide.[34]

Percentage motility less than 30% or complete lack of motility should be investigated further to determine if the sperm are immotile or dead (necrozoospermia). Semen should be mixed with a vital dye such as eosin Y and smeared onto a slide (Fig 3–3). As a control, a second portion of the semen should be mixed with buffered formalin to kill all sperm before staining. Living sperm exclude the dye, and dead sperm stain dark pink. Use of a counterstain such as nigrosin aids detection. The percentage of dead sperm should never be greater than the percentage of motile sperm (dead sperm don't swim!). If the nonmotile sperm are alive, the sample should be fixed and analyzed by means of electron microscopy for ultrastructural flagellar defects.[30]

Some laboratories attempt to grade the forward progression of the sperm, with ranges from no movement to high forward progression.[7,22,24] These measures are highly subjective and almost impossible to control. Using a gridded chamber and defining movement over a specific distance (ie, number of squares) may improve measurement reproducibility, but quality control remains a problem.

Automated systems for assessing motility are available. Computer-assisted sperm analysis systems allow rapid, objective, and reproducible measurement of the percentage of motile sperm and of sperm swimming characteristics that the human eye cannot determine. These kinematic measurements include sperm velocity, amplitude of lateral head displacement, wobble, and beat cross frequency.[35] Although sperm population average values of some kinematic variables have been shown to correlate with fertility,[36-38] multivariate and cluster analyses offer more robust ways to analyze kinematic data. Such statistical techniques can identify specific sperm subpopulations which may better predict fertility outcome.[39-41] Comprehensive discussion of CASA technology is beyond the scope of this chapter and the reviewer is referred to recent reviews for more information.[1,29,35,42]

Sperm Morphology

One of the most predictive components of semen analysis is sperm morphology.[43] Ironically, morphology is one of the most difficult components to standardize because of its highly subjective nature.[44] Part of the disagreement on correct classification of different morphologic forms is that they display continuous variation rather than discrete typologies.[45,46] Adding to the difficulty are the many sperm morphology classification schemes. At least four are in routine use,[22,24,26,43] and all have different standards of normal, leading to considerable confusion, especially when the method in use is not stated on the report. Furthermore, the two most common schemes used in fertility laboratories, the WHO 1992 criteria[22] and the strict criteria[43,47,48] are rarely used in general hospital and reference laboratories, which usually use older, less critical schemes. This difference leads to enormous discrepancies in normal values, as shown in Table 3–3.

The questions raised about the variety of classifications are the following: (1) What is a normal sperm? (2) What impact does abnormal sperm have on reproduction? Older schemes attempted to define normal as an idealized oval form. Researchers examined the number of these forms in putatively fertile individuals, a difficult undertaking because of the extreme heterogeneity of sperm morphology in healthy humans.[49] In contrast, the strict classification was based on a reference population of sperm found in postcoital upper endocervical canal mucus.[47,48] Menkveld et al[47,48] found a remarkably homogeneous population in this location, which is presumably biologically selected for normality. Normal limits were determined by comparison with fertilization in vitro.[43] Nevertheless, no matter which classification scheme is used, morphology can be viewed only as a vector and not as an absolute indicator of fertility versus sterility.[50] This is particularly true since the introduction of intracytoplasmic single-sperm injection (ICSI), in which a single sperm selected from a sample containing no normally shaped sperm may be injected into the cytoplasm of an egg and yield a successful pregnancy.

Preparation of semen smears differs from that of blood films in that a rectangular, even, and thin smear is preferred over a feathered-edge wedge smear.[22] Approximately 10 μL of well-mixed semen is placed onto a clean, labeled glass slide. The edge of another slide is touched to the drop, and the semen is allowed to spread evenly and completely along the edge. With the plain slide held at a 45° angle from the labeled slide, slow, even pressure is used to push the semen until it is spread evenly along the entire length of the slide. If the sperm count is more than 60 $\times 10^6$ per milliliter, a wider angle should be used. If the count is less than 40×10^6 per milliliter, a lesser angle should be used to achieve even distribution.

Papanicolaou stain is preferred by many laboratories because of its ability to show clearly fine cellular details of all regions of the sperm and immature cells, its optical advantages, and its storage stability for future reference. Previous objections to the solvents formerly used in Papanicolaou stains are no longer relevant because of the availability of aqueous nontoxic clearing reagents. The ability to immediately fix the specimen is another distinct advantage of Papanicolaou stain preparations, because artifacts of air drying, such as vacuoles, and alterations of head size are reduced. Many publications erroneously state that the smear should be air dried after preparation. On the contrary, the smear should be immediately and completely covered with aerosol fixative unless using a giemsa-based stain. Although cytologic fixatives can be used with Papanicolaon stains, my laboratory obtains consistent fixation with inexpensive commercial hair spray (AquaNet, regular, not superhold). When the slides are completely dry, they can be stored in the dark until stained. Fixatives interfere with many giemsa-containing staining methods and should be avoided when using these types of stains.

At least 200 sperm should be examined with a 100×

TABLE 3–3. COMPARISON OF SEVERAL COMMONLY USED MORPHOLOGIC CLASSIFICATION SCHEMES

	MacLeod	WHO Second Edition	WHO Third Edition	Strict
Normal lower limit (%)	60–80	50	30	14
Reference population source	Semen; investigator selection	Semen; investigator selection	Semen; investigator selection	Postcoital cervical mucus; biologic selection
Reference population	Heterogeneous	Heterogeneous	Heterogeneous	Homogeneous
Borderline normal forms	Included in normal	Included in normal	Excluded from normal	Excluded from normal

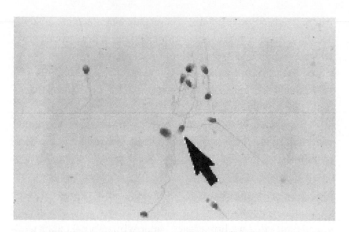

Figure 3–2. Normal sperm. Arrow points to normal spermatozoan by all criteria. Head shape is perfectly oval without tapering. Sperm at the left and lower right are borderline normal spermatozoa according to strict criteria because the heads are not truly oval. Most laboratories that use WHO criteria would classify these sperm as normal.

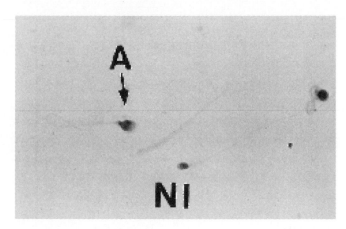

Figure 3–4. Megalocephalic sperm (**A**) indicated with arrow. Normal size head shown for reference (**NI**).

bright-field objective and classified as normal or abnormal. Each type of abnormality should be recorded. Because abnormal sperm may have more than one abnormality, the abnormalities usually are cumulatively higher than 100% and should be expressed as the percentage of the abnormal sperm. Only recognizable sperm should be counted in the differential, including tailless heads scored as midpiece defects, but not including headless tails.

Sperm Classification—World Health Organization

Normal

Normal sperm (Figs 3–2, 3–3) have an oval head (4.0 to 5.5 μm length, 2.5 to 3.5 μm width) with a well-defined acrosomal region composing 40% to 70% of the head area. No neck, mid-

piece, or tail abnormalities are present. If a cytoplasmic droplet is present, it should be smaller than one third of the head area. Some variations are allowed (such as vacuoles if less than 20% of the head space or very slight tapering at top or bottom). Unlike previous recommendations, the latest edition of the WHO manual considers all borderline normal forms to be abnormal.[22]

Abnormal Head Shape and Size

Microcephalic sperm are approximately one half the size of a normal sperm or smaller; megalocephalic sperm are approximately one and a half times the size of a normal sperm or greater (Fig 3–4). Pinhead sperm are not included in the differential, but if more than one pinhead is present per five sperm, the finding should be reported.

Tapered sperm have elongated, cigar-shaped heads and are usually longer than normal sperm (Fig 3–5). Elongated sperm

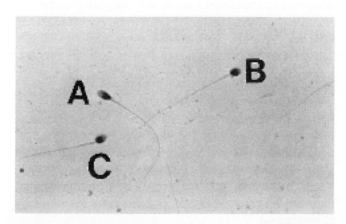

Figure 3–3. A, B. Borderline normal spermatozoa according to strict criteria. **C.** Normal sperm by all criteria.

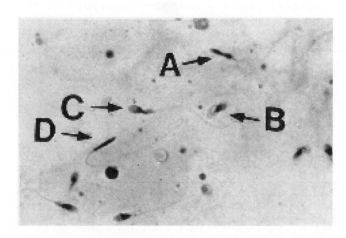

Figure 3–5. A, C. Amorphous head. **B.** Coiled tail. **D.** Tapered head.

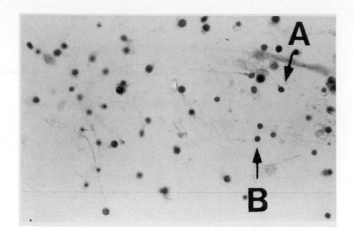

Figure 3–6. A, B. Round head (no acrosome).

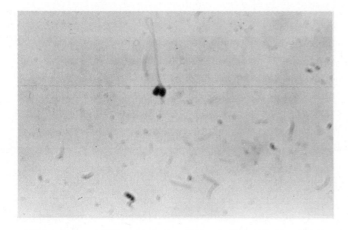

Figure 3–7. Bicephalic sperm with amorphous heads, cytoplasmic droplet, and duplicate tail.

whose heads come to a point are not true tapers but are artifacts usually seen in crowded areas of the slide or where much debris is present. Tapered sperm are often observed in patients with varicocele or recent viral illness.[5]

Round sperm lack an acrosome, making them incapable of fertilization without ICSI (Fig 3–6).

Bicephalic or multicephalic sperm have a developmental abnormality in which two or more heads are joined at the neck or midpiece (Fig 3–7).

Neck or Midpiece Defects

Sperm heads that have no tail, an improperly inserted tail, or a bent tail that forms a 90° angle to the long axis of the head have midpiece defects (Fig 3–8). Other forms in this category include midpieces that are distended, irregular, bent, or abnormally thin (no mitochondrial sheath) or any combination of these forms.

Tail Defects

Sperm in this group may have short, multiple, hairpin, broken (>90° angle), thick, or coiled tails with or without terminal droplets or any combination of these (Fig 3–9). If any one defect predominates, it should be noted on the report. Many coiled tails usually indicate hypoosmotic stress or senescence.

Cytoplasmic Droplet (Remnant)

Cytoplasmic droplets are indicators of incomplete spermiogenesis. They usually are not larger than one third the area of the sperm head. Droplets are usually located in the neck or midpiece region but occasionally appear along the tail (Figs 3–7, 3–9, and 3–10).

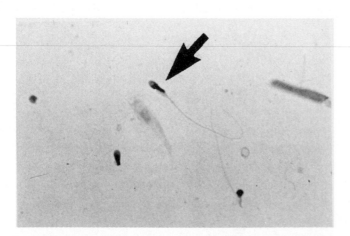

Figure 3–8. Arrow points to spermatozoan with amorphous head and cytoplasmic droplet. Sperm at lower right has midpiece defect resulting in bent tail and amorphous head. Sperm at lower left has midpiece defect resulting in missing tail.

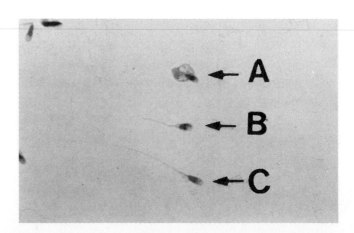

Figure 3–9. A. Coiled tail, amorphous head, cytoplasmic droplet. **B.** Short tail. **C.** Normal tail, amorphous head.

Sperm Classification—Strict Criteria

Normal

Normal sperm have an oval head (for Papanicolaou stain 3 to 5 µm long, 2 to 3 µm wide; for Diff-Quik stain 5 to 6 µm long, 2.5 to 3.5 µm wide) with a well-defined acrosomal region that composes 40% to 70% of the head area (see Fig 3–2). No neck, midpiece, or tail abnormalities are present. Any tapering at the top or bottom of the head is considered abnormal. The midpiece must be axially attached with a width less than or equal to 1 µm and a length 1.5 times the head area. Cytoplasmic droplets are acceptable only if retained in the midpiece and are smaller than half of the sperm head area. The tail should be uniform, slightly thinner than the midpiece, uncoiled, free from bends or twists, and approximately 45 µm in length.

Abnormal

All sperm that do not meet the criteria for normal are considered abnormal, and no further classification is necessary. The scheme allows differentiation between the following.

Slightly Abnormal to Borderline Normal Head Form. This classification includes slightly amorphous sperm that do not meet the strict definition of normal but that do not have a specific abnormality (see Fig 3–3).

Severely Abnormal. All other sperm defects are included in this category.

Nonsperm Morphology

In addition to classifying sperm, the morphologic assessment should evaluate nonsperm cells in the ejaculate. Of particular interest are infectious organisms, immature germinal cells, and leukocytes (Figs 3–11, 3–12). Germinal cells and leukocytes can be confused. With proper training (especially by a hematopathologist), however, one can easily differentiate leukocytes from germinal cells in most Papanicolaou or Giemsa stained preparations. In the routine laboratory setting, benzidine-based histochemical stains are rarely if ever needed to identify leukocytes, eliminating the need for handling carcinogens. Proper identification of the two classes of cells is important. The presence of inflammatory cells such as macrophages and polymorphonuclear neutrophils suggests bacterial infection, whereas the presence of immature germ cells indicates viral infection or exposure to sperm toxicants.[5]

Leukocytes and germinal cells or spermatids are not included in calculations of sperm morphology. The recommended measurement of these nonsperm cells is concentration, which can be derived from the number of cells per sperm. For example, if the sperm count is 10×10^6/mL and the number of leukocytes is 20 sperm per 100, then the total concentration is 2×10^6. The upper limits of normal for leukocyte and germinal cell concentrations are 1×10^6/mL and 5×10^6/mL, respectively.[22,24]

Several atlases provide reference photomicrographs of various morphologic anomalies and their clinical significance.[19,48] These valuable training tools can be augmented with a laboratory slide collection of both typical and unusual slides. It is important to re-read slides periodically to ascertain that normal standards are not changing. At least one laboratory reported a decrease in normal values over time that was attributed to technologists' becoming more strict with their definition of normal morphology (Gerrity M, personal communication, 1994). This phenomenon can be prevented with a quality-control program

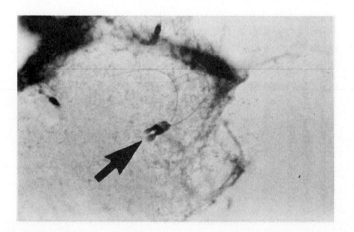

Figure 3–10. Bicephalic sperm with amorphous heads, large cytoplasmic droplet, and duplicate tail.

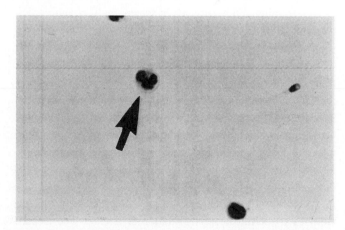

Figure 3–11. Polymorphonuclear leukocyte. Cytoplasmic bridges connect the tri-lobed nucleus.

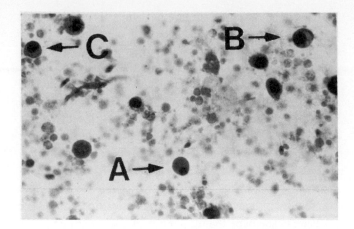

Figure 3–12. A–C. Immature germinal cells.

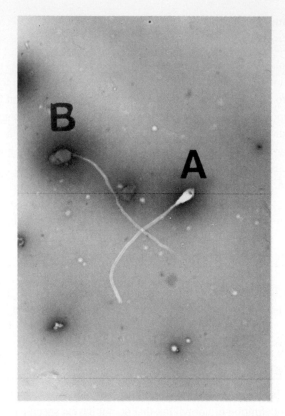

Figure 3–13. Eosin-nigrosin stained smear. **A.** Viable sperm. **B.** Dead sperm.

in which previously analyzed smears are used. Photomicrographs also make good reference and training materials.[51]

Considerable research on application of digital image analysis of sperm has led to the development of computer-assisted morphometric analyzers.[45,52,53] At present, the technology is expensive and relatively slow but clearly represents a method for reducing subjectivity.

HOW TO RECOGNIZE A QUALITY SEMEN ANALYSIS LABORATORY

Semen analysis is almost entirely a manual procedure; accordingly the quality of the personnel performing the procedure is critical. The testing personnel should have a bachelor's degree in a relevant laboratory science and preferably be registered or certified in clinical laboratory medicine. They should have extensive training and experience in semen analysis and participate in continuing medical education. The laboratory director should have board certification in clinical laboratory testing with a specialization in andrology or other comparable credentials.

In many countries, semen analysis performance standards have been set by government regulations. In the United States, the Clinical Laboratory Improvement Act (CLIA) defines laboratory testing categories on the basis of complexity, which determines the personnel education and training requirements and the quality management standards for each test.[54] All laboratories performing semen analysis of any complexity must have a valid CLIA certificate of registration or license. The Department of Health and Human Services permits several accrediting organizations, such as the College of American Pathologists and the Commission on Office Laboratory Accreditation, and

several states to accredit laboratories and to conduct periodic inspections to ensure compliance with the regulation.

Under the CLIA regulation, semen analysis is included in two categories: *moderate complexity* for qualitative semen analysis, which tests only for the presence or absence of sperm, and *high complexity* for quantitative semen analysis in which various components of the semen are enumerated, such as sperm count, percentage motile sperm, and percentage normal forms.[54] Qualitative semen analysis is also included in the recently defined test category *Provider-performed microscopy,* which allows physicians, nurse practitioners, and physician assistants to perform the testing procedure.[55] However, *all* procedures in which sperm are counted or described, motility or morphologic forms are quantified, or biochemical components are measured remain *high complexity* and require rigorous practice of defined laboratory standards. The distinction between these categories has changed several times since the rules were first published, and even some CLIA inspectors are confused about them.

A list of essential laboratory quality procedures is shown in Table 3–2. The CLIA regulation requires laboratories to perform control procedures to monitor the stability of the test method and to assess the accuracy and precision of the results.

Qualitative semen analysis must include a positive and negative control with each run of patient specimens. Quantitative testing must include at least two samples of different concentrations of control materials at least once during each run of patient tests. A *run* is defined as an interval within which the accuracy and precision of a testing system is expected to be stable, but it cannot exceed 24 hours.[54] Statistical process control charts (see Fig 3–1) are useful for displaying and rapidly analyzing data.[56–58]

Control materials for components of quantitative semen analysis are available commercially in unassayed or assayed lots. If using unassayed reagents, the laboratory must establish performance standards by repetitive testing to determine the mean and standard deviation for each lot. Manufacturers' target values for assayed control materials are acceptable performance standards as long as they are verified by the laboratory. Quality control records must be kept for at least 2 years. Laboratories must also undergo proficiency testing at least twice a year, ideally with peer comparison (eg, see Fig 3–14). The American Association of Bioanalysts begins offering semen analysis proficiency testing in 1996, giving laboratories the opportunity to compare their performance with that of their peers.

The regulations outline good laboratory practice. The testing laboratory should be able to document its compliance with these or similar requirements. In addition, the laboratory staff should be able to assist clinicians with interpretation of results and should provide good customer service to patients referred for testing.

LIMITATIONS OF SEMEN ANALYSIS

Semen analysis has many important roles in fertility medicine. Unfortunately, it does not consistently provide definitive and predictive value for the assessment of male fertility potential.[59,60] A number of reasons can account for the discrepancy.

In spite of many workshops, manuals, and tightened federal regulation, semen analysis often is performed poorly. Although requirements for routine quality control and proficiency testing exist, most laboratories that perform semen analysis fail to use these fundamental measures of laboratory quality.[61] Furthermore, standards for semen analysis procedures are not uniform and are not consistently applied, making results highly

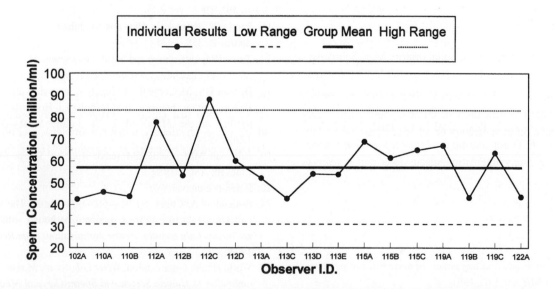

Figure 3–14. Results from a proficiency test conducted by Fertility Solutions in July 1995. Numbers designate laboratories and letters designate observers within the laboratory. One observer's result (112C) was outside the two standard deviation range established from the group answers. The second highest result was from the same laboratory (112A); however, observer B from laboratory 112 had a result that was 40 million per milliliter lower than the laboratory's highest value, suggesting a need for training and internal quality control.

subjective and variable.[51,61–63] Improvements in training and techniques must occur to reduce variation and improve the quality of results of semen analysis. Regulations such as CLIA place semen analysis in a category that requires rigorous quality assessment, providing the opportunity for more reliable results.

Another problem is overinterpretation or overreliance on results of semen analysis. Although semen analysis is an essential and primary test of male fertility, it is not the sole predictor of fertility. Sperm characteristics such as mucus penetration, acrosome reaction, and capacitation are critical fertility functions that are not measured in a routine semen analysis. Given the multifactorial nature of male fertility, the expectation that a single test can help one accurately predict reproductive success is naive.[64]

Finally, the fertility of a man must be taken in context with that of his partner.[65] Many examples exist of couples who have no demonstrable fertility problems in spite of subnormal sperm counts or sperm motility.[66] The female partner must be highly fertile, and the function of existing sperm must be normal. Conversely, even small disturbances of the female partner's reproductive system coupled with minor abnormalities in semen quality can have a multiplicative negative effect on fertility.[67] Other variables, such as duration of infertility have considerable impact on the predictive value of slight abnormalities,[68] which may distract the fertility investigation from the real cause.[67] Until such abnormalities are corrected or technically overcome, for example with ICSI, other causes of infertility in a couple may not be demonstrable.[69]

ACKNOWLEDGMENTS

The author thanks her long-time collaborators Mari Schroeder-Jenkins, MT(ASCP)SH, and Julia Haehn, MT(ASCP), for their invaluable contributions to her understanding of semen analysis. She also thanks her colleagues William C. Baird III, Russell Davis, PhD, David Katz, PhD, Gail Prins, PhD, HCLD, and Steven Schrader, PhD, for sharing their insights and ideas about the topic during many interesting discussions and conversations.

REFERENCES

1. Katz DF: Human sperm as biomarkers of toxic risk and reproductive health. *J NIH Res* 3:63, 1991
2. Schrader SM, Chapin RE, Clegg ED, et al: Laboratory methods for assessing human semen in epidemiologic studies: A consensus report. *Reprod Toxicol* 6:275, 1992
3. Mueller C: The andrology laboratory in an assisted reproductive technologies program: Quality assurance and laboratory methodology. *J Androl* 13:349, 1992
4. Freund M: Interrelationships among the characteristics of human semen and factors affecting semen-specimen quality. *J Reprod Fertil* 4:143, 1962
5. MacLeod J: Human seminal cytology as a sensitive indicator of the germinal epithelium. *Int J Fertil* 9:281, 1964
6. Poland ML, Moghissi KS, Giblin PT, Ager JW, Olson JM: Stability of basic semen measures and abnormal morphology within individuals. *J Androl* 7:211, 1986
7. Sigman M, Lipshultz LI, Howards SS: Evaluation of the subfertile male. In: Lipshultz LI and Howards SS (eds). *Infertility in the Male, Second Edition*. St. Louis, Mosby-Year Book, 1991, 179–210
8. Jouannet P, Czyglik F, David G, et al: Study of a group of 484 fertile men. I. Distribution of semen characteristics. *Int J Androl* 4:440, 1981
9. MacLeod J: Semen examination. *Clin Obstet Gynecol* 8:115, 1965
10. Kaye MC, Schroeder-Jenkins M, Rothmann SA: Impairment of sperm motility by water-soluble lubricants as assessed by computer-assisted sperm analysis. *J Androl* (Suppl) 12:P-52, 1991
11. Keel A: The semen analysis. In: Keel BA, Webster BW (eds), *CRC Handbook of the Laboratory Diagnosis and Treatment of Infertility*. Boca Raton, FL, CRC Press, 1990:27–69
12. Mann T, Lutwak-Mann C: *Male Reproductive Function and Semen*. Berlin: Springer-Verlag, 1981
13. Lilja H, Oldbring J, Rannevik G, Laurell CB: Seminal vesicle-secreted proteins and their reactions during gelation and liquefaction of human semen. *J Clin Invest* 80:281, 1987
14. Amelar RD: Coagulation, liquefaction and viscosity of human semen. *J Urol* 87:187, 1962
15. Ahlgren G, Rannevik GR, Lilja H: Impaired secretory function of the prostate in men with oligo-asthenozoospermia. *J Androl* 16:491, 1995
16. Papp GK, Hoznek A, Hegedus M, Juhasz E: Hematospermia. *J Androl* 15:31S, 1994
17. Zavos PM. Qualitative and quantitative seminal losses during production of ejaculates via masturbation. *Infertility* 9:153, 1995
18. Benson GS, McConnell JA: Erection, emission and ejaculation: Physiologic mechanisms. In: Lipshultz LI, Howards SS (eds), *Infertility in the Male*, ed 2. St. Louis: Mosby–Year Book, 1990:155–176
19. Adelman MM, Cahil EM (eds): *Atlas of Sperm Morphology*. Chicago: ASCP, 1989
20. Reference unavailable
21. Bollendorf A, Check JH, Katsoff D, Fedele A: The use of chymotrypsin/galactose to treat spermatozoa bound with anti-sperm antibodies prior to intra-uterine insemination. *Hum Reprod* 9:484, 1994
22. World Health Organization: *WHO Laboratory Manual for the Examination of Human Semen and Sperm-Cervical Mucus Interactions*, ed 3. Cambridge, England, Cambridge Univ Press, 1992
23. Mortimer D: Semen analysis and sperm washing techniques. In: Gagnon C (ed), *Controls of Sperm Motility: Biological and Clinical Aspects*. Boca Raton, FL: CRC Press, 1990:263–302

24. World Health Organization: *Laboratory Manual for the Examination of Human Semen and Sperm-Cervical Mucus Interactions,* ed 2. Cambridge, England, Press Syndicate of Univ of Cambridge, 1987

25. Rothmann SA, Morgan BW: Laboratory diagnosis in andrology. *Cleve Clin J Med* 56:805, 1989

26. MacLeod J, Gold RZ: The male factor in fertility and infertility. IV. Sperm morphology in fertile and infertile marriage. *Fertil Steril* 2:394, 1951

27. Oates RD, Amos JA: The genetic vasis of congenital bilateral absence of the vas deferens and cystic fibrosis. *J Androl* 15:1, 1994

28. Makler A: A new multiple exposure photography method for objective human spermatozoal motility determination. *Fertil Steril* 30:192, 1978

29. Mortimer D: Objective analysis of sperm motility and kinematics. In: Keel BA, Webster BW (eds), *CRC Handbook of the Laboratory Diagnosis and Treatment of Infertility.* Boca Raton, FL: CRC Press, 1990:99–133

30. McConnell J: Abnormalities in sperm motility: Techniques of evaluation and treatment. In: Lipshultz LI, Howards SS (eds), *Infertility in the Male,* ed 2. St. Louis: Mosby–Year Book, 1990: 254–276

31. Aitken RJ: The role of free oxygen radicals and sperm function. *Int J Androl* 40:183, 1989

32. Aitken RJ, West KM, Buckingham DW: Leukocyte infiltration into the human ejaculate and its association with semen quality, oxidative stress, and sperm function. *J Androl* 15:343, 1994

33. Sikka SC, Rajasekaran M, Hellstrom WJG: Role of oxidative stress and antioxidants in male infertility. *J Androl* 16:464, 1995

34. Weinberg JB, Doty E, Bonaventura J, Haney AF: Nitric oxide inhibition of human sperm motility. *Fertil Steril* 64:408, 1995

35. Boyers SP, Davis RO, Katz DF: Automated semen analysis. *Curr Probl Obstet Gynecol Fertil* 12:165, 1989

36. Barratt CLR, Tomlinson MJ, Cooke ID: Prognostic significance of computerized motility analysis for in vivo fertility. *Fertil Steril* 60:520, 1993

37. Liu DY, Clarke GN, Baker HGW: Relationship between sperm motility assessed with the Hamilton-Thorn Motility Analyzer and fertilization rates in vitro. *J Androl* 12:231–239, 1991

38. Marshburn PB, McIntire D, Carr BR, Byrd W: Spermatozoal characteristics from fresh and frozen donor semen and their correlation with fertility outcome after intrauterine insemination. *Fertil Steril* 58:179–186, 1992

39. Davis RO, Overstreet JW, Asch RH, Ord T, Silber SJ: Movement characteristics of human epididymal sperm used for fertilization of human oocytes in vitro. *Fertil Steril* 56:1128, 1991

40. Davis RO, Drobnis EZ, Overstreet JW: Application of multivariate cluster, discriminate function, and stepwise regression analyses to variable selection and predictive modeling of sperm cryosurvival. *Fertil Steril* 63:1051, 1995

41. Ginsburg KA, Sacco AG, Ager JW, Moghissi KS: Variation of movement characteristics with washing and capacitation of spermatozoa. II. Multivariate statistical analysis and prediction of sperm penetrating ability. *Fertil Steril* 53:704, 1990

42. Davis RO, Katz DF: Operational standards for CASA instruments. *J Androl* 14:385, 1993

43. Kruger TF, Acosta AA, Simmons KF, et al: Predictive value of abnormal sperm morphology in in vitro fertilization. *Fertil Steril* 49:112, 1988

44. Freund M: Standards for the rating of human sperm morphology. *Int J Fertil* 97:97–180, 1966

45. Katz DF, Overstreet JW, Samuels SJ, Niswander PW, Bloom TD, Lewis EL: Morphometric analysis of spermatozoa in the assessment of human male fertility. *J Androl* 7:203, 1986

46. Souchier C, Czyba J, Grantham R: Difficulties in morphologic classification of human spermatozoa. *J Reprod Med* 21:244, 1978

47. Menkveld R, Stander FSH, Kotze TJ, Kruger TF, van Zyl JA: The evaluation of morphological characteristics of human spermatozoa according to stricter criteria. *Hum Reprod* 5:586, 1990

48. Menkveld R, Oettlé EE, Kruger TF, Swanson RJ, Acosta AA, Oehninger S: *Atlas of Human Sperm Morphology.* Baltimore: Williams & Wilkins, 1991

49. Davis RO, Gravance CG: Consistency of sperm morphology classification methods. *J Androl* 15:83, 1994

50. Seibel MM, Zilberstein M: The diagnosis of male infertility by semen quality: The shape of semen morphology. *Hum Reprod* 10:247, 1995

51. Davis RO, Gravance CG, Overstreet JW: A standardized test for visual analysis of human sperm morphology. *Fertil Steril* 63:1058, 1995

52. Garrett C, Baker HWG: A new fully automated system for the morphometric analysis of human sperm heads. *Fertil Steril* 63: 1306, 1995

53. Moruzzi JF, Wyrobek AJ, Mayall BH, Gledhill BL: Quantification and classification of human sperm morphology by computer-assisted image analysis. *Fertil Steril* 50:142, 1988

54. Department of Health and Human Services, Health Care Financing Administration: Clinical Laboratory Improvement Amendments of 1988, Final Rule. Federal Register Part II. 1992; (Friday February 28) 57 no. 40 [42 CFA 405 et al]

55. Department of Health and Human Services, Health Care Financing Administration: Clinical Laboratory Improvement Amendments of 1988. Federal Register. 1995; (Monday April 24): 60 no. 78:2044 [42 CFR 493.19]

56. Amsden RT, Butler HE, Amsden DM: *SPC Simplified: Practical Steps to Quality.* White Plains, NY, 1992

57. Quality America: *SPC: Control Charts Software on CD-ROM.* Tucson, AZ: Quality America, 1996

58. Wheeler D, Chambers D: *Understanding Statistical Process Control,* ed 2. Knoxville, TN: SPC Press, 1992

59. Bartoov B, Eltes F, Pansky M, Lederman H, Caspi E, Soffer Y: Estimating fertility potential via semen analysis data. *Hum Reprod* 8:65, 1993

60. Zaini A, Jennings MG, Baker HWG: Are conventional sperm morphology and motility assessments of predictive value in subfertile men? *Int J Androl* 8:427, 1995

61. Baker DJ, Paterson MA, Klaassen JM, Wyrick-Glatzel J: Semen evaluations in the clinical laboratory: How well are they being performed? *Lab Med* 25:509, 1994

62. Chong AP, Walters CA, Weinrieb SA: The neglected laboratory test: The semen analysis. *J Androl* 4:280, 1983

63. Dunphy BC, Kay R, Barratt CLR, Cooke ID: Quality control during the conventional analysis of semen: An essential exercise. *J Androl* 10:378, 1989

64. Amann RP, Hammerstedt RH: In vitro evaluation of sperm quality: An opinion. *J Androl* 14:397, 1993

65. Steinberger E, Rodroquez-Rigau LJ, Smith KD: The interaction between the fertility potentials of the two members of an infertile couple. In: Frajese G, Hafez ESE, Conti C, Fabbrini A (eds), *Oligozoospermia: Recent Progress in Andrology*. New York, Raven, 1981:9–19

66. Bartoor B, Eltes F, Pansky M, Lederman H, Caspi E, Soffer Y: Estimating fertility potential via semen analysis data. *Hum Reprod* 8:65–70, 1989

67. Jansen RPS: Elusive fertility: Fecundability and assisted conception in perspective. *Fertil Steril* 64:252, 1995

68. Aafjes JH, van der Vijver JCM, Schnenck PE: The duration of infertility: An important datum for the fertility prognosis of men with semen abnormalities. *Fertil Steril* 30:423, 1978.·

69. Sherins RJ, Thorsell LP, Dorfmann A, et al: Intracytoplasmic sperm injection facilitates fertilization even in the most severe forms of male infertility: Pregnancy outcome correlates with maternal age and number of eggs available. *Fertil Steril* 64:369, 1995

70. MacLeod J, Gold RZ: The male factor in fertility and infertility. II. Spermatozoan counts in 1,000 men of known fertility and in 1,000 cases of infertile marriage. *J Urol* 66:436, 1951

71. Rehan NE, Sobrero AJ, Fertig JW: The semen of fertile men: Statistical analysis of 1,300 men. *Fertil Steril* 26:408, 1974

72. Upadhyaya M, Hibbard BM, Walker SM: Use of sputolysin for liquefaction of viscid human semen. *Fertil Steril* 657, 1981

CHAPTER 4

Endocrine Testing in Infertility

SHALOM BAR-AMI

Bioassays: Historical and Present Applications
Indications for Laboratory Hormone Testing
  Women
  Men
Immunochemical Reaction
Nonlabeled Immunoassays
  Agglutination inhibition
  Complement-fixation assay
  Precipitin assay
Tag-labeled Immunoassay
Radiometric Assay

Labeled-hormone immunoassay
Labeled-antibody immunoassay
Type of radiometric labeling
Separation of the labeled complex
Enzyme Immunoassay and Enzyme-linked
  Immunosorbent Assay
Luminescent Immunoassay
  Fluorescence assay
  Chemiluminescent and bioluminescent assays
Automated Immunoassay

The techniques used to evaluate endocrine fluctuation are as old as endocrine research. Early on it became apparent that accurate measurement of biologic constituents is essential for proper evaluation and diagnosis of various diseases. Although many procedures were developed to measure the level of a specific compound, it was the radioimmunoassay developed by Yallow and Berson[1,2] that provided the breakthrough by use of labeled binding assays. Since then, scientific ingenuity has devised a number of assays based on binding the tested compound to antibody. Various methods of endocrine testing for infertility are available each with its advantages and limitations.

BIOASSAYS: HISTORICAL AND PRESENT APPLICATIONS

Evaluation of infertility achieved little progress until the late 19th century when intensive scientific research based on anatomic studies and clinical treatments provided new insights. The concept of blood-borne substances' exerting effects throughout the body can be traced to Berthold's[3] work on testicles of castrated roosters. Implantation of the castrated testicles on the intestines prevented the usual effects of castration. The concept of ductless glands was suggested in 1878 by Claude Bernard,[4] but the definition of endocrine organs was established much later after histologic studies of various tissues, such as the corpus luteum.[5] More complicated investigations of the correlation between the periodic changes in ovarian morphology and the morphology of the vaginal epithelium[6,7] paved the road for research by means of diagnostic bioassays into the endocrinologic function of the reproductive organs.

The development of the pregnancy test is a fascinating example of the establishment of bioassays. The test evolved through the pioneering discovery that removal of the corpus luteum terminated pregnancy.[8] The involvement of internal secretions of the corpus luteum in preparing the endometrium for implantation of the fertilized egg was demonstrated by Bouin and Ancel.[9] Such biologic phenomena were used to purify various hormones and determine their levels. Thus only 20 years later, Corner and Allen[10] described the hormonal activity of the corpus luteum. The discovery of the effect of placental hormones on the preservation of corpus luteum activity established the relationship between the corpus luteum and the fetus. Injection of human placental tissue into a nonpregnant rabbit caused the production and maintenance of corpora lutea.[11] These findings allowed Zondek and Aschheim[12] to develop the pregnancy test. In their test, growth and maturation of ovarian follicles and subsequent formation of hemorrhagic corpora lutea were observed after the urine of pregnant women was injected into female mice. This approach was also successful in rabbits and became known as the rabbit test.[13] These interspecies bioassays were extended even to frogs. A woman's urine was injected into the dorsal lymph sacs of frogs. Extrusion of either sperm by the male or eggs by the female indicated the presence of human chorionic gonadotropin (hCG) secreted by the implanted embryo.[14,15]

Further application of the test was accompanied by many obstacles. The main problem was that the preparation contained other hormones that could exert the same action as the hormone of interest. Thus new techniques were developed to increase the specificity of the test. For example, the bioassay for measuring follicle-stimulating hormone (FSH) required the elimination of possible luteinizing hormone (LH) contamination. Control animals were treated with high amounts of hCG simultaneously with the test preparation. Any possible LH contamination would not show up because of the exposure of all animals to high amounts of hCG.[16]

The desire for more quantitative information led to more biochemical evaluations. For example, quantitative estimation of pituitary hormones was achieved by means of measurement of the depletion of ascorbic acid in the target organ, such as in the adrenal glands by adrenocorticotropic hormone (ACTH)[17] or in the ovary by LH.[18] The test represented only an acute effect, however, and it could be induced by many other hormones. A long list of other hormones such as histamine, serotonin, norepinephrine, and lysine vasopressin could also cause ascorbic acid depletion. Another approach was the absorption of [^{131} I]albumin into the ovary,[19] which replaced the morphologic concept of the Zondek pregnancy test. More specific bioassays were developed to measure specific functions induced by hormones, such as ACTH stimulation of corticosterone secretion by the adrenal glands.[20]

In an attempt to increase specificity, many assays were developed for organ or tissue culture. Raw fluid or an extract of it was added, and the responses of the cultured organ or tissue in terms of cell morphology and biochemical changes were evaluated. For example, the amount of FSH or LH-hCG and FSH were estimated quantitatively by means of measurement of the effect of the test preparation on [^{3}H]thymidin incorporation into cultured mouse ovaries[21] or on progesterone secretion by cul-

tured slices of rat ovary,[22] respectively. To increase specificity, however, bioassays were developed for a single cell type of tissue or cell line. As such, tissue culture systems have been used to obtain precise results that are specific for testing LH with ovarian cells[23] or testicular cells[24] and testing for the amount of FSH with Sertoli cells.[25]

Despite their contribution to endocrine testing and to promoting endocrinology in general, the bioassays lagged behind the desire to improve endocrine testing in at least four aspects. *Specificity* indicates that in a mixture of hormones, the assay should detect the level of only a single hormone. It should not be influenced by the constituents of other samples, and it should not measure levels of other hormones in the preparation. In most bioassays, the biologic effect exerted by a certain hormone also was exerted by a few other hormones that might have been present in the specimen.

Sensitivity refers to the least amount that can be measured by the assay. Sometimes only a small amount of the preparation is available, and sometimes small changes in the hormone levels become significant with respect to interpretation and clinical treatment. It is necessary therefore to have a test with the potential to measure small amounts of the analyte, that is, have higher sensitivity. Most bioassays do not fulfill these demands.

Precision indicates that an assay gives reliable and reproducible data. In many assays, the preexisting differences among animals affect the degree of response and the length of time necessary to obtain this response, whether the system is in vivo or in vitro. Furthermore, the bioassayed variable may represent an acute or a chronic effect. Differences in quantitative estimates existed among the different systems. In addition, sometimes the test required experience, training, and skill on the part of the technicians. As such, they involved subjective evaluation of results and eliminated the development of automation. These factors cause an unacceptable variation within and between assays.

The performance of bioassays is associated with a high *cost* for materials, animals, and equipment (surgical tools, microscopes). In addition, some tests require a long time before the biologic response is evident.

To overcome these limitations, some bioassays were replaced by chemical assays. Hormones or their metabolites were extracted from urine and subjected to chemical analysis, such as fluorometric analysis, or were identified by means of gas-liquid chromatography. These tests were performed until the 1970s,[26] when they were gradually replaced by immunoassays. In the late 1950s and early 1960s, new methods were used. Various serologic approaches were developed to measure the levels of hormones such as growth hormone and gonadotropins. Three of these are the plate technique[27] which later was modified into the complement-fixation test,[28] agglutination inhibition,[29] and precipitin assay.[30] Although they were much more specific and sensitive than bioassays and the results were obtained within a fairly short time, the serologic tests were not adequate for every hormone.

The establishment of radiolabeled immunoassay by Yallow and Berson[1,2] was an important step forward and started a revolution in research and the clinical application of endocrinology. Ekins[31] used natural thyroxine-binding globulin to build a competitive binding assay that worked on principles similar to those of the immunologic test of Yallow and Berson. Ligand-antibody tagging procedures became the mainstay for determination of hormone levels.

Bioassays are still relevant and necessary to assure hormone activity. Although immunoassay can be used to establish amounts of hormones, it is not always sufficient. Sometimes a large discrepancy exists between the immunoreactivity and bioactivity of hormone such as gonadotropins.[32-34] The hormone can be biologically inactive, such as LH in old men[35,36] or in breastfeeding woman.[37] Sometimes it is important to know the in vivo action of a hormone rather than its amount. In such situations rather than immunoassay an in vivo bioassay is necessary to demonstrate the exact function of the hormone in terms of biochemical and anatomic changes.

In the past, mouse breast bioassay to measure serum prolactin[38] was equally reliable as the prolactin radioimmunoassay in both differentiating prolactin from growth hormone (GH) and providing sensitivity.[39] This fact is sometimes extrapolated to hormones in other systems, such as granulocyte colony-stimulating factor.[40] Even today, in well-defined syndromes it is sometimes preferable to determine the altered bioactive level of a hormone to evaluate the cause of infertility.[41] An in vivo bioassay is sometimes necessary to evaluate the half-life of a hormone by means of examination of its chronic effects, as with naturally synthesized FSH[42,43] or even artificially altered FSH.[44] In research, bioassays are used mainly to establish the level of activity in new lots of purified hormones.

The bioassays that were developed in the 1940s or later were used until recently to evaluate possible causes of and therapy for infertility. Among these are the hyperemic response of the ovary to gonadotropin,[45] enhancement of uterine growth by FSH stimulation of ovarian estrogen secretion,[46] or both.[47] These bioassays have been used to determine possible active antihormone antibodies in a patient's serum as a cause of infertility. The serum was injected together with the hormone (e.g., FSH, hCG) of interest. Failure of the hormone to exert its specific effect indicated that the patient's serum contained antihormone antibodies.

Bioassays are used for quantitative assessment of a hormone level in case the hormone is not well defined chemically. In this context, one may consider various factors with documented hormonal activity in the genital system, such as the gonadotropin surge-attenuating factor,[48] the early pregnancy factor,[49] and the embryo toxic factor.[50] Other bioassay tests are performed to evaluate infertility, for example, the sperm-penetration assay[51] or the effect of various toxicans on fertility.[52]

INDICATIONS FOR LABORATORY HORMONE TESTING

Various approaches dictate the type of hormone testing. The practical goal of these measurements is to supply hormone levels to evaluate the causes of infertility. Most of the urinary steroids are metabolites of the steroid of interest, and sometimes the levels are too low to allow proper assessment. For example, pregnanediol, pregnanetriol, and 17-ketosteroids are the urinary metabolites of progesterone, 17-hydroxyprogesterone (17-OHP), and dehydroepiandrosterone (DHEA), respectively. (The level of pregnanediol in urine is about 7% to 20% of the level in blood.[53]) Protein hormones are virtually altered in urine compared with their original chemical structure and composition in blood. For example, intact serum hCG is metabolized into β core, which manifests the β subunits and consists of two polypeptides linked by a disulfide bridge. Sometimes β core can be produced from LH, because it is present in the urine of postmenopausal women.[54] Thus compared with urine tests, testing various hormones in blood usually gives more reliable results and has physiologic relevance to causes of infertility.

An initial approach to the evaluation of infertility is to measure serial blood levels of a hormone. The data are evaluated in reference to changes in physiologic and metabolic status that take place in 24 hours or longer. Table 4–1 represents an accepted range of serum hormone levels for women and men. Deviation from these ranges may suggest an abnormality or a physiologic change.

The hormone level that for decades was presented in various ways, mainly as mass per volume (grams per liter), has been changed to Système Internationale (SI) units. The SI units represent amount per volume, which is usually expressed as moles per liter and sometimes as units per liter. Conventional hormone levels are changed to SI units with a conversion factor (Table 4–2).

The hypothalamic-pituitary-gonadal axis consists of positive and negative feedback of closed loops. A deviation from the normal state is best determined by means of measurement of the secretion of hormones by two glands. Such deviation can be indicative of totally or partially dysfunctional or overfunctional glands. In women, for example, a very low to undetectable serum level of gonadotropins, together with a low level of 17β-estradiol, may suggest a hypogonadotropic-hypogondal syndrome, whereas considerably high levels of FSH (30 IU/L or greater) together with a low to undetectable level of estradiol may suggest dysfunctional or even absent gonads. In men, a low serum testosterone level together with low FSH and LH levels suggest hypogonadotropic-hypogonadal syndrome.

TABLE 4–1. NORMAL RANGES OF SERUM AND PLASMA HORMONAL LEVELS

Hormone	Adult Male	Female Menstrual Cycle				
		ARW	FP	MC	LP	PM
FSH (mIU/mL)	2–14	NA	3–10	6–20	2–10	41–124
LH (MIU/mL)	1.4–7.7	NA	1–8	15–62	ND-8.1	>14
PRL (ng/mL)	2.5–17	3–20	NG	NG	NG	NG
TSH (μIU/mL)	0.4–4	0.4–4	NA	NA	NA	NA
Free T$_4$ (ng/dL)	0.8–1.9	0.8–1.9	NA	NA	NA	NA
E$_2$ (pg/mL)	ND–56	NA	20–266	118–355	26–165	ND–30
P (ng/mL)	ND–2	NA	ND–1.5	NG	2–25	ND–0.7
DHEA-S (μg/mL)	0.8–5.6	0.35–4.3	NA	NA	NA	NA
T (ng/mL)	2.6–15.9	0.02–0.8	NA	NA	NA	0.04–0.61

Hormone levels are the averages achieved with the Immulite automated immunoassay. ARW, average range in women; FP, follicular phase; MC, middle cycle; LP, luteal phase; PM, postmenopause; NA, not applicable; ND, no detected level; NG, not given by the company. In women, the hormone level may be presented only under ARW. This occurs when the level is not dramatically altered during the menstrual cycle. FSH, follicle-stimulating hormone; LH, luteinizing hormone; PRL, prolactin; TSH, thyroid-stimulating hormone; T$_4$, thyroxine; E$_2$, estradiol; P, progesterone; DHEA-S, dehydroepiandrosterone sulfate; T, testosterone.

Sometimes the original measurements must be repeated in the same glands, or other hormones must be quantified to evaluate a cause of infertility. For example, a man with low testosterone, LH, and FSH levels should have his prolactin measured, and even a low testosterone and a normal LH level may be associated with prolactinemia.[55]

The secretion of many hormones is correlated with certain physiologic states. For example, a serum progesterone level less than 32 nmol/L 5 to 10 days before menses may suggest luteal dysfunction and anovulation, whereas at the start or the end of the luteal phase it is acceptable. Hormones are secreted in episodic and diurnal patterns. Thus serial measure-

ments of hormone levels could be an informative way to indicate an abnormality. In women, for example, progesterone secretion is pulsatile and becomes diurnal during the midluteal phase.[56,57] In men, LH and testosterone are secreted in a pulsatile pattern and require several consecutive measurements.[58] Furthermore, the levels should be measured in a pool sample to verify a correlation and establish a proper diagnosis.[59] A single hormone measurement is not always sufficient to indicate a deviation from normal and to determine causes of infertility, even for gonadotropins and steroids. However, frequent measurements are not always practical and thus other approaches are used.

Hormone levels may deviate from normal after infertility treatments or hormone challenge. These procedures should be performed, however, to search for the cause of infertility, for example, amenorrhea (Fig 4–1) or azoospermia or severe oligospermia (Fig 4–2). Both disorders can be associated with inappropriate function of one endocrine gland or more, such as in the hypothalamic-pituitary-gonadal axis or other endocrine glands or with metabolic irregularities.

Women

Figure 4–1 is a suggested algorithm for endocrine tests to evaluate possible causes of amenorrhea. First measured is hCG, especially in women with secondary amenorrhea, to exclude pregnancy. Next FSH and prolactin are measured. Various other hormones such as the steroids progesterone, estradiol, and an-

TABLE 4–2. CONVERSION FACTORS FOR A REPRESENTATIVE LIST OF HORMONES

Hormone	Conventional Value	Conversion Factor	SI Unit
DHEA-S	1 μg/dL	0.0271	0.0271 μmol/L
E$_2$	1 pg/mL	3.671	3.671 pmol/L
FSH	1 mIU/mL	1.0	1 IU/L
LH	1 mIU/mL	1.0	1 IU/L
PRL	1 ng/mL	44.4	44.4 pmol/L
T	1 ng/dL	0.0347	0.035 nmol/L
17-OHP	1 ng/dL	0.03	0.03 nmol/L
T$_4$	1 ng/dL	12.9	12.87 nmol/L
P	1 ng/mL	3.18	3.18 nmol/L
TSH	1 μIU/mL	1.0	1.0 mIU/L

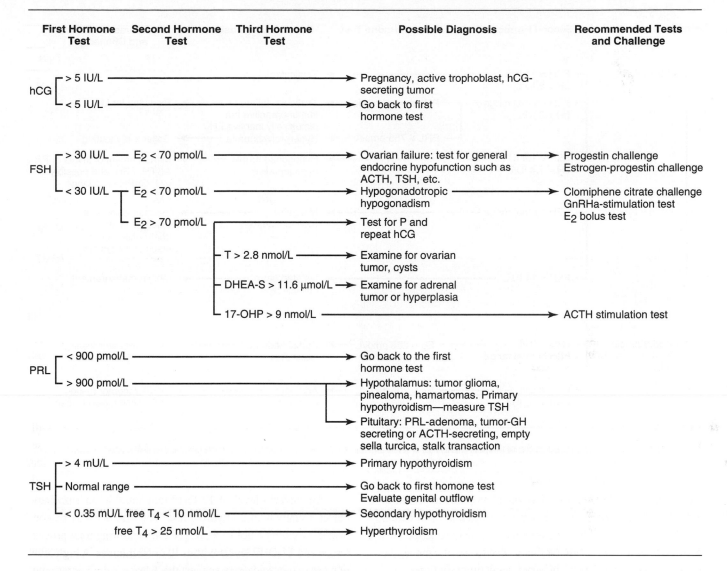

Figure 4–1. Strategy to evaluate various causes of amenorrhea. *(Values were collected from our laboratory and Immulite published data.)*

drogens, including ovarian testosterone and adrenal DHEA sulfate (DHEA-S), are measured to diagnose the activity of a second gland.

In case of hypogonadotropic hypogonadism, hypothalamus-pituitary dysfunction might be assumed and deserves investigation. There are direct and indirect provocative tests to evaluate hypothalamic function. Administration of an estradiol bolus exerts direct positive feedback on the hypothalamus to stimulate gonadotropin-releasing hormone (GnRH) secretion and thereby induce gonadotropin secretion.[60] Treatment with a GnRH agonist is an indirect method of inducing pituitary gonadotropin secretion.[61,62] Thus a marked increase in gonadotropin and possibly steroid secretion may reveal that the levels of the hormones were undetectable because of a dysfunctional hypothalamus. A marked rise in gonadotropin level after a clomiphene citrate challenge may indicate that the

hypothalamic-pituitary axis is not severely dysfunctional. Specific syndromes that cause hypothalamic dysfunction, such as Kallmann syndrome and other congenital disorders, can be evaluated primarily by means of physical examination before endocrine testing.

For women with oligomenorrhea, the initial procedure should be clomiphene citrate treatment. Clomiphene is bound to the estrogen receptors in the hypothalamic-pituitary axis and prevents a possible negative effect of estrogen on gonadotropin secretion. Thus clomiphene citrate is not a drug of choice for hypoestrogenic women with amenorrhea. A progestational challenge is sometimes necessary as the initial step to establish the outflow of the genital system on the basis of physical signs such as bleeding. In rare instances the level of gonadotropins is normal but bleeding does not occur after progestational tests. This discrepancy is sometimes associated with the pituitary hor-

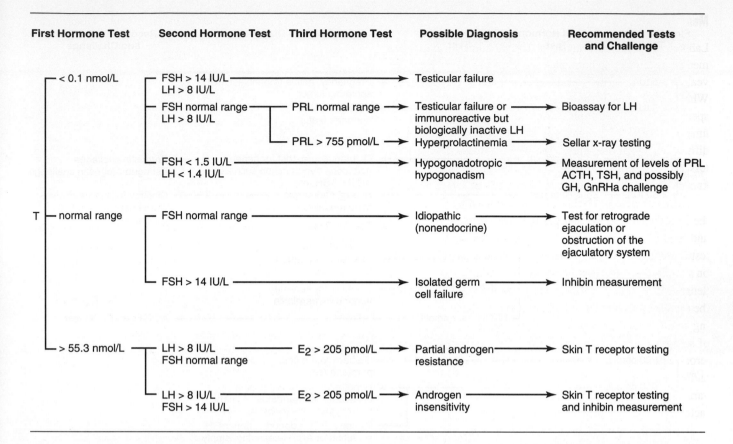

Figure 4–2. Strategy to evaluate endocrine linkage to azoospermia or severe oligospermia. *(Values were collected from our laboratory and Immulite published data.)*

mone with lower bioactivity. Thus gonadotropins are produced with altered biologic activity in terms of induction of follicular growth.[32,42,63] Other causes of oligoamenorrhea are associated with dysfunction of the pituitary gland due to specific metabolic irregularities such as anorexia nervosa and pituitary tumor.

Premature ovarian failure may be a cause of amenorrhea when bleeding does not occur after progestational challenge and levels of gonadotropins are high (FSH >30 IU/L, LH >20 IU/L). Sometimes estrogen treatment for several days followed by gonadotropin treatment causes gonadal activity to resume at least temporarily, although the diagnosis is still ovarian failure.

Ovarian irregularity may be associated with high androgen levels of ovarian (testosterone) or adrenal (DHEA-S) origin. Hirsutism may suggest that the amenorrhea is associated with the high serum androgen level. Sometimes hirsutism is caused by high skin sensitivity to androgens or by high 5α-reductase activity without noticeable change in the values of these androgens.[64] Amenorrhea with high androgen levels also occurs in women with polycystic ovary (PCO) syndrome. High androgen production can be associated with other clinical conditions such as congenital adrenal hyperplasia (CAH), Cushing syndrome, ovarian hyperthecosis, ovarian androgen-producing tumors, and adrenal adenoma.

An elevated level of 17-OHP may point to an enzymatic defect, usually with 21-hydroxylase. The disorder may be confirmed by giving a bolus of ACTH and measuring total progesterone and 17-OHP levels within 30 or 60 minutes. A high level of these two steroids may suggest the disease. Administration of dexamatozone also should cause a reduction in ACTH level and as such prevent overproduction of androgens by the adrenal glands or possibly even elevated production of androgens by the ovaries in PCO syndrome. The condition of most women with ovarian resistance is compatible with biochemical PCO syndrome.[65] A clomiphene citrate challenge may result in high LH levels because of unresponsiveness of the ovaries.[66] A combination of clomiphene citrate and antiandrogens such as spironolactone may cause ovulation to resume and increase pregnancy rate.[67]

Other irregularities that cause amenorrhea may be associated with high levels of prolactin, so prolactin should be measured. Amenorrhea is rarely associated with hypothyroidism, so measuring thyroid-stimulating hormone (TSH) and free and total thyroxine is not the first step. Of course, clinical markers such as goiter and galactorrhea can help one diagnose these irregularities. The increase in prolactin level and galactorrhea can be secondary to hypothyroidism, however.

Men

Laboratory testing to evaluate male-factor infertility includes measuring circulating hormones and semen analysis, which reveal the activity of the gonads, prostate, and seminal vesicles. When semen analysis shows a low quality of seminal fluid and sperm values or when clinical tests indicate small testicular volume or a history of anomalies such as loss of libido or erectile difficulties, endocrine causes should be evaluated. Nevertheless, azoospermia and severe oligospermia are associated with a known endocrine disorder in less than 5% of the population.

The secretion of FSH and LH is regulated by GnRH from the hypothalamus. FSH and LH regulate secretion of steroids and inhibin from the testicles. LH stimulates the secretion of testosterone from Leydig cells. FSH enhances the effect of LH on stimulating testosterone secretion by increasing LH receptor density in Leydig cells. Together with testosterone, FSH acts on the seminiferous tubules to induce sperm production, by exerting an effect on the Sertoli cells. FSH enhances the production of several proteins, including inhibin, by Sertoli cells. Testosterone and inhibin exert negative feedback on secretion of LH and FSH, respectively. The algorithm in Figure 4–2 shows the various tests necessary to evaluate an endocrine basis for male-factor infertility due to azoospermia or severe oligospermia.

A low testosterone level is the best indication of hypogonadism of hypothalamic or pituitary origin. Low testosterone with high LH and FSH levels may indicate testicular failure. Low testosterone with low FSH and LH levels may indicate hypogonadotropic hypogonadism. In such cases, other hormones should be tested, such as ACTH, TSH, and GH. Sometimes secreted LH is detected immunologically but is ineffective biologically.[35,36] The most relevant findings for prolactinemia are low testosterone level without a concomitant decrease in LH level. This suggests that the hypothalamic-pituitary axis failed to respond to the lower testosterone level by increasing LH. In case of a high FSH level but normal LH and testosterone levels, possible Sertoli cell damage and nonproduction of inhibin might be assumed. When LH and testosterone are elevated and FSH is in the normal range, possible androgen resistance may be assumed. In such instances, measurement of estradiol is recommended.[68,69] A history of precocious puberty may imply CAH.[70] Serum levels of 17-OHP and 11-deoxycortisol are elevated in deficiencies of 21-hydroxylase and 11-hydroxylase, respectively.[58]

IMMUNOCHEMICAL REACTION

During the last 35 years many methods used antibodies to measure levels of hormones for clinical and research purposes. These assays are applicable to measure hormone levels either in different biologic fluids such as serum, urine, and saliva or in extracts made from various test preparations such as tissue samples. A short description of the basic elements involved in the immunochemical reaction should enhance the reader's understanding of these techniques.

The immunochemical reaction takes place in aqueous solution and includes the binding of an antigen to a specific antibody. The antibody has two binding sites, both of which are equally specific to a single antigen. The binding affinity of the antibody to the antigen is associated with both stereochemical fitness (as a key fits a specific lock) and chemical forces. The forces are hydrogen, ionic, and van der Waals bonds and hydrophobic interactions.

The γ-immunoglobulin (IgG) antibodies are usually used for an immunoassay. They are raised simply by means of injection of the antigen of one species into other species. Sometimes it is difficult to raise antibodies to a certain molecule because of the low antigenicity or small size and weight of the molecule. In such cases, this molecule is linked to a large carrier molecule such as albumin or hemocyanin to produce a complex with higher antigenicity. It is important that a nonreactive residue of the antigen be linked to the carrier to eliminate the possibility of changing the conformation and stereochemistry of the molecule. It is equally important not to link the antigen at or close to the site that exerts its specific biologic activity. Keeping the latter may cause the raised antibody to detect the antigen near or on its bioactive site. Measuring the amount of antigen by means of immunoassay may also determine the bioactivity of the antigen.

Injection of the carrier-antigen complex results in production of many different antibodies that are specific to different chemical residues on the carrier and on the antigen. Furthermore, the same chemical residue may be detected by more than one specific antibody population that differ in chemical structure and composition. These different antibody populations are called *polyclonal antibodies*. When only one type of IgG is totally identical both in chemical structure and composition and specificity for a given antigen, this antibody population is usually *monoclonal*. Today most immunoassays are based on monoclonal antibodies that give higher specificity and precision than polyclonal antibodies, which are associated with high cross-reactivity with other hormones and compounds. Sometimes a polyclonal immunoassay is preferable, however, because it increases the likelihood of correlation between the immunoreactive and bioactive levels of the antigen.[33]

$$[Ab]+[Ag] \underset{K_{-1}}{\overset{K_1}{\rightleftharpoons}} [Ab\text{-}Ag] \quad K_1=k_1/k_{-1} \quad K=[Ab\text{-}Ag]/[Ab][Ag]$$

Figure 4–3. Immunochemical reaction. The rate of the reaction is described by an association constant (K_1) and a dissociation constant (K_{-1}). Ab, antibody; Ag, antigen; Ab-Ag, antibody-antigen complex.

The immunochemical reaction may be described as a saturation reaction that follows the law of mass action (Fig 4–3). The concentration of the antibody-antigen complex (Ab-Ag) is proportional to the concentration of the antibody (Ab) and the antigen (Ag) and becomes unchangeable at equilibrium, as described by the equation K = [Ab-Ag]/[Ab][Ag]. Thus at a given Ab amount and equilibrium constant value (K), the increase in the amount of Ab-Ag complex depends on increasing the amount of Ag. The affinity of the antibody to its specific antigen could be as high as 10^{-12} M, which makes it the best option for measuring levels of a given hormone with high specificity, sensitivity, and precision.

The immunoassays can be categorized as nonlabeled and labeled. Nonlabeled assays include various serologic tests such as agglutination inhibition, complement fixation, and precipitin reaction. In the last, detection may be visual examination, nephelometric light scattering, or particle counting. The labeled assays are radiometric, enzymatic, and luminescent approaches. Each of these tests may be divided into competitive or noncompetitive types.

NONLABELED IMMUNOASSAYS

The nonlabeled immunoassays are the serologic antibody-antigen reactions such as agglutination, complement fixation, and precipitation (Fig 4–4). The end products of these tests are detected mainly by means of visible expression. To intensify the visible expression of the immunoreaction, other factors are added, such as red blood cells (RBCs) and carriers bound to antibodies or antigen.

Agglutination Inhibition

Agglutination inhibition refers to the aggregation of antibodies and their specific antigen by alternate binding and cross-linking. Usually artificial carriers such as latex particles, colloidal charcoal, or biologic carriers such as erythrocytes or bacteria are added to this reaction. When the test is performed to detect the presence of antibodies, the specific antigen is linked to the carrier. On the other hand, the antibodies are linked to carrier when the purpose is to detect the presence of the specific antigen for these antibodies. The addition of carriers intensifies the reaction because it increases the density of binding sites or the antigens on the small area of the carrier. Presence of the carrier also intensifies the visible expression of the agglutination reaction. This reaction is sensitive to physical conditions, such as temperature, length of incubation, and chemistry, such as pH, ionic composition, and strength, as well as the density of antigen or antibodies on the carrier. Sometimes the agglutination reaction is enhanced by addition of a second antibody or other chemical such as polyethylene glycol or dioxane, which enhances precipitation of the agglutinated antibodies or antigen.

The agglutination reaction is used to detect levels of hormones such as hCG and LH. The hormone of interest is linked to the carriers. With the addition of the antibodies directed to the hormone, the agglutination reaction takes place. However, if the antibodies are initially incubated with patient serum, the agglutination reaction can be inhibited if the serum contains the specified hormone. This approach is able to detect hCG levels of 1500 to 2500 IU/L[71] and can be used to diagnose pregnancy about 3 to 4 weeks after conception.

Complement-fixation Assay

The complement-fixation assay was developed to detect the presence of antibody in serum. This reaction takes place with three elements: sheep RBCs, antibodies (IgG) directed against RBCs, and serum containing complement. When these three components are put together in the right proportions, hemolysin (IgG) is bound to the RBCs, and complement is subsequently bound to the RBC-antibody complex and induces cell lysis. If one of these three components is removed, RBC lysis does not occur. The addition of other antibodies and their specific antigen may cause complement to fix on this antibody-antigen complex instead of binding to the RBC-antibody complex eliminating the expected RBC lysis.

This principle was used in laboratory tests of hormone levels. Antibodies to the hormone were added to a patient's biologic fluid. The presence of the hormone in the specimen resulted in fixation of complement on the antibody-hormone complex. Thus if there was no complement fixation with the RBCs, there was no lysis. This procedure was used successfully to measure very low amounts of hCG.[28] It was improved by performing the reaction in test tubes, measuring hemolysis with a spectrophotometer, and obtaining quantitative results.

Precipitin Assay

When antibodies and their specific antigen are mixed, the cross linking between them produces precipitate mainly when both are in optimal or nearly optimal concentrations. The concentration of the antigen is unknown in the tested sample, so a system was developed in which a gradient of concentrations of both antigen and antibodies is allowed to be produced by diffusion. At the point at which the two gradients are mixed in the right concentration, a precipitate is produced. The precipitation reaction takes place in a semisolid medium such as the neutral gel, for example, agarose. The antibody and antigen are put in separate wells and diffuse in the gel. When they mix in the right proportions, they produce a flocculent precipitate, visible as a band or line. The size and shape of the wells, the distance between them, temperature, and incubation time should be predetermined for best results.

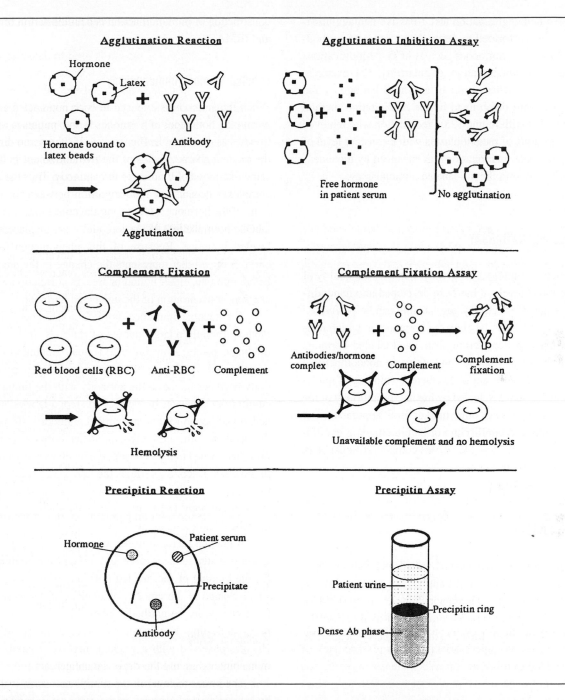

Figure 4–4. Assessment of hormone levels by means of nonlabeled immunoassays. On the left three different serologic processes that are usually used in clinical immunology are described. The utilization of these processes for determining hormone levels is depicted on the right.

This technique was used by McKean[30] to measure hCG. A urine sample was layered over a denser antibody phase in a microtest tube. When hCG was present, a precipitin ring formed at the interface. The time necessary for the appearance of the precipitin ring was correlated with the hCG concentration. When this approach was used to measure highly purified hCG, a concentration of 30 to 60 IU/mL was accurately determined within 2 hours. This time was established as the standard, because with

a patient's urine a longer period could cause the formation of a nonspecific precipitate.

Nonlabeled immunoassays are no longer used to measure hormone levels; however, serologic immunoassays are an integral part of infertility evaluation. Premature ovarian failure is often associated with autoimmune diseases. Ovarian antibodies are sometimes determined by means of serologic procedures such as indirect immunofluorescence, complement-fixation test, or passive hemagglutination test.[72] Passive hemagglutination is sometimes performed to detect the presence of antibodies directed to various hormones such as hCG.[73] Modifications are employed to evaluate causes of infertility. For example, quantitative values such as level of anti-hCG antibodies and their specificity were determined by the precipitation method using hCG labeled with iodine 125. Precipitation was achieved by series of dilutions of patient plasma with a constant level of labeled antigen while precipitation was enhanced by dioxane.[47] This approach is used in the tag-labeled immunoassay.

TAG-LABELED IMMUNOASSAY

The tag-labeled immunoassay[1,2] greatly increases the quality of testing of hormone levels. It has been developed into many different approaches. Collectively, tag labeling can be performed in either of two ways: (1) labeling the hormone, in which nonlabeled hormones (patient serum, urine) and labeled hormone are bound to the antibody in a competitive or noncompetitive manner or (2) labeling the antibody where the binding of nonlabeled hormone is usually selected by linking the antibody or the hormone to a solid phase or other marker. Both approaches can be conducted either to equilibrium or before attaining equilibrium. Whichever is selected, the labeled compounds must be in constant known concentrations.

RADIOMETRIC ASSAY

In a radioimmunoassay (RIA), nonlabeled and radioisotope-labeled hormones are bound to the antibody in a competitive or noncompetitive manner. In an immunoradiometric assay (IRMA), the antibody is labeled by a radioisotope, and usually either the hormone or the antibody is linked to the solid-phase carrier. The

construction of immunoreaction is detailed herein for both RIA and IRMA.

Labeled-hormone Immunoassay

When the antibody is exposed to both nonlabeled and labeled hormones, both types of hormones form complexes with the antibodies as described in Figure 4–5. If there is no difference in the binding characteristics of the two hormones, both have the same likelihood of binding to the antibody. Thus the number of complexes depends on the proportion between the concentrations of the hormones. Increasing the concentration of the nonlabeled hormone results in more and more displacement of the labeled hormone. Because of this phenomenon, a standard curve is drawn that represents the change in the amount of labeled hormone, either bound or free, in correlation with the increasing concentration of the unlabeled hormone.

A sequential immunoassay is a noncompetitive two-step method. Initially, a large amount of antibody (that is, with large binding capacity) is available to a small amount of nonlabeled hormone. In the first step, all the nonlabeled hormone essentially becomes bound to the antibody with the limitation of the equilibrium constant. In the second step, a labeled hormone is added and bound to the unoccupied antibodies. To prevent the dissociation of the antibody–nonlabeled hormone (Ab-H) complex that formed in the first step, the incubation period is shorter in the second step. Sometimes the hormone is labeled in a way that causes a small reduction in the affinity of labeled hormone (H*) to antibody (Ab), attenuating its ability to displace the nonlabeled hormone in the Ab-H complex.

A gradual increase in the amount of nonlabeled hormone in the first step reduces more and more of the binding capacity for the binding of the labeled hormone in the second step. A small change in the amount of nonlabeled hormone causes a large change in the antibody–labeled hormone (Ab-H*) complex, indicating a substantial increase in sensitivity. The changes observed with a gradual increase in nonlabeled hormone binding are used to draw a standard curve.

The hormone level in a patient's specimen is determined by subjecting the specimen to the same assay conditions as the nonlabeled hormone in the standard curve. Thus the patient's serum is added at the first step instead of a known amount of a nonlabeled hormone. The amount of labeled hormone bound to the antibody in the second step is used to provide the concentration of hormone from the standard curve.

Labeled-antibody Immunoassay

Labeling the antibody has a technical advantage in that it eliminates the necessity to develop specific approaches to label each hormone. There are two ways to perform the labeled-antibody

---

Competitive

$$H+H^*+Ab \rightleftharpoons Ab\text{-}H+Ab\text{-}H^*+H+H^*+Ab$$

Noncompetitive

$$(1) \; Ab+H \rightleftharpoons Ab\text{-}H+Ab$$

$$(2) \; Ab\text{-}H+Ab+H^* \rightleftharpoons Ab\text{-}H+Ab\text{-}H^*+H^*$$

Figure 4–5. Competitive and noncompetitive labeled-hormone immunoassays. Ab, antibody; H, nonlabeled hormone; H*, labeled hormone; Ab-H, antibody–nonlabeled hormone complex; Ab-H*, antibody–labeled hormone complex.

(1) $Ab^*+H \quad\quad Ab^*-H+Ab^*$

(2) $Ab^*-H+Ab^*+[H] \Longrightarrow Ab^*-H+Ab^*-[H]$

Figure 4–6. Two-step labeled antibody immunoassay. Ab*, labeled antibody; H, nonlabeled free hormone; [H], nonlabeled hormone linked to solid phase; (Ab*-H), labeled antibody-free hormone complex; Ab*-[H], labeled antibody-solid phase-linked hormone complex.

assay, with one site or two. The first way consists of two steps (Fig 4–6). Initially, the nonlabeled hormone reacts with excess labeled antibody until equilibrium is reached. In the second step, the unreacted labeled antibody is bound to nonlabeled hormone linked to the solid phase. The latter complex (Ab*-[H]) is removed from the system, usually by centrifugation, and the amount that remains in the solution is measured. As the amount of free nonlabeled hormone is increased in the first incubation, the amount of the Ab*-H complex increases. A standard curve is drawn and is used to establish the amount of hormone in patient serum.

The second labeled-antibody assay is also called a *sandwich-labeled assay*. This name is related to the end product of the reaction, which resembles a sandwich. It is a complex built of a single hormone bound to two different antibodies, each directed to a different chemical determinant on the hormone. This is also a two-step reaction (Fig 4–7). In the first step, large amounts of nonlabeled antibody linked to a solid phase are mixed with nonlabeled hormone. When the reaction attains equilibrium, most of the hormone is extracted out of the solution and is bound to the antibody. In the second step, this complex is exposed to labeled antibody that is specific to a second determinant on the hormone. The amount of the bound labeled antibody is directly proportional to the quantity of the nonlabeled antibody hormone complex that was obtained in the first step. When the amount of the nonlabeled hormone increases in the first step, the sandwich complex increases. The standard curve drawn is based on this phenomenon, and it is used to find the amount of hormone in patient serum. With this approach, the sensitivity of the assay increases considerably. It is important to note that this

(1) $[Ab]+H \Longrightarrow [Ab]-H$

(2) $[Ab]-H+Ab^* \Longrightarrow [Ab]-H-Ab^*$

Figure 4–7. Two-site labeled antibody immunoassay. [Ab]; solid-phase–linked primary antibody; Ab*, labeled second antibody; [Ab]-H, solid-phase–linked antibody-hormone complex; [Ab]-H-Ab*, solid-phase–linked antibody-hormone-labeled antibody complex.

assay is performed with large-protein hormones that have several epitopes and allow the production of this large complex.

Type of Radiometric Labeling

Hydrogen 3, carbon 14, and iodine 125 are the most commonly used tracers to label various low-molecular-weight hormones such as steroids. Iodine 125 is used to label proteins, peptides, and steroids.[74] Iodine 125 generally is used to label the antibody in IRMA. The specific activity may be increased by use of a high-DPM (disintegration per minute) isotope such as iodine 125 or by means of an increase in the number of radioactive isotopes per single molecule. After labeling, the final specific activity is estimated after the radioactive-labeled hormone is separated from the nonradioactive-labeled hormone. Increased specific activity usually is associated with increased sensitivity.

Because the labeled hormone is damaged with time, it is recommended that its stability be tested. In an RIA, this is usually done by means of measurement of both the *total bound* labeled hormone in absence of an unlabeled hormone and the *blank* value in the absence of antibodies. A decrease in the total bound value and an increase in the blank value may suggest that the hormone is damaged.

Separation of the Labeled Complex

Once the RIA attains equilibrium, the level of the antibody-labeled antigen complex (Ab-Ag*) can be measured in two ways: (1) absorption of the free nonlabeled and labeled hormones when only Ab-Ag* and Ab-Ag complexes remain in the solution for detection and (2) removal of the Ab-Ag* and Ab-Ag complexes from the solution by various means and discarding the supernatant that contains the free radioactive-labeled hormone. The first method usually is used for low-molecular-weight molecules such as steroids and small peptides; the second is used for polypeptides and protein hormones.

The most commonly used absorbent is dextran-coated charcoal. It is assumed that dextran is attached to the charcoal and coats it. Dextran acts as a sieve; that is, its pore size is sufficiently large to allow small molecules such as free hormone to pass through it and attach to the charcoal. However, large molecules such as the Ab-Ag and Ab-Ag* complexes cannot pass through dextran-coated charcoal and remain in the solution. The charcoal that now contains the free nonlabeled and labeled hormone is sedimented by centrifugation. The supernatant is used to measure the amount of the Ab-Ag* complex. In the second method, the Ab-Ag and Ab-Ag* complexes are precipitated by various means, including a second antibody that is directed toward the primary antibody, that is, the antibody bound to hormone. Precipitation of the primary antibody is further enhanced by centrifugation.

The hormone-antibody complex is removed by means of tagging of the hormone or the antibody with a nonradioactive flag. This includes linking the hormone or the primary antibodies to small beads or even to the wall of the plastic vessel in which the immunoassay is performed. The primary antibody may also be conjugated to a ferric oxide, and the complex is separated by a magnetic field. In this procedure, the immunoreaction is terminated by placing the test tubes into a magnetic tray that has a strong magnet located at the base. After a while, all the test tubes are decanted simultaneously and blotted. The remaining radioactivity in the test tubes is the level of Ab-Ag* complex.

In addition to the high specific activity for the labeled hormone, highly specific and sensitive antibody, and good separation of the Ab-Ag* complex, the quality of the immunoassay should be ensured by determining within-assay and between assay variations.[75] An already known amount of the nonlabeled hormone is available commercially and should be used as quality control to measure both variances and reproducibility. One must be careful about the quality of the water and chemicals used to prepare the buffers and other constituents.[76] Introducing nonspecific factors may disturb the accuracy and reproducibility of data. It is necessary to validate the RIA or IRMA regularly and every time new buffer, new lots of antibody, and hormone (labeled or nonlabeled) are prepared. In our experience, this is the best way to maintain the high quality of these tests.

ENZYME IMMUNOASSAY AND ENZYME-LINKED IMMUNOSORBENT ASSAY

The principles of the immunohistochemical approach to detecting antigen in situ were used by Engvall and Perlmann[77] to develop the first enzyme-linked immunosorbent assay (ELISA). Since then this technique has been used either to detect the presence of specific antibodies[78] or to measure levels of specific antigen and hormones.[79] The principles of the immunochemical reaction using radiolabeled isotopes are not basically different except for a change in enzyme-labeling approach. In this context enzyme immunoassays (EIAs) and immunoenzymatic assays are similar in principle to RIA and IRMA, respectively.

An EIA is advantageous in that it reduces the exposure of laboratory personnel to radioactive isotopes and eliminates the high cost of a radiometric assay. Among the expenses for the radiometric assay are those for the radioisotopes and their disposal and for equipment such as β and γ counters. Furthermore, an EIA is more easily automated than a radiometric assay.

In an EIA, an enzyme is linked to the antibody or to the hormone. There are three ways in which this takes place: the antibody is linked to a solid phase, and free hormone and enzyme-tagged hormone compete for binding to the antibody; the bind-

ing between an enzyme-labeled antibody and a solid-phase linked hormone is inhibited by nonlabeled free hormone; and a two-site sandwich immunoassay is performed in which the primary antibody is linked to the solid phase and the enzyme is bound to the second antibody in the solution, similar to the two-site radiometric assay.

To detect the end product of an EIA, a specific substrate or chromogen is added. The enzymatic reaction occurs with a light emission that includes visible color and a luminescent wave. These signals enable the development of fast, high-quality systems for identification of ELISA results. With a microtest plate with 96 wells and an ELISA plate reader, many samples can be analyzed in short time and with specificity, sensitivity, and precision as accurate as those of radiometric immunoassays. The end products of either of these approaches are detected on the constituents bound to the solid phase, and the other components are washed away. This eliminates the possibility that the quality of the assay may be affected by the nonspecific action of any compound that is present in the sample. The enzymes generally

Antibody-induced inactivation of the enzyme

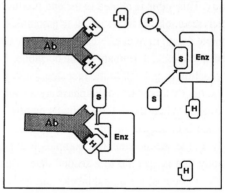

Antibody-induced reactivation of the enzyme

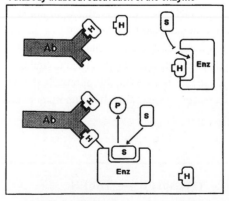

Figure 4–8. Enzyme inactivation (top) and reactivation (bottom) in EMIT. H, hormone; Ab, antibody; Enz-H, enzyme-labeled hormone; S, substrate; P, product. *(Modified from Oellerich M: Enzyme-immunoassay: A review. J Clin Chem Clin Biochem 22:895, 1984.)*

used in an EIA are horseradish peroxidase, β-D-galactosidase, alkaline phosphatase, glucose oxidase, acetylcholesterase, catalase, carbonic anhydrase, and glucoamylase.[80]

The next step in the development of the EIA was to simplify the system by requiring less input on the part of technicians and automating the system. This was achieved by eliminating the separation between bound and free hormone. All the EIA constituents remain in the test vessel, including the sample itself. To eliminate the possible influence of the constituents on the enzymatic reaction, specific enzymes are selected. The most commonly used are glucose-6-phosphate dehydrogenase (G6PD), lysozyme β-D-galactosidase, malate dehydrogenase, and β-amylase. The concept is that binding the enzyme-labeled hormone to the antibody may alter (interrupt, enhance) the degree of enzyme activity. Thus it is not necessary to separate the hormone-antibody complex and free hormone, because binding to the antibody is recovered by a change in enzyme activity.

Figure 4–8 summarizes the two ways that employed to carry on this concept.[81,82] When enzyme activity is interrupted or enhanced by the binding of the hormone tagged with the enzyme, the EIA is defined as an inactivating or a reactivating enzyme multiple-immunoassay technique (EMIT), respectively. In an inactivating EMIT the reduced enzyme activity can be caused by steric hindrance, by conformational change, or by prevention of the required conformational change to activate the enzyme. In a reactivating EMIT, binding of enzyme-tagged hormone to the antibody results in enhanced enzyme activity.[81,83]

In their basic forms, EIA and radiometric assays are comparable in specificity, sensitivity, and precision. A further elaboration of EIA was to increase its sensitivity. This was achieved in two ways: by increasing the number of enzymes tagged per single hormone or antibody molecule (that is, increasing the number of enzyme molecules per hormone-antibody interaction) and by increasing the degree of enzyme activity by means of substitute amplification.[84]

The first approach is performed with an avidin-biotin complex. The avidin-biotin interaction is one of the strongest noncovalent interactions (10^{-15} M) between a protein and a ligand.[85] The antibody can be biotinylated easily, and then avidin is bound to the biotin-labeled antibody.[86] Avidin actually has the capacity to bind four biotin molecules. Because one biotin molecule serves as connector between the avidin and the antibody, the other three molecules are used to bind three enzyme molecules. This increases by three the number of enzyme molecules per single hormone-antibody complex. The number of enzyme molecules is increased to four per single antibody with latex beads (Fig 4–9).[84]

In the other approach, enzyme substrates are replaced with specific substrates that can be regenerated by enzymes in the re-

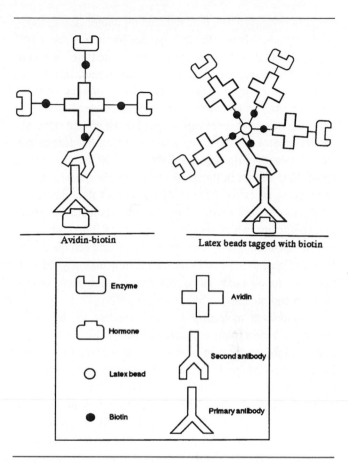

Figure 4–9. Increasing numbers of enzymes are linked to a single antibody molecule by means of an avidin-biotin complex. *(Modified from Nilsson B: Enzyme-linked immunosorbent assays.* Curr Opin Immunol *2:898, 1990.)*

action solutions.[84] In this way, a marked increase in the detected signal is observed. Combining the two techniques tremendously increases the sensitivity of the assay.

LUMINESCENT IMMUNOASSAY

The word *luminescence* refers to light emission from substance. There are three types of luminescence: radioluminescence, photoluminescence, and chemiluminescence. Radioluminescence was the first to be used for immunoassays. The uses of the other two types of light emission are described.

Fluorescence Assay

Absorption of a light photon raises the photoluminescent molecule to an excited state by means of an electron transfer to a higher-energy orbit. This excess energy is released either as nonradiative conversion such as heat, or as radiative transition to a ground state (fluorescence) or a semistable triplet state (phosphorescence). The time required for photon absorption is 10^{-15} seconds, whereas the fluorescence lifetime is about 10^{-8} seconds. This short lifetime allows many more times of excitation, and this intensifies the fluorescence signal, thereby increasing sensitivity. Phosphorescence has a lifetime of up to several parts of a second because the excited electrons stop at intermediate triplet states before reaching the ground state. According to Stokes' law, the emission wavelength is longer than the wavelength of the absorbed light. This shift (Stokes shift) is about 30 to 50 nm in fluorescence, and in phosphorescence it could be in excess of 200 nm. The quality of fluorophore has several more characteristics. The most important are the extinction coefficient, which reflects probability of light absorption, and the quantum yield, which is the ratio between quanta released to quanta absorbed. The optimum quantum yield is 1; that is, the number of released photons is equal to the number of the absorbed photons.

Fluorescent molecules are very sensitive to changes in their environment, such as temperature, pH, oxidation state, polarity, and the presence of quenching groups in the test sample. One can eliminate problems of quenching and autofluorescence in the following ways. The first is to have a fluorescent probe with an absorbed wavelength greater than 500 nm. Such a wavelength reduces the possibility of autofluorescence since the absorbed wavelength in most of the proteins and other specimen constituents is usually between 320 and 350 nm and as high as 430 to 470 nm.[87] The second is to have the antibody or the antigen linked to a solid-phase support. After the immunochemical reaction is completed, the sample constituents can be washed out of the solution before detection. The last way is to have a fluorescent probe with a longer lifetime.[88]

The most commonly selected probes for immunoassay are fluorescein, rhodamine, and umbelliterone. Other probes are fluorescamine, dansylchloride pyrene derivatives, and natural substances such as porphyrins, chlorophils, and phycobiliproteins.[87] In the development of newer fluorophores, several features seem to deserve specific attention: high quantum yield; high Stokes shift (absorption and emission maxima widely spaced); excitation by a common light source; a simple labeling procedure; and a stable fluorophore that does not affect the immunochemical reaction after linking to either the antibody or the antigen.

In a fluorescence immunoassay (FIA), the hormone is labeled; in an immunofluorometric assay (IFMA) the antibody is labeled. The IFMA can be both a one-site and a two-site procedure. Both types include separating (heterogenous) and nonseparating (homogenous) assays. In the separation assay, the methods for detecting binding either by FIA or IFMA are not different from those for RIA or IRMA. Nevertheless, sometimes it becomes important that the labeled material be eluted from the solid phase before measurement.[89] Modifications such as particle-concentration FIA have been introduced.[90]

The nonseparating techniques are based on the phenomenon that the formation of the antibody-antigen complex may be associated with a change in fluorescence properties either as enhancement or quenching FIA. This principle was used to invent many new techniques of quenching or enhancement of fluorescence emission in the antibody-antigen complex, as shown by the next few examples.

Quenching the fluorescent label can be achieved indirectly with antibody directed against the fluorescent conjugate.[91] It is possible to use the different fluorophores in such a way that one can quench the other. With labeling of two different reactants with two of these fluorophores, such as fluorescein and rhodamine, binding results with total quenching of the formed antibody-antigen complex. A combination of FIA and enzyme activity was invented in which fluorescence is observed only after enzymatic action on the labeled molecule. This enzymatic action does not occur when the antibody-antigen complex is formed. Thus data manifest the free reactant of the system.

Other approaches involve the properties of the fluorophore in which excitation with polarized light yields most of the emitted light. In the fluorescence-polarization immunoassay (FPIA), the fluorescence signal is from the antibody-antigen complex that has lowered brownian motion and not from the free-labeled reactant, which has random motion. Many other nonseparation techniques of FIA and IFMA use these principles and increase the sensitivity of the immunoassay.[92]

In the nonseparating assay, polyacrylamide and polystryrene beads are likely to be applicable due to their low fluorescence and light-scattering characteristics. Because of the interference of the sample constituents in the emitted light, the sensitivity of the homogenous fluorescence assay is usually lower than that of the heterogenous one. The nonseparating technique is usually applicable to hormones that are known to be present in large quantities in the tested fluid, about 1 ng/mL.[92] An improvement in the nonseparating assay was achieved with use of better fluorophores, for example, a polyfluorescein or chelated rare earth lanthanides such as europian and terbium, which resulted in lower background, and with improvement in the instrumentation, including optics and detection tools. These improvements increased the sensitivity to even more than that of the radiometric and enzymatic assays. To reduce sample interference and background noise, compounds representing phosphorescence immunoassays are effective.[93] This approach was used in heterogenous and homogenous assays. Phosphorescence probes such as erythrosin have a long life of several microseconds and a long Stokes shift (>150 nm).

Chemiluminescent and Bioluminescent Assays

As with photoluminescence, in chemiluminescence and bioluminescence assays the emission of the light photon is a dissipation of energy from a molecule that is in an electronically excited state. What is special about this type of photon emission is that the energy source is from a chemical reaction and not from the absorption of light photons. Furthermore, the fluorescent molecule is ready for reexcitation when it returns to ground state and thus to its initial form. In chemiluminescence and bioluminescence, the emitting molecule is different from the initial substance and thus cannot be reexcited through another chemical reaction. The reaction depends on its own rate, its efficiency in forming electronically excited state, and the capacity of the excited molecules to produce photons. The overall quantum yield represents the number of photons emitted per number of molecules undergoing the reaction. The average quantum yield for chemiluminescence is 0.001 to 0.01 and for bioluminescence is 0.01 to 1.0.

Luciferin and luciferase, which refer to the substance and the enzyme, respectively, involved in the bioluminescence reaction, were first introduced by Dubois in 1887.[94] So far five distinct types of chemical families of luciferin that result in four different chemical reactions have been described. The bioluminescence reaction requires at least three components, luciferin (substance), luciferase (enzyme), and oxygen or a specific metabolite of oxygen. Other components that might be necessary are metabolites such as reduced nicotinamide-adenine dinucleotide phosphate (NADPH) or adenosine triphosphate (ATP), cations such as Cu^{2+}, Mg^{2+}, or Ca^{2+}, and energy transfer acceptor. The main energy source to generate a photon comes from oxidation of luciferin. Dioxetan is an intermediate substance produced through the oxidation of luciferin. The dioxetan intermediate is also produced in chemiluminescence reactions in which synthetic organic substance is used. Thus O_2 O_2^- or H_2O_2 is added as the oxidant, and emissions result from the excited carbonyl molecule. This type of reaction was used to synthesize stable dioxetan as adamantyldenene adamantane 1,2-dioxetan, which can be decomposed into excited carbon to emit photons by heating.[95] This compound and others, such as

acridinium esters,[96] are used as probes for many purposes including immunoassay, because they are not affected by environmental conditions.

The synthetic chemiluminescence compounds such as isoluminol, acridinium esters, and dioxetanes are detected easily in the range of 10^{-15} to 10^{-19} mol, and with enzyme amplification down to 10^{-21} mol. Radioactive isotopes can be detected down to 10^{-12} to 10^{-15} (hydrogen 3 or carbon 14) or to about 10^{-18} (iodine 125 or phosphorus 32). Other advantages with the luminescence compounds, in addition to safety of laboratory personnel, are a long shelf-life until triggered, the ability to allow analysis in seconds, and the ability to be used in homologous immunoassays. The high sensitivity of chemiluminescence and bioluminescence assays is effective in following various processes within living cells, such as second messengers of various hormonal stimuli, including Ca^{2+}, inositol triphosphate (IP_3), cyclic adenosine monophosphate (c-AMP), and oxygen and its metabolite, NADPH.

Bioluminescence is used to detect levels of hormone or other metabolites in two ways—direct assay and immunoassays. The firefly and bacterial luciferases are most commonly used for these reactions. Firefly luciferase provides an ATP-dependent oxidative decarboxylase reaction, and bacterial luciferase depends on the supply of NADH (Fig 4–10). In the direct assay, any molecule or substance that can be used to generate ATP or NADH can be measured with the appropriate reaction. This system is used to measure 3-, 7-, and 12α-hydroxy steroids. Its efficiency is increased by linking the enzymes to sepharose, which enables the automation of the system by use of a flow cell. The flow cell that contains the immobilized enzyme is used in up to 300 assays.[97] Although the direct assay is limited, it is very efficient and has high precision.

There are many applications of bioluminescence immunoassays: linking luciferin or luciferase to the antigen or antibody; linking the enzyme that generates ATP or NADH to the antigen or antibody; and modifying luciferin into an inactive lu-

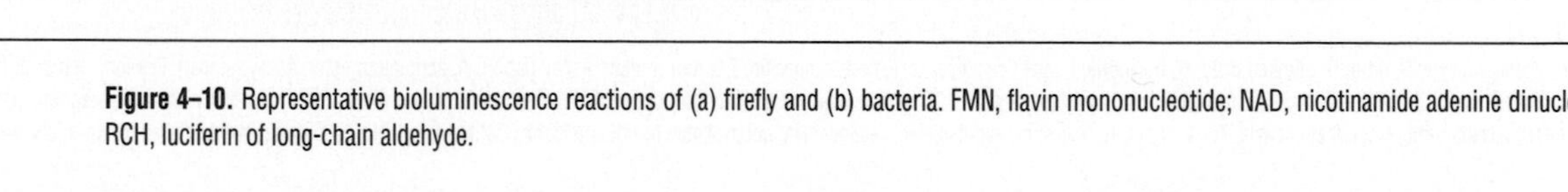

(b) NADH + FMN *reductase* NAD⁺ + FMNH₂
    FMNH₂ + RCHO + O₂ *luciferase* FMN + RCO₂H + H₂O + Light

Figure 4–10. Representative bioluminescence reactions of (a) firefly and (b) bacteria. FMN, flavin mononucleotide; NAD, nicotinamide adenine dinucleotide; RCH, luciferin of long-chain aldehyde.

ciferin and linking the enzyme that can make these luciferin derivatives into active luciferin to a second antibody. Homogeneous bioluminescence assays also have been developed. For example, the reacting components luciferase, oxidoreductase, and antibody are immobilized in close proximity, and monoclonal antibody to the amylate is bound to G6PD. The binding value of this conjugate to the immobilized antibody is proportional to the conjugate concentration. The NADH generated by G6PD is used by oxidoreductase and luciferase to generate light. The possible interference of NADH generated by G6PD in the solution is eliminated by use of parallel oxidation with soluble lactate dehydrogenase and pyruvate.[98]

Chemiluminescence reactions were improved with the development of new chemiluminescent molecules that have low loss of quantum yield when attached to the antigen or antibody. These new molecules can be used in heterogeneous and homogeneous assays. Immunoassays based on the chemiluminescence reaction were developed to detect the levels of various steroids.[99] New models of luminometers increase the sensitivity of the chemiluminescent-bioluminescent approach. The light emitted by the reaction is detected as one-photon, one-event, one-pulse (digital) or photocurrent (analog), both in proportion to light intensity produced by the reaction.

AUTOMATED IMMUNOASSAY

Establishment of an automated system is the goal for each of the techniques described. Automated testing satisfies the demands of new clinical laboratories, which are facing difficulties including limited resources, space conservation, and the need to consolidate. Managed care competition, cost reduction, health care reform, and increased regulation of test laboratories also push for automated immunoassays for endocrine testing. These goals can be achieved if automation reduces costs, requires less labor, and can yield rapid testing. In addition, it reduces sample handling, which is important to avoid possible contamination with viruses that cause hepatitis and acquired immunodeficiency syndrome.

In automated immunoassay, calibration stability is achieved within 2 to 4 weeks. This allows more frequent testing, eliminating the batch concept and daily calibration. The number of

TABLE 4–3. FEATURES OF AUTOMATED IMMUNOASSAY SYSTEMS

System Manufacturer	AxSYM Abbott	OPUS MAGNUM Behring	VIDAS Bio- Merieux	ACS:180 Ciba Corning	IMMULITE Diag. Prod. Corp.	aca Plus DuPont	Immuno 1 Bayer	Cobas Core Roche	ACCESS Sanofi	AIA-1200 DX Tosoh	auto DELFIA Wallac
Automation	C	C	C	C	C	C	C	C	C	C	C
Analyte											
Number	25	30	26	20	30	42	27	16	24	20	20
Type	All	All	H,I	H,T,D*	H,T,D*	H,D,P	All	H,T	H,I,D*	H,T	H,T
Assay											
Homogenous	Y	N	N	N	N	Y	Y	N	N	N	N
Heterogenous	Y	Y	Y	Y	Y	Y	Y	Y	Y	Y	Y
Competitive	Y	Y	Y	Y	Y	Y	Y	Y	Y	Y	Y
Immunometric	Y	Y	Y	Y	Y	Y	Y	Y	Y	Y	Y
Label	E/F	E	E	A	E	E	E/L	E	E	E	F
Signal	F	F	F	L	L	S	S/T	S	L	F	tF
Separation	PF/NA	CF/MF	CT	MP	CB	MP	MP/NA	CB	MP	MP	CW
On-board	20	36	15-30	13	12	1-42	22	10	24	21	8
Sample											
Tray capacity	90	150	15-30	60	72	16-80	78	180	60	100	432
Primary tube	Y	Y	N	Y	N	N	Y	Y	Y	Y	Y
STAT add	Y	Y	Y	Y	Y	Y	Y	Y	Y	Y	Y
Throughput											
Incubation time (m)	10	6-21	20-45	10	30	4.2-15	5,30-45	30-75	10-25	40	60
Time 1st result (m)	15	10-25	20-45	15	40-70	7-30	7,38-50	35-100	15-75	50	75
Time bet. results	0.5-1 m	0.5 m	N/A	20 sec	30 sec	40 sec-2.5 m	30 sec	25 sec	36 sec	0.5 m	NA
Maximum (no. of tests)	60-120	80-120	40-90	90-180	120	60	120	150	50-100	120	192
Calibration											
Stability	4 wk	2-8 wk	2 wk	2 wk	2 wk	8-12 wk	8 wk	4 wk	4 wk	4 wk	L/2

Y, yes; N, no.

Automation: C, continuous access. Analyte: D, drug; D*, limited drug; H, hormone; I, infectious disease; P, protein specific; T, tumor marker. Assay (label); A, acridinium ester; Assay (signal); F, fluorometric; tF, time-resolved fluorometric; L, luminescence; S/T, spectrophotometric turbidimetric; Assay (separation): CB, coated bead; CF, coated filter paper; CT, coated tube; CW, coated well; MF, multilayer film; MP, magnetic particle; P, particle; PF, particle filter; TB, turbidimetric; NA, not applicable, Throughput: h, hours; m, minutes; sec, seconds; NA, not available or not applicable. Calibration: L/No, lot specific/number of calibrators; wk, weeks.

samples that can be loaded on the automated system is important in allowing technicians to spend less time placing samples in the system. No complicated scheduling system is necessary. The total automated system is coupled to computer terminals for data entry, reporting, evaluation, and analysis. The technician becomes a data manager but grows less skillful in performing the assays. This can be risky, especially if malfunction results in total shutdown of the immunoassay.

The automated system is constructed of four parts: a sampling center; a reagent and waste center; a processing center; and an operation and data-reporting center. Some modifications may occur from one system to the other. For example, in some systems all the reagents are supplied in a strip and the tested sample is added to this strip. Thus, there is no reagent center. Other differences are in the ways samples are shuffled from one center to the other, in the positioning of the centers, and in the processing center that sometimes is associated with the type of signal or type of detector. An excellent comprehensive description of automated systems is available elsewhere.[100]

The automated systems are diverse with respect to types of assays (such as homogenous, competitive), types of labels (such as enzyme, fluorometric) and types of signals (such as spectorphotometric, luminescent). Other features include the number of samples that can be tested per hour and number of assays that are available for the system. Table 4–3 presents some automated systems.

Each system uses one of the immunoassay approaches such as EIA, fluorescent, chemiluminescent, or combination of ELISA and fluorescence. For example, in the AxSYM, OPUS, MAGNUM, VIDAS, AIA-1200 DX, and autodisassociation enhancement lanthanide fluoroimmunoassay (DELFIA) systems, the end product is detected with a fluorometric signal but not in the same manner in all the systems.

In the AxSYM system the fluorescent molecule is bound to the antigen in the FPIA, or it is supplied as an inactive molecule in the microparticle enzyme immunoassay (MEIA). As indicated, in the FPIA the measured fluorescence polarization is detected only in the immobilized antibody-antigen complex with the bound tracer. In the MEIA alkaline phosphatase linked to the antibody converts 4-methylumbelliferyl phosphate into the fluorophore methylumbelliferone, which can be detected. In VIDAS and AIA-1200DX, detection is based on enzyme-linked fluorescent immunoassays using alkaline phosphatase as the enzyme, whereas in the auto-DELFIA the assay uses lanthanide compounds, especially europium. Europium, which has a weak fluorescence signal when bound to protein, is released from the protein by means of lowering the pH to detect the fluorescence signal at a higher magnitude. Similar examples are presented for the other automated immunoassay systems.

The future clinical laboratory will have advanced immunoassay automation with all the advantages but in miniature homogeneous assays. Simultaneous measurements may be applied by use of different fluorescent labels with different wavelengths or use of different-sized particles to produce immobilized different amylates and then using flow cytometry to detect the signal at different positions, primarily on the basis of particle size. The design of such systems will be based on users' needs.[100]

ACKNOWLEDGMENTS

I am grateful to Dr. Machelle Seibel for the opportunity and support to write this chapter. I would like to thank Dr. Hui-Zhong Yin for drawing some of the figures and Ms. Nancy Junker for typing this chapter.

REFERENCES

1. Yallow RS, Berson SA: Radiobiology: Assay of plasma insulin in human subjects by immunological methods. *Nature* 184:1648, 1959
2. Yallow RS, Berson SA: Immunoassay of endogenous plasma insulin in man. *J Clin Invest* 39:1157, 1960
3. Berthold AA: Transplantation der hoden. *Arch Anat Physiol Leipzig* 16:42, 1849
4. Bernard CI: *Leçons sur les phénoménes de la vie commune aux animaux et aux végétaux.* Paris, Bailliére, 1878
5. Prenant A: La valeur morphologique du corps jaune: Son action physiologique et thérapeutique possible. *Rev Gen Sci* 9:646, 1898
6. Morau DH: Des transformations épithéliales de la muqueuse du vagin de quelques rongeurs. *J Anat Physiol Paris* 25:277, 1889
7. Lataste MF: Transformation périodique de l'épithélium du vagin des rongeurs rythme vaginal: Compt rend hebdomadaires seances et memoires. *Soc Biol Paris* 44:765, 1892
8. Fraenkel L: Die function des corpus luteum. *Arch Gynaekol* 68:438, 1903
9. Bouin P, Ancel P: Recherches sur les fonctions du corps jaune gestatif. I. Sur le déterminisme de la préparation de l'utérus á la fixation de l'oeuf. *J Physiol Pathol Gener* 12:31, 1910
10. Corner GW, Allen WM: Physiology of the corpus luteum. II. Production of a special uterine reaction (progestational proliferation) by extracts of the corpus luteum. *Am J Physiol* 88:326, 1929
11. Murata M, Adachi K: Über die künstliche erzeugung des corpus luteum durch injektion der plazentarsubstanz aus frühen schwangerschaftsmonaten. *Geburtshilfe Gynakol* 92:45, 1927
12. Zondek B, Aschheim S: Hypophysenvorderlappen und ovarium: Bezichungen der endokrinen drüsen zur ovarialfunktion. *Arch Gynäkol* 130:1, 1927
13. Friedman MH: Humoral mechanisms concerned in ovulation in the rabbit. *Endocrinology* 14:328, 1930
14. Simpson ME: Role of anterior pituitary gonadotropins in reproductive processes. In: Cole HH, Cupps PT (eds), *Reproduction in Domestic Animals.* New York, Academic Press, London 1959: 59–110

15. Hon EH: Biologic tests for pregnancy. In: *A Manual of Pregnancy Testing.* Boston, Little, Brown, 1961:39–52

16. Steelman SL, Pohley FM: Assay of the follicle stimulating hormone based on the augmentation with human chorionic gonadotropin. *Endocrinology* 53:604, 1953

17. Munson PL, Barry AG Jr, Koch FC: A simplified hypophysectomized rat adrenal ascorbic acid bioassay method for adrenocorticotropin (ACTH): Specificity and application to preparative problems. *J Clin Endocrinol* 8:586, 1948

18. Parlow AF: A rapid bioassay method for LH and factors stimulating LH secretion. *Fed Proc* 17:402, 1958

19. Ellis S, Porter J: Assay of luteinizing hormone. *Fed Proc* 16:34, 1957

20. Guillemin R, Clayton GW, Smith JD, Lipscomb HS: Measurement of free corticosteroids in rat plasma: Physiological validation of a method. *Endocrinology* 63:349, 1958

21. How MJ, Chaplin MF, Ryle M: The distribution of [^{14}C] thymidine in mouse ovaries cultured in vitro with and without gonadotrophic hormones. *Biochem Biophys Acta* 213:226, 1970

22. Watson J: Progesterone synthesis in response to luteinizing hormone by rat ovarian tissue in vitro. *J Endocrinol* 49:471, 1971

23. Bajpai PK, Dash RJ, Midgley AR Jr, Reichert LE Jr: Progesterone production by dissociated rat ovarian cells: A sensitive method for quantitation of hormones with luteinizing activity. *J Clin Endocrinol Metab* 38:721, 1974

24. Dufau ML, Catt KJ, Tsuruhara T: A sensitive gonadotropin responsive system: Radio-immunoassay of testosterone production by the rat testis in vitro. *Endocrinology* 90:1032, 1972

25. Padmanabhan V, Chappel SC, Beitins IZ: An improved *in vitro* bioassay for follicle-stimulating hormone (FSH): Suitable for measurement of FSH in unextracted human serum. *Endocrinology* 121:1089, 1987

26. Gold JJ: Endocrine laboratory procedures and available tests. In: Gold JJ (ed), *Gynecologic Endocrinology,* ed 2. Hagerstown, MD, Harper & Row, 1975:647–667

27. Fulton F, Dumbell KR: The serological comparison of strains of influenza virus. *J Gen Microbiol* 3:97, 1949

28. Brody S, Carlstrom G: Estimation of human chorionic gonadotrophin in biological fluids by complement fixation. *Lancet* 2:99, 1960

29. Wide L, Gemzell CA: An immunological pregnancy test. *Acta Endocrinol* 35:261, 1960

30. McKean CM: Preparation and use of antisera to human chorionic gonadotrophin. *Am J Obstet Gynecol* 80:596, 1960

31. Ekins RP: The estimation of thyroxine in human plasma by an electrophoretic technique. *Clin Chim Acta* 5:453, 1960

32. Fauser BCJM, Pache TD, Lamberts SWJ, Hop WCJ, de Jong FH, Dahl KD: Serum bioactive and immunoreactive luteinizing hormone and follicle-stimulating hormone levels in women with cycle abnormalities, with or without polycystic ovarian disease. *J Clin Endocrinol Metab* 73:811, 1991

33. Fauser BCJM, Pache TD, Hop WCJ, de Jong FH, Dahl KD: The significance of single serum LH measurement in women with cycle disturbance: Discrepancies between immunoreactive and bioactive estimate. *Clin Endocrinol* 37:445, 1992

34. Papandreou M-J, Asteria C, Pettersson K, Ronin C, Beck-Peccoz P: Concavalin A affinity chromatography of human serum gonadotropins: Evidence for changes of carbohydrate structure in different clinical conditions. *J Clin Endocrinol Metab* 76:1008, 1993

35. Beitins IZ, Axelrod L, Ostrea T, Little R, Badger TM: Hypogonadism in a male with an immunological active, biologically inactive luteinizing hormone: Characterization of the abnormal hormone. *J Clin Endocrinol Metab* 52:1143, 1981

36. Mitchell R, Hollis S, Rothwell C, Robertson WR: Age related changes in the pituitary-testicular axis in normal men: Lower serum testosterone results from decreased bioactive LH drive. *Clin Endocrinol* 42:501, 1995

37. Serôn-Ferré M, Vergara M, García-Huidobro V, Huhtaniemi I, Díaz S: Diminished luteinizing hormone biopotency in breastfeeding women. *Hum Reprod* 10:2849, 1995

38. Kleinberg DL, Frantz AG: Human prolactin: Measurement in plasma by in vitro bioassay. *J Clin Invest* 50:1557, 1971

39. Frantz AG: Bioassay and radioimmunoassay of prolactin. In: Antoniades HN (ed), *Hormones in Human Blood: Detection and Assay.* Cambridge, MA, Harvard University Press, 1976:449–463

40. Hattori K, Shimizu K, Takahashi M, et al: Quantitative in vivo assay of human granulocyte colony-stimulating factor using cyclophosphamide-induced neutropenic mice. *Blood* 75:1228, 1990

41. Méchain C, Cédrin I, Pandian C, Lemay A: Serum FSH bioactivity and response to acute gonadotrophin releasing hormone (GnRH) agonist stimulation in patients with polycystic ovary syndrome (PCOS) as compared to control groups. *Clin Endocrinol* 38:311, 1993

42. Padmanabhan V, Lang LL, Sonstein J, Kelch RP, Beitins IZ: Modulation of serum follicle-stimulating hormone bioactivity and isoform distribution by estrogenic steroids in normal women and in gonadal dysgenesis. *J Clin Endocrinol Metab* 67:465, 1988

43. Creus S, Pellizzari E, Cigorrage SB, Campo S: FSH isoforms: Bio and immuno-activities in post-menopausal and normal menstruating women. *Clin Endocrinol* 44:181, 1996

44. Galway AB, Hsueh AJW, Keene JL, Yamoto M, Fauser BCJM, Boime I: *In vitro* and *in vivo* bioactivity of recombinant human follicle-stimulating hormone and partially deglycosylated variants secreted by transfected eukoriotic cell lines. *Endocrinology* 127:93, 1990

45. Singh O, Venkateswara L, Gaur A, Sharma NC, Alam A, Talwar GP: Antibody response and characteristics of antibodies in women immunized with three contraceptive vaccines inducing antibodies against human chorionic gonadotropin. *Fertil Steril* 52:739, 1989

46. Platia MP, Bloomquist G, Williams RF, Hodgen GD: Refractoriness to gonadotropin therapy: How to distinguish ovarian failure versus pseudoovarian resistance caused by neutralizing antibodies. *Fertil Steril* 42:779, 1984

47. Claustrat B, David L, Faure A, Francois R: Development of anti-human chorionic gonadotropin antibodies in patients with hypogonadotropin hypogonadism: A study of four patients. *J Clin Endocrinol Metab* 57:1041, 1983

48. Messinis IE, Lolis D, Zikopoulos K, et al: Effect of follicle stimu-

lating hormone or human chorionic gonadotrophin treatment on the production of gonadotrophin surge attenuating factor (GnSAF) during the luteal phase of the human menstrual cycle. *Clin Endocrinol* 44:169, 1996

49. Clarke FM: Identification of molecules and mechanisms involved in the "early pregnancy factor" system. *Reprod Fertil Dev* 4:423, 1992

50. Hill JA, Polgar K, Harlow BL, Anderson DJ: Evidence of embryo and trophoblast-toxic cellular immune response(s) in women with recurrent spontaneous abortion. *Am J Obstet Gynecol* 166:1044, 1992

51. Chang YS, Lee JY, Moon SY, Kim JG, Pang MG, Shin CJ: Factors affecting penetration of zona-free hamster ova. *Arch Androl* 25:213, 1990

52. Xu YE, Wang YI, Lin N, Zhang J-W, Qian SZ: Subcapsular intra-testicular assay: A preliminary screening method for putative male antifertility drugs. *Int J Androl* 18(Suppl): 53, 1995

53. Speroff L, Glass RH, Kase NG: *Clinical Gynecologic Endocrinology and Infertility.* Baltimore, Williams & Wilkins, 1994

54. Iles RK, Lee CL, Howes I, Davies S, Edwards R, Chard T: Immunoreactive β-core-like material in normal postmenopausal urine: Human chorionic gonadotrophin or LH origin? Evidence for the existence of LH core. *J Endocrinol* 133:459, 1992

55. Carter JN, Tyson JE, Tolis G, Van Vliet S, Faiman C, Friesen HG: Prolactin-secreting tumors and hypogonadism in 22 men. *N Engl J Med* 299:847, 1978

56. Filicori M, Butler JP, Crowley WF Jr: Neuroendocrine regulation of the corpus luteum in the human: Evidence for pulsatile progesterone secretion. *J Clin Invest* 73:1638, 1984

57. Syrop CH, Hammond MG: Diurnal variations in midluteal serum progesterone measurements. *Fertil Steril* 47:67, 1987

58. Bardin CW, Paulsen CA: The testes. In: Williams RH (ed), *Textbook of Endocrinology.* Philadelphia, Saunders, 1981: 293–354

59. Goldzieher JW, Dozier TS, Smith KD, Steinberger E: Improving the diagnostic reliability of rapidly fluctuating plasma hormone levels by optimized multiple-sampling techniques. *J Clin Endocrinol Metab* 43:824, 1976

60. Shaw RW, Butt WR, London DR, Marshall JC: The estrogen provocation test: A method of assessing the hypothalamic-pituitary axis in patients with amenorrhoea. *Clin Endocrinol* 4:267, 1975

61. Akande EO, Carr PJ, Dutton A, et al: Effect of synthetic gonadotrophin-releasing hormone in secondary amenorrhea. *Lancet* 2:112, 1972

62. Nakano R, Kotsuji F, Mizuno T, Hashiba N, Washio M, Tojo S: Response to luteinizing hormone releasing factor (LRF) in normal subjects and anovulatory patients. *Acta Obstet Gynecol Scand* 52:171, 1973

63. Lobo RA, Kletzky OA, Campeau JD, diZerega GS: Elevated bioactive luteinizing hormone in women with the polycystic ovary syndrome. *Fertil Steril* 39:674, 1983

64. Horton R, Hawks D, Lobo R: 3α,17β-androstanediol glucuronide in plasma: A marker of androgen action in idiopathic hirsutism. *J Clin Invest* 69:1203, 1982

65. Lobo RA, Gysler M, March CM, Goebelsmann U, Mishell DR Jr:

Clinical and laboratory predictors of clomiphene response. *Fertil Steril* 37:168, 1982

66. Polson DW, Kiddy DS, Mason HD, Franks S: Induction of ovulation with clomiphene citrate in women with polycystic ovary syndrome: The difference between responders and nonresponders. *Fertil Steril* 51:30, 1989

67. Blum I, Bruhis S, Kaufaman H: Clinical evaluation of the effects of combined treatments with bromocriptine and spironolactone in two women with the polycystic ovary syndrome. *Fertil Steril* 35:629, 1981

68. Swerdloff RS, Boyes SP: Evaluation of the male partner of an infertile couple: An algorithmic approach. *JAMA* 247:2418, 1982

69. McClure RD: Endocrine investigation and therapy. *Urol Clin North Am* 14:471, 1987

70. Urban MD, Lee PA, Migeon CJ: Adult height and fertility in men with congenital virilizing adrenal hyperplasia. *N Engl J Med* 299:1392, 1978

71. McArthur JW, Powell DA: Human chorionic gonadotropin. In: Antoniades HN (ed), *Hormones in Human Blood: Detection and Assay.* Cambridge, MA, Harvard University Press, 1976: 517–526

72. Betterle C, Rossi A, Dalla Pria S, et al: Premature ovarian failure: Autoimmunity and natural history. *Clin Endocrinol* 39:35, 1993

73. Hancock RJT, Cockett ATK: Reactions of antisera to hCG with living human spermatozoa. *J Reprod Fertil* 65:125, 1982

74. Butt WR: The iodination of follicle-stimulating and other hormones for radioimmunoassay. *J Endocrinol* 55:453, 1972

75. Rodbard D, Rayford PL, Cooper JA, Ross GT: Statistical quality control of radioimmunoassays. *J Clin Endocrinol Metab* 28:1412, 1968

76. Challand GS, Chard T: Quality control in a radioimmunoassay: Observations on the operation of a semi-automated assay for human placental lactogen. *Clin Chim Acta* 46:133, 1973

77. Engvall E, Perlmann P: Enzyme-linked immunosorbent assay (ELISA): Quantitative assay of immunoglobulin G. *Immunochemistry* 8:871, 1971

78. Vejtorp P: Enzyme-linked immunosorbent assay for determination of rubella IgG antibodies. *Acta Path Microbiol Scand* 86:387, 1978

79. Voller A, Bartlett A, Bidwell DE: Enzyme immunoassay with special reference to ELISA techniques. *J Clin Pathol* 31:507, 1978

80. O'Sullivan MJ, Bridges JW, Marks V: Enzyme immunoassay: A review. *Ann Clin Biochem* 16:221, 1979

81. Oellerich M: Enzyme-immunoassays in clinical chemistry: Present status and trends. *J Clin Chem Clin Biochem* 18:197, 1980

82. Oellerich M: Enzyme-immunoassay: A review. *J Clin Chem Clin Biochem* 22:895, 1984

83. Rubenstein KE, Schneider RS, Ullman EF: "Homogeneous" enzyme immunoassay: A new immunochemical technique. *Biochem Biophys Res Commun* 47:846, 1972

84. Nilsson B: Enzyme-linked immunosorbent assays. *Curr Opin Immunol* 2:898, 1990

85. Green NM: Avidin. In: *Advances in Protein Chemistry,* vol 29. New York, Academic Press, 1975:85–133

86. Guesdon JL, Ternynck T, Avrameas S: The use of avidin-biotin in-

teraction in immunoenzymatic techniques. *J Histochem Cytochem* 27:1131, 1979

87. Hemmilä I: Fluoroimmunoassay and immunofluorometric assays. *Clin Chem* 31:359, 1985

88. Waggoner AS: Fluorescent probes for analysis of cell structure, function, and health by flow and imaging cytometry. In: Taylor DL (ed), *Application of Fluorescence in the Biomedical Sciences.* New York, Liss, 1986:3–28

89. Aalberse RC: Quantitative fluoroimmunoassay. *Clin Chim Acta* 48:109, 1973

90. MacCrindle C, Schwenzer K, Jolley ME: Particle concentration fluorescence immunoassay: A new immunoassay technique for quantitation of human immunoglobulins in serum. *Clin Chem* 31:1487, 1985

91. Nargessi RD, Landon J, Smith DS: Use of antibodies against label in non-separation non-isotopic immunoassay: "Indirect quenching" fluoroimmunoassay of proteins. *J Immunol Methods* 26:307, 1979

92. Barnard G: The development of fluorescence immunoassay. In: Albertson BD, Hazeltine FP (eds), *Non-Radiometric Assays: Technology and Application in Polypeptide and Steroid Hormone Detection.* New York, Liss, 1988:15–37

93. Sidki AM, Landon J: Fluoroimmunoassay and phosphoroimmunoassay. In: Collins WP (ed), *Alternative Immunoassays.* Chichester, England, Wiley, 1985:185–201

94. Dubois R: Note sur la fonction photogénique chez les Pholades: Compt Rend Seances et memoires. *Soc Biol Paris* 4:564, 1887

95. Adam W, Cilento G: Determination of chemiexcitation yields in the thermal generation of electronic excitation from 1,2-dioxetanes. *Chemical and Biological Generation of Excited States.* Academic Press, New York, 1982

96. Weeks I, Sturgess ML, Woodhead JS: Chemiluminescence immunoassays: An overview. *Clin Sci* 70:403, 1986

97. Vellom DC, Kricka LJ: Continuous-flow bioluminescent assays employing sepharose-immobolized enzymes. In: Deluca M, McElroy WD (eds), New York, Academic Press, 1986: 229–237

98. Térouanne B, Nicolas J-C, Crastes de Paulet A: Bioluminescent immunoassay for fetoprotein. *Anal Biochem* 154:132, 1986

99. De Boever J, Kohen F, Bouve J, Leyseele D, Vanderkerckhove D: Direct chemiluminescence immunoassay of estradiol in saliva. *Clin Chem* 36:2036, 1990

100. Chan DW: Summary of automated immunoassay systems. In: Chan DW (ed), *Immunoassay Automation: An Updated Guide to Systems,* San Diego, Academic Press, 1996:9–10

PART II

Endocrinology of Female Infertility

CHAPTER 5

Oocyte Development and Meiosis in Humans

SHALOM BAR-AMI · MACHELLE M. SEIBEL

Gametogenesis and Folliculogenesis During Gestation
Formation of the primary oocyte and primordial follicle
Follicular development during gestation and pubertal life
The Growing Oocyte: Ultrastructure and Molecular Composition
Altered morphologic features in a growing oocyte
Biosynthesis and storage of RNA and protein

Control of Meiotic Maturation
Meiotic competence
Regulation of meiotic resumption
In Vitro Growth of Follicle-Enclosed Oocytes
Explanted oocytes and their growth
Completion of Meiosis, and Beginning of the First Mitotic Divisions
Role of the microtubules and centrosomes
The role of microfilaments
Failure of Meiotic Completion and Oocyte Mitosis in Human Oocyte

Development and meiosis of the female gamete in humans begins early in fetal life and is not completed until fertilization occurs in adult life, often more than two decades later. The main purpose of this process is to provide the means by which a diploid germ cell (2n), which has four times the necessary chromatin (4c), can exchange genetic material and ultimately result in a genetically distinct gamete that is haploid (1n) and contains only the necessary amount of chromatin (1c).

Early in the development of in vitro fertilization (IVF) for humans, it became clear that much of the success in solving various infertility problems depended on the degree of oocyte growth, health, and maturation. Compared with sperm, human oocytes possess a higher rate of chromosomal abnormalities. Thus, various techniques of assisted reproduction have become more and more directed at the basic events that yield a mature healthy oocyte poised to undergo fertilization and develop into a viable normal fetus. Furthermore, on the basis of successes with

rodents, it seems that in vitro full development and maturation of human oocytes starting as primary or even primordial follicles may soon be possible. Therefore, understanding of oocyte meiosis and its regulation becomes indispensable for both scientists and clinicians who deal with gynecology and genetics.

Several excellent reviews have been published on various aspects of oocyte growth and maturation in mammals in this evolving area of research.[1-3] Herein is reviewed the state of the art of the various aspects of oocyte development and meiosis in mammals with special focus on the human oocyte.

GAMETOGENESIS AND FOLLICULOGENESIS DURING GESTATION

The history of a germ cell begins at a very early stage of embryonic life and can be divided into several stages: migration from the extraembryonic region to the genital ridge, an increase in numbers by mitosis, and finally initiation of meiosis. The progression of these processes depends on interaction between germ cells and somatic cells. In a neonatal girl the ovary is populated mostly with primordial follicles.

Formation of the Primary Oocyte and Primordial Follicle

At the 16-somite stage of the human embryo on day 24 after fertilization, the primordial germ cells (PGCs) can be identified in the yolk sac and hindgut near the developing allantois.[4] Figure 5–1[5] depicts the trail of primordial germ cells from their presumable place of formation, that is, posterior to the caudal end of the primitive streak toward the roof of the coelom near the nephrogonadoblastic ridge. PGCs can be traced because of their large size and high content of alkaline phosphatase. In mice, epiblasts isolated from preimplanted blastocysts give rise to germ cells after being injected into host blastocysts.[6] Similarly, primitive ectoderm taken from the caudal end of 7- to 7.5-day mouse embryos are capable of developing PGC-like cells in vitro.[3]

The initial movement of PGCs is passive, but when they approach the hindgut and move along the mesoderm and endoderm of the primitive streak, PGCs acquire active ameboid movement and invasive characteristics.[7,8] The estimated speed of PGC movement is 50 μm per hour.[9] Although PGCs usually degenerate if they fail to reach the genital ridge, occasionally they survive and may develop into teratomas. Such teratomas are usually found in the mediastinum, the sacrococcygeal region, and in the oral region.[5] Interestingly, when ectopic PGCs

reach the adrenal gland, they develop into meiotic oocytes whether their karyotype is XX or XY.[10] It has been demonstrated that PGC movement is regulated by various factors. Their migration and proliferation are impaired in mice bearing the *gcd* (germ cell deficient) mutation.[11] Studies of mice with a mutation at the white-spotting (*W*) and steel (*SL*) loci implicate the involvement of these loci in gametogenesis. Mutations in any of these loci result in equivalent deficiencies in production of either germ cells, melanocytes, or hematopoietic cells.[12] It appears that *W* and *SL* loci encode the c-*kit* receptor and the KL ligand, respectively. The KL ligand is necessary for PGC survival and together with leukemia inhibitory factor stimulates PGC proliferation.[13] Basic fibroblast growth factor (bFGF) together with KL ligand enhances long-term proliferation of PGCs.[13] Studies have demonstrated that the KL ligand and transforming growth factor β_1 (TGF-β_1) are involved in the migration of PGCs toward the genital ridge.

TGF-β_1 is produced in the genital ridge and is implicated as a chemotactic factor that attracts the PGCs there by way of a diffusion gradient.[14] In vitro studies have not suggested a chemotropic effect of KL ligand on primordial germ cell movement.[15] However, the importance of KL ligand is emphasized by the finding that only PGCs moving on course to the gonadal ridge survive, whereas aberrant PGCs not exposed to the KL ligand die.[16]

Studies have suggested a role for KL ligand as an adhesion factor and TGF-β_1 as a chemoattractant.[17] In mice bearing milder mutations in the *W* and *SL* loci, PGCs are colonized in

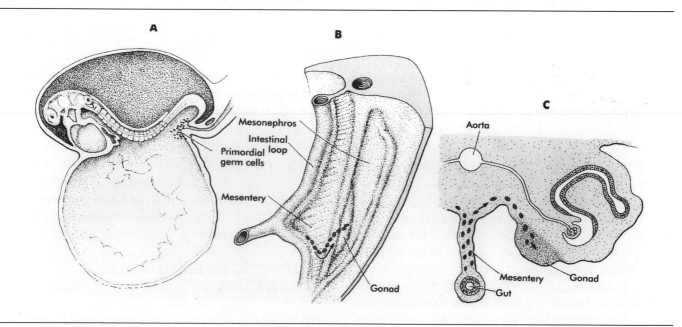

Figure 5–1. Origin and migration of primordial germ cells in the human embryo. **A.** Location in the 16-somite human embryo. **B.** Pathway of migration through the dorsal mesentery. **C.** Cross section showing the pathway of migration through the dorsal mesentery into the gonad. (*From Carlson BM:* Human Embryology and Developmental Biology. *St. Louis, Mosby–Year Book, 1994.*)

the ovary and become primordial follicles but do not grow. Strong evidence suggests that the KL ligand, c-*kit* receptor, and other factors are essential for later stages of oogenesis.[18–20] Once PGCs settle in the genital ridge they increase in number by means of mitotic multiplication of several rounds in mice or for several months in humans. PGCs are defined as oogonia once they settle in the cortex of the genital ridge and are organized in the sex cords.

Oogonia increase in number by increasing mitosis. This is associated with atresia at both primordial germ cells and oogonia. Some of the oogonia degenerate after leaving the ovary, which is crowded with primordial germ cells and oogonia.[21] Oogonia also degenerate in cases of incomplete chromosome pairing[22] and when they are not surrounded by a somatic cell layer.[23] However, the bulk of oogonia death occurs among cells entering first meiotic division at the pachytene stage and is associated with synaptic errors, which suggests some mechanism of selection.[24] The dying oogonia are removed by phagocytes. In this respect it is interesting that PGCs do migrate to the gen-

ital ridge, normally in females with chromosomal abnormalities such as trisomy 21, trisomy 18, or 45XO. However, ovarian development is distorted and in the case of 45XO, oogonia undergo mitosis but fail to enter meiosis, leading to an oocyte-deficient ovary and ovarian failure.[25]

Beginning at about 5 weeks' gestation in humans, some of the oogonia begin replication by means of mitosis. Each of these oogonia is diploid (2n) and contains 46 chromosomes. By 5 to 6 months' gestation this process results in 6 to 7 million oogonia (Fig 5–2). During mitosis, two daughter cells genetically identical to the parent cell are produced. The oogonia undergoing mitosis pass through the four stages of cell life: G_1 (Gap$_1$, the stage in which a cell carries out its primary function), S (synthesis of DNA), G_2 (Gap$_2$), and M (mitosis, including prophase, metaphase, anaphase, and telophase). As a result of DNA synthesis and chromosome replication, each oogonium still has 46 chromosomes but has produced twice the amount of chromatin or DNA in anticipation of dividing into two genetically identical daughter cells during mitosis. Beginning at 11 to

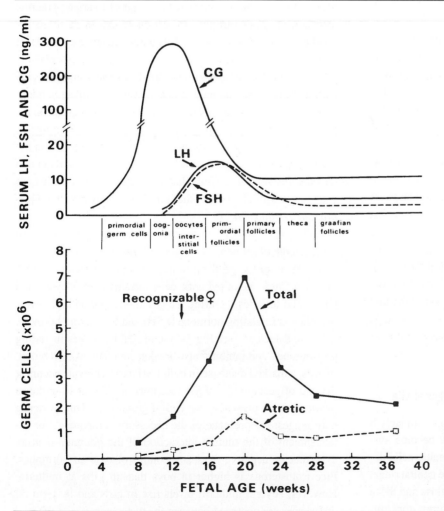

Figure 5–2. Gamete number and follicle maturation and gonadotropin levels at various fetal ages. Gonadotropin values approximate the menopausal range at approximately 16 weeks. CG, chorionic gonadotropin; LH, luteinizing hormone; FSH, follicle-stimulating hormone. (*From Winter JSD, Faiman C, Reyes FL: The gonadotropins of the fetus and neonate: Their pregnancy, function, and regulation. In: Flamigni C, Givens JR (eds), The Gonadotropins: Basic Science and Clinical Aspects in Females. New York, Academic Press, 1982:160.*)

12 weeks' gestation, however, some of the oogonia with twice the amount of chromatin stop entering mitosis and instead enter prophase of the first meiotic division. These oogonia are now called *primary oocytes* and progress through the stages of meiotic prophase (see Fig 5–2).

Meiosis is a form of cell division that occurs only in gametes. It is believed that messages originating from the medullary mesonephros region (rete ovary) are responsible for oocytes' entering the *prophase* of meiosis. Removing the mesonephros tubules may harm ovarian differentiation and formation of the oocyte.[26] The embryonic mesonephros system is assumed to secrete a soluble agent that is a meiosis-inducing substance[26,27] that acts in synergism with forskolin.[28] Several sterols isolated from human follicular fluid have been considered as possible key substances that induce meiosis.[29] In males, anti-müllerian hormone (AMH) together with testosterone causes regression of the müllerian ducts and stabilizes the wolffian structures. Thus, AMH determines the development of the male genital system. It is not produced at this stage of female life. However, AMH is produced by cumulus cells of growing and large graafian follicles and has been found to inhibit resumption of meiosis in fully grown oocytes.[30,31]

During the *leptotene* stage of meiotic prophase, the 46 chromosomes that contain twice the needed DNA are decondensed and appear as 46 single, slender threads. During the next stage, *zygotene,* the homologous chromosomes align parallel to each other in synapse, forming 23 bivalent pairs. Each of the pairs has twice the needed DNA. Therefore, each bivalent pair represents two times (2n) the haploid number of chromosomes and four times (4c) the needed amount of chromatin or DNA. At this point each chromosome splits longitudinally except at points of junction, called *centromeres.* The four chromatids are now called *tetrads.* It is during the ensuing *pachytene* stage that the chromatids break and recombine, resulting in the exchange of genetic material. In the next stage of prophase, *diplotene,* the pairs of chromatids demonstrate mutual repulsion from each other except at the chaismata, where crossing over has occurred. At this point, most of the oocytes have entered the first resting phase, called the *dictyate* or *dictyotene stage.* This stage is exceedingly long and lasts from the time of birth until after puberty, before ovulation occurs.

Follicular Development During Gestation and Pubertal Life

During fetal life the follicle also develops. At approximately 8 weeks' gestation some of the primary oocytes become surrounded by a single layer of spindle-shaped somatic cells derived from mesonephric tissue that migrates to the genital ridge. The cells in this layer are the precursors of granulosa and theca cells. Enclosing the oogonia within these structures stops mitotic activity and results in ultrastructural changes such as re-

duced endoplasmic reticulum and nucleolar complexity.[32] In males these somatic cells are the precursors to the development of tubules and their cellular components including the Sertoli cells.[33] In girls these cells develop cytoplasmic processes that project to the plasma membrane of the oocyte. The oocyte and adjacent granulosa cells become surrounded by a basal lamina, which separates this complex, now called a *primordial follicle,* from the stroma (Fig 5–3).

During the fifth to sixth gestational month some of the spindle-shaped granulosa cells become cuboidal and begin to divide. This unit is called a *primary follicle* and it is the first evidence of recruitment. During this transition the oocyte and surrounding granulosa cells become electrically and metabolically coupled by means of developing between them small gap junctions, which increase in number during this developmental stage and remain throughout the rest of folliculogenesis. In this way the oocyte and its surrounding environment are capable of communicating. Granulosa cell proliferation results in numerous layers of granulosa cells that contribute greatly to an increase in follicle diameter. Although up to four layers of granulosa cell proliferation are believed to be independent of gonadotropin control, and may be the result of ovarian paracrine mechanisms, gonadotropins are definitely necessary to go beyond this point. The oocyte and its early surrounding layers of granulosa cells are called a *secondary follicle.* The cytoplasmic process from the granulosa cells traverses the zona pellucida (ZP) and maintains intimate association with the plasma membrane of the oocyte. At about 7 months' gestation some of the primary follicles form an antrum and thus become known as *tertiary follicles.* The oocyte is located eccentrically within the antrum surrounded by several layers of granulosa cells called the *cumulus oophorus.* Cells that make up the cumulus that are contiguous with the wall of the follicle are known as the *membranum granulosum.*

Only 0.1% to 0.5% of the total follicular population are in some degree of growth. The others are *resting primordial follicles.*[34] Many of the growing follicles manifest varying degrees of atresia (high rate of pyknotic cells and shrunken oocytes) and polyovular follicles.[35] During the gestational period high levels of follicle-stimulating hormone (FSH) and luteinizing hormone (LH) are detected[36] (see Fig 5–2). Gonadal hormones including testosterone[37] and inhibin[38] also are detected in fetal cord blood. In girls, a marked decrease in both FSH and LH levels occurs at the end of gestation.[37,39] FSH receptors are absent in midterm ovaries but are present at the end of gestation.[40] This evidence may suggest the presence of the necessary components for establishment of the mutual interaction of the pituitary–ovarian axis, that is, negative feedback control of ovarian hormones. Free testosterone is higher in boys than in girls at midterm. However, beyond midterm levels rise in girls and by term no differences are observed between the two sexes.[37]

A difference in the dynamic level of pituitary hormones is

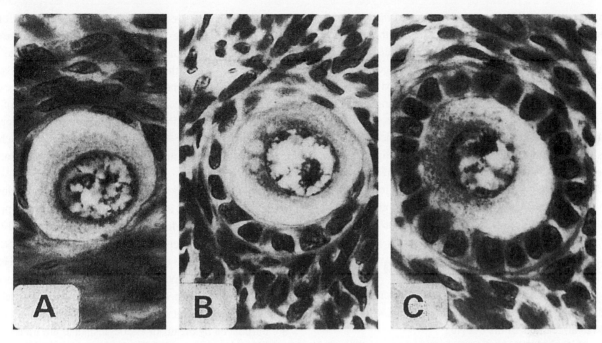

Figure 5–3. Resting follicles in the human ovary, ×570. **A.** Primordial follicle in which the oocyte is surrounded by flattened germ cells. **B.** Intermediary follicle in which the oocyte is surrounded by a mixture of flattened and cuboidal germ cells. **C.** Primary follicle in which the oocyte is surrounded by a single layer of cuboidal germ cells. (*From Góugeon A, Ecochard R, Thalavard JC: Age related changes of the population of human ovarian follicles: Increase in the disappearance of non-growing and early growing follicles in aging women.* Biol Reprod *50:653, 1996.*)

seen when hormonal bioactivity is compared with immunoreactivity levels. For example, at the end of gestation, there is a decrease in immunoreactive FSH levels, which is in contrast to the constant increase in bioactive FSH levels.[37] During the neonatal period primordial follicle formation ends and the ovary is populated with three types of primordial (resting) follicles (see Fig 5–3).[41] It is estimated that at birth the human ovary is populated with 266,000 to 472,000 of these resting follicles.[42,43]

THE GROWING OOCYTE: ULTRASTRUCTURE AND MOLECULAR COMPOSITION

In humans oocyte diameter is about 30 μm in a primordial follicle and increases to 120 μm in a preovulatory follicle, a 64-fold increase in volume. As in gestational life, the commencement of oocyte growth is associated with incipient follicular recruitment and growth. In many respects, the developmental stage of the oocyte correlates with oocyte size. Once the oocyte acquires its full size, it acquires competence to go through full meiotic maturation, from the diplotene stage to metaphase II.

Compared with other cells in the body, the oocyte possesses one of the largest ratios of cytoplasmic volume to plasma membrane area. The metabolic coupling between the oocyte and its surrounding cells overcomes this deficiency by providing a mechanism for nourishment during the period of active oocyte growth. Gap junctions between the oocyte and its surrounding follicular cells provide the cytoplasmic communication between the oocyte and the cumulus cells. Gap junctions have been found in the cumulus cells of various species.[44,45] Uptake of a variety of molecules, including amino acids, is higher among cumulus-enclosed oocytes than among denuded oocytes.[46–49] The deficiency in the energy-dependent A transport system in the oocyte reduces its ability to take up amino acids from its vicinity.[50] One of the most studied metabolic interactions between the oocyte and other follicular cell types is the absence of the glycolytic pathway in the oocyte. Pyruvate is transported to the oocyte via gap junctions and is used as an energy source within the oocyte in the Krebs cycle.[51] This situation continues after fertilization up to the eight-cell stage preembryo, which can use glucose as an energy source.

Mutual regulatory processes exist between the oocyte and the follicular cells. Thus, during follicular growth, the oocyte regulates cumulus cell proliferation[52,53] and the organization and activity of the granulosa cells within the growing follicle.[54] On the other hand, oocyte growth is highly dependent on communication with its surrounding somatic cells. In vitro culture of denuded oocytes results in a lower growth rate than oocytes grown in vivo.[55] In contrast, cultured oocytes enclosed by one or a few layers of follicular cells preserve most of their in vivo growth rate.[56] However, cell types other than granulosa cells such as Sertoli or 3T3 cells coupled to oocytes do not support in vitro oocyte growth,[57] albeit fibroblastic monolayer[58] and 3T3 cells[59] support the acquisition of meiotic competence in denuded mouse oocytes. This finding may suggest that granulosa cell-specific activity is necessary for oocyte growth.

The c-*kit*–KL ligand system has been implicated in the regulation of oocyte growth by granulosa cells. Antibodies directed to c-*kit* indicate the presence of c-*kit* receptors on oocyte surfaces.[60] The KL ligand has been detected in the granulosa cells of growing follicles that possess at least one layer of granulosa cells. However, the KL ligand is not expressed once the oocyte acquires full size.[61] Involvement of the c-*kit*–KL ligand system in inducing oocyte growth has been demonstrated in several ways.[62] This finding may provide an explanation for the failure of oocyte and follicular growth in mice-bearing mild mutations in the *W* and *S* loci.

Altered Morphologic Features in a Growing Oocyte

Oocyte growth in humans results in a 64-fold increase in volume. This remarkable change is associated with structural modifications in all features of the oocyte.

The *nucleus* is the most conspicuous structure within the oocyte. It is designated *germinal vesicle*. In a nongrowing oocyte, the germinal vesicle possesses about 0.12% and 0.17% of the total oocyte volume in mice and humans, respectively. The germinal vesicle increases in volume with oocyte growth but at a much lower rate than the oocyte. The meiotic state of the nucleus is characterized G_0, which is equivalent to G_2 in a somatic cell. The oocyte chromosomes are in diffusable diplolene during oocyte growth but become more condensed when a large antrum is formed.[63] Within the nucleus a prominent nucleolus with some smaller nucleoli may be present. With oocyte growth, the nucleoli grow, become more dense and less fibrillar, and intensively accumulate ribosomal RNA.[64,65]

It is assumed that before initiation of oocyte growth the nucleus is primarily active in maintaining oocyte viability for the possibility of future growth. At this stage, there are few membranous organelles. In primates the various oocyte organelles, including the Golgi apparatus, mitochondria, and lipid droplets have been seen around the nucleus and are usually called the *Balbiani vitelline body* (yolk nucleus). When the oocyte initiates growth, some of these organelles migrate to the oocyte periphery.

In nongrowing oocytes, the *Golgi apparatus* appears as a mounded, bow-like lamella associated with a few other cytoplasmic organelles. With the initiation of oocyte growth, the Golgi apparatus moves from the center of the oocyte toward the periphery. It breaks up into separate units that swell and become vacuolated. The Golgi apparatus becomes noticeable through very active synthesis of glycoproteins such as ZP proteins and because of the contiguity of lipid droplets, granules, and other vesicles.[66,67] As the oocytes approach maturity, Golgi apparatus activity declines.

Mitochondria are elongated, dumbbell-shaped, or oval. Their number increases progressively during oocyte growth; it reaches about 10^5 in the preovulatory oocytes of mice.[68] More oval and round mitochondria are accumulated, and the mitochondria cristae become columnar. In preovulatory oocytes the cristae appear as concentric arches. During the course of oocyte growth the mitochondria are in proximity to the endoplasmic reticulum.[66,67,69] After fertilization, the oocyte mitochondria contribute most if not all of the mitochondrial population to the developing embryo.[70]

Rough *endoplasmic reticulum* (ER) becomes predominant during oocyte growth, and the smooth ER diminishes, probably because it is recycled to other membranous structures. The ER interacts with the Golgi apparatus. In the latter, polysaccharides are processed and also become part of glycoproteins. Heritable virus-like particles have been identified in the ER cisterns in various mammalian species including humans.[71] Oocyte growth depends on a constant supply of nourishment. Some nutrients are introduced by means of endocytosis and are transported by small *cytoplasmic vesicles*. Endocytosis of follicular fluid protein is well documented.[72] Informative material and secreted proteins are transported within these cytoplasmic vesicles by both endo- and exocytosis. Endocytosis was seen in both unfertilized and fertilized human oocytes.[73] In mature human oocytes that failed to become fertilized in vitro, aberrant endocytosis of perivitelline fluid has been observed.[74]

In addition to these membranous organelles, in rodents the ooplasm is filled with other typical particles such as the *fibrous lattice*.[75] The fibrous lattice appears initially in the growing oocyte and constantly increases in amount with oocyte development to about 10% of the volume of the oocyte before gradually disappearing in the developing preembryo. It has been suggested that the fibrous lattice stores a form of mammalian yolk. In humans and nonhuman primates, fibrous lattices are not detected. However, human oocytes fertilized in vitro are capable of developing into preembryos within basal culture medium. Therefore, storage of noninformative material for this in vitro development is assumed. It is possible that some kind of stored material may be found in various other structures, such as the ER.

Ribosome number is increased with oogenesis; in mature mouse eggs, the number of ribosomes increases severalfold.[76] The increase in the ribosome number, which are organized in polysomes, is probably necessary for increased protein synthesis within the growing oocyte. It was assumed that ribosomal RNA is stored in the fibrous lattice,[77–79] although more evidence to support this hypothesis is needed. Despite increased ribosome number, ribosome density decreases with the increase in oocyte volume.

The oocyte plasma membrane, or *oolemma*, undergoes considerable change during oocyte growth. The oolemma appears as a smooth plasma membrane in the small oocyte and with oocyte growth becomes more folded and populated with microvilli that extend into the ZP and sometimes are attached to the corona radiata cells. The oolemma is less active in absorbing molecules beyond its borders. Most absorbed molecules are transferred from the cumulus cells through cell processes that contact the oolemma surface or via pits within the oolemma via gap junctions. The oolemma becomes very active and important when it interacts with the penetrating sperm. Various proteins have been suggested to be involved in this process, such as viral fusion proteins[80] and integrin.[81]

The *cortical granules* appear as refractile, small, spherical bodies of 300 to 500 nm in diameter and are associated with the Golgi apparatus. They are produced at the time the oocyte begins growth.[82] In humans, there are two types of cortical granules that differ in diameter, that is, 350 and 450 nm.[73] It was assumed that cortical granules were derived from the Golgi apparatus and resembled some type of lysosomes. In the mature oocyte, the cortical granules are close to the plasma membrane. Cortical granule content is not identical throughout this population. This heterogeneity may reflect different stages of germ-cell maturation.[3] Cortical granule content has been extensively studied in rodents,[83] and antibodies have been raised to their principal proteins.[84] Nevertheless, the role of cortical granules in the human oocyte is poorly understood. It is known that at fertilization, their expelled content modifies the ZP, preventing polyspermic penetration. Other structures have been identified in most mammalian oocytes, including glycogen granules and lipid droplets. Their content is probably used as an energy source in the fertilized egg for new metabolic activities.

The *zona pellucida* is an extraoocyte matrix composed of proteins synthesized and secreted by the oocyte.[85] It appears initially as patches of fibrillar material that ultimately connect and surround the entire oocyte outside the oolemma. The ZP progressively thickens as the oocyte increases in size. Cytoplasmic processes from the cumulus and granulosa cells traverse the ZP, producing interaction between the oocyte and the somatic cells of the follicle via gap junctions. In fully grown human oocytes, ZP width is approximately 15 μm. Three ZP proteins have been identified in mice; they are designated ZP1, ZP2, and ZP3.[86] These fibrillar glycoproteins possess *N*-linked oligosaccharides. ZP2 and ZP3 also have sides for O-linked glycosylation. ZP proteins have been identified in many other species including pig,[87] cow,[88] and rabbit.[89] In humans, the ZP is composed of three types of glycoproteins.[90,91] The genes that encode the ZP proteins have been characterized in humans and share similarities with mouse genes.[91,92] In ovulated oocytes additional glycoproteins have been isolated from the ZP. These glycoproteins have been designated *oviductins* and have been identified in various species. They are probably absorbed into the ZP from the oviductal lumen.[93–95] Some of these proteins also may be detected in preembryos.[95] In mice ZP2 and ZP3 are present in equimolar amounts, and the amount of ZP1 is much lower than that of the other two proteins.

ZP2 and ZP3 are involved in the fertilization process. The sperm head initially attaches to the ZP3 O-linked oligosaccharide, and the enzyme β-1,4-galactosyltransferase located in the sperm head is bound to the ZP3 *N*-linked oligosaccharide.[96] Next the acrosome-reacted sperm binds to ZP2, which enhances sperm penetration through the ZP. After sperm penetration, a process designated the *zona reaction* takes place and causes the ZP to become insoluble (zonal hardening) and blocks further sperm penetration. In humans, the presence of antibodies against ZP proteins interferes with fertilization.[97] It has been demonstrated that patients with unexplained infertility who undergo IVF may possess anti-zona antibodies in the follicular fluid of some of their follicles. In one study all the corresponding oocytes within the anti-zona antibodies that contained follicles failed to undergo IVF.[98]

Biosynthesis and Storage of RNA and Protein

A mature mouse oocyte contains about 0.3–0.55 ng of RNA in toto. RNA is synthesized and accumulated mainly during early and mid-oocyte growth. Most of the RNA is ribosomal (65%), 5S RNA and transfer RNA (tRNA) (20%). The rest is heterogenous RNA (15%). In fully grown oocytes, RNA is barely synthesized, although even when an oocyte resumes meiosis, RNA is still synthesized.[49,99] Polyadenylated (poly [A]) RNA is the source of gene information. About 70% of it is degraded or loses its poly [A] tail in the mature ovulated oocyte before fertilization.[100] Further degradation of stored RNA occurs in the two-cell embryo. Thus, the embryonic genome does not initiate an active role in RNA transcription until the second cleavage stage and beyond.[101]

After fertilization, poly[A]RNA is steadily increased because of selective polyadenylation of the stored messenger RNA (mRNA).[102] Thus, part of the mRNA is degraded while some is selectively recruited and translated. This kind of regulation occurs in various proteins such as the actin, which is one of the most synthesized proteins in the growing oocyte. Actin transcripts decrease to about 50% in ovulated oocytes and to about 10% in two-cell embryos but return to very high levels in eight-cell embryos.[103] ZP3, however, manifests a pattern similar to that of actin, but its mRNA does not reappear at the eight-cell or later embryonic stage.[104] Many other investigated proteins mimic either pattern, which suggests that most of the stored mRNA of an oocyte is for the oocyte and probably not for the embryo. Nevertheless, during the first 24 hours after fertilization, the mammalian embryo is entirely dependent on the translation of stored mRNA within the oocyte.

The types of transcripts in growing oocytes and mature oocytes are altered constantly, indicating a regulatory mechanism. The aforementioned examples manifest proteins that are synthesized in high quantity in the oocyte and thus are likely to have an important function in the growing oocyte. However, possible regulation of other mRNA molecules that encode other proteins that are at low levels but have a critical role in oocyte and possibly early preembryo life has not been studied.

Some oocyte proteins are introduced by means of endocytosis from the follicular fluid.[72] However, most oocyte proteins are biosynthesized within the oocyte. Some of these proteins are necessary for oocyte growth and differentiation, whereas others are prepared and stored for the future developing embryo. Some oocyte peptides and proteins are involved in interaction between the oocyte and its surrounding somatic cells. It appears that with oocyte growth, there is little change in the type of proteins synthesized, but a great deal of change occurs in the quantitative pattern of the synthesized proteins.[105,106] The rate of protein synthesis decreases considerably with oocyte growth and is lowest in fully grown oocytes.[107] In general, the rate of protein synthesis decreases at dissolution of the nuclear membrane and mixing of nucleoplasm and cytoplasm.[3]

CONTROL OF MEIOTIC MATURATION

In most mammals, resumption of meiosis occurs before ovulation. At the onset of the LH surge the egg is still a primary oocyte. The chromosomes in the germinal vesicle become short and thick. This is called the *diakinesis* stage of meiosis, and the first meiotic prophase becomes complete. The nuclear membrane breaks down and the tetrads align themselves on the equator of the metaphase I plate. The homologous chromosomes are separated into two equal sets of chromosomes. Each set contains twice the necessary chromatin. One of the chromosome sets pinches off in a small cell called the *polar body*. The polar body is located in the perivitelline space and contains one chromosome set (1n) and a double amount of chromatin (2c). The oocyte is now haploid (1n) but contains twice the necessary chromatin (2c). The chromosomes in the oocyte are aligned in metaphase; this stage is called *metaphase II,* and the egg is called a *secondary oocyte*. This is the stage at the time of ovulation (Fig 5–4). Deviation from this scheme is uniquely found in dogs, in which immature oocytes are ovulated.[108]

Metaphase II is the second resting phase of meiosis. The oocyte remains in this stage unless fertilization occurs. Should fertilization occur, the remaining chromosome that contains twice the chromatin (2c) splits longitudinally, and half the chromatin pinches off to the second polar body. The oocyte is now haploid and contains the proper amount of female chromatin (1n, 1c), and a similar amount of the male chromatin of the penetrated sperm. Therefore, the process of meiosis, which begins in the early fetus, becomes complete in adults only when fertilization occurs. The changes that occur in the female gamete and ovary are summarized in Table 5–1.[109]

Regulation of meiotic division in the female gamete in terms of acquisition of meiotic competence and regulation of meiotic resumption are subject to hormonal and paracrine regulation. During the last decade, the regulation of these processes was highlighted by much research. These new findings become highly relevant for the understanding of human oocyte meiosis.

Meiotic Competence

It has been known for some time that oocytes isolated from fully mature follicles possess the capability of resuming meiosis spontaneously in culture.[1] However, failure of the oocyte to resume meiosis spontaneously was described in the mouse in 1972.[110] This phenomenon has been confirmed in many mammalian species, including nonhuman primates[111,112] and humans.[113] It appears that meiotic competence is acquired concomitantly with the increase in oocyte size,[114,115] formation of the antral cavity,[115,116] and sometimes with the increase in follicular size.[111,117,118]

Meiotic competence is acquired in a stepwise manner. Initially the oocyte acquires the ability to resume meiosis up to metaphase I. With further progression in growth the oocyte becomes competent to complete meiosis up to metaphase II in rodents,[114,115] domestic animals,[119] and nonhuman primates.[111] Further oocyte development is necessary for the oocyte to become competent to undergo fertilization and cleavage divisions.[120,121]

Normal development of meiotic competence is reduced in rats hypophysectomized on day 15 postpartum.[115] Administration of pregnant mare serum gonadotropin (PMSG), FSH, or estradiol 17β but not LH, progesterone or androstenedione to rats hypophysectomized on day 15 postpartum restored development of meiotic competence to rat oocytes.[115,122] These studies suggest an in vivo priming action of gonadotropins on meiotic competence. Other studies have shown that in vitro cultures without hormonal supplement support meiotic competence acquisition in mouse oocytes either when inoculated as primary follicles[56] or when enclosed with granulosa cells and cocultured with fibroblastic cell monolayer.[58] Furthermore, meiotic competence was developing in hypogonadal (*hpg*) mouse strain.[123] These findings were contradictory to the possibility that in vitro meiotic competence development is associated with previous in vivo exposure of the primary oocyte to gonadotropins.[124]

These contradictory results have been resolved. Growth and acquisition of meiotic competence in follicle-enclosed oocytes are increased by cyclic adenosine monophosphate (cAMP) in mice.[125] In addition, meiotic competence is en-

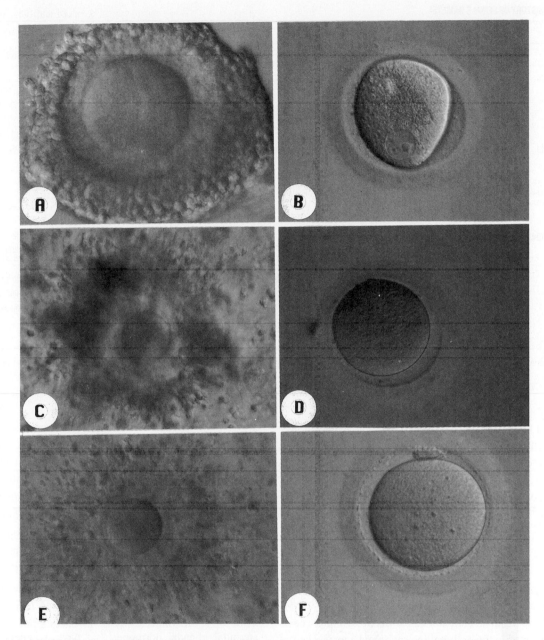

Figure 5–4. Light photomicrograph of human cumulus oocyte complexes of various stages of maturation. The altered morphology of the cumulus mass and oocyte meiosis are depicted on the left and right side, respectively, of immature (**A,B**), intermediate (**C,D**), and mature (**E,F**) complexes.

hanced in mouse oocytes with an increase in cAMP level within the oocytes in culture.[59] Similarly, incompetent rat oocytes cultured within ovarian fragments become competent when cultured for 3 or 6 days in the presence of FSH or isobutylmethylxanthine (IBMX), a substance that increases levels of cAMP.[126] Because cAMP is the second messenger of FSH, the effect of FSH on meiotic competence may be mediated by cAMP elevation. These new findings may explain the involvement of FSH in the acquisition of meiotic competence in rodent oocytes. Nevertheless, the beneficial effect of FSH on the acquisition of meiotic competence has been demonstrated in various mammals and nonhuman primates.[112,127–129]

Administration of PMSG or estradiol 17β to rats hypophysectomized on day 15 postpartum does not induce development of meiotic competence before the normal age (day 20 postpartum) for development of meiotic competence.[130] Similarly, acquisition of meiotic competence of mouse oocytes in vitro closely corresponds to the time required for this developmental state in vivo.[58] The effect of gonadotropins on the development of meiotic competence before the normal age of development has been repeated in intact and hypophysectomized rats. Surprisingly, FSH induced meiotic competence before day 20 postpartum in intact rats. This finding suggests that FSH synergizes with another hypophyseal or hypophysis-dependent hormone.

TABLE 5–1. LIFE HISTORY OF FEMALE GAMETE[a]

| | Formation of Ovum | | | |
Status	Chromatin State	Events	Ovarian Morphology	Known Regulators
Primordial germ cell to oogonium	CN-46; DNA-4C	Multiplication by means of mitosis and migration to the genital ridge	Invasion of cells from mesonephric rudiment and surface epithelium and formation of sex cords	c-*kit*–KL ligand system; TGFβ, bFGF and other growth factors
Oogonium to oocyte	CN-46; DNA-4C	Final DNA synthesis and meiotic prophase initiation: leptotene to diplotene state	Formation of primordial follicle	MIS/MPS
Primary oocyte (growing)	CN-46; DNA-4C	Oocyte growth, meiotic competence	Follicular recruitment and growth up to formation of graafian follicle	c-*kit*–KL ligand system; FSH, estradiol 17β, GH
Primary oocyte (large)	CN-46; DNA-4C	Resumption of meiosis and progression until abstriction of first polar body	Cumulus expansion and change in the steroidogenic pathway	Midcycle surge initiation of FSH and LH
Secondary oocyte	CN-23; DNA-2C	Continuation of meiosis and arrest at metaphase II	Follicular rupture and ovulation	Midcycle surge completion of FSH and LH
Ovum	CN-23; DNA-1C	Sperm penetration and completion of meiosis	Formation of corpus luteum	LH, progesterone
Zygote	CN-46; DNA-2C			

[a] Concomitant changes in the ovarian morphology and the main known regulators. DNA-4C, amount of DNA at G_2 phase; CN, chromosome number; MIS, meiosis-inducing substance; MPS, maturation-promoting factor.

Modified from Biggers JD: Oogenesis. In: Gold JL (ed), Gynecologic Endocrinology. Hagerstown, Md, Harper & Row, 1975:612–620.

It appears that unlike that of FSH, administration of human or rat growth hormone (GH) to hypophysectomized rats induces a marked increase in meiotic competence, and this effect is augmented by FSH (Fig 5–5).

The involvement of GH and possibly other hormones in the development of meiotic competence speaks to the complexity of this developmental process. Removal of one hormone such as FSH in a hypogonadal mouse strain is insufficient to exclude the possible hormonal regulation of meiotic competence. Interestingly, in snell dwarf (*dw*) mice, which have undetectable levels of GH, prolactin, and thyroid-stimulating hormone (TSH), oocytes attain full capability for maturation and full developmental capability after fertilization.[123] However, development of meiotic competence could be exerted by the in vivo presence of FSH. In other words, only the hypophysectomy model[115,122] is appropriate for study of the role of hypophyseal hormones because of more than one hypophyseal hormone and other nonsteroidal gonadal hormones[124,131] have a beneficial effect on meiotic competence.

In one study of human IVF, 8.6% of women treated with gonadotropin yielded one or more oocytes that failed to resume meiosis after stimulation with human chorionic gonadotropin (hCG) and the subsequent 20 hours in culture. When the percentage of incompetent oocytes was equal to or greater than 25%, most of the IVF outcomes for the other oocytes were markedly reduced.[113] These same women manifested lower than expected increases in estradiol 17β levels after hCG administration.[113] Overall, this study suggested a correlation among failure of meiotic competence, the developmental features of other follicles in terms of secretion of estradiol 17β, fertilization, and embryonal competence of the corresponding oocytes.[113]

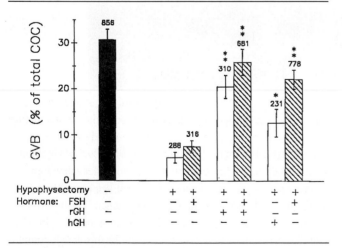

Figure 5–5. Development of meiotic competence in hypophysectomized rats treated with rat growth hormone (rGH) or human growth hormone (hGH). Some of the rats were treated with human FSH (hFSH, 2 IU/day) on days 15–19 postpartum and others were treated with 10 μg daily of either rGH or hGH on days 17–19 postpartum. A third group of rats were coadministered hFSH and either rGH or hGH in the same time period.* p<.05; ** p<.001 vs. hypophysectomized untreated rats. (*Zlotkin et al, unpublished data*).

The cause of failure of meiotic competence has been studied in terms of ultrastructural and molecular deficiencies. It is difficult to identify substantial changes in the ultrastructures of competent compared with incompetent oocytes.[67] Nuclear modification of the nucleus has been found in oocytes that became competent to resume meiosis. At the time of antrum formation, a continuous perinucleolar chromatin sheath is formed.[132] Ultrastructural changes in the nuclear material occur in competent oocytes that are not seen in incompetent oocytes. In monkeys, most of the large antral-enclosed oocytes (competent oocytes) develop perinucleolar encapsulation. This ultrastructural change is not found in most oocytes collected from small follicles that enclose incompetent oocytes.[133] In rodents, the transition of the germinal vesicles from an unrimmed to a rimmed state is coincident with acquisition and expression of meiotic competence.[134]

In the very early stages of the study of oocyte maturation in amphibian oocytes, it is known that injection of aliquots of cytoplasm of mature oocytes into immature oocytes causes germinal vesicle breakdown and resumption of meiosis.[135,136] The cytoplasmic factor involved is called *maturation-promoting factor* (MPF). MPF has been identified as a protein kinase that comprises two protein components—cyclin B and $p34^{cdc2}$. The level of $p34^{cdc2}$ is almost stable, but the level of cyclin is altered in relation to the stage of cell cycle. In the G_1 stage, cyclin level increases and toward the end of this stage, cyclin and $p34^{cdc2}$ are bound together to form MPF. Toward the end of the G_2 stage, MPF is activated by phosphorylation and dephosphorylation of amino acids in cyclin B and $p34^{cdc2}$, respectively. Active MPF induces the breakdown of the nuclear membrane. At the end of the division stage, cyclin level is reduced, and $p34^{cdc2}$ is dephosphorylated. The last event leads the cell to G_1 of the next cycle.

A first attempt to reveal the molecular mechanism that underlies failure of meiotic competence may be related to the finding that fusion of an incompetent immature mouse oocyte with a mature oocyte causes resumption of meiosis in the incompetent oocyte. These findings suggest the transfer of a cytoplasmic stimulator from the maturing to the incompetent oocyte.[137] Further elaboration of meiotic incompetence in growing oocytes in terms of MPF activity was carried out in porcine and rat oocytes. In both rat and porcine incompetent oocytes, the level of $p34^{cdc2}$ was not significantly different from the level in competent oocytes.[138,139] Furthermore, the level of cyclin B and the MPF substrate microtubule-associated protein kinase in swine and rats, respectively, were not different between incompetent and competent oocytes.[138,139] In one study, the level of both $p34^{cdc2}$ and cyclin B appeared not to be the limiting factor in the incompetent oocytes.[140]

Studies have revealed that okadaic acid, which inhibits phosphatases 1 and 2A, can induce resumption of meiosis in

several species even under various inhibitory conditions[141–143] by reducing the phosphorylation state of $p34^{cdc2}$. Addition of okadaic acid to incompetent porcine oocytes also induces meiotic competence, suggesting that meiotic incompetence is a result of an inactive MPF.[138] Normally MPF that induces germinal vesicle breakdown is associated with activation of histone H1-kinase. When okadaic acid induces germinal vesicle breakdown, histone H1-kinase is not activated, indicating that induction of meiosis resumption by okadaic acid is not mediated by MPF activation.[144] However, okadaic acid–induced germinal vesicle breakdown is preceded by induction of microtubule-associated protein kinase (MAPK) p42 ($p42^{MAPK}$), suggesting that induction of germinal vesicle breakdown by okadaic acid bypasses MPF activation and exerts its action directly on $p42^{MAPK}$.[144] Induction of meiosis by okadaic acid in mouse incompetent oocytes has been associated with a statistically significant increase in MAPK 1 and 2 before germinal vesicle breakdown, suggesting that these kinases may promote meiotic competence.[145] Actually, MAPK is detected at very early stages of oocyte growth and throughout growth and acquisition of meiotic competence in mammals. It appears that acquisition of meiotic competence involves phosphorylation of MAPK species. Exposure to okadaic acid also induces phosphorylation of MAPK species. However, in oocytes that do not respond to okadaic acid treatment, okadaic acid does not induce phosphorylation of MAPK species.[146] In rodents, specific changes in the microtubule organizing center occur at acquisition of meiotic competence. Thus, the microtubule organizing center becomes more prominent and localizes in the nuclear periphery.[132] Furthermore, competent oocytes contain phosphorylated centrosomes that nucleate short microtubule arrays, whereas incompetent oocytes contain nonphosphorylated centrosomes and interphase microtubule (long) arrays.[147]

Regulation of Meiotic Resumption

The midcycle gonadotropin surge initiates many processes within the follicle that eventually result in ovulation of a mature cumulus oocyte complex (COC). The ovulated COC has an expanded cumulus mass, and the oocyte is arrested at metaphase II. A similar process can be induced in vitro in follicle-enclosed oocytes exposed to the proper hormonal stimulus. In contrast, cumulus-enclosed or denuded oocytes resume meiosis spontaneously in vitro without hormonal stimulation. It was therefore hypothesized that the oocyte is maintained in the diplotene stage within the follicle by means of inhibitory mechanisms.[148] Follicular fluid inhibits spontaneous meiotic maturation in rabbit isolated COCs in culture.[149] Studies have revealed that inhibition of oocyte maturation is exerted by granulosa cells[150–152] but not by theca cells or ovarian bursa.[150,153,154] High cell density of cumulus cells also inhibits spontaneous meiotic resumption in isolated oocytes.[155] It was assumed that the inhibitory activity was exerted by a factor designated *oocyte maturation inhibitor* (OMI).

The inhibitory action of granulosa cells was similarly observed with use of both granulosa cell extracts[152] and conditioned medium from granulosa cell culture.[156] The latter suggested that granulosa cell inhibitory activity is water soluble and accumulates in the granulosa cell vicinity with time. However, other studies could not demonstrate that granulosa inhibitory activity is soluble in ever-tested mammalian species.[153,154,157] Actually, many studies have shown meiotic resumption to be inhibited in COC–granulosa cell coculture or in COC cultured with portions of follicular wall.[150–154,157,158] Thus, the OMI of granulosa cells is better exerted when contact between COC and granulosa cells is maintained.

Addition of porcine follicular fluid inhibits meiotic resumption in cumulus-enclosed but not denuded oocytes.[159] Furthermore, addition of LH overcomes the inhibitory activity observed in vitro either with follicular fluid or with coculture with granulosa cells.[151,159] The level of OMI activity decreases with follicular growth.[160] A decrease in OMI activity in human follicular fluid is associated with an increase in oocyte fertilizability, a property that demonstrates advanced oocyte development.[161] Collectively these findings indicate that OMI manifests a physiologic role that mimics the in vivo situation.

The chemical nature of OMI is far from being resolved. Various peptides have been suggested to exert OMI action, such as AMH,[162] inhibin,[163] fragments of follistatin,[164] and insulin-like growth factor (IGF) binding protein-3.[165] Other studies have demonstrated a high level of hypoxanthine in follicular fluid. Because hypoxanthine exerts OMI activity in vitro, it was considered an OMI candidate.[166,167] However, although charcoal extraction removes most purines from follicular fluid, follicular fluid still preserves OMI activity.[167] Further investigation revealed that hypoxanthine was not present in bovine follicular fluid, although bovine follicular fluid inhibited spontaneous maturation of bovine oocytes.[168]

In parallel to extensive studies performed on the chemical nature of OMI, it has been demonstrated in mice that increasing ooplasmic cAMP concentrations lead to the inhibition of in vitro resumption of meiosis.[169] This finding has been consistently correct in the oocytes of all mammalian species tested, including rats,[170] domestic animals,[171,172] nonhuman primates,[173] and humans.[174] A drop in cytoplasmic cAMP levels appears necessary for resumption of meiosis.[175,176] The fact that inhibitors of phosphodiesterase, such as IBMX, inhibit the spontaneous resumption of meiosis of isolated oocytes forms the basis for the hypothesis that cAMP is generated by the follicular somatic compartments such as cumulus cells and granulosa cells and is transferred into the oocyte.[170] Actually, hypoxanthine, the presumed OMI, also inhibits phosphodiesterase and thus indirectly

causes accumulation of cAMP within the cumulus mass, which is probably transferred into the oocytes, increasing ooplasmic levels of cAMP.[177,178] It is suggested that cAMP is transferred from the somatic portion of the follicle into the oocyte via the cytoplasmic projections that traverse the ZP and interact with the oolemma via the gap junctions.[179,180]

Meiosis normally occurs after the midcycle surge of gonadotropins. It is widely accepted that most gonadotropin effects are cAMP dependent. This concept holds true for the mechanism that underlies the induction of resumption of meiosis; many agents that induce resumption of meiosis in vitro in follicle-enclosed oocytes also increase cAMP levels within the follicle.[181,182] Direct action of cAMP on resumption of meiosis also was found in vitro in follicle-enclosed oocytes. Thus, resumption of meiosis in follicle-enclosed oocytes can be induced either by injection of a membrane-permeable cAMP derivative[183] or by short exposure to such a cAMP derivative.[184,185]

The dual action of cAMP as both inhibitor and stimulator of resumption of oocyte meiosis was difficult to explain. It appears that induction of resumption of meiosis occurs when cAMP levels are four times higher than the cAMP levels necessary to inhibit meiosis.[186] Thus, the type of cAMP action is concentration dependent. The higher cAMP level necessary to induce meiotic maturation causes biochemical and morphologic changes within the somatic follicular portion. Among these changes reduction in gap junction communication between the oocyte and surrounding cumulus cells appears to be extremely important for control of meiotic maturation of the oocyte. It is conceivable that reduction in this type of communication would generate parallel reduction in cAMP transfer and ultimately oocyte escape from cAMP inhibition.[185] It appears that in some species resumption of meiosis is not preceded by a decrease in oocyte–cumulus cell communication. However, in such species a decrease in communication between the COC and membrane granulosa has been found.[187,188] These findings provide a mechanism for the dissociation of the oocyte as a prerequisite for its release from the inhibitory action of cAMP.

The mutual interaction between the oocyte and its surrounding follicular cells involves other processes before ovulation. The level of cytochrome P-450 side chain cleavage (P-450$_{scc}$) enzyme increases in the surrounding cumulus cells,[189] and cumulus expansion and mucification are induced[190] only when the germinal vesicle of the oocyte is dissolved. Similarly, in vivo hCG treatment is less capable of inducing full cumulus expansion in meiotically incompetent compared with meiotically competent oocytes in humans.[113]

A decrease in ooplasmic cAMP level is followed by commitment of the oocyte to resume meiosis, which usually continues until metaphase II. This type of meiotic dynamic takes place in vitro either in isolated or follicle-enclosed oocytes. However, in many species completion of meiotic maturation (attaining metaphase II) by isolated oocytes is not associated with normal fertilizability and developmental capability in swine,[191] sheep,[192] or rabbits.[193] In contrast, in vitro hormonal stimulation of resumption of meiosis in COC–granulosa cell coculture or in isolated follicles increases oocyte fertilizability and developmental capability in various mammals, such as sheep,[192] cattle,[193a,194] and swine.[191] These observations indicate that normal meiotic maturation is largely associated with proper paracrine regulation by the somatic portion of the follicle. Similar observations have been obtained in studies with nonhuman primate and human oocytes. A lower percentage of germinal vesicle versus metaphase II oocytes (24% vs 73%) mature to metaphase II in culture, and germinal vesicle oocytes that attain metaphase II stage achieve lower IVF rates (0 vs 32%) than metaphase I oocytes that achieve metaphase II. In contrast, 93% of metaphase II oocytes fertilize when collected at that stage of maturity.[195] In humans, oocyte meiotic maturation is completed to metaphase II stage 34 to 36 hours after the start of the LH surge (Fig 5–6).[196] However, higher fertilization rates were found among human oocytes collected 39 as opposed to 34 hours after a preovulatory injection of hCG.[197]

The beneficial effect of the follicular environment on meiotic maturation of an oocyte probably is associated with the local hormonal stimulation of meiotic maturation. In a study with rabbits, inhibition of cholesterol P-450$_{scc}$ enzyme, which inhibits the entire steroidogenic system, did not affect the oocyte meiotic maturation but did reduce oocyte fertilizability.[198] In monkeys, total blockage of steroid biosynthesis by means of inhibition of 3β-hydroxysteroid dehydrogenase had no adverse effect on in vivo meiotic maturation but dramatically hindered oocyte fertilizability.[199] However, inhibition of aromatase during late follicular development reduced the percentage of oocytes that attained metaphase II.[200] A correlation between the degree of 3β-hydroxysteroid dehydrogenase activity, including progesterone secretion, and oocyte fertilizability was found in human oocytes.[201] Estrogen receptor RNA has been detected in human oocytes.[202] The role of estrogen in meiotic maturation of oocytes was further elucidated in the finding that estradiol 17β exerts an effect on the cell surface. It appears that estradiol 17β induces an extracellular Ca^{2+} influx in the maturing human oocyte.[203]

Addition of estradiol 17β does not affect oocyte meiotic maturation but does increase their fertilizability. The evolving pattern of estradiol 17β in the periovulatory period is demonstrated in Fig 5–7.[204] The increased levels of estradiol 17β during metaphase I may suggest a beneficial action. In clomiphene citrate–managed cycles the time necessary for oocytes to reach metaphase I was longer than that occurring in natural cycles. The time necessary for metaphase I oocytes to reach metaphase II was longer in natural cycles.[205] Because clomiphene citrate acts as an antiestrogen, the finding may indicate that the increasing level of estradiol that surrounds metaphase I oocytes is important for the continuation of meiotic maturation within the follicle. In stimulated cycles for IVF embryo transfer (IVF-ET), the level of follicular fluid estradiol 17β is markedly higher in follicles that contain mature cumuli oophori[206] or in women who become pregnant.[207] Nevertheless, completion of meiotic maturation to metaphase II[208] and increased cleavability[209] can occur in follicles that contain very low estradiol or progesterone concentrations.

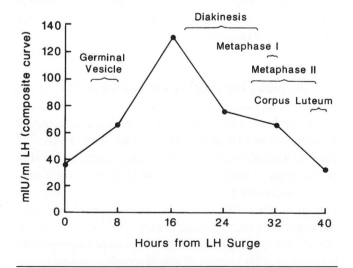

Figure 5–6. Oocyte maturation at various times after the LH surge. (*From Seibel MM, Smith D, Dlugi AM, Levesque L: Periovulatory follicular fluid hormone levels in spontaneous human cycles.* J Clin Endocrinol Metab *68:1073, 1989.*)

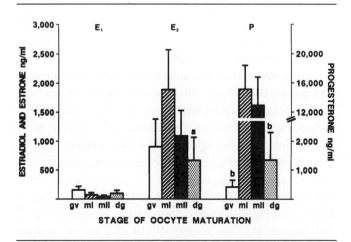

Figure 5–7. Follicle fluid levels of estrone (E$_1$) estradiol 17β (E$_2$), and progesterone (P) at various stages of oocyte maturation in unstimulated cycles. (*From Seibel MM, Smith D, Dlugi AM, Levesque L: Periovulatory follicular fluid hormone levels in spontaneous human cycles.* J Clin Endocrinol Metab *68:1073, 1989.*)

The relation between follicular fluid levels of FSH, LH, and prolactin and oocyte maturity does not present a clear picture. Some studies fail to reveal any correlation between oocyte maturity and gonadotropin levels,[210–212] whereas other studies have demonstrated a statistically significant increase in FSH levels in both mature and fertilizable oocytes compared with immature and unfertilized oocytes.[206,213] Administration of hCG to women in natural cycles as opposed to FSH-managed cycles yields accelerated meiosis in the latter, suggesting that the increasing level of FSH within the follicle generates a positive signal for completion of meiotic maturation.[131] Similar observations have been described in monkey oocytes that mature in vitro.[112] Furthermore, in one study addition of FSH and LH increased the percentage of germinal vesicle breakdown and maturation to metaphase II in cultured monkey oocytes collected in the late follicular phase.[214]

Other peptide hormones have been implicated in normal meiotic maturation of nonhuman primate and human oocytes. These hormones include prolactin, epidermal growth factor (EGF), and IGF-1. It has been shown that follicular fluid prolactin levels increase with oocyte maturation.[204,211] These increases in follicular fluid prolactin level have been associated with higher rates of oocyte fertilization.[212] Nevertheless, a decrease in prolactin levels with advancing follicular growth also has been found.[215] The dynamic increase in the level of follicular fluid FSH, LH, and prolactin with progression of human oocyte meiosis to metaphase II[204] (Fig 5–8) may suggest involvement of these hormones in oocyte meiotic maturation. IGF-1 and EGF have been implicated in cellular differentiation of follicular cell types. The level of these growth factors is altered in follicular fluid collected at IVF-ET. Higher follicular fluid levels of IGF-1 have been detected in follicles yielding mature oocytes,[216] and EGF receptors have been found in human oocytes and their surrounding cumulus cells.[217] Furthermore, meiotic maturation to metaphase II has been induced in human oocytes with EGF and IGF-1 in vitro.[131] According to these findings, it is conceivable that the follicular microenvironment is involved in meiotic maturation, yielding an oocyte with greater fertilizability and developmental competence.

Further investigation into the mechanisms involved in the inhibition and induction of meiosis indicates involvement of protein kinase A. Microinjection of cAMP-dependent protein kinase inhibitor is sufficient to induce meiosis in mouse oocytes cultured under inhibitory conditions.[178] Similarly, various agents that induce protein kinase C activation, such as phorbol ester of diacylglycerol and gonadotropin-releasing hormone (GnRH) also induce in vitro resumption of meiosis in isolated oocytes.[218,219] Resumption of meiosis also is induced by agents that activate tyrosine kinases, such as EGF in rats[220] and humans[131] or by bFGF.[221]

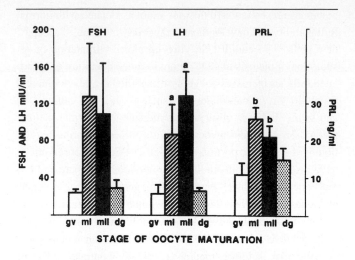

Figure 5–8. Follicle fluid levels of LH, FSH, and prolactin at various stages of oocyte maturation in unstimulated cycles. (*From Seibel MM, Smith D, Dlugi AM, Levesque L: Periovulatory follicular fluid hormone levels in spontaneous human cycles. J Clin Endocrinol Metab 68:1073, 1989.*)

Further insight into the biochemical events of oocyte meiotic maturation is indicated by changes in MPF activity.[222,223] Resumption of meiosis is primarily dependent on activation of MPF, namely dephosphorylation of p34^{cdc2} kinase[224] and its association with cyclin. The continuation of meiosis in terms of stimulating activation of MAPK depends on *mos*.[225]

Cyclin is degraded abruptly after each cell cycle and reaccumulates during the next cycle. When cyclin degradation is inhibited, MPF remains active and eggs remain in metaphase II. Cyclin degradation appears to be blocked, and MPF appears to be reactivated before metaphase II by the proto-oncogene c-*mos* product known as cytostatic factor, which is expressed in germ cells. Relatively high concentrations of c-*mos* mRNA have been confirmed in human eggs.[226]

IN VITRO GROWTH OF FOLLICLE-ENCLOSED OOCYTES

In vitro ovarian culture with a proper response to hormonal stimulation was first demonstrated in the early 1970s.[227,228] Early on it became evident that successful induction of in vitro growth required maintenance of oocyte–granulosa cell contact.[55,56] Successful in vitro growth of oocytes enclosed within primary or primordial follicles has been achieved in various mammals, including hamsters,[229] mice,[56,230,231] pigs,[117] and humans.[232] The growing in vitro follicles developed the capability to respond to FSH in terms of steroid secretion, antrum formation, reduced atresia, induction of oocyte maturation, and ovulation.[233–236] It appears that in addition to FSH and LH, inclusion of various other hormones improves in vitro follicular growth.[237,238] Our current studies on the in vitro culture of primary and small antral follicles in rat ovarian fragments indicate that the addition of IBMX or FSH increases the number of isolated oocytes per fragment and their capability of resuming meiosis after 3 or 6 days in culture.[113]

Isolation and in vitro growth of human primary and primordial follicles has only recently been achieved successfully.[232,239] Figure 5–9 demonstrates a 3-day culture of human oocytes isolated from a perimenopausal woman after aggressive collagenase digestion. Primary follicles isolated from the premenopausal human ovary form an antrum within 5 days in FSH-supplemented culture medium, but the diameter of the oocytes is not altered substantially. More successful results are achieved with primordial follicles isolated at 16 to 20 weeks' gestation, the time in which primordial follicles are formed. After more than 40 days in culture oocytes larger than 80 μm were observed. Extrusion of the first polar body occurs in some of the largest oocytes. Oocytes collected from small antral follicles typically complete meiotic maturation in vitro. However, only a small fraction of them undergo fertilization and continue to the blastocyst stage,[120,121,240] suggesting the need for advanced oocyte development. The same rule should be assumed in humans. Thus, full oocyte growth is necessary before in vitro oocyte growth is used for clinical treatment. Furthermore, this successful model should be attempted in adult women who are at risk of losing their ovaries for various clinical reasons or possibly for instances in which in vivo oocyte and follicular growth are not possible.

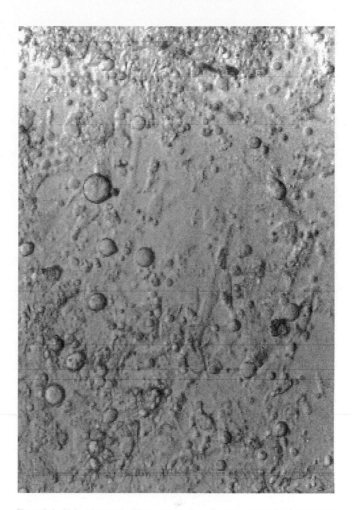

Figure 5–9. Light micrograph of human oocytes and ovarian cells isolated from a 46-year-old woman.

Explanted Oocytes and Their Growth

The grafting of pig ovaries from one individual to another was proved successful in fresh tissue by Castle and Phillips in 1911.[241] Frozen (thawed) mice ovaries grafted to recipients resulted in development of preovular follicles, ovulation, and pregnancies.[242–244] Grafting of primordial or primary follicles in mice resulted in successful oocyte growth with the capability of normal meiotic maturation, fertilization, and development of viable offspring, whether transplanted under the kidney capsule[125,245] or into the ovarian bursa.[246] Similar success with this technique was observed with frozen (thawed) primary and primordial follicles whether or not subjected to initial growth in vitro.[247–249]

Cryopreservation of rodent oocytes produced successful results,[250–252] whereas cryopreservation of human oocytes either at the germinal vesicle stage or at metaphase II has been disappointing. It appears that the human microtubule spindle is labile under reduced temperature conditions and predisposes the oocyte to a variety of chromosomal disorders.[253,254] Addi-

tion of the cryoprotectant dimethylsulfoxide (DMSO) at 4°C has been shown to prevent some of this damage, and a higher rate of survival of normal oocytes can be expected.[255] When oocytes are cooled in propanediol to 0°C at the rate of −3°C per minute and plunged into liquid nitrogen (−1000°C per minute), results are much better.[256] Vitrification of human oocytes, which prevents ice formation, results in a higher rate of normal morphology of thawed oocytes.[257] It appears that freezing oocytes with a germinal vesicle results in better and healthier oocytes.

It seems that normal in vitro growth and maturation of human oocytes is a more approachable task today than it was before. The possibility of grafting human donated small follicles may solve a number of infertility problems in humans. Examples include ovarian conservation before chemotherapy in the treatment of premenopausal women and extending reproductive potential in women in need of delaying child bearing.

COMPLETION OF MEIOSIS, AND BEGINNING OF THE FIRST MITOTIC DIVISIONS

The arrest of the oocyte at metaphase II is probably caused by a cytostatic factor (c-*mos* protooncogene product), which stabilizes MPF.[258] Sperm penetration induces a transient increase in Ca^{2+}, which is probably released from the cortical vesicles of the ER.[259] This process is associated with inactivation of MPF–cytostatic factor and MAPK.[258] The latter event allows the oocyte to escape from metaphase II arrest (Fig 5–10).[260] The degradation of cyclin precedes the inactivation of c-*mos* and MAPK by a few hours.[261,262]

The progression of oocyte meiotic or mitotic events in relation to the motility of chromosomes is a microtubule-dependent process. These events include alignment of the chromosomes along the metaphase I cell equator, migration of the meiotic spindle toward the oocyte cortex, and organization of the meiotic II spindle.[263] The first mitosis involves separate condensation of the maternal and paternal chromosomes, intermixing of the chromosomes at the equator of the barrel-shaped spindle, and alignment in metaphase, which concludes the fertilization process. Understanding of these events in terms of ultrastructural changes together with involvement of the microtubule, microfilaments, and centrosome becomes increasingly relevant for optimization of assisted reproduction treatment of humans.

Role of the Microtubules and Centrosomes

The basic components in the microtubule are the α and β tubulin dimers. These dimers are asymmetric and when bound together produce a string of polarity. Each microtubule contains 13 strings, yielding a microtubule of 25 nm diameter. The microtubule is constantly subjected to assembly and disassembly processes called *dynamic instability*. The microtubule spindle either after extrusion of the first polar body or at the first mitosis is a highly active structure.[264] Its stability depends on post-translational modifications[265] expressed at different parts of the microtubule spindle. There are similarities between modifications at the meiotic and at the mitotic spindles.[265]

At the postmetaphase state, movement of chromosomes to the spindle poles along the shrinking microtubule is a result of disassembly of the tubulin dimers at the end of the microtubule. Many proteins designated *microtubule-associated proteins* are bound to the microtubule. Some of them are structural and increase microtubule stability, and others are the microtubule motor, that is, they are located along the microtubule surface and hydrolize adenosine triphosphate (ATP). Assembly of the microtubules is nucleated from the microtubule organizing center, that is, the centrosome. At interphase, the centrosome is located close to the nuclear membrane, and long microtubules run all over the cell toward its periphery. The important component of the centrosome is the γ-tubulin, which is involved in microtubule nucleation and polymerization. The disassembly and build-up of the microtubule spindle is initiated by the active MPF.

The microtubule is attached to the chromosomal centromere via the kinetochore. This important structure is involved in alignment of the chromosomes at the spindle equator and later in their separation at anaphase. Several proteins involved in the kinetochore centromere complex have been identified[266] and probably function as microtubule binding proteins. Injection of antibodies directed at the kinetochore proteins at prophase may interfere with prometaphase congregation and anaphase segregation. However, later injection of these antibodies at metaphase does not affect the kinetochore-dependent processes.[267]

The centrosome has three main functions—reproduction, microtubule organization, and microtubule nucleation. It is interesting that the centrosome is maximally condensed when the chromosomes are condensed and is maximally decondensed when the chromosomes are in S phase. Thus, it is believed that replication of the centrosome is under cell-cycle control. Although many proteins, enzymes, and other molecules have been

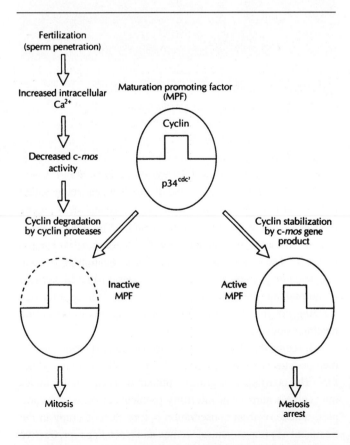

Figure 5–10. Schematic of maturation-promoting factor (MPF). (*From Zilberstein M, Seibel MM: Fertilization and implantation.* Curr Opin Obstet Gynecol *6:184, 1994.*)

found to be integral constituents of the centrosome, much of its composition is still unknown. During gametogenesis various elements of the centrosomes are lost. In sperm, most of the γ tubulin and other proteins defined as γ-some are lost, but in oocytes they are retained in ooplasm during oogenesis. In the oocyte, the centrosome is lost. Thus, as the sperm penetrates the oocyte, both entities join together, which renews centrosome activity. This process manifests parallelism to chromosome activity, in which there is a reduction to haploid set in gametes but renewal of the original situation in the zygote.

The source of the microtubule-organizing center in the oocyte after sperm penetration does not represent a common feature in all mammals. The mouse is the most atypical. The first mitotic spindle poles are organized by maternal centrosomes apparently without a contribution from the sperm.[268] Actually, mouse sperm do not contain a centrosome, and the sperm do not produce an aster after penetration of the ooplasm.[269] Antibodies directed at centrosomal proteins mark both the poles of the meiotic spindle and the cytoplasmic centrosomes.[269] Furthermore, it appears that these cytoplasmic centrosomes are derived from centrosomes of the second meiotic spindle.[270] In other species, including humans, no cytoplasmic centrosomes have been detected. In rabbits, microtubules have been detected at the base of the sperm head,[271,272] and in studies with domestic animals, evidence has been collected to support production of the microtubule aster by the sperm neck.

After sperm penetration, the microtubules begin to assemble around the base of the penetrated sperm head. This process continues to produce a huge aster-like structure that expands in the cytoplasm and makes contact with the maternal pronucleus. It is involved in pronuclear apposition during interphase.[273] In human mitotic oocytes the sperm-derived centrosome is seen in the metaphase spindle poles, which is evidence that it acts as a microtubule-organizing center.[274] Intensive studies of human oocytes subjected to conventional IVF[275] and monkey oocytes subjected to intracytoplasmic single-sperm injection (ICSI)[276] indicate that it is the male centrosome that is involved in the first oocyte mitosis.

Using oocytes from nonhuman primates, *Macaca mulatta,* it appears that the microtubule-organizing center obtained from the sperm is dominantly involved in apposition of the male and female pronuclei.[277] Similarly, in humans, inseminated oocytes treated with nocodazole (a microtubule inhibitor) neither assemble microtubules nor enable pronuclear apposition, which is evidence that microtubules are necessary for pronuclear migration and probably for pronuclear congregation.[278]

The role of the sperm centrosome in determining the spindle structure can be determined from dispermic fertilization. In such cases, a three-pole spindle is produced that leads in two thirds of instances to three daughter blastomeres.[279,280]

By anaphase, the astral formation dramatically increases in size. This process ultimately yields an increased microtubule density that integrates into the cytoplasmic array in the two resulting blastomeres. In studies with domestic animals, evidence has been collected to support microtubule assembly as being organized by the sperm centriolar complex.[281] However, parthenogenic activation of a bipolar spindle is present,[282] suggesting that in domestic animals both paternal and maternal factors in some way share establishment of a centrosome involved in microtubule assembly at fertilization.

In the human oocyte, the only detectable microtubule is in the meiotic spindle. It appears to be astral, radiating to the cell surface and located in the oocyte cortical region.[283,284] The penetrating sperm contributes the centrosome, which is located at the basal body in the base of the sperm head. To evaluate sperm capability to produce an aster, a cell-free system has been developed with *Xenopus* egg extracts. *Xenopus* sperm[285,286] and human sperm pretreated by a disulfide reducing agent[287] can bind γ tubulin from *Xenopus* egg extract. Actually, unlike *Xenopus* oocyte cytoplasm, the mammalian oocyte has disulfide-reducing activity, which naturally primes the sperm basal body to develop into the centrosome and later to bind additional γ tubulin as it is phosphorylated. After these prerequisite events, the centrosome nucleates the microtubules and reassembles them into an aster.

The Role of Microfilaments

Microfilaments are located near the plasma membrane. They participate in the various motion events of the meiotic spindle, such as migration, rotation (in mouse oocytes), and cell division, including polar body extrusion. Microfilaments are involved in fertilization in terms of their assembly in the region of sperm–egg fusion and later in the formation of an incorporation cone after sperm penetration. In mice the migration of the meiotic spindle to the cortical region is associated with deprivation of cortical granules and formation of a microvilli-free area in the eventual location of the meiotic spindle. This location is enriched with submembranous actin.[288,289] This situation persists in the second meiotic arrest. After sperm penetration, the second meiotic spindle rotates and radiates within the plasma membrane to the cell center. In other mammalian species, the second meiotic spindle does not rotate because it is oriented initially perpendicular to the plasma membrane.

The role of microfilaments in nuclear migration in mouse oocytes has gained support in studies with microtubule depolymerization drugs or microfilament inhibitors. Exposure to microtubule depolymerization drugs induces scattering of chromosomes throughout the cortical region. However, addition of microfilament inhibitors such as cytochalasin[268] or latranculin[290] blocks this chromosome scattering. Once a nuclear membrane is formed around either the male or female pronucleus, the microfilament polarization disappears from the pronuclear region.

Microfilament inhibitors prevent extrusion of the second polar body and thus result in formation of two female pronuclei. However, these inhibitors do not prevent sperm-head incorporation. Near the location of sperm entry, an increased assembly of actin occurs[289] that ultimately becomes the incorporation cone that leads to male pronuclei migration. Formation of the incorporation cone, incorporation of the sperm tail, and male pronuclei migration and apposition[290] are prevented by microfilament inhibitors. The effects of these inhibitors are associated with marked reduction of cortical microfilaments.

In contrast to mouse oocyte, oocytes of other mammals distribute an equivalent amount of cortical actin beneath the oocyte plasma membranes. Cortical granule distribution and microvilli have been found uniformly distributed in oocytes of domestic animals,[282,291] primates,[283,293] and humans.[293] Furthermore, in domestic animals, increased microfilament assembly around the first meiotic spindle has not been detected, and the motion events of this spindle are probably not microfilament dependent.[2] However, as in mice, domestic mammals,[294] and primates,[295] formation of the sperm incorporation cone is a microfilament-dependent process.

FAILURE OF MEIOTIC COMPLETION AND OOCYTE MITOSIS IN HUMAN OOCYTE

It is assumed that first and second polar body extrusion, presence of two pronuclei and normal cleavage, that is, two to four to eight cells, and so on, and the presence of a low number of fragments greatly reduces the likelihood that a transferred embryo is defective and will not implant. However, in human IVF, only a small fraction of inseminated oocytes develop into normal implantable embryos. This situation is associated with the many events that occur during oocyte growth, maturation, fertilization, and eventually implantation. In each of these steps, a variety of defects can cause failure to develop a healthy baby.

The presence of a second polar body can be a misleading indication of normal completion of meiotic division because the first polar body is capable of dividing into two polar bodies or even fragmenting. Furthermore, the oocyte may not extrude an entire haploid set of chromosomes to the second polar body. In such instances the resultant embryo bears an aneuploid or even a triploid set of chromosomes, usually resulting in embryo death. There can also be incomplete sperm incorporation sufficient to activate the oocyte to extrude the second polar body but yielding an abnormal embryo. In extreme instances the oocyte may extrude the entire maternal genome into the second polar body, leaving only the sperm genome within the oocyte.[284]

Abnormalities in both first and second polar bodies such as the aforementioned are not uncommon and may lead to abnormal embryos.[296,297] Similar observations have been made about polar bodies tested soon after oocyte retrieval, excluding the possibility that the abnormalities observed were caused by degenerative processes in polar body chromosomes at the time of culture.[298] A molecular basis for the defects in meiosis may be associated with incomplete inactivation of c-mos and MAPK, yielding either a continuation of metaphase II arrest or defects in its completion. It is also possible that defects in the signal transduction intercessions may cause the oocyte, sperm, or both to miscommunicate. Thus, the results are manifested as various defects in these processes. Nevertheless, in sperm, a very low percentage of meiotic abnormalities are detected.[299]

In mice[300] and humans[301–303] sperm penetration into metaphase I oocytes usually results in progression of the oocyte to metaphase II. The sperm nucleus swells and undergoes premature chromosome condensation (PCC) to a chromosome-like structure, skipping the pronucleus stage. Such sperm PCC has been observed in human oocytes fertilized either by means of conventional IVF[284,302,304] or by means of ICSI,[305] and in monkey oocytes.[276] A lower rate of PCC occurs in ICSI-treated versus standard IVF-treated oocytes.[306] The lower rate of PCC among ICSI oocytes might be related to the fact that ICSI is performed only on oocytes that possess a first polar body, presumably at metaphase II. The PCC found in some ICSI-treated oocytes might be associated with a defective ooplasmic process.

When parthenogenetic activation occurs, the viability of the embryo varies according to species. In rabbits[307] or mice[308] these embryos implant and produce small fetuses. In humans, parthenogenetic embryos are arrested at the eight-cell stage,[309] which may be associated with disorderly assembled microtubules that yield nonviable embryos. In one study in which DNA fluorescence and electron microscopy were used, sperm were found in most oocytes defined as unpenetrated by sperm. A single sperm was present in the ooplasm of 22% of oocytes that appeared unfertilized and 52% of those parthenogenetically activated.[310]

One of the main indications of failed in vitro preembryo development is cleavage arrest or sometimes asynchronous karyokinesis and cytokinesis. A diagram of the various possibilities for the latter abnormality is presented in Fig 5–11.[311]

Insemination of apparently normal metaphase II oocytes can result in various failures. Defective cortical architectural systems that include microfilament spectrin or forbin may be associated with incapability of sperm to incorporate completely.[275] Other defective processes may include incomplete sperm aster assembly, detachment of the sperm aster and tail from the male pronucleus, and disarrayed sperm astral organization.[284] Collectively these defects in the oocyte and sperm nuclear activity are mostly associated with the various failures in microtubule assembly and with centrosome insufficiency.

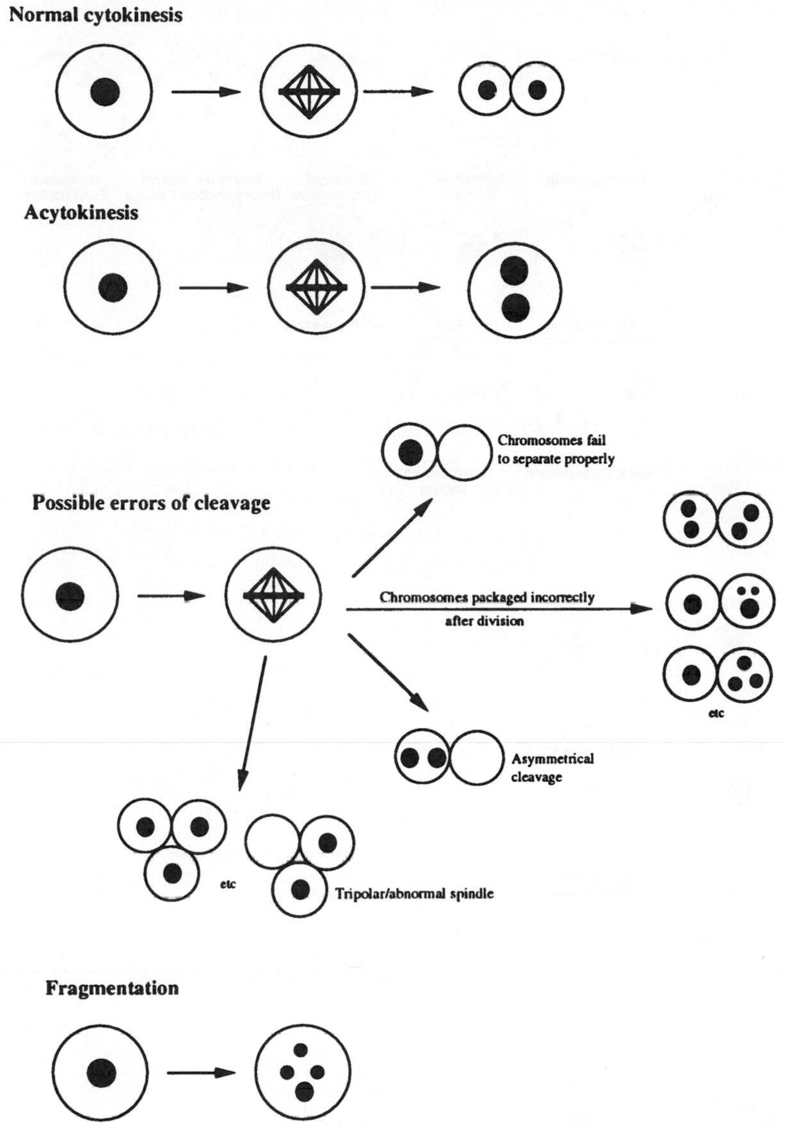

Normal cytokinesis

Acytokinesis

Possible errors of cleavage

Chromosomes fail to separate properly

Chromosomes packaged incorrectly after division

etc

Asymmetrical cleavage

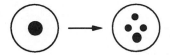

etc   Tripolar/abnormal spindle

Fragmentation

Figure 5–11. Schematic of possible mechanisms that lead to formation of multinucleate blastomeres in human embryos. (*From Pickering SJ, Taylor A, Johnson MH, Braude PR: An analysis of multinucleated blastomere formation in human embryos.* Hum Reprod *10:1912, 1995.*)

Navara et al[312] demonstrated that differences exist in the aster quality of different bull strains. The sperm centrosomes of bull strains with higher fertilizing capability manifest a larger aster (80% of cell volume) and a well-defined focus. Deviations from these configurations, such as a small aster, less defined aster focus or several focuses, and as an extreme example failure of the aster to organize around the male pronucleus, are associated with lower fertilization capability.[312] The study actually indicated that a male factor rather than an oocyte factor is associated with the lower fertilizability. Similar aster defects may occur after IVF in arrested oocytes of humans.[275,284] In such situations donor sperm may fertilize the same woman's oocyte,[284] emphasizing that the sperm is defective in this process.

Defects in microtubule organization may lead to fertilization failures that can be detected in the sperm only after it penetrates the oocyte. Such cases of male fertility defects have been described in lower animals and in rams.[313] Changes or mutations in the proteins that construct the centrosome may be the initial cause of defects in the capability of the centrosome to bind to γ tubulin, to nucleate the microtubule, and to produce normal asters.

Penetration of more than one sperm into an oocyte can manifest as several centrosome defects. Sometimes only one sperm can produce an aster, a result designated *silent polyspermy.* The cause of such developments is not fully understood. It has been suggested that the oocyte cytoplasmic compounds involved in decondensation of the sperm and oocyte

Figure 5–12. Microtubule organization in inseminated oocytes that do not complete fertilization and development in humans. Normal microtubule patterns detected during fertilization in humans. Schematic details of the microtubule configurations are shown on the left (**A–H**). **A.** Fresh, unfertilized human oocytes possess microtubules only in the second meiotic metaphase spindle. **B.** Soon after sperm penetration, microtubules can be detected at the base of the sperm head as the now-activated oocyte completes second meiosis and polar body formation. **C.** As sperm decondensation continues, the sperm aster enlarges while the developing paternal pronucleus moves away from the cortex. **D.** The female pronucleus moves toward the male and the sperm aster becomes asymmetric and bipolar. **E.** By the onset of prophase, the maternal and paternal chromosomes condense separately as the two microtubule arrays establish the beginning of the mitotic spindle apparatus. **F.** The chromosomes intermix along the equator of the anastral metaphase spindle, and one or two small asters associated with the sperm axoneme form at one of the poles. Both the pronuclei and mitotic spindle remain eccentrically positioned within the cytoplasm. **G.** At the initiation of anaphase, the spindle pole asters elongate and interact with the adjacent cortex, inaugurating the cleavage furrow at this site. **H.** Cleavage results in the formation of equal-sized daughter blastomeres. Stages at which human fertilization arrest include failures to complete are (1) meiotic maturation, sperm incorporation, egg activation, and exit from meiosis, producing oocytes with the following phenotypes: androgenetic oocytes; maternal spindle activation failure and male premature chromosome condensation defects; maternal karyomere formation without sperm penetration defect; activated oocyte but failure to fully incorporate the sperm defect; and fertilization of the immature oocyte (**A**); (2) sperm aster microtubule nucleation defects; oocytes with undetected or silent polyspermy; or oocytes displaying multiple sperm penetration (**B**); (3) sperm aster development, giving rise to oocytes with detached asters or sperm axonemes from the base of the sperm heads or truncated microtubule asters (**C**); (4) normal cell cycle events, including the interphase-to-mitosis (**E**) or mitosis-to-interphase (**F**) transitions; and (5) normal embryonic development, resulting in fragmented embryos arrested at various stages of the cell cycle (**H**). (*From Asch R, et al: The stages at which human fertilization arrests: Microtubule and chromosome configurations in inseminated oocytes which failed to complete fertilization and development in humans. Hum Reprod 10:1897, 1995.*)

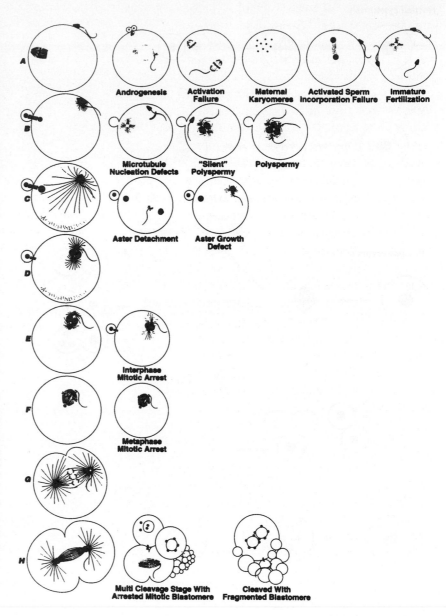

chromosomal material are limited. Therefore, incorporation of more than one sperm into the oocyte leads to sharing of this ooplasmic material between more than one sperm, which leads to development of smaller pronuclei.[314] However, when excessive numbers of spermatozoa enter the oocyte, only some or none develop into sperm pronuclei.[315] It also has been suggested that when oocyte meiosis occurs in the absence of granulosa cells, there is a lower potential for development of sperm pronuclei.[316] It is impossible to determine silent polyspermy in two pronuclei zygotes with conventional light microscopy. Furthermore, in about one fourth of pursued unfertilized oocytes, a silent sperm is present,[275,310] which calls into question the wisdom of reinsemination strategy either by means of conventional IVF or ICSI, especially because it is a strategy that fails most of the time.[317] More complicatioons are related to pursued parthenogenesis, in which 52% of oocytes are actually penetrated by one sperm.[310] The latter may suggest that to identify parthenogenesis, preimplantation genetic diagnosis should be used before these preembryos are discarded.

Although ICSI overcomes the problem of sperm penetration and polyspermy, it does not resolve situations in which the introduced centrosome is defective in its various functions.

Thus, the first mitotic division depends on a well-controlled system in the course of events that lead to development of the sperm centrosome aster.[275] Failure in this process may be associated with defects in nucleating microtubules, microtubule assembly, and pronuclei migration. Defects in microtubule assembly may result in a miniature sperm aster. Furthermore, the presence of impaired microtubule motor protein may result in detachment of the aster from the male pronuclei or migration failure of the pronuclei.[275] These undetected types of male-factor infertility may be evaluated with two different approaches. It has been shown that human sperm centrosomes primed with a disulfide-reducing agent can nucleate microtubules when incubated in *Xenopus* egg extract in a cell-free system.[287] Another approach is to test human sperm aster development in mature oocytes of cows.[273] Failure of aster development as a cause of male-factor infertility should increase motivation for development of techniques for centrosome donation. Exogenous centrosome introduction has resulted in successful results in several animal systems.[282] Thus, it has been suggested that this type of treatment of humans may provide a cure for defective sperm.[273,284] Much research is necessary to introduce a treatment of this nature into infertility practice. A summary of the various defects that may arise in the completion of oocyte meiotic division and commencement of oocyte mitosis is presented in Fig 5–12.[275]

REFERENCES

1. Tsafriri A, Bar-Ami S, Lindner HR: Control of the development of meiotic competence and of oocyte maturation in mammals. In: Beier HM, Lindner JR (eds), *Fertilization of the Human Egg in Vitro.* Berlin, Springer-Verlag, 1983:3–17

2. Thibault C, Szöllosi D, Gerard M: Mammalian oocyte maturation. *Reprod Natur Dev* 27:865, 1987

3. Wassarman PM, Albertini DF: The mammalian ovum. In: Knobil E, Neil JD (eds), *The Physiology of Reproduction.* New York, Raven, 1994:79–122

4. Witschi E: Migration of germ cells of human embryos from the yolk sac to the primitive gonadal folds. *Contrib Embryol Carnegie Inst* 32:67, 1948

5. Carlson BM: *Human Embryology and Developmental Biology.* St. Louis, Mosby, 1994

6. Rich IN: Hemapoietic-initiating cells. *J Perinat Med* 23:31, 1995

7. Stott D, Wylie CC: Invasive behaviour of mouse primordial germ cells in vitro. *J Cell Sci* 86:133, 1986

8. Wylie CC, Stott D, Donovan PJ: Primordial germ cell migration. *Dev Biol* 2:433, 1986

9. Kuwana T, Fujimoto T: Active locomotion of human primordial germ cell in vitro. *Anat Rec* 205:21, 1983

10. Upadhyay S, Zamboni L: Ectopic germ cells: Natural model for the study of germ cell sexual differentiation. *Proc Natl Acad Sci USA* 79:6584, 1982

11. Pellas TC, Ramachandran B, Duncan M, Pan SS, Marone M, Chada K: Germ-cell deficient (*gcd*): An insertional mutation manifested as infertility in transgenic mice. *Proc Natl Acad Sci USA* 88:8787, 1991

12. Williams DE, De Vries P, Namen AE, Widner MB, Lyman SD: The steel factor. *Dev Biol* 151:368, 1992

13. Resnick JL, Bixler LS, Cheng L, Donovan PT: Long term proliferation of mouse primordial germ cells in culture. *Nature* 359:550, 1992

14. Godin I, Wylie CC: TGF β_1 inhibits proliferation and has chemotropic effect on mouse primordial germ cells in culture. *Development* 113:1451, 1991

15. Godin I, Deed R, Cooke J, Zsebo K, Dexter M, Wylie CC: Effects of the steel gene product on mouse primordial germ cell in culture. *Nature* 352:807, 1991

16. Wei G, Mahowald AP: The germline: Familiar and newly uncovered properties. *Ann Rev Genet* 78:309, 1994

17. De Felici M, Pesce M: Growth factors in mouse primordial germ cell migration and proliferation. *Prog Growth Factor Res* 5:135, 1994

18. Coulombre JL, Russell ES: Analysis of the pleiotropism of the W-locus in the mouse and the effect of W and W^v substitution upon postnatal development of germ cells. *J Exp Zool* 126:277, 1954

19. Kuroda H, Terada N, Nakayama H, Matsumoto K, Kitamura Y: Infertility due to growth arrest of ovarian follicles in *sl/sl*^{t} mice. *Dev Biol* 126:71, 1988

20. Huang EJ, Manova K, Packer AI, Sanchez S, Bachvarova R, Basmer P: The murine *steel panda* mutation affects kit-ligand expression and growth of early ovarian follicle. *Dev Biol* 157:100, 1993

21. Motta PM, Makabe S: Elimination of germ cells during differentiation of the human ovary: An electron microscope study. *Eur J Obstet Gynecol Reprod Biol* 22:271, 1986

22. Speed RM: Prophase pairing in a mosaic 18p; iso18q human female foetus studied by surface spreading. *Hum Genet* 72:256, 1986

23. Ohno S, Smith JB: Role of fetal follicular cells in meiosis of mammalian oocytes. *Cytogenesis* 3:324, 1964

24. Burgoyne PS, Baker TG: Meiotic pairing and gametogenic failure. In: Evans CW, Dickinson HG. Controlling Events in Meiosis. *Symp Soc Exp Biol* 38:349, 1984

25. Carr DH, Haggar RA, Hart AG: Germ cells in the ovaries of XO female infants. *Am J Clin Pathol* 19:521, 1968

26. Byskov AG: Does the rete ovarii act as a trigger for the onset of meiosis? *Nature* 252:396, 1974

27. Byskov AG: The role of the rete ovarii in meiosis and follicle formation in the cat, mink and ferret. *J Reprod Fertil* 45:201, 1975

28. Byskov AG, Fenger M, Westergaard L, Andersen CY: Forskolin and the meiosis inducing substance synergistically initiate meiosis in fetal male sperm cells. *Mol Reprod Dev* 34:47, 1993

29. Byskov AG, Andersen CY, Nordholm L, et al: Chemical structure of sterols that activate oocyte meiosis. *Nature* 374:559, 1995

30. Hirobe S, He WW, Gustatson ML, Maclaughlin DT, Donahoe PK: Müllerian inhibiting substance gene expression in the cycling rat ovary correlates with recruited or graafian follicle selection. *Biol Reprod* 50:1238, 1994

31. Takahashi M, Koide SS, Donahoe PK: Müllerian inhibiting substance as oocyte meiosis inhibitor. *Mol Cell Endocrinol* 47:225, 1986

32. Francavilla S, Cordesch G, Properzi G, Concordia N, Cappa F, Pozzi V: Ultrastructure of fetal human gonad before sexual differentiation and during testicular and ovarian development. *J Submicrosc Cytol Pathol* 22:389, 1990

33. McLaren A: Development of the mammalian gonad: The fate of the supporting cell lineage. *Bioessays* 13:151, 1991

34. Kurilo LF: Oogenesis in antenatal development in man. *Hum Genet* 57:86, 1981

35. Peters H, Byskov AG, Grinsted J: Follicular growth in fetal and prepubertal ovaries of humans and other primates. *Clin Endocrinol Metab* 7:469, 1978

36. Winter JSD, Faiman C, Reyes FL: The gonadotropins of the fetus and neonate: Their ontogeny, function and regulation. In: Flamigni C, Givens JR (eds), *The Gonadotropins: Basic Science and Clinical Aspects in Females.* New York, Academic Press, 1982:160–166

37. Beck-Peccoz P, Padmanabhan V, Baggiani AM, et al: Maturation of hypothalamic-gonadal function in normal human fetuses: Circulating levels of gonadotropins, their common alpha-subunit and free testosterone, and discrepancy between immunological and biological activities of circulating follicle stimulating hormone. *J Clin Endocrinol Metab* 73:525, 1991

38. Massa G, de Zegher F, Vanderschueren-Lodeweyckx M: Serum levels of immunoreactive inhibin FSH and LH in human infant at preterm and term birth. *Biol Neonate* 61:150, 1992

39. Voutilainen R: Differentiation of the fetal gonad. *Horm Res* 38(Suppl):66, 1992

40. Huhtaniemi IT, Yamamoto M, Ranta T, Jalkanen J: Hormone receptors appear earlier in primate fetal testes than in the ovary. *J Clin Endocrinol Metab* 65:1210, 1987

41. Góugeon A: Regulation of ovarian follicular development in primates: Facts and hypothesis. *Endocr Rev* 17:121, 1996

42. Forabosco A, Sforza C, de Pol A, Vizzotto C, Marzona L, Ferrario V: Morphometric study of the human neonatal ovary. *Anat Rec* 231:201, 1991

43. Góugeon A, Ecochard R, Thalavard JC: Age related changes of the population of human ovarian follicles: Increase in the disappearance of non-growing and early growing follicles in aging women. *Biol Reprod* 50:653, 1994

44. Anderson E, Albertini DF: Gap junctions between the oocyte and companion follicle cells in the mammalian ovary. *J Cell Biol* 71:680, 1976

45. Gilula N, Epstein M, Beers W: Cell-to-cell communication and ovulation: A study of the cumulus cell–oocyte complex. *J Cell Biol* 78:58, 1978

46. Heller DT, Schultz RM: Ribonucleoside metabolism by mouse oocytes: Metabolic cooperactivity between the fully grown oocyte and cumulus cell. *J Exp Zool* 214:355, 1980

47. Moor RM, Smith MW, Dawson RMC: Measurement of intercellular coupling between oocyte and cumulus cells using intracellular markers. *Exp Cell Res* 126:15, 1980

48. Haghighat N, van Winkle LJ: Developmental change in follicular cell-enhanced amino acid uptake into mouse oocytes that depends on intact gap junctions and transport systems Gly. *J Exp Zool* 253:71, 1990

49. Wassarman PM, Letourneau GE: RNA synthesis in fully grown mouse oocytes. *Nature* 261:73, 1976

50. Colonna R, Cecconi S, Buccione R, Mangia F: Amino acid transport systems in growing mouse oocytes. *Cell Biol Int Rep* 7:1007, 1983

51. Biggers JD: Metabolism of the oocyte. In: JD Biggers and AW Schuetz (eds), *Oogenesis.* Baltimore, University Park Press, 1972:241–251

52. Moriya S, Tanaka T, Okada Y, Kikuchi T, Fujimoro S, Ichinoe K: Influence of the oocyte upon proliferation, differentiation and steroidogenesis of cultured granulosa cells. *Serono Symp Publ* 48:146, 1988

53. Vanderhyden BC, Caron PJ, Buccione R, Eppig JJ: Developmental pattern of the secretion of cumulus expansion enabling factor by mouse oocytes and the role of oocytes in promoting granulosa cell differentiation. *Dev Biol* 140:307, 1990

54. Satoh H, Tanaka T, Takaoka H, et al: Oocyte factors may be involved in the formation of cumulus oophorus. *Serono Symp Publ* 48:216, 1988

55. Bachvarova R, Boran M, Tejblum A: Development of naked growing mouse oocytes in vitro. *J Exp Zool* 211:159, 1980

56. Eppig JJ: A comparison between oocyte growth in coculture with granulosa cells and oocyte with granulosa cell–oocyte junctional contact maintained in vitro. *J Exp Zool* 209:345, 1979

57. Buccione R, Cecconi S, Talone C, Mangia F, Colonna R: Follicle and regulation of mammalian oocyte growth. *J Exp Zool* 242:351, 1987

58. Canipari R, Palombi F, Riminucci M, Mangia F: Early programming of maturation competence in mouse oogenesis. *Dev Biol* 102:519, 1984

59. Chesnel F, Wigglesworth K, Eppig JJ: Acquisition of meiotic competence by denuded mouse oocytes participation of somatic-cell product(s) and CAMP. *Dev Biol* 101:285, 1994

60. Manova K, Nocka K, Besmer P, Bachvarova RF: Gonadal expression of c-kit encoded at the W locus of the mouse. *Development* 110:1057, 1990

61. Manova K, Huang EJ, Angeles M, De Leon V, et al: The expression pattern of the *c-kit* ligand in gonads of mice supports a role for the *c-kit* receptor in oocyte growth and in proliferation of spermatogonia. *Dev Biol* 157:85, 1993

62. Packer AI, Chang Hsu Y, Besmer P, Bachvarova RF: The ligand of the *c-kit* ligand receptor promotes oocyte growth. *Dev Biol* 161:194, 1994

63. McGaughey R, Montgomery D, Richter J: Germinal vesicle configuration and patterns of polypeptide synthesis of porcine oocytes from antral follicles of different size, as related to their competency for spontaneous maturation. *J Exp Zool* 209:239, 1979

64. Mirre C, Stahl A: Ultrastructure organization, sites of transcription and distribution of fibrillar centers in the nucleolus of the mouse oocyte. *J Cell Sci* 48:53, 1981

65. Chouinard L: A light- and electron-microscope study of the nucleolus during growth of the oocyte in the prepubertal mouse. *J Cell Sci* 9:637, 1991

66. Szöllosi D: Changes of some cell organelles during oogenesis in

mammals. In: Biggers JD, Schultz AW (eds), *Oogenesis*. Baltimore, University Park Press, 1972:47–64

67. Wassarman PM, Josefowicz WJ: Oocyte development in the mouse: An ultrastructural comparison of oocytes isolated at various stages of growth and meiotic competence. *J Morphol* 156:209, 1978

68. Piko L, Matsumoto L: Number of mitochondria and some properties of mitochondrial DNA in the mouse egg. *Dev Biol* 49:1, 1976

69. Zamboni L: Comparative studies on the ultrastructure of mammalian oocytes. In: J Biggers, Schultz A (eds), *Oogenesis*. Baltimore, University Park Press, 1972:5–46

70. Gyllensten U, Wharton D, Josefsson A, Wilson AC: Paternal inheritance of mitochondrial DNA in mice. *Nature* 352:255, 1991

71. Yotsuyanagi Y, Szöllosi D: Virus-like particles and related expressions in mammalian oocytes and preimplantation stage embryos. In: Van Blerkom J, Motta PM (eds), *Ultrastructure of Reproduction*. Boston, Martinus Nijhoft, 1984:218–234

72. Glass LE: Transmission of maternal proteins into oocytes. *Adv Biosci* 6:29, 1971

73. Hinduja IN, Kumar A, Anand Kumar TC: Ultrastructure of the cortex in human egg. *Hum Reprod* 5:66, 1990

74. Van Blerkom J: Occurrence and developmental consequences of aberrant cellular organization in meiotically mature human oocytes after exogenous ovarian hyperstimulation. *J Electron Microsc (Tokyo)* 16:324, 1990

75. Weakley BS: Comparison of cytoplasmic lamellae and membranous elements in the oocytes of five mammalian species. *Z Zellforsch* 85:109, 1968

76. Garcia R, Pereyra-Altonso S, Sotelo J: Protein-synthesizing machinery in the growing oocyte of the cyclic mouse. *Differentiation* 14:101, 1979

77. Burkholder GD, Comings DE, Okada TA: A storage form of ribosomes in mouse oocytes. *Exp Cell Res* 69:361, 1971

78. Bachvarova R, De Leon V, Spiegelman I: Mouse egg ribosomes: Evidence for storage in lattice. *J Embryol Exp Morphol* 62:153, 1981

79. Piko L, Clegg KB: Quantitative changes in total RNA, total poly (A) and ribosomes in early mouse embryos. *Dev Biol* 89:362, 1982

80. Blobel CP, Wolfsberg TG, Turck CW, Myles DG, Primakoff P, White JM: A potential fusion peptide and an integrin ligand domain in a protein active in sperm–egg fusion. *Nature* 356:248, 1992

81. Fusi FM, Vignali M, Gailit J, Bronson RA: Mammalian oocytes exhibit specific recognition of the RGD (Arg-Gly-Asp) tripeptide and express oolemmal integrins. *Mol Reprod Dev* 36:212, 1993

82. Gulyas B: Cortical granules of mammalian eggs. *Int Rev Cytol* 63:357, 1980

83. Pierce KE, Siebert MC, Kopf GS, Schultz RM, Calarco PG: Characterization and localization of a mouse egg cortical granule antigen prior to and following fertilization or egg activation. *Dev Biol* 141:381, 1990

84. Pierce KE, Grunvald E, Kopf GS, Schultz RM: Temporal pattern of synthesis of the mouse cortical granule protein, p75, during oocyte growth and maturation. *Dev Biol* 152:145, 1992

85. Fowler RE: An autoradiographic study of gonadotropin regulation of labelled glycoconjugates within preovulatory mouse follicles during the final stages of oocyte maturation, using [3H]glucosamine as the radioactive precursor. *J Reprod Fertil* 83:759, 1988

86. Bleil JD, Wassarman PM: Structure and function of the zona pellucida: Identification and characterization of the proteins of the mouse's zona pellucida. *Dev Biol* 75:185, 1980

87. Hedrick JL, Wardrip NJ: On macromolecular composition of the zona pellucida from porcine oocytes. *Dev Biol* 121:478, 1987

88. Bercegeay S, Allaire F, Jean M, et al: The bovine zona pellucida: Differences in macromolecular composition between oocytes, pre-treated with A23187 or not and embryos. *Reprodo Nutr Dev* 33:567, 1993

89. Wolgemuth DJ, Celenza J, Bundman DS, Dunbar BS: Formation of the rabbit zona pellucida and its relationship to ovarian follicular development. *Dev Biol* 106:1, 1984

90. Shabanowitz RB: Mouse antibodies to human zona pellucida: Evidence that human ZP3 is strongly immunogenic and contains two distinct isomer chains. *Biol Reprod* 43:260, 1990

91. Chamberlin ME, Dean J: Human homolog of the mouse sperm receptor. *Proc Natl Acad Sci USA* 87:6014, 1990

92. Liang L-P, Dean J: Conservation of mammalian secondary sperm receptor genes enables the promoter of the human gene function in mouse. *Dev Biol* 156:399, 1993

93. Araki Y, Kurata S, Oikawa T, et al: A monoclonal antibody reacting with zona pellucida of the oviductal egg but not with that of the ovarian egg of the golden hamster. *J Reprod Immunol* 11:193, 1987

94. Wegner CC, Killian GJ: In vitro and in vivo association of an oviduct estrus-associated protein with bovine zona pellucida. *Mol Reprod Dev* 29:77, 1991

95. Kan FWK, Roux E, Bleau G: Immunolocalization of oviduction in endocytic compartments in the blastomeres of developing embryos in the golden hamster. *Biol Reprod* 48:77, 1993

96. Miller DJ, Macek MB, Shur BD: Complimentary between β surface β-1,4-galactosyl-transferase and egg coat ZP3 mediates sperm–egg binding. *Nature* 357:589, 1992

97. Kamada M, Daitoh T, Mori K, et al: Etiological implication of autoantibodies to zona pellucida in human female infertility. *Am J Reprod Immunol* 28:104, 1992

98. Papale ML, Grillo A, Leonardi E, Giufrida G, Palumbo M, Palumbo G: Assessment of the relevance of zona pellucida antibodies in follicular fluid of in vitro fertilization (IVF) patients. *Hum Reprod* 9:1827, 1994

99. Rodman T, Bachvarova R: RNA synthesis in preovulatory mouse oocytes. *J Cell Biol* 70:251, 1976

100. Bachvarova R, De Leon V, Johnson A, Kaplan G, Paynton B: Changes in total RNA polyadenylated RNA and actin mRNA during meiotic maturation of mouse oocytes. *Dev Biol* 108:325, 1985

101. Flach G, Johnson MH, Braude PR, Taylor RAS, Bolton VN: The transition from maternal to embryonic control in the 2-cell mouse embryo. *EMBO J* 1:681, 1982

102. Clegg KB, Piko L: Quantitative aspects of RNA synthesis and poly-adenylation in 1-cell and 2-cell mouse embryos. *J Embryol Exp Morphol* 74:169, 1983

103. Taylor KD, Piko L: Quantitative changes in cytoskeletal β- and alpha-actin mRNAs and apparent absence of sarcomeric actin in early mouse embryos. *Mol Reprod Dev* 26:111, 1990

104. Roller RJ, Kinloch RA, Hiraoka BY, Li SS-L, Wassarman PM: Gene expression during mammalian oogenesis and early embryogenesis: Quantification of three messenger RNAs abundant in fully grown mouse oocytes. *Development* 106:251, 1989

105. Golbus M, Stein M: Qualitative patterns of protein synthesis in the mouse oocyte. *J Exp Zool* 198:337, 1976

106. Wassarman PM: Oogenesis: Synthetic events in the developing mammalian egg. In: Hartmann J (ed), *Mechanism and Control of Animal Fertilization.* New York, Academic Press, 1983:1–54

107. Schultz R, Letournear G, Wassarman PM: Program of early development in the mammal: Changes in the patterns and absolute rates of tubulin and total protein synthesis during oocyte growth in the mouse. *Dev Biol* 73:120, 1979

108. Yamada S, Shimazu Y, Kawaji H, Nakazawa M, Naito K, Toyoda Y: Maturation, fertilization and development of dog oocytes in vitro. *Biol Reprod* 46:853, 1992

109. Biggers JD: Oogenesis. In: Gold JL (ed), *Gynecologic Endocrinology.* Hagerstown, Maryland, Harper & Row, 1975: 612–620

110. Szybek K: In vitro maturation of oocytes from sexually immature mice. *J Endocrinol* 54:527, 1972

111. Gilchrist RB, Nayudy PL, Nowshari MA, Hodges JK. Meiotic competence of marmoset monkey oocytes is related to follicle size and oocytes–somatic cell association. *Biol Reprod* 52:1234, 1995

112. Yeoman RR, Helvacioglu A, Williams LE, Aksel S, Abee CR: Restoration of oocyte maturational competency during the nonbreeding season with follicle-stimulating hormone stimulation in squirrel monkeys (*Saimiri boliviensis boliviensis*). *Biol Reprod* 50:329, 1994

113. Bar-Ami S, Zlotkin E, Brandes JM, Itskovitz-Eldor J: Failure of meiotic competence in human oocytes. *Biol Reprod* 50:1100, 1994

114. Sorensen RH, Wassarman PM: Relationship between growth and meiotic maturation of mouse oocytes. *Dev Biol* 50:531, 1976

115. Bar-Ami S, Tsafriri A: Acquisition of meiotic competence in the rat: Role of gonadotropin and estrogen. *Gamete Res* 4:463, 1981

116. Erickson GF, Sorensen RA: In vitro maturation of mouse oocytes from late middle and preantral graafian follicles. *J Exp Zool* 190:123, 1974

117. Hirao Y, Nagai T, Kubo M, Miyano T, Miyake M, Kato S: In vitro growth and maturation of pig oocytes. *J Reprod Fertil* 100:333, 1994

118. Martino A, Mogas T, Palomo MJ, Paramio MT: Meiotic competence of pre-pubertal goat oocytes. *Theriogenology* 41:969, 1994

119. De Smedt V, Crozet N, Gall L: Morphological and functional changes accompanying the acquisition of meiotic competence in ovarian goat oocyte. *J Exp Zool* 269:128, 1994

120. Eppig JJ, Schroeder AC, O'Brien MJ: Developmental capacity of mouse oocytes matured in vitro: Effects of gonadotrophic stimulation, follicular origin and oocyte size. *J Reprod Fertil* 95:119, 1992

121. Pavlok A, Lucas-Hahn A, Niemann H: Fertilization and developmental competence of bovine oocytes derived from different categories of antral follicles. *Mol Reprod Dev* 31:63, 1992

122. Bar-Ami S, Nimrod A, Brodie-AMH, Tsafriri A: Role of FSH and oestradiol-17β in the development of meiotic competence in rat oocytes. *J Steroid Biochem* 19:965, 1983

123. Schroeder AC, Eppig JJ: Developmental capacity of mouse oocytes that undergo maturation in vitro: Effect of the hormonal state of the oocyte donor. *Gamete Res* 24:81, 1989

124. Eppig JJ, Schroeder AC: Capacity of mouse oocytes from preantral follicles to undergo embryogenesis and development to live young after growth, maturation and fertilization in vitro. *Biol Reprod* 41:268, 1989

125. Carroll J, Whittingham DG, Wood MJ: Effect of gonadotropin environment on growth and development of isolated mouse primary ovarian follicles. *J Reprod Fertil* 93:71, 1991

126. Bar-Ami S, Zlotkin E, Itskovitz-Eldor J: In vitro induction of meiotic competence in rat oocytes. Presented at the *XTH Ovarian Workshop.* 1994, Bar Harbor, Michigan

127. Singh B, Barbe GJ, Armstrong DT: Factors influencing resumption of meiotic maturation and cumulus expansion of porcine oocyte–cumulus cell complexes in vitro. *Mol Reprod Dev* 36:113, 1993

128. Zelinski-Wooten MB, Hutchinson JS, Hess DL, Wolf DP: Follicle-stimulating hormone alone supports follicle growth and oocyte development in gonadotropin-releasing hormone antagonist-treated monkeys. *Hum Reprod* 10:1658, 1995

129. Younis AI, Sehgal PK, Biggers JD: Antral follicle development and in-vitro maturation of oocytes from macaques stimulated with a single subcutaneous injection of pregnant mare's serum gonadotropin. *Hum Reprod* 9:2130, 1994

130. Bar-Ami S, Tsafriri A: The development of meiotic competence in the rat: Role of hormones and of the stage of follicular development. *Gamete Res* 13:39, 1986

131. Gomez E, Tarin JJ, Pellicer A: Oocyte maturation in humans: The role of gonadotropins and growth factors. *Fertil Steril* 60:40, 1993

132. Mattson BA, Albertini DF: Oogenesis: Chromatin and microtubule dynamics during meiotic prophase. *Mol Reprod Dev* 25:374, 1990

133. Schramm RD, Tennier MT, Boatman DE, Barvister BD: Chromatin configuration and meiotic competence of oocytes are related to follicular diameter in non-stimulated rhesus monkey. *Biol Reprod* 48:349, 1993

134. Johnson LD, Albertini DF, McGinnis LK, Biggers JD: Chromatin organization meiotic status and meiotic competence acquisition in mouse oocytes from cultured ovarian follicles. *J Reprod Fertil* 104:277, 1995

135. Masui Y, Markert CL: Cytoplasmic control of nuclear behaviour during maturation of frog oocytes. *J Exp Zool* 177:129, 1971

136. Smith LD, Ecker RE: The interaction of steroids with *Rana pipiens* oocytes in the induction of maturation. *Dev Biol* 25:232, 1971

137. Balakier H: Induction of maturation in small oocytes from sexually immature mice by fusion with meiotic or mitotic cells. *Exp Cell Res* 112:137, 1978

138. Christmann L, Lung T, Moor RM: MPF components and meiotic competence in growing pig oocytes. *Mol Reprod Dev* 38:85, 1994

139. Goren S, Piont Kewitz Y, Dekel N: Meiotic arrest in incompetent rat oocytes is not regulated by cAMP. *Dev Biol* 166:11, 1994

140. Chesnel F, Eppig JJ: Synthesis and accumulation of p34cdc2 and cyclin B in mouse oocyte during acquisition of competence to resume meiosis. *Mol Reprod Dev* 40:503, 1995

141. Rime H, Ozon R: Protein phosphatases are involved in the in vivo activation of histone H1a kinase in mouse oocyte. *Dev Biol* 141:115, 1990

142. Schwartz DA, Schultz RM: Stimulatory effect of okadaic acid, an inhibitor of protein phosphatases, on nuclear envelope breakdown and protein phosphorylation in mouse oocytes and one-cell embryos. *Dev Biol* 145:119, 1991

143. Kalous J, Kubelka M, Rimkevicova Z, Guerrier P, Motlik J: Okadaic acid accelerates germinal vesicle breakdown (GVBD) and overcomes cyclohexamide and G-imethylaminopurine block in cattle and pig oocytes. *Dev Biol* 157:448, 1993

144. Gavin AC, Cavadore JC, Schorderet-Slotkin S: Histone H1-kinase activity germinal vesicle breakdown and *m*-phase entry in mouse oocytes. *J Cell Sci* 107:275, 1994

145. Chesnel F, Eppig JJ: Induction of precocious germinal vesicle breakdown (GVB) by GVB-incompetent mouse oocytes: Possible role of mitogen activated protein kinase rather than p34cdc2 kinase. *Biol Reprod* 52:895, 1995

146. Harrouk W, Clarke HJ: Mitogen-activated protein (MAP) kinase during the acquisition of meiotic competence by growing oocytes of the mouse. *Mol Reprod Dev* 41:29, 1995

147. Wickramasinghe D, Albertini DF: Centrosome phosphorylation and developmental expression of meiotic competence in mouse oocytes. *Dev Biol* 152:62, 1992

148. Pincus G, Enzmann EV: The comparative behaviour of mammalian eggs in vivo and in vitro. *J Exp Med* 62:655, 1935

149. Chang MC: The maturation of rabbit oocytes in culture and their maturation, activation, fertilization and subsequent development in fallopian tube. *J Exp Zool* 128:378, 1955

150. Foote WD, Thibault C: Recherches experimentales sur la maturation in vitro des ovocytes de truie et de veau. *Ann Biol Anim Biochem Biophys* 9:329, 1969

151. Tsafriri A, Channing CP: An inhibitory influence of granulosa cells and follicular fluid upon porcine oocyte meiosis in vitro. *Endocrinology* 96:922, 1975

152. Sato E, Ishibashi T: Meiotic arresting action of the substance obtained from cell surface to porcine ovarian granulosa cells. *Jpn J Zootech Sci* 48:22, 1977

153. Leibfried L, First NL: Effect of bovine and porcine follicular fluid and granulosa cells on maturation of oocyte in vitro. *Biol Reprod* 23:699, 1980

154. Leibfried L, First NL: Follicular control of meiosis in the porcine oocyte. *Biol Reprod* 23:705, 1980

155. Lefévre B, Góugeon A, Peronny H, Testart J: Effect of cumulus cell mass and follicle quality on in-vitro maturation of cynomolgus monkey oocytes. *Hum Reprod* 3:891, 1988

156. Tsafriri A, Pomerantz SH, Channing CP: Porcine follicular fluid inhibitor of oocyte meiosis: Partial characterization of the inhibitor. *Biol Reprod* 14:511, 1976

157. Racowsky C, Baldwin KV: *In vitro* and *in vivo* studies reveal that hamster oocyte meiotic arrest is maintained only transiently by follicular fluid but persistently by membrane/cumulus granulosa cell contact. *Dev Biol* 134:297, 1989

158. Fleming AD, Kuehl TJ, Armstrong DT: Maturation of pig and rat oocytes transplanted into surrogate pig follicles in vitro. *Gamete Res* 11:107, 1985

159. Tsafriri A, Bar-Ami S: Oocyte maturation inhibitor: A 1981 perspective. *Adv Exp Med Biol* 47:145, 1982

160. Van de Wiel DFM, Bar-Ami S, Tsafriri A, de Jong FH: Oocyte maturation inhibitor, inhibin and steroid concentrations in porcine follicular fluid at various stages of the oestrous cycle. *J Reprod Fertil* 68:247, 1983

161. Winter-Sorgen S, Brown J, Ono T, et al: Oocyte maturation inhibitor activity in human follicular fluid: Quantitative determination in unstimulated and clomiphene citrate- and human menopausal gonadotropin-stimulated ovarian cycles. *J In Vitro Fertil Embryo Transf* 3:218, 1986

162. Ueno S, Manganaro TF, Donahoe PK: Human recombinant müllerian inhibiting substance inhibition of rat oocyte meiosis is reversed by epidermal growth factor in vitro. *Endocrinology* 123:1652, 1988

163. O, W-S, Robertson DM, de Kretser DM: Inhibin as an oocyte meiotic inhibitor. *Mol Cell Endocrinol* 62:307, 1989

164. Buscaglia M, Fuller F, Mazzola T, et al: A new intra-ovarian function for follistain: The inhibition of oocyte meiosis [abstract]. *Proc Endocr Soc USA* 71 (abstract 883), 1989

165. Yoshimura Y, Nagamatsu S, Ando M, et al: Insulin-like growth factor binding protein-3 inhibits gonadotropin-induced ovulation, oocyte maturation, and steroidogenesis in rabbit ovary. *Endocrinology* 137:438, 1996

166. Eppig JJ, Ward-Bailey PF, Coleman DL: Hypoxanthine and adenosine in murine ovarian follicular fluid: Concentrations and activity in maintaining oocyte meiotic arrest. *Biol Reprod* 33:1041, 1985

167. Downs SM, Coleman DL, Ward-Bailey PF, Eppig JJ: Hypoxanthine is the principal inhibitor of murine oocyte maturation in a low molecular weight fraction of porcine follicular fluid. *Proc Natl Acad Sci USA* 82:454, 1985

168. Sirard MA, Bilodeau S: Effects of granulosa cell co-culture on in-vitro meiotic resumption of bovine oocytes. *J Reprod Fertil* 89:459, 1990

169. Cho WK, Stern S, Biggers JD: Inhibitory effect of dibutyryl cAMP on mouse oocyte maturation in vitro. *J Exp Zool* 187:383, 1974

170. Dekel N, Beers WH: Rat oocyte maturation in vitro: Relief of cyclic AMP inhibition by gonadotropins. *Proc Natl Acad Sci USA* 75:3469, 1978

171. Homa ST: Effects of cyclic AMP on the spontaneous meiotic maturation of cumulus-free bovine oocyte cultured in chemically defined medium. *J Exp Zool* 248:222, 1988

172. Rice C, McGaughey RW: Effect of testosterone and dibutyryl cAMP on the spontaneous maturation of pig oocytes. *J Reprod Fertil* 62:245, 1981

173. Warikoo PK, Bavister BD: Hypoxanthin and cyclic adenosine 5′-monophosphate maintain meiotic arrest of rhesus monkey oocytes in vitro. *Fertil Steril* 51:886, 1989

174. Tornell J, Hillensjo T: Effect of cAMP on the isolated human oocyte–cumulus complex. *Hum Reprod* 8:737, 1993

175. Schultz RM, Montgomery RR, Belanoff JR: Regulation of mouse oocyte meiotic maturation: Implication of a decrease in oocyte cAMP and protein dephosphorylation in commitment to resume meiosis. *Dev Biol* 97:264, 1983

176. Vivarelli E, Conti M, De Felici M, Siracusa G: Meiotic resumption and intracellular cAMP levels in mouse oocytes treated with compounds which act on cAMP metabolism. *Cell Differ* 12:271, 1983

177. Downs SM, Eppig JJ: Induction of mouse oocyte maturation in vivo by perturbants of purine metabolism. *Biol Reprod* 36:431, 1987

178. Downs SM, Daniel SAJ, Bornslaeger EA, Hoppe PC, Eppig JJ: Maintenance of meiotic arrest in mouse oocytes by purine. *Gamete Res* 23:323, 1989

179. Racowsky C: Effect of forskolin on the spontaneous maturation and cyclic AMP content of rat oocyte cumulus complexes. *J Reprod Fertil* 72:107, 1984

180. Salustri A, Petrungaros S, de Felici M, Conti M, Siracusa D: Effect of follicle-stimulating hormone on cyclic adenosine monophosphate level and on meiotic maturation in mouse cumulus cell-enclosed oocyte cultured in vitro. *Biol Reprod* 33:797, 1985

181. Lindner HR, Tsafriri A, Lieberman ME, et al: Gonadotropin action on cultured graafian follicles: Mechanism of induction of maturation of the mammalian oocyte. *Recent Prog Horm Res* 30:79, 1974

182. Hillensjö T: Oocyte maturation and glycolysis in isolated preovulatory follicles of PMS-injected immature rats. *Acta Endocrinol* 82:809, 1976

183. Tsafriri A, Lindner HR, Zor U, Lamprecht SA: In vitro induction of meiotic division in follicle-enclosed rat oocytes by LH cyclic AMP and prostaglandin E$_2$. *J Reprod Fertil* 31:39, 1972

184. Hillensjö T, Ekholm C, Ahrén K: Role of cyclic AMP in oocyte maturation and glycolysis in the preovulatory rat follicle. *Acta Endocrinol* 87:377, 1978

185. Dekel N, Lawrence TS, Gilula NB, Beers WH: Modulation of cell-to-cell communication in the cumulus–oocyte complex and the regulation of oocyte maturation by LH. *Dev Biol* 86:356, 1981

186. Dekel N, Galiani D, Sherizly I: Dissociation between the inhibitory and the stimulatory action of cAMP on maturation of rat oocytes. *Mol Cell Endocrinol* 56:115, 1988

187. Motlik J, Fulka J, Flechon JE: Changes in intercellular coupling between pig oocytes and cumulus cells during in vivo and in vitro maturation. *J Reprod Fertil* 76:32, 1986

188. Racowsky C, Baldwin KV, Larabell CA, DeMarais AA, Kazilek CJ: Down-regulation of membrane granulosa cell gap junctions is correlated with irreversible commitment to resume meiosis in gold syrian hamster oocytes. *Eur J Cell Biol* 49:244, 1989

189. Goldschmit D, Kraicer P, Orly J: Periovulatory expression of cholesterol side-chain cleavage cytochrome P-450 in cumulus cells. *Endocrinology* 124:369, 1989

190. Salustri A, Yanagishita M, Hascall VC: Mouse oocytes regulate hyaluronic acid synthesis and mucification by FSH-stimulated cumulus cells. *Dev Biol* 138:26, 1990

191. Mattioli M, Galeati G, Bacci ML, Seren E: Follicular factors influence oocyte fertilizability by modulating the intercellular cooperation between cumulus cells and oocyte. *Gamete Res* 21:223, 1988

192. Staigmiller RB, Moor RM: Effect of follicle cells on the maturation and developmental competence of bovine oocytes matured outside the follicle. *Gamete Res* 9:221, 1984

193. Thibault C: Are follicular maturation and oocyte maturation independent processes? *J Reprod Fertil* 51:1, 1977

193a. Hensleigh HC, Hunter AG: In vitro maturation of bovine cumulus-enclosed primary oocytes and their subsequent in vitro fertilization and cleavage. *J Dairy Sci* 88:1456, 1985

194. Gordon I, Lu KH: Production of embryos in vitro and its impact on livestock production. *Theriogenology* 33:77, 1990

195. Lanzendorf SE, Zelinski-Wooten MB, Stouffer RL, Wolf DP: Maturity of collection and the developmental potential of rhesus monkey oocytes. *Biol Reprod* 42:703, 1990

196. Seibel MM, Smith D, Levesque L, Borten M, Taymor ML: The temporal relationship between the luteinizing hormone surge and human oocyte maturation. *Am J Obstet Gynecol* 142:568, 1982

197. Jamieson ME, Fleming R, Kader S, Ross KS, Yates RW, Coutts JR: In vivo and in vitro maturation of human oocytes: Effects on embryo development and polyspermic fertilization. *Fertil Steril* 56:93, 1991

198. Yoshimura Y, Hosoi Y, Atlas SJ, Bongiovanni AM, Santulli A, Wallach EE: The effect of ovarian steroidogenesis on ovulation and fertilizability in the in vitro perfused rabbit ovary. *Biol Reprod* 35:943, 1986

199. Zelinski-Wooten MB, Hess DL, Wolf DP, Stouffer RL: Steroid reduction during ovarian stimulation impairs oocyte fertilization, but not folliculogenesis, in rhesus monkeys. *Fertil Steril* 61:1147, 1994

200. Zelinski-Wooten MB, Hess DL, Baughman WL, Molskness TA, Wolf DP, Stouffer RL: Administration of an aromatase inhibitor during the late follicular phase of gonadotropin-treated cycles in rhesus monkeys: Effects on follicle development, oocyte maturation, and subsequent luteal function. *J Clin Endocrinol Metab* 76:988, 1993

201. Bar-Ami S: Increasing progesterone secretion and 3β-hydroxysteroid dehydrogenase activity of human cumulus cells and granulosa-lutein cells concurrent with successful fertilization of the corresponding oocyte. *J Steroid Biochem Mol Biol* 51:299, 1994

202. Wu TC, Wang L, Wan YJ: Detection of estrogen receptor messenger ribonucleic acid in human oocytes and cumulus–oocyte complexes using reverse transcriptase-polymerase chain reaction. *Fertil Steril* 59:54, 1993

203. Tesarik J, Mendoza C: Nongenomic effects of 17β-estradiol on maturing human oocytes: Relationship to oocyte developmental potential. *J Clin Endocrinol Metab* 80:1438, 1995

204. Seibel MM, Smith D, Dlugi AM, Levesque L: Periovulatory follicular fluid hormone levels in spontaneous human cycles. *J Clin Endocrinol Metab* 68:1073, 1989

205. Seibel MM, Smith DM: The effect of clomiphene citrate on human preovulatory oocyte maturation in vivo. *J In Vitro Fertil Embryo Transf* 6:3, 1989

206. Suchanek E, Simunic V, Juretic D, Grizely V: Follicular fluid contents of hyaluronic acid, follicle-stimulating hormone and steroids relative to the success of in vitro fertilization of human oocytes. *Fertil Steril* 62:347, 1994

207. Tarlatzis BC, Laufer N, DeCherney AH, Polan ML, Haseltine FP, Behrman HR: Adenosine 3′,5′-monophosphate levels in human follicular fluid: Relationship to oocyte maturation and achievement of pregnancy after in vitro fertilization. *J Clin Endocrinol Metab* 60:1111, 1985

208. Brzyski RG, Hofmann GE, Scott RT, Jones HW: Effects of leuprolide acetate on follicular fluid hormone composition at oocyte retrieval for in vitro fertilization. *Fertil Steril* 54:842, 1990

209. Lee MS, Ben-Rafael Z, Meloni F, Mastroianni L Jr, Flickinger GL: Relationship of human oocyte maturity, fertilization, and cleavage to follicular fluid prolactin and steroids. *J In Vitro Fertil Embryo Transf* 4:168, 1987

210. Jeremy JY, Okonofua FE, Thomas M, et al: Oocyte maturity and human follicular fluid prostanoids, gonadotropins and prolactin after administration of clomiphene and pergonal. *J Clin Endocrinol Metab* 65:402, 1987

211. Bodis J, Hartmann G, Torok A, et al: Relationship between the monoamine and gonadotropin content in follicular fluid of preovulatory graafian follicles after superovulation treatment. *Exp Clin Endocrinol* 101:178, 1993

212. Lindner C, Lichtenberg U, Westhof G, Braendle W, Bettendorf G: Endocrine parameters of human follicular fluid and fertilization capacity of oocytes. *Horm Metab Res* 20:243, 1988

213. Laufer N, Botero-Ruiz W, DeCherney AH, Haseltine F, Polan ML, Behrman HR: Gonadotropin and prolactin levels in follicular fluid of human ova successfully fertilized in vitro. *J Clin Endocrinol Metab* 58:430, 1984

214. Alak BM, Wolf DP: Rhesus monkey oocyte maturation and fertilization in vitro: Roles of the menstrual cycle phase and of exogenous gonadotropins. *Biol Reprod* 51:879, 1994

215. Reinthaller A, Deutinger J, Riss P, et al: Relationship between the steroid and prolactin concentration in follicular fluid and the maturation and fertilization of human oocytes. *J In Vitro Fertil Embryo Transf* 4:228, 1987

216. Roussi M, Royere M, Guillonueau M, Lansac J, Muh JP: Human antral fluid IGF-I and oocyte maturity: Effect of stimulation therapy. *Acta Endocrinol* 121:90, 1989

217. Maruo T, Ladines-Llave CA, Samoto T, et al: Expression of epidermal growth factor and its receptor in the human ovary during follicular growth and regression. *Endocrinology* 132:924, 1993

218. Hillensjö T, LeMaire WJ: Gonadotropin-releasing hormone agonists stimulate meiotic maturation of follicle-enclosed rat oocytes in vitro. *Nature* 287:145, 1980

219. Aberdam E, Dekel N: Activators of protein kinase C stimulate meiotic maturation of rat oocytes. *Biochem Biophys Res Commun* 132:570, 1985

220. Dekel N, Sherizly I: Epidermal growth factor induces maturation of rat follicle-enclosed oocytes. *Endocrinology* 116:406, 1985

221. La Polt PS, Yamoto M, Veljkovic M, et al: Basic fibroblast growth factor induction of granulosa cell tissue-type plasminogen activator expression and oocyte maturation: Potential role as a paracrine ovarian hormone. *Endocrinology* 127:2357, 1990

222. Hashimoto N, Kishimoto T: Regulation of meiotic metaphase by a cytoplasmic maturation-promoting factor during mouse oocyte maturation. *Dev Biol* 126:242, 1988

223. Mattioli M, Galeati G, Bacci ML, Barboni B: Changes in maturation promoting activity in the cytoplasm of pig oocytes throughout maturation. *Mol Reprod Dev* 30:119, 1991

224. Choi T, Aoki F, Mori M, Yamashita M, Nagahama Y, Kohmoto K: Activation of p34^{cdc2} protein kinase activity in meiotic and mitotic cell cycles in mouse oocytes and embryos. *Development* 113:789, 1991

225. Verlhac M-H, Kubiak JZ, Weber M, et al: MOS is required for MAP kinase activation and is involved in microtubule organization during meiotic maturation in the mouse. *Development* 122:815, 1996

226. Pal SK, Torry D, Serta R, et al: Expression and potential function of the c-mos proto-oncogene in human eggs. *Fertil Steril* 61:496, 1994

227. Ryle M: A quantitative in vitro response to follicle stimulating hormone. *J Reprod Fertil* 19:87, 1969

228. Ryle M: The time factor in response to pituitary gonadotropins by mouse ovaries in vitro. *J Reprod Fertil* 25:61, 1971

229. Roy SK, Greenwald GS: An enzymatic method for dissociation of intact follicles from the hamster ovary: Histological and quantitative aspects. *Biol Reprod* 32:203, 1985

230. Torrance C, Telfer E, Gosden RG: Quantitative study of the development of isolated mouse pre-antral follicles in collagen gel culture. *J Reprod Fertil* 87:367, 1989

231. Gore-Langton RE, Daniel SAJ: Follicle-stimulating hormone and estradiol regulate antrum like reorganization of granulosa cells in rat preantral follicle culture. *Biol Reprod* 43:65, 1990

232. Zhang J, Liu J, Xu KP, Liu B, DiMattina M: Extracorporal development and ultrarapid freezing of human fetal ova. *J Assist Reprod Genet* 12:361, 1995

233. Qvist R, Blackwell LF, Bourne H, Brown JB: Development of mouse ovarian follicles from primary to preovulatory stages in vitro. *J Reprod Fertil* 89:169, 1990

234. Eppig JJ: Maintenance of meiotic arrest and induction of oocyte maturation in mouse oocyte–granulosa cell complexes developed in vitro from preantral follicles. *Biol Reprod* 45:824, 1991

235. Boland NI, Humpherson PG, Leese HJ, Gosden RG: The pattern of lactate production and steroidogenesis during growth and maturation of mouse ovarian follicles in vitro. *Biol Reprod* 48:798, 1993

236. Hartshorne GM, Sargent IL, Barlow DH: Meiotic progression of mouse oocytes throughout follicle growth and ovulation in vitro. *Hum Reprod* 9:352, 1994

237. Smyth CD, Gosden RG, McNeilly AS, Hillier SG: Effect of in-

hibin immunoneutralization on steroidogenesis in rat ovarian follicles in vitro. *J Endocrinol* 140:437, 1994

238. Hartshorne GM, Sargent IL, Barlow DH: Growth rates and antrum formation of mouse ovarian follicles in vitro in response to follicle-stimulating hormone, relaxin, cyclic AMP and hypoxanthine. *Hum Reprod* 9:1003, 1994

239. Roy SK, Treacy BJ: Isolation and long-term culture of human preantral follicles. *Fertil Steril* 59:783, 1993

240. Moor RM, Trounson AO: Hormonal and follicular factors affecting maturation of sheep oocytes in vitro and their subsequent development capacity. *J Reprod Fertil* 49:101, 1977

241. Castle WE, Phillips JC: On germinal transplantation in vertebrates. Washington DC, Carnegie Institute, Publ no. 144, 1911

242. Deanesly R: Immature rat ovaries grafted after freezing and thawing. *J Endocrinol* 2:197, 1954

243. Parker AS: Grafting of mouse ovarian tissue after freezing and thawing. *J Endocrinol* 14:xxi, 1956

244. Parrott DMV: The fertility of mice with orthotopic ovarian grafts derived from frozen tissue. *J Reprod Fertil* 1:230, 1960

245. Telfer E, Torrance C, Gosden RG: Morphological study of cultured preantral ovarian follicles of mice after transplantation under the kidney capsule. *J Reprod Fertil* 89:565, 1990

246. Gosden RG: Restitution of fertility in sterilized mice by transferring primordial ovarian follicles. *Hum Reprod* 5:117, 1990

247. Carroll J, Whittingham DG, Wood MJ, Telfer E, Gosden RG: Extra-ovarian production of mature viable mouse oocytes from frozen primary follicles. *J Reprod Fertil* 90:321, 1990

248. Gosden RG: Extra-ovarian production of mature viable mouse oocytes from frozen primary follicles. *J Reprod Fertil* 90:321, 1990

249. Carroll J, Gosden RG: Transplantation of frozen-thawed mouse primordial follicles. *Hum Reprod* 8:1163, 1993

250. Whittingham DG: Fertilization in vitro and development to term of unfertilized mouse oocytes previously stored at −196°C. *J Reprod Fertil* 49:89, 1977

251. Schroeder AC, Champlin AK, Mobraaten LE, Eppig JJ: Developmental capacity of mouse oocytes cryopreserved before and after maturation in vitro. *J Reprod Fertil* 89:43, 1990

252. Carroll J, Wood MJ, Whittingham DG: Normal fertilization and development of frozen-thawed mouse oocytes: Protective action of certain macromolecules. *Biol Reprod* 48:606, 1993

253. Sathanathan AH, Trounson A, Freeman L, Brady T: The effect of cooling human oocytes. *Hum Reprod* 332:724, 1988

254. Pickering SJ, Braude PR, Johnson MH, Cant A, Currie J: Transient cooling to room temperature can cause irreversible disruption of the meiotic spindle in human oocyte. *Fertil Steril* 54:102, 1990

255. Hunter JE, Bernard A, Fuller B, Amso N, Shaw RW: Fertilization and development of the human oocyte following exposure to cryoprotectants, low temperatures and cryopreservation: A comparison of two techniques. *Hum Reprod* 6:1460, 1991

256. Bernard A, Hunter JE, Fuller BJ, Imoedemhe D, Curtis P, Jackson A: Fertilization and embryonic development of human oocytes after cooling. *Hum Reprod* 7:1447, 1992

257. Pensis M, Loumaye E, Psalti I: Screening of conditions for rapid freezing of human oocytes: Preliminary study toward their cryopreservation. *Fertil Steril* 52:787, 1989

258. Masui Y: The role of cytostatic factor (CSF) in the control of oocyte cell cycles: A summary of 20 years of study. *Dev Growth Diff* 33:543, 1991

259. Mehlmann LM, Terasaki M, Jaffe LA, Kline D: Reorganization of the endoplasmic reticulum during meiotic maturation of the mouse oocyte. *Dev Biol* 170:607, 1995

260. Zilberstein M, Seibel MM: Fertilization and implantation. *Curr Opin Obstet Gynecol* 6:184, 1994

261. Verlhac MH, Kubiak JZ, Clarke HJ, Maro B: Microtubule and chromatin behavior follow MAP kinase activity but not MPF activity during meiosis in mouse oocytes. *Development* 120:1017, 1994

262. Schultz RM, Kopf GS: Molecular basis of mammalian egg activation. *Curr Top Dev Biol* 30:21, 1995

263. Longo FJ, Chen DY: Development of cortical polarity in mouse egg: Involvement of meiotic apparatus. *Dev Biol* 107:382, 1985

264. Gorbsky GJ, Simerly C, Schatten G, Borisy GG: Microtubules in the metaphase-arrested mouse oocyte turn over rapidly. *Proc Natl Acad Sci USA* 87:6049, 1990

265. Schatten G, Simerly C, Asai DJ, Szöke E, Cooke P, Schatten H: Acetylated tubulin in microtubules during mouse fertilization and early development. *Dev Biol* 130:74, 1988

266. Pluta AF, Cooke CA, Earnshaw WC: Structure of the human centromere at metaphase. *Trends Biochem Sci* 15:181, 1990

267. Simerly C, Balczon R, Brinkley BR, Schatten G: Microinjected kinetochore antibodies interfere with chromosome movement in meiotic and mitotic mouse oocytes. *J Cell Biol* 111:1491, 1990

268. Maro B, Howlett SK, Houliston E: Cytoskeleton dynamics in the mitotic cycle. *J Cell Sci* 5(Suppl):343, 1986

269. Schatten H, Schatten G, Mazia D, Balczon R, Simerly C: Behavior of centrosomes during fertilization and cell division in mouse oocytes and in sea urchin eggs. *Proc Natl Acad Sci USA* 83:105, 1986

270. Messinger SM, Albertini DF: Centrosome and microtubule dynamics during meiotic progression in the mouse oocyte. *J Cell Sci* 100:289, 1991

271. Longo FJ: Sperm aster in rabbit zygotes: Its structure and function. *J Cell Biol* 69:539, 1976

272. Yllera-Fernandez MDM, Crozet N, Ahmed-Ali M: Microtubule distribution during fertilization in the rabbit. *Mol Reprod Dev* 32:271, 1992

273. Schatten G: The centrosome and its mode of inheritance: The reduction of the centrosome during gametogenesis and its restoration during fertilization. *Dev Biol* 165:299, 1994

274. Sathanathan AH, Osbourne IKJ, Trounson A, Bongso SC, Ng A, Ratnam SS: Centrioles in the beginning of human development. *Proc Natl Acad Sci USA* 88:4806, 1991

275. Asch R, Simerly C, Ord T, Ord VA, Schatten G: The stages at which human fertilization arrests: Microtubule and chromosome configurations in inseminated oocytes which failed to complete fertilization and development in humans. *Hum Reprod* 10:1897, 1995

276. Hewitson LC, Simerly CR, Tengowski MW, et al: Microtubule

and DNA configuration during rhesus intracytoplasmic sperm injection: Successes and failures. 1996 (in press)

277. Wu J-G, Simerly C, Zoran S, Navara C, Gerrity M, Schatten G: Microtubule organization in the rhesus monkey during fertilization, polyspermy and parthenogenesis and in mature human oocytes. *Mol Cell Biol* 4(Suppl):142, 1993

278. Schatten H, Simerly C, Maul G, Schatten G: Microtubule assembly is required for the formation of the pronuclei, nuclear lamin acquisition and DNA synthesis during mouse but not sea urchin fertilization. *Gamete Res* 23:309, 1989

279. Kola I, Trounson A, Dawson G, Rogers P: Tripronuclear human oocytes: Altered cleavage patterns and subsequent karyotypic analysis of embryos. *Biol Reprod* 37:395, 1989

280. Van Blerkom J, Henry G: Dispermic fertilization of human oocytes. *J Electron Microsc Technique* 17:437, 1991

281. Crozet N: Behaviour of the sperm centriole during sheep oocyte fertilization. *Eur J Cell Biol* 53:321, 1990

282. Navara CS, First NL, Schatten G: Microtubule organization in the cow during fertilization polyspermy parthenogenesis and nuclear transfer: The role of the sperm after aster. *Dev Biol* 162:29, 1994

283. Pickering SJ, Johnson MH, Braude PR, Houliston E: Cytoskeletal organization in fresh, aged and spontaneously activated human oocytes. *Hum Reprod* 3:978, 1988

284. Simerly C, Wu G-J, Zoran S, et al: The paternal inheritance of the centrosome, the cell's microtubule-organizing center, in human, and the implications for infertility. *Nature* 1:47, 1995

285. Félix M-A, Antony C, Wright M, Maro B: Centrosome assembly in vitro. *J Cell Biol* 124:19, 1994

286. Stearns T, Kirschner M: In vitro reconstitution of centrosome assembly and function: The central role of γ-tubulin. *Cell* 76:623, 1994

287. Zoran S, Simerly C, Schoff P, Stearns T, Salisbury J, Schatten G: Reconstitution of human sperm centrosome in vitro. *Mol Cell Biol* 5:38a, 1994

288. Ducibella T, Kurasawa S, Rangarajan S, Kopf G, Schultz R: Precocious loss of cortical granules during mouse oocyte meiotic maturation and correlation with an egg-induced modification of the zona pellucida. *Dev Biol* 137:46, 1990

289. Maro B, Johnson MH, Pickering SJ, Flach G: Changes in actin distribution during fertilization of the mouse egg. *J Embryol Exp Morphol* 81:211, 1984

290. Schatten G, Schatten H, Spector I, et al: Latrunculin inhibits the microfilament-mediated processes during fertilization, cleavage, and early development in sea urchins and mice. *Exp Cell Res* 166:191, 1986

291. Kruip TAM, Crar DG, Van Benden TH, Dieleman SJ: Structural changes in bovine oocyte during final maturation in vivo. *Gamete Res* 8:29, 1983

292. Johnson LD, Mattson BA, Albertini DF, et al: Quality of oocytes from superovulated rhesus monkeys. *Hum Reprod* 6:623, 1991

293. Santella L, Alikani M, Talansky BE, Cohen J, Dale B: Is the human oocyte plasma membrane polarized? *Hum Reprod* 7:999, 1992

294. Le Guen P, Crozet N, Huneau D, Gail L: Distribution and role of microfilaments during early events of sheep fertilization. *Gamete Res* 22:411, 1989

295. Sathanathan AH, Trounson AO, Wood C: *Atlas of Fine Structure of Human Sperm Penetration: Eggs and Embryos Cultured in Vitro.* New York, Praeger, 1986

296. Verlinsky Y, Cieslak J, Freidine M, et al: Pregnancies following pre-conception diagnosis of common aneuploidies by fluorescent in-situ hybridization. *Hum Reprod* 10:1923, 1995

297. Dyban A, Freidine M, Severova E, Cieslak J, Ivakhnenko V, Verlinsky Y: Detection of aneuploidy in human oocytes and corresponding first polar bodies by fluorescent in situ hybridization. *J Assist Reprod Genet* 13:73, 1996

298. Munné S, Dailey T, Sultan KM, Grifo J, Cohen J: The use of first polar bodies for preimplantation diagnosis of aneuploidy. *Hum Reprod* 10:1014, 1995

299. Cozzi J, Chevret E, Rousseau S, Pelletier R, Séle B: Human sperm chromosome analysis after microinjection into hamster oocytes. *J Assist Reprod Genet* 12:384, 1995

300. Clarke HJ, Masui Y: Transformation of sperm nuclei to metaphase chromosomes in the cytoplasm of maturing oocyte of the mouse. *J Cell Biol* 102:1039, 1986

301. Calafell JM, Badenas J, Catala V, Egozcue J, Santalo J: Premature chromosome condensation (PCC) as a sign of oocyte immaturity [abstract]. *Hum Reprod* 78(Suppl):(abstract 251), 1990

302. Schmiady H, Kentenich H: Premature chromosome condensation after in vitro fertilization. *Hum Reprod* 4:689, 1989

303. Tesarik J, Kopency V: Developmental control of the human male pronucleus by ooplasmic factors. *Hum Reprod* 4:962, 1989

304. Selva J, Martin-Pont B, Hugues JN, et al: Cytogenetic study of human oocytes uncleaved after in-vitro fertilization. *Hum Reprod* 6:709, 1991

305. Bergere M, Selva J, Volante M, et al: Cytogenetic analysis of uncleaved oocytes after intra-cytoplasmic sperm injection. *J Assist Reprod Genet* 12:322, 1995

306. Plachot M, Crozet N: Fertilization abnormalities in human in vitro fertilization. *Hum Reprod* 7:89, 1992

307. Ozil JP: The parthenogenetic development of rabbit oocytes after repetitive pulsatile electrical stimulation. *Development* 109:117, 1990

308. Kaufman MH, Barton SC, Surani MAH: Normal postimplantation development of mouse parthenogenic embryos to the forelimb bud stage. *Nature* 265:53, 1977

309. Winston N, Johnson M, Pickering S, Brande P: Parthenogenetic activation and development of fresh and aged human oocytes. *Fertil Steril* 56:904, 1991

310. Van Blerkom J, Davis PW, Merriam J: A retrospective analysis of unfertilized and presumed parthenogenetically activated human oocytes demonstrating a high frequency of sperm penetration. *Hum Reprod* 9:2381, 1994

311. Pickering SJ, Taylor A, Johnson MH, Braude PR: An analysis of multinucleated blastomere formation in human embryos. *Hum Reprod* 10:1912, 1995

312. Navara CS, First NL, Schatten G: Program in Cell and Molecular

Biology, Department of Zoology, University of Wisconsin, Madison, WI 53706, USA. Phenotypic variations among paternal centrosomes expressed within the zygote as disparate microtubule lengths and sperm aster organization: Correlations between centrosome activity and developmental success. *Proceedings of the National Academy of Sciences of the United States of America.* 93:5384, May 28, 1996

313. Fukui Y, Glew AM, Gandolfi F, Moor RM: Ram-specific effects on in vitro fertilization and cleavage of sheep oocytes matured in vitro. *J Reprod Fertil* 82:337, 1988

314. Austin CR, Walton A: Fertilization. In: Parks AS (ed), *Marshall's Physiology of Reproduction,* vol I, part 2. London, Longmans Green, 1960:310–416

315. Hirao Y, Yanagimachi R: Development of pronuclei in polyspermic eggs of the golden hamster: Is there any limit to the number of sperm heads that are capable of developing into male pronuclei? *Zool Mag* 88:24, 1979

316. Thibault C, Gerard M: Cytoplasmic and nuclear maturation of rabbit oocytes in vitro. *Ann Biol Anim Biochem Biophys* 13:145, 1973

317. Trounson A, Webb J: Fertilization of human oocyte following reinsemination in vitro. *Fertil Steril* 41:816, 1984

CHAPTER 6

Anovulation and Amenorrhea

JUDITH L. VAITUKAITIS

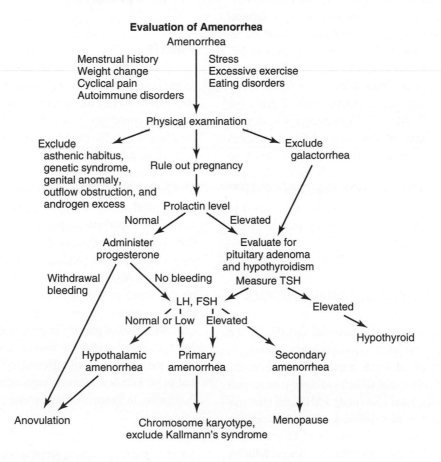

Evaluation of Amenorrhea

Amenorrhea

Menstrual history
Weight change
Cyclical pain
Autoimmune disorders

Stress
Excessive exercise
Eating disorders

Physical examination

Exclude
asthenic habitus,
genetic syndrome,
genital anomaly,
outflow obstruction, and
androgen excess

Rule out pregnancy

Exclude
galactorrhea

Prolactin level

Normal

Elevated

Administer
progesterone

Evaluate for
pituitary adenoma
and hypothyroidism

Withdrawal
bleeding

No bleeding

Measure TSH

LH, FSH

Elevated

Normal or Low

Elevated

Hypothyroid

Hypothalamic
amenorrhea

Primary
amenorrhea

Secondary
amenorrhea

Anovulation

Chromosome karyotype,
exclude Kallmann's syndrome

Menopause

The normal menstrual cycle reflects carefully regulated interactions among the hypothalamus, pituitary gland, and ovaries. Modulators of gonadotropin secretion include sex steroids, secreted by the ovaries, and gonadotropin-releasing hormone (GnRH), a decapeptide synthesized and secreted by hypothalamic peptidergic neurons. In addition, a host of other peptide and biogenic amines modulate GnRH neuron function.[1-3] Nutrition, stress, physical activity, abnormalities of the central nervous system, and systemic illness may adversely affect gonadotropin secretion through poorly defined mechanisms and induce menstrual dysfunction ranging from an irregular menstrual pattern to anovulation to amenorrhea.[4-7]

FETAL OVARIAN DEVELOPMENT

Early in fetal life, germ cells migrate to the primitive ovary and proliferate so that by the tenth week of fetal life the ovary contains 5 to 7 million oogonia. To protect oogonia from accelerated degeneration and atresia, a layer of progranulosa cells must surround the oocyte, forming a primordial follicle. With stimulation by follicle-stimulating hormone (FSH), the layer of flattened granulosa cells becomes cuboidal and forms a structure known as a *primary follicle*. Once follicles are formed, they undergo atresia even with the protective layer of granulosa cells. At birth only 1 to 2 million follicles persist. Atresia continues, so that by the expected time of onset of spontaneous menses, only 300,000 to 400,000 follicles remain. When no gonadotropin-responsive follicles remain in the ovaries, primary gonadal failure results and usually signals menopause.[8,9]

In the Western world, spontaneous menopause occurs in the early to middle 50s. Women with primary ovarian failure before age 40 have premature menopause.[10,11]

ONSET OF HYPOTHALAMIC-PITUITARY-OVARIAN FEEDBACK

Coincident with the formation of primordial follicles by the 20th week of gestation, fetal pituitary gonadotropin synthesis is evident and fetal FSH blood levels approach castrate levels. With differentiation of primordial follicles to those with several layers of granulosa cells, fetal circulating FSH concentrations decline, signaling the onset of negative feedback between the hypothalamic-pituitary axis and the ovaries.[12] Gonadotropin synthesis and secretion decrease thereafter, but ovarian follicles continue to undergo growth and atresia. Fetal ovarian follicular growth depends on fetal gonadotropin stimulation, since ovaries of the anencephalic fetus contain only primordial and primary follicles, reflecting abnormal hypothalamic-pituitary function in the anencephalic fetus.[13]

Cells of ovarian follicles synthesize a host of peptides, which some investigators suggest may modulate pituitary gonadotropin secretion. More than likely, they modulate ovarian function locally through a paracrine mechanism. Those peptides include inhibin, epidermal growth factor (EGF), and GnRH-like peptide.[14-16]

NEONATAL AND PREPUBERTAL GIRL

At birth only 1 to 2 million ovarian follicles remain. For the first 1 to 2 years after birth, girls have slightly elevated levels of circulating gonadotropin and sex steroids.[17] The physiologic mechanism responsible for the increased hypothalamic-pituitary-ovarian activity is unknown. After the first year or two, circulating gonadotropin levels remain tonically low until the onset of puberty.

PUBERTY

In the United States and other Western countries, menarche, or the onset of the first menses, occurs at a mean age of 13.5 years, with 95% confidence limits of 11 to 16 years. If menarche occurs before age 10, an abnormality exists and the patient has precocious puberty. If the onset of menses is delayed beyond the 16th year, the girl has a form of primary amenorrhea. Menarche is one pubertal milestone. Puberty reflects a closely orchestrated series of dynamic physiologic events integrated among the hypothalamic-pituitary axis and higher central nervous system sites. Puberty occurs over 3 to 5 years. The first sign is usually breast budding, normally observed at a mean age of 11 years. Approximately 6 months after breast budding, pubic hair develops. For approximately 20% of healthy girls, pubic hair growth is the first sign of puberty. Table 6–1 summarizes the stages of puberty in girls, with the expected mean age and age range for onset. Whenever a young patient is amenorrheic, the clinician should document Tanner staging[18] of breast and pubic hair development, especially if the girl is a teenager. A disparity in Tanner staging by more than one stage for breast

This chapter was written by Dr. Vaitukaitis in her private capacity. Official support or endorsement by the Division of Research Resources, National Institutes of Health, is not intended, nor should it be inferred.

TABLE 6–1. STAGING OF PUBERTAL EVENTS IN GIRLS

Event	Mean Age(y)	Range
Breast budding	11.2	9–13.5
Pubic and axillary hair growth	11.7	9–14.5
Menarche	13.5	11–16
Adult-pattern pubic hair	14.4	
Adult breast development	15.3	

and pubic hair development may be a clinical clue to an underlying developmental defect of the internal genitalia or a sign of abnormal sex steroid synthesis or action.

With the onset of normal puberty, daytime or nighttime sleep-induced secretion of both FSH and luteinizing hormone (LH) occurs.[19,20] The frequency of LH secretory pulses ranges between 75 and 100 minutes, similar to that for the rapid eye movement–nonrapid eye movement (REM-NREM) sleep cycle[19] (Fig 6–1). The increased gonadotropin levels are the result of increased amplitude and frequency of gonadotropin secretory pulses. The anatomic site of the "neuronal switch" that mediates gonadotropin pulsatile secretion with sleep during puberty is unknown. With completion of puberty sleep-induced release of gonadotropin subsides. That pattern may return with selected pathophysiologic states, for example, anorexia nervosa. Circulating levels of gonadotropin undergo marked changes in peripheral blood levels over short segments of time. That pattern reflects pulsatile gonadotropin secretion and has been called *circhoral* secretion, reflecting the approximately hourly pulses of gonadotropin release into the peripheral circulation. GnRH probably undergoes pulsatile variation in portal blood, as found in studies with nonhuman primates.[21]

MENSTRUAL CYCLE

The normal menstrual cycle is divided into two parts, the follicular and luteal phases. By convention, the follicular phase be-

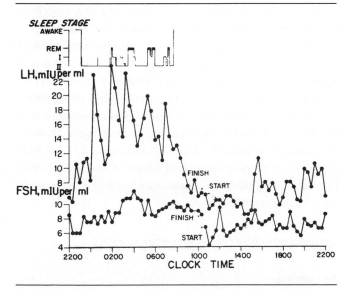

Figure 6–1. Plasma LH and FSH levels sampled during nocturnal sleep and after awakening. Sleep-associated increased gonadotropin secretion is apparent. Sleep stage is indicated at the top of the figure. Note the linking with REM-NREM sleep stage. (*From Boyar RM, et al. Twenty-four hour patterns of plasma luteinizing hormone and follicle stimulating hormone in sexual precocity. N Engl J Med 289:282, 1973.*)

gins with the first day of menses and extends to the midcycle or preovulatory surge of LH. Blood LH levels progressively increase during the follicular phase and culminate in a preovulatory surge that divides the menstrual cycle into the follicular and luteal phases. In contrast, circulating FSH levels increase during the first half of the follicular phase but decrease in the second half. In most healthy women there is a concordant preovulatory or midcycle surge of both LH and FSH. Ovulation occurs 36 to 38 hours after the onset of the midcycle LH surge. On the basis of studies with nonhuman primates, the follicle, destined to become the dominant or graafian follicle, is selected and becomes the primary source of circulating estradiol during the second half of the follicular phase.[22] The rising estradiol blood levels exert a negative feedback effect on pituitary FSH synthesis and secretion, resulting in decreased FSH levels during the second half of the follicular phase. Moreover, the increased estradiol levels observed during the second half of the follicular phase exert a positive feedback effect on gonadotropin secretion and contribute to the midcycle surge of gonadotropin. Other hypothalamic modulators undoubtedly contribute to the preovulatory surge, but the sites of their effects are unknown.

At the time of ovulation, the ovum and its surrounding cells are extruded from the graafian follicle. The remainder of the follicle is subsequently transformed into a corpus luteum, predominantly an organ responsive to LH and human chorionic gonadotropin (hCG). The corpus luteum secretes progesterone, estradiol, and 17-hydroxyprogesterone. As a result of increased secretion of estradiol and progesterone during the luteal phase, circulating levels of both LH and FSH decrease. The luteal phase encompasses that part of the menstrual cycle from the LH preovulatory surge up to the first day of menses. Figure 6–2 characterizes changes in circulating gonadotropin and sex steroid levels during the normal menstrual cycle.[23]

The pulse frequency and amplitude of both immunoreactive and bioactive LH vary during the normal menstrual cycle.[2,24,25] In the follicular phase, pulse frequency varies between 60 and 90 minutes; LH pulse amplitude and frequency increase progressively. Pulse frequency decreases during the luteal phase and ranges from 100 minutes in the early phase to 250 to 300 minutes in the late phase. In general, as pulse frequency decreases, LH pulse amplitude increases. Pulsatile release of both immunoreactive and bioactive LH is similar throughout the menstrual cycle.[24] Both bioactive and immunoreactive LH are secreted in discrete pulsations, but discordance exists between bioactive and immunoreactive pulses. Those relationships are summarized in Fig 6–3.

With the development of the corpus luteum and its concomitant secretion of progesterone, a thermogenic shift in basal body temperature results. Progesterone produces that effect by interacting with a hypothalamic thermoregulatory site. The luteal phase generally lasts between 11 and 15 days; most

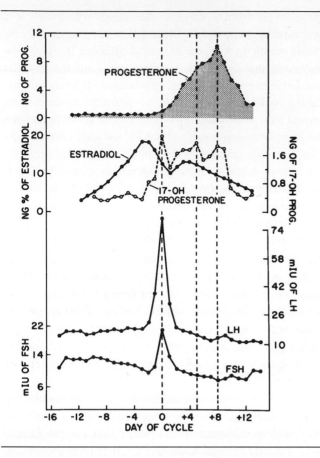

Figure 6–2. Gonadotropin and sex steroid levels during a presumptively ovulatory menstrual cycle. Levels are synchronized about the LH midcycle or preovulatory surge and designated day 0 of the cycle. (*From Vaitukaitis JL, Ross GT: Clinical studies of gonadotropin in the female.* Pharmacol Ther *1:317, 1976.*)

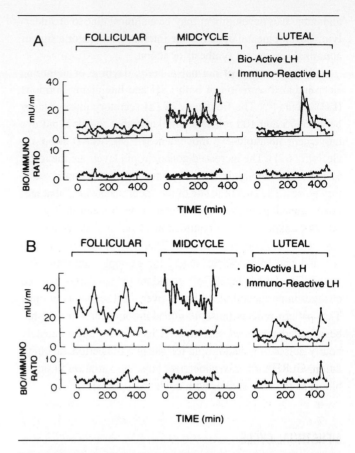

Figure 6–3. Immunoreactive and bioactive LH in samples of two different women who provided samples during the follicular, midcycle, and luteal phases. Note the lack of synchronization of activities for many of the LH pulses. (*From Veldhuis JD, et al: Biologically active luteinizing hormone is secreted in episodic pulsations that vary in relation to stage of the menstrual cycle.* J Clin Endocrinol Metab *58:1050, 1984.*)

women have a luteal phase of 13 to 14 days.[11] It is the luteal phase that is the most contant part of the normal menstrual cycle. In contrast, the follicular phase is variable. With prolonged intermenstrual intervals, the follicular phase is markedly lengthened. Circulating levels of progesterone usually exceed 10 ng/mL (32 nmol/L) 5 to 8 days after the midcycle surge of LH. During the reproductive years, the median intermenstrual interval is approximately 28 days.[11]

The extremes of the reproductive life cycle are accompanied by a higher frequency of anovulatory or inadequate ovulatory cycles. Moreover, the intermenstrual intervals during these extremes vary widely. Postmenarcheal adolescents manifest considerable variability in LH secretory profiles, which contributes to the higher frequency of anovulatory menstrual cycles in this age group.[2,26] Healthy adult women exhibit nocturnal slowing of LH secretory pulses during the follicular phase[2,27] (Fig 6–4). As women approach their late 20s and early 30s, the intermenstrual interval decreases by a few days.

During the several years before permanent cessation of spontaneous menses, there is a disproportionate increase in circulating FSH levels and lower circulating estradiol concentrations during the menstrual cycle compared with earlier reproductive years.[28] Investigators have attributed the increased FSH levels to decreased ovarian inhibin secretion[28]; however, no evidence exists for a direct effect of inhibin on pituitary FSH secretion in a physiologic state. The waning years of the reproductive life span have been referred to as *perimenopause,* but that is a misnomer since it alludes to premenopausal changes. Menopause is characterized by high circulating LH and FSH levels, reflecting primary gonadal failure. A few follicles may be present in the postmenopausal ovary but they are apparently not gonadotropin responsive.

PATHOPHYSIOLOGY OF THE MENSTRUAL CYCLE

Amenorrhea

The word *amenorrhea* simply connotes the absence of menses and does not indicate the anatomic site of a possible abnormality. Classification of amenorrhea as primary and secondary may

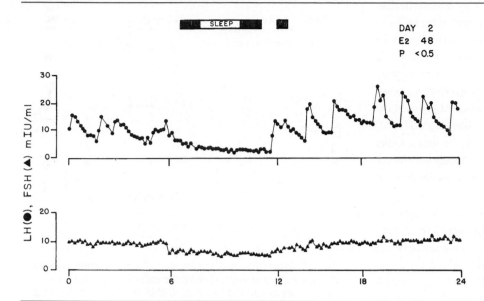

Figure 6–4. Immunoreactive LH levels of a young woman who provided samples over 24 hours. (*From Crowley WFD Jr, et al: The physiology of gonadotropin-releasing hormone (GnRH) secretion in men and women. Recent Prog Horm Res 41:473, 1985.*)

be misleading, since the same abnormalities may induce either the primary or secondary condition. That classification, however, is helpful since patients with primary amenorrhea have a 35% to 40% probability of having either primary ovarian failure or a developmental defect of the fallopian tubes, uterus, or vagina. Primary amenorrhea is characterized by the failure of onset of spontaneous menses by age 16.

Secondary amenorrhea is characterized by the cessation of spontaneous menses for at least 4 consecutive months. The most common cause is pregnancy. Whether a patient has primary or secondary amenorrhea, one can localize the site of abnormality by measuring circulating levels of estradiol and gonadotropin. Measuring FSH alone suffices and is cost effective. Hypothalamic-pituitary abnormalities are characterized by tonically low gonadotropin and estradiol levels, comparable with or lower than those of the normal early follicular phase. Primary gonadal dysfunction is characterized by high gonadotropin levels and low estradiol levels. Whenever a woman is amenorrheic, pregnancy should be excluded by measuring hCG in a specific hCG β-subunit assay. As with any other medical disorder, a careful history and physical examination are important in the differential diagnosis of menstrual dysfunction because the condition is an early warning for systemic illness.[4] Table 6–2 presents the definitions of amenorrhea and the biochemical differences between central and peripheral causes of menstrual dysfunction.

Primary Amenorrhea

The most common cause of primary amenorrhea is gonadal dysgenesis, usually due to a genetic defect. Patients with classic Turner's syndrome have a 45,XO karyotype. Genetic mo-

saicism is common among patients with Turner's syndrome; several different karyotypes may be encountered and may include 45,XO, 46,XX, and ringed X chromosomes. Phenotypically, patients demonstrate linear growth abnormalities resulting in short stature, cardiovascular abnormalities including coarctation of the aorta, developmental abnormalities of the genitourinary tract, high-arched palate, increased freckling, and a shield chest. Of interest, women with Turner's syndrome are endowed with a normal cohort of primordial follicles in utero.[29,30] Those follicles undergo atresia at an accelerated rate, however, so that by the time of menarche, none persist.[30] Consequently, the patients have primary amenorrhea. If the rate of atresia is slower, young girls with Turner's syndrome may have secondary amenorrhea with other classic somatic abnormalities. In fact, some women with Turner's syndrome have conceived and delivered healthy term babies.[29]

The second most common cause of primary amenorrhea is a defect of müllerian duct differentiation that results in aberrant development of the fallopian tubes, uterus, or vagina. Ovarian function remains intact. Consequently, young women with this abnormality have normal secondary sex characteristics, reflect-

TABLE 6–2. TYPES OF AMENORRHEA

Type	Description
Primary	No spontaneous menses by age 16
Secondary	Cessation of spontaneous menses for ≥4 mo
Central	Low basal gonadotropin levels, low blood estradiol concentrations (<50 pg/mL [184 pmol/L])
Peripheral	High basal gonadotropin levels, low estradiol levels (<25 pg/mL [92 pmol/L])

ing normal ovarian function, but have primary amenorrhea because of the absence or incomplete development of the uterus or vagina, or both. Graded developmental abnormalities may be observed. Some affected girls may have monthly abdominal pain but no external genital bleeding because the menstruum cannot be sloughed because of a lack of a vagina or functional connection between the uterus and the vagina. At physical examination, enlarged fallopian tubes (filled with sloughed blood) and an enlarged uterus filled with blood may be found. Other young women may have fully developed secondary sex characteristics and primary amenorrhea because of an imperforate hymen.

Intense exercise begun several years before the expected age of menarche may result in delayed puberty and primary amenorrhea. Swimmers and runners who begin training before the expected onset of menarche are at increased risk for amenorrhea or irregular menses.[31] The effect of training on menses is discussed in more detail later. In general, menarche may be delayed 0.4 years for each year of intense premenarcheal training.[32] A variety of other acquired congenital abnormalities of the hypothalamic-pituitary axis may result in primary amenorrhea, including defects in hypothalamic synthesis of GnRH, together with developmental abnormalities of the olfactory nerve, craniofacial abnormalities that may result in a cleft palate or harelip, and developmental abnormalities of the genitourinary tract. Affected women have the syndrome as olfactogenital dysplasia, the female counterpart of Kallmann's syndrome in males.

Secondary Amenorrhea

Pregnancy must be excluded by means of physical examination or measurement of urinary or blood hCG levels with specific assay before the patient undergoes further testing. Secondary amenorrhea results from primary gonadal dysfunction as well as from abnormalities of the hypothalamic-pituitary axis, or an unresponsive or absent uterus. Hypothalamic amenorrhea is a diagnosis of exclusion and simply reflects a functional defect of the hypothalamic-pituitary axis. It is characterized by absent cyclic gonadotropin secretion and levels of circulating estradiol that are comparable with or lower than those encountered in the early follicular phase of a normal menstrual cycle. Patients with secondary amenorrhea have a high frequency of prolactin secretory abnormalities. Prolactin levels should be determined in blood samples obtained in a truly basal, nonstressed state. When prolactin level is elevated, the patient should be examined for a pituitary adenoma. Hypothyroidism should be excluded with a blood test for thyroid-stimulating hormone (TSH), since with extreme hypothyroidism both serum TSH and prolactin levels are increased. In the presence of normal prolactin levels, elevated nocturnal plasma melatonin levels have been reported in women with

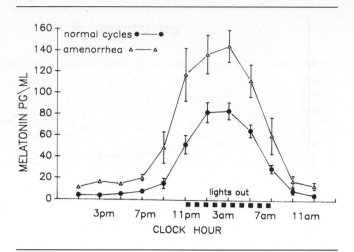

Figure 6–5. Mean (±SE) plasma melatonin levels in 14 healthy women (mean of all 3 study days) and 7 women with hypothalamic amenorrhea. To convert pg/mL melatonin to pmol/L, multiply by 4.31. (*From Brzezinski A, et al: The circadian rhythm of plasma melatonin during the normal menstrual cycle and in amenorrheic women. J Clin Endocrinol Metab 66:891, 1988.*)

secondary hypothalamic amenorrhea, suggesting that the hormone may be involved in the neuroendocrine abnormality underlying this disorder (Fig 6–5).[33] A precise mechanism has not been elucidated.

Among young women in the United States, the most common contributors to hypothalamic amenorrhea are rapid weight loss with or without excessive physical conditioning. Athletes who begin training after menarche may have a 50% frequency of irregular menses, including amenorrhea.[34] It should be remembered, however, that those who have amenorrhea with exercise may have an underlying organic defect. The intensity and duration of physical exercise, independent of body weight, may directly influence the occurrence of amenorrhea. Of interest, amenorrheic athletes may resume menstrual function during states of inactivity, despite little change in weight. Well-designed studies found a higher frequency of anovulatory cycles than previously suspected among women undergoing supervised, graded-intensity training.[35]

Some women undergo voluntary weight loss too rapidly and experience amenorrhea. Those with anorexia nervosa may experience rapid, marked weight loss to levels 50% of their ideal body weight. They may have bradycardia, constipation, lanugolike hair growth on the trunk and legs, leukopenia, and hypothalamic abnormalities that result in altered thermoregulation and partial diabetes insipidus. The partial diabetes insipidus, thermoregulatory alterations, and amenorrhea are hypothalamic abnormalities reversible with weight gain. Restoration toward normal or normalization of hypothalamic function usually occurs after a variable length of time after restoring weight to the ideal range.

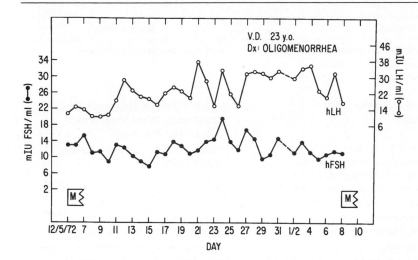

Figure 6–6. The LH and FSH levels of a woman with a prolonged intermenstrual interval. M, menses.

An exciting explanation for the relationship between obesity, starvation, and reproduction has been suggested.[36] A total deficiency in or resistance to the peptide leptin results in obesity, whereas in starvation, leptin concentrations fall. Totally leptin-deficient *ob/ob* mice have neurologic disorders similar to those seen in starvation, suggesting a physiologic role. Preventing the starvation-induced fall in leptin by administering exogenous leptin prevents the starvation-induced delay in ovulation in female mice. However, leptin repletion during periods of starvation has limited if any effect on body weight, blood glucose, or ketones. Leptin receptors have been identified on the choroid plexus and hypothalamus, and neuropeptide Y is a potential mediator of its central effects. The fall in leptin level may represent the critical signal that initiates the neuroendocrine response to starvation, including limiting procreation.

Some women with amenorrhea may need endocrinologic intervention with clomiphene citrate to restore cyclic menses. Others may require more complex therapeutic measures with exogenous GnRH or exogenous gonadotropin stimulation to induce ovulation if they wish to conceive.

Autoimmune disorders may induce transient or permanent ovarian dysfunction; women may have either primary or secondary amenorrhea.[37] The latter is more common. Autoimmune pluriglandular endocrine gland failure may be a familial disorder.[38] Convincing evidence now exists for autoimmune-induced ovarian failure. Perifollicular lymphocytic infiltrates, circulating antibody to components of the ovarian follicle, and the presence of other autoimmune disorders in the same patient constitute that evidence. Patients may have circulating antibody discernible to several endocrine glands—thyroid, adrenal, pancreatic, and ovarian tissues—in addition to antibodies to other tissues, such as the acetylcholine receptor in patients with myasthenia gravis.[37–39] Other associated immunologic disorders include systemic lupus erythematosus, rheumatoid arthritis, and Sjögren's syndrome.

In the early stages of ovarian autoimmune involvement, follicles undergo accelerated atresia, probably as a result of ovarian cytotoxic antibodies. Because affected ovaries may have lymphocytic infiltrates, clinicians have treated some patients with glucocorticoids, but with little therapeutic benefit. Affected women have elevated levels of circulating gonadotropin and low levels of estradiol, consistent with primary gonadal failure. Some of those women resume spontaneous menses with normalization of circulating gonadotropin levels, however. Other women have been treated with oral contraceptive formulations that contain both estrogen and progestins; some have conceived.[40] Similarly, women undergoing systemic chemotherapy, especially alkylating agents, for an underlying malignant disease experience secondary amenorrhea with elevated gonadotropin and low estradiol levels, consistent with primary gonadal failure. After a variable time, sometimes years, they may resume spontaneous cyclic menses and even conceive. Longitudinal studies suggest that women who undergo chemotherapy during their younger reproductive years may experience menopause at a younger age. A wide array of environmental agents may induce transient or permanent primary ovarian failure.[41] Irradiation can also induce secondary amenorrhea. A dose of 150 rad or less is seldom sufficient, but 800 rad results in permanent ovarian failure in nearly all patients.

Anovulation

The word *anovulation* is confusing. In everyday parlance, it is used interchangeably with ovulation of an immature egg from an incompletely developed graafian follicle. Technically, anovulation occurs only when no graafian follicle develops. In-

TABLE 6–3. CAUSES OF MENSTRUAL DYSFUNCTION

Disorder	Comment	Hormone Levels
Hypothalamic amenorrhea	Diagnosis of exclusion. Functional defect of gonadotropin secretion induced by rapid weight loss or gain, systemic illness, intense exercise, stress. May be preceded by luteal phase insufficiency and anovulation.	Gonadotropin tonically low; estradiol low.
Pregnancy	Most common cause of secondary amenorrhea. May be asymptomatic early in gestation.	Specific hCG (β-subunit) assay positive; FSH low or undetectable; LH high because of cross-reactivity with hCG antiserum.
Turner's syndrome	Most commonly causes short stature and primary amenorrhea; may result in secondary amenorrhea. May have congenital developmental anomalies of the genitourinary tract, cardiovascular system, and skeletal system. May be 46, XX/45, XO, ringed X chromosome, or some other genetic variant.	Gonadotropin high and estradiol low, signaling primary gonadal failure.
Polycystic ovary	Most common endocrinologic cause of infertility. May cause regular or irregular menstrual pattern including amenorrhea. Signs of androgen excess.	Gonadotropin may be low or LH may be inappropriately high and FSH tonically low. Androgen may be normal or increased.
Drugs, irradiation	Opiates suppress gonadotropin secretion and may be associated with amenorrhea or irregular menses. Chemotherapeutic agents may induce transient or permanent gonadal failure. Ethanol induces both primary gonadal and hypothalamic defects. Irradiation may destroy ovarian follicles and induce amenorrhea.	Gonadotropin and estradiol low with amenorrhea. Chemotherapeutic agents associated with high gonadotropin and low estradiol. Alcohol may suppress gonadotropin secretion. Irradiation associated with high gonadotropin and low estradiol transiently or permanently.
Congenital abnormalities of vagina, uterus, or fallopian tubes	Secondary sex characteristics normal but women have primary amenorrhea. May have pelvic mass. Normal secondary sex characteristics.	Normal gonadotropin and sex steroid for menstrual cycle.
Premature menopause	Cessation of menses permanently before age 40. May be induced chemically or through an autoimmune mechanism. No genetic abnormality in most. May be familial disorder.	Gonadotropin high, estradiol low.
Pituitary tumor	May cause regular or irregular menses or amenorrhea. If tumor large, may have signs of suprasellar extension (eg, visual field abnormalities, diabetes insipidus). May have signs of hormonal secretion by tumor (eg, Cushing's syndrome, acromegaly).	Gonadotropin usually tonically low, comparable with early follicular phase levels; estradiol low. Prolactin increased in most.
Hypothalamic tumor or cyst	Irregular or absent menses. Young girls may have precocious puberty or delayed menarche or arrested pubertal development.	Gonadotropin and estradiol low.
Infiltrative disorders of pituitary stalk or hypothalamus (tuberculosis, sarcoidosis, histiocytosis X)	Irregular or absent menses. Signs and symptoms of underlying disorder.	Gonadotropin and estradiol low.

adequate gonadotropin stimulation or a defect of steroidogenesis that precludes the synthesis of sex steroids may induce abnormal development of the graafian follicle. If a follicle is underdeveloped, the corpus luteum derived from that structure also is abnormal and secretes lower than normal levels of progesterone. Sufficient levels of progesterone may be secreted, and that amount may induce a marked increase in basal body temperature. In general, many of the acquired causes of amenorrhea also are associated with anovulation. In fact, anovulatory menstrual cycles with or without an irregular menstrual interval may precede the onset of amenorrhea. Women with well-documented irregular intermenstrual intervals may have both ovulatory and anovulatory cycles. The frequency of anovulation is greater among those with intermenstrual intervals of 35 to 40 days than among women with a history of regular intervals.

Figure 6–6 depicts circulating gonadotropin levels in a woman with anovulation and an irregular menstrual interval. The gonadotropin pattern is markedly different from that of a woman with normal cycles.

Table 6–3 provides a summary of the more common causes of menstrual dysfunction and their clinical features.

REFERENCES

1. Vaitukaitis JL: Neuroendocrine control of gonadotropin secretion in women. In: Taymor MD, Nelson JH Jr (eds), *Progress in Gynecology.* New York, Grune & Stratton, 1983:3–19
2. Crowley WF Jr, Filicori M, Spratt DI, Santoro NF: The physiology of gonadotropin-releasing hormone (GnRH) secretion in men and women. *Recent Prog Horm Res* 41:473, 1985

3. Ferrin M, Jewelewicz R, Warren MP: *The Menstrual Cycle.* New York, Oxford University Press, 1993
4. Warren MP: Evaluation of secondary amenorrhea. *J Clin Endocrinol Metab* 81:437, 1996
5. Herzog AG, Seibel MM, Schomer DL, Vaitukaitis JL, Geschwind N: Reproductive endocrine disorders in women with partial seizures of temporal lobe origin. *Arch Neurol* 43:341, 1986
6. Henley K, Vaitukaitis JL: Exercise-induced menstrual dysfunction. *Annu Rev Med* 39:443, 1988
7. Pirke KM, Schweiger U, Laessle RG, et al: Dieting influences the menstrual cycle: Vegetarian versus nonvegetarian diet. *Fertil Steril* 46:1083, 1986
8. Baker TG: A quantitative and cytological study of germ cells in human ovaries. *Proc R Soc Lond* 158:417, 1963
9. Peters H: The human ovary in childhood and early maturity. *Gynecol Reprod Biol* 9:137, 1979
10. MacMahon B, Worcester J: *Age at Menopause: United States 1900–1962.* Washington, DC, U.S. Government Printing Office, 1966
11. Treloar AE, Boynton RE, Behn BG: Variation of the human menstrual cycle through reproductive life. *Int J Fertil* 12:77, 1967
12. Kaplan SL, Grumbach MM, Aubert ML: The ontogenesis of pituitary hormones and hypothalamic factors in the human fetus: Maturation of central nervous system regulation of anterior pituitary function. *Recent Prog Horm Res* 32:161, 1976
13. Baker TG, Scrimgeour JB: Development of the gonad in normal and anencephalic human fetuses. *J Reprod Fertil* 60:193, 1980
14. Li CH, Ramasharma K, Yamashiro D, Chung D: Gonadotropin-releasing peptide from human follicular fluid: Isolation, characterization, and chemical synthesis. *Proc Nat Acad Sci USA* 84:959, 1987
15. Khan-Dawood FS: Human corpus luteum: Immunocytochemical localization of epidermal growth factor. *Fertil Steril* 47:916, 1987
16. Demoulin A, Guichard A, Mignot TM, et al: Inhibin concentration in the culture media of human oocyte–cumulus–corona cell complexes is not related to subsequent embryo cleavage. *Fertil Steril* 46:1150, 1986
17. Swerdloff RS: Physiological control of puberty. *Med Clin North Am* 62:351, 1978
18. Marshall WA, Tanner JM: Variations in patterns of pubertal changes in girls. *Arch Dis Child* 44:291, 1969
19. Boyar R, Finkelstein J, Roffwarg H, et al: Synchronization of augmented luteinizing hormone secretion with sleep during puberty. *N Engl J Med* 287:582, 1972
20. Boyar RM, Finkelstein JW, David R, et al: Twenty-four-hour patterns of plasma luteinizing hormone and follicle-stimulating hormone in sexual precocity. *N Engl J Med* 289:282, 1973
21. Carmel PW, Araki S, Ferin M: Pituitary stalk portal blood collection in rhesus monkeys: Evidence for pulsatile release of gonadotropin-releasing hormone (GnRH). *Endocrinology* 99:243, 1976
22. Goodman AL, Hodgen GD: The ovarian triad of the primate menstrual cycle. *Recent Prog Horm Res* 39:1, 1983
23. Vaitukaitis JL, Ross GT: Clinical studies of gonadotropin in the female. *Pharmacol Ther* 1:317, 1976
24. Veldhuis JD, Beitins I, Johnson ML, Serabian MA, Dufau M: Biologically active luteinizing hormone is secreted in episodic pulsations that vary in relation to stage of the menstrual cycle. *J Clin Endocrinol Metab* 58:1050, 1984
25. Santen RJ, Bardin CW: Episodic luteinizing hormone secretion in man. *J Clin Invest* 52:2617, 1973
26. Apter D, Raisanen I, Ylosalo P, Vihko R: Follicular growth in relation to serum hormonal patterns in adolescent compared with adult menstrual cycles. *Fertil Steril* 47:82, 1987
27. Soules MR, Steiner RA, Cohen NL, Bremner WJ, Clifton DK: Nocturnal slowing of pulsatile luteinizing hormone secretion in women during the follicular phase of the menstrual cycle. *J Clin Endocrinol Metab* 61:43, 1985
28. Sherman BN, West JH, Korenman SG: The menopausal transition of LH, FSH, estradiol and progesterone concentrations during menstrual cycles of older women. *J Clin Endocrinol Metab* 42:629, 1976
29. Nielsen J, Sillesen I, Hansen KB: Fertility in women with Turner's syndrome: A case report and review of the literature. *Br J Obstet Gynaecol* 86:833, 1979
30. Singh RP, Carr DH: The anatomy and history of XO human embryos and fetuses. *Anat Rec* 155:369, 1966
31. Warren MP: The effect of exercise on pubertal progression and reproductive function in girls. *J Clin Endocrinol Metab* 51:1150, 1980
32. Frisch RE, Gotz-Welbergen AV, McArthur JW, et al: *JAMA* 246:1559, 1981
33. Brzezinski A, Lynch HJ, Seibel MM, et al: The circadian rhythm of plasma melatonin during the normal menstrual cycle and in amenorrheic women. *J Clin Endocrinol Metab* 66:891, 1988
34. Warren MP: Amenorrhea in endurance runners. *J Clin Endocrinol Metab* 75:1393, 1992
35. Bullen BA, Skrinar GS, Beitins IZ, et al: Induction of menstrual disorders by strenuous exercise in untrained women. *N Engl J Med* 312:1349, 1985
36. Ahima RS, Prabarkaran D, Mantzoros C, et al: Role of leptin in the neuroendocrine response to fasting. *Nature* 1996
37. Coulam CB: The prevalence of autoimmune disorders among patients with primary ovarian failure. *Am J Reprod Immunol* 4:63, 1983
38. Alper MA, Garner PR, Seibel MM: Premature ovarian failure: Current concept. *J Reprod Med* 31:699, 1986
39. Coulam CB, Kempers RD, Randall RV: Premature ovarian failure: Evidence for the autoimmune mechanism. *Fertil Steril* 36:238, 1981
40. Shangold MM, Turksoy RN, Bashford RA, Hammond CB: Pregnancy following the "insensitive ovary syndrome." *Fertil Steril* 28:1179, 1977
41. Verp MS: Environmental causes of ovarian failure. *Semin Reprod Endocrinol* 1:101, 1983

CHAPTER 7

Polycystic Ovary Syndrome

HOWARD S. JACOBS

Definition
  Multicystic ovaries
  Polycystic ovaries
  Prevalence of polycystic ovaries
Clinical Features of Polycystic Ovary Syndrome
  Endocrine findings
  Heterogeneity of the polycystic ovary syndrome

Etiology of Polycystic Ovary Syndrome
Management of Polycystic Ovary Syndrome
  Infertility
  Hyperandrogenism

Polycystic ovary (PCO) syndrome goes under many names. It is common, and it excites much controversy. As I hope will soon become apparent, differences that have developed in terminology are far outweighed by similarities in the approach to diagnosis and management taken by most groups. Over the last decade the important advances that have occurred in our understanding of the condition have derived from our ability to identify PCOs accurately and in our realization of the importance of genetic factors in the causation of the syndrome.

DEFINITION

After the clinical characterization of the condition by Stein and Leventhal in 1935,[1] workers in this area have either followed a functional definition, speaking of chronic anovulation or functional hyperandrogenism or taken a structural view, placing diagnostic emphasis on anatomic identification of PCOs. It must be instantly clear that these approaches rather than being in conflict are in reality complementary. In this chapter I refer to *polycystic ovary,* as identified during ultrasonography (the structural approach), and to *polycystic ovary syndrome,* as identified on the basis of the association of characteristic ovarian ultrasound features with certain well-recognized symptoms, signs, and endocrine findings (the functional approach). I take it as axiomatic that one cannot have PCO syndrome without having PCOs. On the other hand, PCOs are identified in many more women than those suffering from the syndrome. Identification of the factors that lead to clinical expression of the PCO syndrome is clearly one of the goals of research in this area.

Multicystic Ovaries

It is important at the outset to differentiate *polycystic ovaries,* the kind found in women with the Stein-Leventhal syndrome, from *multicystic ovaries,*[2] that is, the ovarian ultrasound appearance of the healthy pubertal girl, as described histologically in the classic studies of Peters et al.[3] The striking ultrasound features of the latter are the presence of follicles of various size scattered throughout an ovary that has no excess of medullary stroma (Fig 7–1). This appearance is a feature of normal mid-puberty and results from incomplete pulsatile gonadotropic stimulation of the ovaries. When inducing puberty in hypogonadotropic children with pulsatile gonadotropin-releasing hor-

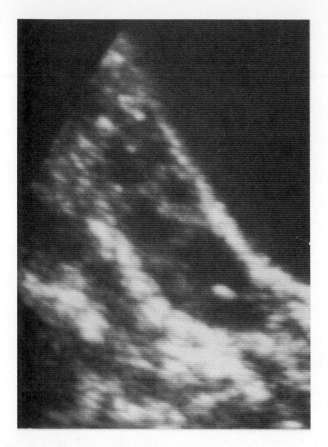

Figure 7–1. Ultrasound scan of multicystic ovary, according to the criteria set out by Adams et al.[2] Transabdominal scan shows cysts up to 8 mm in diameter scattered throughout the ovary with no increase of stroma.

mone (GnRH), Stanhope et al[4] found that the normal immediately premenarchial ovarian appearance of multicystic ovaries was produced when treatment was restricted to less than 24 hours per day. When, however, pulsatile infusion was maintained for the full 24 hours, a single dominant follicle developed followed by suppression of the cohort follicles. The ovaries in these girls with delayed puberty were essentially normal, and the genesis of the problem lay in incomplete gonadotropic control of ovarian follicular development. When normal pulsatile gonadotropin stimulation of the ovary was attained physiologically or through treatment (gonadotropin stimulation that was normal in amplitude, frequency, and duration), the normal intraovarian regulation that underlies establishment of a single dominant follicle was established. The ovarian appearance then returned to normal.

The pathologic correlate of these events occurs in two clinical situations. The first is during treatment of women with hypogonadotropic hypogonadism (HH) when the amplitude or duration of the pulsatile stimulus, that is, the dose of GnRH, is suboptimal. Occasionally this occurs with standard doses given subcutaneously, presumably because in these women absorp-

tion of GnRH is impaired. The ovarian appearance rapidly resolves when the same dose is given intravenously or when the dose of subcutaneous GnRH is raised.

The second situation in which this appearance may be seen is in women recovering from a phase of suppression of endogenous GnRH activity, most commonly women with partially recovered weight loss–related amenorrhea. The importance of the condition is that the ovaries are polyfollicular and have lost the external (pituitary) control that leads to unifollicular ovulation. If these patients are exposed to ovarian stimulation, there is a strong possibility that in the first cycle of treatment they will have multiple ovulation. Therefore, such patients are at risk for multiple conception.

Polycystic Ovaries

Described at an operation as ovaries that are larger than normal with a thickened capsule through which cysts can be seen, these ovaries on cross section reveal thickened stroma with peripherally arranged cysts (Fig 7–2). Concordance between histologic appearance and ultrasound image has been demonstrated.[5] Figure 7–3 shows the characteristic appearance of a PCO on a two-dimensional ultrasound scan performed with a transvaginal probe. Recent studies with three-dimensional ultrasonography of PCOs[6] (Fig 7–4) amplified these findings by showing that the increase in ovarian size is caused by an increase in stromal rather than in cystic volume (Fig 7–5). Using color Doppler studies of blood flow,[7] one can appreciate the considerable vascularity of the stroma at a time when follicular growth is quiescent.

PCOs are indentified on the basis of appearance at transabdominal scanning of stromal thickening with 10 or more cysts 2 to 8 mm in diameter arranged in a "necklace" around the periphery.[2] Using transvaginal ultrasonography most authorities consider it necessary to identify 15 or more cysts to establish the diagnosis. The overall dimensions of the ovary are increased (Table 7–1) although PCOs of normal size may be found in some women who take combined oral contraceptives, in some with gonadotropin deficiency, and in a proportion of girls who have no symptoms before puberty. These situations are discussed later but are mentioned here to emphasize that an increase in overall ovarian volume is not a sine qua non of diagnosis.

PREVALENCE OF POLYCYSTIC OVARIES

Several studies[8] have confirmed the original observation of Polson et al[9] that PCOs can be identified in about 22% of volunteers who do not have symptoms. The same authors also reported PCOs in 85% of women with oligomenorrhea and 95% of women with hirsutism. PCOs are nearly always present in

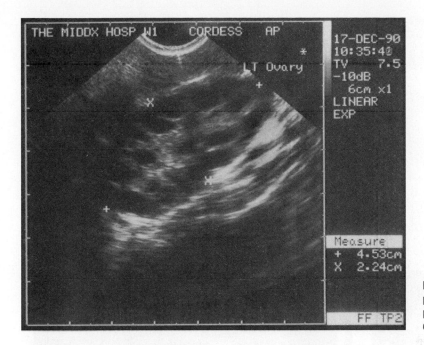

Figure 7–2. Transvaginal, two-dimensional ultrasound scan of ovary of a patient with Stein-Leventhal (polycystic ovary) syndrome. Scan shows peripherally distributed multiple small cysts and thickened, echodense central stroma.

women with severe acne. An important study by Bridges et al[10] established ovarian ultrasound criteria for healthy prepubertal girls and showed a steadily increasing prevalence of PCOs with age (Fig 7–6). PCOs are found in 35% of women with amenorrhea, in 75% of women with congenital adrenal hyperplasia, and in most women with acromegaly and Cushing's syndrome.

The very high rates of detection of PCOs with ultrasound scans of volunteers without symptoms has raised the question of the pathophysiologic significance of the ultrasound finding. Clearly some and perhaps most women whose ovaries fulfill the morphologic criteria of PCOs continue not to have symptoms throughout reproductive life. To investigate the significance of finding PCOs with ultrasonography, my colleagues and I conducted a study that involved women with HH who also had PCOs as detected during ultrasonography.[11] Some of these women had Kallmann's syndrome, and so presumably their ovaries had never experienced any pituitary gonadotropic stimulation. When the patients were treated with exogenous gonadotropins, their ovarian response was indistinguishable from the characteristically exuberant response of patients with classic Stein-Leventhal syndrome. It was different, however, from that of women with gonadotropin deficiency and normal ovarian morphology (Fig 7–7). These observations resonate with the finding that among patients undergoing infertility treatment with in vitro fertilization (IVF), ovarian hyperstimulation syndrome (OHSS) occurs almost entirely in those with (frequently asymptomatic) PCOs.[12]

Although PCOs may be asymptomatic in healthy women, if the reproductive axis is stressed, clinical expression of the condition can be provoked. Second, these findings, together with the observations of Bridges et al[10] of a 6% prevalence of PCOs among children 6 years of age that rises to a plateau in the teen-age years of about 25%, are consistent with the hypothesis that the presence of PCOs is independent of any particular endocrine milieu. This view receives strong support from investigators who conducted in vitro studies that showed steroid accumulation by cultured human thecal cells is much greater in cells obtained from PCOs than in cells from normal ovaries.[13]

CLINICAL FEATURES OF POLYCYSTIC OVARY SYNDROME

Table 7–2 shows the clinical features of more than 1700 women with PCO syndrome treated at the reproductive endocrine clinics of The Middlesex Hospital, London. PCO syndrome was diagnosed according to the aforementioned criteria. The frequency of specific symptoms is compared with that in the classic compilation of data assembled some 30 years earlier by Goldzieher and Green.[14] The differences reflect in part changes in diagnostic method, but they also reflect referral bias, the earlier set of data originating from gynecology clinics, the later from endocrine clinics. Not shown in the table are the 5% of patients with acanthosis nigricans and the 10% with coexisting late-onset adrenal 21 hydroxylase deficiency.

Endocrine Findings

The prevalence of the well-known increase in serum luteinizing hormone (LH) and testosterone concentrations depends on the

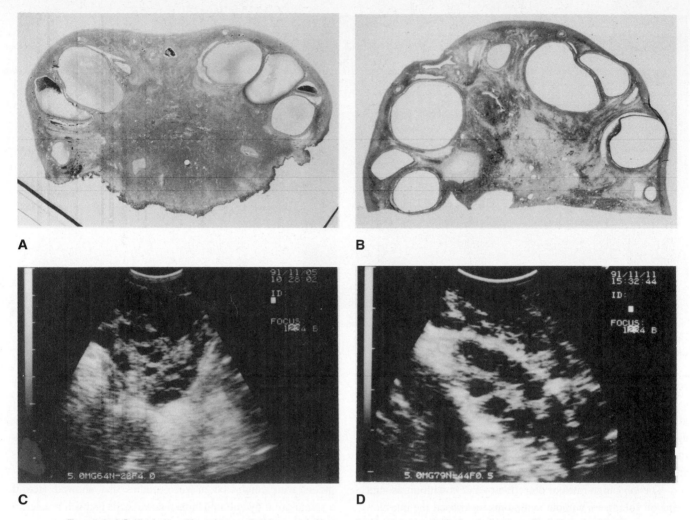

Figure 7–3. A–D. Histologic sections and transvaginal ultrasonographic scans of polycystic ovaries. Histologic and ultrasonographic findings of peripherally arranged cysts correlate with highly echo-dense central stroma. (From Takahashi K, et al: Relationship between ultrasonography and histopathological changes in polycystic ovarian syndrome. *Hum Reprod* 9:2255, 1994.)

diagnostic criteria used. Some groups consider that a diagnosis of PCO syndrome can be made only in the presence of elevated readings. In our series[15] 40% of women with PCO syndrome had serum LH concentrations above the normal range (Fig 7–8). About 30% of women have a raised serum testosterone concentration, but the importance of this figure is uncertain because of the confounding factor of obesity-mediated suppression of sex hormone-binding globulin (SHBG). Figure 7–9 shows the relation of serum total testosterone level to the presence of hirsutism and to body weight. It must be appreciated that these measurements represent a serious underestimation of free testosterone concentration and testosterone production rate.

Hyperprolactinemia occurs among about 15% of patients.[16] In about one third of them, depending on the height of the prolactin concentration, a microadenoma can be identified by means of magnetic resonance imaging (MRI). In about one

third of patients it seems likely that the hyperprolactinemia is a consequence of the hyperestrogenism of the PCO syndrome; in the remaining patients the association is probably coincidental.

Late-onset adrenal 21 hydroxylase deficiency was detected in 5% of our patients. It is likely that this is an underestimation of the true prevalence because we performed adrenocorticotropic hormone (ACTH) stimulation tests and DNA genotyping only for hirsute patients who have not responded to conventional antiandrogen therapy.

Heterogeneity of the Polycystic Ovary Syndrome

The classic description by Stein and Leventhal referred to overweight patients with menstrual disturbances, hirsutism, and infertility. Later the endocrine findings of raised LH and tes-

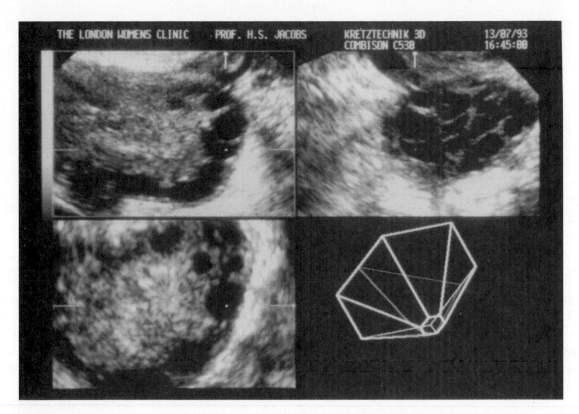

Figure 7–4. Transvaginal, three-dimensional ultrasound scan of a polycystic ovary. In the bottom right-hand panel, shows the splay of ultrasound and the plane in which the image in the top left-hand panel is reconstructed. In this scan the echodense stromal hyperplasia is readily seen, as is the peripheral distribution of the cysts.

tosterone concentrations were added. It is now widely accepted that patients may present with any combination of these features and that the condition is phenotypically heterogeneous. In this respect there has been increasing recognition of the important role of insulin resistance and the adverse effects on the ovary (and the body's metabolism) of the consequent hypersecretion of insulin. There is also evidence that hypersecretion of LH not only is a marker of the syndrome but also may mediate some of the fertility problems experienced by these patients. In my opinion there are at minimum two phenotypic variants of

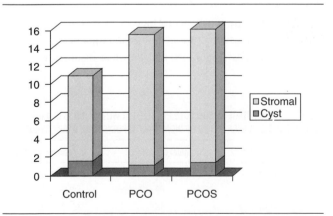

Figure 7–5. Measurements of ovarian volume by means of three-dimensional ultrasonography in women with normal ovaries (control), women with polycystic ovary syndrome (PCOS), and women whose ovaries were polycystic but who had no symptoms of polycystic ovary syndrome (PCO). Increase in ovarian volume is attributable to the increase in stromal volume. Data kindly provided by Amma Kyei-Mensah, MD.

TABLE 7–1. CHARACTERISTICS OF 1741 WOMEN WITH ULTRASOUND-DETECTED POLYCYSTIC OVARIES

Characteristic	No. of Women	Range
Age (years)	31.5	14–50
Ovarian volume (cm^3)	11.7	4.6–22.3
Uterine cross-sectional area (cm^2)	27.5	15.2–46.3
Thickness of endometrium (mm)	7.5	4.0–13.0
BMI (kg/m^2; 19–25)[a]	25.4	19.0–38.6
FSH (IU/L; 1–10)[a]	4.5	1.4–7.5
LH (IU/L; 1–10)[a]	10.9	2.0–27.0
Testosterone (nmol/L; 0.5–2.5)[a]	2.6	1.1–4.8
Prolactin (<350 μg/L)[a]	342	87–917

Values are mean and 5th to 95th percentiles.
BMI, body mass index; FSH, follicle-stimulating hormone; LH, luteinizing hormone.
[a] Normal range.
From Conway GS: Polycystic ovary syndrome: Clinical aspects. Baillieres Clin Endocrinol Metab 10:263, 1996.

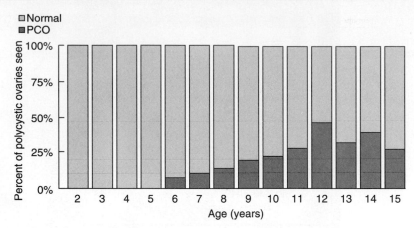

Figure 7–6. Percentage of ovaries with a polycystic appearance in girls between the ages of 2 and 15 years. (From Bridges NA, et al: Standards for ovarian volume in childhood and puberty. *Fertil Steril* 60:456, 1993. Reproduced with the permission of the publisher, the American Society for Reproductive Medicine [The American Fertility Society].)

the PCO syndrome, and these can be linked to disturbances of secretion of insulin and LH.

Hypersecretion of Insulin

The association of acanthosis nigricans with PCO syndrome first alerted clinicians to the potential role of insulin in the dis-

order. It was, however, the demonstration that high serum insulin concentrations can be found in nonobese women with PCO syndrome that led to the extensive investigations of insulin dynamics in these patients.[17] These studies have shown that many women, particularly those who are anovulatory, have resistance to the extrasplanchnic actions of insulin on carbohydrate metabolism. Despite an intense search, mutations in the gene that encodes the insulin receptor do not appear to be the cause.[18] Women with PCO syndrome possess a specific post–receptor-binding defect in insulin action whereby normal insulin-induced tyrosine autophosphorylation (an essential component of transduction of the insulin signal) is replaced by phosphorylation of serine.[19] Transduction of the insulin signal is thereby impaired. The abnormality is thought to be genetic in origin because it can be demonstrated in cells removed from the in vivo environment for generations.[19] In addition, of course, there are also the usual mechanisms of insulin resistance, that is, those related to obesity and diabetes, to be considered in patients with PCO syndrome.

Whatever the mechanism, there is a striking correlation between serum insulin concentrations and the interval between menstrual periods (Fig 7–10) and between insulin and serum

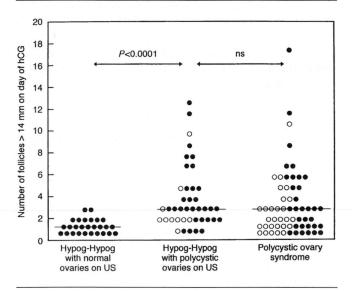

Figure 7–7. Number of follicles greater than 14 mm in diameter on the day of administration of human chorionic gonadotropin (hCG) to three groups of women undergoing induction of ovulation. Left, the characteristic unifollicular response of women with gonadotropin deficiency treated with human menopausal gonadotropin (hMG) (closed circles) or follicle-stimulating hormone (FSH) (open circles). Right, the characteristic multifollicular response of women with polycystic ovary (PCO) syndrome. Center, women with hypogonadotrophic hypogonadism but with PCOs at ultrasound have a response indistinguishable from that of women with PCO syndrome, irrespective of the gonadotropic stimulation used. (Data from Shoham Z, et al: Polycystic ovaries in patients with hypogonadotropic hypogonadism: Similarity of ovarian response to gonadotropin stimulation in patients with polycystic ovarian syndrome. *Fertil Steril* 58:37, 1992. Reproduced with the permission of the publisher, the American Society for Reproductive Medicine [The American Fertility Society].)

TABLE 7–2. PERCENTAGE OF SUBJECTS PRESENTING WITH VARIOUS CLINICAL FEATURES IN TWO LARGE SERIES OF WOMEN WITH POLYCYSTIC OVARY SYNDROME

Finding	Surgical diagnosis[14]	Ultrasound diagnosis[15]
Number of patients	1079	1741
Hirsutism	69	66
Normal menstrual cycle	12	30
Oligomenorrhea	37	47
Amenorrhea	51	19
Infertility	74	23

From Conway GS: Polycystic ovary syndrome: Clinical aspects. Baillieres Clin Endocrinol Metab 10:263, 1996.

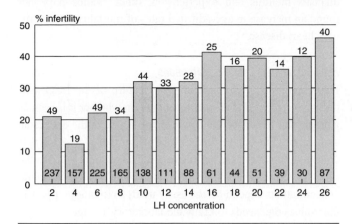

Figure 7–8. Serum luteinizing hormone (LH) concentrations in relation to reported infertility among women with PCO syndrome. The number of reports of infertility increases when serum LH level exceeds 10 IU/L, which with this radioimmunoassay is the upper limit of normal. There is a steady increase in the proportion of women reporting infertility as basal LH concentration rises. *(From Balen AH, et al: Polycystic ovary syndrome: The spectrum of the disorder in 1741 patients.* Hum Reprod *10:2017, 1995.)*

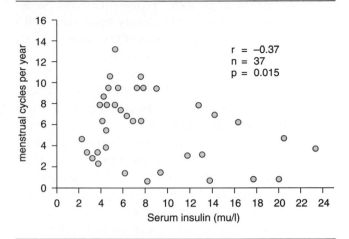

Figure 7–10. Relation of fasting serum insulin concentration to the number of menstrual cycles per year. As insulin concentration rises, the interval between cycles increases and the number per year decreases. *(From Conway GS: Polycystic ovary syndrome: Clinical aspects.* Baillieres Clin Endocrinol Metab *10:263, 1996.)*

androstenedione concentrations (Fig 7–11). The effect on the menstrual cycle is important because the chances of conception are directly related to the rate of ovulation. The relation to androstenedione concentration is important because this steroid is not protein bound and so the confounding effect of insulin-mediated suppression of SHBG does not hamper interpretation. Insulin excess thus increases the secretion of androgen and through an effect on its transport increases its metabolic clearance rate, a result that amplifies its biologic effect. The impact of hypersecretion of insulin is compounded in overweight patients because obesity increases insulin resistance and further increases secretion of insulin.

In addition to its effect on the reproductive process, increased secretion of insulin has adverse effects on cholesterol

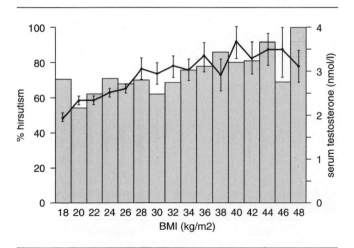

Figure 7–9. Serum testosterone concentrations of women with polycystic ovary syndrome in relation to body mass index (BMI) and to presence of hirsutism. There is a steadily increasing testosterone concentration with obesity, a remarkable finding because of the well-known obesity-mediated suppression of sex hormone-binding globulin. The testosterone production rate among the very obese women is seriously underestimated on the basis of total serum testosterone concentration. *(From Balen AH, et al: Polycystic ovary syndrome: The spectrum of the disorder in 1741 patients.* Hum Reprod *10:2017, 1995.)*

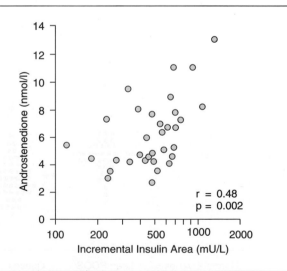

Figure 7–11. Relation of serum androstenedione concentration to incremental insulin area after oral glucose in slim women with polycystic ovary syndrome. As the amount of insulin secreted in response to oral glucose increases, serum androstenedione concentration also increases. *(From Conway GS: Polycystic ovary syndrome: Clinical aspects.* Baillieres Clin Endocrinol Metab *10:263, 1996.)*

metabolism and blood pressure.[20] Figure 7–12 shows the depression of cardioprotective high-density lipoprotein (HDL) cholesterol in anovulatory women with PCO syndrome. The effect is even more marked among overweight patients. In an important follow-up study of histologically verified cases of PCO syndrome, Dhalgren et al[21] found a 15% prevalence of diabetes mellitus and a 40% prevalence of clinically significant hypertension 15 to 20 years after diagnosis.

These nonreproductive effects of excessive secretion of insulin have suggested that these patients represent the female version of Reavan's metabolic syndrome X.[22] By this term one means the aggregation of adverse coronary risk factors that have been described in association with insulin resistance. When, however, patients with PCO syndrome underwent follow-up studies with respect to coronary events rather than surrogate markers of risk, no increase in the rate of fatal or nonfatal myocardial infarction was detected.[23] It appears that women with PCO syndrome, like postmenopausal women receiving hormone replacement therapy, may be protected from the expression of coronary risk markers. The most probable mechanism is extraglandular production of endogenous estrogen, that is, conversion of androgens to estrogens in fat tissue.

To summarize, hypersecretion of insulin by women with PCO syndrome is believed to arise from resistance to the extrasplanchnic actions of the hormone. Hypersecretion of insulin has adverse effects on the reproductive process; it increases androgen secretion and enhances the metabolic clearance rate of testosterone. It is associated with disruption of the ovulatory cycle, contributing to infertility. Hypersecretion of insulin also has adverse effects on cholesterol metabolism and blood pressure. Although follow-up studies have shown an increased risk for

diabetes mellitus and hypertension, other studies have not found an increase in age-adjusted rates of mortality from coronary heart disease.

Hypersecretion of Luteinizing Hormone

Hypersecretion of LH is a familiar feature of the PCO syndrome, the exact prevalence depending on whether it is seen as a diagnostic feature of the condition or as one of the endocrine associations. In our series, 40% of patients had a serum LH concentration above the normal range. The relation of LH to the report of infertility is shown in Table 7–3 and Fig 7–8. Absolute concentrations depend on the assay used, so to interpret particular values one needs to know the laboratory's range.

The neuroendocrinology of hypersecretion of LH has been investigated for many years. It is established that there is an increase in both the rate and amplitude of LH pulses.[24] Hypotheses that relate to changes in neurotransmitter activity, such as reductions in dopaminergic, opioid, and serotonin tone, or to an increase in noradrenergic tone, are summarized in Table 7–4. A reduction in ovarian secretion of gonadotropin surge-attenuating factor has been postulated. In in vitro studies, an increase in the pituitary response to GnRH stimulation has been noted in the presence of insulin, suggesting a role for hyperinsulinism in the increase in LH secretion.

Conway and I recently suggested that there may be involvement of the leptin system in the control of gonadotropin secretion in women with PCO syndrome (in preparation). Leptin is a protein secreted by adipocytes that is involved in the control of food intake. Leptin is believed, among other things, to act on the brain as a satiety signal. Serum leptin levels are high in obesity, suggesting that obesity is a leptin-resistant state. Genetic deficiency of leptin occurs in mice that are homozygous for the *obese* gene. These mice are overweight, infertile, and have low gonadotropin levels. Treatment with recombinant leptin results in a return of fertility, which because it cannot be explained by a reduction in weight, is believed to be mediated by an effect on the hypothalamic control of gonadotropin secretion.[25] In the hypothalamus leptin inhibits synthesis and release

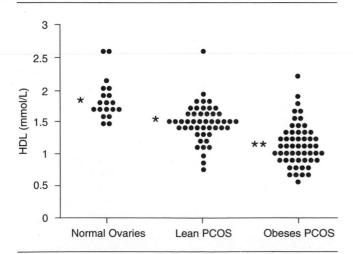

Figure 7–12. Measurements of high-density lipoprotein cholesterol in women with normal ovaries and those with polycystic ovary syndrome. *(From Conway GS, et al: Risk factors for coronary artery disease in lean and obese women with the polycystic ovary syndrome.* Clin Endocrinol 37:119, 1992.)

TABLE 7–3. SERUM LUTEINIZING HORMONE (LH) CONCENTRATION (IU/L) IN RELATION TO FERTILITY STATUS

Status	Concentration
Proven fertility	7.2 ± 2.1
Untested fertility	7.4 ± 2.2
Primary infertility	11.0 ± 2.2[a]
Secondary infertility	9.0 ± 2.0[b]

[a] Different from proved fertile and secondary infertile groups.
[b] Different from proved fertile group.
From Balen AH, et al: Polycystic ovary syndrome: The spectrum of the disorder in 1741 patients. Hum Reprod 10:2017, 1995.

TABLE 7–4. OVERVIEW OF NEUROENDOCRINE DISTURBANCES IN POLYCYSTIC OVARY SYNDROME

Neurotransmitter	Hypothesis	Balance of experimental evidence	Conclusion
Dopamine	Decreased dopaminergic tone	Decreased urinary dopamine metabolites Inconsistently decreased LH after dopamine No effect on dopamine antagonism Failure of disulfiram to decrease LH level Variable response to bromocriptine	Decreased dopaminergic activity of limited importance in PCO syndrome
Opioid	Decreased opioid tone	Increased peripheral levels in PCO syndrome Estrogen replacement causing increased opioid tone Decreased opioid effects on LH in PCO syndrome secondary to progesterone deficiency	Decreased central opioid tone, when present, secondary to chronic anovulation
Norepinephrine	Increased noradrenergic tone	Increased urinary metabolites of norepinephrine No change in LH level after α_1 blockade Failure of disulfiram to decrease LH level	Increased norepinephrine activity of no proved importance in PCO syndrome
Serotonin	Decreased serotoninergic tone	Increased platelet serotonin in PCO syndrome No change in LH level by serotonin antagonism	No evidence for role of decreased serotonin activity in PCO syndrome

From Chehab FF, et al: Correction of the sterility defect in homozygous obese female mice by treatment with human recombinant leptin. Nature Genet 12:318, 1996.

of neuropeptide Y, which is itself an inhibitor of GnRH.[26] The suggestion then is that low levels of leptin result in subnormal gonadotropin secretion by allowing inhibition of GnRH action by neuropeptide Y. Fasting lowers serum leptin levels. It is intriguing to recall that starvation, as of women with anorexia nervosa, causes subnormal gonadotropin secretion, particularly with respect to LH secretion. Perhaps the high levels of leptin anticipated among some (particularly obese) patients with PCO syndrome contribute to increased LH secretion in women with this condition. The leptin system certainly provides an important link between nutrition and reproduction. Given the frequent association of PCO syndrome with obesity and eating disorders such as bulimia,[27] some involvement of the leptin system does seem likely in patients with this disorder.

Reproductive Impact of Hypersecretion of LH. Several studies have shown that high serum LH concentrations are associated with impaired fertility despite a normal rate of ovulation, whether occurring spontaneously or as a result of induction of ovulation.[28] A field study of 200 women with regular menstrual cycles who were attending a preconception clinic showed that among those with elevated serum LH concentrations during the follicular phase, the rate of conception was reduced from 83% to 60% ($P = .015$) over the 2-year period of study. Even more remarkably, among those who did conceive, those who had an elevated LH concentration during the follicular phase anytime in the 2 years preceding conception had a miscarriage rate of 65% versus a rate of 12% among those with normal LH levels.[29]

The striking association of high LH levels with such an adverse fertility outcome raises the question of whether LH is a marker or the mediator of the problem. It may be argued that it is a factor common to hypersecretion of LH and low fecundity (the presence of PCO syndrome itself) that is the cause of impairment of fertility. The point has important therapeutic impli-

cations. At present, although there is much circumstantial evidence implicating LH itself,[30] results of a definitive clinical trial of ovulation induction in the presence and absence of high serum LH levels has not been published. In contrast, findings that have been published from studies with transgenic mice that overexpress LH activity are intriguing and suggestive. These mice have PCOs and are anovulatory and infertile.[31]

To summarize, hypersecretion of LH occurs in a large proportion of patients with PCO syndrome. It is caused by an increase in the rate and amplitude of LH pulses, the underlying neuroendocrine mechanisms of which are not yet known. High follicular-phase LH levels are related to infertility and high miscarriage rates.

ETIOLOGY OF POLYCYSTIC OVARY SYNDROME

Over the years there have been essentially two theories of the cause of PCO syndrome. The first has seen the ovary as victim; that is, the fundamental disturbance is in hypothalamic or pituitary control of gonadotropin secretion, which results in chronic anovulation and the development of PCOs. The second has seen the ovary as culprit; that is, the condition is primarily an ovarian disturbance.

It is apparent from the earlier description of the heterogeneity of the PCO syndrome that neither hypothesis gives a complete account of the condition. There are, for example, data that indicate that the PCO syndrome runs in families,[32] perhaps with a dominant mode of inheritance.[33] There is also the in vitro evidence mentioned earlier of increased androgen secretion by interstitial cells cultured from PCOs. On the other hand, not all women with PCOs express the condition; it can be detected before puberty and in women with HH. It is well known that any factor that provokes insulin secretion (obesity, conditions like acromegaly and Cushing syndrome) can lead to clinical expression of the condition. For the genetic cause of PCOs to express themselves, there must be provoking factors, some of which are themselves genetic (for example, mutations in the gene that encodes the insulin receptor in patients with type A insulin resistance). There also remains the possibility of common pathways that link apparent environmental factors (for example, insulin resistance) with apparent genetic factors (overexpression of androgenic steroid activity). For example, Miller et al[34] showed that 17,20-lyase activity (androgen biosynthetic activity) is increased as a result of serine phosphorylation of the steroidogenic enzyme system cytochrome P450C17α. Serine phosphorylation of the insulin receptor contributes to the insulin resistance of PCO syndrome by reducing autophosphorylation of the tyrosine residue of the insulin receptor.[35]

The hypothesis is that in PCO syndrome, activation of a common pathway results in excessive serine phosphorylation of the insulin receptor in a wide variety of tissues and of cytochrome P450C17 in the adrenal glands and ovary, increasing adrenal and ovarian androgen secretion and decreasing insulin sensitivity. Although the common provoking agent is not known, it is clear that progress in this field requires a combination of refinements in definition of the syndrome, that is, in recognition of the importance of its heterogeneity, and improvements in our understanding of the molecular biologic characteristics of hormone secretion and action.

MANAGEMENT OF POLYCYSTIC OVARY SYNDROME

Infertility

There are essentially two causes of the infertility attributable to PCO syndrome. The first is a reduced rate of ovulation, and the second is hypersecretion of LH. The rate of ovulation among women with PCO syndrome is mainly determined by the degree of hyperinsulinism, so initial advice should focus on control of insulin secretion through diet and exercise. Few women with PCO syndrome and a body mass index (BMI) greater than 30 kg/m^2 can expect to have a regular cycle. Successful weight loss is associated with a return of ovarian cyclicity and an increase in the number of women who respond to treatment with antiestrogens.[36]

For most women the first line of treatment with medication is with clomiphene citrate. It is not possible to give a precise figure for its efficacy because many patients receive it before referral to specialty centers. It is probable that this practice should change because of the recent concern over long-term risks of clomiphene treatment, such as development of tumors of the ovary.[37] At our clinic we advise patients that successful induction of ovulation for 6 months will provide them with a realistic chance of conceiving and that increasing the duration of treatment should only be undertaken after a clear discussion of the risks. This approach certainly places a strong onus on the patient to maximize her response to treatment by controlling her weight and on the doctor to ensure maximum efficacy of clomiphene by undertaking careful surveillance of treatment. We do not administer the drug in doses of more than 100 mg for 5 days because higher doses are frequently associated with an antiestrogenic effect on the lower genital tract.

For women who do not ovulate on clomiphene citrate, the next step depends on serum LH concentrations and whether the patient is obese or slim. If the serum LH level is not raised, we proceed to gonadotropin therapy. At present the gonadotropin preparations available are mainly those depleted of LH, which, it must be accepted, is rarely of much consequence for patients with PCO syndrome. We use a low-dose schedule of administration in which the starting dose is half an ampule (37.5 IU of follicle-stimulating hormone [FSH]) per day, and the dose increment is half an ampule per day every 7 to 10 days.[38] Careful ultrasound surveillance is undertaken.[39] Using this approach one achieves acceptable efficacy with almost no cases of OHSS and few multiple pregnancies.[40] For detailed schedules, the reader is referred to the review by Homburg.[41] Perhaps the most important aspect is the timing of administration of hCG (human chorionic gonadotropin). Administration is withheld if there are six or more follicles 14 mm in diameter or smaller (to avoid OHSS) or three or more follicles 16 mm in diameter or larger (to reduce the risk of multiple pregnancy).[42]

If the patient is slim and has a high follicular-phase serum LH concentration, we recommend ovarian diathermy. Details of the technique of this procedure are given by Amar et al.[43] We recommend not more than four diathermy burns per ovary. In a most useful review of the literature, Donesky and Adashi[44] compiled the results for a total of 947 patients. After the operation, ovulation, either spontaneously or with the addition of clomiphene citrate, occurred in 778 (82.1%) and pregnancy in 561 (59.2%) of the patients, results that compare favorably with those of gonadotropin therapy. The best results are obtained by slim women with elevated follicular-phase LH concentrations, which are usually normalized by the operation. In our experience miscarriage rates among these patients with PCO syndrome intriguingly are not greater than those expected for the patient's age.[45]

The potential advantages of the operation are as follows: no increase in the rate of multiple gestation, elimination of the risk of ovarian hyperstimulation, no need for intensive monitoring, potentially lower rate of miscarriage, multiple ovulatory cycles from a single treatment, and finally, the lower cost of the operation compared with gonadotropin therapy. Donesky and

Adashi[44] do point out in their review that the operation is not free of risk. Adhesions may occur, and there have been reports of postoperative ovarian atrophy, which although rare causes one to caution against occasional surgical procedures and in my opinion are strong arguments for minimal damage to the ovary. At present the mode of action of the procedure is unknown.[46]

If a patient is overweight, we advise against ovarian diathermy, and the options become rather limited. We do offer gonadotropin therapy (pulsatile GnRH therapy is futile for obese patients) but are increasingly reluctant to treat patients with a BMI of 35 kg/m^2 or more because the outcome of treatment at this weight is so poor. Although other investigators have found that for patients with high follicular-phase LH concentrations pretreatment with a GnRH analog to suppress gonadotropin secretion is advantageous,[47] in our experience this approach has been disappointing and we rarely advise it.

To summarize, improvement in fertility is obtained by increasing the rate of ovulation while keeping follicular-phase LH concentrations within normal range. Careful ultrasound and endocrine surveillance is required to ensure that rates of multiple pregnancy and ovarian hyperstimulation are kept to a minimum. With these schedules, cumulative conception and live-birth rates should be normal for the patient's age, and multiple pregnancy rates should not exceed 10%.

Hyperandrogenism

Because the cause of hirsutism, seborrhea, and acne is an increase in testosterone production rate, often amplified by a reduction in testosterone binding because of the insulin-induced inhibition of SHBG synthesis, treatment is aimed primarily at reducing androgen production while local dermatologic measures are applied. The two approaches are complementary because reducing testosterone drive reduces the rate of hair growth but does not make hair fall out, whereas depilation removes hair but does not slow its rate of regrowth.

The central role of insulin in stimulating testosterone secretion by a PCO while reducing SHBG synthesis by the liver means that any program of treatment must incorporate a reduction of insulin secretion through a combination of diet and exercise. Parenthetically, one may note that because adverse effects of obesity-mediated hyperinsulinism are a feature of all aspects of PCO syndrome, the sooner our patients receive advice about this, the sooner they will be able to take preventive measures to reduce clinical expression of the disorder.

Drug regimens are predicated on two principles. The first is that except in patients with coexisting congenital or late-onset adrenal hyperplasia, the source of the excess androgen is the PCO. The second is that treatments that worsen insulin resistance should be eschewed. This means that treatment with glu-

cocorticoids is contraindicated unless there is a specific adrenal disorder.

A combined oral contraceptive is for most patients the medication of choice. In Europe, Dianette (containing 35 μg of ethinyl estradiol and 2 mg of cyproterone acetate) is usually chosen, often supplemented with 50 mg of cyproterone acetate for the first 10 days of each packet of Dianette.[48] There has recently been some concern over liver toxicity of cyproterone acetate, but a review by the Committee on Safety of Medicines of the United Kingdom indicated that the problem was mainly related to the high doses administered to men with prostatic carcinoma.[49] There were 96 reports but only five concerned women, of whom four were using Dianette. Oral contraceptives containing 35 μg ethinyl estradiol in combination with a progestin are used widely in the United States. Contraindications to treatment with Dianette with or without cyproterone acetate are essentially those of oral contraceptives. Most women need treatment for 12 to 18 months; thereafter the dose is gradually lowered to the smallest consistent with the patient's perception of her skin and contraceptive needs.

Spironolactone has been used for 30 years as an antagonist of mineralocorticoids, but it also functions as an antiandrogen.[50] It is a weak gestagen, but unlike cyproterone acetate (particularly when combined with an estrogen) it is not contraceptive. Treatment is therefore optimally scheduled with an effective means of contraception because of the risk that the compound will have an adverse effect on male fetal development. Because spironolactone is capable of lowering serum potassium levels, baseline evaluation of electrolytes is warranted.

Flutamide is a nonsteroidal pure antiandrogen. In a randomized, controlled clinical trial of use to treat patients with moderate to severe hirsutism,[51] the results of treatment for 9 months with flutamide in a dose of 250 mg twice a day every day (28 patients) proved superior to those obtained with spironolactone in a dose of 50 mg twice a day on days 5 to 25 of the cycle (27 patients). Both groups also received treatment with a triphasic oral contraceptive. Two problems with flutamide should be noted. Because it is a pure antiandrogen, it is not contraceptive and so when used alone the risk for unintentional exposure during pregnancy must be recognized. Flutamide therefore should be used in combination with birth control. The second problem is the risk of liver damage: It seems that as many as 0.36% of people who use the drug experience a hepatitic reaction, which can progress to severe necrosis and prove fatal.[52] Certainly liver function tests should be performed before therapy and after 2 and 4 weeks of therapy. Treatment should be discontinued if the patient reports nausea, vomiting, fatigue, jaundice, or other signs and symptoms of liver injury.

Suppression of endogenous gonadotropin secretion with a

superactive analog of GnRH may be used to improve hirsutism. This treatment, which can be combined with an antiandrogen and with small doses of estrogen to avoid systemic deestrogenization, is useful in the occasional patient for whom there are contraindications to the usual regimens.

Finasteride, an inhibitor of the 5α-reductase enzyme that converts testosterone to dihydrotestosterone may be used to treat hirsutism.[53] There are two isoforms of the enzyme. One, which in men is expressed in the prostate, is readily inhibited by finasteride. The other, more widely distributed isoform (for example in skin and scalp hair follicles) has different characteristics and requires development of enzyme inhibitors with properties different from finasteride. It is important to note that the study in question involved patients with only mild hirsutism. It will be surprising if finasteride proves successful in severe cases.

In summary, management of the dermal results of hyperandrogenization requires attention to depilation, to reducing the androgen load on the skin through hygienic lifestyle measures that lower insulin drive, and to specific drug regimens. The various components are complementary. Because the cycle of hair growth is very slow, patients should be warned that efficacy cannot be assessed in less than 1 year. Treatment should not be delayed; the longer the hair follicle is exposed to excessive androgen stimulation, the more difficult it is to return its rate of growth to normal.

REFERENCES

1. Stein IF, Leventhal ML: Amenorrhea associated with bilateral polycystic ovary syndrome. *Am J Obstet Gynecol* 29:181, 1935
2. Adams J, Franks S, Polson DW, et al: Multifollicular ovaries: Clinical and endocrine features and response to pulsatile gonadotropin releasing hormone. *Lancet* 2:1375, 1985
3. Peters H, Byskov AG, Grinsted J: The development of the ovary during childhood in health and disease. In: Coutts JRT (ed), *Functional Morphology of the Human Ovary.* Lancaster, England, MTP Press, 1981:26–33
4. Stanhope R, Adams J, Jacobs HS, Brook CGD: Ovarian ultrasound assessment in normal children, idiopathic precocious puberty and during low dose pulsatile gonadotrophin releasing hormone treatment of hypogonadotrophic hypogonadism. *Arch Dis Child* 60:116, 1985
5. Takahashi K, Ozaki T, Okada M, Uchida A, Kitao M: Relationship between ultrasonography and histopathological changes in polycystic ovarian syndrome. *Hum Reprod* 9:2255–2258, 1994
6. Kyei-Mensah A, Zaidi J, Campbell S: Ultrasound diagnosis of polycystic ovary syndrome. *Baillieres Clin Endocrinol Metab* 10:49, 1996
7. Zaidi J, Pittrof R, Campbell S, Tan SL, Kyei-Mensah A, Jacobs HS: Ovarian stromal bloodflow changes in women with polycystic ovaries: A possible new marker for ultrasound diagnosis? *Hum Reprod* 10:1992, 1995
8. Jacobs HS: Prevalence and significance of polycystic ovaries. *Ultrasound Obstet Gynaecol* 4:3, 1994
9. Polson DW, Wadsworth J, Adams J, Franks S: Polycystic ovaries: A common finding in normal women. *Lancet* 2:70, 1988
10. Bridges NA, Cooke A, Healy MJ, Hindmarsh PC, Brook CG: Standards for ovarian volume in childhood and puberty. *Fertil Steril* 60:456, 1993
11. Shoham Z, Conway GS, Patel A, Jacobs HS: Polycystic ovaries in patients with hypogonadotropic hypogonadism: Similarity of ovarian response to gonadotropin stimulation in patients with polycystic ovarian syndrome. *Fertil Steril* 58:37, 1992
12. MacDougal MJ, Tan SL, Balen AH, Jacobs HS: A controlled study comparing patients with and without polycystic ovaries undergoing in vitro fertilisation. *Hum Reprod* 8:233, 1993
13. Franks S, White D, Gilling-Smith, Carey A, Waterworth D, Williamson D: Hypersecretion of androgens by polycystic ovaries: The role of genetic factors in the regulation of cytochrome P450C17α. *Baillieres Clin Endocrinol Metab* 10:193, 1996
14. Goldzieher JW, Green JS: The polycystic ovary syndrome: Clinical and histological features. *J Clin Endocrinol* 22:325, 1962
15. Balen AH, Conway GS, Kaltsas G, et al: Polycystic ovary syndrome: The spectrum of the disorder in 1741 patients. *Hum Reprod* 10:2107, 1995
16. Conway GS: Polycystic ovary syndrome: Clinical aspects. *Baillieres Clin Endocrinol Metab* 10:263, 1996
17. Conway GS, Jacobs HS: Clinical implications of hyperinsulinaemia in women. *Clin Endocrinol* 39:623, 1993
18. Jacobs HS: Polycystic ovary syndrome: Etiology and management. *Curr Opin Obstet Gynecol* 7:203, 1995
19. Dunaif A: Hyperandrogenic anovulation (PCOS): A unique disorder of insulin action associated with an increased risk of non–insulin dependent diabetes mellitus. *Am J Med* 98:33S, 1995
20. Conway GS, Agrawal R, Betteridge DJ, Jacobs HS: Risk factors for coronary artery disease in lean and obese women with the polycystic ovary syndrome. *Clin Endocrinol* 37:119, 1992
21. Dahlgren E, Janson PO, Johansson S, et al: Women with polycystic ovary syndrome wedge resected in 1956–1965: A long term follow up focusing on natural history and circulating hormones. *Fertil Steril* 57:505, 1992
22. Reaven GM: Role of insulin resistance in human disease. *Diabetes* 37:1595, 1983
23. Pierpoint T, McKeigue PM, Isaacs AJ, Jacobs HS: Mortality of women with polycystic ovary syndrome at long term follow up. (In press)
24. Soule SG: Neuroendocrinology of the polycystic ovary syndrome. *Baillieres Clin Endocrinol Metab* 10:205, 1996
25. Chehab FF, Lim ME, Ronghua L: Correction of the sterility defect in homozygous obese female mice by treatment with the human recombinant leptin. *Nature Genet* 12:318, 1996
26. Stephens TW, Basinski M, Bristow PK, et al: The role of neuropeptide Y in the antiobesity action of the obese gene product. *Nature* 377:530, 1995
27. McCluskey S, Evans C, Lacey JH, Pearce JM, Jacobs HS: Polycystic ovary syndrome and bulimia. *Fertil Steril* 55:287, 1991
28. Balen AH, Tan SL, Jacobs HS: Hypersecretion of luteinising hor-

mone: A significant cause of infertility and miscarriage. *Br J Obstet Gynaecol* 100:1082, 1993

29. Regan L, Owen EJ, Jacobs HS: Hypersecretion of LH, infertility and spontaneous abortion. *Lancet* 336:1141, 1990

30. Shoham Z, Jacobs HS, Insler V: Luteinizing hormone: Its role, mechanism of action, and detrimental effects when hypersecreted during the follicular phase. *Fertil Steril* 59:1153, 1993

31. Risma KA, Clay CM, Nett TM, Wagner T, Yun, Nilson JH: Targeted overexpression of luteinizing hormone in transgenic mice leads to infertility, polycystic ovaries, and ovarian tumors. *Proc Natl Acad Sci USA* 92:1322, 1995

32. Hague WM, Adams J, Reeders ST, Peto TEA, Jacobs HS: Familial polycystic ovaries: A genetic disease? *Clin Endocrinol* 29:593, 1988

33. Carey AH, Chan KL, Short F, Frank S, Williamson R: Evidence for a single gene defect in polycystic ovaries and male pattern baldness. *Clin Endocrinol* 38:653, 1993

34. Zhang L-H, Rodriguez H, Ohno S, Miller WL: Serine phosphorylation of human P450c17 increases 17,20 lyase activity: Implications for adrenarche and polycystic ovary syndrome. *Proc Natl Acad Sci USA* 92:10619, 1995

35. Dunaif A, Xia J, Book CB, Schenker E, Tang Z: Excessive insulin receptor serine phosphorylation in cultured fibroblasts and in skeletal muscle: A potential mechanism for insulin resistance in the polycystic ovary syndrome. *J Clin Invest* 96:801, 1995

36. Kiddy DS, Hamilton-Fairley D, Seppala M, et al: Diet-induced changes in sex hormone binding globulin and free testosterone in women with normal or polycystic ovaries: Correlation with serum insulin and insulin-like growth factor-1. *Clin Endocrinol* 31:757, 1989

37. Rossing MA, Daling JR, Weiss NS, Moore DE, Self SG: Ovarian tumors in a cohort of infertile women. *N Engl J Med* 331:771, 1994

38. Hamilton-Fairley D, Kiddy D, Watson H, Franks S: Low dose gonadotrophin therapy for induction of ovulation in 100 women with polycystic ovary syndrome. *Hum Reprod* 6:1095, 1991

39. Shoham Z, Di Carlo C, Patel A, Conway SG, Jacobs HS: Is it possible to run a successful ovulation induction program based solely on ultrasound monitoring? The importance of endometrial measurements. *Fertil Steril* 56:836, 1991

40. Balen AH, Braat DDM, West C, Patel A, Jacobs HS: Cumulative conception and live birth rates after the treatment of anovulatory infertility: Safety and efficacy of ovulation induction in 200 patients. *Hum Reprod* 9:1563, 1994

41. Homburg R: Polycystic ovary syndrome: Induction of ovulation. *Baillieres Clin Endocrinol Metab* 10:281, 1996

42. Farhi J, West C, Patel A, Jacobs HS: Treatment of anovulatory infertility: The problem of multiple pregnancy. *Hum Reprod* 11:429, 1996

43. Armar NA, McGarrigle HHG, Honour JW, Holownia P, Jacobs HS, Lachelin GCL: Laparoscopic ovarian diathermy in the management of anovulatory infertility in women with polycystic ovaries: Endocrine changes and clinical outcome. *Fertil Steril* 53:45, 1990

44. Donesky BW, Adashi EY: Surgical ovulation induction: Role of ovarian diathermy in polycystic ovary syndrome. *Baillieres Clin Endocrinol Metab* 10:293, 1996

45. Armar NA, Lachelin GC: Laparoscopic ovarian diathermy: An effective treatment for antioestrogen resistant women with the polycystic ovary syndrome. *Br J Obstet Gynaecol* 100:161, 1993

46. Balen AH, Jacobs HS: A prospective study comparing unilateral and bilateral laparoscopic ovarian diathermy in women with the polycystic ovary syndrome. *Fertil Steril* 62:921, 1994

47. Fleming R, Haxton MJ, Hamilton MPR, Coutts JTR: Successful treatment of infertile women with oligomenorrhoea using a combination of an LHRH agonist and exogenous gonadotrophins. *Br J Obstet Gynaecol* 92:369, 1985

48. Miller JA, Jacobs HS: Treatment of hirsutism and acne with cyproterone acetate. *Clin Endocrinol Metab* 15:373, 1986

49. Committee on Safety of Medicines of the United Kingdom: *Curr Probl* 21:1, 1995

50. Shaw JC: Spironolactone in dermatologic therapy. *J Am Acad Dermatol* 24:236, 1991

51. Cusan L, Dupont A, Gomez J-L, Tremblay RR, Labrie F: Comparison of flutamide and spironolactone in the treatment of hirsutism: A randomized controlled clinical trial. *Fertil Steril* 61:281, 1994

52. Gomez J-L, Dupont A, Cusan L, et al: Incidence of liver toxicity associated with the use of flutamide in prostate cancer patients. *Am J Med* 92:465, 1992

53. Moghetti P, Castello R, Magnani CM, et al: Clinical and hormonal effects of the 5α-reductase inhibitor finasteride in idiopathic hirsutism. *J Clin Endocrinol Metab* 79:1115, 1994

CHAPTER 8

Luteal-Phase Inadequacy

STEVEN T. NAKAJIMA · MICHAEL R. SOULES

Overview
Luteal-Phase Physiology
   Corpus luteum
   Endometrium
Luteal-Phase Deficiency
   Prevalence
   Pathophysiology
Confirmation of Luteal Function

Evaluation of the Luteal Phase in the Clinical Setting
   Some tests of luteal function
   Endometrial biopsy
Management of Luteal-Phase Deficiency
   Overview
   Treatment protocols
   Alternative therapies
Summary

OVERVIEW

The luteal phase of the menstrual cycle begins after ovulation of a tertiary ovarian follicle and ends with the onset of menstrual bleeding. During this time, the corpus luteum secretes multiple steroids and peptides, but it is progesterone that primarily leads to endometrial gland maturation and deciduation of the endometrial stroma. If an embryo undergoes successful nidation and experiences implantation into the endometrium, the developing trophoblast secretes human chorionic gonadotropin (hCG), and the life span of the corpus luteum is extended. Without luteal rescue by hCG, the corpus luteum undergoes a programmed demise, and menses ensues. New information has supplemented this simplistic view of luteal function and clarified the importance of normal luteal activity to overall cycle fecundity. New markers of luteal function and data on the duration of endometrial receptivity have added important information about the endometrium and the contributions of the ovary. The primary goal of this chapter is to outline the pathophysio-

logic aspects of the luteal phase and to apply the salient principles to clinical practice (Fig 8–1).

LUTEAL-PHASE PHYSIOLOGY

Corpus Luteum

After ovulation, the remaining granulosa cells of the collapsed follicle hypertrophy increase protein synthesis with subsequent secretion, and become exposed directly to the vascular system (granulosa lutein cells).[1] Both the granulosa and theca cells undergo a shift in structure and function as a result of being vascularized, termed *luteinization*. Luteinized granulosa cells are anatomically larger in diameter (20–30 μm) than the smaller luteinized theca cells (5–20 μm) of the corpus luteum.[2] The luteinized granulosa cells are responsible for the basal luteinizing hormone (LH)–independent secretion of progesterone throughout the luteal phase. During the late luteal phase, the

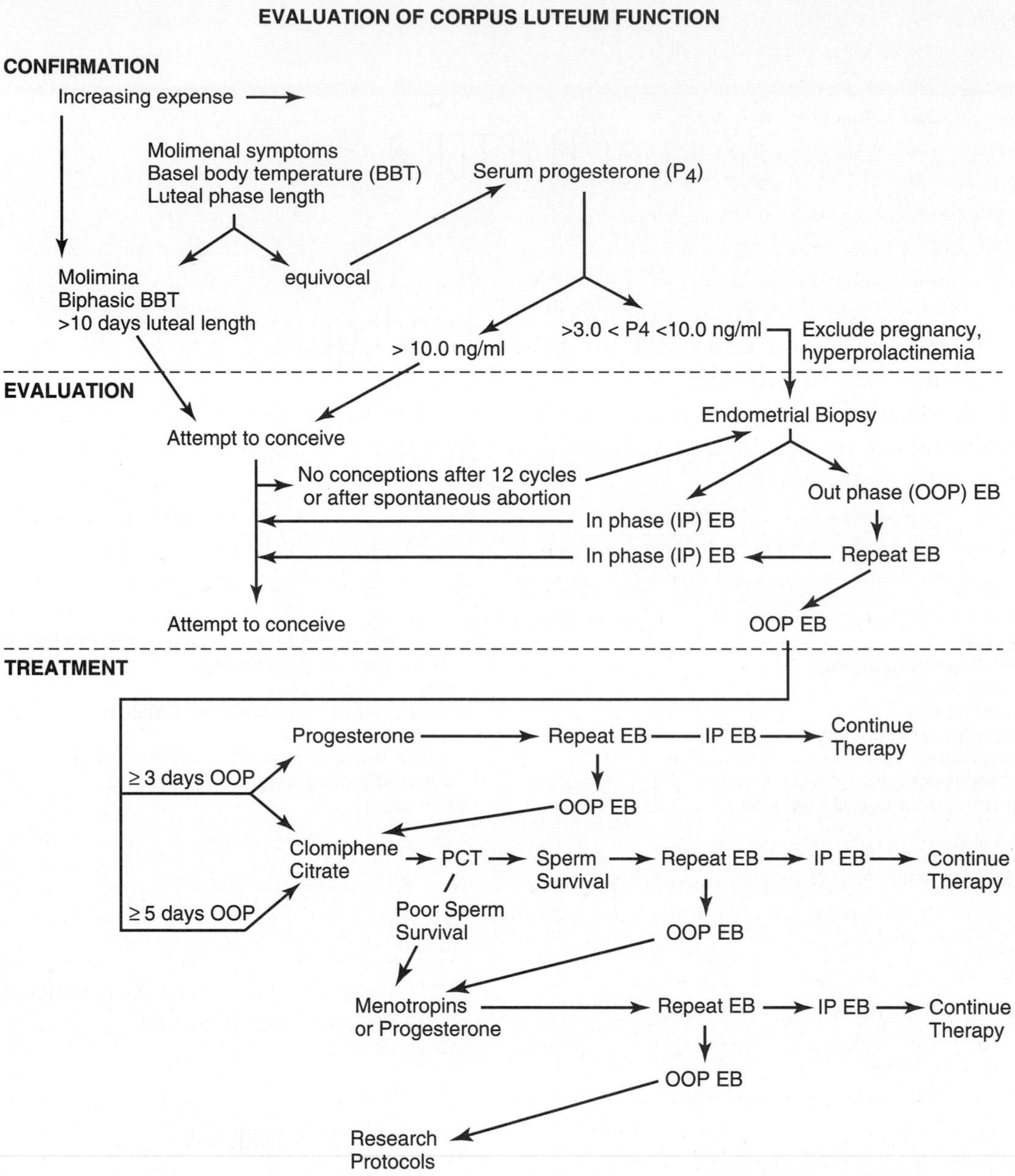

EVALUATION OF CORPUS LUTEUM FUNCTION

CONFIRMATION

Increasing expense ⟶

Molimenal symptoms
Basel body temperature (BBT)
Luteal phase length

Serum progesterone (P$_4$)

Molimina
Biphasic BBT
>10 days luteal length

equivocal

> 10.0 ng/ml

>3.0 < P4 <10.0 ng/ml — Exclude pregnancy, hyperprolactinemia

EVALUATION

Attempt to conceive

Endometrial Biopsy

No conceptions after 12 cycles
or after spontaneous abortion

Out phase (OOP) EB

In phase (IP) EB

In phase (IP) EB ◀ Repeat EB

Attempt to conceive

OOP EB

TREATMENT

Progesterone ⟶ Repeat EB — IP EB ⟶ Continue Therapy

≥ 3 days OOP

OOP EB

Clomiphene Citrate ⟶ PCT ⟶ Sperm Survival ⟶ Repeat EB ⟶ IP EB ⟶ Continue Therapy

≥ 5 days OOP

Poor Sperm Survival

OOP EB

Menotropins or Progesterone ⟶ Repeat EB ⟶ IP EB ⟶ Continue Therapy

OOP EB

Research Protocols

Figure 8–1. Summary of the confirmation (top) and evaluation (middle) of corpus luteum function. Possible treatment options (bottom) for the correction of repetitive endometrial immaturity.

smaller theca lutein cells increase in diameter (<20 μm) and primarily secrete progesterone in response to LH stimulation. These theca lutein cells are believed to be responsible for the episodic secretion of progesterone and the hCG-stimulated increase in progesterone levels during the process of luteal rescue. Other luteal hormones (17-hydroxyprogesterone, inhibin, relaxin) are secreted by the ovary, but these hormones do not appear to be absolutely essential to the implantation process. These observations are based on data from successful embryo transfer procedures performed on patients with underlying gonadal dysgenesis, surgical castration, or deliberate ovarian suppression.[3,4] These hypogonadal patients required only exogenous progesterone supplementation after the endometrium had been initially primed with estrogen.

During the normal luteal phase, discrete LH pulses stimulate the theca lutein cells of the corpus luteum, and progesterone levels acutely increase with a resultant episodic (pulsatile) progesterone secretory pattern.[5,6] This LH-entrained progesterone secretion pattern begins in the midluteal phase and decreases in frequency over the duration of the luteal phase. As the overall progesterone level increases, there is a decrease in LH pulse frequency and an increase in LH pulse amplitude. These LH pulse alterations appear to be directly modulated by endogenous opiate peptides, which are further influenced by increasing levels of progesterone.[7] Coincident with decreasing luteotropic LH stimulation, luteolytic factors, primarily uterine prostaglandins, further oppose corpus luteum activity.[8] If conception and embryo implantation occur, trophoblastic hCG secretion replaces LH secretion as the dominant stimulus to the corpus luteum. This extension of luteal function by hCG stimulation is known as *luteal rescue.* If hCG is not produced, then LH pulses diminish in frequency, leading to inadequate support of the corpus luteum and its eventual demise. Because of decreased luteal progesterone and estradiol secretion, the anatomic integrity of the endometrium collapses, and menses ensues. Despite the relatively small volume of the corpus luteum, peak secretion of progesterone can reach 20 to 40 mg per day. By weight, the corpus luteum at peak function is one of the most active steroidogenic tissues in humans.[1]

Endometrium

During the luteal phase, an orderly progression of changes transforms the endometrium from proliferative to secretory tissue. Noyes et al[9] in 1950 described these histologic changes as an orderly series of steps. In their review of 300 endometrial biopsies, the authors associated distinct histologic changes with discrete periods (days) in the luteal phase. These dating criteria allowed assignment of an idealized menstrual day to an endometrial biopsy specimen. In specimens with a range of histologic changes, the most advanced histologic composition by convention was used to assign a date to the sample. With this tissue dating system, 60% of women had their subsequent menses within 1 day of that predicted with a mid to late luteal-phase endometrial biopsy. Among a subset of 40 women with basal body temperature (BBT) data, 78% of women menstruated within 1 day of predicted menses, counting forward from the day of temperature elevation. Although these biopsy specimens were obtained from a primarily infertile population, the dating criteria of Noyes et al is still used to evaluate luteal function of both fertile and infertile women.

In response to circulating levels of estrogen in the proliferative phase of the menstrual cycle, progesterone receptors form in the endometrium. Garcia et al[10] proposed an alternative endometrial dating system based on the presence of estrogen and progesterone receptors. Because of conflicting findings about the association between hormone receptor status and histologic composition of the endometrium, measurement of hormone re-

ceptor levels for the prediction of luteal adequacy has had limited use. Similarly, daily endometrial prolactin production increases with endometrial maturity and can be used to verify histologic changes in the endometrium.[11] New developments at the level of endometrium have included reports of variations in endometrial placental protein 14 (PP14) levels[12] and the formation of endometrial pinopodes during the luteal phase.[13] Pinopode formation can be detected only with scanning electron microscopy (Fig 8–2). The exact function of these fluctuations in hormone levels or the descriptive changes that occur in the endometrium have not been completely clarified, nor have the findings been used in the routine clinical treatment of infertile patients.

Further evaluation of the endometrium on a molecular level reveals the presence of a family of proteins that may be critical to the events of normal embryo implantation. One protein that may mark the beginning of the implantation window is the αvβ3 vitronectin receptor.[14] This protein is a member of the integrin family of cell adhesion molecules. The integrin αvβ3 appears on the epithelial cells of normal human endometrium on idealized cycle days 19 to 20. The presence of this receptor

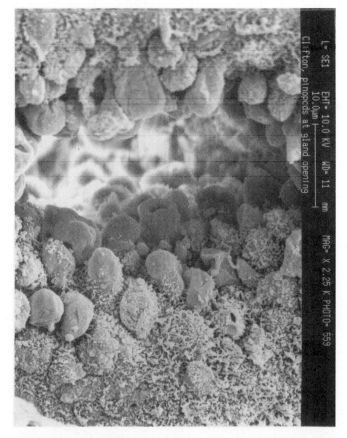

Figure 8–2. Endometrial pinopodes surrounding a gland opening. *(Courtesy of Dr. Richard Paulson.)*

coincides with the optimal midluteal implantation period. Absence of this receptor has been associated with out-of-phase endometrial biopsy specimens dated by the usual histologic criteria. The presence followed by the absence of another integrin, $\alpha4\beta1$, on idealized cycle day 24 marks the end of the period of endometrial receptivity.[15] These observations agree with two other earlier observations on the period of optimal endometrial receptivity. In a classic study of hysterectomy specimens, Hertig et al[16] demonstrated that human embryos undergo endometrial attachment by idealized cycle day 21 to 22. In a more recent review of hCG levels during the periimplantation period, Bergh and Navot[17] extrapolated that hCG production could be detected peripherally as early as idealized cycle day 20 (postovulation day 6). These findings further suggest that the window of implantation begins on idealized cycle day 20 and closes on day 24 and that the presence of the $\alpha v\beta3$ receptor may be synonymous with optimal endometrial receptivity. The application of these concepts is being examined by a number of investigators.

LUTEAL-PHASE DEFICIENCY

Prevalence

The concept of a repetitive corpus luteum deficiency that leads to a defect in endometrial maturation with subsequent infertility or early recurrent abortion is intuitively attractive. Initial work by Jones[18] and Strott et al[19] suggested that there are subgroups of women who consistently have abnormal endometrial maturation or short luteal phases, respectively. These abnormal luteal phases have been collectively categorized as *luteal-phase deficiency* (LPD). After correction of the LPD, many women conceive and have successful pregnancy outcomes. Similar findings have been subsequently reported by others,[20] but the lack of control groups and the small number of treated patients relative to the many different possible causes of LPD have been deficiencies in research. The cited incidence of LPD varies between 8.1% and 17.5% depending on the author's definition of LPD and the sample population,[20,21] but most agree that the incidence of repetitive defects in endometrial maturation is 5% to 10% among referral clinics treating infertility patients. Wild et al[22] reported an incidence of LPD of 10.6% (96 women with LPD among 906 with two biopsy findings more than 2 days out of phase) after they combined the data from two infertility centers. For couples with a history of repetitive pregnancy losses, LPD may be the cause of the losses among 10% to 15% of couples. In some selected series, LPD was the cited cause of 23.0% to 28.3% of recurrent pregnancy losses.[23,24] Again, differences in the definition of LPD, the criteria for the diagnosis of LPD,

and the composition of the referral population account for the wide range in the reported incidence of LPD as a cause of recurrent abortion. Synonymous terms for LPD include *corpus luteum inadequacy, luteal-phase dysfunction, luteal-phase insufficiency,* and *luteal-phase defect.*

Some of the controversy over the prevalence of LPD stems from the inherent variability of the menstrual cycle. Subtle changes in luteal function to frank anovulation can occur from one menstrual cycle to another. Variations in luteal function can, in part, be attributed to alterations in folliculogenesis, inherent variability in the anatomic size of the corpus luteum, or the presence of multiple corpora lutea. Luteal insufficiency can occur more frequently for a short period after a woman's menarche,[25] post partum,[26] postabortion,[27] or during the perimenopausal climacteric period.[25] These specific intervals of time have been called *physiologic luteal dysfunction.*[28] Further alterations in lifestyle or body habitus (strenuous exercise,[29,30] stress,[31] dieting with resulting weight loss[32,33]) also can contribute to decreased luteal function. This concept of varying luteal function has been substantiated by the observations of Davis et al.[34] In this study, the authors performed multiple endometrial biopsies in consecutive menstrual cycles of five previously fertile women. A total of 39 endometrial biopsies were performed. With a commonly applied definition of LPD of a 2 or more day lag in endometrial maturation from expected development, the incidence of two sequential endometrial biopsies demonstrating an endometrial maturation defect was 26.7%. With a more stringent definition for LPD of a 3 or more day lag in endometrial maturation, the incidence of two sequential endometrial biopsies demonstrating an endometrial maturation defect decreased to 6.6%. For two subjects, 10 consecutive menstrual cycles were available for review. For all five women, intervals of abnormal endometrial maturation were interspersed with normal endometrial development (Table 8–1).

In another study, Balasch et al[35] reinforced the concept that a subgroup of women may have a predisposition to repetitive luteal-phase dysfunction. They performed endometrial biopsies in three different menstrual cycles during the course of an infertility investigation. They reported that if the patient had a history of two endometrial biopsies demonstrating inadequate endometrial maturation, there was only a 5.8% likelihood that a third biopsy would have normal endometrial development. The converse of this scenario, in which the first two biopsies were normal followed by an abnormal biopsy, was 4.6%. If the patient's first two biopsies were different, then the third biopsy was abnormal 47% of the time. These findings suggest that there are menstrual cycles in which there is sporadic reversion to an abnormal aberrant endometrial pattern that deviates from the usual and regular maturation process. Because normal periods of endometrial maturation are interspersed with abnormal

TABLE 8–1. INHERENT VARIABILITY IN LUTEAL FUNCTION AS DETERMINED BY ENDOMETRIAL HISTOLOGIC CHANGES FOR TWO FERTILE WOMEN

Biopsy	Idealized Cycle Day by Next Menses	Ideal Histologic Cycle Day	Lag in Development[a] (days)
		Subject B	
1	27	26	1
2	26	24	2
3	26	26	0
4	24	22	2
5	21	Proliferative[b]	>7
6	22	Proliferative[b]	>8
7	Conception	—	—
		Subject E	
1	28	26	2
2	26	23	3
3	19	17	2
4	25	25	0
5	27	22	5
6	24	24	0
7	26	26	0
8	26	26	0
9	23	22	1
10	25	26	—

[a] Idealized cycle day by next menses minus ideal histologic cycle day.
[b] Assigned ideal histologic cycle day 14.
Adapted from Davis OK, et al: The incidence of luteal phase defect in normal, fertile women, determined by serial endometrial biopsies. Fertil Steril 51:582, 1989. Reproduced with permission of the publisher, the American Society for Reproductive Medicine (The American Fertility Society).

intervals, only in cycles in which LPD is present is there a decrease in cycle fecundity. If the occurrence of LPD is infrequent, then a couple's overall cycle fecundity may or may not be decreased.

Pathophysiology

General Concept

It is generally believed that LPD occurs when there is decreased secretion of progesterone by the corpus luteum or when the effect of progesterone is limited at its target tissue, the endometrium. These abnormalities lead to inadequate maturation of the endometrial glands and stroma and biochemical deficiencies intrinsic to implantation. Multiple factors may lead to decreased corpus luteum function, and they can occur during any of three intervals during the menstrual cycle: the follicular phase, luteal phase, or luteal rescue. Within each of these cycle phases, defects in the central trophic stimulus, the ovarian response, or the endometrial response may be defective. It is clear, however, that multiple heterogeneous factors can lead to LPD and that the clinical presentation of LPD may be due to

multiple insults that occur at different times during the menstrual cycle.

Follicular-Phase Events

Because the corpus luteum is derived from the ovarian follicle after ovulation, alterations in folliculogenesis can lead to subsequent inadequate luteal function. Several authors have reported that inadequate levels of follicle-stimulating hormone (FSH) in the follicular phase can lead to LPD. It is informative to review the findings from key studies that addressed this topic. Strott et al[19] observed a lower follicular phase FSH/LH ratio among women with sporadically occurring short luteal phases than among controls. Cook et al[36] reported diminished FSH levels and FSH/LH ratios in the early and midfollicular phases of women with LPD. These findings are supported by both human and animal data showing that FSH levels were temporarily lowered by a gonadotropin-releasing hormone (GnRH) agonist[37] or porcine follicular fluid,[38] respectively, and that luteal function subsequently diminished. The induction of a short luteal phase with porcine follicular fluid suggests that inhibin or an inhibin-like substance may be responsible for LPD. Not all studies have confirmed the presence of lower FSH levels among women with LPD.[39] Among 10 women with LPD whose cycles were intensively studied, Soules et al[39] found no difference in mean follicular phase levels of immunoactive or bioactive FSH, follicular phase length, or ultrasound-determined follicle size compared with these factors in women who did not have LPD. In this same study, mean early and midfollicular immunoreactive inhibin levels were decreased in the LPD cycles compared with controls, suggesting the concept of a suboptimal preovulatory follicle (Fig 8–3). If, however, the previous reports of decreased FSH levels among women with LPD are correct, one would expect an elevation in inhibin levels. Differences in the individual study populations or the need for further refinement of the inhibin assay may be the explanation for the apparent discrepancies in the studies. These conflicting findings suggest that although abnormal folliculogenesis may lead to LPD cycles, it may not be a common cause.

Alterations in LH pulse frequency may be responsible for some instances of LPD. Both Soules et al[40] and Suh and Betz[41] found in separate studies an increased follicular phase LH pulse frequency among women with LPD (Fig 8–4). This hypothesis was substantiated by means of induction of a luteal phase defect in controls with frequent administration of exogenous GnRH during the follicular phase.[42] In contrast, Schweiger et al[43] and Loucks et al[44] in separate studies observed a decreased LH pulse frequency among women with LPD. All four studies showed the pulse abnormalities in the early follicular phase. Subsequent analysis of these studies, however, revealed two different subject populations. The women who participated in the studies by

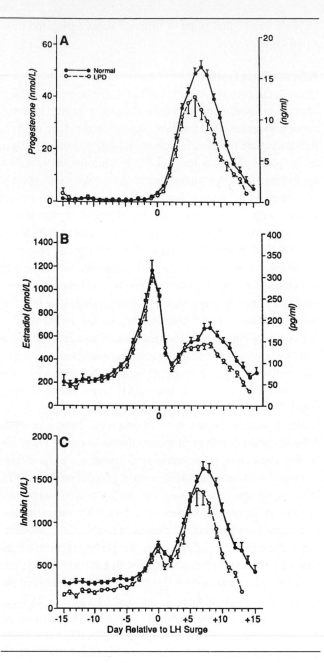

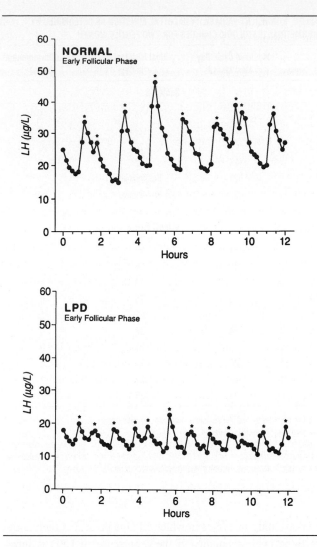

Figure 8–4. The LH secretory pattern of a woman without (top) and a woman with LPD (bottom). Each woman underwent testing for 12 hours with a 10-minute sampling interval. The woman with LPD has more frequent LH pulses of lower amplitude than the woman without LPD. Each identified pulse is indicated by a star. *(From Soules MR, et al: Luteal phase deficiency: Abnormal gonadotropin and progesterone secretion patterns. J Clin Endocrinol Metab 69:813–820, 1989. Reproduced with permission from The Endocrine Society, © 1989.)*

Figure 8–3. The daily mean (±SE) levels of serum progesterone (**A**), estradiol (**B**), and inhibin (**C**) over the menstrual cycle are indicated for the normal (●—●) and LPD (○—○) groups. There was a significant decrease compared with normal values in the luteal-phase integrated levels of these three hormones in the LPD group. There was also a significant decrease in follicular phase (days −12 to −5 relative to the LH surge) mean serum inhibin levels among the LPD group compared with normal values. *(From Soules MR, et al: Luteal phase deficiency: Characterization of reproductive hormones over the menstrual cycle. J Clin Endocrinol Metab 69:804, 1989. Reproduced with permission from The Endocrine Society, © 1989.)*

Soules et al and Suh and Betz were primarily an older, infertile group with biopsy-proved LPD. The women in the studies by Schweiger et al and Loucks et al were younger, exercising, diet-conscious women whose diagnosis of LPD was based on decreased luteal-phase length and lower peak serum progesterone

levels. Despite the discrepancies in the studies, all the investigators may be correct. It may be that any deviation from a normal follicular phase LH pulse frequency might lead to LPD. Alterations in LH pulse frequency may be due to abnormal suprahypothalamic influences on the GnRH pulse generator or an intrinsic GnRH secretory defect. An alteration in LH pulse frequency may be responsible for a suboptimal LH surge. Soules et al[39] documented lower immunoactive and bioactive LH surge levels in LPD cycles compared with normal cycles.

Some data suggest that intrinsic defects might exist in the ovarian follicle or proliferative phase endometrium of women with LPD. Soules et al[39] reported decreased inhibin levels in the early and midfollicular phase of women with LPD compared with controls (see Fig 8–3). Using ultrasound, research groups led by Check[45] and Ying[46] reported a decreased diameter of the dominant follicle among women with LPD. In the study conducted by Ying et al,[46] the investigators demonstrated a significant reduction in the number of small dominant follicles among patients with histologically corrected LPD (P = .04). These ultrasound findings, however, were not confirmed in a larger study of women with LPD.[39] In a study of both proliferative and secretory endometrium for cytosolic and nuclear progesterone receptor concentrations, Jacobs et al[47] found lower proliferative phase endometrial nuclear progesterone receptor concentrations among women with LPD than among women without LPD. The investigators concluded that some women with LPD may have inadequate estrogenic induction of the progesterone receptors. The results of this limited study await confirmation.

Luteal-Phase Events

The secretion of progesterone depends acutely on LH stimulation. When a GnRH antagonist was administered to women in the midluteal phase, progesterone levels decreased and corpus luteum activity quickly diminished.[48] These events led to a shortened luteal phase and premature menstruation. In these same GnRH antagonist–treated subjects, the decline in progesterone levels was reversed by the coadministration of hCG, but not the coadministration of urofollitropin. The luteal rescue due to hCG administration suggests that stimulation of LH receptors, but not FSH receptors, is important for resumption of luteal function. Premature luteolysis has been observed after the disruption of LH secretion by RU486.[49]

Among women with LPD, Soules et al[39] observed lower immuno- and bioactive levels of LH during the mid to late luteal phases compared with controls. Despite short-term negative feedback effects of progesterone on LH secretion,[50] low levels of progesterone do not seem to induce an increase in LH pulse frequency, suggesting an open-loop system. Among women with LPD, the pituitary gland may not compensate and not increase or maintain LH secretion when progesterone levels are low. Further evidence for the importance of LH stimulation on corpus luteum function can be found in the primate model.[51] When LH pulse frequency was decreased to one pulse every 24 hours by a hypothalamic lesion, a short luteal phase occurred.

Central to the pathophysiologic process of LPD is the decreased secretion of progesterone from the corpus luteum over the course of the luteal phase (see Fig 8–3). In LPD cycles, Soules et al[40] demonstrated decreased levels of bioactive LH levels during the midluteal phase (days +6 to +11 relative to the LH surge) and concurrent abnormal fluctuations in circulating progesterone levels over a 24-hour period compared with normal cycles (Fig 8–5). Progesterone pulses in the midluteal

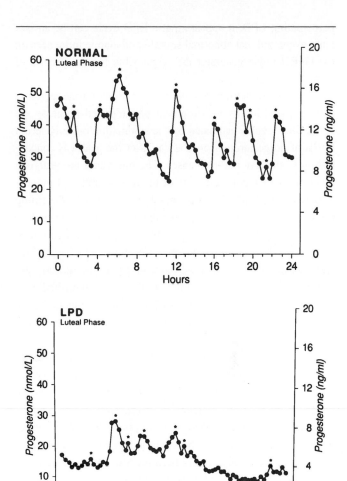

Figure 8–5. The pulsatile patterns of progesterone secretion in the midluteal phase of a normal woman without (top) and a woman with LPD (bottom). Serum progesterone values were determined at 20-minute intervals for 24 hours. Identified pulses are indicated by a star. Note the similar number of progesterone pulses for the two women but the lower progesterone pulse amplitude of the woman with LPD. *(From Soules MR, et al: Luteal phase deficiency: Abnormal gonadotropin and progesterone secretion patterns. J Clin Endocrinol Metab 69:813, 1989. Reproduced with permission from The Endocrine Society, © 1989.)*

phase from LPD cycles were decreased in amplitude (2.5 versus 5.0 ng/mL [8 versus 16 nmol/L]) over a 24-hour period. The mean progesterone level derived from these repetitive samples was similarly lower than among normal cycles (6.3 versus 13.8 ng/mL [20 versus 44 nmol/L]). Similarly, when exogenous pulsatile GnRH was administered during the follicular phase at a supraphysiologic pulse frequency, LPD resulted and low luteal-phase bioactive LH levels were documented.[42] Although low levels of progesterone theoretically may lead to an increased follicular phase LH pulse frequency in the next menstrual cycle, this hypothesis was not confirmed by Soules et al.[52] Instead of perpetuating LPD, it appears that a LPD cycle can be an isolated event and that abnormal suprahypothalamic influences on the GnRH pulse generator are responsible for the genesis of some LPD cycles.

In research settings, the decrease in progesterone secretion can be quantified by measurement of integrated progesterone level. This level is estimated by the summation of daily serum levels of progesterone from the day after the peak LH concentration to the day before menses. The integrated progesterone level provides a good estimate of the total quantity of progesterone secreted. Much debate has been generated concerning the normal luteal-phase range for integrated progesterone levels, but most investigators agree that integrated progesterone levels less than 100 ng·days/mL (318 nmol·days/L) are low, and that levels less than 80 ng·days/mL (254 nmol·days/L) are distinctly abnormal.[53] These lower limits were established from the analysis of progesterone levels from a large number of luteal phases of normal women. The lower limit represents two standard deviations below mean integrated levels.

At the level of the ovary, the human corpus luteum comprises two distinct luteal cell populations derived from the granulosa and theca cells.[2] The granulosa lutein cells appear to be responsible for the basal secretion of progesterone throughout the luteal phase. The theca lutein cells are primarily responsible for the late luteal secretion of progesterone. Specific deficiencies in either cell population have not been reported, but such deficiencies could explain isolated transient abnormalities in endometrial maturation during the luteal phase. In a study by Kusuda et al,[54] in which women underwent both a midluteal and a late endometrial biopsy in the same luteal phase, 32% (27 of 85) of the midluteal biopsies demonstrated a lag in endometrial maturation. Of the 27 abnormal midluteal endometrial biopsies, 52% (14 of 27) of the late luteal biopsies (performed later in the same luteal phase) demonstrated normal appropriate endometrial maturation, whereas 48% (13 of 27) demonstrated persistent endometrial immaturity. It appears that an initially out-of-phase midluteal phase endometrial sample can experience accelerated maturation and appear normal when examined later in the same menstrual cycle. This transient lag in the midluteal phase may be caused by defects in large granulosa lutein cells, and the acceleration in maturity later in the same cycle may be caused by properly functioning small theca lutein cells. Conversely, exclusive defects in the small theca lutein cells may explain the occurrence of a shortened luteal phase. Glandular-stromal asynchrony can be explained by the different luteal cell populations.[21] Because endometrial glandular development predominates in the early luteal phase and stromal maturation occurs primarily in the late luteal phase, glandular-stromal asynchrony (glandular immaturity with normal stromal changes) may be due to a temporal defect in the granulosa lutein cell population.

Evidence for a possible intrinsic defect in the corpus lu-

teum may be attributed to insufficient neovascularization during the luteal phase. Using transvaginal color flow pulsed Doppler ultrasound during both the follicular and luteal phase, Glock and Brumsted[55] demonstrated a significantly increased intraovarian resistance index of the small low-velocity ovarian vessels of the dominant follicle and the subsequent corpus luteum in LPD compared with normal menstrual cycles ($P = .02$). The resistance index is an indicator of downstream vascular resistance. An elevated resistance index is consistent with an absence of maximum capillary penetration and vessel dilatation within the dominant follicle and eventual corpus luteum. This finding was associated with decreased intermittent progesterone levels (obtained during the early, mid, and late luteal phase) at the time of the ultrasound studies. This preliminary finding suggests that an LPD cycle that has been associated with decreased circulating progesterone levels may ultimately result from a poorly vascularized dominant follicle and ensuing corpus luteum. This preliminary finding awaits confirmation in large clinical studies.

Despite adequate levels of circulating progesterone, incomplete endometrial glandular-stromal maturation associated with a marked reduction in endometrial cytosolic high-affinity progesterone binding sites (receptors) was described by Keller et al.[56] Subsequent attempts, however, to correlate the prevalence of progesterone receptors with histologic changes in the endometrium have provided contradictory information.[57–59] Differences in receptor assay method and subject selection probably explain the divergent findings. A series of studies in which prolactin production from explants of endometrial tissue was examined did support the concept of an intrinsic biochemical defect in the endometrium of patients with LPD. Daly et al[11] demonstrated decreased secretion of prolactin in vitro from the endometrium of women with LPD who lagged in expected endometrial maturation compared with control endometrial tissue with the same idealized menstrual dates. Ying et al[60] confirmed these observations and demonstrated that women with corrected LPD with in-phase endometrial biopsy findings secreted appropriate prolactin levels for a given idealized menstrual day.

Luteal Rescue

Defects in the physiologic process of luteal rescue in early pregnancy can occur and lead to diminished cycle fecundity. If trophoblastic hCG production from an intrinsically normal embryo is initially diminished (or late) in stimulating the corpus luteum, failure of luteal rescue can occur. In a study by Stewart et al,[61] daily blood samples obtained from women after therapeutic insemination with donor semen demonstrated elevated levels of ovarian steroids before implantation in conceptive versus conceptive cycles that ultimately aborted and nonconceptive cycles. The women who requested donor insemination had no apparent female factors for their infertility except that they had either an azoospermic or no male partner. In conceptive cycles, levels of estradiol and progesterone were persistently elevated above nonconceptive cycles beginning 6 and 7 days after the LH surge, respectively. This preimplantation elevation in steroid levels occurred before the appearance of detectable serum levels of hCG. The authors suggested that their findings were consistent with preimplantation signaling by the embryo to the corpus luteum. In conceptive cycles that ended in spontaneous abortion, the preimplantation elevation in ovarian steroids was absent and detection of hCG was delayed in comparison with normal conceptive cycles. It should be noted that no findings of diminished hCG bioactivity or an altered hCG secretory pattern during the periimplantation period have been reported to date.[62]

A number of reports over the years have questioned the minimum level of progesterone necessary for the maintenance of early pregnancies.[63–65] Despite very low circulating levels of luteal-phase progesterone, viable pregnancies have been reported in women with the hereditary disorder abetalipoproteinemia.[66] In these women, absence of apoprotein B–containing lipoproteins essential for cholesterol transport causes a marked reduction in progesterone synthesis.[67] In these pregnancies, the minimum threshold level of progesterone may be met by de novo biosynthesis of cholesterol substrate or the presence of another carrier of cholesterol (eg, high-density-lipoprotein subfraction 2).[68] Local increased uteroplacental concentrations of progesterone, not reflected in peripheral levels, may further explain these viable pregnancies. To examine the possible association between lipoprotein levels and circulating ovarian steroid levels, Hansen et al[69] examined the lipid profile of an infertile group of women at the time of endometrial biopsy. They found no difference in total cholesterol or in low- or high-density lipoprotein levels among women with LPD versus women with in-phase histologic changes in the endometrium.

In a study by Azuma et al[70] three women who conceived after assisted reproductive technology treatments all were reported to have low initial circulating serum progesterone levels. None of these pregnancies was supplemented with exogenous progesterone and no episodes of vaginal bleeding occurred. All three pregnancies progressed normally, and all women delivered viable infants. One possible explanation for the successful outcome of these pregnancies may be the elevated follicular phase estradiol levels, which could have induced an increase in the number of endometrial progesterone receptors. In addition to the dramatic examples from Azuma et al[70] another subject in the same study had a progesterone level of 2 nmol/L (0.60 ng/mL) 14 days after oocyte retrieval. This fourth patient did receive progesterone supplementation 4 days later and by 5.5 menstrual weeks had a progesterone level greater than 25 nmol/L (7.8 ng/mL). These findings suggest there may be a grace period 2 to 3 weeks after ovulation during which pregnancies may survive despite very low levels of progesterone.

These findings suggest that corpus luteum-derived or exogenous progesterone may induce formation of a secondary factor that allows maintenance of early pregnancy before progesterone production by the trophoblast.

To establish an ovarian factor as a potential defect in the process of luteal rescue, descriptive studies can establish a normal range for mid and late luteal progesterone levels in conceptive versus nonconceptive cycles.[61] Once the normal periimplantation levels of hCG and progesterone are clearly established, exogenous hCG can be administered to a nonpregnant woman to simulate hCG secretion by an implanting embryo. This process of administering hCG to produce a pseudopregnant condition is similar to other classic endocrinologic provocative tests. Stimulation testing can involve either a physiologic or a pharmacologic dose of hCG. In an initial study of the process of luteal rescue, Batista et al[71] examined the luteal response to a midluteal intramuscular injection of 5000 IU of hCG. They measured serum progesterone and PP14 levels after hCG stimulation in 34 instances. In all cases of hCG stimulation, serum progesterone levels exceeded 11.0 ng/mL (35 nmol/L) 6 hours after hCG stimulation. In contrast, PP14 levels were more variable and inconsistent after hCG stimulation. In light of these findings, the authors suggested that a midluteal serum progesterone level greater than 11.0 ng/mL (35 nmol/L) 6 hours after hCG administration may represent a cutoff limit for normal luteal function.

CONFIRMATION OF LUTEAL FUNCTION

The presence of corpus luteum activity can be determined with history alone. Molimenal symptoms are highly suggestive of circulating ovulatory levels of progesterone. Magyar et al[72] demonstrated that among 40 women with menstrual cycle frequency of 21 to 36 days and molimina 39 (98%) had progesterone levels greater than 3.0 ng/mL (10 nmol/L) in the luteal phase. Many women have one or more premenstrual symptoms (eg, increased tension, headache, backache) that indicate impending menstrual flow. Women without molimina and with subsequent unanticipated vaginal bleeding are likely to be experiencing anovulatory menstrual cycles.

Measurements of BBT and overall luteal length can be helpful in confirmation of the presence of luteal function. Basal temperature increases approximately 1°F (1.8°C) after ovulation has occurred.[18] In a study of 327 luteal-phase lengths, Lenton et al[25] found that the mean luteal-phase length was 14.13 days from the day after the peak serum LH concentration until the day before menses. If luteal-phase length follows a normal frequency distribution, Lenton et al concluded, a luteal-phase length of 9 or fewer days after the peak LH level is abnormal. The incidence of abnormal (short) luteal phases in the sample was 5.2%. Downs and Gibson[73] examined the BBT graphs of 20 women with biopsy-proved LPD and compared the findings with those for 20 infertile women with in-phase endometrial biopsy findings. Neither the slope nor the pattern of the increase in BBT appeared to help the investigators identify the women with out-of-phase biopsy findings. The duration of elevated BBT, however, did appear to be meaningful. Women with LPD had a mean luteal length of 11.8 days, which was significantly shorter than the mean duration of 13.4 days among the women with in-phase findings ($P<.05$). Among the subjects with normal findings, no luteal phase was shorter than 11 days, whereas 6 (30%) of the women with LPD had a luteal-phase duration that lasted less than 11 days.

Serum progesterone measurements can be used for definitive verification of corpus luteum function. Progesterone levels greater than 3.0 ng/mL (10 nmol/L) have generally been accepted as documentation of ovarian progesterone production as opposed to background adrenal progesterone production.[74] Progesterone levels begin to increase immediately before ovulation and reach a peak in the midluteal phase.[28] Progesterone levels return to preovulatory levels and menses begins because of decreasing LH stimulation in the late luteal phase. Because of episodic secretion, hour-to-hour differences in circulating progesterone levels can occur during the mid and late luteal phases.[5] Other activities of daily living (eating a meal) can further influence circulating progesterone levels. An average 34% decrease in circulating progesterone levels was observed to occur 1 hour after meals.[75] This transient decline in progesterone level was attributed to an increase in splanchnic blood flow and increased metabolic clearance of progesterone. Multiple other factors, including circadian variation, assay error, and biologic heterogeneity, have been reported to influence single random serum progesterone measurements.[76]

EVALUATION OF THE LUTEAL PHASE IN THE CLINICAL SETTING

Some Tests of Luteal Function

After cyclic menstrual function has been verified, multiple methods have been proposed to evaluate the luteal phase. The inherent variability of consecutive menstrual cycles, however, makes all these methods imprecise. Research studies led by Davis[34] and Balasch[35] suggested there are intermittent cycles in which deficient luteal function exists. To identify these cycles, one might propose to review prior menstrual cycles and evaluate them retrospectively to predict which women might have a predisposition for repetitively abnormal luteal function. In one study, however, investigators examined luteal-phase length determined from BBT graphs from one cycle and a single midluteal serum progesterone level from a second cycle and were not able to predict the outcome of an endometrial biopsy in a third menstrual cycle.[77]

For adequate comparison of various clinical methods of evaluating the luteal phase, different tests of luteal function must be compared within the same menstrual cycle. In a single intensely monitored luteal phase, Jordan et al[53] compared the methods of calculating luteal-phase length, measuring preovulatory follicle size, performing an endometrial biopsy, and taking a single or summing three serum progesterone measurements. Subjects gave daily samples of venous blood throughout the luteal phase, which enabled the researchers to select randomly the midluteal progesterone levels. The individual sensitivity and specificity of each method in prediction of a deficient integrated progesterone level (<80 ng·day/mL [254 nmol·day/L]) was determined and the selection of random midluteal serum progesterone measurements was performed four different times. In this particular study, a single serum progesterone level less than 10 ng/mL (32 nmol/L) collected 5 to 9 days after the LH surge had a mean sensitivity (86%) and specificity (83%) to allow prediction of an inadequate integrated progesterone level. There was a higher sensitivity (100%) and specificity (86%) if any three randomly selected progesterone levels 5 to 9 days after the LH surge were added together and the sum was less than 30 ng/mL (95 nmol/L). These findings confirmed the earlier concepts of Abraham et al,[78] who obtained daily luteal-phase blood samples from 30 women with normal cycles. The authors found that the sum of any three progesterone levels collected 4 to 11 days before menses consistently exceeded 15 ng/mL. According to the findings of Jordan et al[53] and Abraham et al,[78] if a midluteal serum progesterone level is more than 10 ng/mL (32 nmol/L), it is not unreasonable to observe an infertile couple for a time or investigate other causes of infertility. If the couple does not conceive after 12 cycles of effort, an endometrial biopsy can be performed to verify normal endometrial maturation. If the couple has a history of three spontaneous abortions without a term conception, or if the screening serum progesterone level is between 3.0 ng/mL and 10 ng/mL (10 and 32 nmol/L), an endometrial biopsy should be performed earlier. Progesterone levels between 1.0 and 3.0 ng/mL (3 and 10 nmol/L) reflect either very early or very late luteal activity or anovulation.

Further research in the development of noninvasive methods of assessment of the luteal phase is needed to identify women at increased frequency for abnormal luteal phases. The ideal test is one that can be performed in repetitive cycles with minimal patient discomfort, inconvenience, or expense. Studies examining the utility of daily urine or salivary samples for assessment of the luteal phase demonstrated some promise in identifying patients with possible repetitive endometrial maturational defects.[79-81] Stewart et al[82] reported that serum relaxin levels may be helpful in evaluating the luteal phase.

Millet et al[79] collected daily luteal-phase urine samples from women undergoing endometrial biopsy. The investigators reported decreased excretion of urinary levels of pregnanediol glucuronide (PdG), a metabolite of progesterone, among 9 women with concurrent biopsy-proved delayed endometrial maturation compared with 9 women with normal biopsies. The decreased PdG excretion was most marked and statistically significant in the early luteal phase. During the first 5 days of the luteal phase, PdG excretion among the LPD group was statistically decreased compared with that among the normal biopsy group ($P<.05$). Although total PdG excretion for the first 5 days among the normal group overlapped that of the abnormal group, this study did demonstrate the utility of PdG measurement as a screening test for LPD. Further studies with a larger data set are examining the use of urinary PdG as a screening test.

Daily salivary progesterone levels might reflect an integrated assessment of corpus luteum activity with a less invasive sampling technique than obtaining urine samples.[80,81] Saliva samples are obtained in the morning after a subject has rinsed her mouth with water. The woman collects approximately 5 mL of saliva by drooling or spitting into a container; the sample can be frozen until assayed. Salivary progesterone levels increase in the early luteal phase and parallel serum progesterone levels.[83] In one study, salivary progesterone levels correlated with histologic changes in the endometrium and were reduced in at least half the subjects with LPD.[84] In contrast, luteal-phase salivary progesterone levels did not help identify 46 women with a history of habitual abortion who were undergoing two or three concurrent endometrial biopsies.[85] Among the 8 women (17%, 8 of 46) with biopsy-proved LPD in at least two different endometrial cycles, salivary progesterone levels were not different from those of women with normal endometrial biopsies. Unfortunately, salivary progesterone measurements may be nonspecific in differentiation of endometrial LPD from normal cycles. Research by others is comparing salivary progesterone levels with serum progesterone levels and endometrial histologic findings in a larger data set.

Stewart et al[82] reported that integrated luteal-phase serum relaxin levels were lower in subjects with out-of-phase endometrial biopsy findings. Because relaxin is detectable only in the later half of the luteal phase with current assay technology, lower integrated levels were associated with subjects with short luteal phases and endometrial immaturity detected by means of endometrial biopsy. Although the less stringent definition of a 2-day lag was used to classify an out-of-phase endometrial biopsy finding and the number of subjects was small, this preliminary study suggested that measurement of relaxin may be a promising screening test for LPD. Research is ongoing to evaluate the feasibility of using serum relaxin levels for assessment of the luteal phase.

Endometrial Biopsy

Although endometrial biopsy has multiple shortcomings, it is still one of the best methods of assessment of the luteal phase. Endometrial biopsy is traditionally performed as an office procedure with a Novak curette to obtain a sample of fundal endometrium from either the anterior or a lateral portion of the uterus.[86] Samples from the lower uterine segment are less reliable for histologic dating, and no attempt is made to date abnormal specimens containing polyps, areas of hyperplasia, or chronic endometritis.[9] One modification of the traditional endometrial biopsy technique has been the replacement of the Novak curette with a plastic flexible suction catheter (eg, Pipelle, Unimar, Inc., Wilton, CT).[87] Use of a plastic suction catheter has been found to be less painful and to provide a sufficient sample for evaluation of the histologic changes in the endometrium. In one study, 55 subjects underwent two endometrial biopsies during the same office visit; both the Novak curette and Pipelle catheter were used.[88] The order of use of the instruments was alternated in a randomized manner. Patients reported less pain after an endometrial biopsy with a Pipelle rather than with a Novak curette. Although pathologists tended to prefer evaluating samples obtained with a Novak curette, no discrepancies in diagnosis were made during evaluation of either sample for endometrial hyperplasia or carcinoma.

To prevent performance of an endometrial biopsy in a cycle of conception, some authors have suggested using a rapid office urine pregnancy test to detect occult pregnancy.[89] Biopsies in a cycle of conception not only are emotionally upsetting to a couple, but also the specimen cannot be dated according to the next menses because the patient has conceived. To prevent cycle-of-conception biopsies, authors also have suggested performing the biopsy during a cycle in which abstinence or barrier contraception has been used.[89] Other authors raise less concern about cycle-of-conception biopsies; they cite that the observed clinical pregnancy loss rate is no higher after biopsy than in other cycles.[90] These estimates, however, were made before the increased use of the plastic suction catheter devices. Because the technique of obtaining an endometrial sample using these curettes invariably requires more sampling from different parts of the uterus, a large number of implantation site disruptions might be anticipated. Despite the requirement of a negative urine pregnancy test on the day of endometrial biopsy, we observed disruption of an embryo implantation site with a Pipelle suction catheter (Fig 8–6). Further studies are necessary to clarify if a greater spontaneous loss rate occurs during cycle-of-

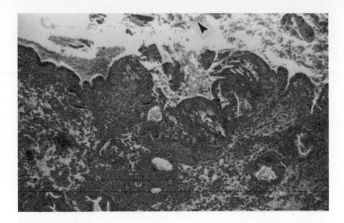

Figure 8–6. Endometrial biopsy specimen containing an embryo implantation site (arrow). The endometrial biopsy was performed with a Pipelle endometrial suction catheter on cycle day 27, 10 days after a nadir in basal body temperature. A urine pregnancy test with a sensitivity of 25 IU/L was negative on the day of the endometrial biopsy. The patient menstruated 4 days after the biopsy. Original magnification, 25×. *(Courtesy of Dr. Richard H. Oi.)*

conception endometrial biopsies with suction catheters as opposed to Novak curettes.

There is a controversy concerning the optimal time in the luteal phase to perform endometrial biopsy. Endometrial biopsy traditionally is performed in the late luteal phase, during which, proponents state, the biopsy findings best reflect the response of the end organ to progesterone throughout the luteal phase. If endometrial maturation is retarded, researchers believe, endometrium is unlikely to support an implanting embryo. Conversely, research endometrial biopsies performed in the midluteal phase have helped identify endometrial proteins uniquely present during the time of embryo implantation.[15] One study suggested that endometrial biopsies demonstrating an absence of the αvβ3 integrin endometrial protein detected at immunohistochemical staining are associated with retarded histologic changes in the endometrium.[14] Midluteal endometrial biopsies have demonstrated initially retarded endometrial development in cycles in which a second late luteal biopsy, performed in the same cycle, demonstrated in-phase histologic changes in the endometrium.[54,91,92] These observations suggest that the endometrium can increase its rate of development during one luteal phase and that a midluteal endometrial maturation defect may represent a cryptic form of LPD. Further research in this area may make a midluteal biopsy more useful than a late luteal biopsy. Although these findings await confirmation in large multicenter clinical studies, these results and concepts are the basis for new methods to assess corpus luteum activity and subsequent endometrial receptivity. Because routine detection of this endometrial integrin is not clinically feasible and the prevalence of isolated retarded midluteal endometrial histologic changes needs further clarification, late luteal

endometrial biopsies for histologic dating are still the standard for initial LPD screening.

Another controversy concerns the reference point for dating the histologic development of the endometrial biopsy specimen. Relating the endometrial histologic changes to the next menses and counting backward from this event to assign an idealized day of endometrial development to the day of the biopsy has been used for more than 40 years. Menses was a convenient physical sign for clinicians who could not accurately determine the day of peak LH concentration or ovulation when endometrial biopsy was first used for the diagnosis of LPD. With the availability of accurate urine monitoring for the LH surge, some researchers have suggested that endometrial development should be dated from this midcycle reference point.[93] Proponents of this technique cite better correlation between histologic changes in the endometrium and LH surge than with use of the next-menses method. One deficiency of the midcycle dating method, however, is erroneous declaration of a short luteal phase of 9 days' duration as in phase if the endometrial biopsy specimen was obtained 8 days after an apparent urinary LH surge and the endometrium was consistent with cycle day 21 development. In contrast, endometrial dating according to next menses would have indicated that the biopsy was 5 days out of phase and further identified this as an LPD cycle (Fig 8–7). Similarly, on the basis of luteal-phase length alone, one might predict that this abnormally short luteal phase would be an abnormal LPD cycle. At present, if an endometrial biopsy is performed in the late luteal phase, the idealized cycle day (for that biopsy) established from the day of next menses is still the standard used by most clinicians for initial LPD screening.

Definition of Abnormal Luteal Phase

An abnormal luteal phase has been defined by most authors as one in which endometrial development lags behind expected development by more than 2 days.[21,94] This deficiency in endometrial maturation is said to be out of phase from expected endometrial development. Some authors used less stringent criteria and inferred that abnormal luteal function exists when the endometrium lags in development by exactly 2 days.[20,24,86] We recommend the more rigorous definition of abnormal endometrial development as 3 or more days out of phase (more than 2 days) to minimize false-positive results. To increase the precision of endometrial dating and further minimize a false-positive diagnosis of LPD, more than one evaluator should date the endometrial samples. In an extensive review of possible contributing factors to error in histologic dating of secretory endometrium, Gibson et al[95] evaluated duplicate endometrial biopsies from 25 women on two separate occasions. They demonstrated that inconsistencies between evaluators (in-

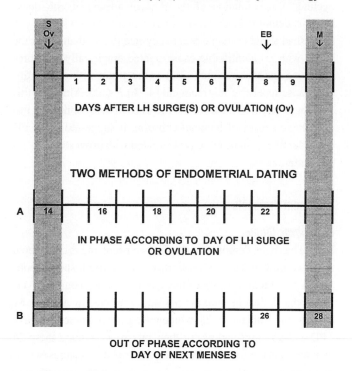

INDEX LUTEAL PHASE

Endometrial Biopsy (EB) Demonstrated Day 21 Histology

DAYS AFTER LH SURGE(S) OR OVULATION (Ov)

TWO METHODS OF ENDOMETRIAL DATING

A

IN PHASE ACCORDING TO DAY OF LH SURGE
OR OVULATION

B

OUT OF PHASE ACCORDING TO
DAY OF NEXT MENSES

Figure 8–7. Endometrial dating by two methods: **A.** Day of LH surge (S) or ovulation (Ov). **B.** Day of next menses (M). An endometrial biopsy (EB) performed 8 days after the LH surge or ovulation demonstrated idealized cycle day 21 histologic changes. The EB would be in phase with dating according to LH surge or ovulation but would be out of phase with dating according to the next menses.

terevaluator variation) accounted for 65% of observed variability and that the same evaluator dating the identical specimen a second time (intraevaluator variation) accounted for 27% of the total observed variability. Regional differences within the uterus were minor (intrauterine variation), accounting for only 8% of the total variability. In clinical practice, endometrial biopsy specimens should be examined by at least two experienced evaluators. If a discrepancy of more than 2 days exists between evaluators, the specimen should be reevaluated and a consensus histologic date obtained.

Because there is cycle-to-cycle variability in luteal function, the endometrial biopsies must be performed in two different menstrual cycles to fulfill the diagnostic criteria of LPD.[86] When two abnormal biopsies were required for the diagnosis of LPD in a group of infertile women, the reported incidence of LPD from two large studies ranged from 8.1% to 17.5% depending on the authors' definition of LPD and the sample population.[20,21]

MANAGEMENT OF LUTEAL-PHASE DEFICIENCY

Overview

Initial therapy for LPD should be aimed at correction of any identified underlying cause of LPD. Correctable causes of LPD may include a persistent oligoovulatory menstrual pattern or persistent low-grade hyperprolactinemia.[96,97] Nonpharmacologic therapies (weight or personal stress reduction) should be used to promote ovulation, and these measures should optimize the patient's inherent folliculogenesis. Although excessive physical exercise[29] and low body weight[32] have been associated with the presence of LPD, a balance between a woman's exercise routine and her mental health must be achieved. Many women find it difficult to alter permanently their daily routine or body habitus, so their inherent suboptimal pattern of folliculogenesis persists. For these patients and others for whom no cause of LPD can be delineated, one can use medical therapies either directed at altering folliculogenesis or supplementing endogenous progesterone levels.

A review of the effect on pregnancy rate of various treatment regimens for LPD revealed no definitive treatment of these infertile patients.[98] In this review of studies performed between 1966 and 1991, only one randomized, controlled trial and three other comparative studies presented enough information to allow comparison of pregnancy rates. It is not surprising that no consensus exists for the management of LPD when the end point of treatment is pregnancy. LPD is a relatively uncommon disorder and not always repetitive from cycle to cycle. Because diagnostic criteria for LPD differ, many studies are not exactly comparable. Because patients with LPD may not undergo complete evaluations for other factors of infertility, pregnancy rates may not be comparable even if studies have the same diagnostic criteria for LPD. Because LPD may be caused by different or a combination of factors, LPD in one woman may be responsive to a particular therapy but not responsive to another. Therapies directed at LPD are meant to increase cycle fecundity and shorten the time to pregnancy. In a long-term follow-up study by Klentzeris et al,[99] women with subtle endometrial maturational defects detected in endometrial samples left untreated had a lower probability of achieving a pregnancy than women without endometrial maturation defects. Furthermore, current clinical therapies are directed at improving the amount of circulating progesterone available to act on the endometrium. Because there are no clinical therapies directed specifically at improving the endometrium, patients with end-organ defects are at a distinct disadvantage when these therapies are used.

When treatment is analyzed by outcome variables other than pregnancy, two studies are notable. In a study examining the response of histologic changes in the endometrium in relation to cycle fecundity by means of life-table analysis, Daly et al[100] treated 33 of 41 patients with LPD with progesterone supplementation for six consecutive cycles. Seventeen patients had correction of LPD documented at repeated endometrial biopsies, and 14 conceived viable pregnancies during therapy with a normal rate of fecundity. The 16 patients with LPD whose endometrial biopsy specimen was refractory to progesterone supplementation took clomiphene citrate for augmentation of folliculogenesis. In the clomiphene-treated group, five patients had correction of LPD documented at repeated endometrial biopsies, and four conceived. Patients whose endometrial biopsy specimen did not correct with clomiphene citrate were treated with additional therapies. Only three patients (7%, 3 of 41) of the total number of women with LPD did not have their endometrial biopsy specimens corrected with any of the treatments. Women with a corrected endometrial biopsy specimen had normal cycle fecundity and an 80% (33 of 41) conception rate. No viable pregnancies occurred without correction of the underlying endometrial maturational defect. Weaknesses of this study included use of the less stringent definition of LPD (≥ 2 days out-of-phase) and exclusion of two noncompliant patients. These factors may explain partially the close approximation of normal cycle fecundity in the corrected endometrial biopsy group.

In a retrospective cohort study by Murray et al,[101] 65 patients with previously diagnosed LPD were treated with either progesterone supplementation or clomiphene citrate. If a repeat endometrial biopsy documented correction of the LPD, patients were continued on their respective therapy. In both treatment groups, patients who achieved normal endometrial histologic findings conceived with a cycle fecundity rate that approached that of an idealized normal population. A strength of this study was the use of the more rigorous definition of LPD of more than 2 days out of phase.

In the studies by Daley et al[100] and Murray et al,[101] the cycle fecundity rate of the normalized treatment group (documented with a repeat endometrial biopsy) exceeded the projected cumulative conception rate calculated by life-table analysis. These findings suggest the presence of a true treatment effect if the endometrial biopsy findings are corrected with therapy.[102]

Therapy for LPD may be analyzed according to indication for therapy rather than the treatment per se. Because LPD causes habitual abortion in a relatively large subgroup of patients, effective therapies that decrease the rate of subsequent abortions may be easier to identify and verify in research studies. Uncontrolled studies[23,103,104] have found a greater than 80% viable pregnancy rate after luteal-phase progesterone supplementation in women with habitual abortions. Despite the lack of randomization, Tho et al[23] conducted a study with 60 women with recurrent pregnancy losses due to either LPD ($n = 23$) or no identifiable cause ($n = 37$). All patients with LPD were treated with progesterone supplementation. Twenty-two of the 37 women in the group with no identifiable cause of the pregnancy loss were treated empirically with progesterone and tetracycline. A reevaluation of the data by means of chi-square analysis demonstrated that the LPD group treated with progesterone had a higher viable pregnancy rate (91%) than either the group with no identifiable cause treated empirically with progesterone and tetracycline (62%) or the group with no identifiable cause receiving no treatment (47%) $P<.05$. Although this study was performed before the use of routine screening for immunologic causes of habitual abortion, it suggested that LPD once identified can be effectively treated with progesterone supplementation.

Treatment Protocols

Clomiphene Citrate

If LPD has been demonstrated to be persistent and is considered to be the probable cause of infertility or recurrent spontaneous abortion, the initial choice of therapy can be based on the severity of the deficit in endometrial development. In a study by Downs and Gibson,[105] 25 women were documented to have LPD and no other factors for their infertility. Among these 25 women, 12 were found to have endometrial deficiencies of 5 or more days out of phase. All 25 women were treated with clomiphene citrate, providing 27 cycles for evaluation. In this subset of women with an out-of-phase endometrial biopsy of 5 or more days, the conception rate was 79% compared with 8.9% among women with a less severe defect ($P<.001$). Clomiphene citrate may exert its beneficial effect by increasing follicular-phase FSH levels, leading to improvement in the quality of the dominant follicle and the subsequent formation of a normal corpus luteum. Although this explanation is intuitively appealing, an increased number of follicles, or quantity rather than quality of the corpus luteum, appears to be responsible for the correction of an out-of-phase endometrium.

In a study performed by Guzick and Zeleznik,[106] 18 women with two previous out-of-phase endometrial biopsies (≥ 3 days out of phase) were given clomiphene citrate, 100 mg/day on cycle days 5 to 9. In this treatment cycle, folliculogenesis was monitored by means of serial pelvic ultrasound examinations, and a late luteal endometrial biopsy was performed. In 80% (8 of 10 women), the endometrial biopsy changes were corrected, and more than one preovulatory follicle was present (>15 mm mean diameter). In contrast, only 25% (2 of 8) women had correction of previously abnormal biopsy findings if only a single preovulatory follicle formed ($P<.05$). These findings suggest that clomiphene citrate is more likely to correct LPD when the medication induces the formation of more than one preovulatory follicle. Although the initial clomiphene citrate dose was 100 mg/day rather than 50 mg/day, this dose may decrease production of cervical mucus and adversely affect cycle fecundity. Because the women were not randomized to clomiphene citrate therapy, some may have corrected their history of LPD without any treatment. As demonstrated by Downs and Gibson,[105] it seems reasonable that increased folliculogenesis would be more effective in women with a profound lag in endometrial maturation and that an abnormal ovulatory pattern similar to intermittent oligoovulation would be most responsive to ovulation induction medication. Clomiphene citrate may also be the medication of choice for patients who have difficulty interpreting their shift in BBT or have poor compliance with the administration of progesterone vaginal suppositories.

Clomiphene citrate is administered in the early follicular phase for 5 days starting on cycle day 3, 4 or 5 to extend the normal elevation in FSH levels present in the early follicular phase of the menstrual cycle. A dose of 50 mg/day is used initially, and a postcoital examination of sperm-mucus interaction should be performed at midcycle. In one study, despite elevated estradiol levels, cervical mucus scores evaluating amount, viscosity and spinnbarkeit were lower among women who used clomiphene citrate (150 mg/day on cycle days 3 to 7) than among controls.[107] After administration of clomiphene citrate, a repeat late luteal endometrial biopsy should be performed to document correction of the out-of-phase endometrium. If the defect is not corrected, increased amounts of clomiphene or menotropins[108] may be administered empirically, but no study has rigorously verified the efficacy of this approach. If the patient experiences poor sperm survival while using clomiphene citrate, she may use either menotropins for increased folliculogenesis and cervical mucus volume or progesterone vaginal suppositories, or intrauterine insemination can be performed for the induced cervical factor.

Ironically, clomiphene citrate has been implicated in the induction of luteal insufficiency.[109] This finding may be flawed, however, because the study was not randomized and it only enrolled subjects who had not conceived after three cycles of clomiphene citrate. These subjects may have represented an inadequate response to therapy. Among patients with LPD who conceived after clomiphene citrate therapy, Soules et al[110] demonstrated that levels of 17-hydroxyprogesterone (17-OHP) were higher than among pregnant controls without LPD. Because elevated 17-OHP levels suggest adequate luteal function, no further exogenous progesterone supplementation should be necessary. In clinical practice, patients who conceive after clomiphene citrate administration for LPD are followed closely without progesterone supplementation.

Progesterone Vaginal Suppositories

Patients with less severe endometrial deficiencies or poor sperm survival after use of clomiphene citrate can use progesterone vaginal suppositories for luteal support. Progesterone suppositories, 25 mg twice a day, are administered 3 days after the BBT shift until the next menstrual period or a positive pregnancy test.[86] Because progesterone suppositories are usually compounded by local pharmacists, marked variability can exist among suppositories. Progesterone solubilized in a polyethylene glycol base has demonstrated higher serum progesterone levels than other commonly used bases.[111] Because of an inadequate treatment response based on endometrial immaturity at repeat biopsy, increasing the daily dose of progesterone (>50 mg per day) and increasing frequency (more than two times a day) have been used.[112] Increasing the amount of exogenous progesterone may prevent menses from occurring in nonconceptive cycles. If menses is delayed, an office urine pregnancy test can be performed before progesterone supplementation is discontinued. Among patients with a diagnosis of LPD, a 69% (9 of 13) conception rate was observed after supplementation with 25-mg progesterone vaginal suppositories twice a day.[20] In the previously mentioned study by Daly et al,[100] an 82% viable pregnancy rate (14 of 17) was observed among patients who corrected their lag in endometrial development with progesterone vaginal suppositories. Unfortunately, both studies classified an out-of-phase endometrial biopsy as a 2 or more day lag dated from next menses. This less demanding criteria for LPD may explain the high corrected biopsy and conception rates.

Progesterone may be administered by other routes and in different preparations. Micronized progesterone capsules (100 mg three times a day) can allow oral administration, but a definitive study examining the use of this preparation for the correction of LPD has not been performed. Although some studies have measured serum progesterone levels after oral administration,[113,114] direct measurement of progesterone included cross-reactivity with its 5α-metabolites, leading to an overestimation of the circulating level of progesterone.[115] If progesterone levels are assessed after oral administration, samples should be subjected to celite column chromatography before measurement with currently available radioimmunoassay kits.[116] Synthetic progestin preparations have been reported to suppress ovarian progesterone production,[117] but Balasch et al[118] reported both similar plasma progesterone levels and a pregnancy rate after treatment of LPD with dehydrogesterone[119] comparable to that after treatment with progesterone vaginal suppositories. In the latter study,[119] patients who were treated with either oral dehydrogesterone or vaginal progesterone had a similar treatment effect, and both treatments were significantly more effective than no treatment of LPD ($P<.001$). Among ten additional infertile patients with normal endometrial maturation documented by means of late luteal biopsy, Balasch et al[118] demonstrated no impairment of endometrial maturation at repeat biopsy after luteal dehydrogesterone therapy. Dehydrogesterone is not approved for use in pregnancy in the United States.

Once progesterone supplementation therapy has been initiated, a repeat endometrial biopsy should be performed to document improvement in endometrial histologic changes. If a lag in development is not corrected, an increased dose of progesterone may be used or treatment with clomiphene citrate may be provided. If patients with LPD conceive after progesterone supplementation, a progesterone level should be measured to document absorption of the preparation. Although a random progesterone level less than 10 ng/mL (32 nmol/L) can be associated with a normal pregnancy,[120] continued progesterone supplementation until 8 weeks after a missed menses should be considered if serial hCG measurements demonstrate a normal initial exponential increase and follow-up ultrasound examinations document a normal pregnancy. After a patient with LPD treated with progesterone supplementation conceives, parenteral progesterone (17-OHP caproate) 250 mg a week is a convenient alternative to daily suppository use.[94] Parenteral progesterone supplementation should overlap the use of vaginal suppositories by 1 week to ensure adequate circulating serum progesterone levels. Progesterone supplementation should be continued until 8 weeks after a missed menses, at which time more than 50% of circulating progesterone is derived from trophoblastic tissue.[121]

Alternative Therapies

Patients with LPD have been successfully treated with the following methods that are known to increase folliculogenesis: human menopausal gonadotropins (hMG) or FSH[108,122–124] with or without hCG, GnRH pulse therapy,[125] epimestrol,[126] tamoxifen,[127] and hCG alone.[128] Menotropin therapy to increase folliculogenesis may be used when poor cervical mucus results after use of clomiphene citrate or a failure to correct a lag in endometrial maturation after either clomiphene citrate or progesterone supplementation. Benadiva and Metzger[129] reported an increased incidence of endometrial gland-stroma dyssynchrony, similar to that for use of clomiphene citrate, after use of hMG for superovulation therapy. The study, however, had design and analysis flaws that may have biased the results. Approximately half of the subjects received supplemental luteal-phase progesterone; endometrial biopsies were not dated uniformly; and the study enrolled subjects after a variable period of one to seven unsuccessful superovulation cycles. Even though the finding of increased endometrial gland-stroma dyssynchrony after menotropins use awaits further confirmation and may not be applicable to LPD, there are other considerations that limit menotropin therapy for LPD. The negative factors of medication expense, increased time commitment, and potential morbidity limit menotropin use to a select group of patients with refractory LPD.

SUMMARY

LPD is an abnormality of luteal function that leads to a lag in endometrial maturation from expected development. It can occur sporadically among women with normal ovulation irrespective of their history of fertility.[34] In a small subgroup of women, LPD may occur repetitively and appears to be responsible for habitual abortion.[23] Among women with a history of infertility, there is some evidence of an association between LPD and decreased cycle fecundity.[35,99] Because LPD can be sporadic in occurrence, with heterogenous causes, and can apparently correct itself spontaneously without therapy, comprehensive diagnostic and treatment recommendations have been difficult to establish.

The classic definition of LPD is the demonstration of retarded endometrial histologic development 3 or more days from expected maturation. The endometrial tissue is obtained from a late luteal endometrial biopsy and dated from the onset of the next menstrual period. Because of the intermittent occurrence of LPD, the defect must be demonstrated in two separate menstrual cycles before therapy is initiated. Variations in the diagnostic criteria have been proposed, but the aforementioned guidelines should be observed initially, because they are followed by most investigators and application of these criteria requires the least amount of ancillary testing. If a patient fulfills these characteristics and does not conceive after standard therapy, more extensive treatment with exogenous gonadotropins can be used or a referral can be made to a center that conducts research into the assessment and treatment of LPD.

REFERENCES

1. Carr BR, MacDonald PC, Simpson ER: The role of lipoproteins in the regulation of progesterone secretion by the human corpus luteum. *Fertil Steril* 38:303, 1982
2. Ohara A, Mori T, Taii S, Ban C, Narimoto K: Functional differentiation in steroidogenesis of two types of luteal cells isolated from mature human corpora lutea of menstrual cycle. *J Clin Endocrinol Metab* 65:1192, 1987
3. Navot D, Laufer N, Kopolovic J, et al: Artificially induced endometrial cycles and establishment of pregnancies in the absence of ovaries. *N Engl J Med* 314:806, 1986
4. Schmidt CL, de Ziegler D, Gagliardi CL, et al: Transfer of cryopreserved-thawed embryos: The natural cycle versus controlled preparation of the endometrium with gonadotropin-releasing hormone agonist and exogenous estradiol and progesterone (GEEP). *Fertil Steril* 52:609, 1989
5. Filicori M, Butler JP, Crowley WF Jr: Neuroendocrine regulation of the corpus luteum in the human. *J Clin Invest* 73:1638, 1984
6. Soules MR, Clifton DK, Steiner RA, Cohen NL, Bremner WJ: The

corpus luteum: Determinants of progesterone secretion in the normal menstrual cycle. *Obstet Gynecol* 71:659, 1988

7. Soules MR, Steiner RA, Clifton DK, Cohen NL, Aksel S, Bremner WJ: Progesterone modulation of pulsatile luteinizing hormone secretion in normal women. *J Clin Endocrinol Metab* 58:378, 1984

8. Maas S, Jarry H, Teichmann A, Rath W, Kuhn W, Wuttke W: Paracrine actions of oxytocin, prostaglandin $F_{2\alpha}$, and estradiol within the human corpus luteum. *J Clin Endocrinol Metab* 74:306, 1992

9. Noyes RW, Hertig AT, Rock J: Dating the endometrial biopsy. *Fertil Steril* 1:3, 1950

10. Garcia E, Bouchard P, DeBrux J, et al: Use of immunocytochemistry of progesterone and estrogen receptors for endometrial dating. *J Clin Endocrinol Metab* 67:80, 1988

11. Daly DC, Maslar IA, Rosenberg SM, Tohan N, Riddick DH: Prolactin production by luteal phase defect endometrium. *Am J Obstet Gynecol* 140:587, 1981

12. Batista MC, Bravo N, Cartledge TP, Loriaux DL, Merriam GR, Nieman LK: Serum levels of placental protein 14 do not accurately reflect histologic maturation of the endometrium. *Obstet Gynecol* 81:439, 1993

13. Psychoyos A, Nikas G: Uterine pinopodes as markers of uterine receptivity. *Assist Reprod Rev* 4:26, 1994

14. Lessey BA, Damjanovich L, Coutifaris C, Castelbaum A, Albelda SM, Buck CA: Integrin adhesion molecules in the human endometrium: Correlation with the normal and abnormal menstrual cycle. *J Clin Invest* 90:188, 1992

15. Lessey BA, Castelbaum AJ, Buck CA, Lei Y, Yowell CW, Sun J: Further characterization of endometrial integrins during the menstrual cycle and in pregnancy. *Fertil Steril* 62:497, 1994

16. Hertig AT, Rock J, Adams EC: A description of 34 human ova within the first 17 days of development. *Am J Anat* 98:435, 1956

17. Bergh PA, Navot D: The impact of embryonic development and endometrial maturity on the timing of implantation. *Fertil Steril* 58:537, 1992

18. Jones GE: Some newer aspects of the management of infertility. *JAMA* 141:1123, 1949

19. Strott CA, Cargille CM, Ross GT, Lipsett MB: The short luteal phase. *J Clin Endocrinol* 30:246, 1970

20. Rosenberg SM, Luciano AA, Riddick DH: The luteal phase defect: The relative frequency of, and encouraging response to, treatment with vaginal progesterone. *Fertil Steril* 34:17, 1980

21. Witten BI, Martin SA: The endometrial biopsy as a guide to the management of luteal phase defect. *Fertil Steril* 44:460, 1985

22. Wild RA, Sanfilippo JS, Toledo AA: Endometrial biopsy in the infertility investigation: The experience at two institutions. *J Reprod Med* 31:954, 1986

23. Tho PT, Byrd JR, McDonough PG: Etiologies and subsequent reproductive performance of 100 couples with recurrent abortion. *Fertil Steril* 32:389, 1979

24. Balasch J, Creus M, Marquez M, Burzaco I, Vanrell JA: The significance of luteal phase deficiency on fertility: A diagnostic and therapeutic approach. *Hum Reprod* 1:145, 1986

25. Lenton EA, Landgren B-M, Sexton L: Normal variation in the length of the luteal phase of the menstrual cycle: Identification of the short luteal phase. *Br J Obstet Gynecol* 91:685, 1984

26. Gray RH, Campbell OM, Zacur HA, Labbok MH, MacRae SL: Postpartum return of ovarian activity in nonbreastfeeding women monitored by urinary assays. *J Clin Endocrinol Metab* 64:645, 1987

27. Nakajima ST, Brumsted JR, Deaton JL, Blackmer KM, Gibson M: Endometrial histology after first trimester spontaneous abortion. *Fertil Steril* 55:32, 1991

28. McNeely MJ, Soules MR: The diagnosis of luteal phase deficiency: A critical review. *Fertil Steril* 50:1, 1988

29. Bullen BA, Skrinar GS, Beitins IZ, vonMering G, Turnbull BA, McArthur JW: Induction of menstrual disorders by strenuous exercise in untrained women. *N Engl J Med* 312:1349, 1985

30. Prior JC, Cameron K, Yuen BH, Thomas J: Menstrual cycle changes with marathon training: Anovulation and short luteal phase. *Can J Appl Sports Sci* 7:173, 1982

31. Schweiger U, Laessle R, Schweiger M, Herrmann F, Reidel W, Pirke K-M: Caloric intake, stress, and menstrual function in athletes. *Fertil Steril* 49:447, 1988

32. Bates GW, Bates SR, Whitworth NS: Reproductive failure in women who practice weight control. *Fertil Steril* 37:373, 1982

33. Pirke KM, Schweiger U, Strowitzki T, et al: Dieting causes menstrual irregularities in normal weight young women through impairment of episodic luteinizing hormone secretion. *Fertil Steril* 51:263, 1989

34. Davis OK, Berkeley AS, Naus GJ, Cholst IN, Freedman KS: The incidence of luteal phase defect in normal, fertile women, determined by serial endometrial biopsies. *Fertil Steril* 51:582, 1989

35. Balasch J, Vanrell JA, Creus M, Marquez M, Gonzalez-Merlo J: The endometrial biopsy for diagnosis of luteal phase deficiency. *Fertil Steril* 44:699, 1985

36. Cook CL, Rao CV, Yussman MA: Plasma gonadotropin and sex steroid hormone levels during early, midfollicular, and midluteal phases of women with luteal phase defects. *Fertil Steril* 40:45, 1983

37. Sheehan KL, Casper RF, Yen SSC: Luteal phase defects induced by an agonist of luteinizing hormone-releasing factor: A model for fertility control. *Science* 215:170, 1982

38. Stouffer RL, Hogden GD: Induction of luteal phase defects in rhesus monkeys by follicular fluid administration at the onset of the menstrual cycle. *J Clin Endocrinol Metab* 51:669, 1980

39. Soules MR, McLachlan RI, Ek M, Dahl KD, Cohen NL, Bremner WJ: Luteal phase defect: Characterization of reproductive hormones over the menstrual cycle. *J Clin Endocrinol Metab* 69:804, 1989

40. Soules MR, Clifton DK, Cohen NL, Bremner WJ, Steiner RA: Luteal phase deficiency: Abnormal gonadotropin and progesterone secretion patterns. *J Clin Endocrinol Metab* 69:813, 1989

41. Suh BY, Betz G: Altered luteinizing hormone pulse frequency in early follicular phase of the menstrual cycle with luteal phase defect patients in women. *Fertil Steril* 60:800, 1993

42. Soules MR, Clifton DK, Bremner WJ, Steiner RA: Corpus luteum insufficiency induced by a rapid gonadotropin-releasing homone–

induced gonadotropin secretion pattern in the follicular phase. *J Clin Endocrinol Metab* 65:457, 1987

43. Schweiger U, Laessle RG, Tuschl RJ, Broocks A, Krusche T, Pirke K-M: Decreased follicular phase gonadotropin secretion is associated with impaired estradiol and progesterone secretion during the follicular and luteal phases in normally menstruating women. *J Clin Endocrinol Metab* 68:888, 1989

44. Loucks AB, Mortola JF, Girton L, Yen SSC: Alterations in the hypothalamic-pituitary-ovarian and hypothalamic-pituitary-adrenal axes in athletic women. *J Clin Endocrinol Metab* 68:402, 1989

45. Check JH, Goldberg BB, Kurtz A, Adelson HG, Rankin A: Pelvic sonography to help determine the appropriate therapy for luteal phase defects. *Int J Fertil* 29:156, 1984

46. Ying YK, Daly DC, Randolph JF, et al: Ultrasonographic monitoring of follicular growth for luteal phase defect. *Fertil Steril* 48:433, 1987

47. Jacobs MH, Balasch J, Gonzalez-Merlo JM, et al: Endometrial cytosolic and nuclear progesterone receptors in the luteal phase defect. *J Clin Endocrinol Metab* 64:472, 1987

48. McLachlan RI, Cohen NL, Vale WW, et al: The importance of luteinizing hormone in the control of inhibin and progesterone secretion by the human corpus luteum. *J Clin Endocrinol Metab* 68:1078, 1989

49. Garzo VG, Liu J, Ulmann A, Baulieu E, Yen SSC: Effects of antiprogesterone (RU486) on the hypothalamic-hypophyseal-ovarian-endometrial axis during the luteal phase of the menstrual cycle. *J Clin Endocrinol Metab* 66:508, 1988

50. Gibson M, Nakajima ST, McAuliffe TL: Short-term modulation of gonadotropin secretion by progesterone during the luteal phase. *Fertil Steril* 55:522, 1991

51. Hutchison JS, Nelson PB, Zeleznik AJ: Effects of different gonadotropin pulse frequencies on corpus luteum function during the menstrual cycle of rhesus monkeys. *Endocrinology* 119:1964, 1986

52. Soules MR, Bremner WJ, Dahl KD, Rivier JE, Vale WW, Clifton DK: The induction of premature luteolysis in normal women: Follicular phase luteinizing hormone secretion and corpus luteum function in the subsequent cycle. *Am J Obstet Gynecol* 164:989, 1991

53. Jordan J, Craig K, Clifton DK, Soules MR: Luteal phase defect: The sensitivity and specificity of diagnostic methods in common clinical use. *Fertil Steril* 62:54, 1994

54. Kusuda M, Nakamura G, Matsukuma K, Kurano A: Corpus luteum insufficiency as a cause of nidatory failure. *Acta Obstet Gynecol Scand* 62:199, 1983

55. Glock JL, Brumsted JR: Color flow pulsed Doppler ultrasound in diagnosing luteal phase defect. *Fertil Steril* 64:500, 1995

56. Keller DW, Wiest WG, Askin FB, Johnson LW, Strickler RC: Pseudocorpus luteum insufficiency: A local defect of progesterone action on endometrial stroma. *J Clin Endocrinol Metab* 48:127, 1979

57. Gautray JP, DeBrux J, Tajchner G, Robel P, Mouren M: Clinical investigation of the menstrual cycle. III. Clinical, endometrial, and endocrine aspects of luteal defect. *Fertil Steril* 35:296, 1981

58. Spirtos NJ, Yurewicz EC, Moghissi KS, Magyar DM, Sundareson AS, Bottoms SF: Pseudocorpus luteum insufficiency: A study of cytosol progesterone receptors in human endometrium. *Obstet Gynecol* 65:535, 1985

59. Saracoglu OF, Aksel S, Yeoman RR, Wiebe RH: Endometrial estradiol and progesterone receptors in patients with luteal phase defects and endometriosis. *Fertil Steril* 43:851, 1985

60. Ying YK, Walters CA, Kuslis S, Lin JT, Daly DC, Riddick DH: Prolactin production by explants of normal, luteal phase defective, and corrected luteal phase defective late secretory endometrium. *Am J Obstet Gynecol* 151:801, 1985

61. Stewart DR, Overstreet JW, Nakajima ST, Lasley BL: Enhanced ovarian steroid secretion before implantation in early human pregnancy. *J Clin Endocrinol Metab* 76:1470, 1993

62. Norman RJ, Buck RH, Kemp MA, Joubert SM: Impaired corpus luteum function in ectopic pregnancy cannot be explained by altered human chorionic gonadotropin. *J Clin Endocrinol Metab* 66:1166, 1988

63. Radwanska E, Frankenberg J, Allen EI: Plasma progesterone levels in normal and abnormal early human pregnancy. *Fertil Steril* 30:398, 1978

64. Kapetanakis E, Pantos KJ: Continuation of a donor oocyte pregnancy in menopause without early pregnancy support. *Fertil Steril* 54:1171, 1990

65. Ben-Nun I, Ghetler Y, Kaneti H, Wolfson L, Fejgin M, Beyth Y: Tubal pregnancy without ovarian hormonal support. *Fertil Steril* 54:351, 1990

66. Parker CR, Illingworth DR, Bissonnette J, Carr BR: Endocrine changes during pregnancy in a patient with homozygous familial hypobetalipoproteinemia. *N Engl J Med* 314:557, 1986

67. Illingworth DR, Corbin DK, Kemp ED, Keenan EJ: Hormone changes during the menstrual cycle in abetalipoproteinemia: Reduced luteal phase progesterone in a patient with homozygous hypobetalipoproteinemia. *Proc Natl Acad Sci USA* 79:6685, 1982

68. Knopp RH, Warth MR, Charles D, et al: Lipoprotein metabolism in pregnancy, fat transport to the fetus, and the effects of diabetes. *Biol Neonate* 50:297, 1986

69. Hansen KK, Knopp RH, Soules MR: Lipoprotein-cholesterol levels in infertile women with luteal phase deficiency. *Fertil Steril* 55:916, 1991

70. Azuma K, Calderon I, Besanko M, MacLachlan V, Healy DL: Is the luteo-placental shift a myth? Analysis of low progesterone levels in successful ART pregnancies. *J Clin Endocrinol Metab* 77:195, 1993

71. Batista MC, Cartledge TP, Nieman LK, Bravo N, Loriaux DL, Merriam GR: Characterization of the normal progesterone and placental protein 14 responses to human chorionic gonadotropin stimulation in the luteal phase. *Fertil Steril* 61:637, 1994

72. Magyar DM, Boyers SP, Marshall JR, Abraham GE: Regular menstrual cycles and premenstrual molimina as indicators of ovulation. *Obstet Gynecol* 53:411, 1979

73. Downs KA, Gibson M: Basal body temperature graph and the luteal phase defect. *Fertil Steril* 40:466, 1983

74. Israel R, Mishell DR Jr, Stone SC, Thorneycroft IH, Moyer DL:

Single luteal phase serum progesterone assay as an indicator of ovulation. *Am J Obstet Gynecol* 112:1043, 1972

75. Nakajima ST, Gibson M: The effect of a meal on circulating steady-state progesterone levels. *J Clin Endocrinol Metab* 69:917, 1989

76. Fujimoto VY, Clifton DK, Cohen NL, Soules MR: Variability of serum prolactin and progesterone levels in normal women: The relevance of single hormone measurements in the clinical setting. *Obstet Gynecol* 76:71, 1990

77. Nakajima ST, Molloy MH, Oi RH, Ohlson KA, Azevedo RA, Boyers SP: Clinical evaluation of luteal function. *Obstet Gynecol* 84:219, 1994

78. Abraham GE, Maroulis GB, Marshall JR: Evaluation of ovulation and corpus luteum function using measurements of plasma progesterone. *Obstet Gynecol* 44:522, 1974

79. Miller MM, Hoffman DI, Creinin M, et al: Comparison of endometrial biopsy and urinary pregnanediol glucuronide concentration in the diagnosis of luteal phase defect. *Fertil Steril* 54:1008, 1990

80. Walker RF, Read GF, Riad-Fahmy D: Radioimmunoassay of progesterone in saliva: Application to the assessment of ovarian function. *Clin Chem* 25:2030, 1979

81. Finn MM, Gosling JP, Tallon DF, Madden ATS, Meehan FP, Fottrell PF: Normal salivary progesterone levels throughout the ovarian cycle as determined by a direct enzyme immunoassay. *Fertil Steril* 50:882, 1988

82. Stewart DR, Cragun JR, Boyers SP, Oi R, Overstreet JW, Lasley BL: Serum relaxin concentrations in patients with out-of-phase endometrial biopsies. *Fertil Steril* 57:453, 1992

83. Riad-Fahmy D, Read GF, Walker RF, Walker SM, Griffiths K: Determination of ovarian steroid hormone levels in saliva: An overview. *J Reprod Med* 32:254, 1987

84. Li TC, Lenton EA, Dockery P, Rogers AW, Cooke ID: The relation between daily salivary progesterone profile and endometrial development in the luteal phase of fertile and infertile women. *Br J Obstet Gynecol* 96:445, 1989

85. Tulppala M, Bjorses UM, Stenman UH, Wahlstrom T, Ylikorkala O: Luteal phase defect in habitual abortion: Progesterone in saliva. *Fertil Steril* 56:41, 1991

86. Jones GS: The luteal phase defect. *Fertil Steril* 27:351, 1976

87. Hill GA, Herbert CM III, Parker RA, Wentz AC: Comparison of late luteal phase endometrial biopsies using the Novak curette or Pipelle endometrial suction curette. *Obstet Gynecol* 73:443, 1989

88. Silver MM, Miles P, Rosa C: Comparison of Novak and Pipelle endometrial biopsy instruments. *Obstet Gynecol* 78:828, 1991

89. Herbert CM, Hill GA, Maxson WS, Wentz AC, Osteen KG: Use of a sensitive urine pregnancy test before endometrial biopsies taken in the late luteal phase. *Fertil Steril* 53:162, 1990

90. Wentz AC, Herbert CM, Maxson WS, Hill GA, Pittaway DE: Cycle of conception endometrial biopsy. *Fertil Steril* 46:196, 1986

91. Gibson M: Clinical evaluation of luteal function. *Semin Reprod Endocrinol* 8:130, 1990

92. Castelbaum AJ, Wheeler J, Coutifaris CB, Mastroianni L Jr, Lessey BA: Timing of the endometrial biopsy may be critical for the accurate diagnosis of luteal phase deficiency. *Fertil Steril* 61:443, 1994

93. Shoupe D, Mishell DR Jr, Lacarra M, et al: Correlation of endometrial maturation with four methods of estimating day of ovulation. *Obstet Gynecol* 73:88, 1989

94. Soules MR, Wiebe RH, Aksel S, Hammond CB: The diagnosis and therapy of luteal phase deficiency. *Fertil Steril* 28:1033, 1977

95. Gibson M, Badger GJ, Byrn F, Lee KR, Korson R, Trainer TD: Error in histologic dating of secretory endometrium: Variance component analysis. *Fertil Steril* 56:242, 1991

96. Del Pozo E, Wyss H, Tolis G, Alcaniz J, Campana A, Naftolin F: Prolactin and deficient luteal function. *Obstet Gynecol* 53:282, 1979

97. Seppälä M, Hirvonen E, Ranta T: Hyperprolactinaemia and luteal insufficiency. *Lancet* 1:229, 1976

98. Karamardian LM, Grimes DA: Luteal phase deficiency: Effect of treatment on pregnancy rates. *Am J Obstet Gynecol* 167:1391, 1992

99. Klentzeris LD, Li T-C, Dockery P, Cooke ID: The endometrial biopsy as a predictive factor of pregnancy rate in women with unexplained infertility. *Eur J Obstet Gynecol Reprod Biol* 45:119, 1992

100. Daly DC, Walters CA, Soto-Albors CE, Riddick DH: Endometrial biopsy during treatment of luteal phase defects is predictive of therapeutic outcome. *Fertil Steril* 40:305, 1983

101. Murray DL, Reich L, Adashi EY: Oral clomiphene citrate and vaginal progesterone suppositories in the treatment of luteal phase dysfunction: A comparative study. *Fertil Steril* 51:35, 1989

102. Cramer DW, Walker AM, Schiff I: Statistical methods in evaluating the outcome of infertility therapy. *Fertil Steril* 32:80, 1979

103. Wentz AC, Herbert CM, Maxson WS, Garner CH: Outcome of progesterone treatment of luteal phase inadequacy. *Fertil Steril* 41:856, 1984

104. Daya S, Ward S, Burrows E: Progesterone profiles in luteal phase defect cycles and outcome of progesterone treatment in patients with recurrent spontaneous abortion. *Am J Obstet Gynecol* 158:225, 1988

105. Downs KA, Gibson M: Clomiphene citrate therapy for luteal phase defect. *Fertil Steril* 39:34, 1983

106. Guzick DS, Zeleznik A: Efficacy of clomiphene citrate in the treatment of luteal phase deficiency: Quantity versus quality of preovulatory follicles. *Fertil Steril* 54:206, 1990

107. Maxson WS, Pittaway DE, Herbert CM, Garner CH, Wentz AC: Antiestrogenic effect of clomiphene citrate: Correlation with serum estradiol concentrations. *Fertil Steril* 42:356, 1984

108. Shapiro AG: New treatment for the inadequate luteal phase. *Obstet Gynecol* 40:826, 1972

109. Cook CL, Schroeder JA, Yussman MA, Sanfilippo JS: Induction of luteal phase defect with clomiphene citrate. *Am J Obstet Gynecol* 149:613, 1984

110. Soules MR, Hughes CL, Aksel S, Tyrey L, Hammond CB: The function of the corpus luteum of pregnancy in ovulatory dysfunction and luteal phase deficiency. *Fertil Steril* 36:31, 1981

111. Price JH, Ismail H, Gorwill RH, Sarda IR: Effect of the supposi-

tory base on progesterone delivery from the vagina. *Fertil Steril* 39:490, 1983

112. Castelbaum AJ, Lessey BA: Insights into the evaluation of the luteal phase. *Infertil Reprod Med Clin North Am* 6:199, 1995

113. Simon JA, Robinson DE, Andrews MC, et al: The absorption of oral micronized progesterone: The effect of food, dose proportionality, and comparison with intramuscular progesterone. *Fertil Steril* 60:26, 1993

114. Chakmakjian ZH, Zachariah NY: Bioavailability of progesterone with different modes of administration. *J Reprod Med* 32:443, 1987

115. Nahoul K, deZiegler D: Letter to the editor. *Fertil Steril* 61:790, 1994

116. Nahoul K, Dehennin L, Scholler R: Radioimmunoassay of plasma progesterone after oral administration of micronized progesterone. *J Steroid Biochem* 26:241, 1987

117. Johansson EDB: Depression of the progesterone levels in women treated with synthetic gestagens after ovulation. *Acta Endocrinol* 68:779, 1971

118. Balasch J, Vanrell JA, Rivera F, Gonzalez-Merlo J: The effect of postovulatory administration of dehydrogesterone on plasma progesterone levels. *Fertil Steril* 34:21, 1980

119. Balasch J, Vanrell JA, Marquez M, Burzaco I, Gonzalez-Merlo J: Dehydrogesterone versus vaginal progesterone in the treatment of the endometrial luteal phase deficiency. *Fertil Steril* 37:751, 1982

120. Nakajima ST, McAuliffe T, Gibson M: The 24-hour pattern of the levels of serum progesterone and immunoreactive human chori-onic gonadotropin in normal early pregnancy. *J Clin Endocrinol Metab* 71:345, 1990

121. Nakajima ST, Nason FG, Badger GJ, Gibson M: Progesterone production in early pregnancy. *Fertil Steril* 55:516, 1991

122. Huang K-E, Muechler EK, Bonfiglio TA: Follicular phase treatment of luteal phase defect with follicle-stimulating hormone in infertile women. *Obstet Gynecol* 64:32, 1984

123. Balasch J, Jove IC, Marquez M, Vanrell JA: Early follicular phase follicle-stimulating hormone treatment of endometrial luteal phase deficiency. *Fertil Steril* 54:1004, 1990

124. Minassian SS, Wu CH, Groll M, Gocial B, Goldfarb AF: Urinary follicle stimulating hormone treatment for luteal phase defect. *J Reprod Med* 33:11, 1988

125. Loucopoulos A, Ferin M: The treatment of luteal phase defects with pulsatile infusion of gonadotropin-releasing hormone. *Fertil Steril* 48:933, 1987

126. Bohnet HG, Hanker JP, Hilland U, Schneider HPG: Epimestrol in treatment of inadequate luteal progesterone secretion. *Fertil Steril* 34:346, 1980

127. Fukushima T, Tajima C, Fukuma K, Maeyama M: Tamoxifen in the treatment of infertility associated with luteal phase deficiency. *Fertil Steril* 37:755, 1982

128. Jones GS, Aksel S, Wentz AC: Serum progesterone values in the luteal phase defects: Effect of chorionic gonadotropin. *Obstet Gynecol* 44:26, 1974

129. Benadiva CA, Metzger DA: Superovulation with human menopausal gonadotropins is associated with endometrial gland-stroma dyssynchrony. *Fertil Steril* 61:700, 1994

CHAPTER 9

Prolactin Disorders in Infertility

RICHARD E. BLACKWELL · KAREN R. HAMMOND · ERIC S. KNOCHENHAUER

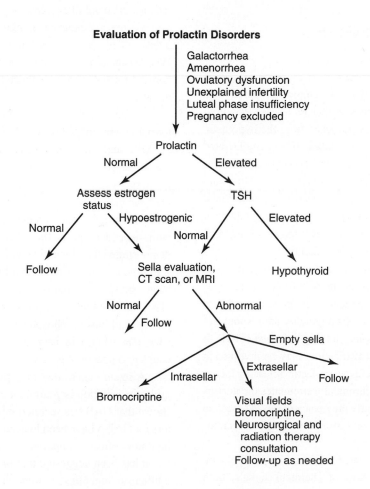

Evaluation of Prolactin Disorders

Galactorrhea
Amenorrhea
Ovulatory dysfunction
Unexplained infertility
Luteal phase insufficiency
Pregnancy excluded

Prolactin

Normal — Elevated

Assess estrogen status — TSH

Normal — Hypoestrogenic — Normal — Elevated

Follow — Sella evaluation, CT scan, or MRI — Hypothyroid

Normal — Follow — Abnormal

Empty sella

Intrasellar — Extrasellar — Follow

Bromocriptine

Visual fields
Bromocriptine,
Neurosurgical and
radiation therapy
consultation
Follow-up as needed

The association between hyperprolactinemia and suboptimal reproductive function has long been recognized in both animals and humans. In the earliest accounts, it was noted that lactating mammals did not conceive as long as intermittent suckling persisted. In 1855, the cases of several women with puerperal atrophy of the uterus, amenorrhea, and persistent lactation were reported in the literature. This condition was redescribed in 1882 and bears the name Chiari-Frommel syndrome. In 1953, a second syndrome, characterized by estrogen insufficiency, galactorrhea, and decreased urinary estrogen levels, was described by Argonz and del Castillo. One year later, Albright and Forbes described the clinical association of galactorrhea, amenorrhea, and low urinary follicle-stimulating hormone levels as a syndrome that bears their names. Although human prolactin could not be measured until 1972, we now know that these disruptions in reproductive function can occur in association with abnormal release of prolactin.

PHYSIOLOGY OF PROLACTIN SECRETION

Hypothalamic-Pituitary Axis

Prolactin once was considered to be unique compared with other anterior pituitary hormones in that its release was governed primarily by an inhibitory influence from the hypothalamus. This concept arose from studies that demonstrated persistent prolactin secretion when the pituitary gland was transplanted in vivo to a site removed from the base of the brain or was maintained in organ culture.[1] It has been thought that a single prolactin-inhibitory factor served as the sole regulator of prolactin secretion. Despite many attempts, however, no such factor has been isolated from the hypothalamus.

Recent observations, however, have suggested that posterior pituitary cells in vitro can stimulate both production and release of prolactin in a specific manner. The coculture of both anterior and posterior pituitary cells augments the responsiveness of lactotrophs to thyrotropin-releasing hormone (TRH). It has been proposed that at least two factors may be involved in this process. One could be the elusive prolactin-releasing factor. Posterior pituitary lobectomy chronically attenuates the nocturnal surge of prolactin seen in early pregnancy in rats. These data support the hypothesis that the posterior pituitary gland secretes a prolactin-releasing factor.[2,3]

The other factor could be a prolactin inhibitor. Prolactin seems to be regulated by a host of chemical signals, both inhibitory and stimulatory, that interact at all levels of the hypothalamic-pituitary axis. The principal inhibitory agent appears to be dopamine. This neurotransmitter inhibits prolactin secretion promptly in vitro and in vivo.[4,5] In vivo studies of rats demonstrated that dopamine produced in the median eminence and secreted into the hypothalamic portal vessels accounts for most of the inhibition. These conclusions were reached after dopamine was measured in hypophyseal portal blood. Those concentrations then were simulated by means of infusion of similar levels of dopamine into rats that had been pretreated with an inhibitor of prolactin synthesis, α-methylparatyrosine. Seventy percent of prolactin secretion was blocked in rats with such pretreatment. The other 30% appeared to arise from the neurohypophyseal lobe. Results of these studies were confirmed with monkeys but not with humans.[6]

Further evidence that dopamine is a principal regulator of prolactin secretion stems from suckling experiments with monkeys and rats. A brief decrease in exogenous dopamine infusion in primates led to a large increase in prolactin secretion. In the rats, a similar small decrease in hypothalamic dopamine secretion was observed during simulated suckling[7,8]; however, simulated sucking results in a limited increase in prolactin level. Whether the transient decline in dopamine level is sufficient to account for the suckling-induced increase in prolactin level is unclear.

At the cellular level, dopamine appears to act on lactotrophs by means of both cyclic adenosine 3′,5′-monophosphate (cAMP) and calcium-dependent mechanisms. High-affinity dopamine receptors have been demonstrated on lactotropic membranes. After establishment of the dopamine receptor complex, the inhibition of adenyl cyclase is believed to occur.[9] Such inhibition brings about a reduction in cAMP production in calcium-dependent prolactin release. Furthermore, it has been demonstrated that dopamine inhibits prolactin synthesis at transcription, and this effect is amplified by cAMP. Calcitonin has been shown to inhibit the thyrotropin-releasing factor (TRF)–induced release of prolactin by acting on calcium mobilization and inositol phosphate generation. Therefore, it is possible that calcitonin acts at the pituitary receptors that are coupled to phospholipase-C in an inhibitory manner.[10]

A second agent that may play a role in the inhibition of prolactin secretion is γ-aminobutyric acid (GABA). It has been shown that GABA is secreted into the portal blood, and receptors for GABA have been located on pituitary lactotrophs.[11] The inhibitory effect of dopamine is far greater than that of GABA, and it has been suggested that these two agents serve different inhibitory functions within the lactotrope. For example, dopamine induces storage of newly synthesized prolactin, which may be rapidly released after the withdrawal of dopamine. Such a response is not seen with GABA.

Although the principal control of prolactin secretion appears to be inhibition, several factors can bring about the short-

R. Jeffery Chang, MD, and Jeffery R. Cragun, MD, helped prepare the first edition of this manuscript.

term release of this hormone. These include TRH,[12] vasoactive intestinal polypeptide (VIP),[13] and angiotensin II.[14] TRH has been shown to stimulate both synthesis and release of prolactin in vitro and in vivo. As a potent stimulator of prolactin release in primates, TRH also provokes a concomitant release of thyroid-stimulating hormone (TSH), and the circulating levels of both triiodothyronine (T_3) and thyroxine (T_4) modify the response. Despite this apparent obligatory interaction, prolactin secretion may be independent of TSH secretion. For example, the short-term release of prolactin after suckling is not accompanied by an increase in TSH secretion.[15] Therefore, although under some clinical conditions, TRH might function as a prolactin-releasing factor, it has a relatively minor role in the normal physiologic control of prolactin.

VIP, purified from porcine duodenum, is a 28–amino acid polypeptide present throughout the nervous system. This hormone has been measured in hypothalamic portal blood samples, and its release appears to be prostaglandin mediated.[16] Studies have demonstrated that VIP may be produced by the pituitary gland. Although a precise role has not been defined, it has been proposed that VIP may serve as an intrahypophyseal regulator of prolactin secretion.

Angiotensin II has been shown to stimulate prolactin release both in vivo and in vitro. That angiotensin II receptors are found on lactotrophs implies a direct action.[17] Angiotensin II is an octapeptide that has been identified throughout the brain. Injection of angiotensin II brings about a rapid release of prolactin that is of far greater magnitude than that produced by TRH. This response has been blocked by the angiotensin II antagonist saralasin.

Several other transmitters appear to be involved in the control of prolactin secretion. Administration of serotonin precursors causes a marked increase in prolactin level, whereas the administration of cyproheptadine, a serotonin antagonist, blocks the prolactin-releasing effect of these precursors.[18] It has been proposed that endogenous opioids modify prolactin secretion by inhibiting dopamine turnover and release. Histamine, a hypothalamic neurotransmitter, has been shown to stimulate prolactin release by binding H1 receptors and to inhibit prolactin release through H2 receptor interaction. Both neurotensin, a tridecapeptide, and substance P, a unidecapeptide, demonstrate a stimulatory effect on prolactin secretion.[19] The precise role of these neuropeptides in controlling prolactin secretion is unclear at present.

Autoregulation and Paracrine Control of Prolactin Secretion

Although the principal regulatory pathway appears to emanate from the median eminence to the pituitary gland, either humorally or by neurotransmission, several intricate mechanisms seem to augment the control of prolactin secretion. First, retrograde flow has been demonstrated in the hypothalamic portal system, which supports the concept that prolactin regulates its own secretion by means of a short feedback loop.[20] For example, an experiment with rats showed that intraventricular injection of prolactin results in an increase in dopamine turnover in the median eminence. A similar high rate of turnover was demonstrated during both lactation and pregnancy; this high rate may be decreased by means of hypophysectomy or treatment with bromocriptine. These data may account for the observation that autographs of prolactin-secreting tumors have been associated with reduced pituitary content of prolactin. Second, intrahypophyseal mechanisms appear to be involved in the self-regulation of prolactin secretion. It was demonstrated that VIP can be synthesized from radiolabeled amino acid added to pituitary cell cultures that can stimulate prolactin release.[21] When antibodies to VIP are introduced into these cultures, prolactin secretion is inhibited. These findings are consistent with those of clinical studies that showed administration of VIP antagonists inhibits the release of prolactin. Thus VIP may function as an autocrine regulator of prolactin synthesis and release.

Several reports have suggested that gonadotrophs may exert a regulatory influence on the secretion of prolactin from lactotrophs in vivo and in vitro. Synthetic gonadotropin-releasing hormone (GnRH) was shown to release prolactin in vitro in rat superfusion and human pituitary monolayer culture systems.[22] Incubation of GnRH with lactotrophs separated from large gonadotrophs did not increase prolactin secretion, whereas coaggregation of these two cell types restored the stimulatory effect of GnRH on prolactin. In human pituitary monolayer cell culture systems, coincubation of a potent GnRH antagonist with native GnRH inhibited the release of prolactin, whereas coincubation of this antagonist with synthetic TRH did not lead to a later release of the hormone.[23] In another study, incubating α-luteinizing hormone (α-LH) with fetal rat lactotrophs stimulated differentiation of these cell types.[24] Incubation of β-LH or follicle-stimulating hormone (FSH) with human pituitary cells in vitro did not stimulate prolactin secretion consistently; however, coincubation of antisera to β-LH and FSH inhibited the GnRH-mediated release of prolactin.[25] GnRH-associated peptide (GAP), a peptide component of the precursor to GnRH, was reported to inhibit prolactin secretion in a rodent model.[26] These observations have not been confirmed. GAP gene sequences in women with hyperprolactinemia have been investigated to determine if mutations of the structural gene are present. No large deletions of the GAP peptide gene appear to be present in these patients; however, small deletions, insertions, or point mutations were not excluded.[27]

In addition to being controlled by endocrine, paracrine, and autocrine mechanisms, juxtacrine control, that is, cell-cell and cell-matrix interactions, appears to occur. The juxtacrine concept pertains to the transmission of information between adjacent cells or between the extracellular matrix and the cell without the apparent exchange of any diffusible substance. The signals appear to be transferred by means of membrane- or matrix-anchored substances that have the capacity to activate receptors on target cells. As an example, the release of prolactin by anterior pituitary cells in vitro seems to be proportional to the density of cells. For example, if the initial density was found to be 30,000 cells per well, prolactin secretion was 10 times greater than that derived from cells plated at 10,000 per well.[28]

Lactotrope and Prolactin Biology

The use of new research techniques, such as monolayer cell culture, evaluation of prolactin with NB2 node rat lymphoma cell cultures, and cell blotting to quantify hormone secretion from individual pituitary cells, has given rise to an entirely different view of pituitary cell populations.[29,30] For example, with the use of dual cytochemical labeling, cell lines have been identified that store adrenocorticotropic hormone (ACTH) with LH, FSH, TSH, or prolactin, implying their multipotential capacity.[31] In addition, populations of lactotrophs have been identified that are resistant to dopamine stimulation in idiopathic hyperprolactinemia.[32] Likewise, with use of the immunoblot technique, subpopulations of rat dopamine-unresponsive lactotrophs have been identified.[33] Further, lactotrophs have been identified that secrete small amounts of prolactin, yet are highly responsive to stimulation with TRH.[34] It has been demonstrated that steroids can modulate the transdifferentiation of prolactin and growth hormone–secreting cells in bovine pituitary cultures.[35] Likewise, there is great heterogeneity of prolactin variance, and these isotypes are found to vary throughout the menstrual cycle and in pregnancy in women with hyperprolactinemia who have normal ovulatory function.[36,37]

Prolactin and growth hormone were thought to evolve from a common ancestral gene. This theory was supported by the fact that they share biologic and immunologic properties, immunoassay sequences, and homologies in nucleic acid sequence.[38] Preprolactin is thought to consist of 914 base pairs in mammals, and the prolactin receptor consists of 830 amino acids in avian species.[39] Prolactin receptors exist in two forms and are members of the prolactin growth hormone cytokine receptor superfamily. DNA cloning experiments have demonstrated a short 300–amino acid and long 600–amino acid form.[40] No clear second messenger for prolactin has been identified, and this may ultimately account for its diversity of biologic action.

The gene for prolactin has been isolated, cloned, and sequenced and has been found to be located on the short arm of chromosome 6. BG/2 polymorphisms have been described, but no mutations have been detected in patients with hyperprolactinemia.[38,41,42] Interactions have been demonstrated between the transcription regulatory regions of prolactin chromatin, estrogen appearing to be a principal enhancer of the interaction.[43]

A discussion of prolactin biology would not be complete without the mention of galanin and granins. Galanin is a widely distributed regulatory peptide that modulates secretion of both prolactin and growth hormone.[44] Galanin is a 29–amino acid peptide secretion which responds strongly to estrogen administration.[45] However, the exact role of galanin is unknown; it is probably a lactotropic growth factor, because galanin immunoneutralization inhibits the mitogenic effects of estrogen. Granins are a family of tyrosine sulfated secretory proteins composed of two members: chromogranin-B and secretogranin-2.[46] These have been found in GH4C1 cell lines that secrete both prolactin and growth hormone. Granins are subject to extensive posttranslational modification, and their function remains the subject of speculation.

Prolactin and Ovarian Function

It has been speculated that the menstrual dysfunction in patients with hyperprolactinemia may be secondary to a direct effect on the ovary in addition to or instead of central inhibition. Possible mechanisms include atresia of the developing dominant follicle, inhibition of interruption of ovulation and normal corpus luteum development, and premature destruction of the corpus luteum. It also appears that suppression of prolactin enhances follicular response and inhibits corpus luteum formation and function. Therefore, the actions of prolactin on follicle and corpus luteum may be different.[47] Such speculation is supported by the finding that in rat fetuses, ovarian interstitial cells contain a single class of specific high-affinity prolactin receptors.[48] In this system, prolactin acts as a potent inhibitor of LH median androgen synthesis. In the porcine model, prolactin not only induces internalization of its own receptor but also causes downmodulation of unoccupied LH receptors. This could account for the diminished ovarian response of patients with chronic hyperprolactinemia. Prolactin also has been shown to inhibit granulosa cell luteinization in Sprague-Dawley rats. The suppression of prolactin by bromocriptine stimulates the aromatization of testosterone to estradiol in women. Therefore, it appears that prolactin participates in the regulation of ovarian steroidogenesis.[49–51] Because most androgen substrate is derived from theca cells, a decrease in its production secondary to hyperprolactinemia could reduce estrogen synthesis. High-affinity prolactin receptors also have been found on the surface membranes of granulosa cells.[52] These receptors have been located near the basal lamina, and it is these same cells that contain aromatase. FSH induces aromatase activity in vitro, and this effect is completely blocked by coincubation of granulosa cells with high levels (100 ng/mL) of prolactin. In vivo prolactin blocks aromatase activity in rat preovulatory follicles. These observations support the hypothesis that prolactin disrupts both synthesis of androgen precursors and induction of aromatase, which results in both decreased estrogen synthesis and reduced induction of FSH receptors. In rats, the oocyte seems to have intracellular prolactin activities.[53] Both prolactin and its receptor are concentrated heavily in the cytoplasm. Whether these findings have a bearing on folliculogenesis and the health of the oocyte is unknown.

A number of clinical studies have evaluated the effect of hyperprolactinemia on the result of in vitro fertilization (IVF).[54–57] These findings suggest that hyperprolactinemia does not affect granulosa cell luteinization, the total number of oocytes, the number of mature oocytes, fertilization, cleavage, or pregnancy rate. Hyperprolactinemia has been demonstrated in as many as 57% of patients undergoing IVF. However, the use of bromocriptine inhibition of the anesthesia-induced hyperprolactinemia response has been touted as having a positive influence on embryonic development after IVF. Other authors have reported that high serum prolactin levels interfere with follicle and oocyte development.

Although prolactin may alter ovarian function in rats, similar evidence in humans is less clear. First, it has been demonstrated that prolactin is present in the microenvironment of follicles in vitro.[58] In the early follicular phase of the cycle, a fourfold to sixfold increase in prolactin level is found in the fluid of developing follicles compared with concentrations in the blood. In one study,[58] most follicles with high concentrations of prolactin were found to have low concentrations of estradiol. Second, in another study, patients with hyperprolactinemia exceeding 100 ng/mL, all follicles in the ovaries were basal; human chorionic gonadotropin (hCG)–stimulated estradiol synthesis occurred in human follicles perfused in vitro.[59] These observations indicate that, in humans, prolactin in excessive amounts may disrupt normal follicular development. Whether this process leads to interruption of ovulation has not been defined.

The role of prolactin in corpus luteum function appears to be even less clear than its role in follicular development. Most evidence has come from experiments with rats. Prolactin both stimulates and inhibits corpus luteum function. On the positive side, it is involved in the induction of LH receptors to stimulate progesterone synthesis.[60] This action of prolactin apparently is necessary for completion of luteinization. In vitro experiments with humans, however, have shown that very high levels of prolactin have an inhibitory effect on both progesterone and estradiol synthesis.[61] Therefore, it is evident that hyperprolactinemia may produce an alteration in normal reproductive function that results in infertility.

Prolactin and Testicular Function

Prolactin has been shown to affect the male hypothalamic-pituitary-gonadal axis. Classic studies demonstrated that crude prolactin extracts decreased testicle size in adult pigeons.[62] In fact, prolactin has been shown to affect almost every aspect of male reproduction, including gonadal function, sexual behavior, seminal plasma, accessory reproductive glands, and the central nervous system. In some species, prolactin is essential in maintaining fertility. Its effect on the central axis has been manifested by impairment of LH release such that the frequency of pulsation is increased and the amplitude is altered. It has been speculated that prolactin alters the presence of basal and GnRH-induced pituitary GnRH receptors.[63] It also has been demonstrated that administration of pulsatile GnRH to hypogonadal men with prolactinomas restores LH pulsatility and normal testosterone concentration.[64]

Although hyperprolactinemia may have a central effect on male reproductive function, prolactin receptors (as in the ovary) have been demonstrated in testicular homogenates.[65] Prolactin receptors were found on Leydig cells in rats, although they have not been documented in human testes. Prolactin receptors also appear to have high affinity and low capacity as in other tissues, and they are subject to both up- and downregulation by prolactin. Luteinizing hormone also has been shown to regulate testicular prolactin receptors; injection of ovine LH was shown to cause an increase in receptor content in rat testes.[66]

LH-stimulated steroidogenesis may be inhibited by chronic hyperprolactinemia, which leads to a decrease in testosterone production in adult animals and humans.[67] It has been proposed that the ability to enhance steroidogenesis is explained by prolactin-induced upregulation of LH receptors in animal models[68]; however, the mechanism by which prolactin inhibits LH-stimulated steroidogenesis is not clear. It appears that in the absence of LH, prolactin has no effect on basal testosterone production. Even with LH, the effect on testosterone production is variable and dose dependent. Similarly, no change in numbers of LH receptors has been demonstrated, suggesting that the inhibitory effect may be at the post–LH receptor–binding site. For instance, in rats, pituitary graft–induced hyperprolactinemia stimulated α-reductase activity but decreased 17-hydroxylase activity.[69] In addition, 5α-reductase activity is reported to be inhibited by sulpiride-induced hyperprolactinemia in humans. Prolactin also has been shown to increase 3β-hydroxysteroid dehydrogenase and accumulation of esterified cholesterol in Leydig cells in mice.

As with Leydig cells, prolactin seems to have an effect on the tubular compartment of the testes.[70] Superphysiologic concentrations are associated with numerous defects in spermatogenesis in human and animal models.[71] These include seminiferous epithelial disorganization, germ cell exfoliation, increased tubule wall thickness, and abnormal lipid content of Leydig cells. Testicular biopsy confirms the presence of tubule wall thickness and Sertoli cell disorganization in humans. It should be noted that no prolactin receptors have been identified in the testes outside the interstitial compartment.

It seems clear that, as in females, prolactin has a substantial impact on male reproduction. Hyperprolactinemia affects prolactin receptors and testicular enzyme activity as well as spermatogenesis. These interactions between prolactin and the gonads, in addition to the central effects discussed previously, help one understand the importance of prolactin in reproductive dysfunction.

Although hyperprolactinemia appears to disrupt sperm production, and treatment with bromocriptine restores this capability, until recently little was known about the effect of these ergoline compounds on sperm motility or viability. In the 1990s, it became fashionable to insert bromocriptine tablets into the vagina to attempt to avoid the emetic effect of these compounds. It was noted that circulating levels of bromocriptine rose more slowly with vaginal delivery but were sustained for a longer period of time. Subsequently, several groups were able to demonstrate that bromocriptine had no adverse effect on sperm survival or motility. In fact, bromocriptine has been shown to reverse the inhibitory effect of macrophages on human sperm motility.[72–76]

Prolactin, Uterine Function, and Infertility

Uterine adenomyosis is a benign lesion that can be characterized by abnormal uterine bleeding, pain, cramps, and infertility. The transplantation of ectopic pituitary isografts in mice has been demonstrated to increase plasma levels of prolactin and induce uterine adenomyosis. It also has been demonstrated that administration of bromocriptine to mice for 1 month beginning at 4 weeks of age suppressed prolactin release and blocked the development of adenomyosis. The relation between hyperprolactinemia and the development of adenomyosis in humans remains to be investigated.[77]

ROLE OF HYPERPROLACTINEMIA IN INFERTILITY

It appears that the main cause of anovulation is an impairment in gonadotropin pulsatility and a derangement of the estrogen positive feedback of LH secretion in the hyperprolactinemic state. Subcutaneous pulsatile GnRH therapy combined with hCG has been shown to compensate for these defects and result in induction of ovulation.[78]

The clinical spectrum of prolactin-related infertility includes galactorrhea, amenorrhea, oligomenorrhea, luteal insufficiency, and possibly subtle follicular dysfunction, all of which occur as a result of hyperprolactinemia.[79] These features are commonly encountered in women with primary disorders of prolactin metabolism, namely, prolactin-secreting pituitary tumors, or prolactinemias.[80] Idiopathic or functional hyperprolactinemia and the empty sella syndrome are also included in this group.

Another form of prolactin-related infertility that might classify as a primary disorder is intermittent or transient hyperprolactinemia. This is an extremely subtle phenomenon, and its precise effect on fertility remains to be elucidated.

Secondary disorders of prolactin-related infertility are those in which the mechanism of infertility is associated with, but not necessarily dependent on, hyperprolactinemia. Examples include polycystic ovary syndrome and primary hypothyroidism.[81] In general, these clinical entities represent the principal disorders of prolactin metabolism. As such they should be considered in the diagnosis and management of hyperprolactinemic infertility.

Prolactinomas and Infertility

Infertility in patients with a prolactinoma generally is a consequence of hyperprolactinemia rather than of tumor size, with the exception of massive lesions. Persistent hyperprolactinemia may act at the level of the gonad or the hypothalamic-pituitary axis to cause infertility. Because hyperprolactinemic infertility generally causes amenorrhea, disruption of pituitary gonadotropin secretion is not necessarily unexpected. In addition to loss of the midcycle gonadotropin surge, attenuation of episodic secretion has been documented. These alterations occurred despite, in some instances, a lack of change in basal LH and FSH concentrations.

Anovulation is likely related to decreased GnRH secretion, as implied by reduced pulsatile gonadotropin release. It has been demonstrated that LH, FSH, and prolactin are released in a copulsatile manner throughout the menstrual cycle. This suggests common regulatory factors might account for these complex temporal patterns. Alterations in GnRH pulse frequency might result in a luteal phase defect. A state of occult hyperprolactinemia has been described in which a dynamic challenge test may help identify patients who would respond to bromocriptine therapy.[82] The presence of a prolactin-secreting neoplasm causes an increase in hypothalamic dopamine level by means of a short loop feedback mechanism. Increased dopamine inhibits the release of GnRH, which is responsible for decreased gonadotropin secretion and anovulation. This concept is supported by the restoration of ovulation after resolution of hyperprolactinemia by means of surgical extirpation of the prolactinoma or administration of bromocriptine.

As with microadenomas, anovulation in patients with macroadenomas commonly results from hyperprolactinemia.[83] On occasion, an extensive lesion occupies or extends beyond the sellar space and destroys the entire pituitary gland, including gonadotrophs. Eradication of such a tumor or resolution of hyperprolactinemia does not restore ovulation; treatment with human menopausal gonadotropin is necessary.

Functional Hyperprolactinemia

Increased prolactin secretion in the absence of a demonstrable pituitary neoplasm is functional or idiopathic. In most patients, serum prolactin levels are minimally or moderately elevated and do not exceed 200 ng/mL. If the patient has amenorrhea, the mechanism of anovulatory infertility is similar to that in women with microprolactinomas. In some instances, however, patients have oligomenorrhea or have regular menstrual cycles. It has been suggested that in these patients infertility may result from an adverse effect of corpus luteum function that leads to a luteal phase defect. In humans, limited clinical evidence supports a direct action of prolactin on the follicle. In contrast, abnormal corpus luteum development may be a direct consequence of prolactin effect or an indirect result of inadequate follicular maturation. A lack of corpus luteum support is reflected by diminished progesterone production and incomplete endometrial development in the luteal phase. This alteration may preclude implantation or lead to increased pregnancy wastage and habitual abortion. A luteal phase defect secondary to hyperprolactinemia is corrected by means of treatment with bromocriptine.[84]

The empty sella syndrome may be viewed as either a primary or a secondary disorder of prolactin metabolism.[85] Not infrequently, this condition is associated with a pituitary tumor. In theory, the lesion has expanded the sella turcica and in doing so has widened the aperture in the sellar diaphragm through which passes the infundibulum. As a result, herniation of the arachnoid membrane into the sellar cavity occurs, and the pituitary gland is displaced to the side. Radiologic evaluation reveals a clear area in the expanded sella, which represents the arachnoid membrane filled with cerebrospinal fluid. The prolactinoma, which may be difficult to detect radiographically owing to a compression effect, continues to release excess prolactin, and anovulation persists. In rare situations, the defect of the sellar diaphragm is congenital, and hyperprolactinemia does not result from a pituitary neoplasm. Instead, the fluid-filled hernial sac impinges on the infundibulum to interrupt the inhibitory control of prolactin, which leads to increased prolactin secretion. If the expansion of the hernia is substantial, compression of the optic chiasm may occur, with compromise of the visual fields.

Intermittent Hyperprolactinemia and Infertility

The concept of intermittent hyperprolactinemia emerged from several studies in which bromocriptine was used to treat unexplained infertility. Although initial impressions suggested that bromocriptine was beneficial in the treatment of these patients, studies to support this contention were lacking. For example, evaluation of follicular phase prolactin levels in 40 ovulatory infertile and 25 fertile women did not demonstrate a significant difference.[86] Two double-blind studies yielded the same results.[87,88] In one of the studies, more pregnancies occurred during the 12-month follow-up period than during treatment cycles with bromocriptine.

In what was perhaps the first study suggesting that intermittent hyperprolactinemia might be associated with infertility, 94% of patients had transient preovulatory hyperprolactinemia.[89] This elevation coincided with the estrogen peak and lasted 1 to 3 days. Forty percent of patients who received bromocriptine conceived within 3 months after beginning therapy compared with 1% before treatment. The relevance of such episodic hyperprolactinemia has to be questioned, since administration of a dopamine antagonist, metoclopramide, for 6 days during the preovulatory period had no apparent detrimental effect on ovulation.[90] If hyperprolactinemia was induced in the early follicular phase, however, ovulation was disrupted in 60% of women. Some investigators noted that patients with sulpiride-induced hyperprolactinemia exhibited similar follicles, with lower estradiol concentrations and higher testosterone levels than euprolactinemic controls with follicles of similar size.

Transient hyperprolactinemia is often associated with ovulation induction and IVF stimulation protocols.[91] It occurs with the use of clomiphene, human menopausal gonadotropin (hMG), or a mixture of the two agents. In IVF programs, preanesthetic serum prolactin levels are correlated with follicular fluid prolactin levels and are inversely related to pregnancy rate. Because the percentage of oocytes fertilized does not correlate with preanesthetic prolactin values, however, any change in pregnancy rate does not appear to be due to disordered fertilization. In monkeys, treatment with hMG increased luteal phase prolactin levels. The administration of bromocriptine suppressed prolactin levels but did not change the length of the menstrual cycle or luteal phase in these animals. Luteal phase progesterone and estrogen levels also are increased in such therapy.[92]

Despite the seeming lack of correlation between intermittent hyperprolactinemia and response to treatment and pregnancy, three subsets of patients might benefit from bromocriptine therapy. First, a variety of heterogeneous forms of prolactin have been described that are present in both healthy persons and patients with hyperprolactinemia.[93] An iso-B–prolactin was described in patients with unexplained infertility; suppression of iso-B–prolactin with bromocriptine resulted in pregnancy in a significant number of these women.[94] Second, in a population of women with high psychologic stress scores associated with intermittent elevations in prolactin level, autogenic training lowered psychologic stress markers.[95] Combined bromocriptine and clomiphene therapy was reported to produce higher pregnancy rates than placebo. Third, women with galactorrhea and euprolactinemia as measured with conventional radioimmunoassay were treated with bromocriptine.[96] This resulted in a significant increase in pregnancy rate than did treatment with clomiphene and vitamin B_6 administered to matched controls. Therefore, subgroups of patients with various forms of hyperprolactinemia might benefit from bromocriptine therapy.[97–99] It appears, however, that empiric treatment of infertile patients with bromocriptine is unwarranted.

Secondary disorders of prolactin metabolism associated with infertility include polycystic ovary (PCO) syndrome and primary hypothyroidism. Serum prolactin levels are reported to be elevated in about 30% of patients with PCO syndrome.[100] In addition, in the absence of overt hyperprolactinemia, prolactin concentrations are increased within the normal range compared with levels in weight-matched ovulatory women.[101] The same study also showed that prolactin response to TRH stimulation in women with PCO syndrome was greater than that of healthy controls. The increased production of prolactin logically has been attributed to the hyperestrogenism associated with this syndrome and possibly a deficiency of hypothalamic dopamine; however, confirmatory evidence of these mechanisms is lacking.

Long-term suppression of estrogen secretion in patients with PCO syndrome treated with a GnRH agonist for 6 months failed to reduce circulating prolactin levels (R. J. Chang, unpublished data). Second, several attempts to document a hypothalamic dopamine deficiency have provided inconclusive results. That hyperprolactinemia is primarily responsible for anovulation in PCO syndrome is unlikely. Available evidence suggests that prolactin has a possible contributory role, and anovulation is a result of a more central disturbance.

An effect of prolactin on adrenal androgen production was suggested in PCO syndrome because of the dehydroepiandrosterone sulfate (DHEAS) response to bromocriptine or dopamine administration.[102] Treatment with bromocriptine decreased prolactin levels and reduced DHEAS level concomitantly. It also was demonstrated that the rate of prolactin production fell and the metabolic clearance rate increased during treatment.[103] It has not been established whether these results are due to changes in prolactin level or to a direct effect of bromocriptine on steroidogenesis. Management of PCO syndrome with bromocriptine has yielded variable results with re-

spect to ovulation and pregnancy.[104] Although this therapy generally reduces prolactin and DHEAS levels, gonadotropin levels and menstrual status are unaltered in all but a small number of patients.[105]

Normal thyroid function has long been thought necessary to maintain synchronous menstrual cycles; however, the precise mechanism of this relationship has not been determined. In thyroid disease, alteration of menstrual cyclicity and disruption of reproductive function have been attributed to abnormal peripheral steroid metabolism.[106] In primary hypothyroidism, irregular vaginal bleeding may occur in part as a result of hyperprolactinemia. In this disorder, elevated TSH levels presumably are stimulated by an increased TRH level, which could account for increased prolactin secretion. Moreover, studies in animals and humans indicate that the prolactin response to TRH is greater than that of TSH, its accepted target hormone. The clinical findings among untreated patients with primary hypothyroidism have not consistently supported this concept. In one study, untreated patients had an exaggerated prolactin response to TRH stimulation that reverted to normal after appropriate thyroid replacement.[107] On the other hand, in one study 15 of 49 patients (30.6%) demonstrated some degree of hyperprolactinemia, whereas only one patient had galactorrhea.[108] In another study, untreated patients had an exaggerated prolactin response to TRH stimulation, which reverted to normal after appropriate thyroid replacement.

These observations suggest that in primary hypothyroidism, an increase of prolactin production may not necessarily be associated with an increase in circulating prolactin levels. The rates of menstrual irregularity and infertility have not been assessed in this condition. Conversely, in infertile couples with menstrual irregularity, the rate of thyroid dysfunction has not been established. Because routine thyroid evaluation for these patients seldom reveals thyroid disease, the prevalence generally has been believed to be low. Despite extensive evidence that thyroid diseases, in particular primary hypothyroidism, can influence prolactin release, the clinical significance of these findings remains in question.

DIAGNOSIS OF HYPERPROLACTINEMIA

A patient with menstrual irregularity or galactorrhea undergoes a serum prolactin determination (see algorithm at beginning of this chapter). If the level is elevated, it should be measured a second time because of the known erratic pattern of secretion. Prolactin is a dynamic hormone whose secretion is influenced by a variety of physiologic stimuli such as stress, exercise, food intake, and sleep.[109] Care must be taken to avoid these confounding features in choosing an optimal time for sampling. For example, the standard has been that blood should be obtained either in the morning after an overnight fast and well removed from awakening or just before lunch provided there has not been a midmorning snack. However, recent prospective trials that evaluated the effect of breast examination on serum prolactin levels in fertile women with normal cycles and the effect of high-protein nutrition on serum prolactin levels in the same group of patients showed no increase in prolactin secretion in any of the women 15, 30, or 45 minutes after the examination (Tables 9–1 and 9–2). Therefore, it behooves us to reevaluate some of our concepts about the measurement of serum prolactin in normal physiologic states. For patients with hyperprolactinemia, T_4 and TSH levels should be measured to rule out the presence of compensated hypothyroidism. In these patients, T_4 levels are often normal while TSH is markedly elevated.[110]

Patients with an abnormal basal body temperature chart, several low midluteal serum progesterone levels, consistent out-of-phase endometrial biopsy findings or poor folliculogenesis patterns as measured with sonography should undergo an evaluation for hyperprolactinemia. It has been reported that as many as 20% of patients with such findings have elevated prolactin levels, although the condition was found in 15 of 130 infertile patients (11.5%) with regular menstrual cycles and no galactorrhea.[111] In the same study, luteal phase levels of progesterone and estrogen were similar in both women with hyperprolactinemia and women with normal prolactin levels. In fact, a larger number of instances of inadequate luteal-phase histologic findings occurred among women with normal prolactin levels than among women with hyperprolactinemia. It was concluded that the role of elevated serum prolactin in patients with apparent luteal phase defects was minimal.

Patients with hyperprolactinemia documented on several occasions should undergo a radiographic examination.[112] When this examination should be performed is controversial. Some reproductive endocrinologists recommend computed tomography (CT) or magnetic resonance imaging (MRI) when any elevation is found. Others proceed depending on a specific maximal concentration of prolactin such as 50 or 100 ng/mL (50 or 100 µg/L). Almost without exception, once a prolactin level of 100 ng/mL (100 µg/L) has been determined on several

occasions, advanced radiologic surveillance is recommended (Fig 9–1). Patients with serum prolactin levels greater than 50 ng/mL (50 µg/L) have a 20% risk for prolactinoma; those with a 100 ng/mL (100 µg/L) value are at 50% risk. Levels greater than 100 ng/mL (100 µg/L) are almost diagnostic for the presence of at least a microadenoma.[113] If prolactinoma is detected, visual-field examinations by means of Goldman perimetry might be undertaken if the lesion is 10 mm or greater in diameter. There is little indication for visual field surveillance, since most subtle defects (superior bitemporal hemianopsia) are not detected until the prolactinoma extends out of the sella and compresses the optic chiasm.

The choice of radiologic procedure has evolved with time. The cone-down view of the sella once was used to detect lesions 10 mm in diameter or larger. This gave way to linear and hypocycloidal tomography, which have been all but abandoned

TABLE 9–1. BREAST EXAMINATION* AND SERUM PROLACTIN LEVELS

Prolactin Level[†]	
Time (min)	(ng/mL)
0	7.17
15	6.59
30	6.84
45	6.45

*Breast examinations performed on 11 women of reproductive age (22%–38%).
[†]Not significant by ANOVA and paired *t* test.

TABLE 9–2. HIGH PROTEIN NUTRITION* AND SERUM PROLACTIN LEVELS

Prolactin Level[†]	
Time (min)	(ng/mL)
0	6.8
15	7.1
30	7.2
45	7.9

*Eleven women of reproductive age (22%–38%) ate a diet high in arginine, tyrosine, and tryptophan.
[†]Not significant by ANOVA and paired *t* test *P* = .0494 .

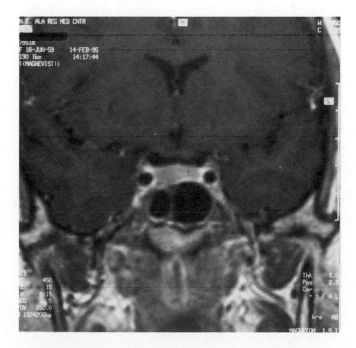

Figure 9–1. Magnetic resonance image demonstrating a pituitary microadenoma.

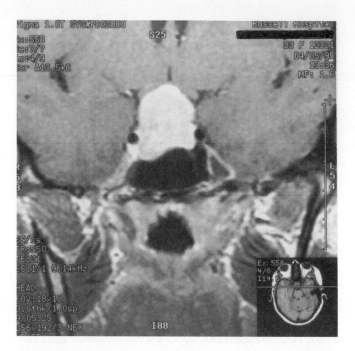

Figure 9–2. Magnetic resonance image demonstrating a pituitary macroadenoma with involvement of the carotid artery.

because they are best used to detect erosion of bone. Unfortunately, a normal sella shows great variation, making the rate of false-positive and false-negative results for adenoma detection high. Computed tomography with metrisemide enhancement can be used to detect lesions as small as 2 mm, and this is currently the most common radiologic technique. Magnetic resonance imaging (MRI) appears to be superior to all previous forms of pituitary surveillance (Fig 9–2). The images generated with MRI performed by a skilled technician and interpreted by an experienced radiologist are vastly superior to CT scans. Moreover, the patient is not exposed to irradiation. Although slower to perform and more expensive than CT, MRI continues to evolve as the state-of-the-art technique for the radiologic evaluation of the pituitary gland in infertile patients with hyperprolactinemia.

MANAGEMENT OF HYPERPROLACTINEMIC INFERTILITY

Historically, radiation and surgical therapy were used exclusively to treat patients with prolactinomas. In the absence of a pituitary lesion, infertile women with hyperprolactinemic anovulation of a functional nature underwent ovulation induction with either clomiphene citrate, hMG, FSH, or GnRH. Patients with microprolactinomas were treated with selective extirpation during a transsphenoidal operation. Consideration of radiation therapy was limited by the risk for hypopituitarism and damage to surrounding structures.

The response to surgical treatment was generally marked

by resumption of ovulatory menses in more than 70% of patients and a corresponding increase in the frequency of pregnancy. Intraoperative complications were minimal, since the tumors were small, and mortality was rare. Initial follow-up studies appeared to justify the surgical management of microadenomas. However, extended long-term follow-up study has revealed a substantial recurrence of hyperprolactinemia and, even more disturbing, reappearance of the tumor.[114] Nevertheless, operative intervention remains one treatment choice.

The development of synthetic dopamine agonists and bromocriptine has been of clear benefit in the management of infertility for patients with microadenoma. Bromocriptine provides at least equivalent clinical responses with respect to ovulation and pregnancy compared with those achieved by means of surgical therapy.[115] In addition, the medication has proved to be well tolerated and has minimal side effects. With the success of dopamine agonist therapy, there seems to be little indication for surgical resection of small pituitary tumors in these patients.

The treatment of the macroadenoma is more complicated and may involve surgical excision, irradiation, the use of a dopamine agonist, or a combination of these therapies. The failure rate after transsphenoidal resection of these lesions has been reported to be as high as 70%. This lack of success is related to tumor size; direct correlation exists between surgical failure and large size of the lesion.[116] Patients with prolactin levels greater than 200 ng/mL (200 µg/L) have a poorer outcome than those with lower levels.[117] It is understandable that surgical resection of a macroadenoma is associated with increased morbidity and mortality compared with operative removal of a microadenoma. Radiation therapy delivered by means of either the linear cobalt or the proton mode has been used as a primary method of managing macroprolactinomas. Most commonly, it is used to treat patients who have undergone an operation and exhibit evidence of persistent disease. Proton beam therapy has posed the risk of panhypopituitarism; the need for hormone replacement as with thyroid hormone, cortisone, sex steroids, or vasopressin must be considered. Dopamine agonists, although not uniformly successful in suppression of growth of prolactinomas, have substantial effects on most large lesions.[118] In 50% to 75% of patients, marked reduction in tumor size has been demonstrated; in 25% to 30%, the neoplasm has resolved totally. The adjunctive use of a dopamine agonist preoperative treatment has been suggested, although clinical benefit has not been evident in all instances.

Several new compounds have been introduced for the management of hyperprolactinemia and prolactinoma. Parlodel SRO (Sandoz, East Hanover, NJ) is a long-acting oral bromocriptine agent with effects that last for 24 hours.[119] It has a similar side effect profile to that of conventional oral Parlodel and is highly effective in the management of hyperprolactinemia. Parlodel LAR is a long-acting injectable form of bromocriptine administered in a 50- to 100-mg dose each month. It has been shown to control prolactin secretion and the growth of macroadenomas.[120] Pergolide mesylate (Permax, Eli Lilly, Indianapolis, IN) has been shown to be as effective as bromocriptine in the treatment of patients with hyperprolactinemia and prolactinoma. It is a nonergoline preparation administered in a dose of 50 to 100 μg per day.[121] Cabergoline (Farmitalia Carlo Erba, Milan, Italy) administered in a dose between 400 and 3000 μg per week inhibits prolactin secretion and shrinks pituitary tumors. It appears to have less severe side effects than other typical dopaminergic compounds.[122,123] Finally, CV205-502 (Sandoz) is a nonergoline dopamine ergoline agonist active in a dose of 40 to 80 μg. It profoundly suppresses prolactin secretion and reduces tumor size in patients unresponsive to other dopamine agonists. This drug has finished U.S. trials, but it has not been brought before the Food and Drug Administratioin (FDA). No estimate can be made about when it will appear on the market. CV205-502 has a 30% better side effect profile than does Parlodel.[124-126]

Pregnancy should be considered for all patients with prolactinoma should therapy result in the return of prolactin levels to normal and resumption of regular ovulatory menses. In the case of a microadenoma, few complications have been reported as a result of tumor expansion during pregnancy.[127,128] At least three large studies examined the development of children exposed in utero to bromocriptine and determined that no abnormalities arose as a result of drug administration.[129] There is no contraindication to breastfeeding by postpartum women with a microadenoma.

In patients with macroadenoma, there is more concern about the side effects of tumor growth. Left untreated, approximately 30% of patients have required medical, surgical, or radiation therapy during pregnancy.[130] This is in contrast to patients with microadenomas, less than 1% of whom need any therapy during gestation. Lactotropic hypertrophy and hyperplasia occur normally in pregnancy as a result of increased estrogen secretion. In most women, the enlargement of the pituitary gland is rarely symptomatic. Preexisting macroadenomas have been known to expand rapidly during pregnancy, however, causing vision disturbances and headaches. It has been suggested that bromocriptine therapy be continued throughout or instituted during pregnancy if clinically indicated. The ability to breastfeed postpartum is contingent on the continued need for bromocriptine therapy.

Precise assessment of tumor size in pregnancy is difficult, because methods of evaluation are limited and indirect. For example, serum prolactin levels rise in a progressive but erratic manner throughout pregnancy, reaching a peak between 200 and 500 ng/mL (200 to 500 μg/L). It is generally accepted that these levels do not provide useful information in pregnancy. Visual field examination with Goldman perimetry has been the most sensitive and noninvasive management technique. Computed tomography during pregnancy is discouraged, and the utility of MRI, with its possible effects of magnetism on the fetus, is as yet unclear. Therefore, the physician is usually faced with making the clinical decision on the basis of limited data.

Despite the problems that can occur with macroadenoma during pregnancy, the long-term effect of a first pregnancy on prolactin secretion results in a marked decrease postpartum when measured from 12 to 150 months since the last delivery.[131] Therefore, first pregnancy leads to a long-term decrease in serum prolactin secretion, lasting at least 12 to 13 years. In addition, there is a differential prolactin response to oral metoclopramide in nulliparous in contrast to parous women. Parous women have a decrease in prolactin response.[132] There also appears to be an augmentation of the metoclopramide prolactin response in nulliparous women that increases with chronologic age. This suggests a gradual decrease in the dopaminergic tone in older women.[133]

NATURAL HISTORY OF HYPERPROLACTINEMIA

It appears that functional (idiopathic) hyperprolactinemia may be a distinct entity from prolactinoma. When 59 women were followed for an average of 5.2 years, 21 (35%) had an improvement in clinical symptoms and only two had any tumor progression. There appears to be a high tendency for spontaneous cure and pregnancy (Fig 9–3).[134-136]

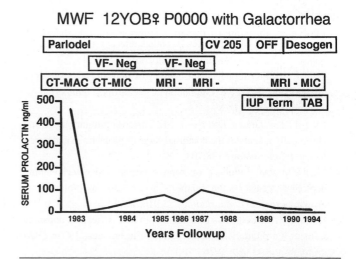

Figure 9–3. Natural history of large suprasellar macroadenoma in an adolescent followed for 11 years. VF, Visual field; MAC, macroadenoma; IUP, intrauterine pregnancy; TAB, therapeutic abortion.

SUMMARY AND CONCLUSION

Hyperprolactinemia is clearly associated with infertility in both men and women. It may effect numerous tissue sites (brain, pituitary gland, ovaries, testes) and alter their physiologic roles in reproduction. As a result, increased prolactin production is associated with a number of pathologic conditions, including PCO syndrome and thyroid and pituitary disease. The cause of hyperprolactinemia must be determined and suppression of one condition carefully confirmed to facilitate appropriate management and eliminate the empiric use of bromocriptine, particularly in infertile patients.

Medical therapy is preferred for both men and women with hyperprolactinemic infertility whether or not a pituitary tumor is present. Reestablishment of normal ovulation predisposes to conception, and during pregnancy, therapy may be discontinued by all patients except those with macroprolactinoma. These patients may need therapy throughout pregnancy.

Evidence indicates no deleterious effects of bromocriptine on mother or fetus. Although bromocriptine is the mainstay of the medical therapy for hyperprolactinemia, a new generation of drugs, both ergoline and nonergoline dopamine agonists, are in the final phases of development. These agents offer once-a-day therapy, have few side effects, and should expand our therapeutic alternatives.

ACKNOWLEDGMENT

I wish to thank Murrill Lynch for her help in the preparation of this manuscript.

REFERENCES

1. Blackwell RE, Guillemin R: Hypothalamic control of adenohypophyseal secretion. *Annu Rev Physiol* 35:357, 1973
2. Dymshitz J, Ben-Jonathan N: Coculture of anterior and posterior pituitary cells: Selective stimulation of lactotrophs. *Endocrinology* 128:2469, 1991
3. Averill RLW, Grattan DR, Norris SK: Posterior pituitary lobectomy chronically attenuates the nocturnal surge of prolactin in early pregnancy. *Endocrinology* 128:704, 1991
4. MacLeod RM: Influence of norepinephrine and catecholamine-depleting agents on the synthesis and release of prolactin and growth hormone. *Endocrinology* 85:916, 1969
5. Leblanc H, Lachelin G, Abu-Fadil S, Yen SSC: Effects of dopamine infusion on pituitary hormone secretion in humans. *J Clin Endocrinol Metab* 43:669, 1976
6. Gibbs OM, Neill JD: Dopamine levels in hypophyseal stalk blood in the rat are sufficient to inhibit prolactin secretion in vitro. *Endocrinology* 102:1895, 1978

7. Plotsky PM, deGreef WF, Neill JD: In situ voltametric microelectrodes: Application to the measurement as median eminence catecholamine release during simulated suckling. *Brain Res* 250:251, 1982
8. Plotsky PM, Neill JD: Interactions of dopamine and thyrotropin-releasing hormone in the regulation of prolactin release in lactating rats. *Endocrinology* 111:168, 1982
9. Schettini G, Cronin MJ, MacLeod RM: Adenosine 3',5'-monophosphate (cAMP) and calcium-calmodulin interrelation in the control of prolactin secretion: Evidence for dopamine inhibition of cAMP accumulation and prolactin release after calcium mobilization. *Endocrinology* 112:1801, 1983
10. Martin TFJ: Calcitonin peptide inhibition of TRH-stimulated prolactin secretion: Additional evidence for inhibitory regulation of phospholipase C. *Trends Endocrinol Metab* 3:82, 1992
11. Grossman A, Delitala G, Yeo T, Besser GM: GABA and muscimol inhibit the release of prolactin from dispersed rat anterior pituitary cells. *Neuroendocrinology* 32:145, 1981
12. Vale W, Blackwell RE, Grant G, Guillemin R: TRF and thyroid hormones on prolactin secretion by rat pituitary cells in vitro. *Endocrinology* 93:26, 1973
13. Matsushita N, Kato Y, Shimatsu A, et al: Effects of VIP, TRH, GABA and dopamine on prolactin release from superfused rat anterior pituitary cells. *Life Sci* 32:1263, 1983
14. Dufy-Barbe L, Rodriguez F, Arsaut J, Verrier D, Vincent JD: Angiotensin II stimulates prolactin release in the rhesus monkey. *Neuroendocrinology* 35:242, 1982
15. Gerhengorn MC: Thyrotropin-releasing hormone: A review of the mechanisms of acute stimulation of pituitary hormone release. *Mol Cell Biochem* 45:163, 1982
16. Shimatsu A, Kao Y, Matsushita N, et al: Effect of prostaglandin E on vasoactive intestinal polypeptide release from the hypothalamus and on prolactin secretion from the pituitary in rats. *Endocrinology* 113:2059, 1983
17. Aguilera G, Hyde CL, Catt KJ: Angiotensin II receptors and prolactin release in pituitary lactotrophs. *Endocrinology* 111:1045, 1987
18. Clemens JA, Roush ME, Fuller RW: Evidence that serotonin neurons stimulate secretion of prolactin-releasing factor. *Life Sci* 22:2209, 1978
19. Knigge U, Dejgaard A, Wollesen F, Thuesen B, Christiansen PM: Histamine regulation of prolactin secretion through H_1-H_2-receptors. *J Clin Endocrinol Metab* 55:118, 1982
20. Bergland R, Page R: Can the pituitary secrete directly to the brain? (Affirmative anatomical evidence). *Endocrinology* 102:1325, 1978
21. Hagen TC, Arnaout MA, Scherzer WJ, Martinson DR, Garthwaite TL: Antisera to vasoactive intestinal polypeptide inhibit basal prolactin release from disbursed anterior pituitary cells. *Neuroendocrinology* 43:641, 1983
22. Denef C, Andries M: Evidence for paracrine interaction between gonadotrophs and lactotrophs in pituitary cell aggregates. *Endocrinology* 112:813, 1983
23. Blackwell RE, Rodgers-Neame NT, Bradley EL, Asch RH: Regulation of human prolactin secretion in gonadotropin releasing hormone in vitro. *Fertil Steril* 46:26, 1986

24. Begeot M, Hemming FJ, DuBois PM: Induction of pituitary lactotrope difference by luteinizing hormone alpha subunit. *Science* 226:566, 1984

25. Blackwell RE, Garrison PN: Inhibition of prolactin secretion by antiserum to the α- and β-subunits of gonadotropin. *Am J Obstet Gynecol* 156:863, 1987

26. Nikolics K, Mason AJ, Szonyl E, Ramachandran JR, Seeburg PH: A prolactin-inhibiting factor within the precursor for human gonadotropin-releasing hormone. *Nature* 316:511, 1985

27. Moretuzzo RW, Layman LC, Tho SPT, Reindollar RH, Gray MR, McDonough PG: Gonadotropin-releasing hormone-associated peptide gene sequences in women with hyperprolactinemia. *Fertil Steril* 58:908, 1992

28. Ben-Jonathan N, Liu JW: Pituitary lactotrophs: Endocrine, paracrine, juxtacrine, and autocrine interactions. *Trends Endocrinol Metab* 3:254, 1992

29. Tanaka T, Shiu RPC, Gout PW, Beer CT, Noble RL, Friesen HG: A new sensitive and specific bioassay for lactogenic hormones: Measurement of prolactin and growth hormone in human serum. *J Clin Endocrinol Metab* 51:1058, 1980

30. Kendall ME, Hymer WC: A new approach to quantify hormone secretion from individual rat pituitary cells. *Endocrinology* 121:2260, 1987

31. Childs GV: Multipotential pituitary cells that contain adrenocorticotropin (ACTH) and other pituitary hormones. *Trends Endocrinol Metab* 2:112, 1991

32. Webb CB, Thominet JL, Barowsky H, Berelowitz M, Frohman LA: Evidence for lactotroph dopamine resistance in idiopathic hyperprolactinemia. *J Clin Endocrinol Metab* 48:1089, 1983

33. Arita J, Kojima V, Kimura F: Identification by the sequential cell immunoblot assay of a subpopulation of rat dopamine-unresponsive lactotrophs. *Endocrinology* 128:1887, 1991

34. Arita J, Kojima Y, Kimura F: Lactotrophs secreting small amounts of prolactin reveal great responsiveness to thyrotropin-releasing hormone: Analysis by the sequential cell immunoblot assay. *Endocrinology* 130:3167, 1992

35. Kineman RD, Faught WJ, Frawley LS: Steroids can modulate transdifferentiation of prolactin and growth hormone cells in bovine pituitary cultures. *Endocrinology* 120:3289, 1992

36. Sinha YN: Prolactin variants. *Trends Endocrinol Metab* 3:100, 1992

37. Larrea F, Escorza A, Valero A, Hernandez L, Cravioto MC, Diaz-Sanchez V: Heterogeneity of serum prolactin throughout the menstrual cycle and pregnancy in hyperprolactinemic women with normal ovarian function. *J Clin Endocrinol Metab* 68:982, 1989

38. Cooke NE, Coit D, Shine J, Baxter JD, Martial JA: Human prolactin; cDNA structural analysis and evolutionary comparisons. *J Biol Chem* 256:4007, 1981

39. Chen X, Horseman ND: Cloning, expression, and mutational analysis of the pigeon prolactin receptor. *Endocrinology* 135:269, 1994

40. Kelly PA, Djiane J, Edery M: Different forms of the prolactin receptor: Insights into the mechanism of prolactin action. *Trends Endocrinol Metab* 3:54, 1992

41. Truong A, Duez C, Belayew A, et al: Isolation and characterization of the human prolactin gene. *EMBO J* 3:429, 1984

42. Myal Y, DiMattia GE, Gregory CA, Friesen HG, Hamerton JL, Shiu RP: A BgIII RFLP at the human prolactin gene locus on chromosome 6. *Nucleic Acids Res* 19:1167, 1991

43. Cullen KE, Kladde MP, Seyfred MA: Interaction between transcription regulatory regions of prolactin chromatin. *Science* 261:203, 1993

44. Hsu DW, El-Azouzi M, McL Black P., Chin WW, Hedley-Whyte ET, Kaplin LM: Estrogen increases galanin immunoreactivity in hyperplastic prolactin-secreting cells in Fisher 344 rats. *Endocrinology* 125:3159, 1990

45. Wynick D, Hammond PJ, Akinsanya KO, Bloom SR: Galanin regulates basal and oestrogen-stimulated lactotroph function. *Nature* 364:529, 1993

46. Hinkle PM, Scammell JG, Shanshala ED: Prolactin and secretogranin-II, a marker for the regulated pathway, are secreted in parallel by pituitary GH_4C_1 cells. *Endocrinology* 130:3503, 1992

47. Kauppila A, Martikainen H, Puistola U, et al: Hypoprolactinemia and ovarian function. *Fertil Steril* 49:437, 1988

48. Magoffin DA, Erickson GF: Prolactin inhibition of LH stimulated androgen synthesis in ocarina interstitial cells cultured in defined medium: Mechanism of action. *Endocrinology* 111:2001, 1982

49. Lane TA, Chen TT: Heterologous down-modulation of luteinizing hormone receptors by prolactin: A flow cytometry study. *Endocrinology* 128:1833, 1991

50. Adashi EY, Resnick CE: Prolactin as an inhibitor of granulosa cell luteinization: Implications for hyperprolactinemia-associated luteal phase dysfunction. *Fertil Steril* 48:131, 1987

51. Martikainen H, Ronnberg L, Puisola U, Tapanainen J, Orava M, Kauppila A: Prolactin suppression by bromocriptine stimulates aromatization of testosterone to estradiol in women. *Fertil Steril* 52:51, 1989

52. Ben-David M, Schenker JG: Human ovarian receptors to human prolactin: Implications in infertility. *Fertil Steril* 38:182, 1982

53. Dunaif AE, Zimmerman EA, Friesen HG, Frantz AG: Intracellular localization of prolactin receptor and prolactin in the rat ovary by localization of prolactin receptor and prolactin in the rat ovary by immunocytobiochemistry. *Endocrinology* 110:1465, 1982

54. Piekos MW, Binor Z, Rawlins RG, Radwanska E: Effects of inducted hyperprolactinemia on in vitro fertilization cycles. *Fertil Steril* 63:371, 1995

55. Hummel WP, Clark MR, Talbert LM: Transient hyperprolactinemia during cycle stimulation and its influence on oocyte retrieval and fertilization rates. *Fertil Steril* 53:677, 1990

56. Sopelak VM, Whitworth NS, Norman PF, Cowan BD: Bromocriptine inhibition of anesthesia-induced hyperprolactinemia: Effect on serum and follicular fluid hormones, oocyte fertilization, and embryo cleavage rates during in vitro fertilization. *Fertil Steril* 52:627, 1989

57. Reinthaller A, Bieglmayer C, Deutinger J, Csaicsich P: Transient hyperprolactinemia during cycle stimulation: Influence on the endocrine response and fertilization rate of human oocytes and effects of bromocriptine treatment. *Fertil Steril* 49:432, 1988

58. Seibel MM, Smith D, Dlugi AM, Levesque L: Periovulatory fol-

licular fluid hormone levels in spontaneous human cycles. *J Clin Endocrinol Metab* 68:1073, 1989

59. McNatty KP: Relationship between plasma prolactin and the endocrine microenvironment of the developing human antral follicle. *Fertil Steril* 32:43, 1979

60. Wang C, Hsueh AJW, Erickson GF: Prolactin inhibition of estrogen production by cultured rat granulosa cells. *Mol Cell Endocrinol* 20:136, 1980

61. Tan GJS, Biggs JSG: Effects of prolactin on steroid production by human luteal cells in vitro. *J Endocrinol* 96:499, 1983

62. Bates RW, Riddle O, Lahr EL: The mechanism of the antigonadal action of prolactin in adult pigeons. *Am J Physiol* 119:610, 1937

63. Marchetti B, Labrie F: Prolactin inhibits pituitary luteinizing hormone (LH)–releasing hormone receptors in the rat. *Endocrinology* 111:1209, 1982

64. Bouchard P, Lagoguey M, Barilly S, Schaison G: Gonadotropin-releasing hormone pulsatile administration restores luteinizing hormone pulsatility and normal testosterone levels in males with hyperprolactinemia. *J Clin Endocrinol Metab* 60:258, 1985

65. Posner BI, Kelly PA, Shiu RPC, Friesen HG: Studies of insulin, growth hormone and prolactin binding tissue distribution, species variation and characterization. *Endocrinology* 94:421, 1974

66. Kelly PA, Seguin C, Cusan L, Labrie F: Stimulatory effect of luteinizing hormone and human chorionic gonadotropin on testicular prolactin receptor levels. *Biol Reprod* 23:924, 1984

67. Murray FT, Cameron DF, Ketchum C: Return of gonadal function in man with prolactin-secreting pituitary tumors. *J Clin Endocrinol Metab* 59:79, 1984

68. Bohnet HG, Friesen HG: Effect of prolactin and GH on prolactin and LH receptors in dwarf mouse. *J Endocrinol Fertil* 48:307, 1976

69. Ngareda T, Takeyama M, Ueda T, et al: Hyperprolactinemia enhances LH-L stimulated 4-ene-5 alpha-reductase activity but inhibits LH-induced 17-hydroxylase activity in testes of hypophysectomized immature rats. *J Steril Biochem* 24:1199, 1985

70. Bartke A, Lloyd CW: Influence of PRL and pituitary isografts on spermatogenesis in dwarf mice and hypophysectomized rats. *J Endocrinol* 46:321, 1982

71. Katovich MJ, Cameron DF, Murray FT, Gunsalus GL: Alterations of testicular function induced by hyperprolactinemia in the rat. *J Androl* 6:179, 1985

72. Vermesh M, Fossum GT, Kletzky OA: Vaginal bromocriptine: Pharmacology and effect on serum prolactin in normal women. *Obstet Gynecol* 172:693, 1988

73. Katz E, Weiss BE, Hassell A, Schran HF, Adashi EY: Increased circulating levels of bromocriptine after vaginal compared with oral administration. *Fertil Steril* 55:882, 1991

74. Chenette PE, Siegel MS, Vermesh M, Kletzky OA: Effect of bromocriptine on sperm function in vitro and in vivo. *Obstet Gynecol* 77:935, 1991

75. Rojas FJ, Djannati E, Rojas IM: The effect of bromocriptine on the motility of human spermatozoa and its capacity to penetrate the cervical mucus. *Fertil Steril* 55:48, 1991

76. Scommegna A, Ye SH, Prins GS: Bromocryptine reverses the inhibitory effect of macrophages on human sperm motility. *Fertil Steril* 61:331, 1994

77. Mori T, Singtripon T, Kawashima S: Animal model of uterine adenomyosis: Is prolactin a potent inducer of adenomyosis in mice? *Am J Obstet Gynecol* 165:232, 1991

78. Matsuzaki T, Azuma K, Irabara M, Yasui T, Aono T: Mechanism of anovulation in hyperprolactinemic amenorrhea determined by pulsatile gonadotropin-releasing hormone injection combined with human chorionic gonadotropin. *Fertil Steril* 62:2254, 1994

79. Blackwell RE: Diagnosis and treatment of hyperprolactinemic syndromes. *Fertil Steril* 43:5, 1985

80. Keye WR, Chang JR, Wilson CB, Jaffe RB: Prolactin-secreting pituitary adenomas. III. Frequency and diagnosis of amenorrhea-galactorrhea. *JAMA* 244:1329, 1980

81. Blackwell RE, Chang RJ: Report of the national symposium on the clinical management of prolactin-related reproductive disorders. *Fertil Steril* 45:607, 1986

82. Inaudi P, Reymond MJ, Rey F, Genazzani AD, Lemarchand-Beraud T: Pulsatile secretion of gonadotropins and prolactin during the follicular and luteal phases of the menstrual cycle: Analysis of instantaneous secretion rate and secretory concomitance. *Fertil Steril* 58:51, 1992

83. Pepperell RJ: Prolactin and reproduction. *Fertil Steril* 35:267, 1981

84. Daly DC, Walters CA, Soto-Albors CE, Riddick DH: Endometrial biopsy during treatment of luteal phase defects unproductive of therapeutic outcome. *Fertil Steril* 45:607, 1983

85. Hsu TH, Shapiro JR, Tyson JE, Leddy AL, Paz-Guevera AT: Hyperprolactinemia associated with empty sella syndrome. *JAMA* 235:2002, 1976

86. Lenton EA, Sobowale OS, Cooke ID: Prolactin concentrations in ovulatory but infertile women: Treatment with bromocriptine. *BMJ* 2:1179, 1977

87. Wright CS, Steele SJ, Jacobs HS: Value of bromocriptine in unexplained primary infertility: A double-blind controlled trial. *BMJ* 1:2037, 1982

88. McBain JC, Pepperell RJ: Use of bromocriptine in unexplained infertility. *J Clin Endocrinol Metab* 55:442, 1983

89. Ben-David H, Schenker JG: Transient hyperprolactinemia: A correctable cause of idiopathic female infertility. *J Clin Endocrinol Metab* 57:442, 1983

90. Ylikorkala O, Kauppila A: The effects on the ovulatory cycle of metoclopramide-induced increased prolactin levels during follicular development. *Fertil Steril* 35:588, 1981

91. Tang LC, Ho PC: Transient hyperprolactinemia in human menopausal gonadotropin induction of ovulation. *Int J Fertil* 29:236, 1984

92. Collins RL, Williams RF, Hodgen GD: Human menopausal gonadotropin-human chorionic gonadotropin-induced ovarian hyperstimulation with transient hyperprolactinemia. Steroidogenesis enhanced during bromocriptine therapy in the monkey. *J Clin Endocrinol Metab* 59:727, 1974

93. Suh HK, Frantz AG: Size heterogeneity of human prolactin in plasma and pituitary extract. *J Clin Endocrinol Metab* 39:928, 1974

94. Ben-David M, Chrambach A: A method for isolation by gel electrophoresis of isohormones B and C of human prolactin from amniotic fluid. *J Endocrinol* 84:125, 1980

95. Harrison FR, O'Moore A, Mosurski K, O'Moore R, Cranny A: Intermittent hyperprolactinemia and the unexplained infertile couple: A placebo-controlled study of combined clomiphene citrate, bromocriptine therapy. *Infertility* 9:1, 1986

96. DeVane G, Guzick D: Bromocriptine therapy in normoprolactinemic women with unexplained infertility and galactorrhea. *Fertil Steril* 46:1026, 1986

97. Huang K, Bonfiglio TA, Muechler EK: Transient hyperprolactinemia in infertile women with luteal phase deficiency. *Obstet Gynecol* 78:651, 1991

98. Soules MR, Bremner WJ, Steiner RA, Clifton DK: Prolactin secretion and corpus luteum function in women with luteal phase deficiency. *J Clin Endocrinol Metab* 72:986, 1991

99. Asukai K, Uemura T, Minaguchi H: Occult hyperprolactinemia in infertile women. *Fertil Steril* 60:423, 1993

100. Corenblum B, Taylor PJ: The hyperprolactinemic polycystic ovary syndrome may not be a distinct entity. *Fertil Steril* 38:549, 1982

101. Shoupe D, Lobo RA: Prolactin response after gonadotropin releasing hormone in the polycystic ovary syndrome. *Fertil Steril* 43:549, 1985

102. Steingold KA, Lobo RA, Judd HL, Lu JKH, Chang RJ: The effect of bromocriptine on gonadotropin secretion in polycystic ovarian disease. *J Clin Endocrinol Metab* 62:1048, 1986

103. Schlebinger RJ, Chrousos GP, Culler GB, Loriaux DL: The effect of serum prolactin on plasma adrenal androgens and the production and metabolic clearance rate of dehydroepiandrosterone sulfate in normal and hyperprolactinemic subjects. *J Clin Endocrinol Metab* 62:202, 1986

104. Suginami H, Hamada K, Yano K, Kuroda G, Matsuura S. Ovulation induction with bromocriptine in normoprolactinemic anovulatory women. *J Clin Endocrinol Metab* 62:899, 1986

105. Seibel MM, Oskowitz S, Kamarara M, Taymor ML: Preliminary observations on the response of low-dose bromocriptine in normoprolactinemic patients with polycystic ovary disease. *Obstet Gynecol* 64:213, 1984

106. Gordon GG, Southren AL, Tochimoto S, Rand JJ, Olivo J: Effect of hyperthyroidism and hypothyroidism on the metabolism of testosterone and androstenedione in man. *J Clin Endocrinol* 29:164, 1969

107. Snyder PJ, Jacobs LS, Utiger RD, Daughaday WH: Thyroid hormone inhibition of the prolactin response to thyrotropin-releasing hormone. *J Clin Invest* 52:2324, 1973

108. Honbo KS, Van Herle AJ, Kellett JA: Serum prolactin levels in untreated primary hypothyroidism. *Am J Med* 65:782, 1978

109. Dollar J, Blackwell R: Diagnosis and management of prolactinomas. *Cancer Metastasis Rev* 5:125, 1986

110. Yamamoto K, Saito K, Takai T, Naito M, Yoshida N: Visual field defects and pituitary enlargement in primary hypothyroidism. *J Clin Endocrinol Metab* 67:283, 1983

111. Vanrell JA, Balasch J: Prolactin in the evaluation of luteal phase in infertility. *Fertil Steril* 39:30, 1983

112. Molitch ME: Evaluation and treatment of the patient with a pituitary incidentaloma. *J Clin Endocrinol Metab* 80:3, 1995

113. Blackwell RE, Boots LR, Goldenberg RE, Younger JB: Assessment of pituitary function in patients with serum prolactin levels greater than 100 ng/mL. *Fertil Steril* 32:177, 1979

114. Serri O, Rasio E, Beauregard H, et al: Recurrence of hyperprolactinemia after selective transsphenoidal adenomectomy in women with prolactinoma. *N Engl J Med* 209:280, 1983

115. Molitch ME, Elton RL, Blackwell RE, et al: Bromocriptine as primary therapy for prolactin-secreting macroadenomas: Results of a prospective multicenter study. *J Clin Endocrinol Metab* 60:698, 1985

116. Domingue JN, Richmond IL, Wilson CB: Results of surgery on 114 patients with prolactin-secreting adenomas. *Am J Obstet Gynecol* 137:102, 1980

117. Faria MA, Tindall GT: Transsphenoidal microsurgery for prolactin-secreting pituitary adenomas: Results in 100 women with the amenorrhea-galactorrhea syndrome. *J Neurosurg* 56:38, 1982

118. Blackwell RE, Bradley EL, Kline LB, et al: Comparison of dopamine agonists in the treatment of hyperprolactinemic syndrome: A multicenter study. *Fertil Steril* 39:744, 1983

119. Weingrill CO, Mussio W, Moraes CRS, Portes E, Castro RC, Lengyel AMJ: Long-acting oral bromocriptine (Parlodel SRO) in the treatment of hyperprolactinemia. *Fertil Steril* 57:331, 1992

120. Ciccarelli E, Miola C, Avataneo T, Camanni F, Besser GM, Grossman A: Long-term treatment with a new repeatable injectable form of bromocriptine, Parlodel LAR, in patients with tumorous hyperprolactinemia. *Fertil Steril* 52:930, 1989

121. Lamberts SW, Quik RFP: A comparison of the efficacy and safety of pergolide and bromocriptine in the treatment of hyperprolactinemia. *J Clin Endocrinol Metab* 72:635, 1991

122. Philosophe R, Seibel MM: Novel approaches to the management of hyperprolactinemia. *Curr Opin Obstet Gynecol* 3:336, 1991

123. Melis GB, Gambacciani M, Paoletti AM, Mais V, Sghedoni D, Fioretti P: Reduction in the size of prolactin-producing pituitary tumor after Cabergoline administration. *Fertil Steril* 52:412, 1989

124. Vance ML, Cragun JR, Reimnitz C, et al: CV205-502 treatment of hyperprolactinemia. *J Clin Endocrinol Metab* 68:336, 1989

125. Shoham Z, Homburg R, Jacobs HS: CV205-502: Effectiveness, tolerability, and safety over 24-month study. *Fertil Steril* 55:501, 1991

126. van der Heijden PFM, Lappohn RE, Corbey RS, de Goeij WBKMV, Brownell J, Rolland R: The effectiveness, safety, and tolerability of CV205-502 in hyperprolactinemic women: A 12-month study. *Fertil Steril* 52:574, 1989

127. Corenblum B: Successful outcome of ergocryptine-induced pregnancies in twenty-one women with prolactin-secreting pituitary adenomas. *Fertil Steril* 32:183, 1979

128. Divers WA, Yen SSC: Prolactin-producing microadenomas in pregnancy. *Obstet Gynecol* 61:425, 1978

129. Turkalj I, Braun P, Krupp P: Surveillance of bromocriptine in pregnancy. *JAMA* 247:1599, 1982

130. Magyar DM, Marshall JR: Pituitary tumors and pregnancy. *Am J Obstet Gynecol* 132:739, 1978

131. Musey VC, Collins DC, Musey PI, Martino-Saltzman D, Preedy JRK: Long-term effect of a first pregnancy on the secretion of prolactin. *N Engl J Med* 316:229, 1987

132. de los Monteros AE, Cornejo J, Parra A: Differential prolactin response to oral metoclopramide in nulliparous versus parous women throughout the menstrual cycle. *Fertil Steril* 55:885, 1991

133. Parra A, Alarcon J, Gavino F, Ramirez A, de los Monteros AE: Age-related changes in the metoclopramide-induced prolactin release in nulliparous women. *Fertil Steril* 60:34, 1993

134. Sluijmer AV, Lappohn RE: Clinical history and outcome of 59 patients with idiopathic hyperprolactinemia. *Fertil Steril* 58:72, 1992

135. Schlechte J, Dolan K, Sherman B, Chapler F, Luciano A: The natural history of untreated hyperprolactinemia: A prospective study. *J Clin Endocrinol Metab* 68:412, 1989

136. Corenblum B, Taylor PJ: Idiopathic hyperprolactinemia may include a distinct entity with a natural history different from that of prolactin adenomas. *Fertil Steril* 49:544, 1988

CHAPTER 10

Thyroid Disorders and Reproduction

JEFFREY GARBER

Physiologic Development
Thyroid Physiology in Pregnancy
Hypothyroidism
   Diagnosis
   Sexual maturation
   Infertility
   Pregnancy
Hyperthyroidism
   Diagnosis
   Sexual maturation
   Female-factor infertility
   Male-factor infertility
   Pregnancy and hyperthyroidism, including non-thyroidal illness, trophoblastic disease, and gestational transient thyrotoxicosis

Neonatal Thyroid Dysfunction
   Neonatal hypothyroidism
   Neonatal hyperthyroidism
Postpartum Thyroid Disease
Thyroid Nodules and Cancer
Autoimmune Thyroid Disease and Miscarriage
   Hypothyroidism
   Hyperthyroidism
Postpartum Thyroiditis
Approach to the Treatment of a Patient
   with Infertility
   Failure to conceive
   Recurrent miscarriage in the setting of positive titers for antithyroid antibodies

Thyroid disorders constitute a group of common diseases that affect fertility, fetal development, and subsequent growth, including the ability to have successful term pregnancies. Many excellent reviews in endocrinology and thyroidology publications discuss various aspects of this topic.[1–6] The initial part of this chapter briefly reviews fetal thyroid development and discusses the physiologic aspects of thyroid hormone economy in pregnancy. This review is followed by a discussion of how thyroid disorders affect conception and pregnancy and how to manage the disorders during pregnancy and the prepartum period, during which obstetric outcome and fertility are the goals. Newer findings such as thyroxine replacement adjustments in pregnancy, gestational transient thyrotoxicosis, the propensity of women with positive antithyroid antibody titers to abort, highly sensitive thyroid-stimulating hormone (TSH) assays, painless thyroiditis, the effect of subclinical hypothyroidism on conception and pregnancy, the impact of iodine[131] on fertility, and the relationship of thyroid dysfunction to male-factor infertility are reviewed.

PHYSIOLOGIC DEVELOPMENT

The fetal thyroid is capable of functioning by 10 to 12 weeks of gestation. Its development is completed by 12 to 14 weeks and is linked to the maturation of the hypothalamic-pituitary axis. It is not until 17 to 19 weeks of gestation, however, that labeled iodothyronines appear in fetal blood following administration of radioiodine to the mother.[7] This finding suggests that the fetus is not making its own thyroid hormone before that. Yet thyroid hormone receptors exist in the brain by approximately 10 weeks of gestation, and thyroid hormone is found in the fetal brain by this time. This finding is evidence for the argument that in early gestation maternal circulation is the source of fetal brain thyroid hormone. Maternal thyroid status may therefore influence early brain development. This hypothesis explains why in areas where iodine deficiency is prevalent and maternal hypothyroidism is regularly encountered in conjunction with congenital hypothyroidism, irreversible mental retardation is often seen in hypothyroid offspring. In contrast, congenital hypothyroidism does not lead to irreversible retardation if maternal hypothyroidism is absent and the newborn is treated promptly and appropriately.[8]

Thyroid hormone produces its impact by means of intracellular binding of triiodothyronine (T_3) to a nuclear receptor. The extent of nuclear exposure to T_3 is generally related to circulating T_3 levels. In the brain and pituitary gland, however, it is largely the result of intracellular T_3 production from intracellular thyroxine, or tetraiodothyronine (T_4). This feature of pituitary thyroid hormone metabolism explains why TSH levels, which in the absence of pituitary and hypothalamic disease are the most sensitive indicators of thyroid status, are more closely linked to circulating T_4 levels than circulating T_3 levels despite the important role of T_3 in cellular metabolism.

Fetal T_4 levels continue to rise between 10 and 30 weeks of gestation in parallel with thyroid hormone binding globulin (TBG) and TSH levels. Subsequently, T_4 levels rise more gradually but are not accompanied by a rise in TBG levels. That is, free T_4 levels rise in conjunction with a drop in TSH levels. The rise in fetal T_4 levels is accompanied by a rise in reverse T_3 (RT_3), a metabolically inactive T_3 produced from T_4. Because T_4 is principally metabolized to RT_3, T_3 levels remain low. Lower T_3 levels presumably allow the fetus to conserve fuel resources without a negative impact on organ development. It is surmised that excessive T_3 exposure in early fetal life may lead to abnormal development.

TSH values peak 30 minutes after delivery and fall to baseline levels 48 to 72 hours postpartum. T_3 levels are initially low. Over the next 24 hours they become transiently elevated and begin to fall by 48 hours postpartum. Some portion of the T_3 surge is the result of cutting the cord and is independent of the neonatal TSH surge. T_4 levels peak 48 hours postpartum. By 3 to 4 weeks postpartum, physiologic neonatal thyroid hyperactivity resolves.

THYROID PHYSIOLOGY IN PREGNANCY

To recognize and treat thyroid dysfunction in pregnancy, one needs a basic understanding of thyroid physiology in pregnancy.

Maternal TBG levels rise in early pregnancy in parallel with the rise in estrogen level. Maternal TBG values generally exceed normal adult levels by 8 weeks of gestation and peak at about 20 weeks. Although originally thought to be the result of an increase in hepatic TBG synthesis, the production of slowly cleared variants is the principal cause of TBG excess. The rise in TBG accounts for the concomitant rise in T_4 levels and the peak immediately after midgestation. In one study, 90% of women in the third trimester had T_4 levels above the upper normal for nonpregnant women. When lower percentages have been reported, iodine deficiency may have been a confounding variable. T_3 is avidly bound to TBG; the rise of T_3 in pregnancy parallels the rise in T_4 level; the ratio of T_3 to T_4 remains normal. Free T_3, free T_4, and TSH levels generally remain within the normal range throughout pregnancy. In early pregnancy, there is a rise in the former two with a concomitant drop in the latter. During the end of pregnancy there is a drop in the former two and an appropriate rise in the latter. Although all of these values generally remain normal, in early pregnancy, a small but important subset become transiently abnormal.

The free T_4 index is a unitless expression calculated by the multiplication of the total T_4 level by the T_3 uptake value. One disadvantage of this index is the nonlinearity of T_3 uptake as an estimate of the percentage of free T_4 and T_3. When T_3 uptake values are very high the percentage of free hormone is underestimated. When T_3 uptake values are very low, the percentage of free hormone is overestimated. In pregnancy T_3 uptake is typically very low because of high TBG values. As a result, the free T_4 index or free T_3 index exaggerates the amount of free hormone present in pregnancy. This in combination with the facts that newer TSH assays are more sensitive than the free T_4 index in picking up mild degrees of either hypothyroidism or hyperthyroidism and that a small change in free T_4 level leads to marked changes in TSH level (negative logarithmic relation) are the arguments for making TSH levels the preferred screening tool for thyroid dysfunction. This is particularly so in pregnancy. Misleadingly low or inappropriately normal (when they should be high) TSH levels caused by unusual cases of hypothalamic or pituitary disease causing secondary hypothyroidism and hyperthyroidism are rarely encountered because of the relatively high incidence of associated hypogonadism and infertility.

There is poor placental passage of T_4 and T_3 from the maternal circulation to the fetus. To transfer biologically significant amounts of either hormone to the fetus, 4 to 10 times maternal physiologic levels must be achieved. When the fetus is athyreotic,[9] the maternal-fetal gradient allows for about one half the maternal level of T_4 to be achieved in the fetus. The poor passage of hormone is a function of both physical barriers and placental Type III deiodinase that degrades thyroid hormone. There are several consequences of poor placental passage. On a positive note, thyrotoxic or hypothyroid mother's thyroid hormone levels have no clinically significant effect on fetal values. On the other hand, fetal hypothyroidism cannot effectively be treated with maternal thyroid hormone ingestion without rendering the mother thyrotoxic.

Human chorionic gonadotropin (hCG) levels double every other day after implantation. They reach their peak near the end of the first trimester. The level of hCG subsequently declines to 5% to 10% of its peak by midgestation. Another rise follows midgestation, but values remain well below peak levels at term. Evidence that hCG is capable of stimulating the thyroid is linked to the neutralization of its effect with anti-hCG antibodies[10] and the inverse relation between hCG and TSH levels; hCG peaks at 10 weeks and TSH reaches its nadir at that point (Fig 10–1). The latter relationship and its pathophysiologic implications for a subset of pregnant women are reviewed later. For most women this relationship is physiologically unimportant. Slight drops in TSH level are noted, but diurnal variation of TSH levels is preserved, an argument against a physiologically significant excess of thyroid hormone.

Renal iodide clearance increases during pregnancy. Serum iodide levels reach their nadir at the end of the second trimester, reaching about one-half normal nongravid values. Iodide diffuses from mother to fetus. Although the radioactive iodine uptake expressed as a percentage may be high, in iodine-sufficient regions the absolute uptake of iodine and urinary iodine excretion is normal. A fetus is particularly vulnerable to excessive or inadequate iodide exposure because its thyroidal autoregulatory capacity is not fully developed. In the United States and other areas without iodine deficiency, pregnancy does not lead to goiter.[11,12] In areas where iodine deficiency exists, even if it is mild, pregnancy is goitrogenic. Although Japan, Scandinavia, Switzerland, and Austria do not have iodine deficiency, other parts of Europe and large components of undeveloped areas continue to suffer from this problem, and it continues to be a serious public health problem.[13]

Levels of thyroglobulin, a protein unique to thyroid tissue, increase during the first trimester and remain so until term.

HYPOTHYROIDISM

Diagnosis

Hypothyroidism has protean clinical manifestations (Table 10–1). Some of these are reviewed in the discussion of pregnancy and hypothyroidism herein. Ultimately, confirmation of the diagnosis is based on laboratory methods that demonstrate, either directly or indirectly, thyroid hormone deficiency.

Most instances of hypothyroidism are related to thyroid gland failure or primary hypothyroidism. Because pituitary TSH secretion rises exponentially when free T_4 levels drop, measurement of serum TSH is more sensitive than an estimate of free T_4 or direct measurement of free T_4 in the detection of early phases of primary hypothyroidism. In fact, TSH elevations are often noted in conjunction with normal free T_4 measurements, a situation referred to as *subclinical hypothyroidism*. Whether such patients truly have no symptoms or simply have normal free T_4 levels in conjunction with features of clinical hypothyroidism cannot always be determined before a trial of thyroid hormone replacement. An additional benefit of thyroid hormone treatment of a patient with subclinical hypothyroidism who has a goiter is prevention of progression of the goiter.

Screening for hypothyroidism can be accomplished with a sensitive TSH assay. Recent refinements in TSH assay methods

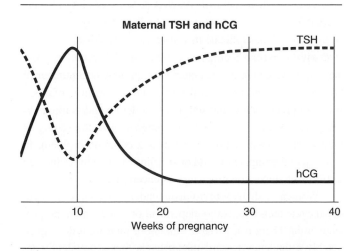

Maternal TSH and hCG

TSH

hCG

10   20   30   40

Weeks of pregnancy

Figure 10–1. Graph shows maternal TSH and hCG levels during pregnancy. (*Redrawn from Speroff L, Glass RH, Kase NG:* Clinical Gynecologic Endocrinology and Infertility, *ed 5. Baltimore, Williams & Wilkins, 1994: chapter 20.*)

TABLE 10–1. CLINICAL FEATURES OF HYPOTHYROIDISM

Mild Disease	Moderate to Severe Disease	Most Severe Disease
Fatigue[a]	Dry, thick skin	Hypothermia
Constipation[a]	Thick, brittle hair	Hypoventilation
Muscle cramps[a]	Hoarse voice, thick tongue	Bradycardia
Fluid retention[a]	Hypertension	Depressed
Menometrorrhagia	Serous effusions	sensorium
Dry skin	Slow thinking and speech	
Cold intolerance	Decreased appetite	
	Delayed reflexes	
	Carpal tunnel syndrome[a]	

[a] Findings that can be caused by pregnancy alone.
Modified from Kaplan MM: Thyroid diseases. In: Gleicher N (ed), Principles and Practice of Medical Therapy in Pregnancy, *ed 2. Norwalk, CT, Appleton & Lange, 1992:321–338.*

and unpublished observations about normal ranges in various clinical laboratories strongly suggest that the upper normal range of serum TSH levels are lower than previously believed.[1] Hence TSH levels alone often are sufficient to help one make the diagnosis of subclinical hypothyroidism. Once TSH levels are shown to be elevated, a measurement of free T_4 is in order. Free T_4 values correlate better with the degree of hypothyroidism than do TSH levels. This is particularly striking in instances in which hypothyroidism is rapidly evolving, as in patients who are taking antithyroid drugs, recently underwent substantial thyroidectomy, received ablative doses of radioactive iodine, or recently discontinued replacement or suppressive treatment with thyroid hormone.

Pitfalls in the use of TSH as a single tool to screen for hypothyroidism include recently evolving hypothyroidism and the unusual instances of secondary hypothyroidism when hypothalamic and pituitary disorders account for hypothyroidism on the basis of failure to produce adequate amounts or normally bioactive TSH. Interference of TSH antibodies with immunoradiometric TSH assays is seldom a problem because the newer TSH kits are designed to adsorb anti-mouse antibodies. Therefore, if a patient is known to have pituitary or hypothalamic disease, measurement of free T_4 in conjunction with TSH level is mandatory. The most commonly overlooked example of this situation is a patient with hyperprolactinemia for whom hypothyroidism is being excluded.

Once the diagnosis of hypothyroidism is established, titers of antibodies to thyroglobulin and thyroid peroxidase, previously called *antimicrosomal antibodies,* are useful in predicting risk for progression of hypothyroidism. However, these titers are not necessary if thyroid hormone replacement is being prescribed.

Therapy for hypothyroidism consists of establishing the proper dose of synthetic T_4 and maintaining replacement therapy over time with the same reputable brand of T_4 to eliminate the possibility of variation in bioavailability from preparation to preparation. Initial dose adjustments can be made every 6 weeks. Once the patient's condition is stable, the interval can be doubled until the patient is seen once a year or sooner in the event of pregnancy.

Sexual Maturation

People with hypothyroidism have normal reproductive systems. Prepubertal hypothyroidism, however, leads to short stature and delayed sexual maturity. Prepubertal hypothyroidism can also, though not often, lead to precocious puberty of both boys and girls. This precocious puberty appears to be caused by the overlap in production of the glycoproteins TSH, follicle-stimulating hormone (FSH), and luteinizing hormone (LH) that accompany prepubertal hypothyroidism.[14] Adrenal androgen production is

not increased, and the process is reversed by means of management of the hypothyroidism.

Infertility

Multiple studies of hypothyroid animals demonstrate a spectrum of abnormalities that can explain infertility in the respective animal model. Rats have irregular menstrual cycles and atrophic ovaries. Litter sizes are reduced because of increased embryo resorption, and more stillbirths occur. Hens have decreased egg production. Sheep have endometrial hyperplasia and smooth muscle hypertrophy. Many clinical impressions about humans are consistent with findings of these controlled animal studies.

Severe and moderate hypothyroidism in humans can clearly cause infertility. Despite the prior empiric use of thyroid hormone,[15] studies have not demonstrated benefit from the administration of thyroid hormone to infertile women in the absence of laboratory evidence of hypothyroidism.[16] When hypothyroidism was diagnosed on the basis of a low basal metabolic rate[17] hypothyroid pregnancies were felt to be rare because of the effect of the condition on fertility. Moreover, when pregnancy occurred in women with hypothyroidism, the miscarriage rate doubled.[18] The fact that subsequent series of patients with moderate to marked hypothyroidism were small reinforced that notion.[19] Daniels[5] commented that the success of empiric therapy with thyroid hormone in the management of infertility and recurrent abortions is unclear and may be a combination of anecdotal reports, placebo effects, therapy for subclinical hypothyroidism, or other actions of thyroid hormone. To what extent mild or subclinical hypothyroidism has an effect on fertility remains conjectural.

Severe hypothyroidism complicating pregnancy is uncommon because 70 percent of affected persons are infertile due to anovulatory cycles.[20] Women are affected more often than men. Some studies indicate that mild hypothyroidism is associated with a favorable pregnancy outcome. Other studies show that hypothyroidism is associated with an increased number of first trimester abortions, stillbirths, and premature infants.[21] Athough pregnancy in the setting of moderate and marked hypothyroidism may be uncommon, pregnancy in the setting of mild or subclinical hypothyroidism is a common problem. In addition to the impact of mild or subclinical hypothyroidism on fertility, the impact on pregnancy is uncertain.

Women with hypothyroidism undergo changes in menstrual cycle length that are independent of associated hyperprolactinemia. There is a variable amount of menstrual flow, most notably a tendency toward menorrhagia that is frequently severe and the result of anovulation and perhaps poor uterine muscle tone and platelet dysfunction.[20,22] Galactorrhea may be a presenting feature and signal the association of hyperprolactinemia. When seen, galactorrhea occurs in the setting of prolonged moderate or severe hypothyroidism.

Hypothyroidism has been suggested as a cause of male-factor infertility. Decreased libido, however, is a nonspecific finding. Early reports of abnormal semen analyses have not been substantiated. Infertile men with hypothyroidism should be examined for secondary hypothyroidism and other causes of infertility.

Although the foregoing statements appear straightforward, several observations raise questions about what constitutes adequate laboratory evidence of hypothyroidism or euthyroid autoimmune thyroid disease. A normal TSH level should be adequate for ruling out primary hypothyroidism or limited thyroid reserve. In one study, however, infertile women who were found to be either oligoovulatory or to have luteal-phase defects had normal basal TSH values but brisk TSH responses to thyrotropin-releasing hormone (TRH) testing. Moreover, the women benefited from administration of thyroid hormone in comparison with controls without abnormal TRH tests.[23] Another study with infertile women found lower spontaneous conception rates among women with brisk TSH responses to TRH when compared with those with normal TRH tests.[24] With current TSH assays, few clinicians see the value of TRH testing in the diagnosis of primary hypothyroidism or the usual causes of hyperthyroidism. These older studies are consistent, however, with the notion that prior upper normal limits of TSH were set too high[1] to identify many cases of subclinical hypothyroidism or limited thyroid gland reserve. What remains to be seen is the relative importance of identifying this subgroup of infertile women with ovulatory dysfunction. There is little evidence to support the role of thyroid hormone treatment or even routine screening of infertile women for thyroid dysfunction in the absence of ovulatory dysfunction.[25]

Intriguing in vitro studies have demonstrated that TSH possesses one fifth the luteotropic effect of hCG.[26] The studies also showed that in vivo human follicular fluid TSH levels at the time of oocyte retrieval after hCG administration are equivalent to simultaneously drawn serum TSH levels. These observations raise the possibility that primary hypothyroidism or cases of secondary hypothyroidism with biologically inactive immunoreactive TSH may affect fertility by means of a direct local action of TSH on the follicle that is independent of the associated hypothyroidism.

The diagnosis of autoimmune thyroid disease in women generally can be confirmed with a determination of antithyroid antibody levels. Antithyroid peroxidase antibody, otherwise known as antimicrosomal antibody, is more sensitive and more specific than antithyroglobulin antibody, but determining levels of both increases the likelihood of identification of patients with autoimmune thyroid disease. Characteristic palpatory findings in women in the reproductive age group and borderline high or frankly elevated TSH values lend further support in the identification of this group. A family history of autoimmune thyroid disease or a history of thyroid dysfunction related to or independent of pregnancy also is suggestive. Although 5% to 10% or more of women with autoimmune thyroid disease in the reproductive age group may not be identified with these methods, further evaluation, such as thyroid imaging techniques with or without thyroid fine-needle aspiration, is not recommended given its low yield, high cost, and uncertain benefit to a patient with normal thyroid function.

Pregnancy

The minimum estimate of the incidence of hypothyroidism that complicates pregnancy after 20 weeks of gestation is 0.6%. Prospective studies reveal an incidence as high as 2.5%[27,28] (Fig 10–2). The incidence is higher among patients with Type I diabetes mellitus. Most patients with hypothyroidism in pregnancy have Hashimoto's thyroiditis or have undergone thyroid ablation for thyrotoxicosis. Hypothyroid patients with Hashimoto's thyroiditis have antibodies against thyroid peroxidase and thyroglobulin (proteins in thyroid follicular cells). They may, however, along with other patients with autoimmune thyroid disease, have immunoglobulins that block the action of TSH on thyroid hormone production and secretion, promote thyroid growth, or prevent thyroid growth. The broad spectrum of immunologic abnormalities contributes to the highly variable thyroid examinations encountered among patients with Hashimoto's thyroiditis whether or not they are pregnant.

Hypothyroidism may have considerable negative impact

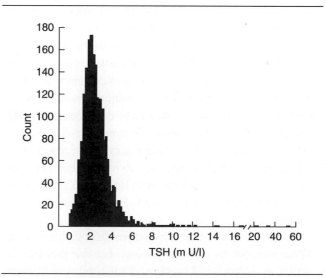

Figure 10–2. Distribution of TSH concentrations in sera of 2000 women at 15 to 18 weeks of gestation. (*Redrawn from Klein RZ et al: Prevalence of thyroid deficiency in pregnant women.* Clin Endocrinol *35:41, 1991.*)

on pregnancy. There is a higher reported incidence of stillbirths, preeclampsia, abruptio placentae, anemia, postpartum hemorrhage caused by uterine atony, and low-birth-weight infants among patients with moderate to severe hypothyroidism. The incidence of these complications is reduced when the hypothyroidism is managed. In one series, pregnant patients with subclinical hypothyroidism had one third the complication rate of patients with clinical hypothyroidism.[20] An intriguing finding by Leung et al[29] suggests that even patients with subclinial hypothyroidism have an increased incidence of hypertension. That this may be related to the underlying thyroid disorder independent of thyroid status is suggested by Lejeune et al,[30] who found hypertension among pregnant patients with autoimmune thyroid disease and normal levels of thyroid hormone. Nonetheless, the lower incidence of hypertension observed when adequate thyroid hormone is administered in pregnancy suggests that thyroidal status remains a key basis for this complication. Maternal mortality, congenital anomalies, and developmental anomalies have not been proved to be the result of hypothyroidism in pregnancy. Although most hypothyroid pregnancies have good outcomes, treatment with thyroid hormone probably increases the likelihood of success and therefore always should be given when hypothyroidism is diagnosed. Moreover, normalization of TSH levels should be considered a goal, although the benefit of this therapy to a patient with subclinical hypothyroidism remains uncertain.

Occasionally one encounters a patient being treated with thyroid hormone whose diagnosis of hypothyroidism is either inconclusive or unavailable. If the patient is pregnant, one should defer investigating whether thyroid hormone is truly required because of both the potential difficulties resulting from induction of hypothyroidism in pregnancy and the possibility that the patient has autoimmune hypothyroidism that is in remission[31] that may resurface postpartum.

Hypothyroidism can be diagnosed on the basis of an elevated serum TSH level in pregnancy unless the patient's history includes high doses of steroids, intravenous dopamine administration, or hypopituitarism. These situations are unusual in pregnancy, but if encountered they make dependence on TSH values less reliable. If the suspicion of hypothyroidism is high or a thyroid examination is consistent with diffuse thyroid disease, an estimate of free hormone and thyroid antibodies is recommended. About 5% of patients with Hashimoto's thyroiditis have negative antibody titers. Total T_3 levels are not useful in this setting.

Treatment of patients with hypothyroidism should be with T_4. Other preparations are nonphysiologic because they lead to excursions in T_3 levels and interfere with the ability to regulate circulating and intracellular T_3 concentrations. Once a diagnosis of hypothyroidism in pregnancy is made, initial treatment with full replacement doses should be entertained unless there are contraindications such as heart disease. One approach is simply to double the anticipated daily dose for 1 week then proceed with the daily dose.[1] Thyroid indices may then be checked in 1 week to assure absorption and compliance. Determinations then are made every 4 weeks until the patient is clinically and biochemically euthyroid and her condition is stable.

Pregnancy increases the dose requirements of patients with hypothyroidism[32–34] for reasons that are not fully understood. When increases in dose requirements do not occur, overreplacement before pregnancy should be suspected. The occasional pregnancy-induced remission of mild hypothyroidism due to Hashimoto's thyroiditis is an infrequent explanation.[31] Older studies indicated normal T_4 production rates when a correction was made for body surface area in pregnancy.[35] Estrogen-induced increases in TBG do not necessarily lead to increased T_4 requirements,[36] yet these two mechanisms are often cited as the basis for the increased dose requirement. In addition, increased intravascular space, placental deiodination of T_4 by placental Type III deiodinase, and impaired absorption because of the iron in prenatal vitamins may be operative. As many as 80% of all patients may require dose adjustments ranging from 10% to greater than 100%. Median increases in prepartum doses range from 30% to 60%.

In iodine-deficient regions the increased demands on the maternal iodine pool are a clear contributor to the observed increase in dose requirement. The initial observation that goiter development and progression are noted in pregnancy in these regions is attributed to the ancient Egyptians. They observed throat enlargement during pregnancy was capable of breaking a snug reed placed around the neck. Markers of thyroidal stimulation and goitrogenesis, such as a relative drop in free T_4 level, preferential T_3 secretion as evidenced by an increased T_3 to T_4 ratio, a rise in TSH values, and a rise in serum thyroglobulin levels also are evident.[6]

Although there is a tendency to emphasize laboratory determinations in the management of thyroid dysfunction, clinical evaluation should remain the key guide to management. Moreover, thyroid hormone levels are not necessarily available at the time patients are being examined, so clinical decision making is at times unavoidable. Clinicians should keep in mind that fatigue, constipation, muscle cramps, and fluid retention are seen in both normal pregnancy and all degrees of hypothyroidism (see Table 10–1). In addition, carpal tunnel syndrome, which can be appreciated in pregnancy, also is a feature of moderate and severe hypothyroidism. Features of mild hypothyroidism that are not attributable to pregnancy are dry skin and cold intolerance. Features of moderate to severe hypothyroidism not attributable to pregnancy are dry, thick skin; thick, brittle hair; hoarse voice, thickened tongue, hypertension, serous effusions, slow thinking and speech, decreased appetite, and delayed reflexes. Features of severe hypothyroidism that necessitate urgent intervention are hypothermia, bradycardia, hypoventilation, and a depressed sensorium. The possibility of hypothyroidism should be kept in mind at the first prenatal visit, when signs and symptoms of thyroid disease should be sought. Hypothyroidism also should be suspected when a goiter is present, there is a history of thyroid disease, the patient is taking medicines with antithyroid action, or there is a family history of autoimmune thyroid disease.

HYPERTHYROIDISM

Diagnosis

Like hypothyroidism, hyperthyroidism has protean clinical manifestations (Table 10–2). Some of these are reviewed in the discussion of pregnancy and hyperthyroidism. Ultimately confirmation of hyperthyroidism requires laboratory methods that directly or indirectly demonstrate an excess of thyroid hormone.

The laboratory diagnosis of hyperthyroidism is alluded to in the discussion of thyroid physiology in pregnancy. The best screening tool for hyperthyroidism is a sensitive TSH assay. Because pituitary TSH secretion falls exponentially when free T_4 levels rise, serum TSH levels are a more sensitive indication of early hyperthyroidism than either free T_4 estimates or direct measures of free T_4. When free T_4 levels are suppressed, they should be complemented with a free T_4 index. If the free T_4 index is normal, a free T_3 index can be used as a confirmatory test because it tends to be disproportionately elevated in most cases of clinically evident thyrotoxicosis. Instances in which TSH levels are suppressed in conjunction with normal free T_4 and free T_3 levels are termed *subclinical hyperthyroidism*. Whether such patients truly have no symptoms or have clinical findings such as thyroid-related bone loss, cardiac difficulty, or diminished fertility often cannot be established without either further evaluation or use of antithyroid therapy that normalizes thyroid indices.

When pregnancy is not an issue, the cause of the thyrotoxic state can be further categorized with measurements of radioiodine uptakes and, in selected instances, imaging of the thyroid gland to evaluate the nature of thyroid nodules in a patient with thyrotoxicosis. Antithyroid antibody titers may help identify autoimmune thyrotoxicosis.

TSH assays alone cannot be used to diagnose hyperthyroidism, because of rare cases of secondary hyperthyroidism in which autonomous secretion of TSH leads to hyperthyroidism. As discussed earlier, TSH antibodies leading to artifactually measurable levels of TSH have become less of a problem with newer TSH kits.

Once hyperthyroidism is diagnosed, its cause should be established. The approach to management is discussed later.

Sexual Maturation

Prepubertal thyrotoxicosis delays sexual maturation. Its documented effects on the reproductive system are discussed in the sections on infertility.

Female-Factor Infertility

The impact of hyperthyroidism on female reproduction was first noted in 1840, when amenorrhea was noted in this setting.[37] A wide range of menstrual disturbances have since been described. Although menometrorraghia is more commonly associated with hypothyroidism, it is also seen in conjunction with hyperthyroidism. Ovulatory, oligoovulatory, and anovulatory cycles with amenorrhea may also be encountered. Elevated LH, FSH, and estradiol levels with a reduction of midcycle LH peak are typical of adversely affected cycles. Elevated levels of sex hormone binding globulin (SHBG) account for elevated estradiol levels and decreased clearance of both estradiol and testosterone. Although it is universally acknowledged that severe hyperthyroidism can cause infertility, authors disagree on the impact of mild to moderate hyperthyroidism.[38]

Male-Factor Infertility

Male fertility also may be affected by hyperthyroidism. Both estradiol and testosterone levels are increased by thyroid hormone–induced SHBG levels, yet the bioavailability of estradiol remains relatively greater because it is less well bound than testosterone. This is certainly in keeping with the clinical observations of relative estrogen excess among some men with thyrotoxicosis. The condition is characterized by gynecomastia, spider angiomas, and decreased libido. The last feature may be nonspecific, because it does not respond to testosterone therapy. In fact, testosterone therapy may make gynecomastia worse. The argument for either absolute or relative testosterone deficiency, despite the preservation of normal free testosterone levels (in conjunction with elevated total testosterone levels attributable to high SHBG levels) is that LH levels are normal to supranormal in both induced and spontaneously occurring hyperthyroidism. Impaired spermatogenesis has been ascribed to some degree of Leydig cell failure. When a euthyroid state is reestablished, SHBG returns to normal, as does reproductive function, including sperm counts.[39] Gynecomastia, particularly when it is mild, also resolves.

TABLE 10–2. CLINICAL FEATURES OF HYPERTHYROIDISM

Intrinsic Hormone Effects	Sympatheticlike Effects	Unique to Graves' Disease
Symptoms		
Fatigue[a]	Palpitation[a]	Irritated, gritty, or sandy feeling in eyes
Increased appetite[a]	Heat intolerance[a]	Diplopia
Weight loss (rarely weight gain)	Excessive sweating[a]	Localized swelling of legs
Muscle weakness	Shortness of breath[a]	
Fine, brittle hair	Increased urinary frequency[a]	
Itching of skin	Nervousness[a]	
Brittle fingernails	Emotional lability[a]	
Oligomenorrhea or amenorrhea[a]	Insomnia	
Increased bowel frequency	Tremor	
Vomiting[a]	Brisk reflexes	
Signs		
Tachycardia[a]	Tachycardia[a]	Diffuse goiter
Atrial fibrillation	Cardiac flow murmur[a]	Exophthalmos
Proximal myopathy	Increased pulse pressure	Periorbital swelling
Fine, warm, moist skin	Systolic hypertension	Extraocular muscle palsy
Onycholysis	Stare, lid lag	Infiltrative dermopathy (pretibial myxedema)
		Lymphadenopathy
		Splenomegaly
		Clubbing of fingers (thyroid acropachy)
Laboratory Findings		
Increased oxygen consumption[a]	Increased oxygen consumption[a]	Thyroid-stimulating IgG
Hypercalcemia		Lymphocytosis
Elevated alkaline phosphatase		Neutropenia
Elevated transaminases		

[a] Findings that can occur due to pregnancy alone. Thyroid enlargement (goiter), either diffuse or localized, is almost always present in young, hyperthyroid patients, regardless of the cause of hyperthyroidism.
Modified from Kaplan MM: Thyroid diseases. In: Gleicher N (ed), Principles and Practice of Medical Therapy in Pregnancy, *ed 2. Norwalk, CT, Appleton & Lange, 1992:321–338.*

Pregnancy and Hyperthyroidism, Including Nonthyroidal Illness, Trophoblastic Disease, and Gestational Transient Thyrotoxicosis

Graves' disease is generally cited as the most common cause of hyperthyroidism in pregnant women. This is certainly the case if gestational transient thyrotoxicosis (GTT) is excluded. Reports of pregnancies that last longer than 20 weeks suggest the incidence of Graves' disease is 2 per 1000 or 0.2%. This is believed to be a low estimate given the exclusion of undiagnosed cases and early abortions. The clinical presentation is characterized by hyperadrenergic features and eye findings. Although eye abnormalities are clinically apparent for only one third of patients, they can be found among patients with Graves' disease when more sophisticated testing also is conducted.

Signs and symptoms of thyrotoxicosis can be confused with the signs and symptoms of second- and third-trimester pregnancy (see Table 10–2). They include fatigue, increased appetite, vomiting, tachycardia, palpitations, heat intolerance, hyperhidrosis, shortness of breath, urinary frequency, nervousness, and perhaps emotional lability. Distinguishing features, however, include goiter, eye signs, weight loss or inadequate weight gain, increased bowel frequency, myopathy, onycholysis, tremor, hyperreflexia, increased pulse pressure, systolic hypertension, pretibial myxedema, acropachy, lymphadenopathy, and splenomegaly.

Hyperthyroidism complicating pregnancy is associated with an increased incidence of first trimester abortions, stillbirths, neonatal death, and two to three times the incidence of low birth weight, maternal congestive heart failure, preeclampsia, and anemia. When hyperthyroidism is diagnosed prepartum, the incidence of thyroid storm may approach 2%, compared with a 20% incidence when it is diagnosed intrapartum. When Graves' disease is moderate or severe, it tends to worsen in the first trimester, improve in the second and third trimesters, and flare postpartum. Mild or subclinical hyperthyroidism has not been shown to contribute to maternal or fetal morbidity.[5]

Therefore it is argued that mild or subclinical hyperthyroidism due to Graves' disease or other causes during pregnancy does not require therapy. This is why achieving mild or subclinical hyperthyroidism serves as a goal of antithyroid drug therapy in pregnancy.

Two forms of hyperthyroidism are unique to pregnancy. They are trophoblastic disease and hyperemesis gravidarum. Trophoblastic disease includes hydatidiform mole and choriocarcinoma. In addition to very high levels of hCG, ranging from 100,000 to 1,000,000 IU/L, alterations in its glycosylation may enhance its potency as a thyroid stimulator. The paucity of clinical findings, including goiter, may be related to the short duration and the relatively low total T_3 levels in comparison with those of patients with Graves' disease. Weight loss and fatigue may be related to the trophoblastic disease and not the alterations in thyroid hormone levels. Discussion of this entity is beyond the scope of this review.

Half of patients with hyperemesis gravidarum have elevated free T_4 levels, and 80% of those have suppressed TSH levels. Like patients with trophoblastic disease, these patients do not typically appear to have thyrotoxicosis. The minimal features of thyrotoxicosis probably also are related to the short duration of the disturbance and the relatively low total T_3 levels compared with those of patients with Graves' disease. Patients with hyperemesis gravidarum with elevated free T_4 indices tend to have low-birth-weight infants. Those with evidence of thyroid hormone excess can be categorized as having GTT.

The incidence of GTT is approximately 2%.[6] This is tenfold greater than the incidence of Graves' disease in pregnancy. Patients with GTT have subnormal TSH levels and supranormal free T_4 indices between 8 and 14 weeks of gestation.[6] Every patient has relatively elevated hCG levels, some exceeding 100,000 IU/L, that remain elevated for several weeks, including a portion of the second trimester. TRH stimulation tests in this group are flat. One half of patients have thyrotoxic symptoms characterized by failure to gain weight, tachycardia, and fatigue. Hyperemesis is seen in those who are most severely symptomatic. Most patients are treated expectantly because all cases appear transient. Resolution parallels the decline in hCG levels. β blockers occasionally are used for up to 2 months, and short-term use of propylthiouracil (PTU) may occasionally be required. Neonates do well. Titers for thyroid-stimulating antibody (TSab) are negative, and Graves' disease does not develop postpartum.

It appears that hCG-associated estradiol production may be the connection between hCG elevations, GTT, and nausea and vomiting, since the severity of the vomiting generally correlates with the degree of hCG elevation, which is correlated with the degree of estradiol elevation. This is also consistent with the finding that hyperthyroidism is generally mild, that vomiting is an unusual complication of hyperthyroidism com-

plicating pregnancy, and that when seen vomiting is generally appreciated in the setting of severe hyperthyroidism. Moreover, 30% of patients with hyperemesis gravidarum do not have hyperthyroidism, and for some patients the hyperthyroidism resolves but the hyperemesis does not.

There are several reasons to differentiate GTT from Graves' disease. GTT is much more common, is self-limited, and usually does not necessitate therapy for the associated thyrotoxicosis.

Two other less frequent forms of hyperthyroidism encountered in pregnancy are toxic adenoma and toxic multinodular goiter. Palpation and the absence of antithyroid antibodies are the key to differentiating them from Graves' disease. Isotope studies, which are contraindicated in pregnancy, may be quite helpful in the diagnosis of these conditions during the nongravid state.

It is almost never necessary to interrupt pregnancy because of coexisting hyperthyroidism. Adequate calories, multivitamins (preferably without iodine), bed rest, and stress avoidance may be necessary, at least initially, to achieve reasonable control of the thyrotoxic state. In the United States PTU is preferred to either carbimazole or methimazole (the active metabolite of carbimazole) because it passes the placenta less efficiently, is not associated with the birth defect aplasia cutis, and blocks conversion of T_4 to T_3. Because of the excellent safety record of methimazole and carbimazole and uncertainty about the teratogenicity of PTU,[40] most clinicians switch patients from PTU to either drug in the event of a minor reaction before recommending surgical treatment.

The goal of treatment with thioamide drugs is to maintain T_4 and T_3 levels at or just above the upper level of normal while TSH levels remain suppressed. When levels become normal, drug doses should be reduced. This approach is associated with minimal risk to a mother who typically tolerates mild degrees of thyrotoxicosis and minimizes fetal exposure to antithyroid drugs. Furthermore, normalization of suppressed TSH levels during maintenance with the same or lower doses of antithyroid drugs establishes ongoing improvement and allows for further dose reductions. How high T_4 and T_3 levels are allowed to gravitate above normal levels should be based on clinical evaluation in conjunction with laboratory assessments of free hormone levels.

Before use of antithyroid drugs is initiated, a baseline white blood cell count and liver indices should be established to determine whether subsequent abnormalities are the result of adverse drug effects, which mandate discontinuation of the drug.

The fetal thyroid cannot escape the effect of iodides on the thyroid. Nonetheless, in the event of a crisis in which rapid control of maternal thyrotoxicosis is mandatory, short-term use of iodides for 7 to 10 days is safe. Because of the slow clearance of iopanoate and sodium ipodate, which serve as organic sources of inorganic iodide, use of these agents should be avoided in pregnancy. Fetal goiter, though quite serious, takes weeks or longer to develop. Low doses of inorganic iodide have been proposed as an alternative to antithyroid drugs, but little experience with this approach has accumulated.[41]

β Blockers, principally when evaluated for use by pregnant women with hypertension, have been associated with intrauterine growth retardation, fetal cardiac distress, neonatal hypoglycemia, and fetal bradycardia. Early labor is another potential adverse effect. Nonetheless, in a crisis, short-term use may become necessary and typically is not associated with major adverse effects.

When patients are allergic to antithyroid drugs or when thyrotoxicosis cannot be controlled with 300 mg or more of PTU or 30 mg or more of methimazole, surgical treatment is recommended. Preoperative preparation is key and may require both iodides and β blockade. The second trimester is often advocated as the stage to perform an operation. However, because fetal outcomes are superior later in pregnancy should premature delivery result from surgical intervention, waiting until the third trimester is preferable if possible.

Thyroid storm requires prompt and aggressive management. This includes high doses of antithyroid drugs (methimazole by suppository if necessary), iodides, β blockers (intravenously if necessary), oxygen, fluid, glucocorticoids, and nonaspirin methods of antipyresis. Because it may contribute to hypermetabolism, aspirin should be avoided in severe thyrotoxicosis.

Opinions vary about the administration of antithyroid drugs once remission takes place in pregnancy. I discontinue antithyroid drugs once the patient is euthyroid with 25 mg of PTU or its equivalent. Other authors argue for maintaining drug therapy throughout pregnancy to reduce the risk for neonatal thyrotoxicosis and to reduce the risk for thyroid storm during labor and delivery, in the event that there is a relapse. One other speculative approach is the addition of T_4 therapy at the time of remission. This approach is based on the belief that with suppression of TSH-mediated thyroid antigen release, the autoimmune trigger that initiates the cascade that leads to flares of Graves' disease will be suppressed, decreasing the risk for relapse.[42]

NEONATAL THYROID DYSFUNCTION

Neonatal Hypothyroidism

The incidence of congenital hypothyroidism in the United States is approximately 1/3500 to 1/4000. Most cases are sporadic and are caused by thyroid dysgenesis, agenesis, or ectopia. Biosynthetic defects are rare (approximately 1/30,000) but are often familial. Congenital pituitary disease as a cause also is

rare. Transient forms are caused by the passage of transplacental blocking antibodies, maternal use of antithyroid drugs, maternal use of iodine in inorganic or organic form, radioiodine therapy, particularly if administered after the first trimester when fetal thyroid development has enabled the gland to trap iodine, and endemic iodine deficiency where the incidence of goitrous hypothyroidism can approach 10%. Respiratory distress syndrome has been associated with abnormal thyroid indices, but these probably reflect alterations in thyroid hormone economy due to nonthyroidal illness rather than transient hypothyroidism. In addition, small-for-dates infants have lower T_4 indices and higher TSH levels than age-matched controls. When hypothyroidism is suspected, assessment of thyroid hormone levels by means of intrapartum funipuncture is superior to sampling amniotic fluid levels. Intrapartum intraamniotic fluid T_4 administration is a therapeutic option.

Screening for congenital hypothyroidism has become routine. When proper treatment is instituted soon after birth, outcomes are excellent.[8]

Neonatal Hyperthyroidism

Neonatal hyperthyroidism is typically the consequence of transplacental passage of stimulatory immunoglobulin G (IgG) from mothers with Graves' disease. The incidence is equal among boys and girls, and the risk is higher if the mother previously delivered an affected child. This condition typically runs a 3- to 12-week course. Presentation is characterized by low birth weight, accelerated bone age, poor growth, weight loss, and premature craniosynostosis. Jaundice, hepatosplenomegaly, and thrombocytopenia have been reported. Minimal brain dysfunction has been recognized as a long-term sequela.

Neonatal hyperthyroidism should be suspected if a mother has Graves' disease (whether or not her thyroid gland has been ablated) when there is unexplained fetal tachycardia that exceeds 160 beats per minute. Ultrasound examination may reveal goiter and cardiomegaly. Administration of PTU to the mother can be used to treat the fetus. T_4 is added if necessary to ensure that the mother stays euthyroid. Thyroid hormone receptor antibody titers are useful to an athyreotic mother whose thyroid was ablated as therapy for Graves' disease. Although one can see high titers without the development of neonatal disease, it is unusual to see disease without a marked titer elevation. Surveillance of the mother for TSab is recommended as of midgestation because that is when the transplacental passage of IgG increases and when evidence of the condition usually first appears. Once elevated titers are found, ultrasound examination for fetal goiter and growth retardation in conjunction with monitoring for fetal tachycardia is recommended. If tachycardia is found, the institution of therapy as outlined earlier should be considered. Confirmation with funipuncture before initiation of therapy has been advocated.

If the mother has an intact thyroid, her thyroid status can generally serve as a bioassay of Graves' disease activity, and immunoglobulin titers contribute little to the treatment of the infant.

POSTPARTUM THYROID DISEASE

Disruption of thyroid function is more frequent peripartum and postpartum than intrapartum. Four entities should be considered in this discussion. The first two are pituitary disorders, which are uncommonly appreciated. The first is postpartum pituitary necrosis, known as *Sheehan's syndrome*. It has become increasingly uncommon as obstetric techniques have improved and hypotension and blood loss at delivery have been reduced. The second rarely recognized postpartum pituitary disorder, lymphocytic thyroiditis, may be more common than the former condition in good obstetric settings. Both these conditions are associated with secondary hypothyroidism and a variable degree of pituitary failure. Lymphocytic hypophysitis, an autoimmune disorder, may be associated with autoimmune primary endocrine gland failure, including primary hypothyroidism.

Graves' disease has a tendency to go into remission intrapartum but often flares postpartum. It is, however, less common than the third of the four autoimmune conditions, postpartum thyroiditis. As many as 25% of patients with Graves' disease who have thyrotoxicosis postpartum may in fact have postpartum thyroiditis. The distinction is best made with a radioiodine uptake test, which may be performed if the patient is not nursing. Graves' disease is characterized by elevated uptake, and the thyrotoxic phase of postpartum thyroiditis is associated with a low uptake, consistent with the leak of thyroid hormone from a typically painlessly inflamed gland.

Postpartum thyroiditis is probably a form of chronic autoimmune thyroiditis, that is, Hashimoto's thyroiditis. Transient hypothyroidism alone, transient thyrotoxicosis alone, and thyrotoxicosis followed by hypothyroidism can be documented with almost equal frequency. The risk for the development of hypothyroidism over time appears to be progressive. Women who appear to recover completely and are not treated with thyroid hormone need to be monitored indefinitely for the development of thyroid dysfunction.

The incidence of postpartum thyroiditis ranges from 3% to 8%, depending on the population studied. Because of the prevalence of postpartum thyroiditis, evaluation of thyroid status 6 weeks to 3 months postpartum is indicated for nervousness, depression, lethargy, emotional lability, and palpitations. In addition, the detection of goiter or the enlargement of preexisting goiter, particularly in patients with Hashimoto's thyroiditis, Graves' disease, or Type I diabetes mellitus (the last also has been associated with a higher incidence of postpartum thyroiditis[43]) should prompt an assessment of thyroid status.

The argument to treat all women with postpartum thyroiditis with T_4 in the event that they have documented instances of TSH elevation and to maintain drug therapy throughout the reproductive years[1,5] is based on the fact that hypothyroidism may be permanent in as many as 25% of instances. Subsequent evaluations for the development of hypothyroidism are minimized during times of vague symptoms or fatigue. Because postpartum thyroiditis is a recurrent condition, preventing the hypothyroid phase of future relapses is accomplished.

THYROID NODULES AND CANCER

Pregnancy is not associated with the progression of thyroid cancer. Even in the presence of newly discovered or preexisting thyroid cancer, interruption of the pregnancy is not necessary unless there is evidence of widespread or progressive disease. Although iodine-131 therapy may be desirable, it can almost always be postponed until after pregnancy and, if necessary, until breast feeding is finished.

An increase in birth defects was not found in most series in which radioiodine was administered to young women with thyroid cancer.[44,45] Notable exceptions, however, have been reported among babies conceived within 1 year of therapy.[46] Hence once iodine-131 therapy is administered for the management of cancer, the results of the study[46] suggest waiting a year before conceiving.

Instances in which sperm counts appear affected by radioiodine therapy have occurred when high doses of iodine-131 have been used. Therefore, when repeated doses of iodine-131 are used to treat men with thyroid cancer, serial sperm counts are advisable.

Although pregnancy has been associated with thyroid growth and increases in both nodule number and nodule size in pregnancy, at least in areas of marginal iodine intake,[47] an aggressive approach to the evaluation and management of thyroid nodules is not mandatory. This fact notwithstanding, many clinicians thoroughly evaluate all newly diagnosed thyroid nodules found in pregnancy, perform fine-needle aspiration, and recommend surgical therapy for aspirates suggestive or diagnostic of malignancy. An alternative approach is to consider watching low-risk nodules that are relatively small and not associated with any features of local invasiveness or spread. This can be accomplished with or without suppressive therapy. As long as the patient's condition remains stable, one can defer further diagnostic procedures until the postpartum period, because pregnancy poses little clinical impact. This is true even if the nodule proves to be a low-stage differentiated malignant tumor of the thyroid, which categorizes most malignant tumors of the thyroid found in young women. When the latter approach is advocated, the patient must fully understand the risks and benefits.

AUTOIMMUNE THYROID DISEASE AND MISCARRIAGE

In 1990 Stagnaro-Green et al,[48] using sensitive detection techniques, reported a doubling of first trimester miscarriage rate among women with positive titers for antithyroid antibodies. The increased incidence continued to be evident when women with marked elevations in TSH level were excluded. These patients were not shown to have a disproportionate incidence of anticardiolipin antibodies, which had previously been shown to be associated with a high incidence of spontaneous miscarriage. Similar findings were noted by Lejeune et al[28,30] in iodine-deficient areas. More recent studies emphasized that antithyroid antibodies are a risk factor for clinical miscarriage. The incidence of biochemical pregnancy loss may not be higher than the control value.[49] At present these findings appear to be markers for autoimmunity-related miscarriage rather than a cause of miscarriage.

PRECONCEPTION PLANNING

Hypothyroidism

Women with hypothyroidism should be examined prepartum, and their thyroid hormone levels should be adjusted to a euthyroid range. Adjustment of free T_4 indices to high normal levels with TSH levels in the low normal range minimizes subsequent intrapartum adjustments. I advise all women with hypothyroidism to have their thyroid indices checked as soon as they learn they are pregnant so that medication adjustments, typically required before 8 to 10 weeks of pregnancy, can be made expeditiously. Prenatal vitamins, iron, and calcium supplements should be taken separately from the thyroid hormone. TSH levels are checked regularly until the indices are both normal and stable. TSH levels are checked within 1 to 2 weeks of the initial dose adjustment to document that TSH values are not rising. Once TSH values begin to drop, evaluation intervals are progressively lengthened. For a patient whose condition is stable marked changes in dose requirement are not generally noted beyond the end of the second trimester. Postpartum requirements typically return to preconception doses.

Hyperthyroidism

Patients with hyperthyroidism due to Graves' disease, toxic multinodular goiter, or toxic adenoma should be rendered euthyroid before pregnancy. I use iodine-131 for this purpose. Experience with this modality of therapy is now 50 years old. The radiation dose to the ovary is comparable to that of a hysterosalpingogram. Experience with children treated for hyperthyroidism[50] or cancer[44–46] with iodine-131 does not show any impairment in fertility. Although I typically advise waiting 1 year after iodine-131 therapy for cancer, in which doses to the ovary are typically higher than those with therapy for hyperthyroidism, 6 months is the typical recommendation for deferring conception after radioiodine therapy for hyperthyroidism. This allows both sufficient time to stabilize thyroid status if the radioiodine is effective and a long enough interval for the acute and subacute effects of radioiodine therapy to occur, retaining open the option to provide more treatment at 6 months.

Surgical intervention is another but rarely needed alternative to accomplish permanent control of thyroid status. In some parts of the world, surgical treatment remains more popular than therapy with radioactive iodine. Ablative therapy minimizes the risk for relapse and allows easier control of maternal thyroid status during subsequent pregnancies.

POSTPARTUM THYROIDITIS

The management of postpartum thyroiditis is discussed earlier, and the rationale for using T_4 therapy at the time hypothyroidism is diagnosed has been reviewed. The cost effectiveness of screening patients at risk for postpartum thyroiditis is not proved. Detection would be increased if obstetricians and primary care providers caring for women of reproductive age were more aware of this entity.

An unusual basis for the aggressive management of recurrent painless thyroiditis in my practice relates to the following three instances: (1) recurrent miscarriages or failure to conceive with well-documented cases of recurrent thyroiditis both independent of and after miscarriage; (2) affective disorder markedly worsened by recurrent episodes of painless thyroiditis; and (3) cardiac disease, particularly if a clinically significant rhythm disorder exists. In these instances an aggressive approach comprises thyroid ablation with radioiodine therapy when the patient is recovering from the hypothyroid phase of a bout of thyroiditis. At that time radioiodine uptake can exceed the normal range and ablation can be readily accomplished. In the two instances in which I used this therapy for indication no. 1, successful pregnancies followed. In one of those instances unassisted success was achieved three times after almost a decade of recurrent failures.

APPROACH TO THE TREATMENT OF A PATIENT WITH INFERTILITY

Failure to Conceive

The role of thyroid hormone–related treatment of an infertile patient is not well documented in the absence of laboratory data establishing thyroid dysfunction.[5] A reasonable but not well established approach has been suggested. When there is failure to conceive without evidence of ovulatory dysfunction, thyroid indices have not proved to be cost effective.[25] When there is evidence of ovulatory dysfunction, thyroid indices should be determined. The possibility of an early phase of premature ovarian failure, particularly in the setting of autoimmune thyroid disease, should be considered. If a patient proves to be clearly hypothyroid, the benefit of treatment is clear. Subclinical hypothyroidism should be treated because there is no negative impact and the patient's well-being may improve, goiter may be prevented, and fertility may be enhanced.

A high index of suspicion is required to diagnose secondary hypothyroidism as a cause of infertility on the basis of thyroid and pituitary hormone abnormalities, such as secondary hypogonadism or hyperprolactinemia with or without an associated prolactinoma. Therefore, an infertile patient with ovulatory dysfunction and an unremarkable physical examination that includes a normal thyroid gland, should always undergo an estimation of free T_4 in conjunction with a TSH level. In the event that the estimate of free T_4 is either frankly low or in the low normal range and TSH level is either low or inappropriately "normal," further evaluation of pituitary function, including a prolactin level should be undertaken. A man with secondary hypothyroidism who is infertile usually has a factor independent of thyroid status to explain the infertility.

If a patient proves to be clearly thyrotoxic, therapy is clearly recommended. The benefit of treating subclinical hyperthyroidism, however, is less certain and not without the hazard of antithyroid drugs or ablative therapy. Nonetheless, if no other basis exists for explaining ovulatory dysfunction in the setting of infertility, establishing a biochemically euthyroid state is advisable. One can proceed with antithyroid drugs and at a later point, if pregnancy is not achieved, decide whether to continue antithyroid drugs or even to proceed with ablative therapy.

Men with abnormal sperm counts, particularly if they have thyrotoxic symptoms, impotence, and clinical evidence of feminization should undergo screening for thyrotoxicosis and be rendered euthyroid. There is no evidence to believe that antithyroid drug therapy interferes with spermatogenesis. In addition, the standard doses of iodine-131 used in the treatment of thyrotoxicosis do not appear to have an adverse effect on spermatogenesis.

In the event that there is ovulatory dysfunction and the patient appears clinically euthyroid with a normal free thyroxine index and a normal TSH level, there are few data to support pursuing therapy with thyroid hormone. The possibility remains, however, that one is overlooking an early phase of hypothyroidism in some infertile patients. This could be the result of the fact that some laboratories use upper limits of TSH assays that are too high. In addition, a normal TSH level in certain settings such as autoimmune thyroid disease, iodine deficiency, and other settings of impaired thyroid reserve, such as the aftermath of a subtotal thyroidectomy, may not allow one to predict sustained normal thyroid function under conditions of increased thyroid hormone demand such as pregnancy, gonadotropin therapy,[51] or the use of anticonvulsant drugs that increase thyroid hormone metabolism. A study by Glinoer et al[52] with patients with autoimmune thyroid disease in the setting of mild to moderate iodine deficiency in

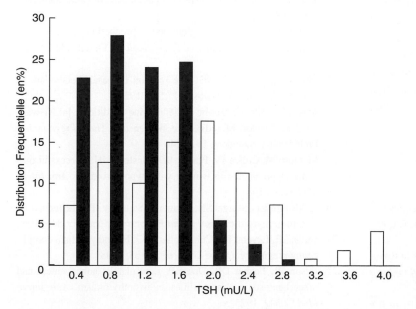

Figure 10–3. Frequency distribution of basal TSH levels at 11 weeks of gestation among women with positive antibodies (□) compared with a group of 550 healthy pregnant women without thyroid antibodies (■) at a similar gestational age. (*Redrawn from Glinoer D et al: Risk of subclinical hypothyroidism in pregnant women with asymptomatic autoimmune thyroid disorders.* J Clin Endocrinol Metab *79:197, 1994.*)

pregnancy identified a euthyroid subgroup that had greater increases in basal TSH level than unaffected controls during the course of pregnancy (Fig 10–3). Although initial TSH levels were normal, the initial mean was higher than that for the control group. This is consistent with the thesis that some patients with primary thyroid disease with limited thyroid reserve may present with normal TSH levels. Prospective identification of a portion of this subgroup can be accomplished with demonstration of positive antithyroid antibody titers and, in the event of a normal clinical thyroid examination, ultrasonographic demonstration of a small thyroid or features of a chronically inflamed or fibrotic one. TRH testing, which has little utility, might help one differentiate some of these patients from healthy controls. Given the theoretic, though unproved, benefit of thyroid hormone therapy for such patients with ovulatory abnormalities, empirically treating those with higher than normal mean TSH values, antithyroid antibodies, or palpable thyroid abnormalities with 50 or 75 μg of T_4 while pursuing other avenues of assisted conception is advisable. Until better data on the benefit or lack of benefit of treating infertile patients with subclinical hypothyroidism, that is, those with above normal TSH levels but normal estimates of free T_4, are available, this approach is defensible though not based on any documentation of efficacy.

Recurrent Miscarriage in the Setting of Positive Titers for Antithyroid Antibodies

A multicenter trial is being organized to evaluate this group of patients (Glinoer, personal communication, 1995). In the interim, this group of patients should be considered candidates for forms of therapy, including immunotherapy, aimed at preventing miscarriage attributable to an immune factor. Because a subset of patients with recurrent spontaneous abortion have limited thyroid reserve and higher, though normal, TSH levels than a control group[52] the potential benefit of empiric use of thyroid hormone should be entertained. This approach will remain defensible until we know more about the thyroid status of these patients at the time of miscarriage and whether this intervention has any documented impact on the rate of miscarriage when studied in a controlled manner.

REFERENCES

1. Kaplan MM: Thyroid diseases. In: Gleicher N. (ed), *Principles and Practice of Medical Therapy in Pregnancy,* ed 2. Norwalk, CT, Appleton & Lange, 1992:321–338
2. Longcope C: The male and female reproductive systems in thyrotoxicosis. In: Braverman LE, Utiger RD (eds), *Werner and Ingbar's The Thyroid,* ed 6. Philadelphia, Lippincott, 1991:828
3. Longcope C: The male and female reproductive systems in hypothyroidism. In: Braverman LE, Utiger RD (eds), *Werner and Ingbar's The Thyroid,* ed 6. Philadelphia, Lippincott, 1991:1052
4. Emerson CH: Thyroid diseases during and after pregnancy. In: Braverman LE, Utiger RD (eds), *Werner and Ingbar's The Thyroid,* ed 6. Philadelphia, Lippincott, 1991:1263
5. Daniels GH: Thyroid disease and pregnancy: A clinical overview. *Endocrinol Pract* 1:287, 1995
6. Glinoer D: The thyroid in pregnancy: A European Perspective. *Thyroid Today* 18:1, 1995
7. Fisher DA: Neonatal thyroid disease in the offspring of women with autoimmune thyroid disease. *Thyroid Today* 9:1, 1986
8. New England Congenital Hypothyroidism Collaborative: Neonatal thyroid screening: Now we are nine. In: Delange F, Glinoer D (eds), *Research in Congenital Hypothyroidism.* New York, Plenum, 1989:291
9. Vulsma T, Gons M, de Vijlder JJM: Maternal-fetal transfer of thyroxine in congenital hypothyroidism due to a total organification defect or thyroid agenesis. *N Engl J Med* 321:13, 1989
10. Kimura M, Amino N, Tamaki H, Mitsuda N, Miyai K, Tanizawa O: Physiologic thyroid activation in normal early pregnancy is induced by circulating hCG. *Obstet Gynecol* 75:775, 1990
11. Levy RP, Newman DM, Rejali LS, Barford DA: The myth of goiter in pregnancy. *Am J Obstet Gynecol* 137:701, 1980
12. Berghout A, Endert E, Ross A, Hogerzell HV, Smits NJ, Wiersinga WM: Thyroid function and thyroid size in normal pregnant women living in an iodine replete area. *Clin Endocrinol* 41:375, 1994
13. Delange F, Dunn JT, Glinoer D: General comments, conclusions, and final recommendations of the International Workshop on Iodine Nutrition in Europe. In: Delange F, Dunn JT, Glinoer D (eds), *Iodine Deficiency in Europe: A Continuing Concern.* New York, Plenum, 1993:473
14. Van Wyk J, Grumbach MM: Syndrome of precocious menstruation and galactorrhea in juvenile hypothyroidism: An example of hormonal overlap pituitary feedback. *J Pediatr* 24:1, 1973
15. Tenney B, Little B: *Clinical Obstetrics.* Philadelphia, Saunders, 1961:189
16. Burrow GN: The thyroid gland and reproduction. In: Yen SSC, Jaffe RB (eds), *Reproductive Endocrinology.* Philadelphia, Saunders, 1986:424
17. Litzenberg JC, Carey JB: The relation of basal metabolism to sterility. *Am J Obstet Gynecol* 17:550, 1926
18. Niswander KR: Metabolic and endocrine conditions. In: Niswander KR, Gordon M (eds), *The Women and Their Pregnancies.* Philadelphia, Saunders, 1972:246
19. Montoro M, Collea JV, Frasier SD, Mestman JH: Successful outcome of pregnancy in women with hypothyroidism. *Ann Intern Med* 94:31, 1981
20. Goldsmith RE, Sturgis SH, Lerman J, Stanbury JR: The menstrual pattern of thyroid disease. *J Clin Endocrinol Metab* 12:846, 1962
21. Davis LE, Leveno KJ, Cunningham FG: Hypothyroidism complicating pregnancy. *Obstet Gynecol* 72:108, 1988
22. Edson JR, Fecher DR, Doe RP: Low platelet adhesiveness and other hemostatic abnormalities in hypothyroidism. *Ann Intern Med* 82:342, 1975

23. Bispink L, Brandle W, Lindner C, Betterdorf G: Preclinical hypothyroidism and disorders of ovarian function. *Geburtshilfe Frauenheilkd* 49:881, 1989

24. Gerhard I, Eggert-Kruse W, Merzoug K, Klinga K, Runnebaum B: Thyrotropin-releasing hormone (TRH) anda metoclopramide testing in infertile women. *Gynecol Endocrinol* 5:15, 1991

25. Shalev E, Eliyahu S, Ziv M, Ben-Ami M: Routine thyroid function tests in infertile women: Are they necessary? *Am J Obstet Gynecol* 171:1191, 1994

26. Wurfel W: Thyroid regulation pathways and its effect on human luteal function. *Gynakol Geburtshilfliche Rundsch* 32:145, 1992

27. Klein RZ, Haddow JE, Faix JD, et al: Prevalence of thyroid deficiency in pregnant women. *Clin Endocrinol* 35:41, 1991

28. Lejeune B, Lemone M, Kinthaer J, Grun JP, Glinoer D: The epidemiology of autoimmune and functional thyroid disorders in pregnancy [abstract]. *J Endocrinol Invest* 15(Suppl 2):77, 1992

29. Leung AS, Millar LK, Koonings PP, Montoro M, Mestman JH: Perinatal outcome in hypothyroid pregnancies. *Obstet Gynecol* 81:349, 1993

30. Lejeune B, Grun JP, de Nayer P, Servais G, Glinoer D: Antithyroid antibodies underlying thyroid abnormalities and miscarriage or pregnancy induced hypertension. *Br J Obstet Gynaecol* 100:669, 1993

31. Nelson JC, Palmer FJ: A remission of goitrous hypothyroidism during pregnancy. *J Clin Endocrinol Metab* 40:383, 1975

32. Mandel SJ, Larsen PR, Seely EW, Brent GA: Increased need for thyroxine during pregnancy in women with primary hypothyroidism. *N Engl J Med* 323:91, 1990

33. Tamaki H, Amino N, Takeoko K, Mitsuda N, Miyai K, Tanizawa O: Thyroxine requirement during pregnancy for replacement therapy of hypothyroidism. *Obstet Gynecol* 76:230, 1990

34. Kaplan MM: Monitoring thyroxine treatment during pregnancy. *Thyroid* 2:147, 1992

35. Dowling JT, Appleton WG, Nicoloff JT: Thyroxine turnover during human pregnancy. *J Clin Endocrinol Metab* 27:1749, 1967

36. Refetoff S, Larsen PR: Transport, cellular uptake, and metabolism of thyroid hormone. In: DeGroot LJ (ed), *Endocrinology,* ed 2, vol 1. Philadelphia, Saunders, 1989:541

37. Von Basedow CA: Exopthalmos durch hypertrophie des Zellgewebes in der Augenhohl. *Wochenschrift Heilk* 6:197, 1840

38. Becks GP, Burrow GN: Thyroid disease and pregnancy. *Med Clin North Am* 75:121, 1991

39. Clyde HR, Walsh PC, English RW: Elevated plasma testosterone and gonadotropin levels in infertile males with hyperthyroidism. *Fertil Steril* 27:662, 1976

40. Van Dijke CP, Heydendael RJ, De Kleine MJ: Methimazole, carbimazole, and congenital skin defects. *Ann Intern Med* 106:60, 1987

41. Momotani N, Hisaoka T, Noh J, Ishikawa N, Ito K: Effects of iodine on thyroid status of fetus versus mother in treatment of Graves' disease complicated by pregnancy. *J Clin Endocrinol Metab* 75:738, 1992

42. Hashizume K, Ichikawa K, Nishii Y, et al: Effect of administration of thyroxine on the risk of postpartum recurrence of hyperthyroid Graves' disease. *J Clin Endocrinol Metab* 75:6, 1992

43. Bech K, Hoier-Madsen M, Feldt-Rasmussen U, Moller Jensen B, Molsted-Pedersen L, Kuhl C: Thyroid function and autoimmune manifestations in insulin-dependent diabetes mellitus during and after pregnancy. *Acta Endocrinol* 124:534, 1991

44. Sarkar SD, Beierwaltes WH, Gill SP, Cowley BJ: Subsequent fertility and birth histories of children and adolescents treated with ^{131}I for thyroid cancer. *J Nucl Med* 17:460, 1976

45. Dottorini ME, Lomuscio G, Mazzucchelli L, Vignati A, Colombo L: Assessment of female fertility and carcinogenesis after iodine-131 therapy for differentiated thyroid carcinoma. *J Nucl Med* 36:21, 1995

46. Smith MB, Xue H, Takahashi H, Cangir A, Andrassy RJ: Iodine 131 Thyroid ablation in children and adolescents: Long-term risk of infertility and birth defects [abstract]. *Ann Surg Oncol* 1:128, 1994

47. Glinoer D, Soto MF, Bourdoux P, et al: Pregnancy in patients with mild thyroid abnormalities: Maternal and neonatal repercussions. *J Clin Endocrinol Metab* 73:421, 1991

48. Stagnaro-Green A, Roman SH, Cobin RH, El-Harazy E, Alvarez-Marfany M, Davies TF: Detection of at-risk pregnancy by means of highly sensitive assays for thyroid autoantibodies. *JAMA* 264:1422, 1990

49. Singh A, Dantas ZN, Stone SC, Asch RH: Presence of thyroid antibodies in early reproductive failure: Biochemical versus clinical pregnancies. *Fertil Steril* 63:277, 1995

50. Hamburger JI: Management of hyperthyroidism in children and adolescents. *J Clin Endocrinol Metab* 60:1019, 1985

51. Mandel SJ, Hornstein M, Rein M, Hill JA: Thyroid function during gonadotropin therapy [abstract]. Presented at the 10th International Congress of Endocrinology, The Endocrine Society, June 12–14, 1996, San Francisco

52. Glinoer D, Riahi M, Grun JP, Kinthaert J: Risk of subclinical hypothyroidism in pregnant women with asymptomatic autoimmune thyroid disorders. *J Clin Endocrinol Metab* 79:197, 1994

PART III

Endometriosis

CHAPTER 11

Pathophysiology and Medical Treatment of Endometriosis-Associated Infertility

IVO A. BROSENS

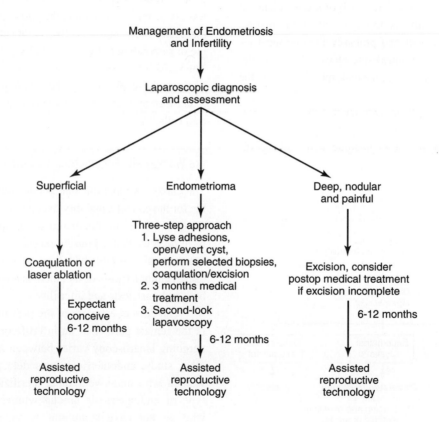

Endometriosis is one of the most comon diseases of menstruating women. Despite the widespread prevalence of the disease, the pathophysiologic features of endometriosis-associated infertility are complex. This chapter explores the pathophysiologic features of endometriosis-associated infertility and describes indications for medical treatment.

PATHOPHYSIOLOGY

Appearance and Hormone Receptors

Three different types of endometriosis have been differentiated.[1] The first type was described as adenomyoma, which was predominantly located in the pelvic support structures and characterized by the presence of bundles of smooth muscle and fibrous tissue with islands of glands and stroma.[2] The second type was hemorrhagic ovarian cyst, which at microscopic examination revealed superficial implants, some of which looked exactly like normal uterine mucosa.[3] The third type was peritoneal endometriosis which has received much interest since it was described in detail by Sampson.[4] Each of these variants of endometriosis ultimately affects management of the disease (Fig 11–1). The development and probably the hormonal response of endometrial tissue outside the uterine cavity are determined as much by location as is the endometrium within the uterus (Fig 11–2).

Implants in an endometrioma are characterized histologically by the presence of either surface epithelium only, surface epithelium studded with stroma, or in some areas full superficial endometrium similar to that in the uterine cavity. Deep nodular implants, on the other hand, are formed by bundles of fibrous and smooth muscle tissue that enclose a variable amount of glands and stroma. This type of nodular endometriosis frequently cannot be differentiated from uterine adenomyosis. Superficial peritoneal implants are covered by mesothelium[5] in contrast to eutopic endometrium, which has a ramified glandular structure.[6] Their protean appearance at laparoscopy has become a source of a colorful terminology (Table 11–1). Implants vary greatly in activity on the basis of their prostaglandin production, hormonal response, and degree of fibrosis. Lesions can spontaneously appear and disappear on the surface, making peritoneal endometriosis a changing phenomenon.[7] Microscopic implants have been described as one type found at scanning electron microscopy. In these implants mesothelium is being replaced by endometrial surface epithelium.[5] A second type consists of glands and stroma covered by mesothelium. It is found at biopsies of normal looking peritoneum.[8]

Most authors agree that estrogen receptors are much more variable in endometriotic tissue than in endometrium and that progesterone receptors are frequently absent. Estrogen receptors are identified in no more than 30% of specimens, indicating that many endometriotic cells are not yet or are no longer capable of responding to the cyclical changes in plasma steroids.[9,10] The variability of steroid hormone receptors in endometriosis is likely to be explained by the heterogeneity of the implants rather than by a difference between endometriotic and endometrial cells.[11]

Are Women with Endometriosis Infertile?

The classic assumptions that pelvic endometriosis is responsible for the patient's inability to conceive and that medical treatment that makes the endometriosis disappear improves fertility have been challenged during recent years. Until a causal relationship can be established, it is just as plausible that infertility causes endometriosis or that there is a primary causal factor for both endometriosis and infertility.

The current estimate of the prevalence of endometriosis in the female partner of an infertile or subfertile couple undergoing laparoscopy varies between 20% and 50%.[12] In another study, endometriosis was detected in 22% of fertile women who underwent tubal sterilization.[13] The dominant type of endometriosis among women of reproductive age who do not have symptoms is superficial peritoneal endometriosis. For this reason infertility associated with endometriosis can best be divided into infertility in women with superficial peritoneal endometriosis alone and infertility in women with mechanical compromise of the reproductive organs in the form of adnexal adhesions, ovarian endometriomas, or tubal obstruction.

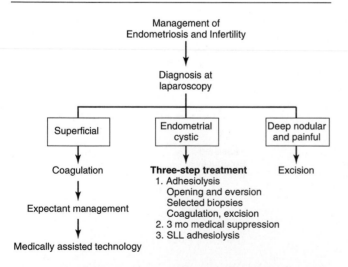

Figure 11–1. Flow chart of the management of endometriosis and infertility. SLL, second-look laparoscopy.

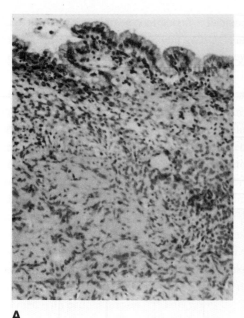
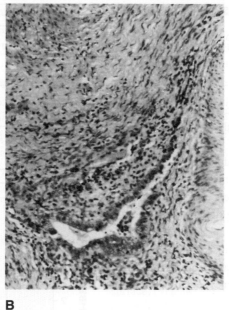

A   **B**

Figure 11–2. Two different types of endometriosis. **A.** Ovarian endometriosis. Superficial endometriosis in ovarian cortex. **B.** Deep endometriosis. Island of endometrial tissue in a fibromuscular nodule.

The association between endometriosis and infertility has been based on data on decreased cycle fecundity in women undergoing therapeutic insemination with donor sperm (TID) because of their partner's severe male-factor infertility. The finding that women without visible endometriosis subsequently achieved higher cycle fecundity with insemination than women with endometriosis[14,15] has not been confirmed by others.[16–18] Performing intrauterine insemination (IUI) for women with minimal endometriosis in both stimulated and spontaneous cycles appears to increase monthly fecundity to rates that approach normal fecundability (Fig 11–3).[19]

In summary, endometriosis-associated infertility is not a

condition of sterility but more properly subfertility. The association between endometriosis and subfertility is not a strong one, and a causal relationship has been questioned. The presence of endometriosis may be an epiphenomenon among patients with otherwise unexplained fertility. The decreased monthly fertility in these women has been related to other factors, such as age and duration of fertility.[20]

TABLE 11–1. TERMINOLOGY USED TO DESCRIBE PERITONEAL ENDOMETRIOSIS

Powder burn, puckered black lesions
Vascularized, glandular papule
Vesicular lesions
    Serous, surrounded by marked vascularization
    Red hemorrhagic
Red flame-like
Petechial peritoneum
Hypervascularized area
Discolored area
    Yellowish brown
    Blue
    White
White scarring
Peritoneal defects
Cribriform peritoneum
Subovarian adhesions

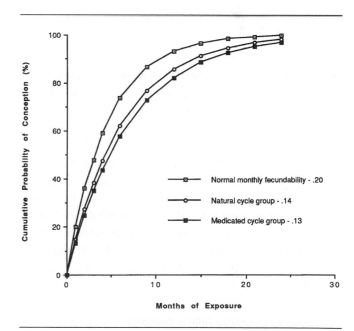

Figure 11–3. Results of intrauterine insemination in stimulated and spontaneous cycles in which hCG was used to trigger ovulation in patients with minimal endometriosis. *(From Serta R, et al: Minimal endometriosis and intrauterine insemination: Does controlled ovarian hyperstimulation improve pregnancy rates?* Obstet Gynecol *80:37, 1992.)*

also been shown to have immunosuppressive properties, including improvement in autoimmune conditions, such as idiopathic thrombocytopenic purpura[59] and systematic lupus erythematosis[60] associated with a fall in the levels of the appropriate autoantibodies. In addition to its hormonally mediated effect on endometriosis, danazol has been shown to have immunosuppressive properties by in vitro inhibition of lymphocyte proliferation[61] and reduction of the total levels of immunoglobulin at the end of treatment.[62] The effect of the immunoregulation and its importance in the treatment of endometriosis have not been fully established.

Doses of danazol of 800 mg per day are frequently used in North America; 600 mg or less per day is the norm in Europe and many other countries. The incidence of amenorrhea increases with increasing doses of danazol.[63] A minimum dose of 400 mg per day seems optimal. This dose inhibits ovulation in more than 95% of women.[64] The 400-mg daily dose appears to be appropriate to begin treatment and is increased if necessary to achieve amenorrhea and relief of symptoms.[65]

The symptomatic side effects of danazol are mainly related to the hyperandrogic state that it produces. Symptoms are dose dependent and include weight gain, oily skin and hair, acne, muscle cramps, and hirsutism. Deepening of the voice is uncommon but of importance because it appears to be irreversible.[66] Other side effects are hypoestrogenic, such as hot flushes, decreased breast size, and decreased libido. Because of the androgenicity of the drug, inadvertent administration of danazol to a pregnant woman may result in masculinization of a female fetus.

Danazol has several metabolic side effects. Therapy produces a rapid reduction in high-density lipoprotein (HDL) cholesterol (particularly in the putative cardioprotective HDL_2 subfraction) coupled with a rise in levels of the proatherogenic low-density lipoprotein (LDL) cholesterol (Fig 11–7). These changes are reversed when use of danazol is discontinued but it is prudent to recognize the potential detriment that may follow these perturbations. Concern is warranted only when therapy is prolonged (>12 months) or the drug is given to patients at high risk for ischemic heart disease.

Gestrinone

Gestrinone is a trienic 19-nosteroid derivation originally studied as an oral weekly contraceptive. In humans it acts as an androgen, progestogen, antiprogestogen, and antiestrogen. Gestrinone acts both centrally and peripherally to reduce estradiol and mean LH levels, obliterate the midcycle LH surge, reduce levels of SHBG, and increase free testosterone levels.[67] Estradiol levels are suppressed only to the early follicular range.[68]

Gestrinone has the advantage of a long half-life when it is given orally, making 2.5 mg twice or three times a week the standard dose. A 1990 study showed that 1.25 mg of gestrinone twice a week is just as effective as the standard dose.[69] Another study looked at the histologic effect of gestrinone 1.25 mg a day for 2 months and found the effect to be similar to the effect seen after 6 months of danazol therapy.[70] The symptomatic and metabolic side effects of gestrinone are androgenic and similar to

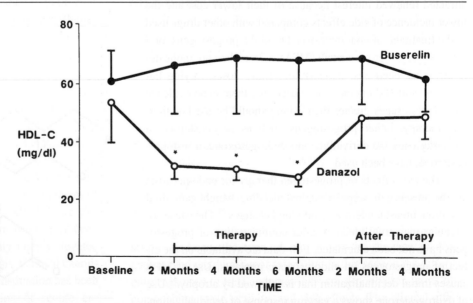

Figure 11–7. Mean plasma high-density lipoprotein (HDL) levels for a group of patients with endometriosis who were treated with buserelin or danazol. *(From Dlugi AM, et al: A companion of buserelin versus danazol on plasma lipids. Fertil Steril 49:913, 1988.[85] Reprinted with permission of the publisher, The American Fertility Society.)*

those of danazol; the hypoestrogenic side effects are less evident.[71]

Gonadotropin-Releasing Hormone Agonists

The suppression or downregulation of the pituitary gland by GnRH agonists that cause suppression of ovarian steroid production and induce medical, reversible pseudomenopause is an established mode of treatment of endometriosis. Various formulations and dosages of GnRH agonists have been used; the drugs are administered by means of injection or nasal spray (Table 11–3). Depot formulations are attractive because of the reduced dosage frequency and because nasal administration can be complicated by variations in absorption rate and problems with patient compliance. The implants produce higher suppression of the pituitary ovarian axis, better laparoscopic scores and more histologic regression of implants than does use of a nasal spray.[72]

The side effects of GnRH agonists are consequent to the hypoestrogenic state (Fig 11–8). Use of depot preparations appears to produce more marked bone loss than does daily use of a nasal spray. Recovery of bone loss may take 6 to 12 months after the end of therapy with considerable individual variations. Patients at high risk for osteoporosis should not undergo GnRH agonist therapy.

Therapy should not be extended longer than 6 months. GnRH agonist therapy may not be suitable for patients who need treatment of early recurrence (within 1 year) or multiple courses of medical therapy because of the potential problem of cumulative repetitive bone loss.[73] In such instances, baseline and follow-up bone densitometry scans should be considered. Currently, various regimens are being investigated to determine to the most appropriate combination to add to the GnRH agonist to counteract bone loss and enable these highly effective drugs to be used in long-term therapy and for repeated courses in recurrent endometriosis.[74]

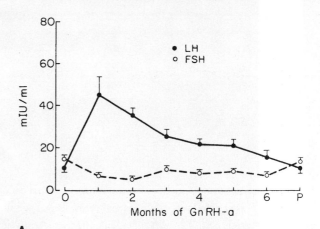

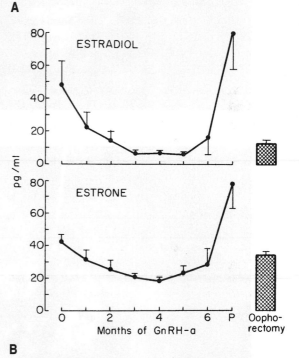

Figure 11–8. A. Levels of LH and FSH before, during, and after 6 months of GnRH therapy. **B.** Mean ± SE levels of estradiol and esterone before, during, and after 6 months of GnRH therapy compared with the concentration in 10 women who had undergone oophorectomy. *(From Steingold KA, et al: Treatment of endometriosis with a long-acting gonadotropin-releasing hormone agonist. Obstet Gynecol 69:403, 1987.)*[86]

TABLE 11–3. CHEMICAL STRUCTURES OF GONADOTROPIN-RELEASING HORMONE AND FIVE GONADOTROPIN-RELEASING HORMONE AGONISTS

Name	Structure
	1 2 3 4 5 6 7 8 9 10
GnRH	ProGlu-His-Trp-Ser-Tyr-Gly-Leu-Arg-Pro-Gly-NH$_2$
Leuprolide	-D-Leu--Pro-NEt
Buserelin	-D-Ser (tBu)- -Pro-NEt
Nafarelin	-D-Nal-
Zoladex	-D-Ser(tBu)- -Aza-Gly-
Lutrelin	-D-Trp- Me-Leu--Pro-NEt

MEDICAL TREATMENT OF ENDOMETRIOSIS-ASSOCIATED INFERTILITY

The clinical efficacy of medical treatment of endometriosis in infertile patients has been assessed by means of laparoscopic evaluation of implants and the subsequent pregnancy rates (Fig 11–9).

52. Moghissi KS, Boyce CR: Management of endometriosis with oral medroxy-progesterone acetate. *Obstet Gynecol* 47:265, 1976

53. Cornillie FJ, Puttemans P, Brosens IA: Histology and ultrastructure of human endometriotic tissues treated with dydrogesterone (Duphaston). *Eur J Obstet Gynecol Reprod Biol* 26:39, 1987

54. Greenblatt RB, Dmowski WP, Mahesh VB, Scholer HFL: Clinical studies with an anti-gonadotropin, danazol. *Fertil Steril* 22:102, 1971

55. Davison C, Banks W, Fritz A: The absorption, distribution, and metabolic rate of danazol in rats, monkeys, and human volunteers. *Arch Int Pharmacodyn Ther* 221:294, 1976

56. Steingold KA, Lu JKH, Judd HL, Meldrum DR: Danazol inhibits steroidogenesis by the human ovary in vivo. *Fertil Steril* 45:649, 1986

57. Barbieri RL: The use of danazol as treatment of endometriosis. In: Thomas EJ, Rock JA (eds), *Modern Approaches to Endometriosis.* London, Kluwer, 1991:239–255

58. Nilsson B, Sodergard R, Damber MG, Damber JE, Von Schouler B: Free testosterone levels during danazol therapy. *Fertil Steril* 39:505, 1983

59. Ahn YS, Harrington WJ, Simon SR: Danazol for the treatment of idiopathic thrombocytopenic purpura. *N Engl J Med* 308:1396, 1983

60. Agnello V, Pariser K, Gell J, Gelfand J, Turksoy RN: Preliminary observations on danazol therapy of systemic lupus erythematosus: Effects on antibodies, thrombocytopenia and complement. *J Rheumatol* 10:682, 1983

61. Hill JA, Barbieri RL, Anderson DJ: Immunosuppressive effects of danazol in vitro. *Fertil Steril* 48:414, 1987

62. El-Roeiy A, Dmowski WP, Gleicher N: Danazol but not gonadotropin-releasing hormone agonist suppresses auto-antibodies in endometriosis. *Fertil Steril* 50:864, 1988

63. Dmowski WP, Kapetanakis E, Scommegna A: Variable effects of danazol on endometriosis at 4 low-dose levels. *Obstet Gynecol* 59:408, 1982

64. Dmowski WP, Scholer HFL, Mastesh VV, Greenblatt RB: Danazol, a synthetic steroid derivative with interesting physiologic properties. *Fertil Steril* 22:9, 1971

65. Wingfield M, Healy DL: Endometriosis: Medical therapy. *Baillieres Clin Obstet Gynaecol* 7:813, 1993

66. Boothroyd CV, Lepre F: Permanent voice change resulting from danazol therapy. *Aust N Z J Obstet Gynaecol* 30:275, 1990

67. Thomas EJ, Mettler L: Gestogens and anti-gestogens as treatment of endometriosis. In: Thomas EJ, Rock JA (eds), *Modern Approaches to Endometriosis.* London, Kluwer, 1991:221–238

68. Thomas EJ, Cooke ID: Impact of gestrinone on the course of asymptomatic endometriosis. *Br Med J* 294:272, 1987

69. Hornstein MD, Gleason RE, Barbieri RL: A randomized double-blind prospective trial of two doses of gestrinone in the treatment of endometriosis. *Fertil Steril* 53:237, 1990

70. Brosens IA, Verleyen A, Cornillie F: The morphologic effect of short-term medical therapy of endometriosis. *Am J Obstet Gynecol* 157:1215, 1987

71. Fedele L, Bianchi S, Viezzoli T, Arcaini L, Candiani GB: Gestrinone versus danazol in the treatment of endometriosis. *Fertil Steril* 51:781, 1989

72. Donnez J, Nisolle-Pochet M, Clerckx-Braun F, Sandow J, Casanas-Roux F: Administration of nasal buserelin as compared with subcutaneous buserelin implant for endometriosis. *Fertil Steril* 52:27, 1989

73. Dawood MY: Hormonal therapies for endometriosis: Implications for bone metabolism. *Acta Obstet Gynaecol Scand* 73(Suppl 159):22, 1994

74. Shaw RW: Evaluation of treatment with gonadotrophin-releasing hormone analogues. In: Shaw RW. *Endometriosis: Current Understanding and Management.* Blackwell Science, Oxford, England, 1995:206–234

75. Evers J: The second look laparoscopy for the evaluation of the results of medical treatment of endometriosis should not be performed during ovarian suppression. *Fertil Steril* 47:502, 1987

76. Hughes EG, Fedorkow DM, Collins JA: A quantitative overview of controlled trials in endometriosis-associated infertility. *Fertil Steril* 59:963, 1993

77. Thomas EJ, Cooke I: Successful treatment of asymptomatic endometriosis: Does it benefit infertile women? *Br Med J* 294:1117, 1987

78. Bayer SR, Seibel M, Saffan DS, Berger MJ, Taymor M: Efficacy of danazol treatment for minimal endometriosis in infertile women. *J Reprod Med* 33:179, 1988

79. Telima S: Danazol and medroxyprogesterone acetate inefficacious in the treatment of infertility in endometriosis. *Fertil Steril* 50:872, 1988

80. Hull ME, Moghissi K, Magyar DF, Hayes MF: Comparison of different treatment modalities of endometriosis in infertile women. *Fertil Steril* 47:40, 1987

81. Badaway SZA, ElBakry MM, Samuel F, Dizer M: Cumulative pregnancy rates in infertile women with endometriosis. *J Reprod Med* 33:757, 1988

82. Pouly JL, Manhes H, Mage G, Canis M, Bruhat MA: Laparoscopic treatment of endometriosis (laser excluded). *Contrib Gynecol Obstet* 16:280, 1987

83. Seibel MM, Berger MJ, Weinstein FG, Taymor ML: The effectiveness of danazol on subsequent fertility is minimal endometriosis. *Fertil Steril* 38:534, 1982

84. Donnez J, Nisolle M, Karaman Y, et al: CO_2 laser laparoscopy in peritoneal endometriosis and in ovarian endometrial cyst. *J Gynecol Surg* 5:361, 1989

85. Dlugi AM, Rufo S, D'Amico JF, Seibel MM: A companion of buserelin versus danazol on plasma lipids. *Fertil Steril* 49:913, 1988

86. Steingold KA, Cedars M, Lu JKH, et al: Treatment of endometriosis with a long-acting gonadotropin-releasing hormone agonist. *Obstet Gynecol* 69:403, 1987

CHAPTER 12

Endometriosis: Surgical Treatment

CAMRAN NEZHAT · FARR NEZHAT · CEANA H. NEZHAT · DANIEL S. SEIDMAN

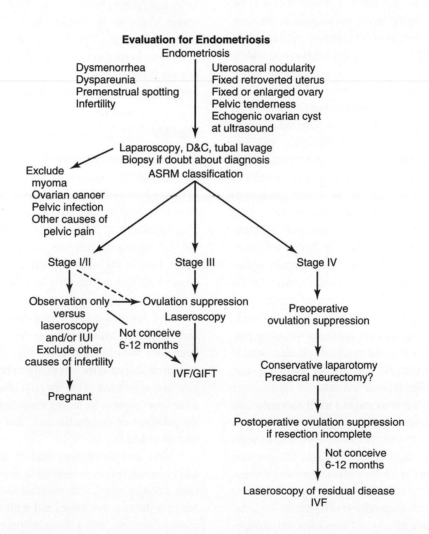

Evaluation for Endometriosis
Endometriosis

Dysmenorrhea
Dyspareunia
Premenstrual spotting
Infertility

Uterosacral nodularity
Fixed retroverted uterus
Fixed or enlarged ovary
Pelvic tenderness
Echogenic ovarian cyst
at ultrasound

Laparoscopy, D&C, tubal lavage
Biopsy if doubt about diagnosis
ASRM classification

Exclude
myoma
Ovarian cancer
Pelvic infection
Other causes of
pelvic pain

Stage I/II

Stage III

Stage IV

Observation only
versus
laseroscopy
and/or IUI
Exclude other
causes of infertility

Ovulation suppression

Laseroscopy

Not conceive
6-12 months

IVF/GIFT

Pregnant

Preoperative
ovulation suppression

Conservative laparotomy
Presacral neurectomy?

Postoperative ovulation suppression
if resection incomplete

Not conceive
6-12 months

Laseroscopy of residual disease
IVF

Endometriosis is one of the most prevalent diseases encountered in gynecology. However, the pathophysiology of endometriosis is not fully understood. Thus the management of endometriosis is usually aimed at the presenting symptom. This chapter discusses surgical treatment of the three most common forms of presentation—pelvic pain, endometrioma, and infertility.

PRESENTATION

Pelvic Pain

The leading symptom of endometriosis is pain. The intensity of menstrual pain is related to the number of endometrial implants.[1] Although medical therapy can reduce the size of endometriotic implant sites, it cannot completely suppress the endometriotic lesions.[2] The effectiveness of hormonal suppressive therapy is believed to be limited because ectopic foci may be autonomous to a certain degree and do not respond in the same manner as uterine endometrial glands.[3] Laparoscopic laser ablation of endometrial deposits and associated adhesions is widely accepted and is associated with a success rate of 60% to 70% in relief of pain associated with endometriosis.[4-6] However, the studies that provided these percentages had limitations in methodology.[7] In a recent prospective, randomized, double-blind trial by Sutton et al,[7] at laparoscopy the authors randomized 63 patients with pain (dysmenorrhea, pelvic pain, or dyspareunia) and minimal to moderate endometriosis to undergo laser ablation of endometriosis with uterine nerve ablation or to undergo expectant treatment. The women were unaware of the treatment allocated, as was the nurse who examined and interviewed them 3 and 6 months postoperatively. Six months postoperatively laser laparoscopy had resulted in statistically significant pain relief compared with expectant management. Of the treated patients, 62.5% (20 of 32) reported improvement or resolution of symptoms compared with 22.6% (7 of 31) in the expectant group. The benefit of surgical treatment was more pronounced in women with mild and moderate disease than in women with minimal disease. No operative or laser complications occurred, and the effectiveness and safety of laparoscopy in alleviating pain in women with stages I to III endometriosis were demonstrated. Patients with severe endometriosis were not included in the study. It was considered unethical to withhold surgical treatment in light of the 80% pain relief among this group of patients, most of whom had not responded to medical therapy.[8] Endoscopic surgical treatment may be more cost effective than therapy with hormonal agents, which are commonly associated with side effects and may offer only temporary pain relief.

Endometriomas

Surgical intervention is considered the most appropriate management of endometriomas because aspiration alone has an unacceptably high recurrence rate[9,10] (Fig 12–1). Management of endometriomas with gonadotropin-releasing hormone (GnRH) agonists after drainage is more effective than drainage alone in reduction of ovarian endometrial cysts, but even this combined approach does not completely suppress the endometriotic tissue.[3] Because the second-look laparoscopic procedure is performed immediately after the GnRH agonist therapy, no long-term follow-up data are available. The ovarian cysts will probably recur.[3]

Surgical management of endometriomas has one important advantage. Cystectomy allows histologic study to verify the diagnosis[11,12] and to rule out atypical changes[13] and malignant tumors.[14-16]

Results after laparoscopic management of endometriomas are comparable to those of laparotomy.[17,18] Many patients have severe adhesions in addition to endometriomas that involve other pelvic organs. For this reason, the safety of laparoscopic procedures is related to the experience of the surgeon. Patients recover from laparoscopy faster than from a laparotomy, so the former may be more cost effective.[19]

Infertility

The precise relationship between endometriosis and infertility is not completely understood. Three entities that may adversely influence fertility include pelvic endometrial implants, development of endometriomas, and adhesion formation (Table 12–1). These entities may influence fertility by a number of mechanical, inflammatory, hormonal, or immunologic factors (Table 12–2). Despite the many possibilities, it is unclear whether endometriosis causes infertility or if an underlying defect is responsible for both infertility and development of the disease. It therefore remains controversial whether patients presenting with infertility without pain or an endometrioma should be treated for mild endometriosis (Fig 12–2). The number of endometrial lesions does not predict pregnancy rate. Other factors are associated with the likelihood that a patient will achieve pregnancy, including the extent and type of adhesions, the presence of endometriomas, and possibly obliteration of the cul-de-sac.[21]

Meta-analysis of more than 25 studies showed that medical treatment results in negligible improvements in pregnancy rates among patients with minimal and mild endometriosis.[21,22] Medical therapy was associated with undesirable side effects, considerable cost, and a delay in conception by the duration of the therapy, usually 3 to 6 months. No treatment, laparoscopy,

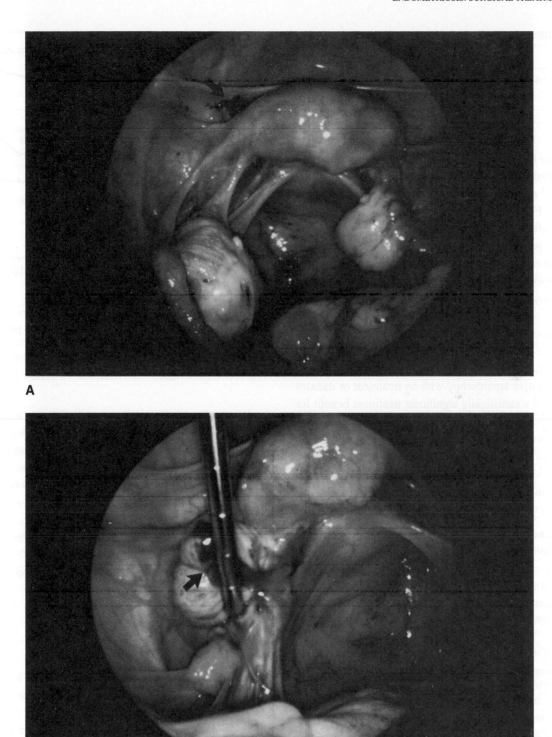

A

B

Figure 12–1. Laparoscopic view of the pelvis shows endometriosis on the anterior bladder flap and in the cul-de-sac. Endometriosis beneath the left ovary cannot be seen with a single puncture. **(A)** but easily seen with the use of a probe through a second puncture **(B)**. *(Courtesy of M. Seibel, MD.)*

Management of Appendiceal Endometriosis

Because approximately 50% of appendiceal lesions are detected at palpation and may be missed at visual inspection, incidental appendectomy is recommended for patients with severe endometriosis or persistent right lower quadrant pain.

A bipolar electrocoagulator and carbon dioxide laser are used sequentially to desiccate and cut the mesoappendix 0.2 to 0.5 cm from the ileocecal area (Figs 12–6 and 12–7). When using the bipolar electrocoagulator, the surgeon should exercise caution to prevent thermal damage to the cecum. Two polydioxanone endosurgical sutures (Endoloops, Ethicon, Somerville, NJ) are passed over the base of the appendix 2 to 5 mm from the cecum and tied, one on top of the other. A third Endoloop suture is applied less than 2 cm distal to the other sutures (Fig 12–8). The appendix is cut between the second and third sutures.

In a subsequent series of 254 laparoscopic appendectomies, there were no serious intraoperative complications.[53] One patient had a transient elevated temperature, one had mild periumbilical ecchymosis, and a third had a pelvic abscess that necessitated surgical intervention and antibiotic therapy.

A modification of this technique uses a single Endoloop suture placed over the base of the appendix 2 to 5 mm from the cecum and tied. The appendix is cut about 5 mm distal to the suture.

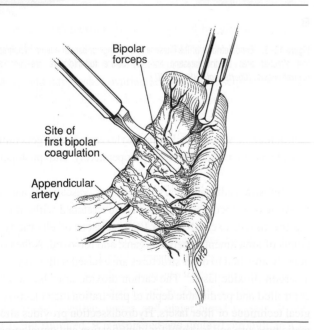

Figure 12–6. The mesoappendix is coagulated with bipolar forceps. *(From Nezhat CR, Nezhat FR, Luciano AA, et al: Complication. In: Operative Gynecologic Laparoscopy: Principles and Techniques. New York, McGraw-Hill, 1995:287-310.)*

Laparoscopic Management of Infiltrative Endometriosis Involving the Rectosigmoid Colon and Rectovaginal Septum

The posterior cul-de-sac is the site most often involved with endometriosis. This area consists of the back of the cervix; the vagina and rectum in the middle; and the pararectal area, uterosacral ligaments and lower portion of the posterior aspect of the broad ligaments laterally. Superficial endometrial implants on the peritoneum in this area can be easily managed with excision or coagulation. Infiltrative lesions, however, are usually proximal to or involve structures such as ureters, uterine and lower pelvic vessels, and rectum. The recognition and thorough management of these implants is challenging and requires surgical skill and familiarity with anatomy, not only to remove the lesions completely but also to manage injuries that may occur during treatment.

Severe and infiltrative lesions cause anatomic distortion of the posterior cul-de-sac. Affected uterosacral ligaments often cause the cervix and ureters to retract medially. Involvement of the posterior broad ligament may result in periureteral fibrosis and stricture, and rarely, partial or complete ureteral obstruction. Partial or complete obliteration of the posterior cul-de-sac occurs when endometriosis of the back of the vagina, pararectal area, and lower rectum is present and there is retraction and attachment of rectum to the uterosacral ligaments, back of the vagina, cervix and uterus laterally or centrally. This attachment usually is associated with different degrees of infiltrative endometrial implants and nodules, which are found after the rectum is separated from the cervix and vagina. The lesions may involve the different layers of the rectal wall and penetrate to the pararectal area below the uterosacral ligaments toward the levator ani muscles or toward the rectovaginal septum. Occasionally they may penetrate the entire vaginal wall.

Technique

The assistant should stand between the patient's legs and perform a rectovaginal examination with one hand. With the other hand, the assistant holds the uterus up with a rigid uterine elevator while both the assistant and the surgeon look at the monitor. For endometriosis of the rectovaginal septum and uterosacral ligament, 5 to 8 mL of dilute vasopressin (10 units in 100 to 200 mL of lactated Ringer's solution) are injected into an uninvolved area with a 16-gauge laparoscopic needle. The peritoneum is opened, and a plane is developed in the rectovaginal septum by means of hydrodissection.

It is imperative that the ureters be located before this procedure continues. Any alteration in the direction of the ureters should be identified. Because ureters are lateral to the uterosacral ligaments, we keep the dissection between the liga-

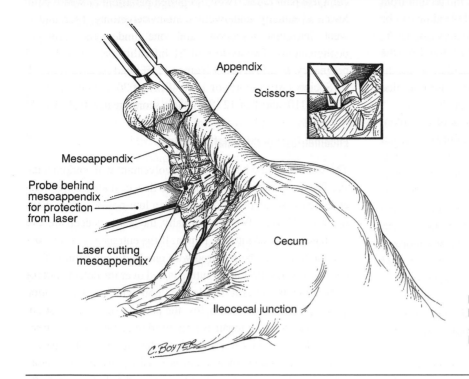

Figure 12-7. The mesoappendix is cut with a carbon dioxide laser or laparoscopic scissors. *(From Nezhat CR, Nezhat FR, Luciano AA, ets al: Complication. In:* Operative Gynecologic Laparoscopy: Principles and Techniques. *New York, McGraw-Hill, 1995:287-310.)*

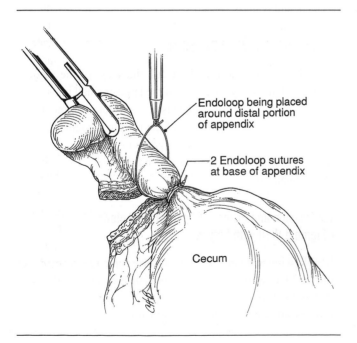

Figure 12-8. Endoloop sutures are placed around the base of the appendix. *(From Nezhat CR, Nezhat FR, Luciano AA, et al: Complication. In:* Operative Gynecologic Laparoscopy: Principles and Techniques. *New York, McGraw-Hill, 1995:287-310.)*

ments as much as possible. Hydrodissection and a relaxing incision lateral to the uterosacral ligament allow the ureters to retract laterally. This increases the protection of the ureters. Ureterolysis often is necessary to free the ureters from the surrounding fibrotic diseased tissue and from endometrial implants. Hydrodissection with a carbon dioxide laser and blunt dissection can be used for ureterolysis, enterolysis, and ovarian resection.

While the assistant examines the rectum, the surgeon completely excises or vaporizes the involved area until the loose areolar tissue of the rectovaginal space and normal muscularis layers of the rectum are reached. In women whose rectum is pulled up and attached to the back of the cervix between the uterosacral ligaments, the uterus is anteflexed sharply, and an incision is made at the right or left pararectal area then extended to the junction of the cervix and the rectum. If the rectal involvement is more extensive and the assistant's finger is not long enough, a sigmoidoscope, a sponge on forceps, or a rectal probe is used. An advantage of the use of a sigmoidoscope is that it helps the surgeon identify the rectum and identify or rule out intestinal perforation because air bubbles can be seen passing from the air-inflated rectum into the posterior cul-de-sac when the latter is filled with irrigation fluid. Insertion of these devices should be gentle and cautious to prevent rectal perforation.

While the assistant guides the procedure with a rectovagi-

60. Franklin RR, Grunert GM: Extragenital endometriosis. In: Nezhat C, Berger GS, Nezhat F, Buttram VC, Nezhat CH (eds), *Endometriosis: Advanced Management and Surgical Techniques.* New York, Springer-Verlag, 1995:127–136

61. Anderson WC, Larsen GD: Endometriosis: Treatment with hormonal pseudopregnancy and/or operation. *Am J Obstet Gynecol* 118:643, 1975

62. Martin DC, Vander Zwaag R: Excisional techniques for endometriosis with the laser laparoscope. *J Reprod Med* 32:754, 1987

63. Nezhat C, Nezhat F, Green B: Laparoscopic treatment of obstructed ureter due to endometriosis by resection and uretero-ureterostomy: A case report. *J Urol* 148:865, 1992

64. Nezhat F, Nezhat C: Laparoscopic segmental bladder resection for endometriosis: A report of two cases. *Obstet Gynecol* 81:882, 1993

65. Bayer SR, Seibel MM, Saffan DS, et al: The efficacy of danazol treatment for minimal endometriosis in an infertile population: A prospective randomized study. *J Reprod Med* 33:179, 1988

PART IV

Male Infertility

CHAPTER 13

Reproductive Physiology of Men

CLARKE F. MILLETTE

Pituitary–Testicular Axis of Spermatogenic Regulation
   Structure and function of Leydig cells
   Androgen biosynthesis
   Testosterone transport and metabolism
   Pituitary–Leydig cell axis: Hormonal
     and local control
Pituitary–Seminiferous Tubule Axis
   Sertoli cells and FSH
   Inhibin
   Paracrine regulation of spermatogenesis

Histologic Aspects of Spermatogenesis
   Spermatocytogenesis
   Meiosis
   Spermiogenesis
   Organization of the seminiferous epithelium
   Duration of spermatogenesis
Sperm Maturation in the Epididymis
Sperm Capacitation and the Acrosomal Reaction
Mechanisms of Sperm–Egg Recognition
Normal Semen Analysis

To assess infertility of men, it is important to appreciate the normal physiologic processes and structural organization of the male reproductive tract. This chapter highlights areas deemed particularly relevant to clinical manifestations of male-factor infertility. Large areas of interest are ignored or underemphasized because of space limitations. For example, the male accessory organs, including the seminal vesicles and prostate, are not discussed, and the processes of epididymal sperm maturation and capacitation are touched on only briefly.

PITUITARY–TESTICULAR AXIS OF SPERMATOGENIC REGULATION

The mammalian testis has a dual role. As an exocrine organ it produces gametes; as an endocrine organ it synthesizes and secretes steroid hormones. These two functions are divided anatomically; the interstitial Leydig cells are necessary for the synthesis of androgens, and the seminiferous tubules contain the various cells involved in spermatogenesis. The anterior pituitary gland plays an important regulatory role, interacting with both Leydig cells and the seminiferous tubules. Two gonadotropins secreted by the pituitary gland act as the key modulators of testicular function. Luteinizing hormone (LH) is primarily involved in the pituitary–Leydig cell axis. Follicle-stimulating hormone (FSH) is responsible for interactions with the Sertoli cells of the seminiferous epithelium. These two hormonal axes are considered in sequence here, but it should be remembered that they exist in close coordination with one another. Moreover, many aspects of the hormonal control of male reproduction, particularly in humans, remain unclear.

Structure and Function of Leydig Cells

The known constituents of the pituitary–Leydig cell axis are the Leydig cells themselves, the hormones gonadotropin-releasing hormone (GnRH), LH, and testosterone, and the blood plasma.

Additional elements, including testosterone-binding proteins and blood estrogens, are important.

Leydig cells are located in the interstitial, connective tissue regions between the seminiferous tubules. They were first described in humans by von Kolliker[1] and in other species by Leydig.[2] Very early, these cells were believed to be the primary source of male sex hormone.[3] Now known to be the most important testicular source of steroid hormones formed de novo from cholesterol, Leydig cells exhibit an ultrastructure consistent with this role.[4] They have large amounts of smooth endoplasmic reticulum, numerous mitochondria that contain tubular cristae, a large Golgi complex, and many lipid droplets. Human Leydig cells also contain specialized crystals in their cytoplasm. Called Reinke crystals, their function has not yet been determined.

Leydig cells are situated in close proximity to blood capillaries of the testicular interstitial stroma. In humans, clusters are scattered randomly in the interstitial space. Because this space contains abundant connective tissue and fluid, the Leydig cells are not always immediately adjacent to a blood vessel. Other species, such as the rodents, have sparse interstitial space with Leydig cells clustered directly around the capillaries and with prominent lymphatic sinusoids. Finally, in yet other mammals, such as boars and some marsupials, Leydig cells fill almost the entire interstitial region, leaving little room for the connective tissue that is present in humans.[5,6]

In humans, the testis begins to differentiate in the sixth week of gestation with a noticeable increase in the numbers of Sertoli cells concomitant with the formation of spermatogenic cords. Fetal Leydig cell precursors arrive among the undifferentiated mesenchymal cells during the eighth week of gestation. Changes in cellular structure begin immediately with increases in cytoplasmic volume and the amount of smooth endoplasmic reticulum and accumulation of lipid related to the eventual functioning of these cells. Newly differentiating Leydig cells are detected until the tenth week of gestation.[7,8] Leydig cell function, however, has already been initiated. Testosterone is present in the fetal testis as early as the sixth or seventh week of development.[9] Testosterone levels continue to increase in tissue, blood and amniotic fluid, reaching maximum levels at 15 to 18 weeks.[10] This increase is accompanied by an increase in the number of differentiated Leydig cells, which by 14 to 15 weeks occupy more than half of the total testicular volume. Plasma levels of human chorionic gonadotropin (hCG) rise concomitantly.

After this initial burst of activity, Leydig cells regress. After about the 16th week of gestation the number of Leydig cells, fetal plasma levels of testosterone, and testicular levels of mRNA for the P450 side-chain cleaving enzyme and P450 17-α-hydroxylase all decrease greatly.[10–12] In fact, at the time of birth the total number of testicular Leydig cells is reduced by 60%, and each individual cell is decreased in volume by one half. These changes are accompanied by a reduction in plasma hCG concentration.[10]

Molecular control of Leydig cell development in humans does not reside with LH generated by the hypophysis, as evidenced by the fact that fetal testicular production of steroid precedes initial LH secretion by 3 to 4 weeks.[10,13,14] In contrast, a regulatory role for hCG is suggested by the close temporal correlation between levels of this hormone and fetal plasma testosterone and the close relation with LH/hCG receptors in testicular tissue.[15,16] In vitro studies have demonstrated that hCG can indeed stimulate steroidogenesis in fetal tissue,[15,17] although some contradictory reports have appeared in the literature.[18] It seems evident that all steroidogenesis by Leydig cells during the first 15 weeks of gestation is mediated by hCG. Later, however, the hypophysis assumes control, as indicated by studies of anencephalic human fetuses, which have a reduced number of Leydig cells and impaired testicular production of testosterone.[8]

Testosterone levels rebound to their eventual adult values after birth with a peak in plasma steroid levels approximately 2 months after birth in humans.[10] The second wave of Leydig cell differentiation occurs during this same time frame.[19–21] Leydig cell number overshoots the eventual steady-state, however, and cells both regress and degenerate until few Leydig cells remain at the conclusion of the initial year of life.[21,22] The final, third-wave development of adult Leydig cells does not occur until the onset of puberty, when undifferentiated mesenchymal cells in the testicular interstitium alter structure and function under the influence of LH. During puberty, Leydig cells increase in number and eventually reach a peak of approximately 5×10^8 cells per testis in men in their twenties.[22] Thereafter cell numbers gradually diminish until they are halved in men older than 60 years.[23] Adult Leydig cells are a relatively stable population, with few mitoses detected at any time. Increased Leydig cell numbers may be caused by the differentiation of other cell types of unclear origin[24,25]; this cellular differentiation depends on both LH and hCG.[26,27]

Without active Leydig cells, androgen-dependent differentiation does not occur. Some rats deficient in Leydig cell function have small testes that remain abdominal and show no androgen-dependent development of internal and external genitalia.[28] Such animals are phenotypic females, are classified as pseudohermaphrodites, and have elevated plasma levels of LH and FSH with very low levels of testosterone. The Leydig cells present do not respond to LH or hCG, and it is thought that they lack specific plasma membrane LH receptors. A similar condition has been described in humans,[29] again indicating the importance of an active Leydig cell population in the testis.

The main response by Leydig cells to LH is the production and secretion of testosterone. Testosterone biosynthesis in the cells results from the binding of LH to specific cell surface receptors. This binding initiates adenylate cyclase catalysis of intracellular cyclic adenosine 3′, 5′-monophosphate (cAMP) synthesis in a process involving three distinct plasma membrane elements: (1) the receptor, which contains the specific LH recognition site; (2) the catalytic unit of adenyl cyclase, which converts adenosine 5′-triphosphate (ATP) to cAMP and pyrophosphate; and (3) the guanyl nucleotide regulatory subunit, which binds guanosine 5′-triphosphate (GTP) and couples the hormone receptor to the adenylate cyclase.[30] Inside the Leydig cell, cAMP releases the regulatory subunit of a protein kinase, which activates the kinase catalytic subunit. The kinase catalytic subunit facilitates conversion of cholesterol to pregnenolone. Although total intracellular cAMP rises after LH binding, maximal testosterone synthesis is achieved with less than a 10% increase in cAMP. In contrast, direct correlation exists between steroid biosynthesis and occupancy by cAMP of the regulatory protein kinase subunits.[31]

The molecular structure of the LH/hCG receptor has, in a variety of species, including humans, been an active area of analysis by means of a number of molecular biologic approaches. Cloning of the mRNA that encodes the human LH receptor has been completed[32]; the receptor structure is homologous to that determined for lower animals. The receptor is similar to other G protein–coupled receptors, which have seven transmembrane domains in addition to a serine- and threonine-rich cytoplasmic domain that carries a presumed phosphorylation site. However, in contrast to other G protein–coupled receptors that also bind low-molecular-weight ligands, the LH/hCG receptor includes an extended extracellular peptide of up to 400 amino acids, which may act as the actual LH hormone binding site. This added extracellular structural domain is also present on the cellular receptors for both thyroid-stimulating hormone (TSH) and FSH, which like LH are glycosylated.[33–35]

The mRNA that encodes the LH receptor is found in the testis and ovary, but also in the brain[36] and thyroid.[37] In the thyroid, most of the transcripts are incompletely spliced. Several transcripts ranging in size from 1.2 to 7.6 kb are detected in the ovary and the testis. The exact size and the relative abundance of these different transcripts varies among species and among organs. It seems that they are the result of variable 3′-noncoding sequences or alternative splicing events. At least 2.1 kb of coding sequence is required to generate a full-length, active LH/hCG receptor molecule. Although transfection experiments have demonstrated that the extracellular domain can itself bind hCG with an affinity equal to that of the intact receptor,[38] it is not yet clear where various truncated forms of the receptor localize within cells. Some studies suggest that truncated molecules that lack the transmembrane domains remain inside the cell.[39,40] Other reports indicate that similar receptor constructs are secreted.[41,42] The cytoplasmic tail of the LH/hCG receptor molecule is, though, a key element in targeting the receptor to the plasma membrane and also in the hormone-induced internalization of the receptor that leads to cAMP production.[43]

Regulation of the plasma membrane LH receptor occurs after binding of exogenous LH. Leydig cells stimulated by LH exhibit a desensitivity that is caused by the downregulation, or loss in numbers, of surface LH receptors. The loss of sensitivity is proportional to the loss of receptors.[44,45] Leydig cells therefore contain substantial reserve numbers of LH receptors, far above those required for maximum stimulation of testosterone secretion. In rats, for example, hormone binding increases until an extracellular concentration of 200 ng/mL is attained, even though steroid synthesis is maximized at hormone levels of only 0.5 ng/mL.[46] As a result of the excess number of LH receptors, complete responsiveness of the adenylate cyclase system can recover faster than the membrane receptors after LH-induced downregulation. In addition, testosterone synthesis remains depressed after Leydig cells have regained their increased cAMP response to LH.[47] These findings are consistent with studies that demonstrate patients with highly elevated levels of hCG have decreased testosterone secretion,[48] since hCG can bind to the membrane receptors targeted for LH.

The time course of LH-mediated downregulation of the LH/hCG membrane receptor varies according to the species and the cell model used for analysis. Murine Leydig cells demonstrate the refractory response quickly, within 20 minutes,[49] whereas rat[44] and porcine[50] Leydig cells exhibit a lag period of several hours before desensitization. Longer lag times may result from the recycling of internalized LH receptors to the cell surface before their eventual degradation. Few if any such analyses have been conducted with human Leydig cells, and the accuracy of extrapolation of the current findings to humans is unknown.

At least two processes other than internalization/degradation, are involved in the regulation of the LH/hCG receptor. Rapid proteolytic cleavage of the receptor causes release of the hormone-binding extracellular domain.[51] Decreases in the levels of receptor mRNA result from treatment with either LH or hCG.[52,53] This decrease in mRNA levels predominantly is due to increased degradation of the message, rather than a reduced rate of RNA transcription, at least in cells of pigs and rats.[54,55] Studies with the murine MA-10 Leydig tumor cell line suggest the reverse.[52] No data are available regarding human Leydig cell LH/hCG receptor mRNA regulation.

LH, or perhaps hCG, is also critical for the regulation of Leydig cell proliferation, as exemplified by three clinical manifestations. First, the absence of Leydig cells in male patients with hypogonadism is caused by a single mutation in the coding sequence of the LHβ chain gene, which abrogates hormone-binding activity.[56] Second, patients with male pseudohermaphroditism and no Leydig cells probably exhibit nonfunctional LH/hCG receptors.[29] Last, studies of the familial male precocious puberty syndrome reveal that affected persons have a single-base change, which replaces a glycine for an asparagine and thus produces a constitutively activated LH/hCG receptor.[59]

Androgen Biosynthesis

Most potent androgens are steroids. It is evident that testosterone is the main androgen synthesized in the testis for secretion into plasma. Although small amounts of other strong androgenic steroids such as dihydrotestosterone (DHT) also are secreted, these substances do not constitute a substantial proportion of total blood androgens in the male humans. Plasma testosterone levels in male humans approximate 7.0 ng/mL (24.3 nmol/L), and only 0.45 ng/mL (1.56 nmol/L) of DHT is detected. Total androgen levels synthesized are 7000 ng/day of testosterone and 300 ng/day of DHT. In female humans, however, DHT is a relatively important circulating hormone; circulating levels are approximately 0.20 ng/mL (0.69 nmol/L), compared with only about 0.45 ng/mL (1.56 nmol/L) of testosterone.

Androstenedione is also secreted by Leydig cells. When secreted, its only known function is to serve as a precursor in plasma for estrogens, although in Leydig cells it is a precursor to testosterone. Still other testosterone anabolites such as 17-hydroxy-progesterone and progesterone are secreted, but have no known physiologic role.

About 95% of the blood testosterone in male humans derives from the Leydig cells of the testis.[58] The principal pathways for its synthesis are shown in Fig 13–1.[58] Although a detailed discussion of the molecular biologic role of each of the key enzymatic steps in testosterone biosynthesis is beyond the scope of this chapter, a recent review has summarized these nicely.[59] Leydig cells either synthesize cholesterol from acetate or use cholesterol formed elsewhere and transported to the testis via the bloodstream. Low-density lipoprotein cholesterol may be used by Leydig cells. The relative proportion of testosterone formed from acetate or imported cholesterol varies among species, but in any case the acetate is first converted to cholesterol, probably as indicated in Fig 13–2. Acetyl coenzyme A (CoA) molecules combine and combine again with acetyl CoA to yield mevalonic acid. Mevalonic acid is then converted and condensed, with accompanying elongation of the carbon chain until squalene is formed. Squalene, which contains 30 carbons, is folded and closed to yield lanosterol, which is finally converted to cholesterol.

The first step necessary in the eventual conversion of cholesterol to testosterone is translocation of the cholesterol into the mitochondria. It has long been understood that the molecular constituents that regulate this transport are labile proteins, but until recently their identity was unclear. During the past few years, however, substantial progress has been made and a num-

ber of candidate cholesterol transport mechanisms have been reported.

First, sterol carrier protein (SCP2) was purified from liver as a 13 kd protein that stimulated the activity of a number of mitochondrial enzymes involved in cholesterol metabolism.[60] SCP2 induces transfer of cholesterol from lipid droplets into mitochondria, weakly enhances adrenal steroidogenesis in mi-

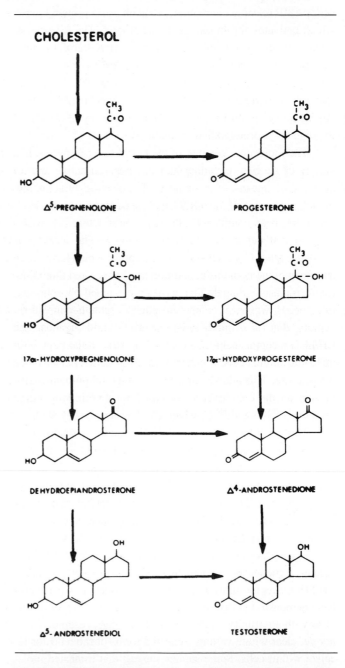

Figure 13–1. The various metabolic pathways from pregnenolone to testosterone. **Right.** delta-4 pathway. **Left.** delta-5 pathway. The conversions from left to right columns use an isomerase and 3β-hydroxysteroid dehydrogenase. Vertically, each pair of conversions involves the same enzyme—17-α-hydroxylase, 17,20-lyase, and 17β-hydroxysteroid dehydrogenase, respectively.

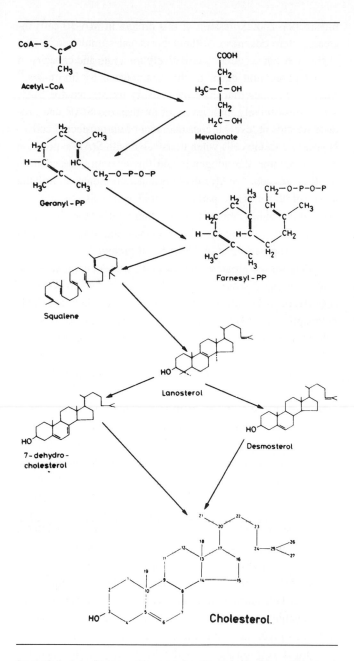

Figure 13–2. A simplified view of the metabolic pathways leading from acetyl coenzyme A to cholesterol.

tochondria, and when overexpressed in COS cells stimulates steroidogenesis in tissue culture.[61] A definitive role for SCP2 in Leydig cell cholesterol metabolism is unlikely. Although the protein is indeed present in Leydig cells,[62] and although hormonal stimulation does alter its intracellular localization, Leydig cell SCP2 does not evidence increased intracellular levels with acute stimulation, nor does it decline abruptly with the inhibition of protein synthesis.[63] It seems likely that in Leydig cells SCP2 alone or in combination with elements of the cytoskeleton[64] modulates transfer of cholesterol to the outer mi-

tochondrial membrane but does not itself regulate intramitochondrial cholesterol transport.

Steroidogenesis activator polypeptide (SAP) is another putative regulator of cholesterol entry into Leydig cell mitochondria.[65,66] SAP is present in all steroidogenic tissues that have been studied; its intracellular levels increase under hormonal stimulation, and this increase precedes the resultant steroidogenic effect. With the inclusion of cycloheximide, SAP levels decrease with a short half-life of not more than 5 to 7 minutes.[67] This is consistent with the proposed labile proteins that modulate cholesterol entry into the mitochondria. Like SCP2, however, SAP is unlikely to be the sole regulator of this process. Whereas SAP does stimulate adrenal mitochondrial cholesterol transport, its total efficacy is not sufficient to account for the overall activation of mitochondrial steroidogenesis in intact Leydig cells. In fact, SAP alone has little effect unless combined with GTP,[64] and SAP probably augments the role of both GTP and SCP2 via alternate pathways.

Definitive roles in modulating cholesterol intake by Leydig cell mitochondria have, instead, devolved on two competing mechanisms that use different proposed labile moieties. The first mechanism to be discussed here is the endogenous polypeptide ligand termed *diazepam-binding inhibitor* (DBI) and the peripheral (mitochondrial) benzodiazepine receptor (PBR).[68] Mitochondrial DBI receptors (MDRs) are abundant in Leydig cells of the testis, adrenal cells, and glial cells and clearly are involved in steroidogenesis.[69,70] Benzodiazepine agonists stimulate steroid production both in intact cells and when added to isolated mitochondria from a variety of relevant cell types.[71–74] Stimulation of isolated mitochondria partially offsets the block induced by cycloheximide and yields higher levels of cholesterol transport from the outer to inner mitochondrial membranes. Also, flunitrazepan, a benzodiazepine that binds to MDR with high affinity but that has little steroidogenic activity inhibits by 50% hormone-stimulated steroidogenesis in both Y-1 adrenal cells and the MA-10 cultured Leydig cell line.

Study of DBI has, concomitantly, added to the complexity of cholesterol transport into mitochondria. The DBI recognizes both central and mitochondrial receptors and is present in many different tissues, but it is especially elevated in Sertoli cells and Leydig cells.[75,76] Mitochondria isolated from adrenal, testicular, and glial cells all demonstrate elevated pregnenolone formation when stimulated by DBI.[71,77] The rate of DBI synthesis and its turnover rate are not altered after acute stimulation of either Y-1 or MA-10 cells by either adrenocorticotropic hormone (ACTH) or hCG,[78] suggesting that it is not the labile protein of importance. Further studies, though, have demonstrated that in rats adrenal ACTH quickly increases processing of DBI to a reactive peptide and that this is effectively blocked by cycloheximide. MDR antagonists also inhibit ACTH steroidogenic effects.[79]

These studies have been extended to demonstrate that both DBI and MDR are present in R2C cells, a rat Leydig tumor constitutive steroid-producing cell line.[80] R2C cells treated with a cholesterol-linked phosphothioate antisense sequence to DBI showed reduced DBI content and a concomitant and dramatic decrease of progesterone production. Sense nucleotide sequences used as controls did not demonstrate this effect. Furthermore, radioligand binding tests identified a single class of PBR-binding site with affinity ten times that of PBR in MA-10 cell mitochondria. Photolabeling experiments indicated that the 18-kd PBR protein was specifically tagged. Chemical cross linking showed that DBI binds directly to the PBR. All in all, these data strongly support the concept that DBI is vital in maintaining constitutive steroidogenesis by binding to the higher-affinity mitochondrial PBR to effect a supply of cholesterol to the inner mitochondrial membrane. Ultrastructural and atomic force microscopic localization studies with MA-10 mitochondria labeled with antibodies that recognize PBR demonstrate, further, that PBR is organized as clusters of four to six molecules with apparent pores identified that can facilitate cholesterol transport across the mitochondrial outer membrane.[81]

Taken together, there are substantial data in support of the following model for the role of DBI and MDR in modulating cholesterol intake by mitochondria.[68] The model is that the interaction of DBI and MDR occurs at contact sites of the inner and outer mitochondrial membranes. This interaction is the signal transducer of both hormone-stimulated and constitutive steroidogenesis in the mitochondria. The affinity of the receptor is regulated by hormone-induced changes in the PBR microenvironment with higher-affinity binding resulting in increased cholesterol transport. It also is postulated that hormone-induced release or processing of a higher-molecular-weight DBI immunoreactive protein from the inner mitochondrial membrane can result in intramitochondrial synthesis of DBI to stimulate directly the loading of the P450 side-chain cleaving enzyme with cholesterol. The combination of both proposed mechanisms would yield efficient delivery and utilization of cholesterol by steroidogenic mitochondria.

Most convincingly, a protein termed *steroidogenic acute regulatory protein* (StAR) has been shown to be involved directly in cholesterol transport into mitochondria.[82,83] Initially, radiolabeling and gel electrophoresis demonstrated in cultured adrenal cells of rats a family of approximately 30 kd polypeptides that appeared rapidly in response to corticotropins and that were cycloheximide sensitive.[84] Later studies revealed that these proteins also are present in Leydig cells.[85,86] These proteins have been examined extensively, purified, cloned, and studied for biofunctionality in the MA-10 mouse Leydig cell line. In particular, the 30-kd mitochondrial polypeptide StAR protein has been identified and characterized by means of both biochemical and molecular biologic approaches. Transient transfection and expression of this protein in MA-10 cells increases steroidogenesis without hormonal stimulation.[87] This expression can account quantitatively for a rate and capacity of steroid production equal to those stimulated by hormones.[82] MA-10 cell lines that have been stably transfected for StAR show constitutively high levels of synthesized StAR and produce steroids at levels higher than that of untransfected cells.[82] Nonsteroidogenic cells when transfected with StAR expression vectors become steroidogenic, and this alteration depends on StAR expression.[83] StAR mRNA is under hormonal control; the levels of this mRNA parallel steroid synthesis. In situ hybridization studies demonstrate that these mRNAs are localized only in cells of the ovary, adrenal glands, and testis, consistent with the proposed function of the StAR protein.[88]

Perhaps the greatest interest in the present context is that studies of the disease congenital lipoid adrenal hyperplasia (LCAH) provide a clear demonstration of the role of the StAR polypeptide. LCAH is lethal disease in which newborn infants exhibit a complete lack of steroidogenesis. Death occurs within days to weeks after birth unless the infant receives replacement hormone therapy. It once was thought that the cause of LCAH was a defect in P450 side-chain cleaving enzyme activity, but levels of this critical enzyme have been shown to be normal in affected infants, as have other possible regulatory constituents, including SAP, SCP2, and the PBR/MDR complex.[89,90] However, testicular tissue from two affected patients and genomic DNA of another have mutations in the gene that encodes StAR that yield truncated StAR protein.[91] Moreover, no precursor forms of StAR are converted to mature protein in cells affected by LCAH. Expression of StAR cDNA from patients with LCAH in nonsteroidogenic COS-1 cells demonstrates that the StAR protein produced is inactive in promoting steroidogenesis,[91] but that the requirement for StAR can be circumvented by providing freely diffusible 20α-hydroxycholesterol as a steroidogenic substrate. Thus studies of LCAH involving human infants have demonstrated a clear and direct relation between the StAR polypeptide and the obligatory transport of cholesterol into Leydig cells required for the synthesis of testosterone.

The proposed mechanism whereby the StAR protein functions is summarized elsewhere.[82] Briefly, in response to hormonal stimulation, a precursor protein is synthesized rapidly in the cytosol and aimed at the mitochondria, where it interacts with a specific receptor on the mitochondrial outer membrane. Contact sites then form between the outer and inner organelle membrane as transfer of the StAR protein to the inner compartment begins. Processing of a 37-kd precursor polypeptide yields the mature 30-kd form, which remains associated with either the inner membrane or the intermembrane compartment of the mitochondrion. It presumably is during the processing step and the concomitant formation of the inner and outer membrane contact sites that cholesterol transfer is effected. Finally, after the completion of StAR precursor processing, the membrane contact sites disassemble, and further steroid transport is blocked. It should be noted, however, that it is not yet known whether cholesterol transport occurs passively or whether the StAR protein acts as an actual cholesterol-binding protein during the transfer process. Nonetheless, the identification, characterization, and functional analysis of the StAR protein represents an important new phase in our understanding of the molecular control of Leydig cell function.

After the successful transfer of cholesterol from the cellular cytosol to the inner mitochondrial membrane, the subsequent steps of testosterone formation occur. The androgenic testicular steroids do not contain a long side chain attached to the 17-carbon atom, as does cholesterol (Fig 13–3). A key early step in the conversion of cholesterol to testosterone is, therefore, cleavage of this side chain to form δ-5-pregnenolone. This reaction requires reduced nicotinamide-adenine dinucleotide phosphate (NADPH). The δ-5-pregnenolone is itself an important precursor to all subsequent reactions in the pathway. In the side-chain cleavage pathway, successive oxidations of cholesterol to 20α-hydroxycholesterol take place before a second hydroxyl group is added to yield 20α-, 20R-dihydrocholesterol. The side chain is finally split off between atoms 20 and 22 by the enzyme C20-C22 lyase to form pregnenolone. It is during

these steps of the testosterone biosynthetic pathway that LH, by way of cAMP and the catalytic subunit of protein kinase, modulates testicular androgen levels.

From pregnenolone there are several pathways by which testosterone may be synthesized (see Fig 13–1). It is likely that important species-specific differences exist in the relative effectiveness of these alternative pathways. The δ-4 pathway, for example, seems most important in rats, whereas in humans the δ-5 pathway predominates.[92,93]

Although LH regulates a key step in testosterone biosynthesis, and its levels are known to oscillate with a frequency of two to four waves every 6 hours, there is little reliable evidence for a corresponding pulsatile secretion of testosterone by Leydig cells. Some data show a daily, that is, circadian, cycle of testosterone secretion with maximum levels at awakening, but the amplitude of the change during each day is small, about 10% to 25%.[94]

Testosterone Transport and Metabolism

Blood transport of testosterone is not a simple process. Because of its highly hydrophobic structure, the steroid is predominantly insoluble in aqueous solutions. Its transport is therefore accomplished by binding to specific plasma proteins. In male humans, one of the most important of these transport proteins is testosterone–estradiol-binding globulin (TeBG). This protein is a different polypeptide from cortisol-binding globulin, which transports cortisol, corticosterone, and progesterone. TeBG has been isolated in an active form from blood plasma.[95] It has a molecular weight of 94,000 and contains 30% carbohydrate by weight. It has two subunits, but only one testosterone-binding site per mole.[96] Under hormonal influence, TeBG levels fluctuate widely. Estrogens increase circulating TeBG concentrations by as much as tenfold, whereas testosterone causes twofold decreases in TeBG levels. In humans, TeBG is responsible for the binding and transport of about 30% of the total plasma testosterone; only approximately 3% is free, the remainder being bound to serum albumin and other blood polypeptides. It is probable that testosterone bound to TeBG is inactive, because metabolism of the steroid by target tissues is usually required for physiologic responses. Moreover, the rate of testosterone metabolism measured in humans is directly proportional to the total of free testosterone plus albumin-bound hormone.[97] Not all mammals exhibit TeBG, suggesting that this transport protein may not play an obligatory role in testosterone function.

Metabolism of testosterone accompanies its irreversible removal from the circulation. This removal may be accomplished by means of steroid entry into a cell followed by metabolic alteration to another steroid form. The metabolite may be less active and be destined for excretion. Alternatively, the metabolized steroid may be more active and may exert a stimula-

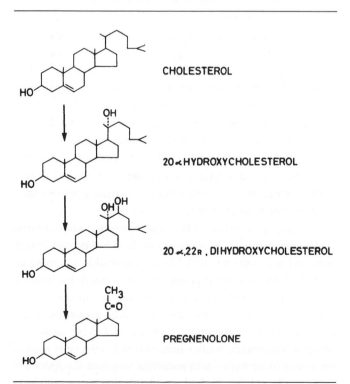

Figure 13–3. The probable pathway for the formation of pregnenolone from cholesterol. Luteinizing hormone stimulation of Leydig cells exerts a strong influence here.

CHOLESTEROL

20 α HYDROXYCHOLESTEROL

20 α,22R , DIHYDROXYCHOLESTEROL

PREGNENOLONE

cleus, the number of lipid inclusions, or the extent of nuclear heterochromatization.

Biochemical responses of Sertoli cells to FSH are exceedingly numerous, involve the synthesis and secretion of both high- and low-molecular-weight moieties, and are undoubtedly critical for the maintenance and regulation of spermatogenesis. A large proportion of the metabolism of Sertoli cells is devoted to the production of glycoproteins in response to FSH. These glycoproteins can be subclassified as (1) transport or bioreactive proteins secreted in high abundance, such as transferrin and ceruloplasmin; (2) proteases and protease inhibitors with the potential to act during the continuous remodeling of the seminiferous epithelium necessitated by germ cell translocation as differentiation proceeds; (3) basement membrane constituents; and (4) regulatory glycoproteins active at relatively low concentrations, such as müllerian inhibiting substance and inhibin.

Although many protein markers for Sertoli cells have been identified, including for example, androgen-binding protein (ABP) and γ-glutamyl transpeptidase, definitive roles for these polypeptide products of FSH stimulation within the seminiferous tubule remain unelucidated. A notable exception, however, is testicular transferrin, an iron-transport protein also synthesized in brain and liver. Sertoli cells contain two forms of transferrin, one apparently identical to the protein detected in serum and another unique to the Sertoli cell itself. Both polypeptides derive from different coding sequences. The Sertoli cell synthesizes its specific form of transferrin to shuttle iron from the bloodstream, at the basal side of the seminiferous tubule, around the highly effective Sertoli cell–Sertoli cell tight junctions. This allows transferrin access into the adluminal compartment of the tubule, providing needed iron to late differentiated germ cells. The Sertoli cells first perform endocytosis on the serum iron–bearing transferrin, dissociate the metal ion, and rechelate it to Sertoli-specific transferrin. This complex is then secreted vectorially, most being aimed above the tight junctional complexes into the lumen of the seminiferous tubule.[123,124] Although virtually all of these steps in the process have been verified adequately by means of in vitro experimentation, the physiologic requirement for such iron transport has best been demonstrated with the study of hypotransferrinemic mice. These animals carry a mutation that results in improper splicing of the transferrin mRNA, such that only 1% to 2% of normal transferrin levels are expressed. Injection of transferrin into the peritoneal cavity of these animals at regular intervals satisfies other bodily needs of these mice but does not result in substantial secretion of transferrin into the testicular adluminal compartment. Morphologic examination of the testes of these mutant animals reveals low sperm counts, large regions of testicular aspermatogenesis, and few sperm stored in the epididymis.[125] The study of Sertoli cell transferrin provides an excellent example of the complexity of the different macromolecular regulatory processes engendered by FSH stimulation of the Sertoli cell surface membrane. Similar results are to be anticipated when additional Sertoli cell secretory products have been analyzed in sufficient detail.

Although present data preclude a well-grounded understanding of the exact roles of FSH- and cAMP-dependent Sertoli cell secretory product function, the issue is confounded further because Sertoli cells also respond to hormonal stimulation by synthesis and secretion of a variety of low-molecular-weight, highly diffusible substances. Prime among these, at least in terms of investigative effort, is intracellular lactate.[126] Differentiation of germ cells in rats and mice depends highly on exogenous lactate and pyruvate for the maximum synthesis of both amino acids and proteins.[127,128] In vitro these cells have been shown to utilize lactate secreted vectorially by Sertoli cells.[129] Isolated populations of human primary pachytene spermatocytes also seem to require exogenous pyruvate for maximal protein synthesis.[130] Although many other cell types produce considerably more total lactate than do Sertoli cells, and although no definitive in vivo genetic model for the obligatory role of Sertoli cell lactate secretion in spermatogenesis has been forthcoming, there seems little doubt that FSH mediation at the level of diffusible secretory compounds is critical in the regulation of spermatogenesis, including testicular function in humans.

The physiologic role of the Sertoli cell and its relation to modulation of hormones produced by the anterior pituitary gland is complex. The key steps in this process may be summarized as follows:

1. FSH binds to specific Sertoli cell plasma membrane receptors and alters adenylate cyclase activity.
2. Intracellular cAMP levels increase because of FSH binding. It should be noted, however, that cAMP levels are also controlled by cAMP phosphodiesterases, which are affected by calcium-dependent calmodulin and other agents.
3. Increased cAMP levels stimulate a cAMP-dependent protein kinase, which phosphorylates a variety of Sertoli cell substrates under the regulation of cytoplasmic phosphokinase inhibitor (PKI).
4. Resultant cellular events include the synthesis and secretion of a large variety of high- and low-molecular-weight compounds, many of which are, or are likely to be, unique to the Sertoli cell. Some, if not all, of these secretory products are involved in the local, paracrine regulation of spermatogenesis. Some Sertoli secretory products, such as inhibin, are also involved in more systemic levels of modulation.
5. Once initiated, most of the FSH-mediated events can be maintained by testosterone alone.

6. Germ cells, testicular myoid cells, and even Leydig cells play important roles in this process, but their importance does not supersede that of the basic FSH-receptor–mediated pathway. Figure 13–4 shows the closely related functioning of the different regulatory levels involved in spermatogenesis within the seminiferous tubule.[131]

Inhibin

A brief discussion of inhibin, a polypeptide secreted by Sertoli cells in response to FSH, is warranted because this is the one important macromolecular component clearly demonstrated to act at the organismic level to provide feedback regulation of spermatogenesis to the pituitary gland. As early as 1932 it was suggested that a water-soluble gonadotropin regulator was produced locally in the testis.[132] Evidence for such a molecule in humans first became apparent in about 1950, when workers reported increases in urinary gonadotropins in men with seminiferous epithelium absent or damaged because of the Sertoli cell-only syndrome, irradiation exposure, and idiopathic oligo-spermia.[133,134] Positive identification of this "inhibin" molecule was, however, long delayed primarily because of technical concerns and problems due to possible contamination by other hormones. Indirect evidence of many types supported the concept that inhibin existed, but biochemical isolation of the molecule was accomplished only in the 1970s.[135,136]

Inhibin consists of two polypeptide chains, of molecular weights 14,000 and 18,000, which may be separated by reduction of interchain bonds. The median effective concentration (EC_{50}) of inhibin is about 0.3 ng/mL (10 pM). Antibodies that recognize the inhibin molecule are able to block its activity in in vitro systems. The gene that encodes inhibin has been cloned and sequenced.[137] This analysis showed that the A chain of inhibin is first synthesized as a large precursor and has glycosylation sites. Across species, comparing humans and pigs, sequence is highly conserved. Few notable differences between the inhibin found in porcine follicular fluid and that secreted by Sertoli cells have been identified. It is firmly established that inhibin is produced by the Sertoli cells and that this represents its only apparent testicular source. The role of inhibin is to feed back negatively on the anterior pituitary gland to maintain func-

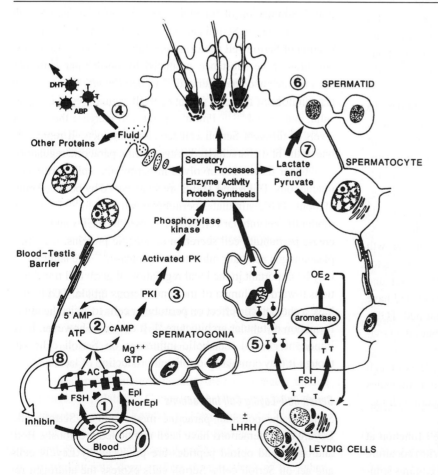

Figure 13–4. Physiologic and structural interrelationships of Sertoli cells and germ cells in the mammalian seminiferous epithelium. Many of the purported paracrine regulatory factors are omitted for clarity. (*Modified from Hansson V: Recent Advances in Male Reproduction: Molecular Basis and Clinical Implications. New York, Raven, 1983.*)

of the primitive germ cells, now termed *gonocytes,* are seen. Until the sixth week of gestation the gonocytes exhibit a round nucleus and a prominent nucleolus. These cells also have sparse mitochondria with tubular cristae and cytoplasma containing numerous microfilaments. A second type of gonocyte that contains extensive cytoplasmic glycogen deposits and many mitochondria disappear by the tenth week of gestation.[195,196]

During the third month of development, fetal spermatogonia are found in humans.[197] The origin of these cells and their relation to the earlier gonocytes is not fully understood. Although in other species many early gonocytes fail to mature,[191,198,199] little is understood in detail for male humans. Investigators have described the proliferation of surviving gonocytic cells,[200] and two populations of germ cells also divide in infant human testis.[201] Quantitative data have been reported on the survival and differentiation of human spermatogonia,[202] but further studies are needed in this area.

Gonocytes differentiate into spermatogonia by means of mitotic division. Spermatogonia continue to undergo rounds of mitosis and form the permanent, renewing stem cell population needed to ensure continuous sperm production during a man's reproductive lifetime. Morphologic studies of human spermatogonia have appeared in the literature.[203–207] Three of four different types can be identified on the basis of morphologic differences in the staining of their cytoplasm, the extent of nuclear heterochromatization, and the cellular position with respect to the basement of the seminiferous tubule. The various spermatogonial populations have been termed *types Ap, Ad, B,* and *AL;* the last type only is discussed by some workers.[204]

Two spermatogonial forms have been described in biopsy specimens of boys 3½ months to 13 years of age.[208,209] Type Ap (type A pale) cells seem most frequent during these ages, and type Ad (type A dark) also are present. Fetal-type spermatogonia are detected up to the age of 4 years. Gonocytes apparently disappear by this age, changing as they do into type Ap spermatogonia. Type A spermatogonia eventually differentiate into type B cells, which are characterized by pale cytoplasm, a spheric nucleus, and clumped, peripheral heterochromatin. In addition, human type B cells may contain a crystal of Lubarsch, a cytoplasmic inclusion composed of packed, parallel, dense filaments and interspersed granules of unknown origin and function.[210] Complete details of the kinetics of spermatogonial proliferation and renewal in animals and humans are not understood, but discussions of this complex problem are available.[211–214]

Meiosis

Type B spermatogonia complete a final mitotic division and then differentiate into primary spermatocytes, initiating meiosis. Meiosis involves two successive nuclear divisions with only one accompanying chromosomal division to achieve haploidy. The first meiotic prophase is long, enabling the processes of chromosomal condensation, pairing, exchange, and separation.

Preleptotene spermatocytes result from the mitotic division of type B spermatogonia. They are characterized by nuclei smaller than those in the type B cells. Preleptotene spermatocytes are located at the periphery of the seminiferous tubule. As they duplicate their DNA, they begin to translocate adluminally, away from the basement membrane regions. The spermatocytes then enter the leptotene stage of meiosis, during which the chromosomes are seen as thin filaments. Leptonema is followed by the zygotene stage, during which synapsis of paired genetic material occurs. The synaptonemal complex is first evident at this stage of development.[191,215–217] Chromosomal thickening, pairing, and exchange continue during the succeeding stage, pachytene spermatocytes. Extensive cell growth occurs during the long pachytene stage, as revealed by both morphometric measurement of overall cell size and biochemical analysis of isolated germ cells in rodents[218–220] and humans.[221,222] After pachynema is complete, spermatocytes enter the diplotene stage, at which time the paired chromosomes begin to separate and chiasmata (chromosomal bridges) may be seen readily. Finally, during diakinesis the chromosomes of each bivalent pair continue to separate as the chiasmata move from the centromeres to the chromosomal telomeres. This completes the first meiotic prophase. Description of detailed spermatocyte morphology during meiosis is published elsewhere.[223]

After diakinesis, the nuclear envelope disintegrates, facilitating alignment of bivalents at the metaphase plate in metaphase I. Anaphase I and telophase I are completed quickly with daughter chromatids moving to opposite poles of the new cells, now called *secondary spermatocytes.* Each secondary spermatocyte contains a haploid number of chromosomes. They are short-lived cells, much smaller than the earlier primary spermatocytes. They are also characterized by spherical nuclei that contain pale, granular chromatin. No DNA synthesis occurs before the second meiotic reduction division. Meiotic interphase II is short, and cells pass rapidly through metaphase II, anaphase II, and telophase II. Completion of these events yields young spermatids, destined to undergo substantial morphologic and biochemical transformation as they develop into testicular spermatozoa.

Spermiogenesis

Spermiogenesis is the process by which a round spermatid transforms morphologically and biochemically into the elongated testicular spermatozoon. This alteration is accomplished without concomitant cell division but involves a host of biochemical changes. Numerous investigators have examined the ultrastructure of spermatozoa in mammals, including humans. Several important reports with emphasis on humans have appeared.[224–233] Differentiating spermatids in humans also have been described in detail.[189,233–236]

The entire process of spermiogenesis is subdivided into four well-described phases: Golgi, cap, acrosome, and maturation. These distinctions are based on the findings of light and electron microscopic morphologic examinations of developing spermatids. During the *Golgi phase,* the new spermatids exhibit an extensive Golgi apparatus in the cytoplasm. The nucleus is spherical, with chromatin condensation not yet initiated. Mitochondria and other normally occurring cytoplasmic organelles are obvious. Soon, proacrosomic granules appear in juxtaposition to the Golgi apparatus. Containing a variety of lytic enzymes, the acrosomal granules fuse, forming a single, large, cytoplasmic compartment called the *acrosomic vesicle.* This vesicle contains a dense granule surrounded by diffusely stained material as seen in electron microscopic examination. The vesicle and granule continue to enlarge, the intracellular position of this structure determining the anterior pole of the differentiating sperm.

Also during the Golgi phase of spermiogenesis, mitochondria leave the perinuclear region and assume positions immediately subjacent to the plasma membrane. The plasma membrane itself seems thickened when examined at the ultrastructural level. Paired centrioles migrate to the nuclear pole opposite that occupied by the acrosomic vesicle as they begin flagellar elongation.

The *cap phase* of spermiogenesis involves continued development of the acrosome, which attaches to the anterior pole of the spermatid nucleus and flattens in close association with the nuclear membrane. Eventually, the acrosomic vesicle covers fully one third to one half of the anterior nuclear surface. This forms the acrosomal cap.

During the *acrosomal phase* of spermatid differentiation the cell nucleus first begins to elongate and condense. The anterior–posterior axis of the cell is well defined, and the cytoplasm is displaced adluminally with respect to the long axis of the entire seminiferous tubule. The anterior nucleus with its associated acrosomal cap becomes closely situated with the overlying plasma membrane as the spermatid nucleus continues elongating. Chromatin condensation also continues until most of the genetic material is involved, and only occasionally do vacuoles remain. These vacuoles often are more pronounced in humans than in other species. The Golgi apparatus detaches from the developing acrosome, and new cytoplasmic organelles appear. The manchette, for example, is composed of microtubules that are aligned parallel to one another and surround the posterior half of the elongating nucleus. Although long postulated to be important in shaping the sperm head, a precise role of the manchette is still unknown. At the site of flagellar attach-

ment to the posterior nucleus, or implantation fossa, organellar structures differentiate to form the eventual neck region of the sperm. From this area, thick, outer, dense fibers develop in concert with the lengthening flagellum. These fibers are characteristic of mammalian spermatozoa. They surround the central microtubular pairs that constitute the flagellar axoneme. The flagellar fibrous sheath is a ribbed structure interposed between the outer dense fibers and the plasma membrane.

Finally, the *maturational phase* of this complex transformation process features the removal and phagocytosis of most residual spermatid cytoplasm by neighboring Sertoli cells. Morphologic details of this event have been reported, but most of the important biochemical events that occur throughout spermiogenesis have not been determined. Much of our current understanding has been reviewed.[191] Figure 13–5 illustrates the important structural steps of human spermiogenesis.[233]

The result of spermiogenesis is a morphologically mature spermatozoon. In humans this cell is about 60 μm long and is subdivided structurally into a head and a tail. The head consists of the nucleus with its associated acrosome and is about 4.5 μm long, 3.0 μm wide, and about 1 μm deep. Human sperm heads have a flattened, oval shape, unlike those of many experimental animals. Joining the head and the tail, the sperm neck

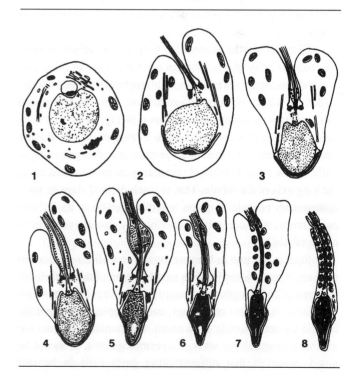

Figure 13–5. The stages of spermiogenesis in humans. (*Modified from Holstein AF: Ultrastructural observations on the differentiation of spermatids in man.* Andrologia 8:157, 1976.)

The overall panoply of changes in sperm motility associated with epididymal maturation have been extensively reviewed.[274,283–289] There are reports that few, but not all, caput epididymal sperm can be stimulated to swim in salt solutions with the addition of egg yolk and caffeine[274] or of defined liposomes.[290] An excellent discussion of the mechanisms involved in inducing motility in caput sperm is available in review.[289] Briefly, egg yolk or phosphatidylcholine liposomes presumably modify the plasma membrane in a way that could alter membrane-bound enzyme activity, ion flux, or substrate transport. Addition of caffeine increases intracellular cAMP level in some of these intact sperm from caput epididymides. It is also possible that throughout the length of the epididymal tract, sperm are in different stages of maturation, which makes some of them capable of fertilization much sooner than the others. However, most sperm gain fertilizing ability when they enter the cauda epididymides. Sperm from the cauda epididymides move with a characteristic flagellar wave, which is different from caput epididymal sperm.[289] Because of data such as these, it may be stated that our knowledge of the biochemistry of sperm maturation is progressing rapidly and that well-defined methods for the improvement of in vitro sperm motility and function should result quickly.

SPERM CAPACITATION AND THE ACROSOMAL REACTION

Epididymal spermatozoa must be capacitated to fertilize. Sperm normally are capacitated as they reside in the female reproductive tract. The exact physiologic and biochemical mechanisms involved in capacitation and the sperm acrosome reaction are still not well-defined for humans. The process in other mammals has been reviewed,[291–293] and therefore complete details are not presented herein. Depending on the particular species being studied, both the timing and the exact events of capacitation vary greatly. Human spermatozoa have been successfully capacitated in a defined tissue culture medium.[294,295] With the advent of human in vitro fertilization (IVF) technology, more workers are conducting clinical trials directed at increasing and maintaining the fertilizing activity of human semen.[296–304] One short review of the varying methods currently being examined in clinical laboratories, including the application of agents such as cytokines, pentoxifylline, phospholipid mediators, and progesterone, provides an excellent starting point for further study of this issue.[305]

On contact with the ovum and its protective investment, the zona pellucida, mammalian sperm undergo the acrosomal reaction during which the acrosome vesiculates, yielding hybrid membrane vesicles composed of acrosomal and plasma membrane components. The process is exocytic and results in exposure of the egg to the lytic enzymes of the acrosome. These enzymes include hyaluronidase, proteinases, glycosidases, lipases, and others. Acrosomal hydroylases are both soluble and attached to the inner acrosomal membranes of the spermatozoon; in either case, they are accessible to the zona pellucida and egg after acrosomal vesiculation.

Regulation of the acrosomal reaction is an important area of research because it is a critical controlling factor in effecting fertilization. Disruption of the acrosomal reaction yields infertility; therefore human sperm have been examined in great detail in attempts to unravel the molecular mechanisms underlying the process of sperm exocytosis. The potential governing factors, however, have proved to be quite complex and elusive.

Ionic regulation is clearly of paramount importance,[291] calcium playing the key role. Current evidence demonstrates that extracellular calcium is absolutely required for both capacitation and acrosomal exocytosis in all mammals. The acrosomal reaction is triggered by an influx of calcium ion, which also promotes sperm membrane potential changes that facilitate fusion with the plasma membrane of the egg.[306,307] It has been demonstrated that mammalian sperm do possess the requisite calcium channels required for the influx of extracellular ion.[308,309] In vitro observations also suggest a role for potassium ion in the regulation of the sperm acrosomal reaction in at least some species, although extracellular potassium per se is not obligatory.[310,311] Na^+,K^+-ATPase may be important in controlling intrasperm concentrations of potassium.[312] Sodium ions also are required for fertilization in both invertebrates and mammals,[291] relatively high concentrations are needed outside the sperm to induce exocytosis of the acrosome. Some extracellular sodium apparently is needed for successful capacitation. As a result of many investigations of the ionic control of sperm acrosomal reactions, the following sequence of events has been proposed: (1) Activation of a sperm sodium–proton exchanger increases intracellular sodium levels. (2) This elevates intracellular pH, which then (3) activates calcium channels to induce a flux of extracellular calcium into the sperm cytoplasm. (4) Elevated levels of intracellular calcium induce exocytosis.

Many other agents are probably important in modulating the human sperm acrosomal reaction and egg-binding events. Bicarbonate, for example, is critical in mediating the progesterone-initiated human sperm acrosomal reaction.[313] Progesterone acts at the level of the sperm membrane,[314] requires increased internal calcium to be effective in inducing sperm exocytosis, involves influxes of chloride ion,[315] and seems to use a unique steroid receptor.[316] It is clear that we still have much to learn regarding the complete control of the sperm acrosomal reaction. The potential clinical relevance of such investigations warrants the effort being expended to elucidate the molecular events that transpire at the time of sperm–egg recognition and fusion.

MECHANISMS OF SPERM–EGG RECOGNITION

After successful transit through the epididymis and release from the successive portions of the male reproductive tract, a fully mature spermatozoon is prepared to bind to the surface of the ovum to initiate fertilization. The molecular mechanisms that govern this specific cell–cell adhesion process are being deciphered, and a limited number of reasonably well-characterized surface receptors and ligands on the plasma membranes of sperm and eggs have been described. This discussion briefly summarizes the current state of knowledge. Sperm surface constituents of potential importance in clinical intervention for fertility–infertility considerations are emphasized. The mechanisms that control sperm–egg binding have been reviewed. The reader is encouraged to pursue these sources for a more complete analysis of this important area of research.[317–319]

The existence of specific sperm and egg surface components responsible for recognition of gamete pairs has been hypothesized since the earliest studies of fertilization conducted by Lillie.[320,321] Investigators have only recently had major success in identifying the relevant molecules, for a variety of technical reasons. In general, plasma membrane constituents are biochemically intractable, being both heavily glycosylated and only sparingly soluble in aqueous solutions. Moreover, the relative lack of abundance of the important macromolecules first necessitated the use of invertebrate animal models, only some of which have apparent relevance to sperm–egg binding mechanisms in mammals, including humans. With the advent of advanced immunologic methods, microanalytical biochemical protocols, and molecular biologic manipulations, however, viable candidate molecules involved in gamete adhesion have been reported.

The situation is perhaps best defined for egg molecules, which act as primary sperm-binding proteins, most initial studies having been conducted with mice. A constituent of the zona pellucida, termed ZP3, is clearly the preeminent sperm-binding element. ZP3 is a glycoprotein of about 83 kd responsible for initial sperm–egg adhesion.[322–324] Its structure is maintained across species, and close homologs have been cloned in humans, guinea pigs, rats, rabbits, hamsters, pigs, and marmosets.[318,325,326] ZP3 is heavily glycosylated with both O- and N-linked oligosaccharides,[327,328] and only about 53% of its molecular weight is attributed to the actual polypeptide chain.[329] Some of these oligosaccharides are critical in mediating the binding of ZP3 to the sperm surface, but it seems that there is a great deal of variation in the exact glycosylation states of ZP3 molecules isolated from different species.[318,319,330] Purified ZP3 binds to sperm and successfully competes for their binding to intact oocytes as well as to isolated zona pellucidae.[331] ZP3 also is able to induce the sperm acrosomal reaction needed before sperm–egg binding.[332,333] According to these and similar findings, ZP3 is believed to be the most important egg constituent in the initial stages of sperm adhesion. Additional egg components, including ZP2 which is also found in the zona pellucida and a number of egg plasma membrane polypeptides, are involved in subsequent secondary interactions between egg and sperm. Although these secondary reactions are necessary for successful fertilization, further discussion is beyond the scope of this chapter. The reader is encouraged to consult reviews for details of these additional gamete adhesion events.

Identification of the sperm surface molecule responsible for direct binding to ZP3 of the oocyte zona pellucida has been problematic. In recent years a small number of candidate molecules have been described and partially characterized. It is entirely possible that more than one sperm-surface molecule is involved in the initial stages of interaction with the zona pellucida, particularly because aggregation of egg ZP3 is a requirement for induction of the sperm acrosome reaction.[329] One or more sperm molecules could be involved in the very first adhesion event, and others might then effect ZP3 aggregation and the acrosomal reaction.

Three prime candidates for sperm receptors for ZP3 are β-1,4-galactosyltransferase (GalTase), which is found on all mammalian spermatozoa[334,335]; a sperm protein, Sp56, which was first purified on the basis of its affinity for ZP3[336,337]; and a sperm polypeptide, p95, first identified because it increased in phosphotyrosine content after binding to ZP3.[338,339]

GalTase has been implicated strongly in the gamete recognition process. Treatment of intact oocytes with N-acetylglucosaminidase inhibits subsequent binding of spermatozoa. This enzyme may be released physiologically from egg cortical granules during formation of the block to polyspermy that occurs during fertilization.[340] ZP3 binds to GalTase unless O-linked oligosaccharides are removed.[341] Transgenic mice which overexpress GalTase undergo precocious acrosome reactions.[342] Many studies demonstrating the receptor/ligand relation between sperm-surface GalTase and egg ZP3 have been reviewed.[334,335]

The sperm protein Sp56 is a homomultimer. As shown with immunohistochemical analysis, it is localized to the outer surface of the sperm head plasma membrane, the correct location for potential involvement in egg binding.[336,343] Cross-linking experiments demonstrate that Sp56 and ZP3 interact using ZP3 O-linked oligosaccharides.[336] However, Sp56 is a peripheral sperm membrane protein; it is not anchored to the underlying membrane lipid bilayer.[318] Therefore, it is unlikely to be the sole mediator of sperm–egg binding.

Finally, sperm polypeptide p95 is localized to the acrosomal region of sperm and clearly serves as a substrate for the tyrosine kinase activity that accompanies the acrosomal reaction.[317] Direct evidence for the molecule–molecule binding of p95 and ZP3 has been difficult to obtain, but synthetic peptides designed to mimic the presumed extracellular domain of p95 are able to inhibit sperm binding to the zona pellucida.[344] It has been shown that p95 is a sperm-specific hexokinase. Amino acid sequence analysis suggests complete homology to a known mouse hexokinase. Antibodies that recognize the mouse hexokinase, moreover, precipitate the p95 moiety.[345] The p95 protein is of definite importance, because no other hexokinases are known to be phosphorylated at tyrosine residues, and because this reaction is triggered by ZP3 activity. The exact role of p95 in sperm–egg adhesion, however, is not yet elucidated.

GalTase, Sp56, and p95 are certainly not the only sperm-surface molecules to be implicated in adhesion to the egg during the beginning stages of fertilization, but they are the molecules that seemingly have the greatest physiologic significance. All of them have been detected on human spermatozoa. Because the formal elucidation of the sperm receptor for ZP3 is critical for possible clinical interventions in infertility, it is expected that investigations of these molecular regulators will proceed rapidly.

NORMAL SEMEN ANALYSIS

Several conditions may result in male-factor infertility. Semen variables that must be considered include abnormal sperm count, sperm motility, fluid volume, fluid viscosity, and the presence of cells other than spermatozoa. Furthermore, one must consider the possible contribution of varicocele, stress, infection, substance abuse, and other similar factors. Both azoospermia and oligospermia may become established because of genetic disorders, endocrinopathies, and other disruptions of either spermatogenesis itself or the ductal system of the male reproductive tract. Subnormal sperm motility may be the result of immunologic causes, infection, morphologic defects in spermatozoa, or poor liquefaction of semen.

Extensive variations in normal semen values always are encountered both among individuals and among samples from particular patients. It is necessary to perform several semen studies (usually three) before a definitive baseline diagnosis is stated. Standard analytic procedures, usually those promulgated by the World Health Organization,[346] have been used so that results may be compared between different laboratories. At least 2 days of sexual abstinence should be required before the collection of sperm by means of masturbation. More extended periods of abstinence usually are not needed and may result in differences in ejaculate volume, which may confound the analysis. Sperm should be stored in a clean glass receptacle and brought to the laboratory within 60 to 120 minutes of collection. Samples must not be exposed to temperature extremes. The time of sperm collection, period of abstinence, and any spillage should

be recorded carefully. To allow for liquefaction, semen should not be examined for at least 30 minutes after ejaculation but should be examined before 2 hours have elapsed. Examination after liquefaction should include determination of viscosity, color, volume, pH, and the persistence of any gel material. An aliquot of raw semen is examined with a light microscope (total magnification $\times 400$ to $\times 600$) and assayed for sperm number, agglutination or aggregation, particulate debris, and round cells. The semen must be well mixed, usually with a vortex mixer, before microscopic study. Samples need not be stained, but if unstained preparations are used, a phase contrast microscope is preferable because of the low inherent contrast of biologic specimens.

Sperm number or concentration should first be estimated to determine a proper dilution for final quantification. That analysis of sperm concentration is not straightforward.[347] With a $\times 40$ objective, the mean number of spermatozoa in several fields is counted. This number multiplied by 10 million provides a rough approximation of the final sperm count. Definitive sperm concentrations may be calculated with a hemocytometer, a Makler counter, or one of several computerized instruments. Low sperm counts should be assessed with a hemocytometer or Makler chamber, as should observations on single samples from which immediate data are required. Samples are diluted as needed in bicarbonate-buffered formalin with gentian violet stain, thoroughly mixed, and examined by means of normal counting protocols. Only spermatozoa that are seemingly mature and that have attached tails are counted. For two different dilutions of the same sample, values should not exceed 10% at low sperm density or 20% at densities greater than 60 million/mL. Concentration is the number of sperm per milliliter of semen; count is the total number of sperm in the ejaculate. Sperm concentrations of 20 to 250 million/mL are usually considered normal, but there are many instances of fertile men with values well below this range. The total number of sperm per ejaculate also varies, but values of 20 million to about 80 million are usually thought to be less than normal (oligospermia). *Azoospermia* means complete absence of spermatozoa in an ejaculate.

Sperm motility is usually assessed by means of microscopic examination. A single drop (2 to 3 mm in diameter) is placed on a slide and covered with an 18-mm^2 coverslip. The sample must be examined immediately to prevent drying artifacts, and the time and temperature conditions during the assay should be standardized. Motility is quantified by means of observation of both motile and immotile cells in at least 10 different randomly chosen fields. A minimum of 100 sperm per field should be observed; the percentage of motile sperm is calculated from the mean value for all fields assayed and adjusted to the nearest 5%. Forward sperm motility is often graded subjectively with one of a number of numerical scales that discrimi-

TABLE 13–1. SHAPES AND FREQUENCIES OF SHAPES OF SPERM HEADS IN NORMAL HUMAN EJACULATES

Morphology	Frequency			
	Mean	*Low*	*High*	*Standard Deviation*
Normal	80.5	48.0	98.0	9.7
Large oval head	0.3	0.0	5.2	0.6
Small oval head	1.4	0.0	13.5	1.8
Tapering head	0.4	0.0	6.2	0.9
Pyriform head	2.0	0.0	21.8	2.8
Duplicate head	1.5	0.0	8.3	1.5
Amorphous head	6.5	0.0	24.9	4.0
Tail defect	5.2	0.0	37.4	4.7
Cytoplasmic droplet	2.2	0.0	14.5	2.1

From Schulze C: On the morphology of the human Sertoli cell. Cell Tissue Res 153:339, 1974.

nate between no, good, or excellent motility. Normal semen samples have 60% or more motile sperm, most of these exhibiting good to excellent forward progression up to 3 hours after ejaculation. Abnormal motility patterns, such as circling movements, should be recorded. Samples with less than 40% motility or impaired forward progression dictate reassessment; both fresh samples and samples taken after prolonged abstinence from either intercourse or masturbation should be used.

The subjective nature of sperm motility measurements has encouraged the recent application of computerized methods to analyze sperm movement in vitro.[348–350] Sophisticated programs facilitate detailed determination of the percentage of motile sperm, their average speed, frequency distributions of velocities, and finely graded quantifiable values for forward progression, including figures that describe the linearity of motion and lateral sperm-head displacement from the forward progression track. These methods have a clear advantage in their relative lack of subjectivity. It is, however, still not evident exactly which of the computerized values are most relevant as predictive factors or what the normal ranges for these values may be. Direct comparisons between computerized determinations and noncomputerized assays on the same samples often produce disconcordant results.[351] As a result, it is difficult to recommend complete reliance on these machines without careful internal standardization of the software with ongoing manual methods already operant in individual laboratories. There is little doubt, however, that the use of computerized technologies will continue to increase and should soon be the method of choice.

Morphologic assessment of spermatozoa and contaminating cells in the ejaculate is an important test of semen normalcy. A freshly smeared slide of the semen sample is usually fixed and stained with fast green stain, Wright's stain, or Giemsa stain. Eosin Y-nigrosin is often used. The total number and percentage of leukocytes or other round cells is easily determined

from light microscopic study of stained samples and hemocytometer counts. Morphology is assayed by means of examination of at least 100 sperm that possess intact tails. Particular attention should be paid to the general shape of the sperm head. The various shapes and their frequencies in normal ejaculates from humans are presented in Table 13–1.[352] As with determinations of sperm motility in vitro, computerized analysis is being developed for measurements of abnormal sperm morphology.[353] These methods are not yet in general clinical application, but rapid progress is expected.

REFERENCES

1. Von Kolliker R: *Beitrage zur Kenntnis der Geschlectsverhaltnisse und der Samenflussigkeit wirbelloser Tiere.* Berlin, 1841

2. Leydig F: Zur Anatomie der mannlichen Geschlechtsorgane und Analdrusen der Saugetiere. *Z Wiss Zool* 2:1, 1850

3. Bouin P, Ancel P: Recherches sur les cellulares interstitielles du testicule des mammiferes. *Arch Zool Exp Gen* 1:437, 1903

4. Christensen AK: Leydig cells. In: Hamilton DW, Greep RD (eds), *Handbook of Physiology. V. Male Reproductive System.* Washington, DC, American Physiological Society, 1975:57–94

5. Fawcett DW, Neaves WB, Flores MN: Comparative observations on intertubular lymphatics and the organization of the interstitial tissue of the mammalian testis. *Biol Reprod* 9:500, 1973

6. Setchell BP: Reproduction in male marsupials. In: Gilmore DP, Stonehouse B (eds), *Marsupials.* London, Macmillan, 1977: 411–457

7. Huhtaniemi I, Pelliniemi LJ: Fetal Leydig cells: Cellular origin, morphology, life span, and special functional features. *Proc Soc Exp Biol Med* 201:125, 1992

8. Rabinovici J, Jaffe RB: Development and regulation of growth and differentiation function in human and subhuman primate fetal gonads. *Endocr Rev* 11:532, 1990

9. Tapanainen J, Kellokumpu-Lehtinen P, Pelliniemi L, Huhtaniemi I: Age-related changes in endogenous steroids of human fetal testis during early and midpregnancy. *J Clin Endocrinol Metab* 52:98, 1981

10. Reyes FI, Winter JSD, Faiman C: Endocrinology of the fetal testis. In: Burger H, de Kretser D (eds), *The Testis,* ed 2. New York, Raven, 1989:119–142

11. Zondek LH, Zondek T: Fetal hilar cells and Leydig cells in early pregnancy. *Biol Neonate* 30:193, 1975

12. Voutilainen R, Miller WL: Developmental expression of genes for the steroidogenic enzymes P450scc (20,22-desmolase), P450c17 (17 α-hydroxylase/17,20-lyase), and P450c21 (21-hydroxylase) in the human fetus. *J Clin Endocrinol Metab* 63:1145, 1986

13. Weniger JP: Steroid secretion by foetal mammal gonads and its regulation by gonadotrophins. *Reprod Nutr Dev* 26:921, 1986

14. Kaplan SL, Grumbach MM, Aubert ML: The ontogenesis of pituitary hormones and hypothalamic factors in the human testis: Maturation of central nervous system—regulation of anterior pituitary function. *Recent Prog Horm Res* 32:161, 1976

15. Molsberry RL, Carr BR, Mendelson CR, Simpson ER: Human chorionic gonadotrophin binding to human fetal testis as a function of gestational age. *J Clin Endocrinol Metab* 55:791, 1982

16. Huhtaniemi IT, Korenbrot CC, Jaffe RB: HCG binding and stimulation of testosterone biosynthesis in the human fetal testis. *J Clin Endocrinol Metab* 44:963, 1977

17. Leinonen PJ, Jaffe RB: Leydig cell desensitization by human chorionic gonadotrophin does not occur in the human fetal testis. *J Clin Endocrinol Metab* 61:234, 1985

18. Word RA, George FW, Wilson JD, Carr BR: Testosterone synthesis and adenylate cyclase activity in the early human fetal testis appear to be independent of human chorionic gonadotrophin control. *J Clin Endocrinol Metab* 69:204, 1989

19. Fouquet J-P, Meusy-Dessolle N, Dang DC: Relationships between Leydig cell morphometry and plasma testosterone during postnatal development of the monkey, *Macaca fascicularis. Reprod Nutr Dev* 24:281, 1984

20. Prince FP: Ultrastructural evidence of mature Leydig cells and Leydig cell regression in the neonatal human testis. *Anat Rec* 228:405, 1990

21. Codesal J, Regadera J, Nistal M, Regadera Rejas J, Paniagua R: Involution of human fetal Leydig cells: An immunohistochemical, ultrastructural and quantitative study. *J Anat* 172:103, 1990

22. Nistal M, Paniagua R, Regadera J, Santomaria L, Amat P: A quantitative morphological study of human Leydig cells from birth to adulthood. *Cell Tissue Res* 246:229, 1986

23. Neaves MB, Johnson L, Porter JC, Parker CR, Petty CS: Leydig cell numbers, daily sperm production and serum gonadotrophin in ageing males. *J Clin Endocrinol Metab* 59:756, 1984

24. Prince FP: Ultrastructure of immature Leydig cells in the human prepubertal testis. *Anat Rec* 209:165, 1984

25. Christensen AK, Peacock KC: Increase in Leydig cell number in testes of adult rats treated chronologically with an excess of hCG. *Biol Reprod* 22:282, 1980

26. Molenaar R, de Rooij DG, Rommerts FFG, van den Hurk R, Wensing CJG: Repopulation of Leydig cells in mature rats after selective destruction of the existent Leydig cell population with ethylene dimethane sulfonate (EDS) is dependent on LH and not FSH. *Endocrinology* 118:2546, 1986

27. Teerds KJ, de Rooij DG, Rommerts FFG, van den Hurk R, Wensing CJG: Proliferation and differentiation of possible Leydig cell precursors after destruction of the existing Leydig cells with ethane dimethyl sulphonate: The role of LH/human chorionic gonadotrophin. *J Endocrinol* 122:689, 1989

28. Bardin CW, Bullock LP, Sherins RJ, Mowszowocz I, Blackburn WR: Androgen metabolism and mechanism of action in male pseudohermaphroditism: A study of testicular feminization. *Recent Prog Horm Res* 29:65, 1973

29. Berthezene F, Forest MJ, Grimaud JA, Claustrat B, Mornex R: Leydig cell agenesis. *N Engl J Med* 295:969, 1976

30. Abramowitz J, Iyengar R, Birnbaumer L: Guanyl nucleotide regulation of hormonally responsive adenyl cyclases. *Mol Cell Endocrinol* 16:129, 1979

31. Catt KJ, Dufua ML: Gonadotrophin receptors and regulation of interstitial cell function in the testis. *Recent Horm Act* 3:291, 1978.

32. Minegishi T, Nakamura K, Takakura Y, et al: Cloning and sequencing of human LH/hCG receptor cDNA. *Biochem Biophys Res Commun* 172:1049, 1990

33. Dohlman HG, Thorner J, Caron MG, Lefkowitz RJ: Model systems for the study of seven transmembrane segment receptors. *Annu Rev Biochem* 60:653, 1991

34. Parmentier M, Libert F, Maenhaut C, et al: Molecular cloning of the thyrotropin receptor. *Science* 246:1620, 1990

35. Sprengel R, Braun T, Nikolics K, Segaloff DL, Seeburg PH: The testicular receptor for follicle stimulating hormone: Structure and functional expression of cloned cDNA. *Mol Endocrinol* 4:525, 1990

36. Lei ZM, Rao ChV, Kornyei JL, Licht P, Hiatt ES: Novel expression of human chorionic gonadotrophin/luteinizing hormone receptor gene in brain. *Endocrinology* 132:2262, 1993

37. Frazier AL, Robbins LS, Stork PJ, Sprengel R, Segaloff DL, Cone RD: Isolation of TSH and LH/CG receptor cDNAs from human thyroid: Regulation by tissue specific splicing. *Mol Endocrinol* 4:1264, 1990

38. Remy JJ, Bozon V, Couture L, Goxe B, Salesse R, Garnier J: Reconstitution of a high-affinity functional lutropin receptor by coexpression of its extracellular and membrane domains. *Biochem Biophys Res Commun* 193:1023, 1993

39. Braun T, Schofield PR, Sprengel R: Amino-terminal leucine-rich repeats in gonadotropin receptors determine hormone selectivity. *EMBO J* 10:1885, 1991

40. Xie YB, Wang H, Segaloff DL: Extracellular domain of lutropin/choriogonadotropin receptor expressed in transfected cells binds choriogonadotropin with high affinity. *J Biol Chem* 265:21411, 1990

41. Tsai-Morris CH, Buczko E, Wang W, Dufau ML: Intronic nature of the rat luteinizing hormone receptor gene defines a soluble receptor subspecies with hormone binding activity. *J Biol Chem* 265:19385, 1990

42. VuHai-LuuThi MT, Misrahi M, Houllier A, Jolivet A, Milgrom E: Variant forms of the pig lutropin/choriogonadotropin receptor. *Biochemistry* 31:8377, 1992

43. Rodriguez MC, Xie YB, Wang H, Collison K, Segaloff DL: Effects of truncations of the cytoplasmic tail of the luteinizing hormone/chorionic gonadotropin (LH/hCG) receptor precursor in a human kidney cell line stably transfected with the rat luteal LH/hCG receptor complementary DNA. *Mol Endocrinol* 6:327, 1992

44. Saez JM, Haour F, Cathiard AM: Early hCG-induced desensitization in Leydig cells. *Biochem Biophys Res Commun* 81:552, 1978

45. Haour F, Sanchez P, Cathiard AM, Saez JM: Gonadotrophin receptor regulation in hypophysectomized rat Leydig cells. *Biochem Biophys Res Commun* 81:547, 1978

46. Catt KJ, Tsuruhara T, Mendelson C, Ketelegers J-M, Dufau ML: Gonadotropin binding and activation of the interstitial cells of the testis. *Curr Top Mol Endocrinol* 1:1, 1874

47. Dufau ML, Catt KJ: Gonadotropin receptors and regulation of steroidogenesis in the testis and ovary. *Vitam Horm* 36:461, 1978.

48. Kirschner MA, Widner JA, Ross GT: Leydig cell function in men with gonadotropin-producing testicular tumors. *J Clin Endocrinol Metab* 30:504, 1970

49. Rebois RV, Fishman PH: Down-regulation of gonadotropin receptors in a murine Leydig tumor cell line. *J Biol Chem* 259:3096, 1984

50. Mather JP, Saez JM, Haour F: Regulation of gonadotropin receptors and steroidogenesis in cultured porcine Leydig cells. *Endocrinology* 110:933, 1982

51. West AP, Cooke BA: Regulation of the truncation of luteinizing hormones receptors at the plasma membrane is different in rat and mouse Leydig cells. *Endocrinology* 128:363, 1991

52. Wang H, Segaloff DL, Ascoli M: Lutropin/choriogonadotropin down-regulates its receptor by both receptor-mediated endocytosis and a cAMP-dependent reduction in receptor mRNA. *J Biol Chem* 266:780, 1991

53. Nelson S, Ascoli M: Epidermal growth factor, a phorbol ester, and 3′,5′-cyclic adenosine monophosphate decrease the transcription of the luteinizing hormone/chorionic gonadotropin receptor gene in MA-10 Leydig tumor cells. *Endocrinology* 130:615, 1992

54. Chuzel F, Schteingart H, Avallet O, Vigier M, Saez JM: LH/hCG induces an increase in the rate of pig Leydig cell receptor mRNA degradation. In: Bartke A (ed), *Function of Somatic Cells in the Testis.* New York, Springer-Verlag, 1992:286–292

55. Lu DL, Peegel H, Mosier SM, Menon MKJ: Loss of lutropin (human choriogonadotropin) receptor messenger ribonucleic acid during ligand-induced down-regulation occurs post-transcriptionally. *Endocrinology* 132:235, 1993

56. Weiss J, Axelrod L, Whitcomb RW, Harris PE, Crowley WF, Jameson JL: Hypogonadism caused by a single amino acid substitution in the β subunit of luteinizing hormone. *N Engl J Med* 326:179, 1992

57. Shenker A, Laue L, Kosugi S, Merendino JS, Minegishi T, Cutler GB: A constitutively activating mutation of the luteinizing hormone receptor in familial male precocious puberty. *Nature* 365:652, 1993

58. Lipsett MB, Wilson H, Kirschner MA, et al: Studies on Leydig cell physiology and pathology: Secretion and metabolism of testosterone. *Recent Prog Horm Res* 22:245, 1966

59. Saez JM: Leydig cells: Endocrine, paracrine, and autocrine regulation. *Endocr Rev* 15:574, 1994

60. Vanhouny GV, Chanderahan R, Noland BJ, Scallen TJ: Cholesterol ester hydroxylase and sterol carrier proteins. *Endocr Res* 10:473, 1985

61. Yamamoto R, Kallen CB, Babalola GO, Rennert H, Billheimer JT, Strauss JF: Cloning and expression of a cDNA encoding human sterol carrier protein 2. *Proc Natl Acad Sci USA* 88:463, 1991

62. Van Noort M, Rommerts FFC, Van Amerougen A, Wirtz KWA: Localisation and hormonal regulation of the nonspecific lipid transfer protein (sterol carrier protein 2) in the rat testis. *J Endocrinol* 109:R13, 1988

63. Hall PF, Almahbori G: The role of the cytoskeleton in the regulation of steroidogenesis. *J Steroid Biochem Mol Biol* 43:769, 1992

64. Xu T, Bowman EP, Glasi DB, Lambeth JD: Stimulation of adrenal mitochondrial cholesterol side-chain cleavage by GTP: Steroidogenesis activator polypeptide (SAP) and sterol carrier protein 2. *J Biol Chem* 266:6801, 1991

65. Pedersen RC, Brownie AC: Cholesterol side-chain cleavage in the rat adrenal cortex: Isolation of a cycloheximide-sensitive activator protein. *Proc Natl Acad Sci USA* 80:1882, 1983

66. Pedersen RC, Brownie AC: Steroidogenesis activator polypeptide isolated from a rat Leydig cell tumor. *Science* 236:188, 1987

67. Meretz LM, Pedersen RC: The kinetics of steroidogenesis activator polypeptide in the rat adrenal cortex. *J Biol Chem* 264:15276, 1989

68. Papadopoulos V, Brown AS: Role of the peripheral-type benzodiazepine receptor and the polypeptide diazepam binding inhibitor in steroidogenesis. *J Steroid Biochem Mol Biol* 53:103, 1995

69. Papadopoulos V: Peripheral-type benzodiazepine/diazepam binding inhibitor receptor: Biological role in steroidogenic cell function. *Endocr Rev* 14:222, 1993

70. Garnier M, Boujrad N, Oke BO, et al: Diazepam binding inhibitor is a paracrine/autocrine regulator of Leydig cell proliferation and steroidogenesis: Action via peripheral-type benzodiazepine receptor and independent mechanisms. *Endocrinology* 132:444, 1993

71. Papadopoulos V, Guarneri P, Krueger KE, Guidotti A, Costa E: Pregnenolone biosynthesis in C6-2B glyoma mitochondria: Regulation by a mitochondrial diazepam binding inhibitor receptor. *Proc Natl Acad Sci USA* 89:5113, 1992

72. Mukhin AG, Papadopoulos V, Costa E, Krueger KE: Mitochondrial benzodiazepine receptors regulate steroid biosynthesis. *Proc Natl Acad Sci USA* 86:9813, 1989

73. Papadopoulos V, Mukhin AG, Costa E, Krueger KE: The peripheral-type benzodiazepine receptor is functionally linked to Leydig cell steroidogenesis. *J Biol Chem* 265:3772, 1990

74. Papadopoulos V, Nowzari FB, Krueger KE: Hormone-stimulated steroidogenesis is coupled to mitochondrial benzodiazepine receptors. *J Biol Chem* 266:3682, 1991

75. Bovolin P, Schlichting J, Miyata J, Ferrarese C, Guidotti A, Alho H: Distribution and characterization of diazepam binding inhibitor (DBI) in peripheral tissues of rat. *Regul Pept* 29:267, 1990

76. Rheaume E, Thonon MC, Smith F, et al: Localization of the endogenous benzodiazepine ligand octadecaneuropeptide in the rat testis. *Endocrinology* 129:1481, 1990

77. Papadopoulos V, Berkovich A, Krueger KE, Costa E, Guidotti A: Diazepam binding inhibitor and its processing products stimulate mitochondrial steroid biosynthesis via an interaction with mitochondrial benzodiazepine receptors. *Endocrinology* 129:1481, 1991

78. Brown AS, Hall PF, Shoyab M, Papadopoulos V: Endozepine/diazepam binding inhibitor in adrenocortical and Leydig cell lines: Absence of hormone regulation. *Mol Cell Endocrinol* 83:1, 1992

79. Cavallaro S, Korneyev A, Guidotti A, Costa E: Diazepam-binding inhibitor (DBI) processing products, acting at the mitochondrial DBI receptor, mediate adrenocorticotropic hormone-induced steroidogenesis in rat adrenal gland. *Proc Natl Acad Sci USA* 89:10598, 1992

80. Garnier M, Boujrad N, Ogwuegbu SO, Hudson JR Jr, Papadopoulos V: The polypeptide diazepam-binding inhibitor and a higher affinity mitochondrial peripheral-type benzodiazepine receptor sustain constitutive steroidogenesis in the R2C Leydig tumor cell line. *J Biol Chem* 269:22105, 1994

81. Papadopoulos V, Boujrad N, Ikonomivic MD, Ferrara P, Vidic B: Topography of the Leydig cell mitochondrial peripheral-type benzodiazepine receptor. *Mol Cell Endocrinol* 104:R5, 1994

82. Stocco DM, Clark BJ: Role of the steroidogenic acute regulatory protein (StAR) in steroidogenesis. *Biochem Pharmacol* 51:197, 1996.

83. Stocco DM, Clark BJ: Regulation of the acute production of steroids in steroidogenic cells. *Endocr Rev* 17:1, 1996

84. Krueger RJ, Orme-Johnson NR: Acute adrenocorticotropic hormone stimulation of adrenal corticosteroidogenesis. *J Biol Chem* 258:10159, 1983

85. Epstein LF, Orme-Johnson NR: Acute action of luteinizing hormone on mouse Leydig cells: Accumulation of mitochondrial phosphoproteins and stimulation of testosterone biosynthesis. *Mol Cell Endocrinol* 81:113, 1991

86. Pon LA, Epstein LF, Orme-Johnson NR: Acute cAMP stimulation in Leydig cells: Rapid accumulation of a protein similar to that detected in adrenal cortex and corpus luteum. *Endocr Res* 12:429, 1986

87. Clark BJ, Wells J, King SR, Stucco DM: The purification, cloning, and expression of a novel luteinizing hormone-induced mitochondrial protein in MA-10 mouse Leydig tumor cells: Characterization of the steroidogenic acute regulatory protein (StAR). *J Biol Chem* 269:28314, 1994

88. Clark BJ, Soo S-C, Caron KM, Ikeda Y, Parker KL, Stocco DM: Hormonal and developmental regulation of the steroidogenic acute regulatory protein. *Mol Endocrinol* 9:1346, 1995

89. Lin D, Gitelman SE, Saenger P, Miller WL: Normal genes for the cholesterol side chain cleavage enzyme, P450scc, in congenital lipoid adrenal hyperplasia. *J Clin Invest* 88:1955, 1991

90. Lin D, Chand YJ, Strauss JF III, Miller WL: The human peripheral benzodiazepine receptor gene: Cloning and characterization of alternative splicing in normal tissues and in a patient with congenital lipoid adrenal hyperplasia. *Genomics* 18:643, 1993

91. Lin D, Sugawara T, Strauss JF III, et al: Role of steroidogenic acute regulatory protein in adrenal and gonadal steroidogenesis. *Science* 267:1828, 1995

92. Yanahara T, Troen P: Studies of the human testis. I. Biosynthetic pathways for androgen formation in human testicular tissue in vitro. *J Clin Endocrinol Metab* 34:783, 1972

93. Yen SSC, Jaffe RB: *Reproductive Endocrinology.* Philadelphia, Saunders, 1986:183

94. Rosner W, Smith RN: Isolation and characterization of the testosterone-estradiol-binding globulin from human plasma: Use of a novel affinity column. *Biochemistry* 14:4813, 1975

95. Musto NA, Larrea F, Cheng S-L, et al: Extracellular androgen binding proteins: species comparison and structure-function relationships. *Ann N Y Acad Sci* 383:342, 1982

96. Vermeulen A, Verdonck L, Van der Straeten M, Orie N: Capacity of the testosterone-binding globulin in human plasma and influence of specific binding of testosterone on its metabolic clearance rates. *J Clin Endocrinol Metab* 29:1470, 1969

97. Bardin CW, Catterall JR: Testosterone: A major determinant of extragenital sexual dimorphism. *Science* 211:1285, 1981

98. Baird DT, Horton R, Longcope C, Tait JF: Steroid dynamics under steady state conditions. *Recent Prog Horm Res* 25:611, 1969

99. Swerdloff RS, Heber D: Endocrine control of testicular function from birth to puberty. In: Burger H, de Kretser D (eds), *The Testis.* New York, Raven, 1981:108–126

100. Connell CJ, Connell GM: The interstitial tissue of the testis. In: Johnson AD, Gomes WR (eds), *The Testis.* New York, Academic Press, 1977:333

101. Risley MS, Tan IP, Roy C, Saez JC: Cell-age and stage-dependent distribution of connexin-43 gap junctions in the testis. *J Cell Sci* 103:81, 1992

102. Kerr JB, Sharpe RM: Follicle-stimulating hormone induction of Leydig cell maturation. *Endocrinology* 116:2592, 1985

103. Odell WD, Swerdloff RS, Jacobs HS, Hercox MA: FSH induction of sensitivity to LH: One cause of sexual maturation in the male rat. *Endocrinology* 92:160, 1973

104. Moger WH, Murphy PR: Reevaluation of the effect of follicle-stimulating hormone on the steroidogenic capacity of the testis: The effects of neuraminidase-treated FSH preparations. *Biol Reprod* 26:422, 1982

105. Vihko KK, LaPolt P, Nishimori K, Hsueh AJW: Stimulatory effects of recombinant follicle-stimulating hormone on Leydig function and spermatogenesis in immature hypophysectomized rats. *Endocrinology* 129:1926, 1991

106. Russell LD, Corbin TJ, Borg KE, de Franca LR, Grasso P, Bartke A: Recombinant human follicle-stimulating hormone is capable of exerting a biological effect in adult hypophysectomized rat by reducing the numbers of degenerating germ cells. *Endocrinology* 133:2062, 1993

107. Sharpe RM: Paracrine control of the testis. *Clin Endocrinol* 15:185, 1986

108. Saez JM, Perrard-Sapori MH, Chatelain PG, Tabone E, Rivarola MA: Paracrine regulation of testicular function. *J Steroid Biochem* 27:317, 1987

109. Bergh A: Local differences in Leydig cell morphology in the adult rat testis: Evidence for a local control of Leydig cells by adjacent seminiferous tubules. *Int J Androl* 5:325, 1982

110. Tabone E, Benahmed M, Reventos J, Saez JM: Interaction between immature porcine Leydig and Sertoli cells in vitro: Ultrastructural and biochemical study. *Cell Tissue Res* 237:357, 1984

111. Reventos J, Perrard-Sapori MH, Chatelian PG, Saez JM: Leydig cell and extracellular matrix effects on Sertoli cell function: Biochemical and morphologic studies. *J Androl* 10:359, 1989

112. Verhoeven G, Cailleau J: Influence of coculture with Sertoli cells on steroidogenesis in immature rat Leydig cells. *Mol Cell Endocrinol* 71:239, 1990

113. Verhoeven G, Cailleau J: Rat tumor Leydig cells as a best system for the study of Sertoli cell factors that stimulate steroidogenesis. *J Androl* 12:9, 1991

114. Lejeune H, Skalli M, Sanchez P, Avallet O, Saez JM: Enhance-

191. Bell
sis.
vol l

192. Bust
Revi
nesis
ence

193. Wits
the
Publ
1948

194. Wag
Testi
Univ

195. Wart
prana
nenn
Gonc
wick

196. Wart
gisch

197. Gonc
the h

198. Aller
I. An
rats a

199. Ross
natal

200. Manc
the g
Cytol
136:4

201. Vilar
adole
Testis

202. Roos
sperm

203. Clern
gonia

204. Rowl
types

205. Fuku
the fe

206. Warte
germ

207. Schul
stem

208. Segue
suchu
zur p
95:13

209. Hadzi
uber
der g
1976

115. Vornberger W, Prins G, Musto NA, Suarez-Quian CA: Androgen receptor distribution in rat testis: New implications for androgen regulation of spermatogenesis. *Endocrinology* 134:2307, 1994

116. Zirkin BR, Awoniyi C, Griswold MD, Russell LD, Sharpe R: Is FSH required for adult spermatogenesis? *J Androl* 15:273, 1994

117. Fritz I: Sites of actions of androgens and follicle stimulating hormone on cells of the seminiferous tubule. In: Litwack D (ed), *Biochemical Actions of Hormones.* New York, Academic Press, 1978:249–278

118. Steinberger E: Hormonal control of mammalian spermatogenesis. *Physiol Rev* 51:1, 1971

119. Means AR, Vaitukaitus J: Peptide hormone "receptors": Specific binding of 3H-FSH to testis. *Endocrinology* 90:39, 1972

120. Rabin D: Binding of human FSH and its subunits to rat testis. In: Dufau ML, Means AR (eds), *Hormone Binding and Target Cell Activation in Testis.* New York, Plenum, 1974:221–236

121. Dym M, Madhwa Raj HG: Response of adult rat Sertoli cells and Leydig cells to depletion of luteinizing hormone and testosterone. *Biol Reprod* 17:676, 1977

122. Chemes HE, Dym M, Madhwa Raj HG: Hormonal regulation of Sertoli cell differentiation. *Biol Reprod* 21:251, 1979

123. Sylvester SR, Griswold MD: The testicular iron shuttle: A "nurse" function of Sertoli cells. *J Androl* 15:381, 1994

124. Sylvester SR, Griswold MD: Molecular biology of iron transport in the testis. In: de Kretser D (ed), *Molecular Biology of the Male Reproductive System.* San Diego, Academic Press, 1993: 311–327

125. Griswold MD: Interactions between germ cells and Sertoli cells in the testis. *Biol Reprod* 52:211, 1995

126. Jutte NHPM, Jansen R, Grootegoed JA, Rommerts FFG, van der Molen HJ: FSH stimulation of the production of pyruvate and lactate by rat Sertoli cells may be involved in hormonal regulation of spermatogenesis. *J Reprod Fertil* 68:219, 1983

127. Nakamura M, Hino A, Yasumasu I, Kato J: Stimulation of protein synthesis in round spermatids from rat testis by lactate. *J Biochem (Tokyo)* 89:1309, 1981

128. Mita M, Hall PF: Metabolism of round spermatids from rats: Lactate as the preferred substrate. *Biol Reprod* 26:445, 1982

129. Jutte NHPM, Jansen R, Grootgoed JA, et al: Regulation of survival of rat pachytene spermatocytes by lactate supply from Sertoli cells. *J Reprod Fertil* 65:431, 1982

130. Nakamura M, Ishida K, Waku M, Okinaga S, Arai K: Stimulation of protein synthesis in pachytene primary spermatocytes from the human testis by pyruvate. *Andrologia* 17:561, 1985

131. Hansson V: *Recent Advances in Male Reproduction: Molecular Basis and Clinical Implications.* New York, Raven, 1983

132. McCullagh DR: Dual endocrine activity of testis. *Science* 76:19, 1932

133. Del Castillo EB, Trabucco A, de la Balze FA: Syndrome produced by absence of the germinal epithelium without impairment of the Sertoli or Leydig cells. *J Clin Endocrinol* 7:493, 1947

134. McCullagh EP, Schaffenberg CA: Role of the seminiferous

ment of testosterone secretion by normal adult human Leydig cells by co-culture with enriched preparations of normal adult human Sertoli cells. *Int J Androl* 16:27, 1993

tubules in the production of hormones. *Ann N Y Acad Sci* 55:674, 1952

135. Scott RS, Burger HG, Quigg H: A simple and rapid bioassay of inhibin for inhibin. *Endocrinology* 107:1536, 1980

136. Rivier J, Spiess J, McClintock R, Vaughan J, Vale W: Purification and partial characterization of inhibin from porcine follicular fluid. *Biochem Biophys Res Commun* 13:120, 1985

137. Mayo KE, Cerelli GM, Spiess J, et al: Inhibin-A-subunit cDNAs from porcine ovary and human placenta. *Proc Natl Acad Sci USA* 83:6849, 1986

138. Steinberger A, Dighe RR, Diaz J: Testicular peptides and their endocrine and paracrine functions. *Arch Biol Med Exp* 17:267, 1984

139. Rivier C, Rivier J, Vale W: Inhibin-mediated feedback control of follicle-stimulating hormone secretion in the female rat. *Science* 234:205, 1986

140. Skinner MK: Cell-cell interactions in the testis. *Endocrin Rev* 12:45, 1991

141. Jegou B: The Sertoli-germ cell communication network in mammals. *Int Rev Cytol* 147:25, 1993

142. Ritzen EM: Chemical messengers between Sertoli cells and neighboring cells. *J Steroid Biochem* 19:499, 1983

143. Tres LL, Smith EP, Van Wyk JJ, Kierszenbaum AL: Immunoreactive sites and accumulation of somatomedin-C in rat Sertoli-spermatogenic cell co-cultures. *Exp Cell Res* 162:33, 1986

144. Vannelli BG, Barni T, Orlando C, Natali A, Serio M, Balboni GC: Insulin-like growth factor-I (IGF-I) and IGF-I receptor in human testis: An immunohistochemical study. *Fertil Steril* 49:666, 1988

145. Feig LA, Klagsbrun M, Bellve AR: Mitogenic polypeptide of the mammalian seminiferous epithelium: Biochemical characterization and partial purification. *J Cell Biol* 97:1435, 1983

146. Bellve AR, Feig LA: Cell proliferation in the mammalian testis: Biology of the seminiferous growth factor (SGF). *Recent Prog Horm Res* 40:531, 1984

147. Buch JP, Lamb DJ, Lipshultz LI, Smith RG: Partial characterization of a unique growth factor secreted by human Sertoli cells. *Fertil Steril* 49:658, 1988

148. Skinner MK, Takacs K, Coffey RJ: Cellular localization of transforming growth factor-alpha gene expression and action in the seminiferous tubule: Peritubular cell-Sertoli cell interactions. *Endocrinology* 124:845, 1989

149. Skinner MK, Moses HL: Transforming growth factor-beta gene expression and action in the seminiferous tubule: Peritubular cell-Sertoli cell interactions. *Mol Endocrinol* 3:625, 1989

150. Khan SA, Soder O, Syed V, Gustafsson K, Lindh M, Ritzen EM: The rat produces large amounts of an interleukin-1-like factor. *Int J Androl* 10:495, 1987

151. Syed V, Stephan JP, Gerard N, et al: Residual bodies activate Sertoli cell interleukin-1 alpha (IL-1 alpha) release, which triggers IL-6 production by an autocrine mechanism, through the lipoxygenase pathway. *Endocrinology* 136:3070, 1995

152. Pollanen P, Soder O, Parvinen M: Interleukin-1 alpha stimulation of spermatogonial proliferation in vivo. *Reprod Fertil Dev* 1:85, 1989

153. Okuda Y, Bardin CW, Hodgskin LR, Morris PL: Interleukins-1

alpha an
Sertoli c
154. O'Brien
mediate
phospha
Endocri

155. Ireland
tein pho

156. Schteing
paracrin
Sertoli c

157. Le Mag
in the re
ture rat
Commu

158. Le Mag
cells by
teractior

159. Le Mag
matocyt
Res Con

160. Le Mag
germ ce
J Endoc

161. Stallard
transfer

162. Djakiew
Sertoli

163. Hutson
ciency
culture.

164. Holmes
secretio
sence
59:1058

165. Camero
toli cell
fibrobla

166. Janecki
androge
cellular
tion. M

167. Ailenbe
toli cell
cells an

168. Skinner
tein und
Proc N

169. Skinner
paracrin
that mo

170. Skinner
paracrin
tions be
Cell En

tion and choice of preparation media: Comparison of Percoll and Accudenz discontinuous density gradients. *J Androl* 17:61, 1996.

305. Naz RK, Minhas BS: Enhancement of sperm function for treatment of male infertility. *J Androl* 16:384, 1995

306. Harrison RAP, Roldan ERS: Phosphoinositides and their products in the mammalian sperm acrosome reaction. *J Reprod Fertil Suppl* 42:51, 1990

307. Thomas P, Meizel S: An influx of extracellular calcium is required for initiation of the human sperm acrosome reaction induced by human follicular fluid. *Gamete Res* 20:397, 1988

308. Fraser LR: Calcium channels play a pivotal role in the sequence of ionic changes involved in initiation of mouse sperm acrosomal exocytosis. *Mol Reprod Dev* 36:368, 1993

309. Florman HM, Corron ME, Kim TD-H, Babcock DF: Activation of voltage-dependent calcium channels in mammalian sperm is required for zona pellucida-induced acrosomal exocytosis. *Dev Biol* 152:304, 1992

310. Boldt J, Casas A, Whaley E, Creazzo T, Lewis JB: Potassium dependence for sperm-egg fusion in mice. *J Exp Zool* 257:245, 1991

311. Mrsny RJ, Meizel S: Potassium ion influx and Na$^+$,K$^+$-ATPase activity are required for the hamster sperm acrosome reaction. *J Cell Biol* 91:77, 1981

312. Mrsny RJ, Siiteri JE, Meizel S: Hamster sperm Na$^+$,K$^+$-adenosine triphosphate: Increased activity during capacitation in vitro and its relationship to cyclic nucleotides. *Biol Reprod* 30:573, 1984

313. Sabeur K, Meizel S: Importance of bicarbonate to the progesterone-initiated human sperm acrosome reaction. *J Androl* 16:266, 1995

314. Meizel S, Turner K: Progesterone acts at the plasma membrane of the human sperm. *Mol Cell Endocrinol* 11:R1, 1991

315. Malendrez CS, Meizel S: Studies of porcine and human sperm suggesting a role for a sperm glycine receptor/Cl$^-$ channel in the zona pellucida-initiated acrosome reaction. *Biol Reprod* 53:676, 1995

316. Turner KO, Meizel S: Progesterone-mediated efflux of cytosolic chloride during the human sperm acrosome reaction. *Biochem Biophys Res Commun* 213:774, 1995

317. Saling PM: How the egg regulates sperm function during gamete interaction: Facts and fantasies. *Biol Reprod* 44:246, 1991

318. Foltz KR: Sperm-binding proteins. *Int Rev Cytol* 163:249, 1995

319. Wassarman PM: Towards molecular mechanisms for gamete adhesion and fusion during mammalian fertilization. *Curr Opin Cell Biol* 7:658, 1995

320. Lillie FR: Studies of fertilization. VI. The mechanisms of fertilization in *Arbacia*. *J Exp Zool* 16:523, 1914

321. Lillie FR: *Problems in Fertilization*. Chicago, Univ Chicago Press, 1919

322. Wassarman PM: Zona pellucida glycoproteins. *Annu Rev Biochem* 57:415, 1988

323. Wassarman PM: Profile of a mammalian sperm receptor. *Development* 108:1, 1990

324. Ward CR, Kopf GS: Molecular events mediating sperm activation. *Dev Biol* 104:287, 1993

325. Chamberlin ME, Dean J: Human homolog of the mouse sperm receptor. *Proc Natl Acad Sci USA* 87:6014, 1990

326. Shabanowitz RB, O'Rand MG: Characterization of the human zona pellucida from fertilized and unfertilized eggs. *J Reprod Fertil* 82:151, 1988

327. Florman HM, Wassarman PM: O-linked oligosaccharides of mouse egg ZP3 account for its sperm receptor activity. *Cell* 41:313, 1985

328. Bleil JD, Wassarman PM: Galactose at the non-reducing terminus of O-lnked oligosaccharides of mouse egg zona pellucida glycoprotein ZP3 is essential for the glycoprotein's sperm receptor activity. *Proc Natl Acad Sci USA* 85:5563, 1988

329. Litscher ES, Wassarman PM: Carbohydrate-mediated adhesion of eggs and sperm during mammalian fertilization. *Trends Glycosci Glycotechnol* 5:369, 1993

330. Moller CC, Bleil JD, Kinloch RA, Wassarman PM: Structural and functional relationships between mouse and hamster zona pellucida glycoproteins. *Dev Biol* 137:276, 1990

331. Bleil JD, Wassarman PM: Mammalian sperm-egg interaction: Identification of a glycoprotein in mouse egg zona pellucida possessing receptor activity for sperm. *Cell* 20:873, 1980

332. Kinloch RA, Mortillo S, Stewart CL, Wassarman PM: Embryonal carcinoma cells transfected with ZP3 genes differentially glycosylate similar polypeptides and secrete active mouse sperm receptor. *J Cell Biol* 115:655, 1991

333. Beebe SJ, Leyton L, Burks D, et al: Recombinant mouse ZP3 inhibits sperm binding and induces the acrosome reaction. *Dev Biol* 151:48, 1992

334. Shur BD: Glycosyltransferase as cell adhesion molecules. *Curr Opin Cell Biol* 5:854, 1993

335. Miller DJ, Shur BD: Molecular basis of fertilization in the mouse. *Semin Dev Biol* 5:255, 1994

336. Bleil JD, Wassarman PM: Identification of a ZP3-binding protein on acrosome-intact mouse sperm by photoaffinity crosslinking. *Proc Natl Acad Sci USA* 87:5563, 1990

337. Bookbinder LH, Cheng A, Bleil JD: Tissue- and species-specific expression of sp56, a mouse sperm fertilization protein. *Science* 268:86, 1995

338. Leyton L, Saling P: 95-KD sperm proteins bind ZP3 and serve as tyrosine kinase substrates in response to zona binding. *Cell* 108:2163, 1989

339. Leyton L, LeGuen P, Bunch D, Saling PM: Regulation of mouse gamete interactions by a sperm tyrosine kinase. *Proc Natl Acad Sci USA* 89:11692, 1992

340. Miller DJ, Gong X, Shur BD: Sperm require β-*N*-acetylglucosaminidase to penetrate through the egg zona pellucida. *Development* 118:1279, 1993

341. Miller DJ, Macek MB, Shur BD: Complementarity between sperm surface β-1,4-galactosyltransferase and egg coat ZP3 mediates sperm-egg binding. *Nature* 357:589, 1992

342. Youakim A, Hathaway HJ, Miller DJ, Gong X, Shur BD: Overexpressing sperm surface β-1,4-galactosyltransferase in transgenic mice affects multiple aspects of sperm-egg interactions. *J Cell Biol* 126:1573, 1994

343. Suzuki-Toyota F, Maekawa M, Cheng A, Bleil JD: Immunocolloidal gold labeled surface replica, and its application to detect sp56, the egg recognition and binding protein, on the mouse spermatozoon. *J Electron Microsc* 44:135, 1995

344. Burks DJ, Carballada R, Moore HD, Saling PM: Interaction of a tyrosine kinase from human sperm with the zona pellucida at fertilization. *Science* 269:83, 1995

345. Kalab P, Visconti P, Leclerc P, Kopf GS: p95, the major phosphotyrosine-containing protein in mouse spermatozoa, is a hexokinase with unique properties. *J Biol Chem* 269:3810, 1994

346. World Health Organization: *WHO Laboratory Manual for the Examination of Human Semen and Sperm-Cervical Mucus Interaction,* ed 3. Cambridge, England, Press Syndicate of Univ of Cambridge, 1992

347. Berman NG, Wang C, Paulsen CA: Methodological issues in the analysis of human sperm concentration data. *J Androl* 17:68, 1996

348. Davis RO, Bain DE, Seimers RJ, Thai DM, Andrew JA, Gravance CG: Accuracy and precision of the CellForm-Human automated morphometry instrument. *Fertil Steril* 58:763, 1992

349. Davis RO, Gravance CG: Consistency of sperm morphology classification criteria. *J Androl* 15:83, 1994

350. Davis RO, Katz DF, Gravance CG, Osorio AM: Sperm morphology abnormalities among lead-exposed battery plant workers. *Fertil Steril* 60 (Suppl):178, 1993

351. Gravance CG, Davis RO: Automated sperm morphometry analysis (ASTHMA) in the rabbit. *J Androl* 16:88, 1995

352. Bel+sey MA, Eliasson R, Gallegos AJ, et al: *Laboratory Manual for the Examination of Human Semen and Semen-Cervical Mucus Interaction.* Singapore, Press Concern, 1980: 30–42

353. Moruzzi JF, Wyrobek AJ, Mayhill BH, et al: Quantification and classification of human sperm morphology by computer-assisted image analysis. *Fertil Steril* 50:142, 1988

TABLE 14–3. FREQUENCY DISTR...
FERTILE MEN

Sperm Count (million/mL)
< 20
20–39
40–59
≥ 60

From Rehan N, Sobrero AJ, Fertig JW:
til Steril 26:492, 1975.

Studies Indicating that L...
May Be Compatible with...

In 1974 workers reported
sperm counts less than 2...
had counts greater than 6...
sperm counts are quite...
deed, a count less than...
male-factor problem. An...
men who requested vase...
findings: 23% of fertile...
lion/mL and only 40%...
Among infertile couples...
preconception whether i...
lem, 42% (twice as man...
million and 29% had co...
spection of all the data su...
likelihood that a couple...
count greater than 10 mi...
less than 10 million that...
vestigators did conclude...
nonessential in determin...
is greater than 10 million...
direct relation of numeric...
couple will become preg...

TABLE 14–4. FREQUENCY DISTRI...
FERTILE MEN

Motility Sperm (%)
< 20
20–39
40–59
60–79
80–100

Men with >40% motile sperm made up 8...
From Rehan N, Sobrero AJ, Fertig JW:
Fertil Steril 26:492, 1975.

CHAPTER 14

Relationship of Abnormal Semen Values to Male-Factor Infertility

SHERMAN J. SILBER

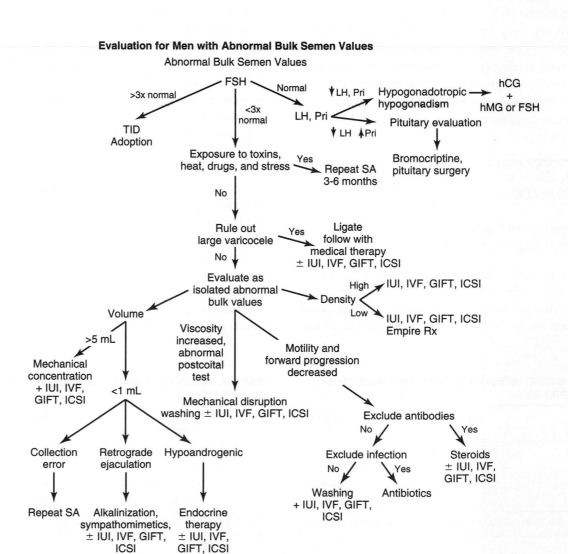

Evaluation for Men with Abnormal Bulk Semen Values

SEMEN ANALYSIS

The time-honored method
has been semen analysis (
that if a man's sperm count
imum, he is infertile, and tl
nancy is caused by his ir
1970s it was believed that
lion/mL meant that men v
these couples a dire progno
occur, it was ascribed to wl
istered to the "infertile" hu
pose. Since the early 198
indicate infertility has bee
group, however, reported p
50,000 sperm per milliliter.
were all carefully blood ty
termined to be 99.99% sur
the father.[1]

Today, with the remarl
in vitro fertilization (IVF)
injection (ICSI), even th
thenospermia may be ove
these men with severe oli
partners naturally, whereas
values may not achieve fe
This chapter discusses the r
male-factor infertility.

LITERATURE REVIEW

Studies Indicating that Low
Indicate Male-Factor Inferti

The original correlation of s
a study of 1000 fertile and
The results clearly indicate
sperm counts for the vast

**TABLE 14-1. FREQUENCY DISTRIBUT
AND 1000 INFERTILE MEN**

Sperm Count (million/mL)	
< 20	
20–39	
40–59	
≥ 60	

From MacLeod J, Gold RZ: The male factor
known fertility and in 1000 cases of infertile

CHAPTER 15

Pathogenesis and Medical Management of Male Infertility

STEPHEN J. WINTERS

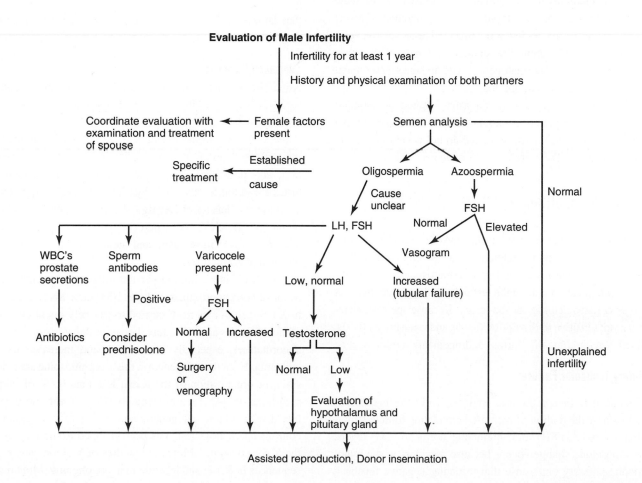

Male factors have been estimated to contribute to infertility in 25% to 50% of infertile couples.[1] Therefore, a screening evaluation for the man is now an early component of the infertility evaluation. Ideally the evaluation should include a medical history, physical examination, and a direct sperm count. This information, together with a similar noninvasive evaluation for the female partner can be used to direct efforts at diagnosis and therapy. It is useful for the andrologist and the gynecologist to interview both partners. This approach facilitates a free exchange of information and the acquisition of important clinical details concerning both partners. Interviews with both partners can help identify psychologic and sexual strain in a marriage.

Male infertility is not one disorder but is a syndrome that results from many congenital and acquired illnesses. Infertile men are most often healthy, have no symptoms, and have few physical findings. However, infertility sometimes is the initial manifestation of a serious systemic illness. Most infertile men have oligospermia (reduced sperm output), asthenospermia (poor sperm motility), and teratospermia (sperm with abnormal morphology), indicating that spermatogenesis is both quantitatively and qualitatively abnormal. Until the causes of male infertility are known, any classification is incomplete. Nevertheless it is necessary to develop a practical approach to evaluation for an infertile male that entails awareness of disorders associated with hypospermatogenesis and an honest assessment of the available treatment options.

Ejaculated sperm may be abnormal because of testicular dysfunction or impaired stimulation of an otherwise normal testis or because the sperm produced do not develop normally or are damaged in the extratesticular male genital tract.

PATHOLOGIC CONDITIONS

Testicular abnormalities may cause Leydig cell dysfunction, which causes androgen deficiency, and seminiferous tubule dysfunction, which produces hypospermatogenesis. The complex communication among the testicular cell types predisposes to a generalized disorder of the testis.[2] Because spermatogenesis is more sensitive to disruption than is androgen biosynthesis, infertility with clinically normal androgenization often occurs.

Primary Testicular Failure

Pronounced testicular damage may be readily recognized in adult men by the finding of increased circulating follicle-stimulating hormone (FSH) and luteinizing hormone (LH) levels. These hormone changes occur because receptors in the hypothalamic-pituitary unit sense that testicular negative feedback signaling is impaired. These feedback signals are the gonadal steroid hormones, testosterone and estradiol, and almost certainly the seminiferous tubular glycoprotein, inhibin. Disorders

TABLE 15–1. DISORDERS THAT PRODUCE PRIMARY TESTICULAR FAILURE

Congenital
Klinefelter's syndrome (47,XXY and variants)
XYY male
Cryptorchidism
Congenital anorchia (vanishing testis syndrome)
Noonan's syndrome
Myotonic muscular dystrophy
Sickle cell disease

Acquired
Orchitis: mumps pyogenic, traumatic
Malignant neoplasm: germ cell, leukemia, lymphoma
Torsion
Varicocele
Spinal cord injury
Liver disease
Renal failure
Retroperitoneal fibrosis
Drugs
Irradiation
Aging

that damage the testes directly can be classified as congenital or acquired (Table 15–1).

Congenital Disorders

Klinefelter's syndrome and its sex chromosomal variants affect 0.21% of men.[3] In one series, Klinefelter's syndrome was found in 4% of infertile men and 11% of azoospermic men. Klinefelter's syndrome is characterized clinically by the findings of small testes, gynecomastia, incomplete androgenization, and infertility.[4] The typical histologic findings in the testes are seminiferous tubule hyalinization and an apparent increase in the density of Leydig cells. A peripheral blood karyotype is 47,XXY. Ten percent of these patients have 46,XY/47,XXY mosaicism and generally have less severe physical abnormalities.

47,XYY is a common sex chromosome abnormality that occurs among approximately 1 per 1000 men. Spermatogenesis in XYY men ranges from normal to severely impaired.[5] Other clinical features are tall stature, behavioral disturbance, skeletal abnormalities, especially of the jaw, and increased risk for leukemia. Even though genes on the Y chromosome are responsible for organization of the testis, less than 0.5% of infertile men have structural rearrangements of the Y chromosome detected with routine cytogenetic studies.[3] A genetic region that controls spermatogenesis has been mapped to the long arm of the Y chromosome.[6] Molecular studies of Y chromosome gene sequences in fertile and infertile men are ongoing. Mutations of the gene that encodes the androgen receptor, located on the X chromosome, have been reported to cause infertility in phenotypic males,[5] but are probably rare causes of male infertility.

Various autosomal abnormalities including translocations, inversions, and extra marker chromosomes occur with increased frequency among infertile men. Only about 1% to 2% of infertile men, however, have identifiable autosomal abnormalities.[3] Cytogenic errors during meiosis may explain as much as 8% of male infertility.[3]

Testicular dysfunction occurs in many congenital disorders, including Noonan's syndrome, Prader-Willi syndrome, Laurence-Moon-Bardet-Biedl syndrome, myotonic muscular dystrophy, adrenoleukodystrophy, Kennedy disease (X-linked spinal and bulbar muscular atrophy), and sickle cell disease. Germinal aplasia (Sertoli-cell-only syndrome) is a histologic diagnosis that defines the complete absence of germ cells in the seminiferous tubules. Men with this syndrome have azoospermia and increased FSH levels. Many cases of the syndrome are idiopathic, although this finding also occurs after chemotherapy and in XYY men, Y chromosomal abnormality, and chronic renal failure, among other disorders.

Cryptorchidism was found in 6.4% of men attending a large infertility clinic. Although patients with sex chromosomal abnormalities, hypogonadotropic hypogonadism, or androgen resistance may also have cryptorchidism, there is generally no clear explanation for why the testis fails to descend into the scrotum. The extent of damage to the seminiferous tubules with cryptorchidism is quite variable. A high rate of infertility is found among men with bilateral cryptorchidism; men with one undescended testis are much more likely to be fertile.[8] Although surgical treatment of cryptorchidism is recommended for boys 1 to 2 years of age, the impact of early surgical treatment on fertility remains to be established.[8]

Acquired Disorders

Testicular trauma and inflammation are recognized causes of hypogonadism. Thirty percent of adult men who have mumps have clinical orchitis; in two thirds of these men the orchitis is unilateral. Before the age of 10 years, however, mumps is rarely accompanied by orchitis. The extent of subsequent adult testicular dysfunction varies from azoospermia and marked androgen deficiency to no fertility disturbance.

Testicular torsion is an acute twisting of the testis that occludes the blood supply. If the patient is not treated, testicular atrophy occurs. Some patients later have abnormal sperm counts, suggesting an underlying testicular disorder or damage to both testes.

Epididymo-orchitis may result from sexually transmitted disease and ascending spread of urethritis. *Neisseria gonorrhoeae* and Chlamydia trachomatis are the commonly associated organisms.[9] Men with the infection experience rapid onset of pain and swelling of the epididymis. In one study testicular biopsy revealed that spermatogenesis was impaired in 20 of 28 patients.[10]

Hypogonadotropic Hypogonadism

Testicular dysfunction in men with hypogonadotropic hypogonadism results from inadequate gonadotropin stimulation of the testis. Table 15–2 lists many of the important causes of this condition. Abnormalities within the pituitary gland, or a disturbance in gonadotropin-releasing hormone (GnRH) secretion by the hypothalamus, can result in gonadotropin deficiency. Men with hypogonadotropic hypogonadism usually seek medical attention for androgen deficiency. Serum levels of testosterone are reduced, and LH levels are low or in the low-normal range.

Congenital Hypogonadotropic Hypogonadism. Congenital hypogonadotropic hypogonadism generally is identified in teenagers who do not enter puberty.[11] They are phenotypic males because maternal human chorionic gonadotropin (hCG) stimulated the fetal testis to produce testosterone with resultant masculinization of the genitalia. These boys produce little or no GnRH, however, so LH secretion does not increase, and testicular function remains prepubertal. Approximately 50% of these patients have midline defects such as anosmia, and the condition is designated Kallmann's syndrome. Many affected kindreds have been described, most demonstrating an autosomal dominant mode of inheritance with incomplete penetrance. There is evidence that a gene coding a factor that stimulates the migration of neurons during fetal development is abnormal in some people, preventing the normal migration of GnRH neurons to the hypothalamus.[12]

Some men with congenital eunuchoidism seek treatment later in life with subnormal testicular growth, partial pubertal development, and reduced circulating testosterone levels. Some

TABLE 15–2. DISORDERS THAT PRODUCE HYPOGONADOTROPIC HYPOGONADISM

Congenital

Isolated hypogonadotropic hypogonadism
Kallmann's syndrome
Prader-Willi syndrome
Fertile eunuch syndrome

Idiopathic hypopituitarism: partial and complete

Acquired

Pituitary adenomas
Nonfunctional chromophobe adenomas
Prolactinomas
Cushing's syndrome
Acromegaly

Hypothalamic tumors and cysts

Others

Head trauma	Hemochromatosis
Meningitis	Vasculitis
Cerebritis	Irradiation
Sarcoidosis	Anorexia nervosa
Acute illness	Autoimmune hypophysitis
Histiocytosis	

of these men have reduced spontaneous LH secretory pulse frequency or LH pulses of reduced amplitude.[13] This variant, which has been called the fertile eunuch syndrome, may be more common among certain ethnic groups.[14] Hypogonadotropic hypogonadism may also occur together with deficiency of other pituitary hormones, especially growth hormone–deficient dwarfism.

Acquired Hypogonadotropic Hypogonadism. Any mass lesion, infiltrative process, or trauma that damages the hypothalamus-pituitary unit can interfere with the secretion of gonadotropins and other tropic hormones. Tumors may be functional, as in acromegaly, or nonfunctional, as in craniopharyngioma. Men with sellar and parasellar tumors may have headaches and visual disturbances.

Gonadotropin secretion can be altered by the effects of other hormones. Men with prolactin-producing tumors may experience delayed puberty, poor androgenization, impotence, and infertility. In addition to the mass effect of the prolactinoma on the surrounding normal pituitary gland, hyperprolactinemia impairs pulsatile LH (and presumably GnRH) secretion. The impairment can be reversed by bromocriptine treatment.[15] The gonadotropin deficiency seen in men with Cushing's syndrome[16] probably results from cortisol hypersecretion, since treatment with a glucocorticoid antagonist[17] restores serum testosterone levels to normal. Men with inadequately treated congenital adrenal hyperplasia may have disturbed gonadotropin secretion and infertility, although the pathophysiologic process remains unclear.[18]

Systemic Illnesses Associated with Testicular Dysfunction

Testicular function is frequently abnormal in men with acute and chronic systemic illnesses.[19] Weight loss, malnutrition, and stress contribute to these changes. Specific endocrine syndromes have been associated with certain clinical disorders.

Chronic liver disease is often associated with infertility, sexual dysfunction, and reduced androgenization.[20] Alcoholic liver disease leads to testicular damage, alteration in the hypothalamic-pituitary unit, increased hepatic production of sex hormone–binding globulin, and increased adrenal steroid production. These effects are believed to result from cirrhosis and the toxic effects of alcohol.[20] Serum FSH and LH levels are often increased, but they may be normal. In contrast, hemochromatosis produces hypogonadotropic hypogonadism because of iron deposition in the hypothalamus and pituitary gland; it also produces cirrhosis, diabetes mellitus, and cardiomyopathy.[21]

Gonadal dysfunction is common in men with chronic renal failure.[22] Reduction in libido, sexual dysfunction, reduced muscle mass, and impaired androgenization all contribute to a poor quality of life for these patients. Testosterone levels are often low, and LH and FSH levels are either normal or elevated. LH pulsatile secretion is markedly attenuated in part because LH metabolic clearance is prolonged. Prolactin levels may increase. Oligoasthenospermia is common even during dialysis, but it generally improves after successful renal transplantation.

Human immunodeficiency virus (HIV) infection affects the male reproduction tract. HIV is often present in semen even when the infection is asymptomatic, but men with early acquired immunodeficiency syndrome (AIDS) appear to have normal sperm output, motility, and morphology.[23] In contrast, men with advanced AIDS (fewer than 200 CD4+ cells/mm^3 may have pronounced pyospermia, a marked decrease in sperm output and motility, and increased abnormal sperm forms.[24] Zidovudine (AZT) treatment reduces semen white blood cell (WBC) concentrations and appears to improve findings at semen analysis. In one study, low testosterone levels were found in 8 of 28 men (29%) with AIDS,[25] perhaps because of weight loss and poor nutrition. The testes of men dying with AIDS demonstrate severe hypospermatogenesis and lymphocyte infiltration.[26]

The reproductive disturbances that occur in women who participate in stressful physical conditioning programs are widely recognized. In men, serum testosterone levels decline transiently after intense exercise[27] and during fasting[28] because these stresses decrease gonadotropin secretion. Libido may also decline. However, two surveys of male athletes that focused primarily on long distance runners revealed normal testosterone levels[29] and normal sperm production[30] in most of the men surveyed. In another study, however, 2 of 20 runners were underweight and had low testosterone levels and oligospermia.[31] The profound weight loss characteristic of anorexia nervosa results in hypogonadotropic hypogonadism in men as well as in women.

Hypogonadism is often suspected in obese men, because androgen deficiency is associated with an increased fat mass and decreased muscle mass. Serum testosterone levels in obese men are subnormal in proportion to body mass index.[32] The principal determinant of the low total testosterone levels is a reduction in serum sex hormone binding globulin (SHBG) concentration.[33] The free testosterone levels of men with morbid obesity also may be low.[32] Serum estrone levels may be elevated because fat tissue aromatase level is increased, and high circulating estrogen levels may decrease testosterone production by suppressing gonadotropin secretion.[34] In fact, serum estrone levels fall and testosterone levels rise when morbidly obese men lose weight.[35] The information available about sperm density and motility in obese men is quite limited but suggests no severe disturbance in spermatogenesis.[32]

Men with thyrotoxicosis may have gynecomastia, suppressed libido and potency,[36] or oligoasthenospermia.[37] Hyperthyroxinemia stimulates SHBG production, increasing serum total testosterone levels, although free testosterone levels are normal. Circulating estradiol levels are often increased in men with hyperthyroidism partly because peripheral conversion of androgenic precursors is increased. Circulating LH levels also may be increased, stimulating Leydig cell aromatase and progesterone production.[38] Testicular disturbances also may occur in men with hypothyroidism.[39] Unsuspected hyper- and hypothyroidism, however, are rare among infertile men.

Aging is associated with a gradual decline in sexual performance and testicular function, although the age at which these changes occur varies.[40] The total number of Leydig cells and spermatogenesis decline as men age.[41] Mean testosterone levels in men in the sixth to seventh decade of life are generally in the low-normal range for young adults; very low levels suggest an additional disorder. Most studies have found increased FSH levels in elderly men, indicating primary testicular dysfunction. Serum LH levels are less affected, however, perhaps because GnRH secretion also appears to decline as men age.[42] Sperm count and quality begin to decrease after the age of 50 years.[43]

Complete androgen insensitivity (testicular feminization) is an X-linked disorder in which genotypic males with testes have a female phenotype.[7] A more limited form of androgen resistance that becomes apparent clinically with variable ambiguity of the external genitalia and impaired peripheral androgenization has been termed *incomplete androgen insensitivity*. These disorders are now known to result from mutations in the gene that codes for the androgen receptor. These mutations cause defective hormone binding by the receptor or failure of the activated receptor to bind to the regulatory region of androgen-responsive genes. Partly because Sertoli and myoid cells of the testis contain androgen receptors, androgen resistance is usually associated with infertility. Rarely, infertile men with normal external genitalia and normal secondary sex characteristics have reduced androgen receptor binding to skin fibroblast and androgen receptor mutations.[44] The finding of a high serum LH level with increased free or bioavailable testosterone levels, implying impaired testosterone negative feedback control, suggests this disorder.

Drugs and Toxins That Affect Testicular Function

Exposure to drugs or toxic substances may explain some cases of male infertility (Table 15–3). Prescription and street drugs can impair testicular function directly or suppress gonadotropin secretion, producing androgen deficiency or spermatogenic arrest. Some experts relate the suggestion that the prevalance of male infertility is increasing, and that mean sperm output is declining due to environmental factors.[45] Drugs may also produce infertility by interfering with erection and ejaculation.

TABLE 15–3. DRUGS AND TOXINS THAT ALTER REPRODUCTIVE FUNCTION

In Utero
Diethylstilbestrol
Antiandrogens

Occupational exposure
Carbon disulfide
Lead
Estrogens
Chlordectone
Ethylene glycol

Prescription drugs associated with reproductive dysfunction
Chemotherapeutic agents
Sulfasalazine
Androgens

Drugs that alter male sexual function

Testosterone biosynthesis inhibitors
Spironolactone
Ketoconazole
Cyproterone acetate

Androgen antagonists
Spironolactone
Cyproterone acetate
Flutamide
Cimetidine

Inhibitors of erectile function and ejaculation
Antihypertensives: methyldopa, reserpine, β-blockers, clonidine
Neuroleptics: phenothiazines, butyrophenone, lithium
Antidepressants: tricyclics, monoamine oxidase inhibitors
Anticholinergics

Recreational drugs
Ethanol
Marihuana
Opiates
Cigarettes

Prescribed Drugs

In utero exposure to diethylstilbestrol (DES) may be associated with the presence of epididymal cysts and functional sperm abnormalities.[46] Spironolactone[47] and ketoconazole[48] impair testosterone biosynthesis, and spironolactone,[47] cimetidine,[49] and flutamide[50] bind to androgen receptors and block androgen action. These drugs can cause genital abnormalities in male fetuses and are contraindicated for use by pregnant women. Each of these drugs has produced gynecomastia in adult men, but detrimental effects on spermatogenesis have not been reported. The androgens abused by athletes for anabolic properties suppress gonadotropin secretion and produce hypospermatogenesis.[51]

Young adult men with cancer are surviving their illness in increasing numbers, but the treatments used commonly damage spermatogenesis. Chemotherapeutic agents, particularly mechlorethamine (Mustargen, Merck, West Point, PA), cyclophosphamide, and procarbazine kill spermatogonia,[52] although the mechanism for this damage is not known. Azospermia is common during treatment. FSH levels rise and germinal aplasia is found at biopsy of the testis. Dose and duration of chemotherapy determine the severity of injury and the potential for recovery. Radiation therapy also damages spermatogenesis, and its effects are additive to those of chemotherapy.[53] There are no reliable methods for prevention of this testicular toxicity.[54] Although sperm banking offers the potential for fertility,[55] results are variable because the results of semen analysis often are abnormal for men with malignant disease even before treatment.[56]

Sulfasalazine, a conjugate of 5-aminosalicylic acid used in the treatment of ulcerative colitis, has been associated with a reduction in sperm motility and sperm density that may reverse after discontinuation of treatment.[57] Although cyclosporine inhibits testosterone synthesis in rats, there is no evidence so far of an adverse effect in men.

Street Drugs

Chronic alcohol use is associated with a reduction in testis size, seminal plasma volume, and sperm density, motility, and morphology.[58] These abnormalities may improve if alcohol use is discontinued.[59,60] Although acute ethanol administration reduces testosterone production in healthy men, moderate alcohol consumption does not appear to depress sperm quality or production.[61]

Opiate abuse, like chronic alcoholism, may produce an abnormal ejaculate.[62] Opiate drugs inhibit gonadotropin secretion and reduce serum testosterone levels.[63] The observation that opiate antagonists increase LH secretion suggests a physiologic role for endogenous opiates in the regulation of gonadotropin secretion in men.[64] Malnutrition and associated acute and chronic illness may contribute to the effects of chronic ethanol and opiate abuse. Results of a study in mice suggest that marihuana interferes with gonadotropin secretion and directly inhibits testosterone biosynthesis. The results also showed that maternal cannabinoid exposure may influence testicular function in offspring.[65] Marihuana also may impair sperm motility directly. Controlled studies with human subjects are not possible, and the data available are insufficient to allow any meaningful conclusions.

Environmental and Occupational Toxins

Although concerns abound, few environmental or occupational agents have been shown to impair fertility.[66,67] Carbon disulfide, a solvent used in the production of rayon, produces neurotoxicity and has been associated with testicular damage. Dibromochloropropane, added to soil to kill nematodes, is mutagenic and is cytotoxic to the testis. The sale and distribution of this agent were banned in the United States in 1979. Central nervous system, hepatic, and testicular toxicity occurred in a group of workers exposed to the chlorinated hydrocarbon chlordecone, an insecticide and fungicide. Overall, agricultural workers may be at higher risk for infertility than are other workers.[68] Reproductive dysfunction in both men and women also occurs from toxic lead exposure. Smelters, painters, battery workers, and those exposed to lead-containing fuels are at risk. The metabolites of ethylene glycol, an antifreeze, are also known to be toxic to germ cells.

Cigarette smoking by the male partner does not appear to reduce a couple's fertility, and there is no apparent difference in the semen analysis of smokers compared with that of nonsmokers.[69] However, male smokers who also have a varicocele may be at increased risk for impaired semen quality.

Genital Tract Obstruction

Genital tract obstruction has been reported to occur in 3% to 13% of infertile men.[70] This diagnosis should be suspected in men with azoospermia who have normal-sized testes and normal serum FSH levels. These findings are not entirely specific, however, and may be present in men with azoospermia who have seminiferous tubular dysfunction. To differentiate these possibilities, vasography is performed to identify obstruction. It is followed with testicular biopsy to confirm that spermatogenesis is normal. If it is, microsurgical reconstruction may be recommended.

The absence of a palpable vas deferens at physical examination suggests congenital absence of the vas. Some of these men have variant forms of cystic fibrosis, and all should undergo sweat chloride testing followed with genetic counseling if the test is positive.[71] Obstructive azoospermia also occurs in patients with mucociliary transport disorders that produce bronchitis and bronchiectasis (Young's syndrome[72]), gonococcal and nongonococcal epididymitis, tuberculosis, surgical trauma, and various tropical diseases.

Immotile Sperm

Immotile-cilia syndrome is a rare disorder caused by a defect in the axoneme of the cilia in the respiratory tract and sperm tail. Men with this disorder produce sperm that are immotile but normal in density and morphology. These men are uniformly sterile. Additional clinical findings include situs inversus, chronic sinusitis, and bronchiectasis (Kartagener's syndrome[73]).

Ejaculatory Dysfunction

Retrograde ejaculation and failure of ejaculation are relatively unusual findings among infertile men. The most common cause is probably diabetes mellitus.[74] Neurologic, vascular, and psychophysiologic factors are believed to contribute to this ejaculatory dysfunction, but endocrine testicular function is generally normal in men with diabetes.[75] Drugs such as narcotics, sedatives, psychotropics, and antiadrenergics may produce anejaculation. Other causes include operations on the pelvic retroperitoneal area and prostatectomy. Men with spinal cord injuries are generally infertile because of ejaculatory failure, genital duct obstruction, and seminiferous tubular dysfunction.[76] Ejaculatory impotence and infertility may be psychophysiologic, and can be treated with sex therapy. Sometimes the semen volume is less than 1 mL. A small semen volume suggests androgen deficiency but is often due to incomplete collection of the ejaculate. Idiopathic low semen volume is associated with poor-quality ejaculate.[77]

Male Infertility of Unknown Causation

Unfortunately, there is no specific diagnosis for most men with oligospermia or asthenospermia. If a testicular biopsy is performed, hypospermatogenesis is almost always found. However, the genetic or biochemical defects in these men are unknown. The following selected additional disorders remain controversial causes of infertility in the male.

Varicocele

Dilatation of the veins of the pampiniform plexus of the scrotum is believed to result from congenital incompetence of the valves of the spermatic veins. The predilection for varicocele on the left side has been explained by the asymmetry in renal-gonadal venous anatomy. Gonadal venography, however, indicates that right and bilateral varicoceles also occur.

Whether varicocele causes male infertility and whether treatment influences the pregnancy rate are controversial.[78] Recent data support affirmative answers to both questions. In a multicenter study of almost 9000 men who underwent infertility evaluations, 25.4% had varicocele,[79] about twice the prevalence among fertile men.[80] Although many men with varicocele are fertile, fertile men with varicocele have an abnormal semen analysis, but the disturbance is less severe than among infertile men with varicocele.[81]

Most studies of therapy for varicocele-associated infertility have been retrospective and inadequately controlled, nonrandomized, insufficiently powered, or have used changes in semen analysis rather than pregnancy rate as the end point. In a prospective, randomized study of men with oligospermia (5 to 20 million sperm/mL) and varicocele, one group underwent high ligation of a varicocele, and surgical intervention was postponed 12 months for the control group.[82] The pregnancy rates were 44.4% (8 of 25) and 10% (2 of 20), respectively, providing the best evidence to date that varicocele repair is effective. It is now known that varicocele generally appears in adolescence.[83] Longitudinal studies of teenagers[84] and adults[85] have revealed progression of the testicular disturbance if the varicocele remains untreated. Treatment failure among certain adult men may be due in part to delaying treatment into adulthood when infertility is recognized. A prospective study of the impact of varicocele treatment of adolescents on adult testicular function and fertility is needed.

Genitourinary infection has been proposed to cause male infertility, since it is reasonable that inflammation of the genital ducts might alter seminal plasma and render sperm abnormal. Antibiotics have been used to treat oligospermia, asthenospermia, elevated semen pH, semen leukocytes, and poor semen liquefaction. Many contradictory reports can be found in the literature. Most of these studies are difficult to interpret because there is no placebo control group, duration of therapy is short, eradication of infection is uncertain, and study design is neither prospective nor randomized. Particular interest surrounds the possible role of infections with *Mycoplasma* species (*Ureaplasma urealyticum*[86]) and *C trachomatis,*[87] because these organisms are recognized pathogens in the female genital tract. The finding of *U urealyticum* in semen is generally unrelated to the results of the semen analysis, however, and the detection of *C trachomatis* has been technically difficult.

Sperm Antibodies

Many studies have sought to determine whether antibodies directed against sperm antigens play a role in male-factor infertility, but results have been conflicting.[88] Sperm antibodies are proposed to impede sperm transport in the female genital tract and to interfere with sperm-egg interaction, but not all antibodies detected influence sperm motility or pregnancy rate. Most current investigations focus on immunoglobulin (IgA) antibodies in semen or bound to sperm membranes, as determined with the mixed antiglobulin reaction (MAR) test or the immunobead test, respectively. Estimates of the prevalence of sperm antibodies among infertile men have ranged from 3% to 20%; they approach 75% of men with vasectomy and vasovastomy.[89] The examination of longitudinal samples sometimes produces inconsistent results.[90] Nevertheless, among men with vasectomy reversal, the finding of IgA on 100% of sperm was highly correlated with infertility.[89] Although the cause of immune infertility is unknown, one hypothesis is that infection and inflammation of the testes and epididymis render sperm antigens immunogenic.

Effects of Temperature on the Testis

The temperature within the scrotum is normally 2 to 3 degrees less than ambient body temperature. It is generally believed that this lower temperature is necessary for normal testicular function. Results of experiments in which the testes of experimental animals were heated support this hypothesis. A higher than normal scrotal temperature has been proposed as the explanation for infertility in men with cryptorchidism and varicocele.[91] The possibility that scrotal hyperthermia might contribute to idiopathic male infertility has been considered.[92] Prolonged exposure in hot saunas has been reported to reduce the sperm count in healthy men[93] and should be discouraged. However, the role of wearing briefs as opposed to boxer shorts, wearing athletic supporters, and moderate use of hot baths and saunas in causing male infertility remains unproved. The temporary decrease in sperm output that follows a febrile illness is probably caused by impaired gonadotropin secretion.

Endocrine Dysfunction

Healthy anovulatory women may have a disturbance in pulsatile LH secretion, which has been designated *hypothalamic amenorrhea*. A similar disturbance has been sought in infertile men. A slight decrease in LH pulse frequency was reported in a group of men with oligospermia and elevated serum FSH levels,[94] but this finding has not been confirmed. Instead, LH pulse frequency is usually normal in infertile men with selective increases in circulating FSH levels, although LH pulse amplitude may be increased.[95] Rarely, infertile men have normal virilization and normal LH and testosterone levels but undetectable serum FSH concentrations.[96] Isolated FSH deficiency due to a mutation in the FSH β-subunit gene leading to a termination codon has been reported in a hypogonadal woman[97] and may also be present in men.

CLINICAL EVALUATION OF INFERTILITY OF MEN

A complete medical history should be taken and a physical examination should be performed for all infertile men. As in many areas of medicine, a chronologic approach to the medical history is useful (Table 15–4). Maternal illness and drug use (such as use of DES) have been associated with infertility in offspring. The presence at birth of ambiguous genitalia, microphallus, cryptorchidism, or inguinal hernia suggests congenital hypogonadism. Most chronic illnesses in childhood cause delayed growth and impaired sexual development. Precocious puberty may indicate congenital adrenal hyperplasia. Delayed puberty and incomplete pubertal development may result from either primary testicular failure or gonadotropin deficiency.

Hypogonadal adult men may report a decrease in libido, sexual dysfunction, gynecomastia, or symptoms of a sellar or suprasellar mass, such as headache or visual disturbance. Men with varicocele may report scrotal aching. Chronic prostatitis

TABLE 15–4. QUESTIONNAIRE FOR USE IN THE INTERVIEW WITH AN INFERTILE MAN

Childhood history
Maternal health while pregnant with patient
Maternal use of medications
Testicular abnormalities at birth: undescended testis, hernia
Penile abnormalities
Childhood illnesses
Medications taken often in childhood
Pubertal development: age at onset, breast swelling or tenderness, age first shaved beard
Testicular injury

Adult medical history
Duration of marriage
Duration of infertility
Frequency of intercourse
Pregnancies with previous partners
Occupation
Medical illness
Medications taken
Smoking history
Alcohol use
Exposure to hydrocarbons, lead, temperature extremes
Problems with erection or ejaculation
Testicular injury
Testicular infections
Change in testis size
Testicular pain

may cause painful ejaculation, nocturia, and dysuria. Orchitis, testicular torsion, and epididymitis are characterized by a sudden onset of pain and swelling of the scrotal contents. An occupational and recreational history is important, since environmental toxins have been implicated in some cases of male infertility. The list of medications should be reviewed. Alcohol and street drugs may impair testicular function. A coital history should identify the timing and technique of intercourse. In the evaluation for a man with a borderline ejaculate, it is important to learn whether the patient had children from a previous relationship. Systemic illnesses such as kidney disease and gastrointestinal disorders are associated with testicular dysfunction.

Exact measurement of the length and width of the testis is important, and is easily accomplished. The testis can be compared in volume with a series of precalibrated ovoids. Median testis length among healthy men approximates 5.0 cm, equivalent to 25 mL in volume. Although testes that measure 4.0 cm in length may be normal, the testes of many men with hypospermatogenesis are 4 cm or more long.

A varicocele may be visible or palpable when the patient assumes the upright posture. Palpability increases with the Valsalva maneuver and decreases when the patient is recumbent. A reduction in the size of the left testis is common among men with varicocele. Gynecomastia is a frequent finding among men with severe testicular dysfunction. The prostate should be examined for fullness. WBC in expressed prostatic secretions can be detected by means of microscopic examination.

Laboratory Evaluation

Semen Analysis

Despite its limitations, routine semen analysis is a simple, inexpensive screening test with which to begin the laboratory evaluation for male infertility. The medical history and physical examination of infertile men often are normal. Therefore, a semen analysis is almost always indicated. Because sperm output varies, three ejaculates should be obtained to provide a representative sample.

If the medical history, physical examination, and semen analysis are normal, attention should be directed to the female partner before evaluation for the man continues (see algorithm at the beginning of the chapter). In couples with unexplained infertility, direct semen analysis may be normal but a disorder of sperm function may still be present. Conversely, direct sperm count may incorrectly identify certain men with borderline sperm output or motility as abnormal.[98] Functional sperm assays, such as the zona-free hamster egg penetration assay and the hemizona assay, may be better indicators of male fertility. These tests, although difficult to perform, may provide useful information in selected instances.

Testosterone

Serum or plasma testosterone level should be measured if hypogonadism is suspected on the basis of clinical evidence or if hypospermatogenesis is detected. Commercial kits for the direct assay of testosterone in unextracted serum with the use of iodine-125-labeled testosterone are relatively simple to use, precise, and accurate. Testosterone is present in serum largely bound to SHBG, a high-affinity protein produced by the liver, and to albumin. Changes in circulating SHBG concentrations influence the measured total testosterone concentration. For example, obese men have low SHBG and total testosterone levels but usually have normal non-SHBG (bioavailable) and free testosterone concentrations.

Gonadotropins

The pituitary gonadotropins LH and FSH are the principal regulators of testicular function. Elevated FSH and LH levels indicate primary testicular failure. High FSH levels indicate seminiferous tubule dysfunction and probably result from a deficiency in the secretion of inhibin and sex steroids. High FSH but normal LH levels are often found among infertile men and suggest that Leydig cell function is relatively preserved compared with seminiferous tubule function.[72] Men with elevated FSH levels may have pituitary tumors. These tumors secrete FSH inefficiently and are usually large when FSH levels are increased, producing headaches, visual disturbances, and low LH and testosterone concentrations. LH levels are rarely increased in men without a concomitant increase in FSH levels. LH and FSH levels generally are normal in infertile men, even with severe oligospermia. Because of overlap between healthy men and men with gonadotropin deficiency, the diagnosis of gonadotropin deficiency in infertile men should not be made by means of measurement of gonadotropin levels alone. The finding of a low testosterone level with a low or normal LH concentration suggests a disturbance in gonadotropin secretion. Pulsatile gonadotropin secretion may be abnormal even when random LH levels are well within the range of normal. Because the proposed clinical approach is to identify recognizable causes of male infertility that are either manageable or unmanageable, the suggestion by some experts that little is gained from measuring gonadotropin levels in infertile men seems counterproductive.

Prolactin

Measurement of prolactin in serum is of great importance in the examination of men with sexual dysfunction, impaired libido, low semen volume, or a possible pituitary tumor. Among men with prolactinomas, circulating testosterone levels are usually low but may be normal.[99] Prolactin levels may be elevated slightly among men with testicular failure[100] but are rarely elevated among otherwise healthy men with oligospermia. Both the stress of venipuncture and chest wall stimulation may increase serum prolactin levels. Prolactin deficiency is rare and is without known sequelae among men.

Estrogens

Estradiol and estrone are present in low levels in the sera of healthy men. Commercial assays, which are optimized to measure levels in women, frequently overestimate the concentration of estrogens in the serum of men. Gonadal and adrenal tumors may secrete estradiol and estrone. Patients with these tumors generally have gynecomastia, decreased libido, and low circulating testosterone levels.[101] Circulating estrone levels are often elevated among men with alcoholic cirrhosis and obese men. The increased secretion of androstenedione by the adrenal glands during stress and the presence of aromatase in fat tissue may contribute to these findings. Estradiol levels are often elevated in men with hCG-producing tumors. Measurement of estrogens is not worthwhile for infertile men who have no signs of feminization and normal testosterone levels.

Functional Endocrine Tests

Response to hCG

Stimulation of testosterone secretion by hCG is a method of assessment of Leydig cell function in prepubertal boys who secrete little endogenous gonadotropin. In contrast, men with Leydig cell failure have elevated circulating LH levels. Administration of hCG to these men increases circulating testosterone levels less than in men with normal Leydig cell function. Short-term administration of hCG also produces an attenuated increase in serum testosterone levels among men with go- nadotropin deficiency because the Leydig cells have been chronically understimulated by LH. In these men, the coexis- tence of low LH and testosterone levels indicates that go- nadotropin secretion is abnormal. Therefore, clinically useful information is rarely gained from an hCG test of a man.

Response to Gonadal-Steroid Hormone Antagonists and Inhibitors

Administration of the estrogen antagonist clomiphene citrate or tamoxifen increases circulating gonadotropin levels in healthy men by blocking the negative feedback effect of estradiol.[102] This is a dose- and time-dependent effect, and several weeks of treatment are needed before consistent changes occur. This test is of limited clinical diagnostic usefulness and provides little additional information beyond basal hormone levels. Similarly, LH levels rise when testosterone production is blocked by steroidogenesis inhibitors such as ketoconazole[103] or antiandro- gens such as flutamide.[58]

GnRH Test

Synthetic GnRH has been used extensively as a research tool. In general, the incremental rise in LH and FSH levels after ad- ministration of GnRH is proportional to basal hormone level. Thus peak gonadotropin levels are higher than normal among men with primary testicular failure. Patients with less severe testicular failure may have basal FSH levels within the range of normal but an exaggerated FSH response to GnRH. Among pa- tients with either pituitary or hypothalamic disease, the release of gonadotropins after stimulation with GnRH is usually re- duced but may be normal. Thus the response to GnRH does not differentiate these two possibilities. For patients with GnRH deficiency and a normal pituitary gland, however, repetitive administration of GnRH may restore gonadotropin secretion.[104] Although repetitive stimulation with GnRH may be useful in the identification of men with gonadotropin deficiency who may be candidates for GnRH therapy, at present the GnRH test has little practical utility in the evaluation of male infertility.

Radiologic Investigation

Magnetic resonance imaging (MRI) of the sella and suprasellar region with gadopentetate dimeglumine enhancement is indi- cated when clinical and biochemical findings suggest hypo- gonadotropic hypogonadism. Careful diagnostic consideration of the many systemic disorders in which suppressed go- nadotropin secretion occurs reduces the number of normal stud- ies performed. Vasography is usually recommended when the diagnosis of genital tract obstruction is entertained. Because va- sography is an invasive and expensive modality, a noninterven- tional method would be useful. Transrectal ultrasonography can

be used to identify absent or obstructed seminal vesicles and may provide evidence of chronic prostatic infection.[105] Vasogra- phy is needed, however, when surgical repair is considered. The presence of varicocele has been determined with noninvasive methods such as Doppler ultrasonography, thermography, and Tc (technetium) radionuclide scanning and with spermatic venography. Only the last technique is accepted as final proof of varicocele, although false-negative results may be obtained. Subclinical varicocele is not known to improve with therapy, however, so these diagnostic tests are often unnecessary.

Testicular Biopsy

Histologic examination of testis tissue from infertile men al- most always reveals abnormalities of the seminiferous tubules, including decreased tubular diameter, incomplete germ cell de- velopment, sloughing of germ cells into the tubular lumen, and peritubular hyalinization. These histologic findings provide lit- tle insight into the pathophysiologic processes of infertility, however, and do not affect therapy. Therefore, routine testicular biopsy is not recommended. For men with azoospermia and normal serum FSH levels, testicular biopsy, including fine nee- dle aspiration, are used to identify men with obstructive azoospermia who may be candidates for microsurgical treat- ment.[106] On the other hand, azoospermic men with elevated serum FSH levels have severe seminiferous tubular dysfunction and should not undergo biopsy.

MEDICAL MANAGEMENT OF MALE INFERTILITY

The cause and pathogenesis of most male infertility remains un- certain; consequently, treatment is often unsatisfactory. Never- theless, there are some infertile men for whom medical or surgical treatment may restore fertility.

Seminiferous Tubule Failure

Primary testicular failure and elevated serum FSH levels due to orchitis, Klinefelter's syndrome, cryptorchidism, varicocele, or unknown causes are not amenable to therapy for infertility. Azoospermia or severe oligospermia are generally found, and additional endocrine diagnostic tests are unnecessary. Andro- gen deficiency is most practically treated with long-acting par- enteral[107] or transdermal[108] testosterone preparations.

Gonadotropin Deficiency

Men with congenital or acquired gonadotropin deficiency can be treated with gonadotropins.[109,110] Most often they are treated with testosterone until fertility is desired. Therapy is then changed to hCG in doses of 1500 to 2000 units intramuscularly or subcutaneously two to three times a week to stimulate Leydig cell function and increase intratesticular testosterone levels and other factors. Selected patients may produce sperm and impregnate their partners when they undergo treatment with hCG alone.[111] It is likely that these patients have some endogenous FSH secretion. Twelve to 18 months of treatment may be needed before sperm begin to appear in the ejaculate. After approximately 1 year of hCG therapy, FSH (LMG) is added to the regimen. Most investigators have used doses of 75 IU intramuscularly or subcutaneously three times a week, although higher doses may be used. Because maturation of spermatogonia to mature sperm takes 72 days, several months of treatment are needed before sperm are produced. Treatment should not be considered a failure until at least 12 months of this regimen have elapsed. Patients with cryptorchidism, with or without orchidopexy, respond poorly to therapy.[112]

Men with congenital GnRH deficiency (Kallmann's syndrome) may be treated with GnRH, since these men have a defect in synthesis or release of GnRH and otherwise normal pituitary function. An infusion pump is used to deliver pulses of GnRH into the subcutaneous tissue of the abdomen.[14,113] Doses of 2 to 8 μg per pulse every 90 to 120 minutes have been used to stimulate gonadotropin secretion. Serum testosterone levels generally rise into the normal range, and sperm begin to appear in the ejaculate 1 to 12 months after the beginning of treatment. As with therapy with hCG or human menopausal gonadotropin (hMG), testis growth precedes the onset of complete spermatogenesis. The highest sperm counts are achieved by patients whose pretreatment testis size is greater than 4 mL, suggesting that they have partial gonadotropin deficiency.[113] Studies suggest that the results of hCG/hMG or GnRH therapy are roughly equivalent, although spermatogenesis may increase more rapidly with GnRH therapy.[114] Patients can be taught to self-administer these medications, and compliance rates are high. Costs and convenience of therapy favor the hCG/hMG regimen.

Idiopathic Oligospermia and Asthenospermia

Various medical therapies have been advocated for idiopathic oligospermia. Unfortunately, most studies are insufficiently powered, suffer from a lack of an appropriate control group, and produce results that cannot be confirmed. Clinical trials for male infertility are complex because the appropriate controls may not be known, coexistent subfertility in the female partner influences outcomes, and a substantial number of couples ultimately conceive with no treatment. For example, in one study that involved 1145 infertile couples, pregnancy occurred in 191 of 548 untreated couples (34.8%) followed for 2 to 7 years.[115] This included 75 of 122 men (61.5%) with sperm den-

sity of less than 20 million/mL and sperm motility less than 40% on two occasions.

Probably the most frequently prescribed male fertility drugs have been the estrogen antagonists clomiphene and tamoxifen. If given in sufficient doses, these drugs increase LH and FSH secretion by blocking the physiologic negative feedback inhibition of the hypothalamus and pituitary gland by estrogens.[102] The rationale is to stimulate spermatogenesis by increasing the gonadotropin drive to testes. The implied but unproved hypothesis is that some men are subtly deficient in gonadotropin secretion, which results in infertility. A second notion is that testicular estrogens impair spermatogenesis directly and that antiestrogens prevent this change. Several carefully performed studies did not show any benefit of clomiphene therapy.[116-118] A multicenter, randomized, placebo-controlled trial of clomiphene, 25 mg a day for 6 months, was conducted with 141 men with sperm concentrations less than 20 million/mL. The cumulative life-table pregnancy rate of 8.6% was identical in both groups. There was no change in sperm motility or morphology, although the motile sperm concentration rose equally in both groups.[118] Several pilot studies of the aromatase inhibitor testolactone suggested that the drug increased sperm output.[119] One randomized, placebo-controlled study of testolactone revealed no effect on semen quality, but this study has been criticized because there also was no change in the hormone profile.[120] Mesterolone, a synthetic androgen, is used in Europe to stimulate spermatogenesis, but appears to be ineffective.[121] Hormonal therapy with hCG/hMG and GnRH and its agonistic analogs is also without effect.[122] In testosterone-rebound therapy, testosterone is administered to suppress gonadotropin secretion and inhibit spermatogenesis. When treatment is discontinued, the hypothesis is that normal spermatogenesis will occur. This approach is unproved.

Kallikreins are a family of serine proteases found in plasma and in a variety of tissues. Kallikrein has been administered orally outside the United States to increase sperm density. A double-blind, placebo-controlled trial, however, demonstrated no effect of kallikrein on sperm count, motility, or quality and no increase in pregnancy rate.[123] Conflicting evidence that the xanthine phosphodiesterase inhibitor, pentoxifylline, increases sperm motility in vitro has led to oral administration of the drug to infertile men. There appears to be no increase in sperm motility or subsequent pregnancy rate,[124] but more studies are needed.

Glucocorticoids have been used to alter the immune response in infertile men with sperm antibodies. In an often quoted placebo-controlled trial,[125] prednisolone at a dose of 20 mg twice a day on days 1 to 20 of the spouse's menstrual cycle for 9 months produced a pregnancy rate of 30% compared with 10% for a group who received a placebo. The findings at semen analysis were not appreciably changed, however. In an earlier, open-label study by the same investigators,[126] 25 of 76 women (33%) whose husbands were treated with prednisolone for antisperm antibodies conceived over a 9-month period. Antisperm antibody titers decreased similarly in the pregnant and nonpregnant groups, however, and 11 of 25 women who eventually conceived were treated for ovulatory dysfunction. Two other double-blind, placebo-controlled studies of prednisolone treatment of infertile men with sperm-associated immunoglobulins found treatment to be ineffective.[127,128] Thus the effectiveness of glucocorticoids in male infertility remains controversial. In addition, glucocorticoids have dangerous side effects, such as aseptic necrosis of the hip, peptic ulcer disease, hyperglycemia, and hypertension.

The possible role of chronic prostatitis in male infertility of unknown causation often leads to treatment with antibiotics. In a multicenter study coordinated by the World Health Organization,[129] only 160 of 2871 men (5.6%) who requested an evaluation of infertility fulfilled the criteria for male accessory gland infection. Of these, 34 couples in whom no other potential cause for infertility was found participated in a double-blind, placebo-controlled study of use of doxycycline. Treatment averaged 5 months; there were two pregnancies in the doxycycline group and one in the placebo group. These data suggest that genital tract infection is rarely the only factor predisposing to male infertility and that doxycycline is of limited use by these patients. The quinolone antibiotics, such as ofloxacin, which are concentrated in prostate tissue and seminal plasma, may be more effective, but have not been studied.

Assisted methods of reproduction have become the dominant method of management of male-factor infertility when no manageable cause is identified or treatment is unsuccessful. Because of cost considerations, donor insemination is often recommended.

REFERENCES

1. Jones HW Jr, Toner JP: The infertile couple. *N Engl J Med* 329:1710, 1993
2. Risbridger GP, de Kretser DM: Paracrine regulation of the testis. In: Burger H, de Kretser D (eds). *The Testis*. New York, Raven, 1989:255
3. De Braekeleer M, Dao T-N: Cytogenetic studies in male infertility: A review. *Hum Reprod* 6:245, 1991
4. Wang C, Baker HWG, Burger HG, De Kretser DM, Hudson B: Hormonal studies in Klinefelter's syndrome. *Clin Endocrinol* 4:399, 1975
5. Skakkebaek NE, Hulten M, Jacobsen P, Mikkelsen M: Quantification of human seminiferous epithelium. II. Histologic studies in eight 47,XYY men. *J Reprod Fertil* 32:391, 1973
6. Ma K, Sharkey A, Kirwch S, et al: Towards the molecular local-

7. Griffin JE: Androgen resistance: The clinical and molecular spectrum. *N Engl J Med* 326:611, 1992
8. Chilvers C, Dudley NE, Gough MH, Jackson MB, Pike MC: Undescended testis: The effect of treatment on subsequent risk of subfertility and malignancy. *J Pediatr Surg* 21:691, 1986
9. Zenilman JM: Update on bacterial sexually transmitted disease. *Urol Clin North Am* 19:25, 1992
10. Wolin LH: On the etiology of epididymitis. *J Urol* 105:531, 1971
11. Lieblich JM, Rogol AD, White BJ, Rosen SW: Syndrome of anosmia with hypogonadotropic hypogonadism (Kallmann syndrome). *Am J Med* 73:506, 1982
12. Bick D, Franco B, Sherins RJ, et al: Brief report: Intragenic deletion of the Kalig-1 gene in Kallmann's syndrome. *N Engl J Med* 326:1752, 1992
13. Spratt DI, Carr DB, Merriam GR, Scully RE, Rao PN, Crowley WF Jr: The spectrum of abnormal patterns of gonadotropin-releasing hormone secretion in men with idiopathic hypogonadotropic hypogonadism: Clinical and laboratory correlations. *J Clin Endocrinol Metab* 64:283, 1987
14. Shargil AA: Treatment of idiopathic hypogonadotropic hypogonadism in men with luteinizing hormone-releasing hormone: A comparison of treatment with daily injections and with the pulsatile infusion pump. *Fertil Steril* 47:492, 1987
15. Winters SJ, Troen P: Altered pulsatile secretion of luteinizing hormone in hypogonadal men with hyperprolactinemia. *Clin Endocrinol* 21:257, 1984
16. Luton JP, Thieblot P, Valcke JC, Mahoudeau JA, Bricaire H: Reversible gonadotropin deficiency in male Cushing's disease. *J Clin Endocrinol Metab* 45:488, 1977
17. Nieman LK, Chrousos GP, Kellner C, et al: Successful treatment of Cushing's syndrome with the glucocorticoid antagonist RU 486. *J Clin Endocrinol Metab* 61:536, 1985
18. Bonaccorsi AC, Adler I, Figueiredo JG: Male infertility due to congenital adrenal hyperplasia: Testicular biopsy findings, hormonal evaluation, and therapeutic results in three patients. *Fertil Steril* 47:664, 1987
19. Semple CG, Gray CE, Beastall GH: Male hypogonadism: A nonspecific consequence of illness. *Q J Med* 64:601, 1987
20. Boyden TW, Pamenter RW: Effects of ethanol on the male hypothalamic-pituitary-gonadal axis. *Endocr Rev* 4:389, 1983
21. Cundy T, Bomford A, Butler J, Wheeler M, Williams R: Hypogonadism and sexual dysfunction in hemochromatosis: The effects of cirrhosis and diabetes. *J Clin Endocrinol Metab* 69:110, 1989
22. Handelsman DJ: Hypothalamic-pituitary gonadal dysfunction in renal failure, dialysis and renal transplantation. *Endocr Rev* 6:151, 1985
23. Krieger JN, Coombs RW, Collier AC, et al: Fertility parameters in men infected with human immunodeficiency virus. *J Infect Dis* 164:464, 1991
24. Politch JA, Mayer KH, Abbott AF, Anderson DF: The effects of

ization of the AZF locus: Mapping of microdeletions in azoospermic men within 14 subintervals of interval 6 of the human Y chromosome. *Hum Mol Genet* 1:29, 1992 disease progression and zidovidine therapy on semen quality in human immunodeficiency virus type 1 seropositive men. *Fertil Steril* 61:922, 1994

25. Raffi F, Brisseau JM, Planchon B, Remi JP, Barrier JH, Grolleau JY: Endocrine function in 98 HIV-infected patients: A prospective study. *AIDS* 5:729, 1991
26. Pudney J, Anderson D: Orchitis and human immunodeficiency virus type 1 infected cells in reproductive tissues from men with the acquired immune deficiency syndrome. *Am J Pathol* 139:149, 1991
27. Kujala UM, Alen M, Huhtaniemi IT: Gonadotropin-releasing hormone and human chorionic gonadotropin tests reveal that both hypothalamic and testicular endocrine functions are suppressed during acute prolonged physical exercise. *Clin Endocrinol* 33:219, 1990
28. Cameron JL, Weltzin TE, McConaha C, Helmreich DL, Kaye WH: Slowing of pulsatile luteinizing hormone secretion in men after forty-eight hours of fasting. *J Clin Endocrinol Metab* 73:35, 1991
29. Rogol AD, Veldhuis JD, Williams FA, Johnson ML: Pulsatile secretion of gonadotropins and prolactin in male marathon runners. *J Androl* 5:21, 1984
30. Bagatell CJ, Bremner WJ: Sperm counts and reproductive hormones in male marathoners and lean controls. *Fertil Steril* 53:688, 1990
31. Ayers JWT, Komesu Y, Romani T, Ansbacher R: Anthropomorphic, hormonal and psychologic correlates of semen quality in endurance-trained male athletes. *Fertil Steril* 43:917, 1985
32. Zumoff B, Strain GW, Miller LK, et al: Plasma free and non-sex-hormone-binding-globulin-bound testosterone are decreased in obese men in proportion to their degree of obesity. *J Clin Endocrinol Metab* 71:929, 1990
33. Strain GW, Zumoff B, Kream J, et al: Mild hypogonadotropic hypogonadism in obese men. *Metabolism* 31:871, 1982
34. Vermeulen A, Kaufman JM, Desylpere JP, Thomas G: Attenuated luteinizing hormone (LH) pulse amplitude but normal LH pulse frequency, and its relation to plasma androgens in hypogonadism of obese men. *J Clin Endocrinol Metab* 76:1140, 1993
35. Stanik S, Dornfeld LP, Maxwell MH, Viosca SP, Korenman SG: The effect of weight loss on reproductive hormones in obese men. *J Clin Endocrinol Metab* 53:828, 1981
36. Kidd GS, Glass AR, Vigersky RA: The hypothalamic-pituitary-testicular axis in thyrotoxicosis. *J Clin Endocrinol Metab* 48:798, 1979
37. O'Brien IAD, Lewin IG, O'Hare JP, Corral RJM: Reversible male subfertility due to hyperthyroidism. *BMJ* 285:691, 1982
38. Nomura K, Suzuki H, Saji M, et al: High serum progesterone in hyperthyroid men with Graves' disease. *J Clin Endocrinol Metab* 66:230, 1988
39. Wortsman J, Rosner W, Dufau ML: Abnormal testicular function in men with primary hypothyroidism. *Am J Med* 82:207, 1987
40. Davidson JM, Chen JJ, Crapo L, Gray GD, Greenleaf WJ, Catania JA: Hormonal changes and sexual function in aging men. *J Clin Endocrinol Metab* 57:71, 1983
41. Neaves WB, Johnson L, Porter JC, Parker CR Jr, Petty CS: Leydig

cell numbers, daily sperm production, and serum gonadotropin levels in aging men. *J Clin Endocrinol Metab* 59:756, 1984
42. Kaufman JM, Deslypere JP, Giri M, Vermeulen A: Neuroendocrine regulation of pulsatile luteinizing hormone secretion in elderly men. *J Steroid Biochem Mol Biol* 37:421, 1990
43. Check JH, Shanis B, Bollendorf A, Adelson H, Breen E: Semen characteristics and infertility in aging. *Arch Androl* 23:275, 1989
44. Eil C, Gamblin GT, Hodge JW, Clark RV, Sherins RJ: Whole cell and nuclear androgen uptake in skin fibroblasts from infertile men. *J Androl* 6:365, 1985
45. Auger J, Kunstmann JM, Czyglik F, Jouannet P: Decline in semen quality among fertile men in pairs during the past 20 years. *N Engl J Med* 332:281, 1995
46. Wilcox AJ, Baird DD, Weinberg CR, Hornsby PP, Herbst AL: Fertility in men exposed prenatally to diethylstilbestrol. *N Engl J Med* 332:1411, 1995
47. Loriaux DL, Menard R, Taylor A, Pita JC Jr, Santen R: Spironolactone and endocrine dysfunction. *Ann Intern Med* 85:630, 1976
48. Sonino N: The use of ketoconazole as an inhibitor of steroid production. *N Engl J Med* 317:812, 1987
49. Winters SJ, Banks JL, Loriaux DL: Cimetidine is an antiandrogen in the rat. *Gastroenterology* 76:504, 1979
50. Gooren L, Spinder T, Spiikstra JJ, et al: Sex steroids and pulsatile luteinizing hormone release in men: Studies in estrogen-treated agonadal subjects and eugonadal subjects treated with a novel nonsteroidal antiandrogen. *J Clin Endocrinol Metab* 64:763, 1987
51. Schurmeyer T, Knuth UA, Belkien L, Nieschlag E: Reversible azoospermia induced by the anabolic steroid 19-nortestosterone. *Lancet* 1:417, 1984
52. Schilsky RL, Lewis BJ, Sherins RJ, Young RC: Gonadal dysfunction in patients receiving chemotherapy for cancer. *Ann Intern Med* 93:109, 1980
53. Pryzant RM, Meistrich ML, Wilson G, Brown B, McLaughlin P: Long-term reduction in sperm count after chemotherapy with and without radiation therapy for non-Hodgkin's lymphomas. *J Clin Oncol* 11:239, 1993
54. Morris ID, Shalet SM: Endocrine-mediated protection from cytotoxic-induced testicular damage. *J Endocrinol* 120:7, 1989
55. Redman JR, Bajorunas DR, Goldstein MC, et al: Semen cryopreservation and artificial insemination for Hodgkin's disease. *J Clin Oncol* 5:233, 1987
56. Vigersky RA, Chapman RM, Berenberg J, Glass AR: Testicular dysfunction in untreated Hodgkin's disease. *Am J Med* 73:482, 1982
57. Consentino MJ, Cyhey WY, Takihara H, Cockett ATK: The effects of sulfasalazine on human male fertility potential and seminal prostaglandins. *J Urol* 132:682, 1984
58. Kucheria K, Saxena R, Mohan D: Semen analysis in alcohol dependence syndrome. *Andrologia* 17:558, 1985
59. Van Thiel DH, Gavaler JS, Sanghvi A: Recovery of sexual function in abstinent alcoholic men. *Gastroenterology* 84:677, 1982
60. Brzek A: Alcohol and male fertility: Preliminary report. *Andrologia* 19:32, 1987
61. Dunphy BC, Barratt CL, Cooke ID: Male alcohol consumption

and fecundity in couples attending an infertility clinic. *Andrologia* 23:219, 1991

62. Ragni G, De Lauretis L, Gambaro V, et al: Semen evaluation in heroin and methadone addicts. *Acta Eur Fertil* 16:245, 1985

63. Azizi F, Vagenakis AG, Longcope C, Ingbar SH, Braverman LE: Decreased serum testosterone concentration in male heroin and methadone addicts. *Steroids* 22:467, 1973

64. Veldhuis JD, Rogol AD, Somojlik E, Ertel NH: Role of endogenous opiates in the expression of negative feedback actions of androgen and estrogen on pulsatile properties of luteinizing hormone secretion in man. *J Clin Invest* 74:47, 1984

65. Dalterio SL, DeRooij DG: Maternal cannabinoid exposure: Effects on spermatogenesis in male offspring. *Int J Androl* 9:250, 1986

66. Schrag SD, Dixon RL: Occupational exposures associated with male reproductive dysfunction. *Ann Rev Pharmacol Toxicol* 25:567, 1985

67. Lamb EJ, Bennett S: Epidemiologic studies of male factors in infertility. *Ann N Y Acad Sci* 709:165, 1994

68. Strohmer H, Boldizsar A, Plockinger B, Feldner-Busztin M, Feichtinger W: Agricultural work and male infertility. *Am J Ind Med* 24:587, 1993

69. Marshburn PB, Sloan CS, Hammond MG: Semen quality and association with coffee drinking, cigarette smoking, and ethanol consumption. *Fertil Steril* 52:162, 1989

70. Jequier AM, Holmes SC: Aetiological factors in the production of obstructive azoospermia. *Br J Urol* 56:540, 1984

71. Durieu I, Bey-Omar F, Rollet J, et al: Diagnostic criteria for cystic fibrosis in men with congenital absence of the vas deferens. *Medicine* 74:42, 1995

72. Handelsman DJ, Conway AJ, Boylan LM, Turtle JR: Young's syndrome: Obstructive azoospermia and chronic sinopulmonary infections. *N Engl J Med* 310:3, 1984

73. Afzelius BA, Eliasson R: Male and female infertility problems in the immotile-cilia syndrome. *Eur J Respir Dis* 64(suppl 127):144, 1983

74. Yavetz H, Yogev I, Hauser R, Lessing JB, Paz B, Homonnai ZT: Retrograde ejaculation. *Hum Reprod* 9:381, 1994

75. Murray FT, Wyss HU, Thomas RG, Spevack M, Glaros AG: Gonadal dysfunction in diabetic men with organic impotence. *J Clin Endocrinol Metab* 65:127, 1987

76. Ver Voort SM: Infertility in spinal-cord injured male. *Urology* 29:157, 1987

77. Dickerman Z, Sagiv M, Savion M, Allalouf D, Levinski H, Singer R: Andrological parameters in human semen of high (greater than or equal to 6 ml) and low (less than or equal to 1 ml) volume. *Andrologia* 21:353, 1989

78. Nilsson S, Edvinsson A, Nilsson B: Improvement of semen and pregnancy rate after ligation and division of the internal spermatic vein: Fact or fiction? *Br J Urol* 51:591, 1979

79. World Health Organization: The influence of varicocele on parameters of fertility in a large group of men presenting to infertility clinics. *Fertil Steril* 57:1289, 1992

80. Kursh ED: What is the incidence of varicocele in a fertile population? *Fertil Steril* 48:510, 1987

81. Nagao RR, Plymate SR, Berger RE, Perin EB, Paulsen CA: Comparison of gonadal function between fertile and infertile men with varicoceles. *Fertil Steril* 46:930, 1986

82. Madgar I, Weissenberg R, Lunenfeld B, Karasik A, Goldwasser B: Controlled trial of high spermatic vein ligation for varicocele in infertile men. *Fertil Steril* 63:120, 1995

83. Haans LC, Laven JS, Mali WP, te Velde ER, Wensing CJ: Testis volumes, semen quality, and hormonal patterns in adolescents with and without a varicocele. *Fertil Steril* 56:731, 1991

84. Okuyama A, Nakamura M, Namiki M, et al: Surgical repair of varicocele at puberty: Preventive treatment for fertility improvement. *J Urol* 139:562, 1988

85. Chehval MJ, Purcell MH: Deterioration of semen parameters over time in men with untreated varicocele: Evidence of progressive testicular damage. *Fertil Steril* 57:174, 1992

86. Gump DW, Gibson M, Ashikaga T: Lack of association between genital mycoplasmas and infertility. *N Engl J Med* 310:937, 1984

87. Greendale GA, Haas S, Holbrook K, Walsh B, Schachter J, Phillips RS: The relationship of *Chlamydia trachomatis* infection and male infertility. *Am J Public Health* 83:996, 1993

88. Jude-Harris AA: Male subfertility due to sperm antibodies: A clinical overview. *Obstet Gynecol Surv* 48:1, 1992

89. Meinertz H, Linnet L, Fogh-Andersen P, Hjort T: Antisperm antibodies and fertility after vasovasotomy: A follow-up study of 216 men. *Fertil Steril* 54:315, 1990

90. Paschke R, Schulze Bertelsbeck D, Bahrs S, Heinecke A, Behre HM: Seminal sperm antibodies exhibit an unstable spontaneous course and an increased incidence of leucocytospermia. *Int J Androl* 17:135, 1994

91. Kandeel FR, Swerdloff RS: Role of temperature in regulation of spermatogenesis and the use of heating as a method of contraception. *Fertil Steril* 49:1, 1988

92. Zorgniotti AW, Cohen MS, Sealfon AI: Chronic scrotal hypothermia: Results in 90 infertile couples. *J Urol* 135:944, 1985

93. Procope BJ: Effect of repeated increase of body temperature on human sperm cells. *Int J Fertil* 19:333, 1965

94. Gross KM, Matsumoto AM, Southworth MB, Bremner WJ: Evidence for decreased luteinizing hormone–releasing hormone pulse frequency in men with selective elevations of follicle-stimulating hormone. *J Clin Endocrinol Metab* 60:197, 1985

95. Wu FC, Taylor PL, Sellar RE: LHRH pulse frequency in normal and infertile men. *J Endocrinol* 123:149, 1991

96. Mozaffarian GA, Higley M, Paulsen CA: Clinical studies in an adult male patient with "isolated follicle stimulating hormone (FSH) deficiency." *J Androl* 4:393, 1983

97. Matthews CH, Borgato S, Beck-Peccoz P, et al: Primary amenorrhea and infertility due to a mutation in the β-subunit of follicle-stimulating hormone. *Nat Genet* 5:83, 1993

98. Seibel MM, Zilberstein M: The shape of semen morphology. *Hum Reprod* 10:247–8, 1995

99. Winters SJ: Diurnal rhythm of testosterone and luteinizing hormone in hypogonadal men. *J Androl* 12:185, 1991

100. Spitz IM, Zylber E, Cohen H, Almaliach U, Leroith D: Impaired

prolactin response to thyrotropin-releasing hormone in isolated gonadotropin deficiency and exaggerated response in primary testicular failure. *J Clin Endocrinol Metab* 48:941, 1979

101. Veldhuis JD, Sowers JR, Rogol AD, Klein FA, Miller N, Dufau ML: Pathophysiology of male hypogonadism associated with endogenous hyperestrogenism: Evidence for dual defects in the gonadal axis. *N Engl J Med* 312:1371, 1985

102. Winters SJ, Troen P: Evidence for a role of endogenous estrogen in the hypothalamic control of gonadotropin secretion in men. *J Clin Endocrinol Metab* 61:842, 1985

103. Glass AR: Ketoconazole-induced stimulation of gonadotropin output in men: Basis for a potential test of gonadotropin reserve. *J Clin Endocrinol Metab* 63:1121, 1986

104. Snyder PJ, Rudenstein RS, Gardner DF, Rothman JG: Repetitive infusion of gonadotropin-releasing hormone distinguishes hypothalamic from pituitary hypogonadism. *J Clin Endocrinol Metab* 48:864, 1979

105. Jarow JP: Transrectal ultrasonography of infertile men. *Fertil Steril* 60:1035, 1993

106. Bergmann M, Behre HM, Nieschlag E: Serum FSH and testicular morphology in male infertility. *Clin Endocrinol* 40:133, 1994

107. Bhasin S: Androgen treatment of hypogonadal men. *J Clin Endocrinol Metab* 74:1221, 1992

108. Koreman SG, Viosca S, Garza D, et al: Androgen therapy of hypogonadal men with transcrotal testosterone systems. *Am J Med* 83:471, 1987

109. Winters SJ, Troen P: Hypogonadotropic hypogonadism: Gonadotropin therapy. In: DT Krieger, CW Bardin (eds), *Current Therapy in Endocrinology and Metabolism.* Toronto, BC Decker, 1985:152

110. Finkel DM, Phillips JL, Snyder PJ: Stimulation of spermatogenesis by gonadotropins in men with hypogonadotropic hypogonadism. *N Engl J Med* 313:651, 1985

111. Burris AS, Rodbard HW, Winters SJ, Sherins RJ: Gonadotropin therapy in men with isolated hypogonadotropic hypogonadism: The response to human chorionic gonadotropin is predicted by initial testicular size. *J Clin Endocrinol Metab* 66:1144, 1988

112. Kirk JM, Savage MO, Grant DB, Bouloux PM, Besser GM: Gonadal function and response to human chorionic and menopausal gonadotropin therapy in male patients with idiopathic hypogonadotropic hypogonadism. *Clin Endocrinol* 41:57, 1994

113. Spratt DI, Finkelstein JS, O'Dea LS, et al: Long-term administration of gonadotropin-releasing hormone in men with idiopathic hypogonadotropic hypogonadism. *Ann Intern Med* 105:848, 1986

114. Schopoh J, Mehltretter G, von Zumbusch R, Eversmann T, von Werder K: Comparison of gonadotropin-releasing hormone and gonadotropin therapy in male patients with idiopathic hypothalamic hypogonadism. *Fertil Steril* 56:1143, 1991

115. Collins JA, Wrixon W, Janes LB, Wilson EH: Treatment-independent pregnancy among infertile couples. *N Engl J Med* 309:1201, 1983

116. Ronnberg L: The effect of clomiphene citrate on different sperm parameters and serum hormone levels in preselected infertile men: A controlled double-blind cross-over study. *Int J Androl* 3:479, 1980

117. Sokol RZ, Steiner BS, Bustillo M, Petersen G, Swerdloff RS: A controlled comparison of the efficacy of clomiphene citrate in male infertility. *Fertil Steril* 49:865, 1988

118. World Health Organization: A double-blind trial of clomiphene citrate for the treatment of idiopathic male infertility. *Int J Androl* 15:299, 1992

119. Vigersky RA, Glass AR: Effects of delta 1 testolactone on the pituitary–testicular axis in oligospermic men. *J Clin Endocrinol Metab* 52:897, 1981

120. Clark RV, Sherins RJ: Clinical trial of testolactone for treatment of idiopathic male infertility (abstract). *J Androl* 4:31, 1983

121. World Health Organization: Mesterolone and idiopathic male infertility: A double-blind study. *Int J Androl* 12:254, 1989

122. Bals-Pratsch M, Knuth UA, Honigl W, Klein HM, Bergmann M, Nieschlag E: Pulsate GnRH therapy in oligozoospermic men does not improve seminal parameters despite decreased FSH levels. *Clin Endocrinol* 30:549, 1989

123. Keck C, Behre HM, Jockenhovel F, Nieschlag E: Ineffectiveness of kallikrein in treatment of idiopathic male infertility: A double-blind, randomized, placebo-controlled trial. *Hum Reprod* 9:325, 1994

124. Tournaye H, van Steirteghem AC, Devroey P: Pentoxifylline in idiopathic male-factor infertility: A review of its therapeutic efficacy after oral administration. *Hum Reprod* 9:996, 1994

125. Hendry WF, Hughes L, Scammell G, Pryor JP, Hargreave TB: Comparison of prednisolone and placebo in subfertile men with antibodies to spermatozoa. *Lancet* 335:85, 1990

126. Hendry WF, Treehuba K, Hughes L, et al: Cyclic prednisolone therapy for male infertility associated with autoantibodies to spermatozoa. *Fertil Steril* 45:249, 1986

127. Hass GG Jr, Manganiello P: A double-blind, placebo-controlled study of the use of methylprednisolone in infertile men with sperm-associated immunoglobulins. *Fertil Steril* 47:295, 1987

128. Bals-Pratsch M, Doren M, Karbowski B, Schneider HP, Nieschlag E: Cyclic corticosteroid immunosuppression is unsuccessful in the treatment of sperm antibody related male infertility: A controlled study. *Hum Reprod* 7:99, 1992

129. Comhaire FH, Rowe PJ, Farley TMM: The effect of doxycycline in infertile couples with male accessory gland infection: A double blind prospective study. *Int J Androl* 9:91, 1986

CHAPTER 16

Surgical Management of Male-Factor Infertility

SHERMAN J. SILBER

Diagnosis and Treatment of Obstructive Azoospermia
Vasectomy reversal
Microsurgical vasoepididymostomy
Evaluation of obstruction not caused by vasectomy
Inguinal disruption of vas deferens
after herniorrhaphy

Obstruction of the ejaculatory duct
Congenital absence of vas deferens
Microsurgery for Undescended Testicle
Rationale for testicular autotransplantation
Microsurgical techniques
Conclusions

DIAGNOSIS AND TREATMENT OF OBSTRUCTIVE AZOOSPERMIA

Vasectomy Reversal

Vasectomy is the most common cause of obstructive azoospermia. There are four major aspects of vasectomy reversal. The first concerns techniques for obtaining a reliable reanastomosis of the vas deferens. With modern microsurgical techniques, accurate reanastomosis should be achievable in almost every instance. The second aspect relates to the detrimental secondary effects of vasectomy, such as pressure-induced epididymal damage. The third aspect concerns microsurgical bypass of this secondary epididymal obstruction. The fourth aspect is freezing of epididymal sperm for later use with intracytoplasmic single-sperm injection (ICSI) as a backup procedure if the reversal operation should fail.[1]

Microsurgical Approach

It is advisable that one practice on animals before performing vasectomy reversal on humans.[2–12] For the best mucosal approximation in humans, in whom lumina are of different diameter (because of chronic obstruction and increased pressure), I recommend a nonsplinted, two-layer approach (Fig 16–1). A one-layer anastomosis provides poorer mucosal approximation when luminal diameters differ. A splint of any kind should never be used. Use of a splint is only an excuse for not being certain one has obtained a good anastomosis. It results in sperm leakage, inflammation, and more scarring.

It is not necessary to determine preoperatively what type of vasectomy was performed. Often a very large segment has been removed, and in most instances, the vasectomy has extended well into the convoluted portion. Such vasectomies would have been considered impossible to correct with conventional techniques. With microsurgical techniques, they merely require a little more dissection but essentially no change from a standard routine.

The preparation of the two ends of the vas deferens microscopic anastomosis is best performed with $\times 2\frac{1}{2}$ loupe magnification. The healthy ends above and below the fibrosis are freed several centimeters and often more than that if a large

sence of sperm was caused not by a disruption of spermatogenesis but by epididymal ruptures and secondary blockage.

Patients who have azoospermia or oligospermia and poor motility more than 1 year after vasovasostomy usually are found to have complete or partial blockage either at the vasovasostomy site or in the epididymis. Although blockage is usually clinically obvious, Rodriguez-Rigau and I developed a simplified quantitative testicular biopsy for cases in which findings are uncertain.[15] If surgical technique was careful, adequate sperm numbers will be found in the ejaculate. Patients who are found to be azoospermic can undergo ICSI if sperm were frozen at the time of the microsurgical procedure.

Quantitative Interpretation of Findings at Testicular Biopsy

Testicular biopsy has been used by most clinicians in a non-quantitative manner only. This has severely limited its usefulness and has led to many errors in interpretation.[22–25] A simplified quantitative evaluation of the results of testicular biopsy is helpful in the assessment of male-factor fertility. It is based on the normal histologic composition and kinetics of spermatogenesis in humans.[26] With radioactive tracers it was determined that the rate of spermatogenesis in humans, or in any species, is constant, even when sperm production is reduced. Reduced production is always caused by lower numbers of sperm "on the assembly line," not diminished speed of production. Therefore the quantity of sperm being produced by a testicle at any given time is reflected by the results of testicular biopsy.

According to this principle, investigators developed a method of quantitative interpretation of the findings at testicular biopsy.[27,28] Initial applications of the technique involved a small number of patients and were limited to making a precise correlation with sperm count. Furthermore, the technique was elaborate and time consuming. In 1978 the same investigators counted all components of spermatogenesis and found good correlation with sperm count.[29] The difficulty remained, however, that the method was time consuming, and very few fertility specialists had an inclination to put that much effort into photographing and analyzing every biopsy specimen.

A simple method can be performed in 10 to 15 minutes. Testicular biopsy specimens of patients with oligospermia and patients with normal sperm counts were analyzed and found to be predictive of mean sperm count. Furthermore, comparing the results of quantitative testicular biopsy with sperm count allowed one to document whether oligospermia was caused by a partially obstructed anastomosis or poor semen transport as opposed to simply deficient spermatogenesis.

Patients with severe oligospermia after structured vasovasostomy become fertile after microsurgical reanastomosis. Thus, we know that obstruction in the ductal system can cause oligospermia and poor motility. In fact, most cases of poor sperm motility and low sperm count after vasectomy reversal have been found to be due to obstruction. When a patient's prior fertility is not known, or when documentation is necessary before a questionable operation is performed, a testicular biopsy should clarify whether or not blockage, or just poor spermatogenesis, is causing the poor semen quality.

The biopsy is performed with careful no-touch atraumatic technique and general anesthesia. The tunica albuginea is sharply incised with a scalpel. The protruding seminiferous tubules are excised with wet, extremely sharp, microiris scissors and allowed to fall into Zenker's solution without being handled. Specimens are carefully fixed, cut in thin sections, and stained with hematoxylin and eosin. The technique of biopsy is important. If the specimen is handled roughly or fixed in formalin, it is difficult to identify accurately the cellular components of the seminiferous tubule.

A testicular biopsy is performed bilaterally, and at least 10 seminiferous tubules are included in the count on each side. Only the mature spermatids (stages I, II, V, and VI) need to be counted (Fig 16–7), that is, the oval-shaped cells with dark, densely stained chromatin. Previous studies have shown that these cells have the greatest correlation with sperm count and are the easiest ones to recognize. All of the steps of spermatogenesis from spermatogonia through resting, leptotene, zygotene, and pachytene spermatocytes and early spermatids, are excluded from consideration. The number of mature spermatids in a minimum of 20 tubules is summed and divided by the number of tubules.

Patients without obstruction with a sperm count fewer than 10 million/mL always have fewer than 20 mature spermatids per tubule. Those with a sperm count of more than 20 million/mL usually have greater than 20 mature spermatids per tubule. The number correlates closely with sperm count.

With an exponential curve (Fig 16–8) the number of mature spermatids per tubule can be used to predict the anticipated sperm count. In the absence of obstruction the correlation is remarkably close. For example, if the patient has 40 mature spermatids per tubule, the sperm count should be just under 60 million/mL; if there are 45 mature spermatids, the sperm count should be just over 85 million. A patient with a sperm count of only 3 million would be expected to have only 6 to 10 mature spermatids per tubule.

The postoperative sperm count of patients who undergo microscopic vasovasostomy or vasoepididymostomy correlates with the findings at quantitative testicular biopsy. A constantly low count is usually caused by continuing obstruction. One can determine this objectively by comparing the mature spermatid count in the testicular biopsy specimen with the sperm count in the semen. For example, if a patient is simply not manufacturing many sperm, his count could be low without continuing obstruction. The semen usually have adequate motility because the low count does not reflect a pathologic condition but rather a low rate of production.

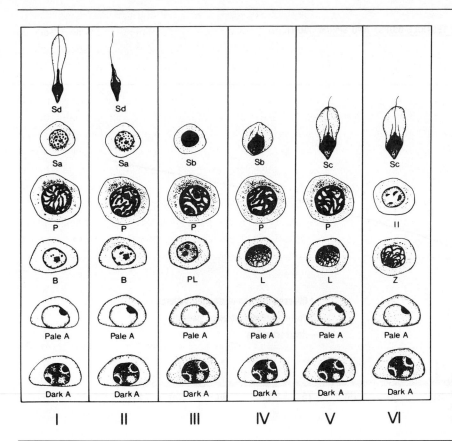

Figure 16–7. Six stages of human spermatogenesis. Mature spermatids are seen only in stages I, II, V, and VI. They are the easiest cells to identify and require very little time for quantification.

Quantitative testicular biopsy can allow a firm diagnosis of obstruction before scrotal exploration that could otherwise require a great deal of guesswork about the presence of epididymal blockage. In addition, it ensures that unwarranted medical therapy is not haphazardly administered to patients who have obstruction.

Patients frequently undergo inappropriate vasoepididymostomy because the pathology report indicates normal spermatogenesis. The readings often are not quantitative but are qualitative impressions that tubules are filled with spermatocytes and some mature sperm. This method of reporting results had led to vasoepididymostomy on many men who do not have obstruction. If the biopsy shows thick tubules with large numbers of spermatocytes but only two or three mature spermatids per tubule, obstruction is not the cause of the patient's "azoospermia."

Some clinicians have attempted to use serum follicle-stimulating hormone (FSH) level to monitor the amount of spermatogenesis: An elevated level in an azoospermic patient would supposedly indicate obstruction. Unfortunately, the correlation is very poor.[30] Patients with maturational arrest that causes azoospermia have a normal FSH level. The level correlates most closely with the total number of spermatogonia and with testicular volume but not with the number of mature

sperm. The feedback mechanism is not tuned finely enough for serum FSH level to reflect what the sperm count should be (Setchel B., personal communication, 1980).

It is ironic that the scattered mosaic arrangement of the various stages of spermatogenesis in the human seminiferous tubule (as opposed to an orderly wave moving across the tubule in most other species) makes quantifying the results of testicular biopsy of humans so simple. In rats a cut through any particular seminiferous tubule shows only one particular stage (Fig 16–9A). In humans, a cut through any area of the testicle reveals a scattered array of all the various stages of spermatogenesis (Fig 16–9B). Thus, in humans it requires only 20 tubules for a good statistical sample of the total range of spermatogenesis in the entire testicle.

Microsurgical Vasoepididymostomy

Technique

The epididymis is a single, 20-foot-long, coiled tubule with myriad intricate convolutions (Fig 16–10). It is squeezed into 2-inch lengths like the pleats of an accordian. Because the epididymis is so tiny, even by microsurgical standards, the results with conventional surgical techniques in repair of obstruction have been very poor.[31–34] The procedure used by Hanley and de-

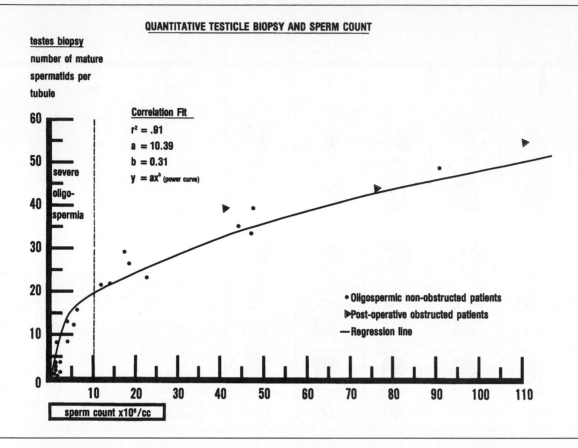

Figure 16–8. Graph demonstrates the relationship between the total number of mature spermatids per tubule at testicular biopsy and the actual sperm count per milliliter. This is an exponential relationship, as one would expect, because the testicular biopsy specimen is two-dimensional. The sperm count relates to a volumetric function of the testicle. (*From Silber SJ, Rodriguez-Rigau LJ: Quantitative analysis of testicle biopsy: Determination of partial obstruction and prediction of sperm count after surgery for obstruction.* Fertil Steril *36:480, 1981. Reprinted with permission of the publisher, the American Society for Reproductive Medicine [The American Fertility Society]).*

scribed by Hotchkiss[35] formed the basis for the usual conventional vasoepididymostomy that is still performed by many urologists. Although it was the best that could be performed in the 1950s, modern microsurgical facilities have rendered the operation obsolete. These patients can now be given a much better prognosis with extremely exacting microsurgical procedures.

The microsurgical specific-tubule technique of vasoepididymostomy was described in 1978.[8–21] After the scrotal sac is entered, the tunica vaginalis is opened and the testis and epididymis are everted from the hydrocele sac. The dilated epididymal tubule is usually about 0.1 to 0.2 mm in diameter. The epididymal duct is extraordinarily delicate, with a wall thickness of about 30 μm. The conventional approach, in which a deep longitudinal incision is made into the outer epididymal tunic, reveals what look like as many as 20 or 30 tiny tubules (Fig 16–11). Without the benefit of microscopic observation, there is an illusion that sperm fluid is welling up from all of these tubules, but in truth the fluid is coming from only one of them. The other tubules are simply blind loops disconnected from

continuity with the testis by this incision. The ideal approach for reestablishment of continuity of the ductal system is to perform an end-to-end anastomosis between the inner lumen of the vas deferens and the one, specific epididymal tubule.

In the past, rather than making a conventional longitudinal incision, one made a *transverse* transaction of the epididymis at the most distal point, that is, at the junction of the cauda and corpus epididymis (Fig 16–12). With this approach one sliced off portions of the epididymis more and more proximally until sperm were recovered at the most distal possible level but proximal to the area of obstruction. I no longer transect the entire epididymis; I prefer a simpler, specific tubular approach that avoids epididymal dissection.

Under an operating microscope, 3 to 10 cut tubules are usually visible on the transected surface of the epididymis, and all are carefully examined for efflux of sperm fluid. This cut surface of the epididymis is smeared on a slide, which is observed under a standard laboratory microscope or phase-contrast microscope for the presence and quality of sperm. Sometimes no

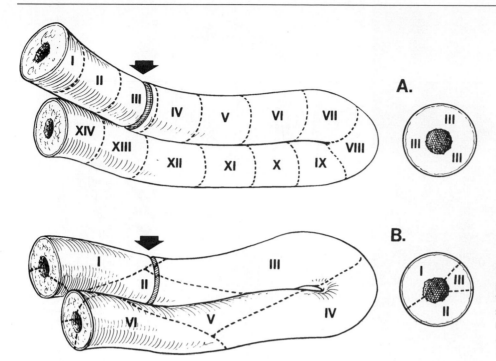

Figure 16–9. A. In most animals, spermatogenesis proceeds in an orderly wave across the seminiferous tubule from one stage to another. **B.** In humans, spermatogenesis has a mosaic, scattered arrangement that does not proceed in an orderly wave. (*From Silber SJ:* Reproductive Microsurgery. *Baltimore, Williams & Wilkins, 1984.*)

fluid at all is observed, in which case transection must be continued proximally. The presence of fluid does not necessarily mean the presence of sperm. One must wait for the report on the fluid before deciding whether to perform the anastomosis at that point or to transect more proximally. The anastomosis is performed at the distalmost level at which normal sperm are found in the epididymal fluid. This allows for the maximum possible length of epididymis.

The original technique is carried out as follows. For the first stitch the epididymis is held between the thumb and the forefinger, facing the microscope. A slight milking action may sometimes be necessary to promote continual efflux of fluid to continue to see which is the correct tubule to anastomose. Monofilament 10-0 nylon on a V-75 taper-cut 75-μm needle is used for the inner layer and 9-0 nylon an a V-100 vas cutting needle for the outer layer. The first suture is placed from the outside to the inside of the specific epididymal tubule that is leaking sperm fluid. Once the suture is placed, the epididymis is put into one jaw of the Silber vasovasostomy clamp, and the vas is inserted into the other jaw. A piece of blue plastic is then placed under the epididymis and vas, which are held in the two jaws of the vasovasostomy clamp. From this point on, the anastomosis of the vas lumen to the epididymal tubule can be performed in a manner somewhat similar to vasovasostomy (Figs 16–13 and 16–14).

The first stitch is placed in the clamp before the epididymis is placed in the clamp because it is extremely difficult to locate the specific tubule leaking the fluid in any other way. The gen-

tle milking action that the thumb and forefinger can provide is helpful in making sure that the fluid is continuing to flow from the tubule that is selected to suture. After the first suture is placed, the tubule is easily identified at all times. An alternative technique, which yields equal results, is to open the outer tunic and make a tiny cut in the epididymal tubule. The posterior muscle layer of the vas is then sutured to the posterior epididymal tunic. The inner mucosa of the vas is sutured end to side to the opening on the epididymal tubule.

Fertility After Vasoepididymostomy

What can be expected of sperm that have not progressed completely through the epididymis? It is well known that sperm from the cauda epididymis are mature and quite capable of fertilizing the ovum; however, it was formerly thought that a large percentage of sperm from the corpus epididymis were incapable of fertilization. Studies with animals revealed that sperm obtained from the head of the epididymis could not achieve maturity or directional motility and thus could not achieve fertilization. We now know differently.

In the human, sperm from anywhere along the corpus epididymis that pass into the vas deferens and into the ejaculate can fertilize an ovum. If the anastomosis is successful anywhere within the corpus epididymis, pregnancy occurs 73% of the time.[36–38] The prognosis is not as good when anastomosis is performed in the head of the epididymis to bypass the obstruction. Among my patients, 43% have attained pregnancy. Pregnancy has even resulted in several instances in which the anastomosis

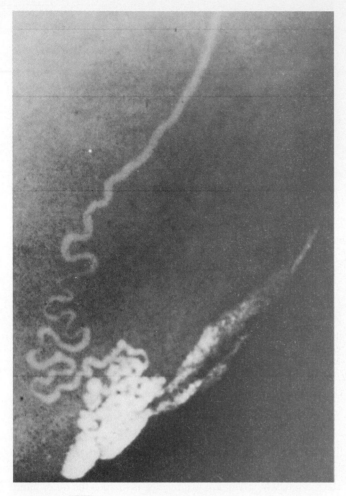

Figure 16–10. Retrograde vasogram of the vas deferens and epididymis shows that the epididymis is simply one long, intricately coiled tube that is continuous with the convoluted region of the vas.

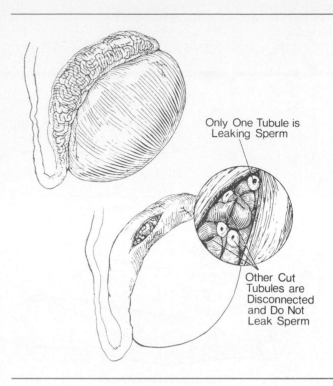

Only One Tubule is Leaking Sperm

Other Cut Tubules are Disconnected and Do Not Leak Sperm

Figure 16–11. In the first stage of a conventional approach to vasoepididymostomy the longitudinal slit is made in the tunic of the epididymis. One epididymal tubule is cut in so many different places that it looks like many cut tubules. Only one of the tubules is leaking sperm. (*From Silber SJ:* Reproductive Microsurgery. *Baltimore, Williams & Wilkins, 1984.*)

had to be performed to the vasa efferentia, meaning the sperm never traversed any portion of the epididymis.

All of the animal data on sperm maturity in the epididymis come from studies in which sperm were sampled from an otherwise functioning epididymis that was intact along its entire length. The question of how well remaining segments of epididymal tubule and vas deferens would be able to promote sperm maturation in the physiologic context of vasoepididymostomy could not be answered with any of the animal experiments that form the basis of our understanding of epididymal function.

For example, in rabbits, spermatozoa were sampled from the seminiferous tubules, the ductuli efferentes, and various levels of the epididymis to determine their intrinsic motility and fertilizing capability.[39] Spermatozoa from the seminiferous tubules and ductuli efferentes showed only weak vibratory movements with no forward progress. Spermatozoa from the proximal head of the epididymis showed very irregular, erratic motility with no forward progression. Traversing the corpus

epididymis, however, increasing numbers of spermatozoa began to show forward movement with proper longitudinal rotation as they progressed distally toward the cauda epididymis. Similar studies with rabbits have been performed by others.[40,41]

In an effort to see whether the increase in maturity was merely a function of the time required for sperm to pass through the epididymis or whether it depended on specific areas of the epididymis, various authors ligated different portions of the epididymis in rabbits and examined samples of the spermatozoa from each portion at intervals.[42–44] After interruption of sperm flow, epididymal spermatozoa that had been poorly motile in the caput region of the epididymis showed increased motility. Because of the pathologic nature of the chronic obstruction made by means of such an experimental model, however, all of these sperm once again lost their motility by 3 weeks. These researchers believed that it was possible for spermatozoa to mature at any level of the epididymal duct, but their experimental approach produced such an abnormal environment that this hypothesis could not be tested adequately. Obstruction to the flow

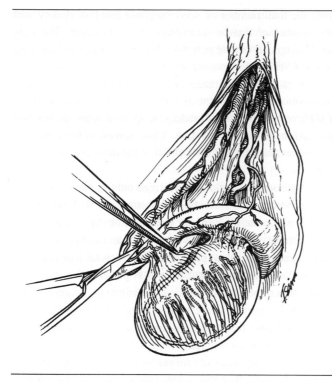

Figure 16–12. The epididymis is freed without damage to the blood supply in preparation for transverse sectioning before a specific tubule-to-tubule vasoepididymostomy. (*From Silber SJ:* Reproductive Microsurgery. *Baltimore, Williams & Wilkins, 1984.*)

of spermatozoa within the epididymis has been shown clearly to result in stagnation of epididymal spermatozoa. Thus, the increased time allowed for maturation in the experiment was counterbalanced by the abnormal obstructed environment.

Orgebin-Crist[45] first suggested that in humans, it was theoretically possible that sperm might be mature and be fertile after vasoepididymostomy even to proximal portions of the epididymis. The remaining epididymal tubule might undergo compensatory changes, or spermatozoa might have more time to mature after coming out of proximal regions of the epididymis than they would in the previously described experimental models. My results with humans who underwent vasoepididymostomy for proximal epididymal obstruction indicated that sperm do not necessarily have to transit all or even part of the epididymis to mature sufficiently for fertilization. They only require sufficient time to mature, and this can occur in the vas deferens as well as the epididymis. It is clear nonetheless that the pregnancy rate is higher with corpus epididymis anastomosis than with caput anastomosis.

In most patients undergoing vasoepididymostomy, the most proximal obstruction is somewhat in the corpus region. I have seen no statistically significant difference in pregnancy rates at any particular point along the corpus epididymis. Among 78% of patients treated with this technique, semen analysis reveals a

sperm count of greater than 10 million/mL and adequate directional motility. About 60% of these patients impregnate their partners within 2 to 3 years. It is too early to know what the eventual pregnancy rate will be because it does seem that fertilizing capability per monthly cycle of sexual exposure is somewhat less among these patients than among the healthy population. Thus, it takes 5 years of follow-up study before it can be stated with assurance how high the pregnancy rate will eventually be. My impression, however, is that the results with vasoepididymostomy will parallel those with vasovasostomy.

Evaluation of Obstruction Not Caused by Vasectomy

The diagnosis of obstruction should really be quite simple; however, it is sometimes approached in a confusing way that can lead to embarrassing situations, such as attempting to do a vasoepididymostomy on a patient who has no obstruction. Ad-

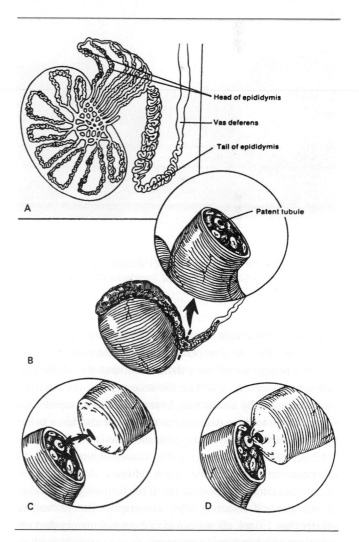

Figure 16–13. A–D. Diagram of the specific tubule technique for vasoepididymostomy first described in 1978. (*From Silber SJ:* Reproductive Microsurgery. *Baltimore, Williams & Wilkins, 1984.*)

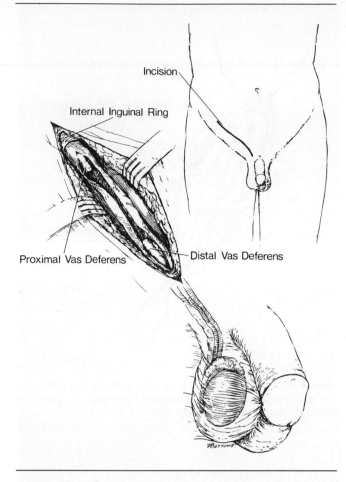

Figure 16–16. Crossover vasovasostomy or vasoepididymostomy. (*From Silber SJ: Reproductive Microsurgery. Baltimore, Williams & Wilkins, 1984.*)

geon and the patient than trying to go through the area of the previous herniorrhaphy to bridge the gap of the missing vas deferens.

Obstruction of the Ejaculatory Duct

A rare cause of azoospermia is congenital obstruction of the ejaculatory duct. This diagnosis is made when the patient has a palpable vas deferens, azoospermia, and a normal testicular biopsy in the presence of low-volume semen with no fructose. A very low semen volume in a patient undergoing assessment of epididymal obstruction should result in a high index of suspicion for ejaculatory duct obstruction. Vasography, which should always be performed routinely at the time of surgical intervention, is the only definitive way to make this diagnosis.

If normal sperm are detected in the vas fluid and the vasogram shows ejaculatory duct obstruction, the patient is placed in the lithotomy position and undergoes transurethral resection of the ejaculatory duct orifice. If the patient has no sperm in the vas fluid, he may have already suffered a rupture in the epididymis from this long-standing obstruction. In that event, a

vasoepididymostomy is first performed and the incision closed before the patient is put in lithotomy position for transurethral resection of the ejaculatory duct.

Transurethral resection of the ejaculatory duct is not difficult for a competent resectionist to perform; however, unless one has had considerable experience with transurethral prostatectomy, it is best not to attempt this procedure.[46,47] First, a resectoscope is inserted through the urethra and the prostatic fossa is inspected. A rectal sheath is used to allow an index finger in the rectum to palpate the posterior floor of the prostatic urethra. With the finger as a guide, a hole is cut sharply into the floor of the prostatic urethra on either the right or the left side just proximal to the verumontanum but distal to the internal sphincter. Less experienced urologists have resected the "verumontanum" in the belief that the ejaculatory duct empties there; it is simply the embryologic remnant of the müllerian duct—the fetal uterus and upper vagina. The ejaculatory duct does not enter it.

It is important not to damage the internal sphincter; the ejaculate must go out the urethra rather than retrograde into the bladder. The external sphincter must not be damaged so as to prevent the complication of postoperative urinary incontinence. If the first tissue bite does not reveal the ejaculatory duct, one can continue to resect deeper. If it is truly a case of a blocked ejaculatory duct orifice, fairly soon after the first few bites one should come across a dramatically large, dilated opening with an equally dramatic efflux of translucent seminal fluid.

Semen volume and fructose level return to normal rapidly after this procedure. One of the ancillary benefits is that patients now have a reasonable volume of ejaculate. Sperm count is normal with good motility within 3 to 8 months, and these patients are fertile. One problem is that they are more susceptible to the possibility of epididymitis because of urinary reflux up the vas deferens. At the slightest hint of prostatitis or epididymitis the patient should be treated aggressively with antibiotics. Adhering to this precaution, I have had success treating this obstruction despite its rarity.

The diagnosis usually is not made definitively before surgical treatment but becomes evident when vasography is performed while the patient is undergoing exploration for probable epididymal obstruction and low semen volume. One can suspect ejaculatory duct obstruction when the patient has normal spermatogenesis at testicular biopsy, azoospermia, a palpable vas deferens, and low semen volume with absent fructose.

Congenital Absence of Vas Deferens

Congenital absence of the vas deferens is a rare condition that until recently has been associated with a poor prognosis for future fertility. Since the first successful use of epididymal sperm aspiration and IVF was reported in two couples,[48] this form of treatment has enormously improved the reproductive potential for men with uncorrectable obstructive azoospermia. With conventional IVF techniques, most patients (81%) achieve poor or no fertilization, and pregnancy rates are consistently less than 10%. The men undergo scrotal exploration immediately after their partners undergo oocyte aspiration. Under ×10 to ×40 magnification with an operating microscope, a 0.5-cm incision is made with microscissors into the epididymal tunic to expose the tubules in the most proximal portion of the congenitally blind-ending epididymis. Sperm are aspirated with a No. 22 Medicut needle (0.7 mm/22 mm; Cook Urological, Spencer, IN) on a tuberculin syringe directly from the opening in the epididymal tubule. Great care must be taken not to contaminate the specimen with blood, and precise hemostasis is achieved with microbipolar forceps. The specimens are immediately diluted in HEPES-buffered Earle's medium, and a tiny portion is examined for motility and quality of progression. If sperm motility is absent or poor, another aspiration is made 0.5 cm more proximally. Sperm are obtained from successively more proximal regions until progressive motility is found. Motile sperm are usually not obtained until the most proximal portion of the caput epididymis is reached. Once the area of motile sperm is found, epididymal fluid is aspirated during a period of 10 to 15 minutes.

When no sperm are found in the epididymis or the entire scrotum is massively scarred, testicular biopsy is performed to obtain sperm for ICSI. A 1-cm horizontal incision is made in the scrotal skin and through the tunica vaginalis. The tunica albuginea is then incised and a small piece of extruded testicular tissue is excised and placed into a small Petri dish with 3 mL of HEPES-buffered Earle's medium. Closure of the tunica albuginea is achieved with 3-0 polyglactin 910 intracuticular stitches. The testicular tissue is finely minced in HEPES-buffered Earles' medium, transferred to a 5-mL tube, and centrifuged for 5 minutes at 300g. A Pasteur pipette is used to remove the supernatant, and the pellet is then resuspended in 0.1–0.2 mL of Earle's medium and incubated in 5% oxygen, 5% carbon dioxide, and 90% nitrogen until the ICSI procedure is performed.[49–51]

The application and inclusion of ICSI in the management of obstructive azoospermia is now an essential component of the care of patients with this condition. In addition, some men who have Sertoli-only syndrome or maturational arrest have a few mature spermatids identified in testicular biopsy samples that can be used for ICSI. Therefore, almost every patient treated for obstructive azoospermia is now a candidate for attempted microsurgical repair, and if failure occurs, for ICSI.

MICROSURGERY FOR UNDESCENDED TESTICLE

Rationale for Testicular Autotransplantation

Considerable discussion has taken place over how best to localize a nonpalpable cryptorchid testis (spermatic venography,

electromagnetic imaging scan, or spermatic arteriography) as well as over proper surgical management for a testis that is high and intraperitoneal.[52–57] There is little need for controversy. Laparoscopy is the simplest, safest, and most reliable method of localizing high intraabdominal testes.[58] For surgical management, the spermatic vessels must be divided for the testicle to be brought into the scrotum, but the collateral blood supply from the deferential artery is not reliable, and this procedure usually results in atrophy unless the spermatic vessels are revascularized.[55]

I originally reported on seven patients with bilateral intraabdominal testes who underwent division of the spermatic vessels with microsurgical reanastomosis to the inferior epigastric vessels on one side, and on the other side simple division without reanastomosis.[59,60] On the side on which revascularization of the spermatic vessels was performed, the testis retained its normal size and texture. On the other side, partial or complete testicular atrophy occurred.

The danger of unrecognized cancer in an intraabdominal testicle certainly provides one motive for placing such a testicle in the scrotum or possibly removing it.[61,62] It was generally assumed in previous years that a cryptorchid testicle suffered only loss of spermatogenic function; hormonal function was supposedly unaltered. Studies have demonstrated that the abdominal environment also affects the endocrine function of the testis and results in premature loss of testosterone production. Patients with cryptorchidism have impaired intratesticular androgen production. An adult with untreated bilateral cryptorchidism has an elevated LH level and premature loss of testosterone secretion.[54,58,63] Experimental studies with rats demonstrated that when scrotal testes are transferred to the abdomen, an immediate and dramatic elevation in FSH level corresponds to rapid deterioration of spermatogenesis.[64] Over a longer period of time, however, LH levels begins to increase gradually, indicating later loss of endocrine function of cryptorchid testes. The intraabdominal environment is detrimental not only to spermatogenesis but also to hormone production. It simply takes longer for this aspect of testicular function to deteriorate.

The question of whether transplanting these testes to the scrotum during childhood allows the development of fertility has been answered. Evidence is overwhelming that making a testicle cryptorchid diminishes spermatogenesis and that replacing a cryptorchid testicle into the scrotum allows spermatogenesis to recover.[65–69] There are documented case reports of adults 16 to 25 years of age with azoospermia with bilateral simple cryptorchidism who after orchidopexy had normal spermatogenesis and reasonable sperm counts.[70,71] Although these patients did not have intraabdominal testicles, the results support the idea that cryptorchid testes can make sperm if they are transferred to the scrotum. We now have very well-documented reports that even intraabdominal testes have normal spermato-

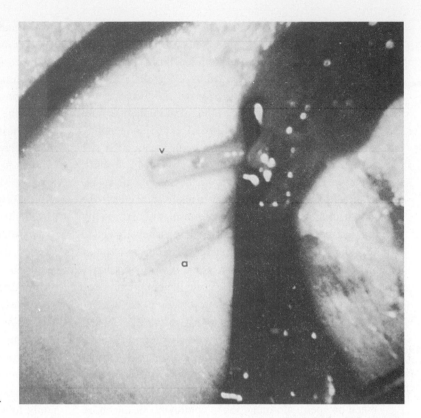

Figure 16–17. The divided spermatic vein (top) and artery (bottom).

genesis after puberty if they are properly transferred to the scrotum without damage to the blood supply.[72]

What is the safest method for transferring the high intraperitoneal testis into the scrotum? The procedure of simply dividing the internal spermatic vessels was first recommended in 1903,[73] and good results were reported.[74] Some authors, however, reported uniformly poor results with this operation.[75–77]

It was first demonstrated in 1963 that by dividing the internal spermatic vessels high and not dissecting their attachment to the cord, it was sometimes possible to preserve collateral circulation by way of the deferential artery.[55] The spermatic vessels could be clamped first and testicular biopsy performed to determine the adequacy of collateral blood flow. Almost half of the patients experienced some testicular atrophy,

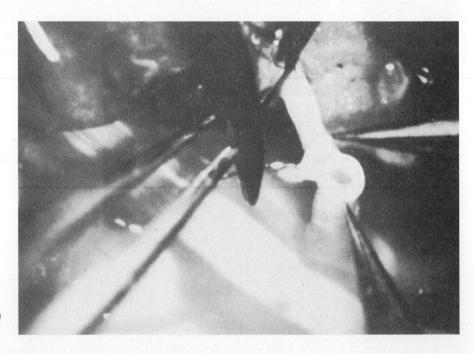

Figure 16–18. Venous anastomosis after the first 120° have been sutured.

however, and among one third it was rather severe. Furthermore, the original diagrams demonstrate that this technique was most valuable in the management of a so-called long-looped vas, in which the testis is really located at the level of the internal inguinal ring and the vas loops down in the canal toward the external ring and then comes back to the testis at the internal ring. By avoiding dissection in the inguinal canal, the collateral circulation can be preserved. It should be noted that most of the cases these authors described did not involve severely high intraabdominal testes. Other authors have used the procedure for high intraperitoneal testes.[54,56,60] Favorable results are reported in the literature, but my observations leave no doubt that atrophy is caused by all groups who use this approach.

In my experience one cannot rely on the deferential blood supply to the testicle. Reports of good results of division of the spermatic vessels without reanastomosis are very overoptimistic. It was demonstrated in fresh autopsy dissections that the sum of the diameters of the deferential and cremasteric arteries was equal to the diameter of the testicular artery only one third of the time, indicating that adequate functional collateral circulation to the testis is by no means universal.[69,78]

Microsurgical Techniques

Microvascular Scoville-Lewis, Schwartz, or Heifetz neurosurgical clips are placed on the deep inferior epigastric artery and both superficial and deep inferior epigastric veins inferiorly. These vessels are then tied off superiorly. The inferior epigastric vessels are each divided and the lumina examined. The spermatic vessels are then brought into the area for anastomosis (Fig 16–17).

For the microvascular anastomosis, 9-0 or 10-0 nylon on a BV-6 or BV-2 needle is ideal. Interrupted sutures are absolutely critical. Continuous suturing results in a purse string effect that will at best bunch and at worst obstruct the anastomosis site. The interrupted sutures should be tied down and cut as one goes, rather than leaving them to be tied down at the end. With the latter, one will have an impossible puppet show in which the spider-web thin sutures become entangled with each other before even half of them have been placed. No attempt should be made to perform the arterial anastomosis until the spatulation has been performed, because the discrepancy between the lumina is otherwise too great.

The technique of venous anastomosis is somewhat simpler than the arterial anastomosis. Because the vessel sizes generally match, spatulation is not necessary. One can perform a standard anastomosis by placing two anterior stitches 120° apart. Several sutures are placed between these two initial stay sutures, and the entire vessel is rotated 18° so that the posterior 240° that have not been sutured yet are facing anteriorly (Fig 16–18). Another stay suture is placed halfway, producing two 120° segments, each of which requires several sutures to complete the anastomosis (Fig 16–19). The clamps on the inferior epigastric vein and then the artery are removed. The testicle has now been completely revascularized; it can be placed into the scrotal sac without any tension (Fig 16–20). Adequacy of blood flow to the testis both intraoperatively and postoperatively is monitored with a Doppler probe. In instances in which I reanastomosed the divided spermatic vessels on one side but relied on collateral circulation through the vas deferens on the other side, I have always wished that I had simply revascularized both sides.

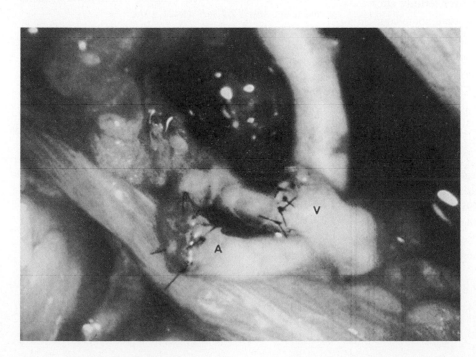

Figure 16–19. Completed arterial and venous anastomoses.

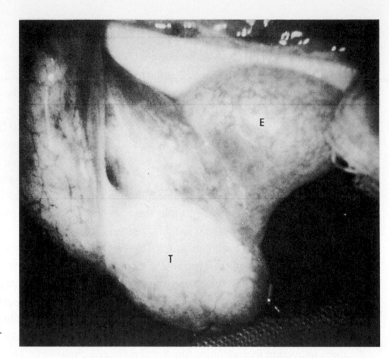

Figure 16–20. The blanched testicle (T) before the vascular clamps are removed. It lies on the groin but is now free to be transferred to the scrotum, epididymis.

Conclusions

Preoperative diagnosis and localization of a high intraabdominal testis is most reliably and easily accomplished at laparoscopy. These high testicles are best placed into the scrotum by means of division of the spermatic vessels. Microsurgical reanastomosis to the inferior epigastric vessels is recommended to prevent partial or complete testicular atrophy and to maximize the eventual prospect for fertility. Because we know that adults with bilateral cryptorchidism can recover fertility after the testes are placed in the scrotum, it is important not to compromise blood supply in the mistaken notion that these testicles are not very good anyway. There certainly is some hope for fertility if orchidopexy is performed with proper attention to blood supply.

REFERENCES

1. Silber SJ, Devroey P, Tournaye H, Van Steirteghem AC: Fertilizing capacity of epididymal and testicular sperm using intracytoplasmic injection (ICSI). *Reprod Fertil Dev* 7:281, 1995
2. Silber SJ: Microscopic technique for reversal of vasectomy. *Surg Gynecol Obstet* 143:630, 1976
3. Silber SJ, Galle J, Friend D: Microscopic vasovasostomy and spermatogenesis. *J Urol* 117:299, 1977
4. Silber SJ, Crudop J: Kidney transplantation in inbred rats. *Am J Surg* 125:551, 1973
5. Silber SJ, Crudop J: A three kidney rat model. *Invest Urol* 11:466, 1974
6. Silber SJ, Malvin RL: Compensatory and obligatory renal growth in rats. *Am J Physiol* 226:114, 1974
7. Silber SJ: Growth of baby kidneys transplanted into adults. *Arch Surg* 111:75, 1976
8. Silber SJ: Transplantation of rat kidneys with acute tubular necrosis into salt-loaded and normal recipients. *Surgery* 77:487, 1975
9. Silber SJ: Successful autotransplantation of an intra-abdominal testicle to the scrotum using microvascular anastomosis. *J Urol* 115:452, 1976
10. Silber SJ: Compensatory and obligatory renal growth in babies and adults. *Aust N Z J Surg* 44:421, 1974
11. Silber SJ: Microscopic vasectomy reversal. *Fertil Steril* 28:1191, 1977
12. Silber SJ: Vasectomy and vasectomy reversal. *Fertil Steril* 29:125, 1978
13. Silber SJ: *Reproductive Microsurgery.* Baltimore, Williams & Wilkins, 1984
14. MacLeod J, Gold RZ: The male factor in fertility and infertility. IV. Sperm morphology in fertile and infertile marriage. *Fertil Steril* 2:394, 1951
15. Silber SJ, Rodriguez-Rigau LJ: Quantitative analysis of testicle biopsy: Determination of partial obstruction and prediction of sperm count after surgery for obstruction. *Fertil Steril* 36:480, 1981
16. Silber SJ: Epididymal extravasation following vasectomy as a cause for failure of vasectomy reversal. *Fertil Steril* 31:309, 1979
17. Bedford JM: Adaptations of the male reproductive tract and the fate of spermatozoa following vasectomy in the rabbit, rhesus monkey, hamster and rat. *Biol Reprod* 14:118, 1976
18. Silber SJ: Microscopic vasoepididymostomy, specific microanastomosis to the epididymal tubule. *Fertil Steril* 30:565, 1978

19. Silber SJ: Vasoepididymostomy to the head of the epididymis: Recovery of normal spermatozoa motility. *Fertil Steril* 34:149, 1980

20. Silber SJ: Reversal of vasectomy in the treatment of male infertility. *J Androl* 1:261, 1980

21. Silber SJ: Reversal of vasectomy in the treatment of male infertility: Role of microsurgery, vasoepididymostomy, and pressure-induced changes of vasectomy. *Urol Clin North Am* 8:53, 1981

22. Charny CW: Testicular biopsy: Its value in male sterility. *JAMA* 115:1429, 1940

23. Nelson WO: Interpretation of testicular biopsy. *JAMA* 151:1449, 1953

24. Mannion RA, Cottrell TLC: Correlation between testicular biopsy and sperm count. *J Urol* 85:953, 1961

25. Albert A: The mammalian testis. In: Young WC (ed), *Sex and Secretions,* ed 3. Baltimore, Williams & Wilkins, 1961:305–365

26. Heller CG, Clermont Y: Kinetics of the germinal epithelium in man. *Recent Prog Horm Res* 20:545, 1964

27. Steinberger E, Tjioe DY: A method for quantitative analysis of human seminiferous epithelium. *Fertil Steril* 19:960, 1968

28. Tjioe DY, Steinberger E, Paulsen CA: A simple method for quantitative analysis of seminiferous epithelium in human testicular biopsies. *J Albert Einstein Med Center* 15:56, 1967

29. Zuckerman Z, Rodriquez-Rigau LJ, Weiss DB, et al: Quantitative analysis of the seminiferous epithelium in human testicular biopsies, and the relation of spermatogenesis to sperm density. *Fertil Steril* 30:448, 1978

30. DeKretser DM, Burger HG, Hudson B: The relationship between germinal cells and serum FSH levels in males with infertility. *J Clin Endocrinol Metab* 38:787, 1974

31. Schoysman R: Operative treatment of ductal obstruction and/or agenesis. Presented at the 33rd Meeting of the American Fertility Society, April 12–16, 1977, Miami Beach, Florida

32. Schoysman R, Drouart JM: Progrès récents dans la chirurgie de la stérilité masculine et feminine. *Acta Clin Belg* 71:261, 1972

33. Amelar RD, Dubin L: Commentary of epididymal vasostomy, vasovasostomy and testicular biopsy. In: *Current Operative Urology.* New York, Harper & Row, 1975:1181–1185

34. Hanley HG: The surgery of male sub-fertility. *Ann R Coll Surg* 17:159, 1955

35. Hotchkiss RS: Surgical treatment of infertility in the male. In: Campbell MF, Harrison HH (eds), *Urology,* ed 3. Philadelphia, Saunders, 1970:671–686

36. Silber SJ: Pregnancy caused by sperm from vasa efferentia. *Fertil Steril* 49:373, 1988

37. Silber SJ: Results of specific tubule vasoepididymostomy: The role of epididymis in sperm maturation. *Human Reprod* 4:xx, 1989

38. Silber SJ: Apparent fertility of human sperm from the caput epididymis. *J Androl* 10:263, 1989

39. Gaddum P: Sperm maturation in the male reproductive tract: Development of motility. *Anat Rec* 161:47, 1969

40. Bedford JM: Development of the fertilizing ability of spermatozoa in the epididymis of the rabbit. *J Exp Zool* 163:312, 1966

41. Orgebin-Crist MC: Sperm maturation in rabbit epididymis. *Nature* 216:816, 1967

42. Glover TD: Some aspects of function in the epididymis: Experi-

mental occlusion of the epididymis in the rabbit. *Int J Fertil* 14:215, 1969

43. Gaddum P, Glover TD: Some reactions of rabbit spermatozoa to ligation of the epididymis. *J Reprod Fertil* 9:119, 1965

44. Paufler SK, Foote RH: Morphology, motility and fertility in spermatozoa recovered from different areas of ligated rabbit epididymis. *J Reprod Fertil* 17:125, 1968

45. Orgebin-Crist MC: Studies of the function of the epididymis. *Biol Reprod* 1:155, 1969

46. Silber SJ: *Transurethral Resection.* New York, Appleton-Century-Crofts, 1977

47. Porch PP Jr: Aspermia owning to obstruction of distal ejaculatory duct and treatment by transurethral resection. *J Urol* 119:141, 1978

48. Silber SJ, Asch R, Ord T, Borrero C, Balmaceda J: New treatment for infertility due to congenital absence of vas deferens. *Lancet* 2:850, 1987

49. Sperm Microaspiration Retrieval Techniques Study Group: Results in the United States with sperm microaspiration retrieval techniques and assisted reproductive technologies. *J Urol* 151:1255, 1994

50. Silber SJ, Van Steirteghem AC, Liu J, Nagy Z, Tournaye H, Devroey P: High fertilization and pregnancy rate after intracytoplasmic sperm injection with spermatozoa obtained from testicle biopsy. *Hum Reprod* 10:148, 1995

51. Silber SJ: Epididymal and testicular spermatozoa and intracytoplasmic sperm injection. *Assist Reprod Dev* 6:45, 1996

52. Levitt SB, Kogan SJ, Engel RM, et al: The impalpable testis: A rational approach to management. *J Urol* 120:515, 1978

53. Weiss RM, Glickman MG, Lytton B: Clinical implications of gonadal venography in the management of the non-palpable undescended testis. *J Urol* 121:745

54. Clatworthy NW, Hallenbaugh RS, Grosfeld JL: The long-louped vas orchidopexy for the high undescended testis. *Am Surg* 38:69, 1972

55. Fowler R, Stephens FD: The role of testicular vascular anatomy in the salvage of high undescended testes. In: Stephens FD (ed), *Congenital Malformations of the Rectum, Anus, and Genital Urinary Tract.* London, Livingstone, 1963:306–320

56. Gibbons MD, Cromie WJ, Duckett JW Jr: Management of the abdominal undescended testicle. *J Urol* 122:76, 1979

57. Martin DC: The undescended testis: Evolving concepts in management. *Urol Dig* 1977

58. Cohen R, Silber SJ: Laparoscopy for cryptorchidism. *J Urol* 124:928, 1980

59. Silber SJ: The intra-abdominal testis: Microvascular autotransplantation. *J Urol* 125:329, 1981

60. Silber SJ, Kelly J: Successful auto-transplantation of an intra-abdominal testis to the scrotum by microvascular technique. *J Urol* 115:452, 1976

61. Campbell HE: Incidence of malignant growth of the undescended testicle: A critical and statistical study. *Arch Surg* 44:353, 1942

62. Martin DC, Menck HR: The undescended testis: Management after puberty. *J Urol* 114:77, 1975

63. Atkinson PM, Epstein MT, Rippon AE: Plasma gonadotropins and androgens in the surgically treated cryptorchid patient. *J Pediatr Surg* 10:27, 1975

64. Altwein JE, Gittes RF: Effect of cryptorchidism and castration on FSH and LH levels in the adult rat. *Invest Urol* 10:167, 1972

65. Hadziselemovic F, Herzag B, Seguchi H: Surgical correction of cryptorchidism at two years: Electron microscopic and morphologic investigations. *J Pediatr Surg* 10:19, 1975

66. Kiesewetter WB, Shull WR, Fetterman GH: Histologic changes in the testis following the anatomically successful orchidopexy. *J Pediatr Surg* 4:59, 1969

67. Mengel W, Hienz HA, Sippe WG Jr, Hecker WC: Studies on cryptorchidism: A comparison of histologic findings in the germinative epithelium before and after the second year of life. *J Pediatr Surg* 9:445, 1974

68. Nelson WO: Mammalian spermatogenesis, effect of experimental cryptorchidism in the rat, and nondescent of the testis in man. *Recent Prog Horm Res* 6:29, 1951

69. Sohval AR: Testicular dysgenesis as an etiologic factor in cryptorchidism. *J Urol* 72:693, 1954

70. Britton BJ: Spermatogenesis following bilateral orchidopexy in adult life. *Br J Urol* 47:464, 1975

71. Comhaire F, Derom F, Vermeulen L: The recovery of spermatogenesis in an azoospermic patient after operation for bilateral undescended testes at age of 25 years. *Int J Androl* 1:117, 1978

72. Silber SJ: Recovery of spermatogenesis after testicle autotransplantation in an adult male. *Fertil Steril* 38:632, 1982

73. Bevan AD: The surgical treatment of undescended testicle: A further contribution. *JAMA* 41:718, 1903

74. Moschowitz AV: The anatomy and treatment of undescended testes, with special reference to the Bevan operation. *Ann Surg* 52:821, 1910

75. Mixter EG: Undescended testicle: Operative treatment and end results. *Surg Gynecol Obstet* 39:275, 1924

76. Wangensteen OH: Undescended testes: Experimental and clinical study. *Arch Surg* 14:653, 1927

77. McCollum DW: Clinical study of spermatogenesis of undescended testicles. *Arch Surg* 31:290, 1935

78. Silber SJ: Transplantation of human testis for anorchia. *Fertil Steril* 30:181, 1978

CHAPTER 17

Assisted Reproductive Treatments of Oligospermia

JOEL H. BATZOFIN · ERIC K. SEAMAN · LARRY I. LIPSHULTZ

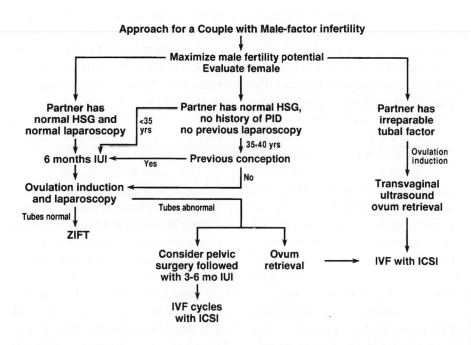

Since the mid 1970s, there have been dramatic advances in our understanding of reproductive biology and the clinical applications of this knowledge. The coordinated efforts of scientists and clinicians have resulted in new therapeutic options for infertile and subfertile couples. It is generally agreed that infertility affects 15% to 20% of couples who are attempting conception.[1] Thorough evaluation of both partners shows the male factor to be the sole cause of the problem, or a substantial contributing factor, in approximately 50% of couples with reproductive dysfunction. Several therapeutic treatments can be offered to infertile couples with an associated male-factor problem.

Since the initial successful reports of conception following intracytoplasmic single-sperm injection (ICSI) by Palermo et al[2] in 1992, there has been a massive explosion of these therapeutic modalities for ever increasing degrees of severity of male-factor subfertility. These frontiers have evolved to such a degree that Tesarik et al[3] reported that successful pregnancies were established by means of injection of round spermatids (the youngest male germ cells to have a set of haploid chromosomes) into the ooplasm. This success was duplicated by Sofikitis et al,[4] who successfully established pregnancies with round spermatid nuclei injected into the oocyte in a series of patients with late maturation arrest disorder.

These micromanipulation alternatives are so powerful that their successful application prompted a keynote speaker at the World Congress on In Vitro Fertilization and Assisted Reproduction, Vienna, Austria, April 1995, to mention, "We have now reached a point where the need for the workup of the male may no longer be necessary."[5] Rather, having all these reproductive alternatives available, the physician might simply begin treatment and "keep going" until sperm are obtained, whether from epididymis or testicle and even from early forms of sperm within the testicle (spermatids), thereby "avoiding the need for a workup." It remains impractical and unwise, however, to treat patients without a clear understanding of the diagnosis. Furthermore, not all clinical units are equipped to effectively treat all severe forms of male-factor infertility. It is the intent of this chapter to briefly review the fundamental male-factor infertility evaluation and allude to the high-technology approaches when they are appropriate. The chapter also discusses new and simplified approaches to sperm aspiration for patients with obstructive azoospermia.

For the male partner, a thorough history and physical examination are the initial steps in any infertility evaluation. Three semen analyses and determination of serum gonadotropin concentrations (luteinizing hormone [LH] and follicle-stimulating hormone [FSH]), serum testosterone levels, and, when appropriate, serum prolactin levels are the primary laboratory tests. Three semen analyses are required because of the between-sample variability that is known to occur in some men.

TABLE 17–1. SEMEN CHARACTERISTICS AND ACCEPTED NORMAL VALUES

Characteristics	Normal Value
Volume	1.5 to 5.0 mL
Color	Whitish gray
Liquefaction	Within 30 minutes
Density	20 to 200 million/mL
Motility	
Quantitative	>60%
Qualitative	Forward progression >2+ (scale 1 to 4)
Morphology	>60% normal
Clumping	Minimal
Leukocytes	<1 million/mL
Immature forms	1 million/mL

The important semen characteristics and normal values are listed in Table 17–1.

After the semen analyses and the appropriate hormone tests, it can be determined whether the male values are completely normal or whether an element of subfertility exists that necessitates additional testing or treatment. All initial steps in working with the couple are directed toward maximizing fertility potential and may ultimately not be therapeutic in and of themselves. Although some therapies may produce a condition in which the man is capable of initiating a pregnancy spontaneously, many therapies merely enhance fertility potential; consequently the couple may still require additional treatment to initiate a pregnancy.

The initial diagnostic and therapeutic steps may halt or reverse a pathologic process that is detrimental to sperm production or function, but the patient remains relatively subfertile because of persistent oligospermia, asthenospermia, or diminished fertilizing capacity of the spermatozoa. In such situations, the clinician must resort to what are known as assisted reproductive treatments (ARTs). At present, for male-factor infertility, these treatments include intrauterine insemination (IUI) with processed spermatozoa, in vitro fertilization (IVF), and zygote intrafallopian transfer (ZIFT).[6] Before a discussion of the treatments per se, clarification of the role of the sperm penetration assay is important. We believe that when performed in an optimal manner this test remains an accurate test of sperm fertilizing capability and provides information useful in deciding the best method of sperm processing for ARTs.

SPERM PENETRATION ASSAY

Men with abnormalities of sperm production (oligospermia or asthenospermia) frequently have concomitant disorders of sperm function manifested as defective oocyte penetrability. Abnormalities in sperm function also may occur in men with normal bulk semen values (count, motility, and morphology). It has long been appreciated that the functional competence of spermatozoa is not necessarily reflected by results obtained in a conventional semen analysis.[7] In efforts to analyze sperm competence, several laboratory tests have been developed and have received critical attention. Three of these are the zona-free hamster egg sperm penetration assay (SPA), computer-assisted analysis of sperm movement, and measurement of sperm adenosine triphosphate (ATP) concentrations. Of these, only the SPA has had a substantial impact on clinical management.

Species specificity of ovum fertilization is lost after enzymatic removal of the cumulus and zona pellucida from mouse, rat, and hamster ova. Heterologous combinations of spermatozoa and zona-free oocytes from guinea pig, mouse, rat, and hamster have demonstrated sperm chromatin decondensation within the egg cytoplasm, indicating that heterologous fusion had occurred.[8,9] Zona-free hamster oocytes demonstrate fusibility with spermatozoa from several species, including humans.[10,11]

Successful fertilization by means of micromanipulation has posed questions regarding the mechanisms of fertilization that, to a large extent, remain unanswered. It was previously believed that gamete membrane fusion occurred only if the spermatozoa had been capacitated and had undergone the acrosome reaction. Therefore, fusion served as a useful end point in determining the occurrence of these two phenomena. It has been demonstrated that heterologous fusion and the postfusion events of chromatin decondensation apparently do not differ from those in homologous fertilizations. Consequently, the use of this heterologous system provided a useful model for diagnostic evaluation of sperm function. Results from several laboratories indicate that the outcome of the SPA is highly correlated with results obtained in human IVF systems, in which fertilization occurred without micromanipulation methods (Fig 17–1). Furthermore, several different sperm processing or sperm enhancing procedures can be analyzed with a SPA, and the results can be compared with those obtained when the test is performed in the standard manner. In this way, information regarding optimization of sperm function can be obtained and used in subsequent treatment cycles involving ART. Therefore, although the SPA is not definitive with regard to the likelihood of fertilization, the lack of fertilization in the SPA should prepare the clinician for the need to use micromanipulation and to discuss this ahead of time with the patients.

Factors that influence results of the SPA have been outlined by several authors.[12–15] Unfortunately, no consensus exists on the specific protocol used in the various laboratories, so valid comparison of results among different centers frequently is not possible. It becomes extremely important, therefore, that for any given laboratory the test be reproducible and sensitive enough to avoid false-negative results (failure to penetrate hamster oocytes but ability to penetrate human oocytes). Results should correlate well with data obtained from the human IVF program when fertilization is achieved by conventional IVF methods.

There are several different methods for reporting results of SPA. In an optimized assay system, the sperm of pregnancy-proved donors penetrates 100% of the ova at sperm concentra-

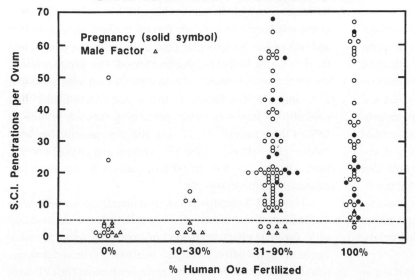

Figure 17–1. Correlation between results obtained in the sperm penetration assay (SPA) and human *in vitro* fertilization (IVF) program (Baylor College of Medicine, Houston, TX). Sperm capacitation index (SCI) is an expression of the mean number of penetrations per ovum. The dotted line at 5 penetrations per ovum represents the sensitivity of this assay system, below which no pregnancies occurred among the 138 patients who participated in the analysis. Note the strong (but not perfect) correlation between results obtained with the SPA and ovum fertility rates in the human IVF program. (*From Batzofin JH, Marrs RP, Serafini PC, et al: Assisted reproductive treatments for male factor infertility.* Probl Urol *1:430,1987*)

tions of 3 to 5 million/mL. In addition, extensive polyspermy (often as high as 90 penetrations per ovum) is detected. Because some patients with infertility also achieve penetration scores of 100% but demonstrate no polyspermy, the results should be considered in terms of the degree of polyspermy and not only in terms of the number of ova penetrated. The sperm capacitation index (SCI) is an expression of the mean number of penetrations per ovum. If the assay is sufficiently sensitive and reproducible, SPA data can be analyzed and correlated with the IVF data, and a cutoff point can be established (for example, 5 penetrations per ovum at a fixed concentration of motile sperm), above which the patient is considered fertile and below which the patient is considered subfertile (see Fig 17–1). Many clinicians and investigators assert that there is no longer a place for the SPA. However, because there is a somewhat poor correlation between bulk semen parameters and sperm function, it remains our contention that the assay is a useful tool to rapidly identify which patients have a defect in sperm fertilizing capacity and would benefit from more advanced forms of treatment. In the age of cost-conscious delivery of health care, it is as imprudent to conduct a series of IUI cycles for a couple with deficient sperm fertilizing capacity as it would be to perform IVF or ICSI for a couple who would be successful with IUI. The SPA, therefore, is useful to facilitate selection of appropriate therapy from all available alternatives.

METHODS FOR SEPARATING SPERMATOZOA FROM SEMINAL PLASMA AND IMPROVING GAMETE EFFICIENCY

Several methods exist for separating motile spermatozoa from the male ejaculate. The most commonly used include direct swim-up separation, two-step washing with swim-up penetration, and Percoll discontinuous gradient-separation techniques (Table 17–2). These three methods have various advantages and disadvantages. For the most part, direct swim-up allows collection of a highly motile fraction of sperm. The number of sperm recovered, however, is considerably less than with the other two techniques. When increased numbers of abnormal or immature forms are present in the ejaculate, or white blood cell count and ejaculate debris concentration is high, swim-up techniques provide a reasonable mechanism for isolation of normal motile spermatozoa; nevertheless, the motile sperm may carry ejaculate debris into the swim-up suspension. The two-step washing procedure provides the highest sperm recovery rate, but nonviable sperm and debris also are collected. Two-step washing, combined with sperm swim-up from the final sperm pellet, yields a highly motile sperm fraction with decreased debris, white cells, and nonviable forms.

Of these three methods, the two-step wash with swim-up is most frequently used. The Percoll gradient technique is used most commonly for men with normal sperm density and very low motility. Because ejaculates with increased concentrations of white blood cells or immature forms can benefit from Percoll separation, this is the method of choice to facilitate the collection of a highly motile sperm fraction.

In essence, the goal of sperm processing is to select for a fraction of highly motile, morphologically normal sperm as free as possible of white blood cells and other debris. In this way, the most functional subpopulation of spermatozoa is collected. An equally important consideration is whether sperm processing procedures are able to improve sperm function and penetrability when these mechanisms are defective.

The pathophysiologic basis of defective sperm function is highly complex. As noted previously, for successful nonoperative ovum fertilization to occur, sperm must undergo capacitation and the acrosome reaction. For the most part, the specifics of these events are unclear. In efforts to determine whether sperm function can be enhanced by separation or coincubation techniques, several alternatives have been examined. The most commonly used methods are Percoll gradient separation, the addition of human follicular fluid to the culture medium, and the TEST yolk buffer incubation method. Our experience has shown that approximately 5% to 10% of men with abnormal SPAs improve after Percoll treatment and that follicular fluid coincubation improves sperm penetrating function in 40% to 50% of these patients. TEST yolk buffer preparation has been extensively evaluated in the SPA system, and clinical correlation indicates that 50% to 60% of patients benefit from this method of sperm processing.

Figure 17–2 summarizes clinical indications for SPA. With the addition of the aforementioned techniques to the standard SPA, the most effective method of improving sperm function can be identified before a couple's treatment cycle, and that particular method can be used in sperm penetration for IVF with embryo transfer (ET), ZIFT, or IUI. The documentation of com-

TABLE 17–2. SUMMARY OF THE USE OF SPERM SEPARATING TECHNIQUES

Semen Factor	Two-Step	Two-Step with Swim-Up	Percoll	Swim-Up
Oligospermia	+	++		+
Asthenospermia		+	++	+
Oligoasthenospermia		+		++
Increased abnormal spermatozoa			+	
Increased white blood cells or debris or both			+	
Normal semen with abnormal penetration			++	+

The method chosen for sperm processing depends on evaluation of both bulk semen values and sperm fertilizing capacity determined by the sperm penetration assay (SPA).
+, Satisfactory; ++, best method; blank, not applicable.

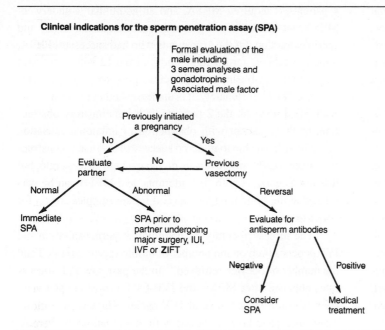

Figure 17-2. Clinical indications for the sperm penetration assay (SPA).

plete lack of fertilization in the SPA or a severe decrease in fertilization compared with a fertile donor control in the same assay, allows the clinician to counsel patients for the need to progress beyond insemination to achieve fertilization in vitro by means of ICSI if necessary.

METHODS OF SPERM HARVESTING

For most patients masturbation is the method of choice for collection of sperm. For patients with severe oligospermia, we have previously incorporated short-term sperm banking for 1 or 2 months before the ART cycle. With this practice sperm counts can be increased. It is recognized, however, that many of these patients' ejaculates do not tolerate freezing and thawing, and counts have been improved by only marginal increments. Furthermore, the sperm requirements for ICSI are so low that it is now our approach to enroll these patients directly into the ICSI program. Some of our patients have had successful outcomes when the man has had fewer sperm in the ejaculate than the woman has had oocytes.

For patients with obstructive azoospermia due to vasectomy, congenital absence of the vas, or prior infection with outflow obstruction, there are now new and simple approaches to sperm retrieval. The anticipated low yield of sperm for such approaches necessitates that the partner be treated with controlled ovarian hyperstimulation (COH) and egg retrieval and that fertilization be achieved with ICSI.

Until recently, the treatment of obstructive azoospermia relied on surgical reconstruction, such as vasovasostomy or epi-

didymovasostomy, to obtain sufficient numbers of sperm to initiate a pregnancy. Historically, patients who could not undergo reconstruction, such as those with congenital bilateral absence of the vas deferens (CBAVD) have been treated by means of construction of an alloplastic spermatocele; however, this technique has met with little success.[16] With newer techniques of assisted reproduction and microsurgery, these patients may now be offered more treatment options and with greater success than in the past in achieving successful pregnancies.

Microsurgical epididymal sperm aspiration (MESA) was first reported in conjunction with IVF in 1985.[17] MESA is usually performed with general anesthesia, especially if performed in conjunction with epididymovasostomy, but it may be performed with local anesthesia and sedation. A vertical scrotal incision is made and carried down to the tunica vaginalis, which is then opened. With the aid of an operating microscope, the epididymis is inspected for a site of obstruction, above which sperm aspiration may be performed. A tubule is microsurgically isolated, and a longitudinal microsurgical slit or controlled puncture site developed. Fluid is aspirated with a 24F Angiocath and a 1 cc tuberculin syringe containing 0.1 cc of modified human tubal fluid (HTF) buffer. As an alternative, a micropipette with gentle suction can be used after micropuncture of the tubule. In general, tubules with dark yellow, thick-appearing fluid are chronically obstructed and do not contain full, intact sperm. Tubules with lighter, transparent or translucent, opalescent fluid often provide substantial numbers of well-formed, motile sperm sufficient for IVF. Additional aspirated sperm may be frozen for later use and, therefore, it is rare to have to perform repeat MESA. MESA also offers the advantage of being a possible adjunct to a reconstructive surgical procedure. If MESA is unsuccessful, testis biopsy may be performed in the same setting for testicular sperm extraction. Postoperative complications or morbidity are exceedingly uncommon. The only substantial disadvantage of MESA is that it must be performed in an operating suite.

Experience with percutaneous epididymal sperm aspiration (PESA) has been reported. Several reports have been published on the results of PESA in patients in whom reconstruction either was not feasible or had failed in the past and in patients with CBAVD.[18–20] The technique is as follows (Fig 17–3). A 21-gauge butterfly needle is connected to a syringe and directed into either the head or corpus of the epididymis after immobilization by holding the testis stable beneath the thumb and index finger. Suction is applied to the syringe, and the needle is withdrawn gradually until segments of fluid from the epididymis are seen entering the tubing of the microeffusion set. The microtubing is clamped before the needle is withdrawn. The aspirate is then washed out of the needle and tubing into a sterile tube containing IVF culture medium.[19] The technique is performed with local anesthesia, often in conjunction with intravenous sedation. The sample is inspected; if the sample is insufficient, additional percutaneous attempts are made. Craft et al[19] reported using this technique for 20 patients: 12 had undergone failed vasectomy reversal, 5 had CBAVD, 2 had inflammatory obstruction, and 1 had obstruction of unknown etiology. Sufficient sperm was recovered in 16 patients. Of the remaining

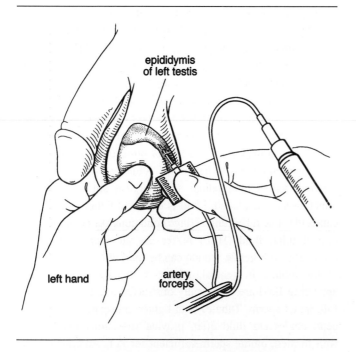

Figure 17–3. Percutaneous epididymal sperm aspiration.

4 patients, 2 required MESA, and an additional 2 underwent MESA that failed. These 2 patients needed testicular biopsy and sperm extraction. Of the 16 patients who had successful PESA, 4 did not achieve fertilization, and 3 of the 12 with successful fertilization established pregnancies (pregnancy per transfer rate of 25%). Unfortunately, it is unclear whether the 12 patients with failed reversal, the 2 patients with inflammatory obstruction, or the 1 patient with obstruction of unknown causation might have been able to undergo successful surgical reconstruction. Redo vasectomy reversals do have a high success rate, but it is not as good as with first attempts, and MESA can be performed at the same time and several semen samples frozen for later use.

The success of combined epididymal sperm aspiration and IVF depends both on the number of motile sperm aspirated and the number of oocytes retrieved.[21] In the past, low IVF success rates obtained after MESA and IVF-ET for most couples with CBAVD necessitated several IVF cycles. Higher fertilization rates since have been achieved with combinations of MESA, IVF, and ICSI. Tournaye et al[22] reported a 58% fertilization rate with a 35.7% pregnancy rate with this combined technique. The fertilizations in the series treated by Craft et al[19] were achieved with ICSI-IVF. When sperm cannot be successfully aspirated from the epididymis, sperm can be extracted, in most instances, directly from the testicle.

Testicular sperm extraction (TESE) involves mincing of testicular tissue in HEPES buffered medium and processing of the effluent. The fluid is centrifuged and the pellet gently resuspended. Individual sperm are then selected for microinjection.[23,24] Several authors have reported pregnancies with this technique.[23,24] Silber et al[24] reported on 12 patients who required TESE. When ICSI was used, the cited fertilization rate of 45% was similar to that with MESA and ICSI for a similar cohort group.

Testicular tissue can be obtained by means of open testis biopsy, percutaneous biopsy, or aspiration. The quality of tissue obtained at open biopsy has been compared with that of tissue obtained at percutaneous biopsy. Hoekstra et al[25] found that although specimens from percutaneous biopsies were generally of inferior quality to those from open biopsies, they usually yielded sufficient tissue in cases of obstructive azoospermia. In cases of hypospermatogenesis, open biopsy is usually required to harvest sufficient sperm-containing tissue.

For patients whose testes do not make sperm because of a defect in the maturation process of spermatogenesis, the technique of round spermatid nuclear injection (ROSNI) may hold hope for the future. This technique has been performed on rabbit oocytes, producing successful fertilizations.[26] To date, no human pregnancies have been carried to term with this procedure.

ASSISTED REPRODUCTIVE TREATMENTS: TREATMENT SELECTION

Perhaps the single biggest challenge confronting clinicians is selection of a treatment modality. As has been already discussed, it is imperative that the couple undergo evaluation as a pair. On occasion, it is obvious how the couples should be treated. For example, if the man has obstructive azoospermia and requires sperm aspiration, IUI is inappropriate. Because of the anticipated low yield of sperm, ICSI is the preferred approach. After measures have been taken to maximize the fertility potential of both partners, the couple frequently needs additional therapy by means of an ART that involves IUI, IVF-ET, or ZIFT with or without micromanipulation. Choice of treatment is a complex decision that involves a thorough evaluation for both partners. If a woman needs laparoscopy, diagnostic and therapeutic steps may be combined with recognition of the fact that this approach may compromise satisfactory tubal assessment if chromotubation cannot be performed at zygote transfer. However, improved pregnancy rates have been reported when laser vaporization of endometriosis is performed at laparoscopy for patients undergoing ART.[27,28] The ideal treatment is the one that carries the highest success rate and is the least invasive. To achieve these goals, decisions are based on many factors. The most important of these include (1) relative severity of the male-factor infertility, (2) associated pathologic conditions in the woman, (3) age of the woman, (4) establishment of previous pregnancies by the patients together and how conception occurred, (5) how long the couple has been in treatment, and (6) financial considerations.

Relative Severity of the Male-Factor Infertility

A man with a sperm density of 10 million/mL and 20% motility presents a much different problem than a patient with a count less than 1 million per ejaculate. In practice, if the processed sample yields fewer than 1 million total motile sperm, IUI is unlikely to be successful. The couple should therefore be treated with either IVF or ZIFT. As already discussed, the need for micromanipulation can be anticipated, in part, by results obtained at SPA.

Associated Pathologic Conditions in the Woman

A known female factor that is likely to decrease the monthly fecundity rate should move the clinician to aggressive treatment. Endometriosis, when more advanced than minimal, is known to have a negative influence on conception rate. Pelvic adhesions, when present, can interfere with pelvic anatomy and architecture, minimizing the likelihood of successful gamete fusion. IUI is less likely to be successful, making IVF a logical therapeutic option.

Age of the Woman

This is a critical factor in the decision-making process. It has long been appreciated that there is a female age-related decline in fertility that begins at 30 years of age, accelerates at 35 years, and becomes severe beyond 40 years.[29,30] This has been confirmed by numerous studies of success rates of ART and how they decline with advanced maternal age. Likewise, with ICSI, successful pregnancies and deliveries depend highly on the age of the oocyte.[31] Therefore, the older the woman, the more prudent it is to not maintain a couple for too long in a treatment program with a low success rate. For a couple in which the woman is younger than 35 years, six cycles of IUI, with appropriate ovarian stimulation, constitutes an adequate trial.[32,33] For couples in which the woman is older than 35 years, three to four cycles represents an adequate insemination regimen.

Establishment of Previous Conceptions

If a couple has successfully reproduced together, the method of initiating a prior pregnancy should be a guide for the clinician. In general, if the previous conception occurred by means of assisted insemination, a longer trial of insemination may be appropriate. However, the clinician should remain cognizant of the age-related decline in fertility associated with advanced maternal age.

Length of Treatment

As is well appreciated, infertility places a tremendous emotional, physical, and financial burden on a couple.[34] It remains important for the physician to minimize burn-out for the couple. It is therefore important to keep improving treatment in the face of repeated failure. This is particularly important if there are unanswered issues, such as, can the sperm fertilize the eggs, or what is the status regarding ovum pick-up in the case of suspected fimbrial phimosis? In such situations, IVF or ZIFT not only may provide critical answers but also may afford a higher probability of conception.

Financial Considerations

This issue is critical in the age of cost consciousness. Everyone has a finite budget, and it is necessary for the physician to be cognizant of this fact. It is particularly important (but not less relevant) for a couple who is paying for their treatment themselves as opposed to using a third-party payment plan. Assuming a cycle of IUI with stimulation costs at least $700, with an attendant pregnancy rate of 10% to 15% per cycle, the cost of six cycles can be $4200, for a cumulative pregnancy rate of 20% to 30%. This can take as long as 8 months to accomplish if the couple does not conceive sooner. A single cycle of IVF (depending on individual centers) costs $5000 to $6000 and may yield a pregnancy rate up to 40% in one cycle. The financial issues are complex and must be carefully considered and presented to the couple.

Summary

With the foregoing guidelines in mind, the clinician is able to formulate a comprehensive management plan for the couple with male-factor subfertility. Depending on the age and reproductive status of the female partner, diagnostic and therapeutic steps may be performed simultaneously. It is important to emphasize, however, that although this management plan can serve as a guideline, much remains to be learned about all of the ARTs. As new information becomes available, the clinical approach for infertile couples will require modification.[35]

TREATMENT AND RESULTS

Intrauterine Insemination

As indicated previously, IUI is offered as a treatment for male-factor subfertility when the degree of subfertility is relatively minor, the woman is younger than 40 years, there is no associated pathologic condition in the woman, excluding minimal endometriosis, and the couple has not undergone numerous prior IUI treatment cycles. It is important that the processed sample of sperm consistently yield more than 1 million motile sperm. When the criteria are satisfied and the woman is younger than 35 years and has regular menstrual cycles, an attempt is made in an unstimulated cycle and the woman undergoes an ultrasound examination when an ovulation prediction kit demonstrates a change in color. Insemination is performed 24 to 48 hours after the initial kit change, provided a mature graafian follicle is seen at ultrasound examination and is associated with a good endometrial pattern (triple-line and optimal uterine biophysical index).[36] On occasion, a single intramuscular dose of 5000 U human chorionic gonadotropin (hCG) is administered to trigger ovulation and to enhance the ovulatory process. Insemination is performed with either a Tomcat or a Shepherd catheter. If conception does not occur without ovarian stimulation or if there is any ovulatory dysfunction, we institute treatment with either clomiphene citrate or gonadotropins alone or in combination. Ovulation is triggered with hCG, and IUI is performed either once or twice in a cycle.

Luteal support is provided with progesterone administered orally, as intravaginal suppositories, or by means of intramuscular injection.

An analysis of 400 treatment cycles involving 82 couples in whom the men had a semen analysis with fewer than 20 million/mL and associated asthenospermia yielded 24 term pregnancies for a pregnancy rate of 6% per treatment cycle. These data underscore the importance of an adequate therapeutic trial for such couples.

In one study,[37] pregnancy rates resulting from IUI were compared with those of timed intercourse for men with moderate and with severe semen defects. For the group with moderate semen defects (10 to 40×10^6 sperm/mL, 30% to 44% motility, and 30% to 40% normal forms), the pregnancy rate per IUI treatment cycle was 8.8% (17 of 193) and for timed intercourse was 4.5% (6 of 133). This comparison demonstrates no statistically significant difference and suggests that success among couples with moderate sperm defects who are treated with IUI may be due to accurate timing of insemination rather than IUI per se. On the other hand, for patients with severe semen defects (counts less than 10×10^6/mL, motility less than 30%, and morphology less than 30% normal), pregnancy rates with IUI were significantly better (9 of 103, or 8.7%) than those resulting from timed intercourse alone (0 of 80). These data indicate that couples with severe semen defects benefit substantially from IUI. The improvement in pregnancy rates is most probably attributable to the fact that the insemination procedure bypasses some of the natural barriers of the woman's reproductive tract, principally the cervix.

IVF-ET and ZIFT

In the past, with conventional IVF procedures (100,000 motile sperm per oocyte) we expected and counseled patients with male-factor infertility to anticipate fertilization rates 50% less than those experienced by couples without male-factor infertility (34% compared with 70%). However, since the introduction of micromanipulation and with the tendency to apply such procedures with more leniency, this is no longer the case. We analyzed fertilization rates after delayed micromanipulation (day 2) after failed fertilization on day 1. The embryos produced did not increase pregnancy rates substantially and the spontaneous abortion rate was higher than day 1 fertilization. Therefore, if male-factor infertility is documented or highly suspect, we believe it is important to perform micromanipulation on the day of egg retrieval. This practice is supported by the findings of other investigators.[38]

In one series, we treated 284 couples (300 cycles) with micromanipulation. The female partners ranged in age from 30 to 42 years. There were 1850 metaphase II oocytes, and monospermic fertilization of 761 oocytes was achieved, an overall fertilization rate of 41%. In this series of 249 couples who had at least one embryo for transfer, 64 (25.7%) achieved a pregnancy; 49 live births resulted (19.7%). As we have refined the techniques further and gained experience, the monospermic fertilization rate with ICSI has risen to 60%, and the pregnancy rate per transfer is 50%. However, the live birth rate per transfer has risen to 32%. This implies a high spontaneous abortion rate, which we have observed to be highly age-dependent. In a review of spontaneous abortions following treatment with ICSI, 14 of 23 patients experienced a spontaneous abortion, whereas 7 of 9 of the ongoing or delivered pregnancies occurred among couples in which the women were younger than 35 years. These data on the one hand underscore the fact that micromanipulation procedures are extremely powerful, resulting in gametes that would ordinarily have no chance of achieving fertilization. These fertilizations have presumably occurred despite possible inherent biochemical or karyotypic abnormalities in the gametes. Furthermore, it is apparent that the age of the oocyte is of paramount importance in the success of this procedure, lending further support to the concept that it is inappropriate to maintain patients for long periods of time in less productive treatments while losing the competitive advantage of the woman's younger age.

We also analyzed fertilization and pregnancy rates as a function of whether the semen analysis had one, two, or three defects by World Health Organization criteria. We were surprised to see consistent fertilization and pregnancy rates irrespective of defects. Palermo et al[39] reported their data and the outcome for couples treated by means of ICSI and IVF. In 227 cycles, the couples achieved an ongoing pregnancy rate of 37%. This was compared with an ongoing pregnancy rate of 32.9% for IVF patients treated over the same time. These results underscore the success and utility of micromanipulation procedures. It is not our intent to review the extensive experience of Van Steirteghem et al[40] as the pioneers and leaders in the field of micromanipulation. Suffice it to say, however, that these authors' reported pregnancy rate of approximately 35% per cycle over an extensive series of patients with severe sperm defects is a tribute to their efforts and confirms the importance of these procedures.

Whether transcervical embryo transfer (IVF) or laparoscopic tubal transfer (ZIFT) is the preferred method of embryo transfer once fertilization is achieved is a complex issue. Clearly, it is simpler to perform transcervical embryo transfer and avoid laparoscopy, general anesthesia, and the attendant costs. Again, we have found a strong correlation with maternal age in this regard. Among couples in which the woman is younger than 35 years, there appears to be little difference between the two approaches, so we tend to favor IVF-ET for these patients. However, when the woman is older than 40 years, we have observed a higher pregnancy and delivery rate when the

laparoscopic approach (ZIFT) rather than the transcervical approach is used.[41] Therefore, each case should be individualized. If there is associated pelvic pain or one wishes to use the procedure for a limited pelvic assessment, laparoscopic transfer can be performed. However, for older patients it seems to be far more important to perform tubal transfer. These data suggest that the tubal milieu may be important in "rescuing" marginal embryos in older patients. Ours was a relatively small series and clearly needs further study to definitively conclude that tubal transfer should be routinely recommended to all patients because of the higher morbidity and cost associated with this form of treatment. Newer, office-based laparoscopic ZIFT procedures or nonsurgical (tubal) ZIFT[42] will undoubtedly minimize the need for hospital-based procedures. Such procedures have the advantages of lower morbidity and cost, but they retain the therapeutic advantage of tubal transfer.

CONCLUSION

There is little question that ART is used successfully for many couples with male-factor infertility, including severe forms of testicular failure. Although opening the zona pellucida by means of chemical, mechanical, or photoablation methods has enhanced fertilization rates, bypassing optimal sperm penetration when conventional procedures of in vitro insemination have failed, these procedures are limited by the requirements for many functional spermatozoa with good progressive motility and the presence of a normal acrosome. The capability of injecting sperm directly into the cytoplasm of a human oocyte, bypassing the zona pellucida and the oolemma, achieving sperm decondensation and male pronucleus formation, has offered new possibilities for male gametes with poor motility and abnormal or absent acrosomes. These techniques have offered new hope to couples heretofore deemed "hopeless" and whose only alternative for reproduction was with donor sperm. Now, donor insemination remains truly a treatment of last resort and should be presented to a couple only within the entire context of treatment alternatives, inclusive of the use, when appropriate, of either epididymal or testicular sperm. Selection of a specific course of treatment for a given couple is a complex decision that can be made only after all factors for both members of the couple are evaluated. It is imperative that urologists, gynecologists, and reproductive biologists collaborate closely so that treatment can be tailored to the needs of each couple.

In this age of cost-conscious medical care, it is imperative that couples not waste precious resources on treatments that are unlikely to be productive or may waste time and expose the patient to unnecessary medications. Some research has implicated the use of ovary-stimulating agents in subsequent ovarian cancer.[43] Although no conclusive evidence exists in this regard, the implications are impressive. All too often, patients seek advanced treatment having been treated by a primary physician for 1 to 2 years with clomiphene citrate–induced cycles combined with artificial insemination.

Since the advent and successful application of micromanipulation procedures within clinical practice, the role of the SPA in terms of the predictive value for ART is unclear. However, if the assay can be performed in a reliable, reproducible, and sensitive manner that enables assessment of different methods of sperm processing, this test can be of considerable assistance in directing management and patient counseling. Although it was once believed that it was necessary for sperm to traverse the epididymis to enable successful fertilization, it is now known that this is not essential. It has been clearly demonstrated that sperm collected after epididymal aspiration and sperm exposed to confounding conditions during collection, such as electroejaculation or cryopreservation, perform as well with intracytoplasmic sperm injection as sperm collected by means of masturbation. Furthermore, the reports of successful pregnancies with round spermatids implies that in the future even couples with extreme cases of spermatogenic maturational arrest may be able to have their own biologic children if they so desire. Now more than ever, it is imperative that patients receive counseling that delineates all options before they are told that their only alternative is donor insemination.

FUTURE CONSIDERATIONS

Although much remains to be learned about the pathophysiologic mechanisms underlying disorders of male fertility, until these mechanisms are better understood, much of the data we obtain from clinical investigations will be perplexing. It is clear that adequate sperm production with normal bulk semen values is not necessarily associated with normal sperm fertilizing capability. The scientific and technologic advances relating to gamete accessibility and handling have reached a level of sophistication that has resulted in successful treatments heretofore believed to be impossible. Researchers now have a unique opportunity to perform investigations and undertake therapeutic measures. Although great strides have been made in the treatment of infertile men, much remains to be learned. As our knowledge increases, other options will become available for these patients. Researchers are addressing issues such as alternative forms of gamete union, including electrofusion and nuclear or pronuclear transfer of DNA. With the great accessibility of gametes and early embryos and improved tissue culture techniques, the stage seems set for more sophisticated investigations into the mechanisms that control reproductive processes. Molecular biologists and geneticists are making great progress in unraveling the genetic bases of many biologic

phenomena. The result will be that our understanding of and therapies for deficits of the reproductive processes will continue to improve.

REFERENCES

1. Hull MGR, Glazeuer CMA, Kelly NJ, et al: Population study of causes, treatment, and outcome of infertility. *Br Med J* 291:1693, 1985
2. Palermo G, Joris H, Devroey P, Van Steirteghem AC: Pregnancies after intracytoplasmic injection of single spermatozoa into an oocyte. *Lancet* 1:826, 1992
3. Tesarik J, Mendoza C, Testart J: Viable embryos from injection of round spermatids into oocytes. *N Engl J Med* 333:525, 1995
4. Sofikitis N, Miyagawa I, Sharlip I, Hellstrom W, Mekras G, Mastelou E: Human pregnancies achieved by intrao-ooplasmic injections of round spermatids (RS) nuclei isolated from testicular tissue of azoospermic men. *J Urol* 153:302A (abstract 368), 1995
5. Silber S, Nagy Z, Liu JJ, et al: The use of epididymal and testicular sperm for ICSI. Presented at the IXth World Congress on In Vitro Fertilization and Assisted Reproduction, April 1995, Vienna, Austria
6. Batzofin JH, Marrs RP, Serafini PC, et al: Assisted reproductive treatments for male factor infertility. *Probl Urol* 1:430, 1987
7. Smith D, Rodriguez-Rigau LJ, Steinberger E: Relation between indices of semen analysis and pregnancy rate in infertile couples. *Fertil Steril* 28:1314, 1977
8. Hanada A, Chang MC: Penetration of zona-free eggs by spermatozoa of different species. *Biol Reprod* 6:300, 1972
9. Yanagimachi R: Penetration of guinea pig spermatozoa into hamster eggs in vitro. *J Reprod Fertil* 28:477, 1972
10. Barros C, Leal J: In vitro fertilization and its use to study gamete interactions. In: Hafez ESE, Semm K (eds), *In Vitro Fertilization and Embryo Transfer.* Lancaster, England, MTP Press, 1982:37
11. Yanigimachi R: Mechanisms of fertilization of mammals. In: Mastrioianni L, Biggers JD (eds), *Fertilization and Embryonic Development In Vitro.* New York, Plenum Press, 1981:81
12. Barros C, Gonzalez J, Herrera E, et al: Human sperm penetration into zona-free hamster oocyte as a test to evaluate the sperm fertilizing ability. *Andrologia* 11:197, 1979
13. Johnson AR, Syms AJ, Lipshultz LI, et al: Conditions influencing human sperm capacitation and penetration of zona-free hamster ova. *Fertil Steril* 41:603, 1984
14. Rogers BJ, Perrearlt S, Bentwood BJ, et al: Variability in the human hamster ova in vitro assay for fertility evaluation. *Fertil Steril* 39:204, 1983
15. Syms AJ, Johnson AR, Lipshultz LI, et al: Effect on aging and cold temperature storage of hamster ova as assessed in the sperm penetration assay. *Fertil Steril* 43:766, 1985
16. Turner TT: On the development and use of alloplastic spermatoceles. *Fertil Steril* 49:387, 1988
17. Temple-Smith PD, Southwick GJ, Yates CA, et al: Human pregnancy by in vitro fertilization (IVF) using sperm aspirated from the epididymis. *JIVFET* 2:850 1985

18. Shrivastav P, Nadkarni P, Wensvoort S, et al: Percutaneous epididymal sperm aspiration for obstructive azoospermia. *Hum Reprod* 9:58, 1994

19. Craft I, Tsirigotis M, Vennett V, et al: Percutaneous epididymal sperm aspiration and intracytoplasmic sperm injection in the management of infertility due to obstructive azoospermia. *Fertil Steril* 63:1038, 1995

20. Tsirigotis M, Pelekanos A, Boulos S, et al: Experience with percutaneous epididymal sperm aspiration and intracytoplasmic sperm injection in azoospermic patients (abstract). Paper Presentation No. P-178. 51st Annual Meeting of the American Society of Reproductive Medicine, October 7–12, 1995, Seattle, WA

21. Silber SJ, Balmaceda J, Borrero C, et al: Pregnancy with sperm aspiration from the proximal head of the epididymis: A new treatment for congenital absence of the vas deferens. *Fertil Steril* 50:525, 1988

22. Tournaye H, Devroey P, Liu J, et al: Microsurgical epididymal sperm aspiration and intracytoplasmic sperm injection: A new effective approach to infertility as a result of congenital bilateral absence of the vas deferens. *Fertil Steril* 62:1045, 1994

23. Bourne H, Watkins W, Speirs A, et al: Pregnancies after intracytoplasmic injection of sperm collected by fine needle biopsy of the testis. *Fertil Steril* 64:433, 1995

24. Silber SJ, Van Steirteghem AC, Liu J, et al: High fertilization and pregnancy rate after intracytoplasmic sperm injection with spermatozoa obtained from testicle biopsy. *Hum Reprod* 10:148, 1995

25. Hoekstra T, Richard JE, Massey JB, et al: The yield of testicular sperm from open excisional biopsy versus percutaneous needle biopsy. Paper Presentation No. 0-098. 51st Annual Meeting of the American Society for Reproductive Medicine, October 7–12, 1995, Seattle, WA

26. Sofikitis N, Zavos P, Koutselinis A, et al: Achievement of pregnancy after injection of round spermatid nuclei into rabbit oocytes and embryo transfer: A possible mode of treatment of men with spermatogenic arrest at the spermatid stage. *J Urol* 151:311 (abstract 334), 1994

27. Batzofin J, Tran C, Tan T, et al: Laser laparoscopy as an adjunct to assisted reproduction treatments in women with pelvic adhesions and endometriosis. *J Gynecol Surg* 5:273, 1989

28. Serafini P, Mota E, Nelson J, et al: Laseroscopy at the time of GIFT improves pregnancy rates in women with stage I and II endometriosis-associated subfertility. Proceedings of 4th World Congress on Endometriosis, May 16–18, 1994, Bahai, Brazil, 77–83

29. Scott RT Jr, Hofmann GE: Prognostic assessment of ovarian reserve. *Fertil Steril* 63:1, 1995

30. Maroulis, GB: Effect of aging on fertility and pregnancy. *Semin Reprod Endocrinol* 9:165, 1991

31. Batzofin J, Tran C, Tan T, et al: Microfertilization: Observations and lessons from a successful program. Poster 273. Presented at the 51st Annual Meeting of the American Society for Reproductive Medicine, October 7–12, 1995, Seattle, WA

32. Dodson WC, Whiteside DB, Hughes CL Jr, et al: Superovulation with intrauterine insemination in the treatment of infertility: A possible alternative to gamete intrafallopian transfer and in vitro fertilization. *Fertil Steril* 48:441, 1987

33. Yeh J, Seibel NM: Artificial insemination with donor sperm: A review of 108 patients. *Obstet Gynecol* 70:313, 1987

34. Boivin J, Hemmings R, Takefman J: The relationship between treatment distress and embryo quality in predicting pregnancy rate with IVF. Prize Paper Presentation No. 112. 51st Annual Meeting of the American Society for Reproductive Medicine, October 7–12, 1995, Seattle, WA

35. Adamson GD, Martin MC, Sharlip I, et al: Treating infertility takes more than technology. *Contemp Obstet Gynecol* 39:71, 1994

36. Serafini P, Nelson J, Batzofin J, et al: Preovulatory sonographic uterine receptivity index (SURI) usefulness as an indicator of pregnancy in women undergoing assisted reproductive treatments. *J Ultrasound Med* 14:751, 1995

37. Kerin J, Quinn P: Washed intrauterine insemination in the treatment of oligospermic infertility. *Semin Reprod Endocrinol* 5:23, 1987

38. Tsirigotis M, Nicholson N, Taranissi M, et al: Late intracytoplasmic sperm injection in unexpected failed fertilization in vitro: Diagnostic or therapeutic? *Fertil Steril* 63:816, 1995

39. Palermo GD, Cohen J, Alikani M, et al: Intracytoplasmic sperm injection: A novel treatment for all forms of male factor infertility. *Fertil Steril* 63:1231, 1995

40. Van Steirteghem AC, Tournaye H, Devroey P: Microfertilization: The Belgium experience. Presented at the 51st Annual Meeting of the American Society for Reproductive Medicine, October 7–12, 1995, Seattle, WA

41. Batzofin J, Tran C, Tan T, et al: A comparison of clinical pregnancy and delivery rates between IVF and ZIFT in women over 40 years of age. Poster No. 227, presented at the 9th World Congress on In Vitro Fertilization and Assisted Reproduction, April 1995, Vienna, Austria

42. Hurst BS, Schlaff WD: Assisted reproduction: What role for ZIFT? *Contemp Ob Gyn* 39:9, 1994

43. Rossing MA, Daling JR, Weiss NS, et al: Ovarian tumors in a cohort of infertile women. *N Engl J Med* 331:771, 1994

CHAPTER 18

Therapeutic Insemination

MARY G. HAMMOND · LUTHER M. TALBERT

Evaluation for Therapeutic Insemination with Husband's Sperm (TIH)

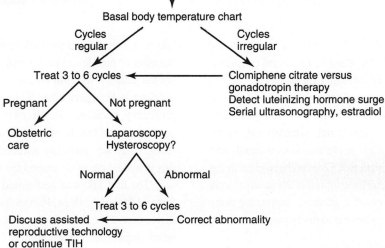

TIH

Semen stored before chemotherapy,
 surgery or radiation therapy
Impotence or vaginismus
Hypospadias
Severe cervical factor
Retrograde ejaculation
Poor results of semen analysis
Antisperm antibodies
*Unexplained infertility
*Mild endometriosis

History and physical examination of woman
History and physical examination of man
Hysterosalpingogram
Discuss procedure, cost, success rates,
 medicated versus unmedicated cycles, and
 informed consent

*Laparoscopy recommended

Basal body temperature chart

Cycles
regular

Cycles
irregular

Treat 3 to 6 cycles

Clomiphene citrate versus
 gonadotropin therapy
Detect luteinizing hormone surge
Serial ultrasonography, estradiol

Pregnant

Not pregnant

Obstetric
care

Laparoscopy
Hysteroscopy?

Normal

Abnormal

Treat 3 to 6 cycles

Discuss assisted
reproductive technology
or continue TIH

Correct abnormality

Evaluation for Therapeutic Insemination with Donor Sperm (TID)

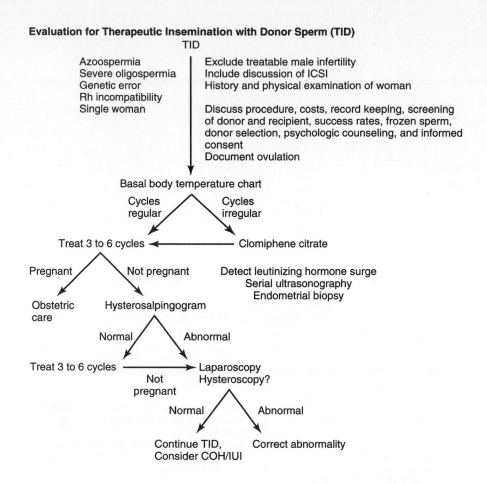

Therapeutic insemination with the husband's semen (TIH) and therapeutic insemination with donor sperm (TID) are the principal modalities in contemporary infertility management.[1] Semen or washed sperm has been recommended for a number of reasons for many decades. Depending on where the sperm is injected, the insemination may be called intravaginal, intracervical, or intrauterine. Recently, intrauterine insemination combined with controlled ovarian hyperstimulation (COH) has been used to improve conception rates in several types of infertility in which conventional management has proved ineffective. Increasing numbers of controlled studies report benefit to many patients.

HISTORY

Therapeutic insemination has been described as early as biblical times. John Hunter (1728–1793) is believed to be the first person in recent history to offer therapeutic insemination. Some time in the late 1770s, Hunter was consulted by a London cloth merchant with hypospadias. Hunter advised the patient to collect his ejacu-

late in a warmed syringe and deposit it into his wife's vagina. Whether or not Hunter performed the insemination is unknown, but the patient's wife did conceive.[2] In the United States, J. Marion Sims in 1866 performed 55 inseminations in six women; one pregnancy occurred. In all cases, the semen samples were deemed normal but the wives had a cervical abnormality. Sims's success rate was probably reduced in part because he believed that ovulation occurred around the time of the menses.[3]

The first TID was performed by William Pancoast of Jefferson Medical College, Philadelphia, in 1884.[4] However, little discussion of the procedure was found until half a century later, when Sophia Kleegman in the United States[5] and Margaret Jackson in England[6] advanced public and medical awareness of the subject. In 1953, Bunge and Sherman[7] reported the first pregnancies following treatment with cryopreserved semen. This experience opened the door to current medical treatment.

The following decades witnessed considerable evolution in the general acceptance of therapeutic insemination. Discussions have ranged from ethical, legal, and religious considerations to concern about transmission of sexually transmitted diseases, including human immunodeficiency virus (HIV) and hepatitis, and donor selection processes.[8] Guidelines have been developed by the American Society for Reproductive Medicine [(ASRM), formerly the American Fertility Society] and have been updated several times. The most recent standards were published in 1994.[9]

INSEMINATION WITH HUSBAND'S SPERM

Indications

Through the years a number of indications for TIH have been proposed (see the algorithm at the beginning of this chapter). These include insemination with semen stored before chemotherapy, an operation, or radiation therapy; and situations in which intercourse or intravaginal deposition of semen is not possible (ie, impotence, hypospadias), severe cervical factor, retrograde ejaculation, and low semen volume (1 mL or less).

With the introduction of COH to increase the number of oocytes available for therapeutic insemination, new indications have been added. These include treatment of oligospermia (reduced number of spermatozoa), asthenospermia (decreased sperm motility), teratozoospermia (increased number of sperm with abnormal morphology), unexplained infertility, mild endometriosis, and antisperm antibodies.

In some instances, the use of a split ejaculate may be beneficial. The first portion of the ejaculate contains the sperm-rich fraction and prostatic fluid. The seminal vesicles contribute most of the remaining ejaculate. The split-ejaculate method provides a specimen of high sperm density and motility. One collects the ejaculate by holding or taping two jars together and collecting the first few drops in one jar and the rest of the ejaculate in the other jar. In 90% of instances the specimen in the first jar is superior; in 5% the specimen in the second jar is superior. In 5% no difference is found between the specimens, and in such instances this method is of no benefit.[1]

Evaluation for Insemination

Evaluation of the Female Partner

Because insemination is time consuming and potentially expensive, even in situations of clear indications of male-factor infertility, we believe an evaluation of the female partner is essential. This should include documentation of ovulation by means of progesterone level, ovulation prediction kits, or endometrial biopsy and of tubal patency by means of hysterosalpingography. Before intrauterine insemination (IUI) for empirical therapy for unexplained infertility or after 6 months of failed therapeutic insemination for any reason, laparoscopy may be indicated and hysteroscopy should be considered. At that time,

any adhesions should be transected and endometrial implants ablated.

Evaluation of the Male Partner

Serial semen analyses should be performed to determine the degree of semen abnormality. At least 10 to 20 million motile sperm per ejaculate are preferred for insemination, since many washing and separation techniques result in yields as low as 10 to 15% of the raw values. There appears to be no benefit to storing several samples, since freezing destroys many sperm. However, two samples can be obtained an hour or so apart, combined, processed, and inseminated as a single specimen. This often doubles the number of sperm for insemination.[10]

Timing of Insemination

Cycles of intracervical insemination can be monitored quite adequately with basal body temperature, checks of cervical mucus, or ovulation prediction kits. If cycles are irregular, problems in collection occur. If the number of specimens is limited, more careful monitoring may be warranted. If adequate stores of semen are available, two inseminations per cycle may speed the time to conception.[11] Postinsemination mucous evaluations may be helpful 12 to 24 hours after insemination to determine sperm penetration and survival. If sperm numbers are low, IUI may be indicated.

IUI is usually performed with stringent control of ovulation. Superovulation with clomiphene or gonadotropins usually is recommended. Standard regimens include clomiphene 50 or 100 mg on days 3 to 7 of the menstrual cycle, commercial home luteinizing hormone (LH) monitoring and insemination on the day of or the day after the LH surge, or ultrasound monitoring with human chorionic gonadotropin (hCG) administration. Insemination is performed 36 hours after hCG administration.

With the advent of controlled ovarian hyperstimulation for in vitro fertilization (IVF), many similar ovarian stimulation protocols have been adopted for TIH. These include clomiphene 100 mg on days 3 to 7 of the menstrual cycle followed in sequence with hMG or initiating hMG from day 3 onward. Protocols such as these require monitoring with ultrasound and estrogen levels until mature follicles are seen. hCG is then administered, and insemination is performed 36 hours later.[12,13]

Semen Preparation for Insemination

Inseminations can be performed by the intracervical or the intrauterine route (Fig 18–1). For many indications in which semen quality and quantity are normal and good-quality cervical mucus is present, intracervical insemination is recommended for the first few cycles. Doing so eliminates the necessity for facilities to process semen and also reduces the need for precise timing of ovulation or controlled ovarian hyperstimulation.

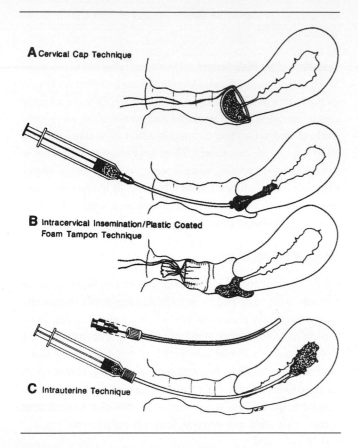

A Cervical Cap Technique

B Intracervical Insemination/Plastic Coated Foam Tampon Technique

C Intrauterine Technique

Figure 18–1. A. Plastic cervical cap. **B.** Acorn-tip catheter and syringe and plastic-covered foam tampon. **C.** Shepard intrauterine catheter.

For intracervical insemination, fresh semen is obtained by means of masturbation into a sterile container. Insemination is performed directly after liquefaction, which requires approximately 30 minutes. If the man has difficulty obtaining a semen sample with masturbation, special nonspermicidal condoms can be used to collect the sample by means of intercourse. We use a cervical cup to protect the specimen from vaginal secretions. Stored frozen samples of the sperm should be handled with care. If the semen is transferred from another laboratory, that laboratory's thawing instructions should be used. In such instances, it is also prudent to develop a consent form stating that because the semen was frozen elsewhere and shipped, the facility performing the insemination cannot be responsible for the condition of the thawed sample. A formal analysis is performed to determine the number of viable sperm. The ideal is about 30 million motile sperm per insemination. It may be necessary to combine several samples to achieve this concentration. The protocol for IUI sperm preparation is summarized in Table 18–1.

Washing the specimen eliminates seminal fluid, which contains prostaglandins that could cause uterine contractions, and concentrates the specimen. Sperm washing may also speed

capacitation of the sperm. Although concerns have been raised about the possibility that IUI leads to formation of antisperm antibodies, the data are far from conclusive.

The "swim-up" procedure eliminates contaminates such as white blood cells (WBCs) and dead sperm. This is accomplished by means of overlayering the washed specimen pellet with medium and allowing the sperm to swim out of the pellet. Unfortunately, the swim-up technique reduces the yield of motile sperm to about 10% of the untreated specimen, or lower in many men with male-factor infertility. Some investigators have hoped that the reduction or elimination of WBCs from the semen specimen would eliminate the risk for transmission of HIV in couples who know the man has HIV infection. This method cannot prevent HIV transmission, however, because the virus is free and not confined exclusively to the WBCs.[14]

Discontinuous Percoll (Pharmacia AB, Stockholm, Sweden) gradient centrifugation ranging from 30% to 95% Percoll has been reported to produce a higher sperm yield than swim-up techniques. Most motile sperm overcome the increasing concentration gradient. Values as high as 60% of the original have been reported.[15]

Commercial preparation methods are available. Sperm Select, in which sodium hyaluronate is used, provides high-quality sperm but can produce low yields. One study reported a 75% yield of motile sperm with the conventional washing technique compared with a 10% yield after processing with Sperm Select.[16]

Obtaining a semen specimen may be both challenging and difficult in some circumstances. Men with retrograde ejaculation must have sperm collected from their bladder. To determine if a man with retrograde ejaculation is a candidate for treatment with artificial insemination, urine specimens are evaluated after masturbation. If more than 1 million sperm are identified, consideration should be given to performing several cycles of TIH with this method. The urine must first be alkalinized by means

TABLE 18–1. PROTOCOL FOR IUI SPERM PREPARATIONS

1. Semen is collected under sterile conditions by means of masturbation into a sterile cup and is allowed to liquefy at 37°C. This usually requires 30 min.

2. A standard semen analysis is performed. The specimen is then centrifuged for 10 min at 1500 rpm in a standard desk-top clinical centrifuge.

3. The supernatant is removed immediately, and the pellet is suspended in 2 mL of commercially prepared medium.

4. The specimen is incubated for 5 min at 37°C and spun 5 min at 1700 rpm.

5. The supernatant is immediately removed, the pellet is mixed with 0.5 to 0.4 mL of medium, and the sperm are counted.

6. The specimen is loaded into a catheter for insemination.

7. For "swim-up," the pellet is overlayered at step 5 with 1 mL of medium and incubated at 37°C for 1 hr. Supernatant is removed, and insemination is performed.

of ingestion of sodium bicarbonate to prevent the acidic urine from killing the sperm, and the bladder must be emptied. The man is then asked to masturbate and urinate again. The sperm are separated, and insemination is performed.[17]

Electroejaculation has been necessary for men with certain neurologic conditions, such as paraplegia. A rectal probe is used, and general anesthesia is often required. Epididymal aspirations are required in cases of congenital absence of the vas or after failed vasovasotomy reversal. In such instances, very small numbers of sperm are available, and consideration should be given to IVF and intracytoplasmic single-sperm injection (ICSI) rather than IUI. Procedures such as these must be coordinated carefully with the woman's treatment cycle.

Insemination Techniques

Intracervical Techniques

A bivalved speculum stored on a heating pad to keep it warm increases patient comfort. Only warm water is used as a lubricant to avoid the potential spermicidal effects of lubricants such as jellies. The semen sample should be less than 2 hours old. The portio vaginalis is wiped with a cotton ball to remove secretions. The closed tip of a long forceps is placed into the external ostium of the uterus. The forceps is allowed to open, turned 180°, and closed to grasp a sample of cervical mucus. A tuberculin syringe may be used for this purpose. The mucus is placed on a clean glass slide, and spinnbarkeit and degree of ferning are established. We then place 0.2 mL of liquefied semen into the endocervical canal and the rest into a cervical cup. The patient remains supine for 15 minutes and then returns to her normal activities. The cup is removed at bedtime. Because the cap forms suction with the cervix, the patient must reach into her vagina to dislodge it. She can remove the cap easily by pulling on the string or tube as if she were removing a tampon. Patients should be warned that the sperm rise into the uterus, but seminal plasma, mucus, and occasionally tinges of blood come out with the cap. The cap should be rinsed under warm running tap water without soap, detergents, or antiseptics that could leach into the plastic and harm the sperm at future inseminations.

Other practitioners place 0.2 mL of liquified semen into the endocervical canal through an acorn-tip cannula (see Fig 18–1B) and hold it in place for 1 minute to ensure adequate sperm-mucus interaction. When the speculum is loosened, the excess semen pools in the posterior vaginal vault that covers the external ostium of the uterus. The patient remains on the examining table for approximately 10 minutes, after which time a plastic-covered foam tampon (see Fig 18–1B) is inserted, more to control leakage than as a fertility aid. The patient is asked to remove the tampon and dispose of it approximately 2 hours after insemination.

Intrauterine Technique

For IUI the cervix is visualized and wiped clean of secretions. A plastic catheter is introduced through the external ostium of the uterus and into the uterine cavity. Many catheters are available for this purpose. A Tomcat catheter (Monoject Sherwood Medical, St Louis, MO) is among the most versatile and the least expensive. If difficulties occur passing the catheter, repositioning the speculum or applying a tenaculum to straighten the canal may help. A transcervical introducer has been developed (Cook OB/GYN, Spencer, IN). The washed sperm is injected slowly. The patient rests supine for 5 to 15 minutes and then returns to normal activity. Some patients experience mild discomfort or uterine cramping. Unwashed sperm should never be injected into the uterine cavity because of an increased risk for infection and the likely occurrence of severe uterine cramping. In rare instances, anaphylaxis and death have been reported after intrauterine injection of unwashed sperm.

The volume of sperm with which the woman is inseminated depends on the technique. Sperm volumes of 0.5 to 1.0 mL remain in the uterine cavity. Some physicians recommend tubal perfusion with up to 4 mL of washed specimen to force sperm into the fallopian tubes.[18] The benefits of one technique over the other have not been clarified.

Other techniques for insemination include transtubal insemination at laparoscopy and direct intraperitoneal insemination through the cul-de-sac.[19,20] The latter techniques have resulted in some pregnancies but are used far less commonly than IUI.

Complications of Therapeutic Insemination with Husband's Sperm

Potential problems with IUI include endometritis or salpingitis from agents introduced into the uterus at the time of cannulation. Severe uterine contractions and vasomotor symptoms are uncommon with washed semen but do occasionally occur. They are far more common with overzealous intracervical injection of aliquots of whole, unprepared ejaculate. Many centers screen anonymous and known donors for syphilis, gonorrhea, HIV infection, hepatitis, and *Chlamydia* infections. We have not done so with cohabiting couples who have similar risks with intercourse. We do, however, use infection precautions in our laboratory when handling sperm.

An additional risk of IUI is the formation of antisperm antibodies. One study demonstrated that antibodies developed in 2 of 41 patients during therapy.[21] Nevertheless, the risk for development of antisperm antibodies after IUI appears to be low.

The most important complication of COH and IUI is increased risk for multiple embryos. Unlike IVF, in which embryo numbers are controlled, all the ovulated oocytes have potential for implantation after IUI. In many patients, large numbers of follicles are recruited to increase the likelihood of conception in any one cycle. Multiple gestations occur more frequently in patients in whom there are underlying ovulatory disturbances. This has led to some concern for the outcome of these pregnancies and their cost.[22]

Success Rates

Studies report per cycle pregnancy rates of 5% to 50%. Most practitioners informally report rates of 10% to 15% per cycle for COH and IUI in a mixed patient population. Delivery rates as low as 1% to 5% are not uncommon in women older than 40 years.

A variety of factors will affect pregnancy rates with COH and IUI. The most important is the cause of infertility. One of the more important problems in assessing early reports of pregnancies with TIH is the heterogeneity of patients treated. Most studies had small numbers and cannot be subdivided by diagnosis.[23] Even in recent reports, only a few studies have control groups or control cycles as part of the study design.

Male-factor infertility is an important indication for IUI. Several reports have addressed pregnancy rates in this broad diagnostic category.[24–29] Hull et al,[24] Hughes et al,[25] and Ho et al[27] reported no pregnancy in 14, 63, and 114 cycles, respectively, of IUI in spontaneous cycles monitored according to LH surge. Friedman et al[28] reported a 6.5% per cycle rate in 276 spontaneous cycles. Martinez[26] reported four pregnancies in 24 cycles with IUI versus no pregnancies in 25 cycles with intercourse. Pregnancies were equally divided between those with spontaneous and those with clomiphene-induced cycles. Chaffkin et al[29] reported mean cycle fecundity rates of 15.3% for hMG and IUI, 7.9% for hMG, and 5.1% for IUI in spontaneous cycles. Dodson and Haney[22] reported a 15% cycle fecundity rate for male-factor infertility with hMG and IUI. These data support an approximately 5% to 7% per cycle success rate for IUI alone and 15% with COH.

Pregnancy rates reported for cervical-factor infertility are higher. Unstimulated cycles with IUI resulted in pregnancy rates of 12.2%,[17] 5%,[24] and 5.1%[29] in unstimulated cycles and 26.3%[29] and 20%[22] in COH-IUI cycles.

In patients with unexplained infertility, fecundity varies between 6.3%[28] in spontaneous cycles and 20.1%,[30] 15%,[22] and 32.6% in COH-IUI cycles. Data for endometriosis are similar. Serta et al[31] compared the IUI success rate among patients with minimal endometriosis with and without ovarian stimulation. The cumulative probabilities of conception for the first, second, and third cycles were 0.13, 0.26, and 0.38 among the natural-cycle group and 0.12, 0.25, and 0.34 among the medicated-cycle group (P>.05). Monthly fecundity was 0.14 for the natural-cycle group and 0.13 for the medicated-cycle group (P>.05), suggesting that ovarian stimulation did not improve

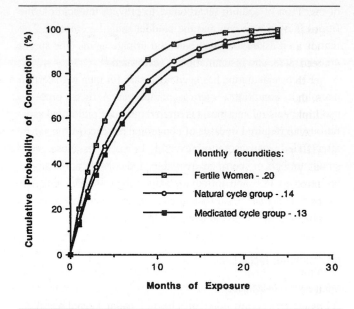

Figure 18–2. Life-table analysis demonstrating the cumulative probability of conception versus months of exposure in patients treated for 3 months with intrauterine insemination. *(From Serta RT, Rufo S, Seibel MM: Minimal endometriosis and intrauterine insemination: Does controlled ovarian hyperstimulation improve pregnancy rates? Obstet Gynecol 80:37, 1992.)*

IUI success rates over natural cycles (Fig 18–2). Some authors[22,29] reported similar pregnancy rates (12.8% and 13%) with COH and IUI.

Two studies controlled for other fertility factors in addition to IUI. Chaffkin et al[29] compared COH, COH with IUI, and IUI and demonstrated that the combination of COH and IUI is more effective than either modality alone. Aboulghar et al[30] used a control period. Patients were treated for 2 months and not treated for 10 months. The pregnancy per cycle rate was less than 1% in the nontreated group compared with a 20% pregnancy rate per cycle during the medicated cycle. Some authors demonstrated a beneficial effect of COH on pregnancy rate per cycle over IUI alone.[32,33] Martinez et al, however, found no benefit to using COH with IUI.[34]

Semen variables have been considered. The importance of sperm motility is suggested by the finding that motility greater than 30% in the original sample and 70% in the swim-up specimen yield higher pregnancy rates.[35] Abnormal morphology greater than 50% in combination with reduced numbers of motile sperm also reduced success rates.[36] Total motile sperm count has been associated with increasing pregnancy rates when numbers exceed 20 million per inseminate.[37] The threshold for pregnancy appears to be about 3 million, although occasional pregnancies are reported with lower values.

Several investigators have evaluated the effect of follicle number, serum estradiol levels, and patient age on TIH success rates. These studies suggest that there are more multiple embryos if more than four mature follicles are seen. Higher pregnancy and delivery rates also are observed when estradiol levels exceed 500 pg/mL. Delivery rates are lower among women older than 35 years (12.7% vs 5.8%). In one study of 779 cycles, there was a 20% spontaneous abortion rate and a 22.3% multiple-embryo rate (4% triplets).[32]

A number of variations have been described in regard to the IUI procedure. These include two inseminations per cycle, tubal perfusion,[18] and direct intraperitoneal insemination.[19] Controlled studies suggest no benefit to multiple inseminations[38] or intraperitoneal inseminations.[20] Tubal perfusion has not been subjected to controlled study.

For the most part physicians must draw their own conclusions about the cost-to-benefit ratio for their patients. We are confident in offering IUI treatment to couples with poor or absent cervical mucus, low semen volume, and ejaculatory problems as long as other conventional treatment has been offered and has failed. For patients with mechanical problems or banked sperm, additional cycles up to 10 are reasonable. We believe the results in unexplained infertility, endometriosis, and male-factor infertility may be beneficial, but our personal approach is to limit treatment to three to four cycles.[28] For empirical therapy, additional cycles are likely to be unproductive, and IVF should be discussed.[39]

For many couples, some form of COH and IUI represents their most sophisticated therapy and their final therapeutic step. IVF may be either too expensive or too invasive, and at the completion of three to four cycles of COH and IUI, the physician should be prepared to recommend closure with the couple, which includes a discussion of other options such as TID, adoption, and child-free living.[40]

TIH for Sex Selection

There has been a long and avid interest in controlling the sex of offspring.[41] For many couples, the incentive is a desire for a child of a particular sex for personal ideals of both number and sex of children. However, of the approximately 6000 heritable defects in humans, only about 370 are known to be X-linked.[42] Because X-linked diseases are typically expressed by sons of carrier mothers who inherit the genetically defective X chromosome, the ability to separate X from Y chromosome–bearing spermatozoa to favorably bias female offspring could greatly reduce the probability of conceiving male offspring affected with diseases such as various muscular dystrophies, hemophilia, and glucose-6-phosphate dehydrogenase deficiency.

Several techniques for sperm separation have been developed to preselect the sex of human offspring. These include using gel filtration,[43] passage through mucus[44] or albumin,[45] electrophoresis,[46] and centrifugation techniques.[47] An albumin gradient technique[45] for Y-sperm enrichment and a Sephadex (Pharmacia AB, Stockholm, Sweden) G-50 gel chromatography method[48] used to concentrate X chromosome–bearing sperm have shown the greatest successes. More recently, human X and Y chromosome–bearing spermatozoa have been separated according to DNA content by means of modified flow cytometric cell sorting technology.[49] All these techniques are time consuming and labor intensive, and they achieve the desired outcome in at most 75% to 80% of instances. Therefore, patients who choose these techniques must be advised that results cannot be guaranteed.

THERAPEUTIC INSEMINATION WITH DONOR SPERM

Therapeutic insemination with donor sperm has become common therapy for specific categories of infertility. In fact, more infertile couples build their families by means of TID than with newborn adoption. Improved understanding of the genetic transmission of some disease and the widespread prevalence of sexually transmitted diseases has made donor selection and screening a rigorous process. This chapter addresses these and other issues involved in the use of donor sperm.

Indications

The most common indication for TID is azoospermia or severe oligospermia in the male partner. Other indications include severe Rh incompatibility or the potential for genetically transmitted disease (eg, Tay-Sachs disease, Huntington's disease). An increasingly common indication is the desire of a single woman to bear a biologic child. Guidelines for TID have been proposed by the ASRM.[9] A modification of those guidelines is presented in Table 18–2.[50]

Donor Selection and Screening

Sperm donors must have semen characteristics consistent with a high rate of fecundity in the recipient woman. The American Society for Reproductive Medicine recommends that the donor's semen specimen have a minimum 1-mL volume, more than 50 million motile sperm per milliliter, and greater than 60% motility in the entire specimen. There must not be an excessive number of abnormal forms, and more than 50% of the sperm must survive freezing.[9] Because pregnancy rate is affected by the number of viable sperm in the specimen, our center requires 40 million viable sperm in the thawed specimen used for insemination.

Genetic screening is an extremely important aspect of donor selection. The donor should be free of any genetically transmittable disease and should be generally healthy. This finding should be confirmed with a complete history and physical

TABLE 18–2. GUIDELINES FOR THERAPEUTIC DONOR INSEMINATION: SPERM

I. Indications

   A. The male partner has irreversible azoospermia.

   B. The male partner has obstruction of the reproductive tract, either acquired or congenital, that cannot be repaired, or the male partner does not want surgical treatment.

   C. The male partner has severe oligospermia or severely impaired semen findings and does not want to use intracytoplasmic single-sperm injection (ICSI) or other assisted reproductive technologies for conception, or these techniques have failed.

   D. The male partner possesses a known inherited or genetic disorder such as Huntington's disease, hemophilia, or chromosomal abnormality that places a biological offspring at risk.

   E. The male partner has noncorrectable ejaculatory dysfunction.

   F. An Rh-negative female partner has severe Rh isoimmunization, and the male partner is Rh-positive.

   G. The male partner has had a positive test for the human immunodeficiency virus (HIV).

   H. A single woman wants to conceive.

II. Preparation

   A. Couples or individuals interested in pursuing TID should receive detailed explanation of the procedure and its benefits and risks, including the risk for infection, the need for recipient and donor screening, and out-of-pocket expenses.

   B. Couples or individuals should understand how and where donors are selected, how they are screened, and how they are matched and any days, if any, that TID is not performed (eg, weekends, holidays).

   C. Informed consent forms should be signed by the couple or the woman if she is single.

   D. The need to obtain and store additional semen samples if the couple or individual anticipates a desire for subsequent pregnancies should be discussed.

   E. Psychologic counseling should be provided to the couple or individual by a trained mental health professional to minimize emotional risk and to explore such issues as whether to discuss the procedure with other people and the child and when to discuss it.

   F. Both partners should be tested for HIV I-II antibody, hepatitis B surface antigen (HBsAg), hepatitis C antibody, and syphilis.

   G. The female recipient should undergo tests for blood type and Rh factor, cervical cultures for gonorrhea and chlamydial infection, and rubella titers (vaccination should be offered to patients without immunity).

   H. The female recipient should be examined and evaluated for potential infertility factors before treatment if there is evidence of a female-factor history or within 3 months of initiation of TID if there is no female-factor history and pregnancy has not occurred.

III. Donor Selection

   A. Donors for TID should be of good general health, should not possess a genetic abnormality or a strong family history for abnormality, and should be between legal age and 40 years of age.

   B. Established fertility is desirable but not an absolute requirement.

   C. Anonymous donors are recommended but not required.

   D. If known donors are used, they should undergo the same examination and treatment as anonymous donors, including quarantine of specimens for 6 months.

   E. Owners, operators, physicians, or employees of a facility performing TID should not be a donor for that program or for patients treated in that program.

IV. Donor Screening

   A. Donors should be found to have normal semen samples on several occasions, and the samples should have a cryosurvival rate of ≥50% of initial motility.

   B. Genetic screening is important, including a pedigree to exclude hereditary and familial diseases, but chromosome analysis is not mandatory.

   C. Donors should be of good general health and not be at risk for HIV infection (intravenous drug use or a sexual partner who uses intravenous drugs) or have multiple sexual partners.

   D. Donors should undergo a complete medical examination with special attention to exclude urethral discharge, genital warts, or ulcers.

   E. Laboratory testing includes Rh factor testing and blood type initially, serum HBsAg, and hepatitis C antibody, serologic tests for syphilis, semen or urethral cultures for gonorrhea and chlamydial infection, and cytomegalovirus (CMV) antibody testing initially and at 6-month intervals. Sperm from CMV antibody–positive donors should be used only with antibody–positive recipients.

   F. Donors should be tested initially for HIV antibodies. If the test is negative, the specimens should be cryopreserved, quarantined for 6 months, and released only if a repeat HIV antibody test is negative.

   G. Donors should sign a form denying any known risk factor for HIV.

   H. Donors should be willing to provide nonidentifying information about themselves that can be made available to the recipient and resulting offspring.

From Seibel MM. Therapeutic donor insemination. In: Family Building through Egg and Sperm Donation. MM Seibel and SL Crockin (eds). Jones and Bartlett, Sudbury, MA, 1996. Modified from ASRM Guidelines for therapeutic donor insemination: Sperm Fertil Steril *62:101 1994. Reprinted with permission of the publisher.*

examination, including examination of the genital organs. At a minimum, a three-generation genetic history should be obtained, and several forms have been devised for that purpose.[51] A modified version of these guidelines is shown in Table 18–3. The donor should not carry an autosomal recessive gene common in his ethnic group (eg, Tay-Sachs disease, thalassemia,

sickle cell disease) and should not have any serious malformation. There should not be a family history of serious malformations or mendelian disorders. The latter include autosomal dominant or X-linked disorders or a high probability for or documentation that the person is a carrier of an autosomal recessive disorder. Men with first-degree relatives with severe polygenic disorders such as diabetes and hypertension should not be allowed to donate sperm. Most sperm banks test for carrier states for some genetic abnormalities, such as thalassemia, cystic fibrosis, sickle cell disease in African Americans, and Tay-Sachs disease in Ashkenazi Jews.

The present widespread prevalence of sexually transmitted diseases, especially HIV infection, has made extensive microbiologic testing essential. Because a person may have HIV infection and transmit the virus for as long as 3 to 6 months before antibody-based tests become positive, the use of fresh semen is no longer permissible.[52] The risk for infection after insemination with semen from an infected donor is reported to be about 3.5%. Several women contracted infections before the present policy of freezing and quarantine was initiated.[53] Therefore, donors undergo extensive testing for sexually transmitted diseases, and the semen specimens are frozen and quarantined for 6 months, after which time the donor again undergoes testing. The semen specimen is released for use only if the donor again has a negative test for sexually transmitted diseases. Tests performed initially and at each subsequent testing session are described in Table 18–3.

Only after semen has been quarantined for 6 months and the donor again has negative tests for infections can the semen be released for use. It is of great importance that sperm-bank personnel maintain a close relationship with donors and that any changes of sexual partners or high-risk behavior be reported so that appropriate testing can be conducted. Known donors, requested by a few patients, undergo the same testing and quarantine procedures as anonymous donors.

Although no absolute rules can be made, most programs limit each donor to approximately 10 pregnancies. This figure may be relaxed somewhat if the distribution of specimens is over a wide geographic area.

Matching Donor to Recipient

Most couples desire that the donor be as close a match to the husband's physical characteristics as possible. Requested characteristics usually include height, eye color, hair color, and general body characteristics. Some couples also request that blood type and Rh factor be matched.

Examination of the Female Recipient Before Treatment

Our views have undergone rather marked evolution over the past several years. In previous years, we recommended that, at minimum, the patient undergo a hysterosalpingogram, serum progesterone determination to prove ovulation, cervical mucus testing, and 2 or 3 months' temperature charting before starting treatment. One of our own studies, however, showed that the hysterosalpingogram was of little value to women with a history that did not suggest tubal disease.[54] Our present pretreatment evaluation consists of a complete history and physical examination and a serum luteal-phase progesterone determination to document ovulation. Postcoital testing is done after the first insemination, the timing of insemination being based on urine dipstick LH testing. Two inseminations per cycle are recommended: the day of the LH surge and the second the following day. If conception has not occurred after four or five cycles, further evaluation, including a hysterosalpingogram, is recommended. Some patients at this time opt to undergo COH with IUI.

Timing of Insemination

Sperm are deposited at the time of ovulation. The most common method for timing ovulation is urine testing for the LH surge, although at least one study suggested that this method is not superior to basing the time of insemination on prior temperature charts.[55] Some studies have suggested that two inseminations per cycle may give higher pregnancy rates than a single insemination. Centola et al,[11] for example, reported a monthly fecundity rate of 6% among women undergoing one insemination compared with 21% among women who had two procedures.

Semen may be simply placed in the upper vagina, or intracervical or intrauterine insemination may be performed. One well-designed study[56] compared intracervical insemination with IUI and found the fecundity rate to be 3.9% with intracervical and 9.7% with intrauterine insemination. Intratubal insemination appears to negate the value of intrauterine placement of sperm.[57]

Pregnancy Rates

Several studies have found that the monthly fecundity rate falls with advancing age of the recipient woman[58,59] and that other fertility factors in the woman may compromise pregnancy rate.[60] Any estimate of fecundity must take into account the age of the woman and any complicating problems. In a population of women who have no female infertility factors, a monthly fecundity rate between 10% and 15% may be expected. Most

---

TABLE 18–3. TESTS PERFORMED INITIALLY AND AT EACH SUBSEQUENT TESTING

1. Serologic test for syphilis.
2. Serum hepatitis B antigen and hepatitis C antibody
3. Urethral or semen culture for *Neisseria gonorrhoeae.*
4. Urethral swab or urine test for *Chlamydia.*
5. Serum antibody tests for cytomegalovirus (immunoglobulin G). The American Society for Reproductive Medicine guidelines suggest that semen from donors with positive immunologic tests for CMV by used only in women who also have positive tests.
6. Serum antibody tests for HIV. If positive, confirmation with a Western blot test is required.

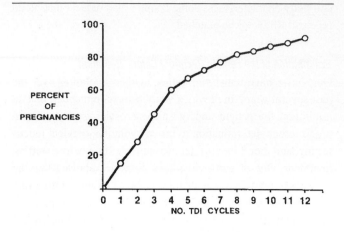

Figure 18–3. Cumulative success rate among patients achieving pregnancy. *(From Yeh J, Seibel MM: Artificial insemination with donor sperm: A review of 108 patients.* Obstet Gynecol *70:313, 1987.)*

women who become pregnant by means of TID do so by the end of the sixth cycle (Fig 18–3).[61] Women older than 35 years typically require more cycles to achieve comparable results.

Legal Aspects

A woman who undergoes TID should be informed of the indications, the nature of the procedure, the risks, and treatment alternatives.[50] Her partner's consent is required if he is to be legally recognized as the father. At least 12 states mandate that the executed consent be filed with a record-keeping body, and 31 states have laws concerning TID.

A consent form should be signed by the sperm donor to affirm his medical, genetic, and sexual history; to maintain confidentiality; to define the terms of donor compensation (if any); to limit liability of the TID program; and to delineate the uses of the donor semen.

CONCLUSIONS

Insemination with both husband and donor sperm continues to offer benefit to a large number of couples.[62] Pregnancy rates are highest among couples with azoospermia who receive donor sperm, and those with cervical factor or coital problems treated with husband insemination. Pregnancy rates among couples with oligospermia or asthenospermia, unexplained infertility, and advanced female age are lower. TIH and TID should be offered for 4 to 10 cycles depending on indications. The cycles should be closely monitored, and all other fertility factors

should be addressed. If success is not obtained, other treatments such as IVF or termination of care should be advised.

REFERENCES

1. Loy RA, Seibel MM: Therapeutic insemination. In: MM Seibel (ed), *Infertility: A Comprehensive Text.* Norwalk, CT, Appleton & Lange, 1990:201
2. Sigler SL: *Fertility in Women.* Philadelphia, JB Lippincott, 1944:403
3. Sims JM: *Uterine Surgery.* New York: William Wood, 1873:365
4. Hard AD: Artificial impregnation. *Med World* 27:163, 1909
5. Kleegman SJ: Therapeutic donor insemination. *Fertil Steril* 5:7, 1954
6. Arny M, Quagliarello JR: History of artificial insemination: A tribute to Sophia K. Leegman, M.D. *Semin Reprod Endocrinol* 5:1, 1987
7. Bunge RG, Sherman JK: Fertilizing capacity of frozen human spermatozoa. *Nature* 172:767, 1953
8. Seibel MM, Crockin S: *Donor Gametes for Family Building.* Boston, Jones & Bartlett, 1995
9. American Fertility Society: Guidelines for Therapeutic Donor Insemination: Sperm. *Fertil Steril* 62:101s, 1994
10. Tur-Kaspa I, Dudkiewicz A, Confino E, Gleicher N: Pooled sequential ejaculates: A way to increase the total number of motile sperm from oligospermic men. *Fertil Steril* 1990:54, 1990
11. Centola GM, Mattox JH, Raubertas RF: Pregnancy rates after double versus single insemination with frozen donor semen. *Fertil Steril* 54:1089, 1990
12. Dodson WC, Whitesides DB, Hughes CL Jr, Easley HA III, Haney AF: Superovulation with intrauterine insemination in the treatment of infertility: A possible alternative to gamete intrafallopian transfer and in vitro fertilization. *Fertil Steril* 48:441, 1987
13. Sher G, Knutzen VK, Stratton CJ, Montakkhab MM, Allenson SG. In vitro sperm capacitation and transcervical intrauterine insemination for the treatment of refractory infertility: Phase I. *Fertil Steril* 41:260, 1984
14. Kiessling AA: Human immunodeficiency virus in semen. *Curr Opin Urol* 4:60, 1994
15. Pardo M, Barri PN, Bancello N, et al: Spermatozoa selection in discontinuous Percoll gradients for use in artificial insemination. *Fertil Steril* 49:505, 1988
16. Zimmerman ER, Robertson KR, Kim H, Drobnis EZ, Nakajima ST: Semen preparation with the Sperm Select system versus a washing technique. *Fertil Steril* 61:269, 1994
17. Urry RL, Middleton RG, McGavin S: A simple and effective technique for increasing pregnancy rates in couples with retrograde ejaculation. *Fertil Steril* 46:1224, 1986
18. Kahn JA, Sunde A, von During V, Sordal T, Molne K: Treatment of unexplained infertility: Fallopian tube sperm perfusion. *Acta Obstet Gynecol Scand* 72:193, 1993
19. Crosignani PG, Ragni G, Finzi GCL, DeLaurtis L, Olivares MD,

Perotti L: Intraperitoneal insemination in the treatment of male and unexplained infertility. *Fertil Steril* 55:333, 1991

20. Hovatta O, Kurunmaki H, Tiitinen A, Lahteenmaki P, Koskimies AI: Direct intraperitoneal or intrauterine insemination and superovulation in infertility treatment: A randomized study. *Fertil Steril* 54:339, 1990

21. Moretti-Rojas I, Rojas FJ, Leisure M, Stone SC, Asch RH: Intrauterine inseminations with washed human spermatozoa does not induce formation of antisperm antibodies. *Fertil Steril* 53:180, 1990

22. Dodson WC, Haney AF: Controlled ovarian hyperstimulation and intrauterine insemination for treatment of infertility. *Fertil Steril* 55:457, 1991

23. Allen NC, Herbert CM, Maxson CM, Rogers BJ, Diamond MP, Wentz AC: Intrauterine insemination: A critical review. *Fertil Steril* 44:569, 1985

24. Hull ME, Magyar DM, Vasquez JM, Hayes MF, Moghissi KS: Experience with intrauterine insemination for cervical factor and oligospermia. *Am J Obstet Gynecol* 154:1333, 1986

25. Hughes EG, Collins JP, Garner PR: Homologous artificial insemination for oligoasthenospermia: A randomized controlled study comparing intracervical and intrauterine techniques. *Fertil Steril* 48:278, 1987

26. Martinez AR, Bernardus RE, Voorhorst FJ, Vermeiden JPW: Intrauterine insemination does and clomiphene citrate does not improve fecundity in couples with infertility due to male or idiopathic factors: A prospective, randomized, controlled study. *Fertil Steril* 53:847, 1990

27. Ho P, Poon IML, Chan SYW, Wang C: Intrauterine insemination is not useful in oligoasthenospermia. *Fertil Steril* 51:682, 1989

28. Friedman AJ, Juneau-Norcross M, Sedensky B, Andrews N, Dorfman J, Cramer DW: Life table analysis of intrauterine insemination pregnancy rates for couples with cervical factor, male factor and idiopathic infertility. *Fertil Steril* 55:1005, 1991

29. Chaffkin LM, Nulsen JC, Luciano AA, Metzger DA: A comparative analysis of the cycle fecundity rates associated with combined human menopausal gonadotropin and intrauterine insemination versus either HMG or IUI alone. *Fertil Steril* 55:252, 1991

30. Aboulghar MA, Mansour RT, Serour GI, Amin Y, Abbas AM, Salah IM: Ovarian superstimulation and intrauterine insemination for the treatment of unexplained infertility. *Fertil Steril* 60:303, 1993

31. Serta RT, Rufo S, Seibel MM: Minimal endometriosis and intrauterine insemination: Does controlled ovarian hyperstimulation improve pregnancy rates? *Obstet Gynecol* 80:37, 1992

32. Dickey RP, Olar TT, Taylor SN, Curole DN, Rye PH, Matulich EM: Relationship of follicle number, serum estradiol and other factors to birth rate and multiparity in human menopausal gonadotropin induced intrauterine insemination cycles. *Fertil Steril* 56:89, 1991

33. Corsan GH, Kemmann EK: The role of superovulation with menotropins in ovulatory infertility: A review. *Fertil Steril* 55:468, 1991

34. Martinez AR, Bernardus RE, Voorhorst FJ, Vermeiden JPW, Schoemaker J: Pregnancy rates after timed intercourse or intrauterine insemination after human menopausal gonadotropin stimulation of normal ovulatory cycles: A controlled study. *Fertil Steril* 55:258, 1991

35. McGovern P, Quagliarello H, Arny M: Relationship of within patient semen variability to outcome of intrauterine insemination. *Fertil Steril* 51:1019, 1989

36. Francavilla F, Pomano R, Santucci R, Poccia G: Effect of sperm morphology and motile sperm count on outcome of intrauterine insemination in oligozoospermia and/or asthenozoospermia. *Fertil Steril* 53:892, 1990

37. Brasch JG, Rawlins R, Tarchala S, Radwanska E: The relationship between total motile sperm count and the success of intrauterine insemination. *Fertil Steril* 62:150, 1994

38. Ransom MX, Blotner MB, Bohrer M, Corsan G, Kemmann E: Does increasing frequency of intrauterine insemination improve pregnancy rate significantly during superovulation cycles? *Fertil Steril* 61:303, 1994

39. Peterson CM, Hatasaka HH, Jones KP, Poulson AAM, Carrell DT, Urry RL: Ovulation induction with gonadotropins and intrauterine insemination compared with in vitro fertilization and no therapy: A prospective, nonrandomized, cohort study and meta analysis. *Fertil Steril* 62:535, 1994

40. Haas GG, Seibel MM: Human menopausal gonadotropins for ovulation induction, intrauterine insemination and assisted reproduction. In: Seibel MM, Blackwell RE (eds), *Ovulation Induction.* New York, Raven, 1994:117–134

41. Seibel MM, Seibel SG, Zilberstein M: Gender distribution—not sex selection. *Hum Reprod* 9:569, 1994

42. McKusick VA: *Mendelian Inheritance in Man,* ed 8. Baltimore, Johns Hopkins University Press, 1992:1733.

43. Quinlivan WLG, Preciado K, Long TL, Sullivan H: Separation of human X and Y spermatozoa by albumin gradients and Sephadex chromatography. *Fertil Steril* 37:104, 1982

44. Broer KH, Winkhaus I, Sombroek H, Kaiser R: Frequency of Y-chromatin–bearing spermatozoa in intracervical and intrauterine post coital tests. *Int J Fertil* 21:181, 1976

45. Ericsson RJ, Langevin CN, Nishino M: Isolation of fractions rich in human Y sperm. *Nature* 246:421, 1973

46. Sirai M, Matsuda S: Galvanic separation of X- and Y-bearing human spermatozoa. *Jpn J Fertil Steril* 37:104, 1982

47. Rhode W, Porstmann T, Prehn S, Dorner G: Gravitational patter of the Y-bearing sperm using Percoll density gradient centrifugation. *Fertil Steril* 40:661, 1983

48. Steeno O, Adimoelja A, Steeno J: Separation of X- and Y-bearing spermatozoa using the Sephadex-gel-filtration method. *Andrologica* 7:95, 1975

49. Johnson LA, Welch GR, Keyvanfar K, Dorfmann A, Fugger EF, Schulman JD: Gender preselection in humans? Flow cytometric separation of X and Y spermatozoa for the prevention of X-linked diseases. *Hum Reprod* 8:1733, 1993

50. Seibel MM: Therapeutic donor insemination. In: Seibel MM, Crockin S (eds), *Family Building through Egg and Sperm Donation.* Boston, Jones & Bartlett, 1995: 62:115(S)

51. American Fertility Society. Minimal genetic screening for gamete donation. *Fertil Steril* 1994

52. Hazeltine WA: Silent H.I.V. infections. *N Engl J Med* 320:1487, 1989

53. Araneta MRG, Mascola L, Eller A, et al: H.I.V. transmission through donor artificial insemination. *JAMA* 273:854, 1995

54. Stovall DW, Christman GM, Hammond MG, Talbert LM: Abnormal findings on hysterosalpingography: Effects on fecundity in a donor insemination program using frozen semen. *Obstet Gynecol* 80:249, 1992

55. Barratt CLR, Cooke S, Chauhan M, Cooke ID: A prospective randomized controlled trial comparing urinary luteinizing hormone dipsticks and basal body temperature charts with time donor insemination. *Fertil Steril* 52:394, 1989

56. Byrd W, Bradshaw K, Carr B, Edman C, Odom J, Ackerman G: A prospective randomized study of pregnancy rates following intrauterine and intracervical insemination using frozen donor sperm. *Fertil Steril* 53:521, 1990

57. Hurd WW, Randolph JF, Ansbacher R, Menge AC, Ohl DA, Brown AN: Comparison of intracervical, intrauterine, and intratubal techniques for donor insemination. *Fertil Steril* 59:339, 1993

58. Stovall DW, Toma SK, Hammond MG, Talbert LM: The effect of age on female fecundity. *Obstet Gynecol* 77:33, 1991

59. Schwartz D, Mayaux MJ: Female fecundity as a function of age: Results of artificial insemination in 2193 nulliparous women with azoospermic husbands. *N Engl J Med* 306:404, 1982

60. Hammond MG, Jordan S, Sloan CS: Factors affecting the pregnancy rates in a donor insemination program. *Am J Obstet Gynecol* 155:480, 1986

61. Yeh J, Seibel MM: Artificial insemination with donor sperm: A review of 108 patients. *Obstet Gynecol* 70:313, 1987

62. Hummel WP, Talbert LM: Current management of a donor insemination program. *Fertil Steril* 51:919, 1989

PART V

Specific Categories
of Infertility

Nearly 5 million American women 15 to 44 years of age report difficulty or delay in achieving a livebirth, and 1.3 million receive medical advice or treatment in a given year.[1] The infertility is unexplained in approximately 20% of cases, because numerous reproductive defects are undetectable with current methods.[2] Although diagnostic capability is limited, many advances in treatment technology now provide a range of therapy options to be considered by each couple. This chapter addresses the approach to the management of unexplained infertility, which depends on knowledge of the baseline prognosis and the extent to which treatment alters the baseline prognosis. Although treatment planning usually dominates clinical consultations, couples with unexplained infertility also require information that addresses additional questions. These questions include: How can infertility remain unexplained in this age of scientific achievement? Would any further diagnostic test be useful? Which treatment is best? Each couple has distinctive family and cultural values and characteristic approaches to risk-taking that help to shape their final choices about treatment. Attention to all these details is necessary in conditions such as unexplained infertility, in which the efficacy of treatment is just one of many considerations in the clinical decisions.

HISTORY OF INFERTILITY INVESTIGATION

Before 1900, virtually all cases of infertility were unexplained because of the lack of clinical tests. Innovations between 1900 and 1940 made possible considerable improvement in the diagnosis of tubal, seminal, and ovulatory problems. In 1920, Rubin[3] described oxygen insufflation as a test of tubal patency, which made possible the diagnosis of tubal disease without resorting to diagnostic laparotomy. Within a year, there was a shift to carbon dioxide as the insufflation medium, instituting a diagnostic test that survives to the present era in some countries.[4,5]

In 1928, Macomber and Sanders[6] reported pregnancy results for a group of infertile men who were the subjects of the first study in which spermatozoa were methodically counted. The orderly counting of living sperm in the ejaculate and the associated pregnancy results defined a new understanding of male reproductive factors in which not only azoospermia but also oligospermia were found to cause infertility; these authors proposed a normal cutoff at 60 million sperm/mL.

By the late 1930s, the understanding of endometrial and basal temperature responses to progesterone in the luteal phase clarified some ovulatory causes of infertility, which had previously depended on a history of amenorrhea.[7,8] Notwithstanding these advances, a relatively large proportion of infertility remained unexplained after deployment of state-of-the-art investigational methods in 1960. In a thoughtful discussion, Southam[9] considered whether this represented a "misfortune due to the laws of chance, or a limitation in our knowledge."

Although diagnosis has improved vastly since 1960, clinical experience and the literature confirm that unexplained infertility remains a problem almost a century after the beginning of the modern era.

EPIDEMIOLOGY OF UNEXPLAINED INFERTILITY

Prevalence

For many reasons, the prevalence of unexplained infertility as reported in the literature is variable. Among the studies shown in Table 19–1, the proportion of cases of infertility that are unexplained ranges from 0 to 31%.[10–26] In most studies, however, the range is from 15% to 25% (Table 19–1, Fig 19–1). The apparent variability in the percentage of unexplained infertility during three decades disappears when the two studies with the highest and lowest percentages of unexplained infertility are excluded from the aggregate results.

Contributing Factors

Unexplained infertility exists for one of two reasons: because an extremely long delay in conception occurs by chance in otherwise healthy couples, or because underlying defects cannot be detected with current clinical tools. In the former situation, the duration of infertility should be shorter than with any other infertility diagnosis, because healthy couples would be expected to conceive more quickly. That is not the case, however, because the duration of infertility is equivalent in unexplained infertility and other diagnostic groups[27] (Fig 19–2). Declining fertility among older female partners is a further reason for unexplained infertility. If the female partner is more than 30 years of age, the likelihood of having unexplained infertility rather than any other infertility diagnosis is 1.6 times higher than with younger female partners.[28]

Otherwise healthy couples may appear to be infertile by chance alone because in any normal population, a small proportion of healthy couples have low fecundity, and thus do not conceive within 1 year.[9,29,30] The definition of infertility is arbitrary, therefore all such couples would fulfill the definition. Provided the diagnostic test results are not falsely abnormal, healthy couples would be included in the group with unexplained infertility after diagnostic assessment. Although their fecundity is low, it is within the normal range, and the long-term prognosis should be excellent. After 1 year, theoretically more than 50% of such couples conceive within the next year.[30] Because they have such a good prognosis, few would reach medical attention after a prolonged period (about 3 or 4 years) of infertility. If healthy couples constituted a large portion of

TABLE 19–1. PROPORTION OF COUPLES WITH UNEXPLAINED INFERTILITY[10–26]

Decade	Authors	N	Number Unexplained	Percentage Unexplained	Lower 95% CI	Upper 95% CI
1950–69	Frank, 1950	134	17	12.7	7	18
	Johansson, 1957	658	33	5.0	3	7
	Southam and Buxton, 1957	1437	446	31.04	29	33
	Anderson, 1968	183	11	6.0	3	9
	Raymont et al, 1976	500	65	13.0	10	16
Aggregate		2912	572	19.64		
1970–79	Cocev, 1972	744	26	3.5	2	5
	Newton et al, 1974	644	142	22.0	19	25
	Cox, 1975	900	158	17.6	15	20
	Ratnam et al, 1976	709	157	22.1	19	25
	Dor et al, 1977	512	92	18.0	15	21
	Gunaratne, 1979	393	0	0	0	0
Aggregate		3902	575	14.74		
1980–89	Sorensen, 1980	196	35	17.8	12	23
	Thomas and Forrest, 1980	291	17	5.8	3	9
	Insler et al, 1981	583	8	1.4	0	2
	West et al, 1982	400	124	31.0	26	36
	Verkauf, 1983	141	16	11.3	6	17
	Kliger, 1984	493	127	25.8	22	30
	Hull et al, 1985	708	170	24.0	21	27
	Collins et al, 1986	1297	219	16.88	15	19
	Harrison, 1986	1020	0	0	0	0
Aggregate		5129	716	13.96		
1990–95	Dhaliwal et al, 1991	455	99	21.8	18	26
	Thonneau et al, 1991	1318	135	10.24	9	12
	Collins et al, 1995	2198	562	25.57	24	27
Aggregate		3971	796	20.04		
TOTAL		15,914	2659	16.71		

CI, confidence interval.

couples with unexplained infertility, one would expect the average duration of infertility among couples with unexplained infertility to be shorter than the average duration among couples with other infertility diagnoses. As mentioned previously, however, the typical duration of infertility is similar in all diagnostic groups.[27]

From the available evidence, then, unexplained infertility appears to arise mainly from undetectable reproductive defects, some of which may be associated with an age-related decline in fertility. An alternative view is that unexplained infertility represents failure to make sufficient use of the available diagnostic tests. That issue is discussed in the section on diagnosis.

HOW CAN INFERTILITY REMAIN UNEXPLAINED?

It is important to raise this question early in the infertility management process, because uncertainty about causation may distort the decisions couples make about diagnostic tests and treatment. Many couples do not realize that the complexity of fertilization and implantation cannot be evaluated within the narrow scope of the current diagnostic assessment. For example, tubal patency tests can be used to evaluate only one aspect of tubal transport functions and provide no information about the role of the fallopian tube in harboring the fertilized oocyte for 3 or 4 days. Nor does this mechanical test provide information about the complex system that senses secretions from the embryo and initiates early maternal recognition of pregnancy. Also, the most comprehensive semen analysis cannot define the fertilizing capacity of one ejaculate. Although semen analysis can be used to confirm that there is a redundancy of normal motile sperm, no test can accurately evaluate whether the sperm can endure storage in the cervix, undergo transportation to the site of fertilization, or achieve the reactions necessary for penetration of the oocyte membranes. Furthermore, although endometrial receptivity during the implantation window is crucial to successful conception, results of endometrial biopsy are not reliably associated with conception. It is not surprising that infertile couples have high expectations of the diagnostic assessment for their problem. It is natural for them to expect that advances in the diagnostic process have matched those that have been so notable in the technology of infertility treatment. Unfortunately, however, advances in treatment technology have outpaced advances in

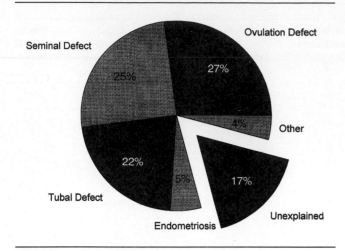

Figure 19–1. Diagnostic assignment for 15,914 infertile couples reported in 23 studies listed in Table 19–1.

the diagnostic assessment. As a result, there is a high proportion of unexplained infertility.

PROBLEMS DEFINING UNEXPLAINED INFERTILITY

The optimum assessment for an infertile couple depends on an orderly evaluation of the fertility potential of both partners. An extensive set of diagnostic tests is available to complement the clinical history and physical findings, including assessment of seminal fluid and the properties and function of sperm cells, ovulatory function, and genital tract integrity, and detection of associated disorders such as infectious diseases. Additional tests required in specific instances to search for the underlying cause of infertility-associated disorders such as azoospermia, amenorrhea, and hyperprolactinemia are discussed in other chapters of this book. Such investigations are not applicable among couples with unexplained infertility who have no apparent abnormality.

In practice, numerous factors influence the extent of the diagnostic investigation. These include duration of infertility, travel time, and the wishes of the couple. It is not surprising that the extent of diagnostic testing required before the label of unexplained infertility may be applied is the subject of much debate.[31,32] As a result, our understanding of this condition is hampered by variability in the diagnostic protocols that contribute to the published clinical experience. The tests stipulated for defining unexplained infertility in several follow-up studies in the literature are shown in Table 19–2.[9,29,33–40] Laparoscopy was not a uniform requirement, even in recent publications, provided that tubal patency had been evaluated with hystero-

salpingography. Postcoital tests and the evaluation of sperm-directed antibody also were not included in some of the investigation protocols. Decision making about whether to include these and other procedures in clinical protocols is discussed herein.

Although unexplained infertility is simply defined as a lack of abnormal findings after a comprehensive diagnostic protocol, it is difficult to achieve consensus on the definition of a comprehensive protocol. Published recommendations range from conservative (semen analysis, mid–luteal phase progesterone assay, and tubal patency testing)[41] to liberal (these three benchmark tests and supplementary tests such as evaluations of cervical mucus, endometrial maturation, and immunity to sperm).[2] There are many diagnostic tests in addition to those shown in Table 19–2. One approach is to judge the value of tests only according to the outcome of interest. The outcome of primary interest to the infertile couple is pregnancy, and the value of diagnostic tests lies in their ability to help predict this outcome. In outcome-based clinical decision making, a diagnostic test result should either alter the probability of pregnancy or lead to use of effective therapy, which can increase the likelihood of pregnancy. An abnormal result must predict a lower pregnancy rate with a high level of confidence. By judging diagnostic tests on their association with the outcome in this way, the most commonly used diagnostic tests fall naturally into three categories.

A. The test result is fairly reliable: semen analysis, tubal patency test, and mid–luteal phase progesterone determination

B. The test result is less than fairly reliable: sperm penetration assay, mucus penetration tests, hysteroscopy, *Chlamydia* antibodies

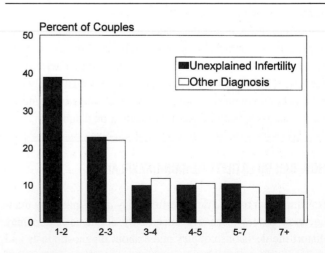

Figure 19–2. Duration of infertility with unexplained infertility and other infertility diagnoses.[27]

TABLE 19–2. DIAGNOSTIC TESTS REQUIRED TO HAVE NORMAL RESULTS IN REPORTED STUDIES OF UNEXPLAINED INFERTILITY

Semen Analysis	Ovulation Confirmation	HSG	Laparoscopy	Postcoital Test	Sperm Antibody
Yes	EB	Yes	Yes	Yes	No[33]
Yes	BBT	Yes	No	Yes	No[34]
Yes	NA	Yes	No	No	Yes[29]
Yes	BBT	Yes	No	No	No[35]
Yes	P4	Yes	Yes	Yes	No[36]
Yes	EB	Yes	No	No	No[9]
Yes	P4	No	Yes	No	No[37]
Yes	EB	Yes	Yes	Yes	No[38]
Yes	P4	Yes	Yes	Yes	No[39]
Yes	P4	Yes	Yes	Yes	No[40]

HSG, hysterosalpingogram; EB, endometrial biopsy; BBT, basal body temperature shift; NA, not available; P4, midluteal progesterone concentration.

C. The meaning of the test result remains uncertain: endometrial dating, postcoital test, antisperm antibody tests, varicocele assessment, salpingoscopy

There are other views on the approach to the diagnostic process. Although the proposed view accepts only diagnostic tests that are unquestionably associated with the outcome, a more liberal view would pursue deviations from the normal reproductive process even if they are less clearly associated with pregnancy rates among infertile patients. In this chapter, outcome-based evidence that the diagnostic test result is an accurate predictor or that it helps identify effective therapy is preferred. According to this kind of evidence, the tests in category B and category C do not aid in clinical decisions.

An additional problem in defining unexplained infertility lies in the use of different cutoffs for the normal range of semen analysis variables and progesterone concentration. If different standards were to be applied, two otherwise similar groups of subjects would appear to include different proportions of unexplained infertility. For example, values of 5, 10, 20, 40, and 60 million sperm/mL have been suggested as the threshold for subfertile sperm density.[42–46] Different criteria also exist for motility and morphology of sperm.[47–49] The number of different standards is due in part to the lack of an absolute association between semen analysis results and pregnancy rates, thus there is an overlap in results recorded among fertile and infertile groups.[50]

When different cutoff values are chosen, the sensitivity and specificity of a diagnostic test mutually fluctuate. Lower cutoffs lead to decreased sensitivity and increased specificity; higher cutoffs increase sensitivity and decrease specificity. Plotting the sensitivity and specificity throughout the range of possible cutoffs produces a receiver operating characteristic (ROC) curve that can be used to access the predictive value of a test.[51] The ROC curves for semen analysis variables reveal that, with respect to the prediction of pregnancy, there is little to choose among the various cutoffs proposed in the literature.[52] Selection of a specific cutoff value by consensus would have a minimal effect on the clinical interpretation of the test and could lead to wider agreement with respect to the definition of unexplained infertility. It makes sense to adhere to international consensus recommendations, such as those in the laboratory manual of the World Health Organization for the examination of semen and semen–cervical mucus interactions.[53]

The definition of unexplained infertility is complicated by the existence of different diagnostic protocols, various definitions of a normal test result, and the limited scope of the diagnostic assessment. The definition also is affected by the inclusion criteria for studies. If a couple conceives before undergoing a test such as laparoscopy, to what category should they be allocated? The choice here is a trade-off between uncertainty and overselection. Requiring laparoscopy increases the certainty of being correct about the unexplained diagnosis, but any infertile group that includes only couples who have undergone laparoscopy no longer represents typical infertile couples. It is evident that the orderly study of unexplained infertility will require much discussion to reach a consensus on the arbitrary decisions needed to refine the definition of this clinical state.

CLINICAL DECISIONS ABOUT DIAGNOSTIC TESTS

Couples with unexplained infertility are under constant pressure to investigate the problem. Other infertile couples, well-meaning relatives, and the news media only too freely offer ideas for new tests and treatment. Should tests with previously normal results be repeated? Will new tests lead to conception? In clinical decision making, the value of tests lies in their ability to help one predict a specific outcome.[54] In the case of infertility, the outcome of interest is pregnancy. The best available diagnostic tests are those that allow accurate prediction of conception.

Which Additional Tests Should Be Performed?

Although the minimum assessment of semen analysis, confirmation of luteinization, and a test of tubal patency are a sufficient diagnostic protocol, information about additional tests may be requested. This section uses four diagnostic tests as examples: the postcoital test, a well-defined, traditional assessment; sperm-directed antibody (SDA), another traditional test for which new methods are available; endometrial biopsy, a long-standing test of endometrial function; and laparoscopy as a routine procedure if tubal patency has been demonstrated with a hysterosalpingogram. The discussion focuses not on the method, but on the application of diagnostic principles on the basis of predictive value of a given test result.

Postcoital Test

Few clinicians question that disorders of cervical function may lead to infertility. The cervix appears to serve both a filtering and a storage function and thus contributes to maintaining a supply of live spermatozoa for a period of 3 to 5 days after deposition.[55] The debate focuses on whether the postcoital test can be used to detect disorders in cervical function. The issue is whether the postcoital test correctly identifies cervical dysfunction rather than whether cervical mucus secretion is critical to fertilization. Cervical mucus characteristics, when judged at midcycle, seem uniformly good to excellent.[56,57] Scoring tends to reveal uniformly high-quality cervical mucus when the test is timed correctly in association with ovulation. Postcoital tests also enumerate the motile sperm in the mucus, and the results appear to correlate with total motile sperm counts in the ejaculate.[58] Abnormal tests are defined by a choice of cutpoints ranging from 0 to 10 sperm per high-power field.[58–65] Postcoital test results show a weak association with pregnancy, which is explained in part by the association with sperm count. This is less evident with larger sample sizes, which may be more representative of the typical results in clinical practice[62,63,66–69] (Fig 19–3). The test does not help identify a disorder that can be treated with effective therapy.[70] In a 1995 survey of European clinics, abnormal results were followed by numerous, but different treatments.[59]

The most important reason for not making use of the postcoital test, however, is the frequency of meaningless abnormal results. In six clinical studies, 45% of the test results were abnormal.[70] Postcoital tests are simple to perform and interpret, and they are used in most North American clinical practices. Nevertheless, the test is a harrowing performance evaluation for infertile couples, and for those with abnormal results there is an emotional impact that is unwarranted by the questionable value of the test results. Because of its low discriminatory power, in clinical practice the postcoital test may be indicated only as an elective choice for couples who understand its limitations.

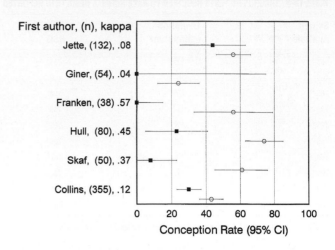

Figure 19–3. Predictive value of postcoital test results.[62,63,66–69] (Heterogeneity χ square = 15.7, five degrees of freedom, P = .0075.) CI, confidence interval.

Sperm-Directed Antibody Test

It has been theorized that immunity to spermatozoa may cause infertility through several mechanisms, including reduced sperm motility, agglutination, and complete immobilization.[71] Sperm-associated antibodies may be evaluated with conventional assays on the basis of observation of an antibody function such as agglutination or immobilization of sperm. Techniques that make use of an intermediate marker such as immune-imprinted micropellets enable identification of specific immunoglobulin types on the sperm surface and in seminal plasma, cervical mucus, and either partner's serum.[72] Although a single assay method has not yet been selected as superior to all others, several techniques for identifying immunoglobulins show highly correlated results.[73–77] The prevalence of abnormal antibody titers appears to be higher among both male and female infertile partners than among fertile individuals; in some but not all studies, the prevalence is especially increased among couples with unexplained infertility.[73,78,79] Nevertheless, the test should be judged primarily on the basis of its correlation with the outcome, which is conception.

The degree of correlation among the methods appears to justify grouping together the results of studies that report on the occurrence of pregnancy during follow-up care. The relevant studies in which antibody presence was assayed in serum, but not in semen, are summarized in Figs 19–4 and 19–5. Pregnancy rates appear to be lower in the presence of antibody detected either on the sperm surface or in the man's serum (Fig 19–4).[80–85] Sperm antibody presence in the male partner is associated with a typical odds ratio (0.60, 95% confidence interval [CI] 0.46, 0.67), which implies a statistically significant 40%

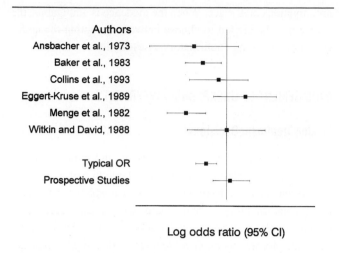

Figure 19–4. Studies evaluating presence of sperm antibody in infertile male partners and conception.[80-85] (Heterogeneity χ square = 13.8, five degrees of freedom, *P* = .017.) OR, odds ratio; CI, confidence interval.

reduction in fertility. The typical estimate is unreliable, however, because the individual odds ratios are significantly heterogeneous (χ square = 13.8, *P* = .017).[82] This apparent association and the lack of agreement among the studies may arise in part from methodologic shortcomings. Considering only the more recent prospective studies, the results are homogeneous, and an association of sperm antibody presence in the male partner with fertility is unproved. Further studies are needed to confirm the impression based on these results.

With respect to sperm antibody presence in the female partner, the typical odds ratio (0.44, 95% CI 0.32, 0.60) also im-

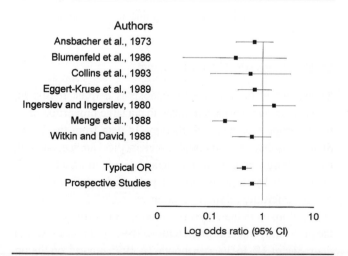

Figure 19–5. Studies evaluating presence of sperm antibody in infertile female partners and conception.[80,82-87] (Heterogeneity χ square = 28.8, six degrees of freedom, *P* < .0001.) OR, odds ratio; CI, confidence interval.

plies a statistically significant reduction in fertility associated with sperm antibody presence (Fig 19–5).[80,82-87] These odds ratios also are significantly heterogeneous, however (χ square = 28.8, *P* < .0001), and in these conditions the estimate may be unreliable. In the prospective studies, the revised estimate of the odds ratio is not significant (0.63, 95% CI 0.38, 1.14), and the results of this smaller group of studies were not heterogeneous (χ square = 0.78, *P* = 0.86).[82]

Sperm antibody presence in either partner may be associated with impaired fertility, but the case remains unproved, as judged by present-day standards of evaluation. There is a need for further studies with adequate sample size and follow-up period. Antibody-free control groups are needed to test the null hypothesis, because sperm antibody synthesis in either partner could be a normal response to sperm antigen or a reaction to errors in spermatogenesis. In the management of unexplained infertility in typical clinical settings, unless there is a specific indication for this test, such as obstruction or infection of the male ductal system, routine use of the SDA does not appear to offer useful information.

Endometrial Biopsy

Successful implantation must depend at least in part on optimal endometrial development and function. Since the 1940s reasonably accurate dating of the endometrium has been used to evaluate the chronologic development of the endometrium according to histologic criteria.[88] A delay of endometrial maturation by more than 2 days in two endometrial biopsy reports is characterized as a luteal-phase defect. The observation may be a chance occurrence, however, because histologic dating of the endometrium is subject to measurement error and biologic variability.[89] For this reason, the frequency of delayed maturation is quite variable, and the results of a second biopsy often differ from those of the first.[90] Even when repeated biopsy results show delayed endometrial maturation, pregnancy rates and pregnancy losses are not affected among untreated individuals.[90,91] Furthermore, the value of luteal-phase support, such as progesterone suppositories or human chorionic gonadotropin (hCG) injections has been demonstrated only in cycles of in vitro fertilization (IVF).[92] Endometrial biopsy is therefore not useful for the assessment of infertility. Endometrial receptivity during the window of blastocyst implantation must be critical to successful conception; regrettably, histologic dating of the endometrium is not a useful marker for this essential endometrial function.

Laparoscopy

If a hysterosalpingogram shows bilateral tubal patency, is there any need for laparoscopy, with the attendant cost, inconvenience, and risks of an operative procedure? The predictive value of a normal hysterosalpingogram (NPV) is 96%

when the prevalence of bilateral tubal obstruction is 10%, a typical rate of severe tubal disease among infertile couples.[93] Laparoscopy is required to make a diagnosis of endometriosis or adnexal adhesions, but in the presence of tubal patency, these lesions are of lesser clinical significance. Management of endometriosis does not improve pregnancy rates,[94] and surgical adhesiolysis has not been evaluated in a randomized clinical trial. In these circumstances, undergoing laparoscopy should be determined by patient preference rather than the clinician's wish to define unexplained infertility in a more precise manner.

Should Tests With Previously Normal Results Be Repeated?

With persistent unexplained infertility, the frustration of not having a reason for the infertility and the desire to ascertain current status are powerful stimulants to repeat tests the results of which previously were reported as normal. The components of semen analysis (sperm density, progressive motility, and morphology) are subject to considerable observer variability[95] and also to inherent variability within a person.[96–98] Because of this, during the initial evaluation it is important to repeat abnormal tests as often as necessary to establish a true range. If the results are within the normal range, however, it is not clinically useful to repeat the semen analysis unless a new exposure factor arises. If results of the initial evaluation are unavailable, incomplete, or outdated, a new test is necessary to establish the current condition.

No studies report the findings of a repeat laparoscopy during otherwise uneventful follow-up therapy for infertility. In the search for an explanation for long-standing infertility, however, an as yet undetectable cause seems far more likely to be the case than a clinically "silent" change in the status of a previously normal pelvis. When laparoscopy has been performed after 2 to 3 years of infertility, and the pelvis has been described reliably as normal, the probability of a new pathologic condition after another year or two must be extremely low. Thus laparoscopy should be repeated only if doubt exists about earlier findings or there has been a substantial change in clinical risk for endometriosis or tubal disease.

Clinical biology can render certain types of repeated tests unnecessary. One common question concerns whether or not ovulation is occurring regularly. When the menstrual intervals are 25 to 35 days, there is 95% confidence that ovulation, as documented with luteinization, is occurring.[99,100] It is important to repeat tests when previous results are ambiguous. Biologic variability, recall errors on the part of referring physicians, and occasional slips in the laboratory all contribute to confusing results. The chart for each couple should include copies of operative notes and actual laboratory reports regardless of where the investigations took place. When the evidence is ambiguous, the couple may be invited to choose between accepting the ambiguity or undergoing confirmatory assessments.

MANAGEMENT OF UNEXPLAINED INFERTILITY

Making Treatment Decisions

Medical practice is both more successful and more satisfying when rational, effective therapy is available to correct specific defects and lead to a desirable outcome. Unexplained infertility is a special dilemma, because there is no specific defect. Although couples may intellectually appreciate the importance of a rationale for treatment, many feel compelled to take some action. Thus there is a need to fall back on empiric therapy. If the published data are representative, a large proportion of these couples continue to be childless; for many, no alternative such as adoption exists. Therefore, it is important to explore the available clinical data to help them choose among the treatment options.

Although therapy is empiric, it is not without logic. It depends on the possibility that the recruitment of multiple follicles or the use of a procedure for bringing oocytes and spermatozoa into proximity will increase the likelihood of fertilization. There is little high-quality evidence, however, because few randomized clinical trials exist. Furthermore, the price paid for treatment may be high, the adverse effects may be serious, and considerable time will be lost from normal activities. Which choice is right for a couple depends on many factors, including the intensity of their feelings with respect to childlessness, their approach to risk taking, their finances, and the time they have available for visits to the infertility clinic. In each case the advice of the physician will be most useful if the untreated prognosis is considered to be the baseline for the calculation of treatment effects.

Baseline Prognosis Without Treatment

Knowledge of the untreated prognosis is helpful in advising couples, because surveys indicate that a large proportion of infertile couples do not seek therapy. In data from the United States, less than 50% of couples seek medical advice, and only half of those who consult physicians decide to undergo treatment.[101] The baseline prognosis in published reports was excellent for infertility of short duration[17,20,21,26,31,34,36,37,40,102–107] (Fig 19–6). With more than 3 years' duration of infertility, however, the probability of conception without therapy is much lower, in the range of 1% to 3% per month.[2] A 1995 report[26] on the untreated prognosis for 2198 couples included 562 couples with unexplained infertility. Their duration of infertility was 3.5

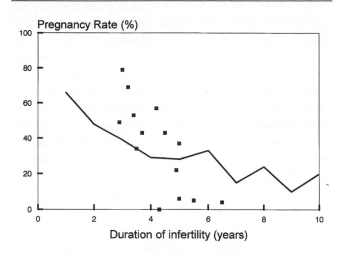

Figure 19–6. Duration of infertility and pregnancy rates in published reports[17,20,21,26,31,34,36,37,40,102–107] and the Canadian Infertility Therapy Evaluation Study.[26]

years, and the mean female partner age was 30 years. The length of the follow-up period averaged 17 months without treatment. The group with unexplained fertility experienced 119 live births (21%) (95% CI 18% to 25%). The cumulative rates of conception leading to livebirth were 4%, 8%, and 14% after 3, 6, and 12 months.[26] Livebirth was 1.8 times more likely (95% CI 1.2 to 2.7) if the couple had secondary infertility, 1.7 times more likely (95% CI 1.1 to 2.5) if the duration of infertility was less than 3 years, and 1.5 times more likely (95% CI 1.1 to 2.2) if the female partner was younger than 30 years.

With unexplained primary infertility of 3 years' duration and a female partner who is 34 years of age, the likelihood of livebirth is similar to that for the aforementioned typical rates—4%, 8%, and 14% after 3, 6, and 12 months. With unexplained infertility of 2 years' duration, the 12-month rate of conception leading to livebirth would be 24% (14% × 1.7). With unexplained infertility of 2 years' duration and a female partner who is less than 30 years of age, the 12-month live birth conception rate would be 36% (14% × 1.7 × 1.5).

The baseline prognosis for a given couple can be used to estimate their likelihood of success with a given treatment. The relative likelihood of conception reported from clinical trials is multiplied by the calculated baseline prognosis for the couple during the number of months under consideration in the treatment plan. For example, with unexplained primary infertility of 4 years' duration and a 32-year-old female partner, the livebirth conception rate after 6 months without treatment is 8%. In clinical trials to evaluate clomiphene therapy for unexplained infertility, the typical duration of the trials was 6 months. The effect of clomiphene treatment on pregnancy was approximately two or more times greater than the placebo effect.[103,108,109] Thus the predicted prognosis would be 16% after 6 months of clomiphene therapy.

Judging Effectiveness of Treatment

Side effects, costs, and personal choice all are considered in making infertility treatment decisions, but the effectiveness of a given treatment compared with other options is the foremost issue. The effectiveness of a given treatment can be judged fairly only in randomized clinical trials because a baseline conception rate occurs without treatment. Thus there is a need for randomization, which isolates the effects of treatment from the effects of other variables that might affect conception rates. With non-random allocation methods, the baseline characteristics of the historical or contemporary control groups may account for the pregnancy rates that are thought to be due to a treatment effect. Moreover, long-standing infertility does not remove the need for controlled studies, because conceptions may occur without treatment even when the infertile state is of long duration.[26,110] Therefore, case series without control groups have little value in establishing the true effect of a given treatment.

In ranking publications by the quality of the evidence, randomized clinical trials represent the best evidence from individual studies, followed at some distance by cohort studies. Case series are much lower in the hierarchy.[111] The use of meta-analysis to combine the results of randomized clinical trials may allow a more precise estimate of the treatment effect than that available from individual studies. If the difference in treatment effects from study to study is statistically significant, as indicated by a test for heterogeneity, one would place less confidence in both the combined and individual results. The publications selected for the treatment sections that follow are those that represented the highest level of clinical evidence; meta-analysis of randomized clinical trials, individual randomized clinical trials, and cohort studies.

BROMOCRIPTINE

Bromocriptine has been used in empiric therapy for unexplained infertility for women with normal concentrations of serum prolactin. Three randomized trials of use of bromocriptine compared with placebo revealed no measurable difference in observed pregnancy rates[107,112,113] (Fig 19–7). Although the studies had small sample sizes, no results of subsequent trials have been published. Bromocriptine has distinct side effects, is not effective, and therefore does not have a role in therapy for unexplained infertility.

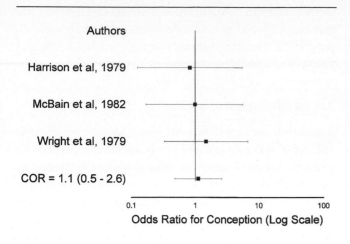

Figure 19–7. Controlled studies of bromocriptine use in unexplained infertility.[107,112,113] (Test for association = .002; P = .96. Test for homogeneity = .32; P = .98.) COR, odds ratio for conception.

Danazol

Two studies evaluated danazol in the management of unexplained infertility.[36,104] Both studies were small, and there was not a statistically significant improvement in pregnancy rate. The expense of danazol and its prolonged contraceptive effect indicate that this drug would be a poor choice in empiric therapy for unexplained infertility.

Clomiphene Citrate

Clomiphene citrate is used in therapy for anovulation, but if the drug is given to ovulatory women, there is a dose-dependent rise in the number of ovarian follicles. The rationale for use of clomiphene in unexplained infertility is that this increase in oocytes numbers will increase the likelihood of fertilization.

Five randomized clinical trials to date have addressed this application of ovulation induction.[103,108,109,114,115] Only one trial made use of central randomization and a double blind design.[103] The remaining trials used a cross-over design, and it was possible to extract data from the first treatment period from only two of the four remaining studies.[108,109] One trial included patients with surgically treated endometriosis in the category of unexplained infertility,[108] and one trial included only patients with primary infertility.[103] Co-interventions were not excluded: luteal phase hCG was administered in clomiphene and placebo cycles in one trial,[103] one trial evaluated use of clomiphene with IUI in a latin square design,[115] and another included IUI in all cycles.[108] The duration of the studies was 4 to 6 months. Four studies used 100 mg of clomiphene daily for 5 days, and one used 50 mg daily.[108]

The aggregate pregnancy rate in these trials was 2.8% (21 of 747) in placebo cycles and 6.8% (50 of 738) in clomiphene

cycles. The typical odds ratio for pregnancy rate per cycle was 2.5 (95% CI 1.5 to 4.3) (Fig 19–8). Although there were clinical differences in the samples and interventions, the Breslow-Day test for heterogeneity revealed no statistically significant heterogeneity, suggesting that despite these clinical differences, a consistent effect of clomiphene was observed. Extensive monitoring and higher clomiphene doses (100 mg daily) did not improve the pregnancy rate. In one trial the greatest relative increase in conception rates occurred when clomiphene was given to women who had been infertile for more than 3 years.[109]

Adverse effects of clomiphene among ovulatory women are similar to those among women with anovulation. They include ovarian cyst formation, multiple-gestation pregnancies, hot flashes, and visual symptoms. Multiple pregnancy occurs in 8% to 10% of clomiphene conceptions. In Canada, 20 of 163 clomiphene-associated multiple pregnancies were higher order (triplet, quadruplet, and quintuplet pregnancies).[116] Other adverse effects include hot flashes in as many as 11% of patients, and visual symptoms, including blurring of vision and diplopia in 1% to 3% of patients. When they occur, these symptoms are transient and usually do not require discontinuation of therapy. An association between fertility drugs and ovarian cancer has been reported, although the initial studies did not quantify the risk for individual drugs.[117] A recent observational study reported no adverse risk with clomiphene use for less than 1 year, but use for longer than 12 months was associated with increased risk for ovarian cancer.[118]

Although the aforementioned trials manifest some design shortcomings, the evidence appears to be consistent. Clomiphene therapy has been widely used among women with infertility due to ovulation disorders. With more than two decades of experi-

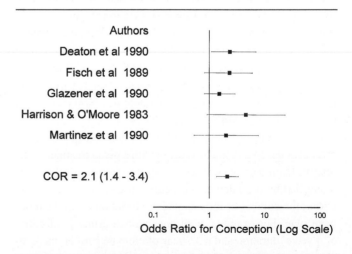

Figure 19–8. Controlled studies of clomiphene use in explained infertility.[103,108,109,114,115] (Test for association = 10.5; P = .001. Test for homogeneity = 1.4; P = .66.) COR, odds ratio for conception.

ence, its benefits and adverse effects are reasonably predictable. The use of clomiphene citrate is uncomplicated and inexpensive and therefore is indicated for about 6 months by women with unexplained infertility. Continuing benefit after 6 months has not been demonstrated, but there may be an increased risk for ovarian cancer with long-term use; therefore prolonged use is not recommended.[118]

Intrauterine Insemination

Another simple therapy is IUI of a concentrated, washed, suspension of the husband's sperm during normal unstimulated ovulation cycles. The rationale arises from the expectation that a concentrated suspension of sperm closer to the oocyte at a critical time after ovulation will improve the likelihood of fertilization.

In two trials of this therapy in unexplained infertility the pregnancy rates were very low. Nevertheless, the pregnancy rate was about two times higher with IUI than with timed intercourse (combined odds ratio [OR] 2.0, 95%CI 0.7 to 6.1.[115,119] This result was not statistically significant, however, and more trials are needed (Fig 19–9). Treatment with IUI is more expensive than clomiphene therapy, but there are very few side effects. The evidence is not conclusive, but IUI is worth considering if a clomiphene trial has been unsuccessful, unless the couple feels pressured to move on to more intensive treatment.

Human Menopausal Gonadotropin and Intrauterine Insemination

The use of human menopausal gonadotropin (hMG) to induce multifollicular recruitment and bring multiple follicles to maturity is generally combined with mechanisms for bringing oocytes and spermatozoa into proximity, such as IUI of pre-

pared spermatozoa, with the intent of improving fertility. The treatment is expensive and time-consuming, and adverse effects such as multiple gestation and hyperstimulation syndrome are potentially serious. Nevertheless, an aggregate of the uncontrolled results from case series suggests that the treatment has promise.[121]

Only two trials have addressed the use of hMG and IUI in unexplained infertility. The trials compared hMG and IUI with hMG therapy alone[122] or IUI alone,[123] and neither study had an untreated control group. To estimate the effect of hMG and IUI therapy compared with no treatment in unexplained infertility, it was necessary to use trials in a variety of diagnostic groups that addressed the use of IUI with or without hMG or clomiphene as augmentation therapy. Thirteen trials included data that could be combined to estimate the independent effects of hMG, clomiphene, and IUI therapy compared with no treatment.[108,115,120,122–131] The common element in this meta-analysis was IUI treatment. All trials either compared IUI treatment with no therapy, or IUI treatment was the active control treatment; the use of clomiphene and hMG varied among the trials.[132] The logistic regression included indicator variables for diagnosis (tubal defect, endometriosis, ovulation defect, and seminal defect as defined by World Health Organization standards) with unexplained infertility as the reference category. Thus it was possible to estimate the independent effects of each therapeutic modality while adjusting for diagnostic group.

The unadjusted aggregate pregnancy rates are shown in Table 19–3. The pregnancy rate was 3% in cycles of observation with timed intercourse, 6% in hMG cycles, and 14% in cycles of hMG and IUI. In the logistic regression analysis, the effects of IUI and hMG treatment were similar: each treatment increases the likelihood of conception approximately two times, and this increase is statistically significant (Table 19–4). The clomiphene treatment effect also was statistically significant although slightly smaller (adjusted OR = 1.7, 95% CI 1.1 to 2.7). The interaction term for hMG and IUI was not significant. This indicates that the effects of hMG and IUI are independent, according to the results of this group of studies. The presence of a seminal defect reduced the likelihood of conception by nearly one half, a statistically significant difference. A diagnosis of en-

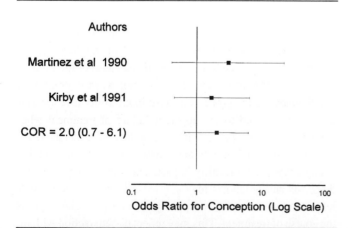

Figure 19–9. Controlled studies of intrauterine insemination during natural cycles as therapy for unexplained infertility.[115,120] (Test for association = .91; P = .34. Test for homogeneity =. 24; P = .62.) COR, odds ratio for conception.

TABLE 19–3. AGGREGATE PREGNANCY RATES IN 13 RANDOMIZED CLINICAL TRIALS OF INTRAUTERINE INSEMINATION (IUI) THERAPY FOR PERSISTENT INFERTILITY[108,115,120,122–131]

Ovulation Stimulation	Number of Pregnancies/Number of Cycles (%)	
	IUI	*No IUI*
None	61/1102 (6%)	25/963 (3)
Clomiphene	27/249 (11%)	5/54 (9)
Gonadotropin	90/625 (14%)	21/331 (6)

TABLE 19–4. RELATIVE LIKELIHOOD OF CONCEPTION IN THE MANAGEMENT OF PERSISTENT INFERTILITY[108,115,120,122–131]

Treatment or Diagnostic Group	Relative Likelihood of Conception (95% CI)[a]
Intrauterine insemination	2.10 (1.52, 2.91)
Gonadotropins	2.01 (1.45, 2.79)
Clomiphene	1.72 (1.10, 2.70)
Seminal defect	0.55 (0.40, 0.77)

[a]Adjusted odds ratio (95% confidence interval) derived from logistic regression model. Variables not in the final model were study, ovulation defect, tubal infertility, endometriosis, and the interaction term for use of gonadotropin and intrauterine insemination.

dometriosis tended to reduce the likelihood of conception, but this term was not statistically significant and did not enter the final model.

Although complications of IUI are rare, adverse effects are associated with the use of gonadotropins for the induction of ovulation. These include ovarian hyperstimulation syndrome, multiple-gestation pregnancies, and an increased rate of early pregnancy loss. Ovarian hyperstimulation with marked ovarian enlargement and lower abdominal pain occurs in 3% to 5% of the initiated cycles. The severe form of this condition (which includes ascites, pleural effusions, hypercoagulability, and risk for thromboembolism) necessitates admission to a hospital. This occurs with less than 1% of cycles. The overall risk of multiple gestation associated with gonadotropin therapy is about 25%, and about one third of these multiple-gestation pregnancies are triplets or higher-order gestations. The possible association between clomiphene and ovarian cancer has caused some concern about the use of gonadotropins, which are potent pharmacologic stimulants of follicular growth. The risk associated with use of gonadotropins has not been quantified or confirmed.[118]

The data indicate that ovulation stimulation together with IUI may be beneficial in therapy for long-standing unexplained infertility. Decisions about this therapy vary from couple to couple and depend on their motivation, attitudes toward risks, ability to arrange for the necessary time commitment, and their ability to pay. The average cost is $1200 per cycle, and the pregnancy rate in long-standing infertility is 7% per cycle.[121] The typical woman undergoes fewer than three cycles,[133] and it is unlikely that the same pregnancy rate applies to the third and subsequent cycles, because a high proportion of the "good responders" have been removed from the cohort by their success in earlier cycles.

IN VITRO FERTILIZATION TECHNIQUES

Some couples who have tried simpler therapy for unexplained infertility without success consider IVF a final step. Techniques include oocyte retrieval and IVF with embryo transfer to the uterus, or transfer of the zygote to the fallopian tube (ZIFT). Retrieved oocytes also may be returned to the fallopian tube in a suspension with spermatozoa (gamete intrafallopian transfer; GIFT). Although the initial purpose of IVF was to circumvent tubal obstruction, the rationale in unexplained infertility depends on the greater likelihood of successful implantation that should follow from the availability of numerous mature oocytes, the relatively high IVF rates, and the return of more than one embryo to the uterus. Thus IVF techniques are widely used in long-standing infertility arising from virtually any infertility diagnosis.

Pregnancy rates with IVF appear to be equivalent whether the diagnosis is unexplained infertility or tubal disease.[134,135] It seems reasonable to use a recent assembly of international registry data, which presents aggregate results for all diagnoses.[136] The livebirth rate was 12.9% in approximately 160,000 IVF cycles initiated in 31 countries. The livebirth rate for approximately 10,000 cycles of GIFT was 19.7%. The higher rates associated with GIFT procedures may represent superior baseline prognostic factors in the GIFT patients. The European trial in unexplained infertility and two other trials with broader inclusion criteria found no advantage of GIFT over IVF.[122,137,138]

IVF procedures are expensive and time consuming, and therefore they tend to be the last step in the treatment plan for unexplained infertility. Pregnancy while waiting for an IVF cycle is not uncommon. Treatment-independent pregnancies occur after unsuccessful IVF and embryo transfer among couples with apparent tubal occlusion as well as with unexplained infertility.[139–141] Couples who contemplate undergoing IVF and similar programs have a real need for continuing support and should be advised to undergo counseling.

COUNSELING

Although psychologic factors may contribute to the cause of unexplained infertility, the stress observed among these couples appears to be a consequence rather than a cause of the infertile condition.[142] Couples respond in different ways to continuing childlessness, to the procedures used in infertility investigation and treatment, and to the apparent failure of treatment when childlessness persists.[143,144] It is important to understand the possible sources of anxiety and stress among infertile couples. With unexplained infertility in particular, uncertainty about the diagnosis and prognosis may aggravate tension. Couples with long-standing infertility frequently change physicians during the course of treatment. This may reflect dissatisfaction with the treatment plan, but more likely it is due to the couple's perception of the attitude of the physician or other members of the clinical team. To offset misunderstandings, conventional counseling can be an important service.[145] It is provided in many IVF programs, and many hospital-based infertility clinics have ready access to knowledgeable counseling by psychologists, social workers, and psychiatrists. For each couple, the type of support needed should be individualized. After diagnosis and treatment are completed, counseling should help couples deal with some of the serious negative emotional and social effects of infertility that have been observed after infertility therapy.[144]

Not all couples need specialized counseling, but virtually all those with long-standing, persistent infertility need extended discussions with clinical personnel. For these discussions to be effective, it is essential that a detailed discussion of biologic and clinical information about infertility be presented in a straightforward way. The prognosis for pregnancy is the chief interest. It is prudent for clinicians to ensure that couples understand their prognosis, using data from the literature when possible. This review leads naturally to questions about the biologic aspects of reproduction, and the answers to such questions should be adapted to the knowledge of each couple. With unexplained infertility in particular, the discussion should include an unvarnished description of the limitations of the diagnostic assessment and the potential for undetectable defects in reproduction that may cause infertility.

REFERENCES

1. Mosher WD, Pratt WF: Fecundity and infertility in the United States: Incidence and trends. *Fertil Steril* 56:192, 1991
2. Guideline for Practice: *Unexplained infertility.* Birmingham, Alabama, The American Fertility Society, 1992:1–4
3. Rubin I: The nonoperative determination of patency of fallopian tubes: By means of intra-uterine inflation with oxygen and the production of an artificial pneumoperitoneum. *JAMA* 75:661, 1920
4. Rubin IC: Subphrenic pneumoperitoneum: Produced by intra-uterine insufflation of oxygen as a test of patency of the fallopian tubes in sterility and in allied gynecological conditions. *Am J Roentgenol* 8:120, 1921
5. World Health Organization: Comparative trial of tubal insufflation, hysterosalpingography, and laparoscopy with dye hydrotubation for assessment of tubal patency. *Fertil Steril* 46:1101, 1986
6. Macomber D, Sanders MB: The spermatozoa count: Its value in the diagnosis, prognosis, and treatment of sterility. *N Engl J Med* 200:981, 1929
7. Rubinstein BB: The relation of cyclic changes in human vaginal smears to body temperatures and basal metabolic rates. *Am J Physiol* 119:635, 1937
8. Rock J, Bartlett MK: Biopsy studies of human endometrium: Criteria of dating and information about amenorrhea menorrhagia and time of ovulation. *JAMA* 108:2022, 1937
9. Southam AL: What to do with the "normal" infertile couple? *Fertil Steril* 11:543, 1960
10. Frank R: A clinical study of 240 infertile couples. *Am J Obstet Gynecol* 60:645, 1950
11. West CP, Templeton AA, Lees MM: The diagnostic classification and prognosis of 400 infertile couples. *Infertility* 5:127, 1982
12. Southam AL, Buxton CL: Factors influencing reproductive potential. *Fertil Steril* 8:25, 1957
13. Belsey MA, Ware H: Epidemiological, social and psychosocial aspects of infertility. In: Insler V, Lunenfeld B (eds), *Infertility: Male and Female.* New York, Churchill Livingstone, 1986:631–647
14. Raymont A, Arronet GH, Arrata WSM: Review of 500 cases of infertility. *Int J Fertil* 14:141, 1969
15. Newton J, Craig S, Joyce D: The changing pattern of a comprehensive infertility clinic. *J Biosoc Sci* 6:477, 1974
16. Dor J, Homburg R, Rabau E: An evaluation of etiologic factors and therapy in 665 infertile couples. *Fertil Steril* 28:718, 1977
17. Sorensen SS: Infertility factors: Their relative importance and share in an unselected material of infertility patients. *Acta Obstet Gynecol Scand* 59:513, 1980
18. Thomas AK, Forrest MS: Infertility: A review of 291 infertile couples over eight years. *Fertil Steril* 34:106, 1980
19. Verkauf BS: The incidence and outcome of single-factor, multifactorial, and unexplained infertility. *Am J Obstet Gynecol* 147:175, 1983
20. Kliger BE: Evaluation, therapy, and outcome in 493 infertile couples. *Fertil Steril* 41:40, 1984
21. Hull MGR, Glazener CMA, Kelly NJ, et al: Population study of causes, treatment, and outcome of infertility. *BMJ* 291:1693, 1985
22. Collins JA, Rand CA, Wilson EH, Wrixon W, Casper RF: The better prognosis in secondary infertility is associated with a higher proportion of ovulation disorders. *Fertil Steril* 45:611, 1986
23. Harrison RF: Pregnancy successes in the infertile couple. *Int J Fertil* 25:81, 1980
24. Dhaliwal LK, Khera KR, Khall GI: Evaluation and two-year follow-up of 455 infertile couples: Pregnancy rate and outcome. *Int J Fertil* 36:222, 1991
25. Thonneau P, Marchand S, Tallec A, et al: Incidence and main causes of infertility in a resident population (1 850 000) of three French regions (1988–1989). *Hum Reprod* 6:811, 1991
26. Collins JA, Burrows EA, Willan AR: The prognosis for live birth among untreated infertile couples. *Fertil Steril* 64:22, 1995
27. Collins JA, Rowe TC: Age of the female partner is a prognostic factor in prolonged unexplained infertility: A multicentre study. *Fertil Steril* 52:15, 1989
28. Collins JA, Crosignani PG: Unexplained infertility: A review of diagnosis, prognosis, treatment efficacy and management. *Int J Gynecol Obstet* 39:267, 1993
29. Koninckx P, Muyldermans M, Brosens IA: Unexplained infertility: "Leuven" considerations. *Eur J Obstet Gynecol Reprod Biol* 18:403, 1984
30. Leridon H, Spira A: Problems in measuring the effectiveness of infertility therapy. *Fertil Steril* 41:580, 1984
31. Templeton AA, Penney GC: The incidence, characteristics, and prognosis of patients whose infertility is unexplained. *Fertil Steril* 37:175, 1982

32. Blackwell RE: Patients with unexplained infertility. *Fertil Steril* 38:261, 1982

33. Rousseau S, Lord J, Lepage Y, Van Campenhout J: The expectancy of pregnancy for "normal" infertile couples. *Fertil Steril* 40:768, 1983

34. Barnea ER, Holford TR, McInnes DRA: Long-term prognosis of infertile couples with normal basic investigations: A life-table analysis. *Obstet Gynecol* 66:24, 1985

35. Lenton EA, Weston GA, Cooke ID: Long-term follow-up of the apparently normal couple with a complaint of infertility. *Fertil Steril* 28:913, 1977

36. van Dijk JG, Frolich M, Brand EC, van Hall EV: The "treatment" of unexplained infertility with danazol. *Fertil Steril* 31:481, 1979

37. Aitken RJJ, Best FSM, Warner P, Templeton A: A prospective study of the relationship between semen quality and fertility in cases of unexplained infertility. *J Androl* 5:297, 1984

38. Collins JA, Wrixon W, Janes LB, Wilson EH: Treatment-independent pregnancy among infertile couples. *N Engl J Med* 309:1201, 1983

39. Haxton M, Black WP: The aetiology of infertility in 1162 investigated couples. *Clin Exp Obstet Gynecol* XIV:75, 1987

40. Trimbos-Kemper GC, Trimbos JB, van Hall E: Pregnancy rates after laparoscopy for infertility. *Eur J Obstet Gynecol Reprod Biol* 18:127, 1984

41. Crosignani PG, Collins J, Cooke ID, Diczfalusy E, Rubin B: Unexplained infertility. *Hum Reprod* 8:977, 1993

42. Bostofte E, Serup J, Rebbe H: Relation between sperm count and semen volume, and pregnancies obtained during a twenty-year follow-up period. *Int J Androl* 5:267, 1982

43. Zuckerman Z, Rodriguez-Rigau L, Smith K, Steinberger E: Frequency distribution of sperm counts in fertile and infertile males. *Fertil Steril* 28:1310, 1977

44. MacLeod J, Gold RZ: The male factor in fertility and infertility. II. Spermatozoa counts in 1000 men of known fertility and in 1000 cases of infertile marriage. *Br J Urol* 66:436, 1951

45. Aafjes J, van der Vijver J, Burgman F, Schenck P: Double-blind cross over treatment with mesterolone and placebo of subfertile oligozoospermic men value of testicular biopsy. *Andrologia* 15:531, 1983

46. Smith KD, Rodriguez-Rigau LJ, Steinberger E: Relation between indices of semen analysis and pregnancy rate in infertile couples. *Fertil Steril* 28:1314, 1977

47. Bostofte E, Serup J, Rebbe H: Relation between number of immobile spermatozoa and pregnancies obtained during a twenty-year follow-up period immobile spermatozoa and fertility. *Andrologia* 16:136, 1984

48. Fredricsson B, Sennerstam R: Morphology of live seminal and postcoital cervical spermatozoa and its bearing on human fertility. *Acta Obstet Gynecol Scand* 63:329, 1984

49. Seibel MM, Zilberstein M: What is the shape of semen morphology. *Hum Reprod* 10:247, 1995

50. Hargreave TB, Elton RA: Fecundability rates from an infertile male population. *Br J Urol* 58:194, 1986

51. Hanley J, McNeil B: The meaning and use of the area under a receiver operating characteristic (ROC) curve. *Radiology* 143:29, 1982

52. Peng H-Q, Collins JA, Wilson EH, Wrixon W: Receiver-operating characteristics curves for semen analysis variables: Methods for evaluating diagnostic tests of male gamete function. *Gamete Res* 17:229, 1987

53. World Health Organization: WHO Laboratory manual for the examination of human semen and semen-cervical mucus interaction. ed 3. Cambridge, UK, Cambridge University Press, 1992:1–42

54. Schechter MT, Scheps SB: Diagnostic testing revisited: Pathways through uncertainty. *Can Med Assoc J* 132:755, 1985

55. Gould JE, Overstreet JW, Hanson FW: Assessment of human sperm function after recovery from the female reproductive tract. *Biol Reprod* 31:888, 1984

56. Pandya IJ, Mortimer D, Sawers RS: A standardized approach for evaluating the penetration of human spermatozoa into cervical mucus in vitro. *Fertil Steril* 45:357, 1986

57. Schats R, Aitken RJJ, Templeton AA, Djahanbakhch O: The role of cervical mucus–semen interaction in infertility of unknown aetiology. *Br J Obstet Gynaecol* 91:371, 1984

58. Boivan J, Takefman JE: Stress level across stages of in vitro fertilization in subsequently pregnant and nonpregnant women. *Fertil Steril* 64:802, 1995

59. Oei SG, Keirse MJNC, Bloemenkamp KWM, Helmerhorst FM: European post-coital tests: Opinions and practice. *Br J Obstet Gynaecol* 102:621, 1995

60. Hamilton CJCM, Evers JLH, de Haan J: Ultrasound increases the prognostic value of the postcoital test. *Gynecol Obstet Invest* 21:80, 1986

61. Harrison RF: The diagnostic and therapeutic potential of the postcoital test. *Fertil Steril* 36:71, 1981

62. Jette NT, Glass RH: Prognostic value of the postcoital test. *Fertil Steril* 23:29, 1972

63. Hull MGR, Savage PE, Bromham DR: Prognostic value of the postcoital test: Prospective study based on time-specific conception rates. *Br J Obstet Gynaecol* 89:299, 1982

64. Samberg I, Martin-du-pan R, Bourrit B: The value of the postcoital test according to etiology and outcome on infertility. *Acta Eur Fertil* 16:147, 1985

65. Santomauro AG, Sciarra JJ, Varma AO: A clinical investigation of the role of the semen analysis and postcoital test in the evaluation of male infertility. *Fertil Steril* 23:245, 1972

66. Giner J, Merino G, Luna J, Aznar R: Evaluation of the Sims-Huhner postcoital test in fertile couples. *Fertil Steril* 25:145, 1974

67. Franken DR, Slabber CF: The postcoital test: A preliminary report. *S Afr Med J* 58:899, 1980

68. Skaf R, Kemmann E: Postcoital testing in women during menotropin therapy. *Fertil Steril* 37:514, 1982

69. Collins JA, So Y, Wilson E, Wrixon W, Casper RF: The postcoital test as a predictor of pregnancy among 355 infertile couples. *Fertil Steril* 41:703, 1984

70. Griffith CS, Grimes DA: The validity of the postcoital test. *Am J Obstet Gynecol* 162:616, 1990

71. Bronson RA, Cooper GW, Rosenfeld D: Sperm antibodies: Their role in infertility. *Fertil Steril* 42:171, 1984

72. Haas GG: Clarifying antibody-mediated infertility. *Am J Reprod Immunol Microbiol* 7:148, 1985

73. Hjort T, Johnson PM, Mori T: An overview of the WHO international multi-centre study on antibodies to reproductive tract antigens in clinically defined sera. *J Reprod Immunol* 8:359, 1985

74. Meinertz H, Hjort T: Detection of autoimmunity to sperm: Mixed antiglobulin reaction (MAR) test or sperm agglutination? A study on 537 men from infertile couples. *Fertil Steril* 46:86, 1986

75. Adeghe J-H, Cohen J, Sawers SR: Relationship between local and systemic autoantibodies to sperm, and evaluation of immunobead test for sperm surface antibodies. *Acta Eur Fertil* 17:99, 1986

76. Francavilla F, Catignani P, Romano R, et al: Immunological screening of a male population with infertile marriages. *Andrologia* 16:578, 1984

77. Jennings MG, McGowan MP, Baker HWG: Immunoglobulins on human sperm: Validation of a screening test for sperm autoimmunity. *Clin Reprod Fertil* 3:335, 1985

78. Clarke GN, Elliott PG, Smaila C: Detection of sperm antibodies in semen using the immunobead test: A survey of 813 consecutive patients. *Am J Reprod Immunol Microbiol* 7:118, 1985

79. Hargreave T: Incidence of serum agglutinating and immobilizing sperm antibodies in infertile couples. *Int J Fertil* 27:90, 1982

80. Ansbacher R, Keung-Yeung K, Behrman SJ: Clinical significance of sperm antibodies in infertile couples. *Fertil Steril* 24:305, 1973

81. Baker HWG, Clarke GN, Hudson B, McBain JC, McGowan MP, Pepperell RJ: Treatment of sperm autoimmunity in men. *Clin Reprod Fertil* 2:55, 1983

82. Collins JA, Burrows EA, Yeo J, Young Lai EV: Frequency and predictive value of antisperm antibodies among infertile couples. *Hum Reprod* 8:592, 1993

83. Eggert-Kruse W, Christmann M, Gerhard I, Pohl S, Klinga K, Runnebaum B: Circulating antisperm antibodies and fertility prognosis: A prospective study. *Hum Reprod* 4:513, 1989

84. Menge AC, Medley NE, Mangione CM, Dietrich JW: The incidence and influence of antisperm antibodies in infertile human couples on sperm-cervical mucus interactions and subsequent fertility. *Fertil Steril* 38:439, 1982

85. Witkin S, David S: Effect of sperm antibodies on pregnancy outcome in a subfertile population. *Am J Obstet Gynecol* 158:59, 1988

86. Blumenfeld Z, Gershon H, Makler A, Stoler J, Brandes JM: Detection of antisperm antibodies: A cytotoxicity immobilization test. *Int J Fertil* 31:207, 1986

87. Ingerslev HJ, Ingerslev M: Clinical findings in infertile women with circulating antibodies against spermatozoa. *Fertil Steril* 33:514, 1980

88. Noyes RW, Hertig AT, Rock JA: Dating the endometrial biopsy. *Fertil Steril* 1:3, 1950

89. Li T-C, Dockery P, Rogers AW, Cooke ID: How precise is histologic dating of endometrium using the standard dating criteria? *Fertil Steril* 51:759, 1989

90. Balasch J, Fabregues F, Creus M, Vanrell JA: The usefulness of endometrial biopsy for luteal phase evaluation in infertility. *Hum Reprod* 7:7:973, 1992

91. Driessen F, Holwerda P, Putte S, Kremer J: The significance of dating an endometrial biopsy for the prognosis of the infertile couple. *Int J Fertil* 25:112, 1980

92. Soliman S, Daya S, Collins JA, Hughes EG: The role of luteal phase support in infertility treatment: A meta-analysis of randomized trials. *Fertil Steril* 61:6:1068, 1994

93. MaGuiness SD, Djahanbakhch O, Grudzinskas JG: Assessment of the fallopian tube. *Obstet Gynecol Surv* 47:9:587, 1992

94. Paulson JD, Asmar P, Saffan DS: Mild and moderate endometriosis: Comparison of treatment modalities for infertile couples. *J Reprod Med* 36:151, 1991

95. Jequier A, Ukomber E: Errors inherent in the performance of a routine semen analysis. *Br J Urol* 55:434, 1983

96. Baker HWG, Burger HG, de Kretser DM, Lording DW, McGowan P, Rennie GC: Factors affecting the variability of semen analysis results in infertile men. *Int J Androl* 4:609, 1981

97. Sherins RJ, Brightwell D, Sternthal PM: Longitudinal analysis of semen of fertile and infertile men. In: Troen P, Nankin HR (eds), *The Testis in Normal and Infertile Men*. New York, Raven, 1977:473–488

98. Tjoa W, Smolensky M, Hsi B, Steinberger E, Smith K: Circannual rhythm in human sperm count revealed by serially independent sampling. *Fertil Steril* 38:454, 1982

99. Rosenfeld DL, Garcia CR: A comparison of endometrial histology with simultaneous plasma progesterone determinations in infertile women. *Fertil Steril* 27:1256, 1976

100. Orrell KGS, Wrixon W, Irwin AC: The clinical prediction of ovulation. *Nova Scotia Med Bull* 59:119, 1980

101. Wilcox LS, Mosher WD: Use of infertility services in the United States. *Obstet Gynecol* 82:1:122, 1993

102. Daly DC: Treatment validation of ultrasound-defined abnormal follicular dynamics as a cause of infertility. *Fertil Steril* 51:51, 1989

103. Fisch P, Casper RF, Brown SE, et al: Unexplained infertility: Evaluation of treatment with clomiphene citrate and human chorionic gonadotropin. *Fertil Steril* 51:828, 1989

104. Iffland CA, Shaw RW, Beynon JL: Is danazol a useful treatment in unexplained primary infertility? *Eur J Obstet Gynecol Reprod Biol* 32:115, 1989

105. Rousseau S: Antisperm antibodies and infertility. *Fertil Steril* 40:549, 1983

106. Welner S, DeCherney AH, Polan ML: Human menopausal gonadotropins: A justifiable therapy in ovulatory women with long-standing idiopathic infertility. *Am J Obstet Gynecol* 158:111, 1988

107. Wright CS, Steele SJ, Jacobs HS: Value of bromocriptine in unexplained primary infertility: A double-blind controlled trial. *BMJ* 1:1037, 1979

108. Deaton JL, Gibson M, Blackmer KM, Nakajima ST, Badger GJ, Brumsted JR: A randomized, controlled trial of clomiphene citrate and intrauterine insemination in couples with unexplained infertility or surgically corrected endometriosis. *Fertil Steril* 54:1083, 1990

109. Glazener CMA, Coulson C, Lambert PA, et al: Clomiphene treatment for women with unexplained infertility: Placebo-controlled study of hormonal responses and conception rates. *Gynecol Endocrinol* 4:75, 1990

110. Eimers JM, te Velde ER, Gerritse R, Vogelzang ET, Looman CWN, Habbema JDF: The prediction of the chance to conceive in subfertile couples. *Fertil Steril* 61:44, 1994

111. U. S. Preventive Services Task Force: Appendix A: Task force ratings. In: Fisher M, Eckart C (eds), *Guide to Clinical Preventive Services: An Assessment of the Effectiveness of 169 Interventions.* Baltimore, William & Wilkins, 1989:387–396

112. Harrison RF, O'Moore RR, McSweeney J: Idiopathic infertility: A trial of bromocriptine versus placebo. *J Ir Med Assoc* 72:479, 1979

113. McBain JC, Pepperell RJ: Use of bromocriptine in unexplained infertility. *Clin Reprod Fertil* 1:145, 1982

114. Harrison RF, O'Moore RR: The use of clomiphene citrate with and without human chorionic gonadotropin. *Ir Med J* 76:273, 1983

115. Martinez AR, Bernardus RE, Voorhorst FJ, Vermeiden JPW, Schoemaker J: Intrauterine insemination does and clomiphene citrate does not improve fecundity in couples with infertility due to male or idiopathic factors: A prospective, randomized, controlled study. *Fertil Steril* 53:847, 1990

116. Compendium of Pharmaceuticals and Specialties. ed 29. Ottawa: Canadian Pharmaceutical Association, 1994: 261

117. Whittemore AS, Harris R, Itnyre J, Collaborative Cancer Group: Characteristics relating to ovarian cancer risk: Collaborative analysis 12 U.S. case-control studies. II. Invasive epithelial cancers in white women. *Am J Epidemiol* 136:1184, 1992

118. Rossing MA, Daling JR, Weiss NS, Moore DE, Self SG: Ovarian tumours in a cohort of infertile women. *N Engl J Med* 331:771, 1994

119. Kerin JF, Peek J, Warnes GM, et al: Improved conception rate after intrauterine insemination of washed spermatozoa from men with poor quality semen. *Lancet* 1:533, 1984

120. Kirby CA, Flaherty SP, Godfrey BM, Warnes GM, Matthews CD: A prospective trial of intrauterine insemination of motile spermatozoa versus timed intercourse. *Fertil Steril* 56:102, 1991

121. Peterson CM, Hatasaka HH, Jones KP, Poulson AM, Carrell DT, Urry RL: Ovulation induction with gonadotropins and intrauterine insemination compared with in vitro fertilization and no therapy: A prospective, non-randomized, cohort study and meta-analysis. *Fertil Steril* 62:535, 1994

122. Crosignani PG, Walters DE, Soliani A: The ESHRE multicentre trial on the treatment of unexplained infertility: A preliminary report. *Hum Reprod* 6:953, 1991

123. Zikopoulos K, West CP, Thong PW, Kacser EM, Morrison J, Wu FCW: Homologous intra-uterine insemination has no advantage over timed natural intercourse when used in combination with ovulation induction for the treatment of unexplained infertility. *Hum Reprod* 8:563, 1993

124. Arici A, Byrd W, Bradshaw K, Kutteh WH, Marshburn P, Carr BR: Evaluation of clomiphene citrate and human chorionic gonadotropin treatment: A prospective, randomized, crossover study during intrauterine insemination cycles. *Fertil Steril* 61:314, 1994

125. Evans JH, Wells C, Gregory L, Walker S: A comparison of intrauterine insemination, intraperitoneal insemination, and natural intercourse in superovulated women. *Fertil Steril* 56:1183, 1991

126. Ho P-C, Poon IML, Chan SYW, Wang C: Intrauterine insemination is not useful in oligoasthenospermia. *Fertil Steril* 51:682, 1989

127. Ho PC, So WK, Chan YF, Yeung WS: Intrauterine insemination after ovarian stimulation as a treatment for subfertility because of subnormal semen: A prospective randomized controlled trial. *Fertil Steril* 58:995, 1992

128. Karlstrom PO, Bergh T, Lundkvist O: A prospective randomized trial of artificial insemination versus intercourse in cycles stimulated with human menopausal gonadotropin or clomiphene citrate. *Fertil Steril* 59:554, 1993

129. Martinez AR, Bernardus RE, Voorhorst FJ, Vermeiden JPW, Schoemaker J: Pregnancy rates after timed intercourse or intrauterine insemination after human menopausal gonadotropin stimulation of normal ovulatory cycles: A controlled study. *Fertil Steril* 55:258, 1991

130. Nulsen JC, Walsh S, Dumez S, Metzger DA: A randomized and longitudinal study of human menopausal gonadotropin with intrauterine insemination in the treatment of infertility. *Obstet Gynecol* 82:780, 1993

131. teVelde ER, van Kooy RJ, Waterreus JJH: Intrauterine insemination of washed husband's spermatozoa: A controlled study. *Fertil Steril* 51:182, 1989

132. Collins JA, Hughes EG: Pharmacological interventions for the induction of ovulation. *Drugs* 50:480, 1995

133. Dodson WC, Haney AF: Controlled ovarian hyperstimulation and intrauterine insemination for treatment of infertility. *Fertil Steril* 55:457, 1991

134. Navot D, Schenker J: The role of in vitro fertilization in unexplained and immunological infertility. *Contrib Gynecol Obstet* 14:160, 1985

135. Leeton J, Mahadevan M, Trounson A, Wood C: Unexplained infertility and the possibilities of management with in vitro fertilization and embryo transfer. *Aust N Z J Obstet Gynaecol* 24:131, 1984

136. International Working Group for Registers on Assisted Reproduction: World Collaborative Report 1993. Montpellier, France: International Federation of Fertility Societies, 1995:1–43

137. Tanbo T, Dale PO, Abyholm T: Assisted fertilization in infertile women with patent Fallopian tubes: A comparison of in-vitro fertilization, gamete intra-fallopian transfer and tubal embryo stage transfer. *Hum Reprod* 5:266, 1990

138. Leeton J, Rogers P, Caro C, Healy D, Yates C: A controlled study between the use of gamete intrafallopian transfer (GIFT) and in vitro fertilization and embryo transfer in the management of idiopathic and male infertility. *Fertil Steril* 48:605, 1987

139. Jarrell JF, Gwatkin RBL, Lumsden B, et al: An in vitro fertiliza-

tion and embryo transfer pilot study: Treatment-dependent and treatment-independent pregnancies. *Am J Obstet Gynecol* 154: 231, 1986

140. Ben-Rafael Z, Mashiach S, Dor J, Rudak E, Goldman B: Treatment-independent pregnancy after in vitro fertilization and embryo transfer trial. *Fertil Steril* 45:564, 1986

141. Haney AF, Hughes CL Jr, Whitesides DB, Dodson WC: Treatment-independent, treatment-associated, and pregnancies after additional therapy in a program of in vitro fertilization and embryo transfer. *Fertil Steril* 47:634, 1987

142. Seibel M, Taymor M: Emotional aspects of infertility. *Fertil Steril* 37:137, 1982

143. Mahlstedt PP: The psychological component of infertility. *Fertil Steril* 43:335, 1985

144. Lalos A, Lalos O, Jacobsson L, von Schoultz B: The psychosocial impact of infertility two years after completed surgical treatment. *Acta Obstet Gynecol Scand Suppl* 64:599, 1985

145. Rosenfeld DL, Mitchell E: Treating the emotional aspects of infertility: Counseling services in an infertility clinic. *Am J Obstet Gynecol* 135:177, 1979

CHAPTER 20

Immunology

RICHARD A. BRONSON

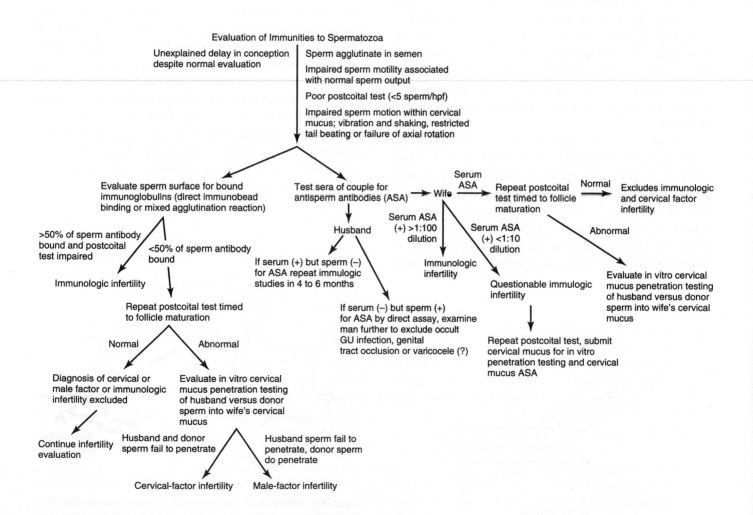

Evaluation of Immunities to Spermatozoa

Unexplained delay in conception despite normal evaluation

Sperm agglutinate in semen

Impaired sperm motility associated with normal sperm output

Poor postcoital test (<5 sperm/hpf)

Impaired sperm motion within cervical mucus; vibration and shaking, restricted tail beating or failure of axial rotation

Evaluate sperm surface for bound immunoglobulins (direct immunobead binding or mixed agglutination reaction)

>50% of sperm antibody bound and postcoital test impaired

<50% of sperm antibody bound

Immunologic infertility

Repeat postcoital test timed to follicle maturation

Normal

Abnormal

Diagnosis of cervical or male factor or immunologic infertility excluded

Evaluate in vitro cervical mucus penetration testing of husband versus donor sperm into wife's cervical mucus

Continue infertility evaluation

Husband and donor sperm fail to penetrate

Husband sperm fail to penetrate, donor sperm do penetrate

Cervical-factor infertility

Male-factor infertility

Test sera of couple for antisperm antibodies (ASA)

Husband

If serum (+) but sperm (−) for ASA repeat immulogic studies in 4 to 6 months

If serum (−) but sperm (+) for ASA by direct assay, examine man further to exclude occult GU infection, genital tract occlusion or varicocele (?)

Wife

Serum ASA

Serum ASA (+) >1:100 dilution

Immunologic infertility

Serum ASA (+) <1:10 dilution

Questionable immunologic infertility

Repeat postcoital test, submit cervical mucus for in vitro penetration testing and cervical mucus ASA

Repeat postcoital test timed to follicle maturation

Normal

Excludes immunologic and cervical factor infertility

Abnormal

Evaluate in vitro cervical mucus penetration testing of husband versus donor sperm into wife's cervical mucus

IgG and IgA antibodies in a semiquantitative way. Comparative studies between MAR and immunobead binding indicates a lower degree of sensitivity for the detection of IgA with MAR (H. Meinertz and R.A. Bronson, unpublished observations).

The sperm-panning test uses xenogenic antibodies raised against human immunoglobulins, which are then coated on microtiter wells.[44] Antibody-bound sperm bind to the wells. This assay is suitable for screening but does not provide information for individual spermatozoa, nor does it allow assessment of regional binding of immunoglobulins on the sperm surface (eg, head versus tail).

Immunobead binding (Irvine) uses polyacrylamide spheres to which rabbit antihuman antibodies are covalently linked.[45] These antibodies are isotype specific, differentiating IgG, IgA, and IgM. Spermatozoa are washed free of seminal fluid. A suspension of motile sperm is mixed with a drop of the immunobead suspension and observed with phase-contrast optics. As spermatozoa swim through the suspension, immunobeads adhere to the surface of spermatozoa that are immunoglobulin bound. The clustering of beads over different regions provides clinically useful information such as the proportion of spermatozoa in an ejaculate that are coated with immunoglobulins over their surfaces (Fig 20-3).

When the seminal fluid concentration of antisperm antibodies is high, agglutinates of sperm may appear that are large enough to form a grossly visible flocculation. In most instances, agglutination is limited, and most sperm remain motile. Immunobead binding has demonstrated that these motile sperm are often antibody bound.

Spermatozoa that carry antibody over most of their surface may be completely motile in semen and are unable to enter the cervical mucus, as shown both on postcoital testing and in vitro.[46-48]

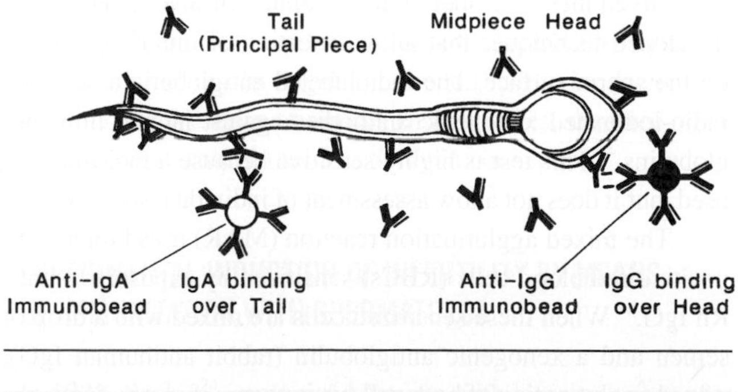

Immunobead binding is highly specific. The indirect assay also appears to be highly sensitive compared with sperm agglutination and complement-dependent immobilization assays.[49] This conclusion was reached after a multicenter, international study in which a large group of clinically defined sera were distributed as unknowns to participating laboratories under the auspices of the World Health Organization (WHO) Reference Bank for Reproductive Immunology (Tables 20-2 and 20-3).

Flow cytometry has been applied to the detection of antisperm antibodies in sera following antibody labeling. This method offers the advantage that many thousands of sperm can be analyzed rapidly in an automated system. Results were initially disappointing, in that Haas et al[50] documented a poor correlation between immunobead binding and antibody detection by fluorescence-activated cell sorter (FACS). Subsequent studies[51,52] documented the reliability of flow cytometry.

Do sperm-reactive antibodies that remain in seminal fluid reflect the cell-bound immunoglobulins present on the sperm surface? To answer this question, a comparison of sperm-bound versus sperm-free antibodies in the semen of 26 men with autoimmunity to sperm was carried out.[53] Spermatozoa were centrifuged from fresh ejaculates, washed, and analyzed by means of direct immunobead binding. Matched sperm-free seminal fluids were studied by means of addition of antibody-free sperm from known fertile donors. After incubation in seminal fluid, the sperm were washed and allowed to react with immunobeads in an indirect assay (Fig 20-4).

In the aforementioned study, the diagnosis of autoimmunity to sperm would have been confirmed by analysis of the seminal fluid of 25 of 26 men. In only 4 of the 26 ejaculates studied, however, was there no difference between sperm-bound and seminal fluid antisperm antibodies. In 22 of the men (85%), neither the isotypes detected nor their regional binding specificities were reflective of the immunoglobulins detected on the sperm surface. Head-directed antibodies were absent from the seminal fluid in 12 men (46%) but present on sperm. This finding is critical because antibodies present over the sperm

Figure 20-3. Schematic of the immunobead test. Anti-IgA or anti-IgG covalently linked to polyacrylamide beads binds to IgA or IgG bound to the sperm surface. Quantification of antisperm antibody is by means of visualization of beads bound to the sperm surface.

TABLE 20-2. COMPARISON OF RESULTS BETWEEN IMMUNOBEAD BINDING AND GEL AGGLUTINATION TESTS IN 129 MALE SERA

Gel Agglutination Titer	Immunobead Binding Level			
	Negative	Low	Intermediate	High
Negative	73	25	6	3
4–8	1	0	0	2
16–32	1	0	1	7
≥64	0	0	0	10

From Bronson RA, et al: Antisperm antibodies, detected by agglutination, immobilization, microtoxicity, and immunobead binding assays. J Reprod Immunol 8:279, 1985.

TABLE 20–3. COMPARISONS OF RESULTS (TITER) WITH FOUR METHODS OF DETECTING ANTISPERM ANTIBODY IN 14 MALE SERA ALL STRONGLY POSITIVE BY IMMUNOBEAD BINDING

Gel Agglutination (macro)	Tray Agglutination (micro)	Complement-Dependent Sperm Immobilization	Passive Hemagglutination
0	0	0	2
16	4	1	8
0	8	0	4
128	128	2	2
256	128	2	2
256	128	2	4
32	16	0	16
4	32	0	8
64	64	1	8
32	64	1	4
64	64	8	8
64	16	0	8
64	16	8	4
32	16	0	8

From Bronson RA, et al: Antisperm antibodies, detected by agglutination, immobilization, microtoxicity, and immunobead binding assays. J Reprod Immune 8:279, 1985.

head could alter direct gamete interaction and impair sperm transport.

It is necessary to determine immunoglobulin isotype. IgA, IgG, and IgM antibodies are structurally different molecules that interact with complement in different ways and have different effects on spermatozoa.[54]

Immune Complement

The complement system consists of a cascade of more than 20 plasma proteins.[55] In association with IgM, IgG1, or IgG2, the final steps in the cascade led to generation of a membrane attack complex (MAC) that is capable of producing a discontinuity in

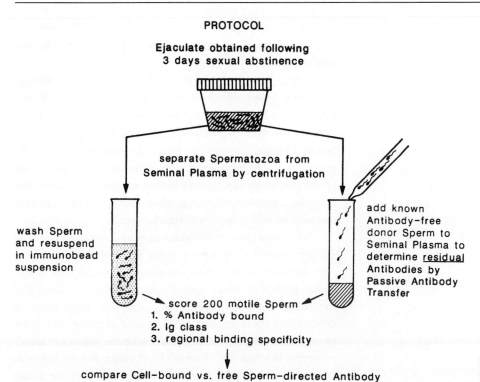

PROTOCOL

Ejaculate obtained following 3 days sexual abstinence

separate Spermatozoa from Seminal Plasma by centrifugation

wash Sperm and resuspend in immunobead suspension

add known Antibody-free donor Sperm to Seminal Plasma to determine <u>residual</u> Antibodies by Passive Antibody Transfer

score 200 motile Sperm
1. % Antibody bound
2. Ig class
3. regional binding specificity

compare Cell-bound vs. free Sperm-directed Antibody

Figure 20–4. Comparison of direct (cell-bound) vs. indirect (free) immunobead binding techniques.

the plasma membrane, leading to cell lysis.[56] IgM antibodies are more efficient than IgG immunoglobulins in mediating hemolysis.[57,58] On the other hand, unaggregated IgA immunoglobulins do not interact with complement and cannot promote generation of the MAC.

The ability of antisperm antibodies of different isotypes to interact with complement, leading to sperm plasma membrane damage, has been studied.[59,60] Sera containing sperm head-directed IgA had no effect on sperm motility or sperm ultrastructure in the presence of complement. In contrast, IgG antibody directed against the principal piece of the tail did mediate complement-dependent immobilization. There is a direct correlation between the extent of immunoglobulin attachment along the sperm tail, as reflected by immunobead binding, and the degree of immobilization. In antibodies that bind solely to the tip of the sperm tail, no change in motility was noted. As the tail surface becomes immunoglobulin bound, however, spermatozoa rapidly lose motility in the presence of complement (Fig 20–5). These results are quite similar to those previously recorded on hemolytic dose-response curves. When RBCs are sensitized with trinitrophenol (TNP), the number of hemolytic sites varies directly with the TNP antigen density and the concentration of anti-TNP IgG.[61] That is, both greater amounts of antigen on the RBC membrane and greater antibody concentra-

tion led to an increased number of plasma membrane–lytic sites.

Because seminal fluid contains complement inhibitors, spermatozoa of men with autoimmunity to sperm retain their viability in the ejaculate despite the presence of sperm-directed immunoglobulins on their sperm surface.[62] On entering the female reproductive tract, however, such sperm become liable to complement-mediated membrane damage.[63]

As anticipated from these studies, the Isojima test, a commonly used complement-dependent method of detecting immunity on the basis of sperm immobilization, would be expected not to detect sperm-directed immunoglobulins of the IgA class.[64]

Other Antibody Tests

Several enzyme-linked immunosorbant assays (ELISAs) have been developed to detect the presence of sperm-reactive antibodies in serum or semen, but dissatisfaction with this approach has increased. The presence of low-titer, naturally occurring antisperm antibodies is detectable with immunofluorescence in most sera of men and women of all ages.[65,66] These antibodies are absorbed by both spermatozoa and testicular extracts but not by other tissues. Sera possessing antiacrosomal antibodies, when absorbed with lyophilized bacteria (*Escherichia coli* and *Staphylococcus, Pseudomonas,* and *Klebsiella* species) as well as *C albicans* no longer react with sperm in indirect immunofluorescence studies. Of special importance, these sperm-reactive, naturally occurring antibodies do not react with the surface of viable sperm in suspension but only after methanol fixation. Hence, these antibodies appear to be directed against subsurface antigens.

The high frequency of naturally occurring sperm-reactive antibodies poses the problem of immunologic background noise for the ELISA. The method of fixation of spermatozoa is critical in determining which antigens are presented to the test serum. Denaturation and loss of surface antigens might be expected to occur during fixation. In addition, breakdown of the sperm plasma membrane may lead to exposure of intracellular antigens. Therefore, this assay allows detection of antibodies that play no role in impaired reproduction.

The importance of differentiating antibodies reactive with surface antigens from those reactive with subsurface antigens was documented in a WHO-sponsored workshop on monoclonal antibodies raised against sperm antigens.[67] Given that monoclonal antibodies are directed against a single antigenic determinant, these reagents could be used as probes to test the premise that only antibodies reactive with the sperm surface alter sperm function. Of 49 monoclonal antibodies studied with immunobead testing, 27 exhibited reactivity with the living sperm surface. Thirty-six of these monoclonal antibodies were

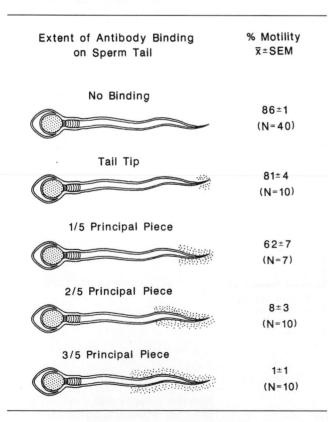

Extent of Antibody Binding on Sperm Tail	% Motility $\bar{x} \pm SEM$
No Binding	86±1 (N=40)
Tail Tip	81±4 (N=10)
1/5 Principal Piece	62±7 (N=7)
2/5 Principal Piece	8±3 (N=10)
3/5 Principal Piece	1±1 (N=10)

Figure 20–5. Schematic of immunobead binding.

studied to determine their influence on the ability of motile spermatozoa to penetrate bovine cervical mucus in vitro. A correlation was found between the degree of reactivity of each monoclonal antibody with motile sperm and their ability to penetrate cervical mucus. Antibodies directed against subsurface antigenic determinants failed to alter sperm cervical mucus penetration (Table 20–4).[68]

When spermatozoa were fixed with different methods, a variation in the ability of an ELISA to detect sperm-reactive antibodies detected with immunobead binding also was documented. Typical methods of fixation were air drying to wells, glutaraldehyde fixation, reaction with test serum while living, and freeze-thaw (Table 20–5).[69] No correlation was found in the results of participating laboratories with the clinically defined sera provided by the WHO Reference Bank for Reproductive Immunology.[70] A correlation was found with results of indirect immunobead binding only when spermatozoa were first allowed to react with test serum and subsequently with enzyme-linked second antibody.

Antisperm Antibodies in Women

To gain an idea of the frequency of immunity to sperm among women, a review of the indirect immunobead binding test results was conducted with 728 women who had experienced a delay in conception in association with an abnormal postcoital test. The husband's spermatozoa were first demonstrated to be free of antibodies and then were exposed to the wife's serum. Three hundred ninety-nine (54.8%) of these women were totally free of detectable antisperm antibodies. A weakly positive result (more than 20% but less than 50% of sperm-binding immunobeads after serum exposure at 1:10 dilution) was recorded for 200 of the 728 women (27.5%), whereas 94 women (12.9%) had intermediate levels of antisperm antibodies (immunobead-binding levels greater than 50% but less than 90%). Only 4.8%

TABLE 20–4. RELATIONSHIP BETWEEN THE EXTENT OF BINDING OF MONOCLONAL ANTIBODY TO MOTILE SPERMATOZOA AND THEIR ABILITY TO PENETRATE A COLUMN OF BOVINE CERVICAL MUCUS IN VITRO

Mab Reactivity as Judged by % Sperm Binding Immunobeads[a]	No. of Samples	Location of Vanguard Spermatozoa (mm) $\times \pm SD^b$
100%	11	17.5 ± 6.2
50 < 100%	7	27.3 ± 11.8
<50%	6	33.0 ± 11.7
None	12	37.4 ± 5.8

[a]A population of nearly 100% motile spermatozoa obtained by swim-up were incubated with monoclonal antibody (Mab), then washed free of ascitic fluid or culture supernatant, and exposed to immunobeads.
[b]After 90-min incubation at 37°C.
From Bronson RA, et al: Correlation between regional specificity of antisperm antibodies to spermatozoan surface and complement-mediated sperm immobilization. Am J Reprod Immunol 2:222, 1982.

of the women (35 samples) possessed high levels of circulating antisperm antibodies. This finding was based on the observation that nearly all sperm were antibody bound after serum exposure at greater than 1:10 dilution.

A study of a large group of clinically defined sera supplied by the WHO Reference Bank for Reproductive Immunology provided insight into the nature of antisperm antibodies in women.[71] Low levels of antisperm antibody were found in 15.6% to 35% of 57 sera from groups of women known to be fertile (low as defined by the previous immunobead-binding criteria). Levels were intermediate in 3% to 9% of these sera. In contrast, high levels were not detected in these sera (high was defined as 80% or more of spermatozoa-bound immunobeads after exposure to sera at 1:4 dilution). From these results, it is apparent that the presence of antisperm antibodies in the serum of a woman takes on clinical significance only if results of the test approach 100% at serum titers greater than 1:10.

Two provisos must be given in attempts to establish clinical guidelines for interpretation of tests of antisperm antibodies in women. The immune system of a woman is capable of local secretion of immunoglobulins. Antisperm antibodies are present in vaginal-cervical secretions or solubilized cervical mucus in the absence of humoral antisperm antibodies in 3% to 10% of women. For this reason there is a need to study cervical mucus in the event of poor sperm survival despite negative serologic results for antisperm antibodies.[72] Finally, the presence of low-level immunity to sperm may be a marker that the cellular arm of the immune system has also been sensitized to spermatozoa; few studies have attempted to deal with this aspect of immune infertility.[73]

Evaluation of a Poor Postcoital Test

Poor penetration and survival of sperm in cervical mucus may be associated with immunity to spermatozoa, although not invariably. The period of time during which spermatozoa may populate the female reproductive tract varies among women and indeed among cycles of the same woman. Absolute amounts of mucin present in human cervical mucus are similar throughout the reproductive cycle and only slightly elevated at midcycle.[74] Functional changes in the viscoelasticity of mucus and penetrability to sperm appear to be caused by an increased degree of hydration by transudated water, which is caused by alterations in the endocervical microvasculature in response to circulating estradiol.[75] The threshold of estradiol exposure at which mucus is formed by the mucus-secreting cells of the cervical crypts varies among women and may be influenced by cervicitis, in utero exposure to diethylstilbestrol, and prior operations on the cervix. Depending on the set point of the hypothalamic-pituitary axis to positive feedback, the rapidity of the rise of estradiol concentration before initiation of the

by intact antibody become entrapped in cervical mucus, whereas sperm exposed to only Fab fragments show no reduction in mucus penetration.[47] Immunoglobulin-bound sperm treated with IgA1 protease (which releases the Fc portion of the immunoglobulin molecule) displayed a normal cervical mucus-penetrating ability. Antisperm IgA and IgG have both been shown to impair sperm motion within cervical mucus, although the former displays a greater degree of sperm entrapment than the latter.[48]

To determine whether the proportion of antibody-bound sperm in the ejaculate influences fertility, results of immunobead-binding tests on the ejaculate were compared with the number of motile sperm identified in cervical mucus at standard postcoital testing.[46] The total number of motile sperm in the ejaculate ranged from 42 to 638 million. When 100% of sperm were antibody bound, only rarely were more than 0 to 3 sperm per high-power field (hpf). A small increase (often less than five

motile sperm/hpf) in the number of penetrating spermatozoa within cervical mucus occurred when binding levels were less than 100% but greater than 50%. Conversely, as immunobead-binding levels dropped to less than 50%, postcoital test results improved substantially. In several instances, 15 to 30 or 40 sperm/hpf were seen (Table 20–7).

The prognostic significance of the percentage of antibody-bound sperm in ejaculates was determined in a study of the pregnancy outcome of 108 couples in which the men had autoimmunity to sperm.[86] Immunobead-binding levels less than 50% were associated with pregnancy rates of 43.3%, as observed retrospectively during a 2-year period when only the women were treated. When more than 50% of sperm were bound, the pregnancy rate was halved to 21.8% ($P<.05$) (Table 20–8).

Results were even more dramatic when the patient population was divided according to clinical status. For couples in whom the presence of autoantibodies to sperm was the only abnormality in the fertility evaluation, pregnancy rates were 15.3% when more than 50% of sperm were bound compared with 66.7% when less than 50% of sperm were antibody bound ($P<.005$).

It is important to acknowledge that these results refer to spontaneous pregnancy rates among couples in which the husbands manifested antisperm autoimmunity in the absence of treatment. The wide variation in pregnancy rates again emphasizes the need to document the proportion of sperm that are antibody bound. In addition, that pregnancies do occur without treatment indicates the need for placebo-controlled studies to determine the efficiency of any treatment.

Sperm-Zona Interaction

To establish whether antisperm antibodies alter the ability of sperm to bind to the zona pellucida, aliquots of motile sperma-

TABLE 20–7. CORRELATION BETWEEN EXTENT OF AUTOIMMUNITY AND NUMBER OF MOTILE SPERMATOZOA IN CERVICAL MUCUS AT POSTCOITAL TESTING[a]

% Antibody-bound Sperm in Ejaculate Detected by Immunobead Binding	Total No. of Motile Sperm in Ejaculate × 10⁶	No. of Motile Sperm/hpf in Postcoital Cervical Mucus[b]
100	42	0–3[c]
	45	0–3
	69	0–1
	80	0–4
	82	0–4
	127	0
	157	0–8
	176	0–1
	345	0
	472	0
	638	7
>50 but <100	15	15
	35	3
	45	2–7
	49	3
	49	0–1
	63	6–15
	67	4
	715	8
<50	94	7
	118	15–40
	150	12
	153	15–26
	158	15–30

[a]Cervical mucus was examined within 48 hr preceding the thermal shift, 8 to 12 hrs after coitus.
[b]Wives were free of sperm-directed antibodies.
[c]Spermatozoa in cervical mucus are listed as the average observed or as a range in each hpf (x400).
From Bronson RA, et al: Auto-immunity to spermatozoa: Effects on sperm penetration of cervical mucus as reflected by post coital testing. Fertil Steril 41:9, 1984.

TABLE 20–8. PREGNANCY OUTCOME AMONG 198 COUPLES WHEN HUSBANDS MANIFESTED AUTOIMMUNITY TO SPERMATOZOA

Clinical Category	Proportion of Couples Pregnant		Level of Significance[b]
	More than 50% Sperm Antibody Bound[a]	Less than 50% Sperm Antibody Bound*	
Fertile men and women	4/26	6/9	.005
Fertile men and infertile women	6/16	13/31	NS
Infertile men and fertile women	0/6	3/4	.01
Infertile men and women	2/7	1/9	NS
All groups	12/55	23/53	.05

[a]As determined by immunobead binding of sperm washed free of seminal fluid.
[b]χ-square analysis. NS, not significant.
From Ayvaliotis B, et al: Conception rates in couples where autoimmunity to sperm is detected. Fertil Steril 43:739, 1985.

tozoa from a fertile donor were labeled with sperm head–directed antibodies by means of incubation in positive sera.[87] Spermatozoa from the same ejaculate were incubated in the same panel of sera, but after absorption with sperm, to lower antibody titers. Nonviable human eggs, which had been retrieved from surgical specimens and salt stored, were exposed to these sperm. The number of sperm bound to the zona pellucida was studied after insemination in vitro, incubation, and serial washing.

Sperm that were antibody labeled exhibited impaired ability to bind to the zona pellucida, and no more than five or so sperm were observed on the zona. That these zonae pellucidae were capable of binding sperm and that the impaired binding was associated with the presence of antisperm antibodies on the surface of a spermatozoon was confirmed with a second challenge with sperm incubated with absorbed sera; more than 100 sperm attached to the surface of the zona in these cases. A wide variation in the degree of inhibition was noted between sera tested despite the fact that all sperm were labeled with antibody, as judged by immunobead binding.[88]

To our surprise, each of these same sera that contained antisperm antibodies promoted rather than inhibited the penetration of zona-free hamster eggs. Hence, penetration frequencies for sperm incubated in antibody-negative sera were 76%, with 1.4 ± 0.27 sperm per penetrated egg. After exposure to antisperm antibody, nearly 100% of eggs were penetrated with two to nine sperm per egg.

These results are important in indicating that the locus of impaired gamete interaction for men with autoantibodies to sperm is at the level of the zona pellucida and not at the egg surface. Whether all antisperm antibodies block zona penetration has not been determined. Indeed, these results also emphasize the need to identify the antigens to which sperm antibodies are directed. This is important because the effects of antibody binding to the sperm surface depend on their antigenic targets.

Antibodies directed against epitopes on or near the zona pellucida would be expected to block zona attachment. Antibodies to other antigens might have effects on oolemmal fusion and on sperm cervical mucus transport. Indeed, this was the case in studies of the effects of different monoclonal antibodies on sperm function in different laboratory animals.[89,90] There is no satisfactory method to differentiate antisperm surface antibodies directed against fertilization-related antigens from those unrelated to fertilization.

In the future, it should be possible to identify and purify specific antigens, which will substantially improve diagnostic capabilities. The availability of such antigens will lead to specific ELISAs for each one, and determining the relative amounts of antibodies directed against different antigens should allow more specific diagnoses. The generation of polyclonal antisera to each antigen also might act as probes of the sperm surface during capacitation, allowing one to differentiate fertilization-related from antigens not related to fertilization. Such sera may allow determination of shared antigenicity among sperm, fertilized eggs, and preimplantation embryos.

EFFECTS OF AUTOIMMUNITY TO SPERM ON SPERM PRODUCTION

Despite the presence of high levels of antisperm antibodies in the reproductive tract, most men with this autoimmunity do not exhibit impairment of sperm production. Their sperm concentration in the ejaculate is similar to that of infertile men in the absence of such antibodies.

A blood-testis barrier exists between Sertoli cells as tight, junctional complexes and divides the seminiferous tubule into the basal and adluminal compartments.[91] Naturally occurring orchitis in dark minks is associated with the breakdown for these junctions, suggesting that the blood-testis barrier can become defective during seasonal regression of the testis.[92]

Experimental immunization of guinea pigs with testis extracts containing specific autoantigens has been associated with the development of immune orchitis.[93] In humans, however, the question is unresolved whether autoimmunity to spermatozoa can imapir spermatogenesis. After vasectomy, there is no evidence of the development of clinical orchitis.[94] In one study, a man with prostatic cancer who was to undergo orchiectomy underwent immunization with spermatozoa, and the testis was examined for evidence of orchitis.[95] Only focal lesions were seen, suggesting that the antigens present on mature spermatozoa would not be expressed during the development of precursor sperm in the testis. However, the cancer itself may have altered the man's immune responsiveness to sperm antigens.

Spontaneously occurring sperm-reactive antibodies have been demonstrated in the serum of an infertile man with normal semen values that cross reacted with intratesticular sperm in frozen, unfixed sections of human testis.[96] The presence of IgG deposits was shown on the seminiferous tubule wall, in germ cells, and in the interstitium of testis biopsy specimens from infertile patients.[97] Immunoelectron microscopy revealed immune complexes on the seminiferous tubule basement membrane in association with orchitis.[98] Antibodies induced experimentally against laminin (a basement membrane component) in rats were shown to alter Sertoli cell ultrastructure and spermatogenesis.[99]

Cause of Immunity to Spermatozoa

At the onset of spermatogenesis in puberty, new antigens make their appearance on the sperm surface.[100] Because tolerance of self-antigens is established in the neonatal period, these antigens may be immunogenic. It has been theorized that sequestration by the blood-testis barrier of spermatozoa during spermatogenesis and subsequent spermiation in the lumen of the seminiferous tubule prevents the generation of autoantibodies to sperm. This concept has been challenged, and the theory has been proposed that some testicular autoantigens are accessible to circulating antibodies and are immunogenic.[103]

Large numbers of lymphocytes ($\sim 1000 \times 10^6$/L) have been identified in the semen of healthy heterosexual men.[102] A population of intraepithelial suppressor T lymphocytes also was identified in the epididymis by means of immunoperoxidase staining with monoclonal probes to T-cell antigens.[103] These suppressor T cells may play a role in preventing the development of autoimmunity to sperm.

Additional evidence suggests that the absence of autoimmunity to sperm may result from continuous active suppression by suppressor T cells. A diminished number of suppressor T cells reactive to helper T cells was found in approximately one third of men with autoimmunity to sperm.[104]

Humoral antisperm antibodies are present in more than one half of men who have undergone vasectomy.[105] Several studies have documented that the likelihood of pregnancy is diminished in men who have undergone vasovasostomy. The likelihood diminishes despite the presence of spermatozoa in the ejaculate of men with antisperm antibodies detected within the reproductive tract.[106–108] Men with bilateral congenital absence of the vas deferens and seminal vesicles, as occurs in cystic fibrosis, have been found to have an autoimmunity to sperm.[109] Both congenital and acquired obstruction to sperm egress may play a role in the genesis of autoimmunity to sperm, perhaps by allowing entrance of sperm antigens into the circulation. The question has been raised whether cryptic unilateral intratesticular or extratesticular obstruction could lead to formation of antisperm antibody.[110] In fact, when mice undergo unilateral vas ligation, these autoantibodies develop in association with diminished fertility.[111]

Among 80 men with spontaneous infertility in whom unilateral testicular obstruction was confirmed at exploratory scrototomy, 40 had severe oligospermia, with sperm counts less than 5 million/mL, even though testicular biopsies showed adequate spermatogenesis and despite the presence of an unobstructed contralateral testis.[112] Sixty of these men (75%) had antisperm antibodies in their plasma. The most common sites of obstruction were the tail of the epididymis and the vas deferens. The investigators proposed that unsuspected unilateral disease might affect testicular sperm output through the development of immune-mediated orchitis.

As mentioned earlier, naturally occurring orchitis leading to infertility occurs in dark minks after seasonal regression of the testis.[94] An experimental immune orchitis that leads to as-

permatogenesis was induced in guinea pigs after immunization with testis extracts.[93] It should be emphasized, however, that most men from infertile couples with autoimmunity to sperm manifest no clinical evidence of orchitis or suppression of spermatogenesis. It could be that sperm antigens associated with autoimmunity to sperm in most men do not appear in the testis during spermatogenesis but rather at a later stage of sperm maturation. Alterations in sperm surface moieties resulting from secretory products of the epididymis have been documented. Antisperm antibodies may also be directed against sperm-associated antigens that are surface-coating glycoproteins derived from secretions of the accessory glands at the time of ejaculation.[113] A tissue-specific antigen of ejaculation that binds to spermatozoa at the time of ejaculation and is secreted by the seminal vesicles has been identified in rats. Cooper and I have noted, however, that epididymal sperm derived from men undergoing orchiectomy for a malignant tumor of the prostate exhibit an unaltered binding pattern of immunoglobulins to the surface compared with ejaculated sperm exposed to antisperm antibodies. This observation suggests that some sperm antigens to which antisperm autobodies are directed are expressed on epididymal sperm before ejaculation (R.A. Bronson and G.W. Cooper, 1981, unpublished observations).

It has been hypothesized that during infection of the genital tract, macrophages and lymphocytes may encounter antigens on sperm to which the immune system is not tolerant. An increased frequency of antisperm antibodies was noted among men who were unresponsive to antibiotics who had repeatedly positive semen *Ureaplasma* cultures.[114] A subsequent study, however, did not corroborate this association.[115] Three hundred twenty-four semen specimens were tested for the presence of autoantibodies to sperm, leukospermia, and *Ureaplasma urealyticum*. Autoantibodies were detected on the sperm surface by means of immunobead binding in 46 of the ejaculates. Of the 46 that were antibody positive, five (10.9%) cultured positive for *Ureaplasma,* and seven (15.2%) were found to have more than 1 million polymorphonuclear leukocytes (PMNs)/mL. This compared with 79 positive results for the 278 antibody-negative ejaculates (28.4%), in which 30 (10.8%) possessed more than 1 million PMNs/mL. It is hoped that additional evidence will help determine whether acute or chronic genital tract infection can cause autoimmunity to sperm.

Experimental exposure of spermatozoa to the gastrointestinal tract results in the development of antisperm antibodies.[10,115] This has been demonstrated in mice orally immunized and rabbits rectally immunized with spermatozoa. A high frequency of antisperm antibodies also has been documented in the sera of homosexual men.[116–118] The distribution of immunoglobulin isotypes of antisperm antibodies in these sera is different from that in heterosexual men from infertile couples.[116] Whereas tail-directed antibody of the IgG class, and to a lesser extent IgA antibodies, predominate in the latter group, sperm head–directed IgM is more frequently detected in the sera of homosexual men. Given the increasing evidence for the existence of a common mucosal immune system in humans, it is probable that lymphocytes in Peyer's patches or the colonic submucosa could become sensitized to spermatozoa and then return to the male genital tract and locally secrete antisperm antibodies.

Cause of Immunity to Sperm Among Women

Although women are inoculated intravaginally with spermatozoa during coitus, this usually is not associated with the development of immunity to sperm. This observation contrasts with the fact that the female reproductive tract of primates is not immunologically privileged, as demonstrated by the intravaginal inoculation of rhesus monkeys with T4 coliphage and a glycopolysaccharide of *Salmonella typhi*.[16] The intravaginal inoculation of women with polio virus also leads to the formation of locally produced antiviral antibodies in vaginal secretions.[11]

An immunoinhibitory substance has been detected and partially isolated from seminal plasma.[119] A relative lack of antigenicity was observed after epididymal mouse sperm were incubated in seminal fluid as opposed to saline solution.[120] Murine germ cells obtained from testicular suspensions and injected into syngeneic recipients yielded evidence of immunosuppression.[121] Although there has been some controversy about the specificity of immune modulation by seminal plasma, a broad spectrum of immunosuppressive effects on lymphocyte function in vitro has been documented.[122] These effects include blocking proliferation of T cells stimulated by mitogen, antigen, and allogeneic cells. Complement activity also is reduced by seminal plasma, possibly by several of the protease inhibitors known to be present.[123]

Could nature provide the means to prevent the development of immunity to sperm in women through concomitant exposure at coitus to seminal fluid immunosuppressors? Conversely, would a lack of immunosuppressive activity of seminal fluid lead to development of antisperm antibodies? A pilot study was designed to answer these questions. The immunosuppressive activity of seminal plasma obtained from men in couples determined to be free of antisperm antibodies was compared with that of men whose wives manifest high- or low-level immunity to sperm.[23] Third-party peripheral blood lymphocytes were exposed to phytohemagglutinin, a mitogen that stimulates lymphoblast formation in the presence of various dilutions of seminal fluid. Although a wide range in immunosuppressive activity of semen was observed between the two groups of men, no statistically significant difference was found between semen

samples of husbands whose wives were highly sensitized to sperm as opposed to those who were not immune.

REFERENCES

1. Goodman JW: Immunoglobulins' structure and function. In: Stites DP, Stobo JD, Wells JV (eds), *Basic and Clinical Immunology*, ed 6. Norwalk, CT, Appleton & Lange, 1987:27–36
2. Nossal GV: The basic components of the immune system. *N Engl J Med* 316:132, 1987
3. Wira CR, Sullivan DA: Sex steroid hormone regulation of IgA and IgG in rat uterine secretions. *Nature* 268:534, 1977
4. Sullivan DA, Wira CR: Hormonal regulation of immunoglobulins in the rat uterus: Uterine response to multiple estradiol treatments. *Endocrinology* 114:650, 1984
5. Sullivan DA, Wira CR: Hormonal regulation of immunoglobulins in rat uterus: Uterine response to a single estradiol treatment. *Endocrinology* 112:260, 1983
6. Wira CR, Sullivan DA, Sandoe CP: Estrogen-mediated control of the secretory immune system in the uterus of the rat. *Ann N Y Acad Sci* 409:542, 1983
7. Parr MB, Parr EL: Immunochemical localization of immunoglobulins A, G, M in the mouse female genital tract. *J Reprod Fertil* 74:361, 1985
8. Wira CR, Stern JE, Colby E: Estradiol regulation of secretory complement in the uterus of the rat: Evidence for involvement of RNA synthesis. *Immunology* 133:2624, 1984
9. Sullivan DA, Richardson GS, MacLaughlin DJ, Wira CR: Variations in the levels of secretory component in human uterine fluid during the menstrual cycle. *J Steroid Biochem* 20:509, 1984
10. Wira CR, Sandoe CP: Specific IgA and IgG antibodies in the secretions of the female reproductive tract: Effects of immunization and estradiol on expression of this response in vivo. *J Immunol* 138:4159, 1987
11. Ogra PL, Ogra SS: Local antibody response to polio vaccine in the human female genital tract. *J Immunol* 110:1307, 1973
12. Allardyce RA: Effect of ingested sperm on fecundity in the rat. *J Exp Med* 159:1548, 1984
13. Chodirker WB, Tomasi TB Jr: Gamma-globulin: Quantitative relationships in human serum and nonvascular fluids. *Science* 142:1080, 1963
14. Waldman RH, Cruz JM, Rowe DS: Intravaginal immunization of humans with *Candida albicans*. *J Immunol* 109:662, 1972
15. Schumacher GFB: Humoral immune factors in the female reproductive tract and their changes during the cycle. In: Dhindsa D. Schumacher GFB (eds), *Immunologic Aspects of Infertility and Fertility Regulation*. New York, Elsevier, 1980:93–142
16. Yang SL, Schumacher GFB: Immune response after vaginal application of antigens in the rhesus monkey. *Fertil Steril* 32:588, 1979
17. Lippes J, Ogra SS, Tomasi TB Jr, Tourville OR: Immunohistological localization of G, A, M secretory piece and lactoferin in the female genital tract. *Contraception* 1:163, 1972

18. Tourville DR, Ogra SS, Lippes J, Tomasi JB Jr: The human female reproductive tract: Immunohistological localizing of A, G, M secretory piece and lactoferin. *Am J Obstet Gynecol* 108:1102, 1970

19. Schumacher GFB, Holt JA, Reale F: Approaches to the analysis of human endometrial secretion. In: Baller FK, Schumacher GFB (eds), *Biology of the Fluids of the Female Genital Tract.* New York, Elsevier–North Holland, 1971

20. Tauber PF: Biochemical components of the human endometrium. In: Baller FK, Schumacher GFB (eds), *Biology of the Fluids of the Female Genital Tract.* New York, Elsevier–North Holland, 1979: 131–150

21. Lippes J, Enders RG, Pragay DA, Bartholomew WR: The collection and analysis of human fallopian tubal fluid. *Contraception* 5:85, 1972

22. Lippes J: Applied physiology of the uterine tube. *Obstet Gynecol Annu* 4:119, 1975

23. Bronson RA: Immunologic abnormalities of the female reproductive tract. In: Gondos B, Riddick DH (eds), *Pathology of Infertility.* New York, Theime, 1987:13–28

24. Baskin MJ: Temporary sterilization by the injection of human spermatozoa: A preliminary report. *Am J Obstet Gynecol* 24:892, 1932

25. McLaren A: Immunological control of fertility in female mice. *Nature* 201:583, 1964

26. Edwards RG: Immunologic control of fertility in female mice. *Nature* 203:50, 1964

27. Seki M, Mettler L: Influence of spermatozoal antibodies in the reproduction of mice. *Am J Reprod Immunol* 2:225, 1982

28. Katsh S: Infertility in female guinea pigs induced by injection of homologous sperm. *Am J Obstet Gynecol* 78:276, 1959

29. Tung KSK, Okada A, Yanagimachi R: Sperm autoantigens and fertilization. I. Effects of antisperm antibodies on rouleaux formation, viability and acrosome reaction of guinea pig sperm. *Biol Reprod* 23:877, 1980

30. Yanagimachi R, Okada A, Tung KSK: Sperm autoantigens and fertilization. II. Effects of anti-guinea pig sperm antibodies on sperm-ovum interactions. *Biol Reprod* 24:512, 1981

31. Menge AC, Peegel H, Riolo ML: Sperm factors responsible for immunologic induction of pre- and post-fertilization infertility in rabbits. *Biol Reprod* 20:93, 1979

32. Lee CYG, Wong E, Zhang JH: Inhibitory effects of monoclonal sperm antibodies on the fertilization of mouse oocytes in vitro and in vivo. *J Reprod Immunol* 9:261, 1986

33. Rumke PH, Hellinga G: Autoantibodies against spermatozoa in sterile men. *Am J Clin Pathol* 32:357, 1959

34. Rumke P, Van Amsterl N, Messa EN, Rezemar PD: Prognosis of fertility of men with sperm agglutinins in the serum. *Fertil Steril* 24:305, 1973

35. Franklin RR, Dukes CD: Antispermatozoal antibody and unexplained infertility. *Am J Obstet Gynecol* 89:6, 1964

36. Beer AE, Neaves WB: Antigenic status of semen from the viewpoints of the female and male. *Fertil Steril* 29:3, 1978

37. Bell EB: An immune-type agglutination of mouse spermatozoa by *Pseudomonas maltophilia. J Reprod Fertil* 17:275, 1968

38. Rose NR, Hjort T, Rumke P, et al: Techniques for detection of iso- and auto-antibodies to human spermatozoa. *Clin Exp Immunol* 23:175, 1976

39. Shulman S, Jackson H, Stone M: Antibodies to spermatozoa. V. Comparative studies of sperm-agglutinating activity in groups of infertile and fertile women. *Am J Obstet Gynecol* 123:139, 1975

40. Pavia CS, Sites DP, Bronson RA: Reproductive immunology. In: Stites DP, Stebo JD, Wells JV (eds), *Basic and Clinical Immunology,* ed 6. Norwalk, CT, Appleton & Lange, 1987:609–613

41. Clarke GN, Elliott PG, Smaila C: Detection of sperm antibodies in semen using the immunobead test: A study of 813 consecutive patterns. *Am J Reprod Immunol Microbiol* 7:61, 1985

42. Haas GG, Cives DB, Schreiber AD: Immunologic infertility: Identification of patients with antisperm antibody. *N Engl J Med* 303:722, 1980

43. Jager S, Kremer J, Van Slochteren-Draaisma T: A simple method of screening for antisperm antibodies in the human male: Detection of spermatozoal surface IgG with the direct mixed agglutination reaction carried out in untreated fresh human semen. *Int J Fertil* 23:12, 1978

44. Hancock RJT, Farakis S: Detection of antibody-coated sperm by panning procedures. *J Immunol Methods* 66:149, 1984

45. Bronson RA, Cooper GW, Rosenfeld DL: Membrane-bound sperm specific antibodies: Their role in infertility. In: Vogel H, Jagiello G (eds), *Bioregulators in Reproduction.* New York, Academic Press, 1981:526–527

46. Bronson RA, Cooper GW, Rosenfeld DL: Auto-immunity to spermatozoa: Effects on sperm penetration of cervical mucus as reflected by post coital testing. *Fertil Steril* 41:9, 1984

47. Jager S, Kremer J, Kuiken J, et al: Induction of the shaking phenomenon by pretreatment of spermatozoa with sera containing antispermatozoal antibodies. *Fertil Steril* 36:784, 1981

48. Bronson RA, Cooper GW, Rosenfeld DL, et al: The effect of IgA_1 protease on immunoglobulins bound to the sperm surface and sperm cervical mucus penetrating ability. *Fertil Steril* 47:985, 1987

49. Bronson RA, Cooper G, Hjort T, et al: Antisperm antibodies detected by agglutination, immobilization microtoxicity and immunobead binding assays. *J Reprod Immunol* 8:279, 1985

50. Haas GG, D'Cruz OJ, DeBault LE: Comparison of the indirect immunobead, radiolabelled and immunofluorescence assays for immunoglobulin G serum antibodies to human sperm. *Fertil Steril* 55:377, 1991

51. Rasanen ML, Hovatta OL, Agrawal YP: Detection and quantitation of sperm-bound antibodies by flow cytometry of human semen. *J Androl* 13:55, 1992

52. Sinton EB, Reiman DC, Ashton ME: Antisperm antibody detection using concurrent cytofluometry and indirect immunofluorescence microscopy. *Am J Clin Pathol* 95:242, 1991

53. Bronson RA, Cooper GW, Rosenfeld DL: Seminal fluid antisperm antibodies do not reflect those present on the sperm surface. *Fertil Steril* 48:505, 1987

54. Rapp HJ, Borsos T: *Molecular Basis of Complement.* New York, Appleton-Century-Crofts, 1970

55. Cooper NR: The complement system. In: Stites DP, Stobo JD, Wells JV (eds), *Basic and Clinical Immunology,* ed 6. Norwalk, CT, Appleton & Lange, 1987

56. Fortin P, Babai F: Ultrastructural visualization of the membrane attack complex of the complement and its insertion in the glycocaly of the red cell using ruthenium red. Presented at the Sixth International Congress of Immunology, July 6–11, 1986, Toronto

57. Humphrey JH, Dourmashkin RR: Electron microscope studies of immune cell lysis. In: Wolstenholme GEW, Knight J (eds), *CIBA Foundation Symposium on Complement*. Boston, Little, Brown, 1965:175–189

58. Colten HR, Boros T, Rapp HJ: Titration of the first component of complement on a molecular basis: Suitability of IgM and unsuitability of IgG hemolysins as a sensitizer. *Immunochemistry* 6:461, 1969

59. Bronson RA, Cooper GW, Rosenfeld DL: Correlation between regional specificity of antisperm antibodies to the spermatozoan surface and complement-mediated sperm immobilization. *Am J Reprod Immunol* 2:222, 1982

60. Bronson RA, Cooper GW, Phillips D: Ultrastructural-physiologic correlates of human sperm egg penetrating ability. Presented at the 12th annual meeting of the American Society of Andrology, March 6–7, 1987, Denver

61. Kratz HJ, Borsos T, Isliker H: Mouse monoclonal antibodies and the red cell surface. II. Effect of hapten density on complement fixation and activation. *Mol Immunol* 22:229, 1985

62. Brooks GF, Lammel CJ, Petersen BH, et al: Human seminal plasma inhibition of antibody complement-mediated killing and opsonization of *Neisseria gonorrhoeae* and other gram-negative organisms. *J Clin Invest* 67:1523, 1981

63. Price RJ, Boettcher B: The presence of complement in human cervical mucus and its possible relevance to infertility in women with complement-dependent sperm immobilizing antibodies. *Fertil Steril* 32:61, 1979

64. Isojima S, Tsuchiya K, Koyama K, Tanaka C: Further studies on sperm immobilizing antibody found in sera of unexplained cases of sterility in women. *Am J Obstet Gynecol* 112:199, 1972

65. Tung KSK, Cooke WD Jr, McCarthy TA, Robitaille P: Human sperm antigens and antisperm antibodies. II. Age-related incidence of antisperm antibodies. *Clin Exp Immunol* 25:73, 1976

66. Hjort T, Hansen RB: Immunofluorescent studies on human spermatozoa. I. The detection of different spermatozoal antibodies and their occurrence in normal and infertile women. *Clin Exp Immunol* 8:9, 1971

67. Mettler L, Czuppon AB, Alexander N, et al: Antibodies to spermatozoa and seminal plasma antigens detected by various enzyme-linked immunosorbent (ELISA) assays. *J Reprod Immunol* 8:301, 1985

68. Bronson RA, Cooper GW: Effects of sperm-reactive monoclonal antibodies on the cervical mucus penetrating ability of human spermatozoa. *Am J Immunol Microbiol* 14:59, 1987

69. Bronson RA, Cooper GW, Witkin SS: Detection of spontaneously occurring sperm-directed antibodies in infertile couples by immunobead binding and enzyme-linked immunosorbent assay. *Ann N Y Acad Sci* 438:504, 1984

70. Hjort T, Johnson PM, Mori T: An overview of the WHO international multi-center study on antibodies to reproductive tract antigens in clinically defined sera. *J Reprod Immunol* 8:539, 1985

71. Bronson RA, Cooper GW, Rosenfeld DL: Sperm antibodies: Their role in infertility. *Fertil Steril* 42:171, 1984

72. Bronson RA, Cooper GW, Rosenfeld DL: Factors affecting the population of the female reproductive tract by spermatozoa: Their diagnosis and treatment. *Semin Reprod Endocrinol* 4:387, 1986

73. McShane PM, Schiff I, Trentham MD: Cellular immunity to sperm in infertile women. *JAMA* 253:3555, 1985

74. Wolf DP, Sokoloski J, Khan M, Litt M: Human cervical mucus. III. Isolation and characterization of rheologically active mucin. *Fertil Steril* 28:53, 1977

75. Nicosia SV: Physiology of cervical mucus production. *Semin Reprod Endocrinol* 4:313, 1986

76. Bronson RA: Sperm dysfunction: A new understanding of male infertility. *Sci Am* (in press)

77. Peterson RN, Hunt WP, Henry LH: Interaction of boar spermatozoa with porcine oocytes: Increase in proteins with high affinity for the zona pellucida during epididymal transit. *Gamete Res* 14:57, 1986

78. Moore HDM, Hartman TD, Pryor JP: Development of oocyte-penetrating capacity of spermatozoa in the human epididymis. *Int J Androl* 6:310, 1983

79. Rogers BJ: The sperm penetration assay: Its usefulness reevaluated. *Fertil Steril* 43:821, 1985

80. Alexander NJ: Antibodies to human spermatozoa impede sperm penetration of cervical mucus and hamster eggs. *Fertil Steril* 41:433, 1984

81. Haas GG Jr, Ansmanus M, Culp L, Tureck RW, Blasco L: The effect of immunoglobulin occurring on human sperm in vivo on the human sperm hamster ova penetration assay. *Am J Reprod Immunol* 7:109, 1985

82. Bronson RA, Cooper GW, Rosenfeld DL: Ability of antibody-bound human sperm to penetrate zona-free hamster ova in vitro. *Fertil Steril* 36:778, 1981

83. Bronson RA, Cooper GW, Rosenfeld DL: Complement-mediated effects of sperm head-directed human antibodies on the ability of human spermatozoa to penetrate zona-free hamster eggs. *Fertil Steril* 40:91, 1983

84. Bronson R, Cooper G, Rosenfeld D: Reproductive effects of sperm surface antibodies. In: Lobl T, Hafez ESE (eds), *Male Fertility and Its Regulation*. Boston, MTP Press, 1985:417–436

85. Dravland E, Josh MM: Sperm coating antigens secreted by the epididymis and seminal vesicle of the rat. *Biol Reprod* 25:649, 1981

86. Ayvaliotis B, Bronson R, Cooper G, Rosenfeld D: Conception rates in couples where autoimmunity to sperm is detected. *Fertil Steril* 43:739, 1985

87. Bronson RA, Cooper GW, Rosenfeld DL: Sperm-specific iso-antibodies and auto-antibodies inhibit the binding of human sperm to the human zona pellucida. *Fertil Steril* 38:724, 1982

88. Mahoney MC, Blackmore PF, Bronson RA, Alexander NJ: Inhibition of human sperm–zona pellucida tight binding in the presence of antisperm antibody positive polyclonal patient sera. *J Reprod Immunol* 19:287, 1991

89. Saling PM, Irons G, Waibel R: Mouse sperm antigens that participate in fertilization. I. Inhibition of sperm fusion with egg plasma membrane using monoclonal antibodies. *Biol Reprod* 33:515, 1985

90. Saling PM, Lakoski KA: Mouse sperm antigens that participate in fertilization. II. Inhibition of sperm penetration through zona pellucida using monoclonal antibodies. *Biol Reprod* 33:527, 1985

91. Dym M, Caviacchia JC: Further observations on the blood-testis barrier in monkeys. *Biol Reprod* 17:390, 1977

92. Tung KSK, Ellis L, Teuscher C, et al: The black mink (*Mustela vision*): A natural model of immunologic male infertility. *J Exp Med* 154:1016, 1981

93. Teuscher C, Wild GC, Tung KSK: Experimental allergic orchitis: The isolation and partial characterization of an aspermatogenic polypeptide (AP3) with an apparent sequential disease-inducing determinant(s). *J Immunol* 130:2683, 1983

94. Massey FJ, Bernstein GS, Fallon WM, et al: Vasectomy and health: Results from a large cohort study. *JAMA* 252:1023, 1984

95. Mancini RE, Andrada JA, Sarceni D, et al: Immunological and testicular response in a man sensitized with human testicular homogenate. *J Clin Endocrinol Metab* 25:859, 1965

96. Haas GG Jr, D'Cruz G, DeBault LE: The distribution of HLA-ABC and Dr antigens in normal human testis. Presented at the 20th Annual Meeting of the Society for the Study of Reproduction, July 20–23, 1987, Urbana, IL

97. Lehmann D, Temminck B, DaRugna D, et al: Role of immunological factors in male infertility: Immunohistochemical and serological evidence. *Lab Invest* 57:21, 1987

98. Salomon F, Saremaslani P, Jakob M, Hedinger CF: Immunocomplex orchitis in infertile men: Immunoelectron microscopy of abnormal basement membrane structures. *Lab Invest* 47:555, 1982

99. Lustig L, Doncel GF, Berenstein E, Denduchis B: Testis lesions, cellular and immune response induced in rats by immunization with laminin. *Am J Reprod Immunol Microbiol* 14:123, 1987

100. O'Brien DA, Millett CF: Immunochemical identification of multiple cell surface antigens appearing during specific stages of mouse spermatogenesis. *Gamete Res* 13:199, 1986

101. Tung KSK, Yule TD, Mahi-Brown CA, Listrom MD: Distribution of histopathology and Ia positive cells in actively induced and passively transferred experimental immune orchitis. *J Immunol* 138:752, 1987

102. El-Demiry MIM, Hargreave TB, Busmittil A, et al: Lymphocytic subpopulations in the male genital tract. *Br J Urol* 57:769, 1985

103. Ritchie AWS: Intraepithelial lymphocytes in the normal epididymis: A mechanism for tolerance to sperm auto-antigens? *Br J Urol* 56:79, 1984

104. Witkin SS: Phenotypic characterization of seminal lymphocytes and their relations to sperm antibody production. Presented at the 43rd Annual Meeting of the American Fertility Society, Sept 28–30, 1987, Reno, NV

105. Shulman S, Zappi E, Ahmed U, Davis J: Immunologic consequences of vasectomy. *Contraception* 5:269, 1972

106. Linnet L, Hjort T, Fogh-Anderson D: Association between failure to impregnate after vasovasostomy and sperm agglutinins in semen. *Lancet* 1:117, 1981

107. Alexander NJ: Antibody levels and immunologic infertility. In Isojima S, Billington WD (eds), *Reproductive Immunology*. New York, Elsevier, 1983:207–214

108. Wicklynd R, Alexander NJ: Vasovasostomy: Evaluation of success. *Urology* 13:532, 1979

109. Girgis SM, Eklandroas EM, Iskander R, El-Dokhly R, Girgis RN: Sperm antibodies in serum and semen in men with bilateral congenital absence of the vas deferens. *Arch Androl* 8:301, 1982

110. Hendry WF: Surgery for testicular obstruction. *Recent Adv Urol Androl* 4:313, 1987

111. Kessler DL, Smith WD, Hamilton MS, Berger RE: Infertility in mice after unilateral vasectomy. *Fertil Steril* 43:308, 1985

112. Hendry WF, Parslow JM, Stedronska J: Exploratory scrotomy in 168 azoospermic males. *Br J Urol* 55:785, 1983

113. Isojima S, Kameda K, Tsuji Y, et al: Establishment and characterization of a human hybridoma secreting monoclonal antibody with high titers of sperm immobilizing and agglutinating activities against human seminal plasma. *J Reprod Immunol* 10:67, 1987

114. Toth A, Lesser ML, Brooks C, Labriola D: Subsequent pregnancies among 161 couples treated for T-mycoplasma genital tract infection. *N Engl J Med* 308:505, 1983

115. Bronson R, Cooper G, Rosenfeld D: Lack of correlation between seminal fluid ureaplasma status, leukospermia and auto-immunity to spermatozoa. Presented at the 30th Annual Meeting of the Society for Gynecologic Investigation, March 17–20, 1983, Washington, DC

116. Bronson R, Cooper G, Rosenfeld D, et al: Comparison of anti-sperm antibodies in homosexual and infertile men with auto-immunity to spermatozoa. Presented at the 30th Annual Meeting of the Society for Gynecologic Investigation, March 17–20, 1983, Washington, DC

117. Witkin SS, Sonnabend J: Immune response to spermatozoa in homosexual men. *Fertil Steril* 39:337, 1983

118. Wolff H, Schill WB: Antisperm antibodies in infertile and homosexual men: Relationship to serologic and clinical findings. *Fertil Steril* 44:673, 1985

119. Lord EM, Sensabaugh GF, Stites DP: Immunosuppressive activity of human seminal plasma: Inhibition of in vivo lymphocyte activation. *J Immunol* 118:1704, 1977

120. Anderson DJ, Tarter TH: Immunosuppressive effects of mouse seminal plasma components in vivo and in vitro. *J Immunol* 128:535, 1982

121. Hurtenbach U, Shearer GM: Germ cell induced immune suppression in mice: Effect of inoculation of syngenic spermatozoa on cell-mediated immune responses. *J Exp Med* 155:1719, 1982

122. James K, Hargreave TB: Immunosuppression by seminal plasma and its possible clinical significance. *Immunol Today* 5:357, 1984

123. Petersen BH, Lammel CJ, Stites DP, Brooks GF: Human seminal plasma inhibition of complement. *J Lab Clin Med* 96:582, 1980

CHAPTER 21

Infections

GILLES R. G. MONIF

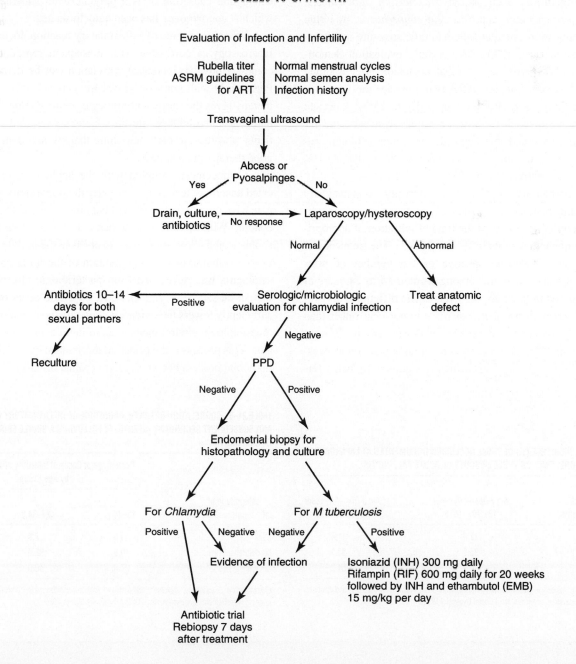

Evaluation of Infection and Infertility

Rubella titer | Normal menstrual cycles
ASRM guidelines | Normal semen analysis
for ART | Infection history

Transvaginal ultrasound

Abcess or Pyosalpinges

Yes / No

Drain, culture, antibiotics —— No response —→ Laparoscopy/hysteroscopy

Normal / Abnormal

Antibiotics 10–14 days for both sexual partners ←— Positive —— Serologic/microbiologic evaluation for chlamydial infection

Treat anatomic defect

Reculture

Negative

PPD

Negative / Positive

Endometrial biopsy for histopathology and culture

For *Chlamydia*   For *M tuberculosis*

Positive / Negative   Negative / Positive

Evidence of infection

Isoniazid (INH) 300 mg daily
Rifampin (RIF) 600 mg daily for 20 weeks
followed by INH and ethambutol (EMB)
15 mg/kg per day

Antibiotic trial
Rebiopsy 7 days
after treatment

The quest for the microbiologic cause of infertility can be subdivided according to anatomic site. Theoretically, microbiologic organisms can function at the cervical, endometrial, and fallopian tube levels and negatively affect fertilization or implantation. Other infections such as human immunodeficiency virus (HIV) and cytomegalovirus (CMV) that are not direct causes of infertility may have an indirect impact on reproduction. This chapter discusses an approach to infection and infertility.

FALLOPIAN TUBE INFERTILITY

Pathophysiology

Certain organisms, such as *Mycobacterium tuberculosis, Chlamydia trachomatis,* and *Neisseria gonorrhoeae,* by virtue of their replication can alter fallopian tube structure and function.[1–3] In the early 1970s, laparoscopic evaluation demonstrated a 12.8% frequency of tubal occlusion after a single episode of acute salpingitis. After two episodes the figure increased to 35.5% and after three episodes to 75%.[2] A decade later, when improved therapeutic techniques were used, the impact of one, two, and three episodes of acute salpingitis revealed the frequency of tubal occlusion to be 11.4%, 23.1%, and 54.3%, respectively (Table 21–1).[4]

The probability of secondary infertility is statistically linked to age, number of antecedent episodes of acute salpingitis, and severity of disease at the time of initiation of appropriate antibiotic therapy (Tables 21–2 and 21–3). The frequency of infertility was lowest irrespective of the number of prior episodes of acute salpingitis among women 15 to 24 years of age as opposed to those 25 to 34 years. The difference may reflect the increased prevalence of overt gonorrheal rather than chlamydial infection among the younger group. Women younger than 25 years of age who previously had gonococcus-associated salpingitis had a statistically significantly better fer-

tility prognosis than those who previously had so-called nongonococcal salpingitis. Nongonococcal salpingitis usually has a chlamydial causation or is a polymicrobial superinfection in which *N gonorrhoeae* has been autoeliminated.[5]

When the degree of inflammatory reaction documented at laparoscopy is correlated with subsequent reproductive outcomes, a positive increased correlation can be demonstrated. Particularly with gonococcal disease, early effective antibiotic therapy gives the shortest erythrocyte sedimentation rate (ESR) half-time.[6] Involuntary infertility is greatly reduced among patients who receive early antibiotic therapy and demonstrate a good therapeutic response.

Culdocentesis coupled with the application of sophisticated anaerobic techniques provides the opportunity to investigate what could be construed as both the front and the back of a conduit. With the information derived, it is possible to make a sophisticated guess about what happens in the middle. The concept of polymicrobial superinfection of the initial gonococcal salpingitis was developed from bacteriologic observations of the cul-de-sac.[7–10] *N gonorrhoeae,* by virtue of its replication, sufficiently lowers the oxidation-reduction potential of the local microbiologic environment so as to initiate anaerobic progression. This process is the principal mechanism by which a monomicrobial process becomes polymicrobial disease.[11]

TABLE 21–2. PERCENTAGE OF CASES OF SECONDARY INFERTILITY AFTER SALPINGITIS IN DIFFERENT AGE GROUPS

Number of Infections	Percentage of Cases of Infertility after Salpingitis by Age Group		
	15–24 y	24–34 y	Total
1	9.4	19.2	11.4
2	20.9	31.0	23.1
3	51.6	60.0	54.3

From Westrom L: Incidence, prevalence and trends of acute pelvic inflammatory disease and its consequences in industrialized countries. Am J Obstet Gynecol *138:880, 1980.*

TABLE 21–1. INCIDENCE (%) OF TUBAL OCCLUSION DOCUMENTED AT LAPAROSCOPY FOLLOWING ONE, TWO, OR THREE EPISODES OF ACUTE SALPINGITIS

Number of Episodes of Acute Salpingitis	Am J Obstet Gynecol 121:707, 1975	Am J Obstet Gynecol 138:880, 1980
1	12.8	11.4
2	35.5	23.1
3	75	54.3

From Westrom L: Incidence, prevalence and trends of acute pelvic inflammatory disease and its consequences in industrialized countries. Am J Obstet Gynecol *138:880, 1980.*

TABLE 21–3. CORRELATION BETWEEN MAGNITUDE OF INFLAMMATORY CHANGE AND SUBSEQUENT SECONDARY INFERTILITY FOLLOWING A SINGLE EPISODE OF SALPINGITIS

Magnitude of Inflammatory Change	Percentage of Cases of Infertility after Salpingitis by Age Group		
	15–24 y	24–34 y	Total
Mild	5.8	7.8	6.1
Moderately severe	10.8	22.0	13.4
Severe	27.3	40.0	30.0

From Westrom L: Incidence, prevalence and trends of acute pelvic inflammatory disease and its consequences in industrialized countries. Am J Obstet Gynecol *138:880, 1980.*

As progressive changes in the microbiologic environment select for the more microaerophilic organisms (class II anaerobes), *N gonorrhoeae* undergoes autoelimination. This process occurs in the cul-de-sac and then sequentially in the fallopian tubes, endometrium, and endocervix. Ultimately the gonococcus cannot be recovered from either end of the conduit. When nonrecovery of *N gonorrhoeae* can be excluded because of technical problems (such as delayed plating, use of cold Thayer-Martin plates, or absence of initial ambient carbon dioxide), absence of the gonococcus has come to imply either infection caused by *C trachomatis* or advanced disease as a result of anaerobic superinfection of initial gonococcal salpingitis.

Therapeutic Staging of Acute Salpingitis

Because pelvic infection can lead to secondary infertility, ectopic pregnancy, and in some instances tubo-ovarian complexes, optimization of treatment is highly desirable. One accomplishes this by devising a staging system that allows a more objective application of treatment. The Gainesville staging system (Table 21–4) was developed in conjunction with direct observation of acute salpingitis at laparoscopy. There is greater than 82% correlation between clinical stage and laparoscopic findings. Nonetheless staging must be viewed only as a guideline for the initiation of therapy and development of a treatment plan. Should the anticipated therapeutic response not occur, clinical management should be reassessed and more aggressive therapy initiated.

Stage I: Acute Salpingitis Without Peritonitis

Stage I disease affects patients without peritonitis who have no underlying structural damage to the fallopian tubes, no penicillinase-producing strains of *N gonorrhoeae* and no intrauterine device (IUD) in place. Such patients respond well to penicillins or tetracyclines. Outpatient treatment is sufficient for patients who are anticipated to be compliant. Nevertheless, hospitalization may be beneficial if the patient intends to preserve future fertility, because intravenous antibiotics may reach therapeutic levels quicker. Any patient with an IUD in place and stage I disease should be hospitalized.

Stage II: Acute Salpingitis with Peritonitis

Stage II disease is clinically similar to stage I disease with the exception that the patient exhibits bilateral lower quadrant rebound tenderness. The goal of therapy for stage II disease is to preserve fallopian tube structure and function. The diagnosis of stage II disease is confirmed with the finding of peritonitis at physical examination. For patients with stage II disease who are found to have gonococcus as part of their polymicrobial bacterial flora, the probability of achieving the anticipated therapeutic response is approximately 60%. In the absence of gonococcus, the probability of successful treatment is 30%. It is believed that the gonococcus is an important biologic marker of the status of the microbiologic environment and is in part responsible for inducing the progression of the microenvironment from aerobic to anaerobic. The addition of cefoxitin to the therapeutic regimen increases the therapeutic potential to 90% if the gonococcus is present and to 80% if it is not.

TABLE 21–4. GAINESVILLE STAGING OF ACUTE SALPINGITIS

Stage	Therapeutic Goal	Therapy
I—Acute salpingitis without peritonitis (ES)	Eradication of symptoms and ineffectivity	Doxycycline, 200 mg loading dose then 100 mg every 12 hours; route of administration: intravenous. Once clinical amelioration is achieved, conversion to oral route should be implemented.
II—Acute salpingitis with peritonitis (ESP)	Preservation of fallopian tube structure and function	
		and
		Cefoxitin, 2 g loading dose then 2 g every 6 hours. Once anticipated therapeutic response is achieved, parenteral drug administration can be discontinued.
		When administering a bacteriostatic-bactericidal antibiotic combination, it is prudent to administer the bactericidal antibiotic 1/2 hour before beginning the bacteriostatic drug.
III—Acute salpingitis with evidence of tubal occlusion or tubo-ovarian complex	Preservation of ovarian function	Triple Therapy: Penicillin, 2–5 million units every 6 hours; clindamycin, 600 mg every 6 hours; and tobramycin on mg/kg basis; route of administration: intravenous
IV—Ruptured tube-ovarian complex	Preservation of life	Triple therapy and surgical removal of diseased organ

From Monif GRG: Acute salpingitis. In: Monif GRG (ed), Infectious Diseases in Obstetrics and Gynecology. ed 3. Omaha, IDI, 1993: 79–99.

Selecting the best antibiotic therapy for stage II disease is benefited by knowing the type of polymicrobial infection that is present. The combination of cefoxitin and doxycycline allows these two medicines to offset their relative deficiencies. In combination, however, these medications are inadequate to cover enterococci. If only one organism is present, the three primary infecting organisms most likely are *N gonorrhoeae,* the penicillinase-producing strains of *N gonorrhoeae,* and *C trachomatis.* If a polymicrobial bacterial superinfection occurs, the traditional four-category coverage of the Gainesville classification is necessary.

The presence of tubal occlusion or a tubo-ovarian complex increases the disease to stage III, and antibiotic therapy with penicillin, clindamycin and an aminoglycoside (triple therapy) is implemented. Ultrasound examination of the pelvis is useful to help establish the presence of a tubo-ovarian complex.

Stage III: Suspected Tubal Occlusion or Tubo-ovarian Complex

Tubal occlusion may occur as a result of interstitial inflammation and secondary edema. The occlusion may occur proximally, distally, or in combination. When occlusion is both proximal and distal, the inflammatory exudate cannot drain into the peritoneal cavity through the distal end or into the endometrial cavity through the proximal opening. Because of the volume, intraluminal pressure is exerted that increases the diameter of the fallopian tube. The resulting pressure may lead to focal submucosal fibrosis and progression of the disease. If the occlusions remain permanent, a tubo-ovarian abscess develops.

The presence of tubal occlusion or a tubo-ovarian complex defines stage III disease and provides an anatomic marker for its progression. In this setting, preservation of fallopian tube function is diminished. To reduce the risk of surgical intervention, triple therapy (penicillin, clindamycin, and an aminoglycoside) is necessary. The goal is prevention of progression from aerobic to anaerobic infection. Aminoglycoside therapy rarely is needed for more than 72 hours. Parenteral therapy is typically discontinued 24 hours after the abatement of monitored evidence of infection. In stage III disease, transvaginal aspiration and drainage may be effective in reducing morbidity, accurately identifying the pathogens, and shortening hospital stay.

Stage IV: Ruptured Tubo-ovarian Complex

Stage IV disease is defined by rupture of a tubo-ovarian complex. This event represents an extremely serious medical condition, and the therapeutic goal is preservation of life. If rupture occurs from a location in the fallopian tube, omentum or intestine may ultimately close the defect and allow medical therapy to be successful. However, when rupture occurs at an ovarian site, there is an increased probability of associated septic thrombophlebitis. Unless surgical intervention is initiated, death is the likely outcome. Stage IV disease is a surgical condition that necessitates removal of the site of rupture in the presence of appropriate antibiotic coverage. Triple therapy (penicillin, clindamycin, and an aminoglycoside) should be administered to reduce postoperative infectious complications. Drainage should be strongly considered postoperatively and septic thrombophlebitis should be excluded.

Duration of Antimicrobial Therapy for Acute Salpingitis

The definition of adequate antimicrobial therapy remains a debated topic. The optimal duration of antibiotic therapy for acute salpingitis is unknown. Resolution of the signs and symptoms of disease within a 4-day period combined with nonprogression to a tubo-ovarian complex is considered a good therapeutic response. One can anticipate lysis of fever, disappearance of peritoneal inflammatory signs, and a marked reduction in organ tenderness within 36 hours. Failure of these events to occur suggests a complicating factor such as presence of an IUD, substantial prior structural damage, or tubal occlusion. The white blood cell (WBC) count usually falls to less than $10,000/mm^3$ within 48 hours after the onset of therapy. The total duration of therapy depends on the patient's clinical symptoms: her sense of well-being, her decline in WBC count, her comfort at abdominal and pelvic examination, and her return to afebrile status. One should monitor ESR in stage III disease to decide when to discontinue therapy. For optimal results, oral medication should be continued 7 to 10 days after discontinuation of intravenous antibiotics and improvement in clinical response.

Clinical Follow-up Care

On the basis of therapeutic efficacy of single-drug therapy for acute salpingitis among subgroups of patients with gonococcal salpingitis (determined by bacteriologic characterization of cul-de-sac aspirates), monomicrobial disease is relatively easy to manage with new-generation tetracyclines. Patients exhibit lysis of fever in 24 to 36 hours, marked amelioration of signs of peritoneal irritation and deep organ tenderness in 36 to 48 hours, and normal WBC count in 48 hours. Even when the initial WBC count is within normal limits, a marked decrease can be demonstrated in the first 48 hours of therapy.

The ability to achieve the anticipated therapeutic response observed for monomicrobial disease is altered in patients with advanced polymicrobial superinfection. When *N gonorrhoeae* is a constituent of a polymicrobial peritonitis, some patients have what are called secondary febrile spikes. After an initial reduction of temperature to less than 37.68°C, there is a secondary elevation to 388°C or greater, which is sustained for 4 hours. Other patients do not exhibit amelioration of physical findings and have a persistently elevated WBC count 48 hours after the initiation of therapy. The presence of a resistant anaerobic bacterial species in the cul-de-sac does not preclude duplication of the response of patients with monomicrobial disease. When an altered therapeutic response is observed, however, invariably one or more class II or III anaerobic bacteria are present and are beyond the therapeutic efficacy of the drug used.

Once basement membrane destruction has been achieved by either anaerobic bacteria or *C trachomatis,* the only resolution is healing by means of fibrosis, with its permanent alterations of fallopian tube function. Because tubal occlusion is not an invariable consequence of clinically overt salpingitis associated with *N gonorrhoeae* or *C trachomatis* infection (alone or in conjunction with the anaerobic progression) other clinically discernible factors may allow one to predict the probability of structural damage leading to infertility.

In his study of acute salpingitis, Heynemann[12] demonstrated that if antibiotic treatment is started early and adnexal tumors do not have time to form, the reproductive prognosis for these women is very good. If palpable adnexal masses develop, the prognosis for fertility is only about 18% to 20%.[12] Hedberg and Anberg[13] demonstrated that risk for infertility varied roughly with the duration of disease before treatment. Similarly, Falk[14] demonstrated that the interval between the onset of pain and medication with antibiotics was an important factor in prognostication about ability or inability to become pregnant at a future date. The higher the ESR or the larger the adnexal swelling, the poorer was the prognosis for subsequent reproductive outcomes.

Hedberg and Spetz[15] reviewed 216 cases of acute salpingitis. Cultures for *N gonorrhoeae* were positive for 96 and negative for 120 patients. The investigators found a better prognosis for fertility among women who had experienced gonococcal salpingitis than among those from whom gonococcus was not isolated. Viberg[16] surveyed a group of women about voluntary infertility and surgical intervention 2½ to 5 years after discharge from hospitalization for acute salpingitis. The incidence of pregnancy was better for patients with gonococcal versus nongonococcal salpingitis. The findings of these studies, which were conducted in the 1950s and 1960s, correlate well with our current understanding of the pathogenesis of acute gonococcal salpingitis.[17] In the absence of concomitant presence of *C trachomatis,* gonococcal salpingitis is initially monomicrobial. With alteration of the oxidation-reduction potential, anaerobic progression is initiated. The current theory is that anaerobic bacteria are primarily responsible for basement membrane destruction and healing by means of fibrosis within the fallopian tube. Early monoetiologic gonococcal salpingitis is associated with relatively limited elevation in ESR (20–45 mm/hr). With secondary

anaerobic bacterial superinfection, levels of 60 mm/hr or greater usually indicate the presence of tubal occlusion or the presence of tubo-ovarian complex.

Pelvic ultrasonography is being used with increased frequency in the evaluation and management of acute pelvic inflammatory disease.[18] Ultrasonographically guided transvaginal aspiration of any tubo-ovarian abscess or pyosalpinges can be performed at the time of diagnosis and the fluid sent for culture and sensitivity. When local and systemic administration of antibiotics is initiated at the time of the procedure, the response is effective for most patients, and laparotomy and laparoscopy can be avoided.

The ability to achieve what has been termed the anticipated therapeutic response had the best correlation with subsequent reproductive success. When acute salpingitis is exclusively due to *N gonorrhoeae* infection, there is a predictable clinical response, as follows: afebrile in 24 to 36 hours, loss of peritoneal signs and most deep organ tenderness in 36 to 48 hours, and a normalization of the WBC count within 24 to 48 hours.[10] When *N gonorrhoeae* is present as part of polymicrobial peritonitis or has undergone autoelimination and replacement by an anaerobic isolate, the probability of an altered therapeutic response is greatly enhanced.

When these two groups of patients were followed longitudinally, predicated on their ability to achieve or not achieve the "anticipated therapeutic response," a good therapeutic response resulted in a reproductive potential not grossly different from that of matched controls. An altered therapeutic response correlated in a statistically significant manner with ensuing negative reproductive outcomes.

An inverse correlation exists between duration of disease after initiation of effective therapy and subsequent reproductive outcome.[12,13] The therapeutic window is defined as the time from onset of disease to the initiation of appropriate therapy. The therapeutic window may be limited to as little as 25 hours between onset of clinical overt disease and therapy.

C trachomatis is an obligate, intracellular, gram-negative organism that contains both RNA and DNA. Failure to supply the organism with essential growth factors can lead to a state of latency, which is recognized as a common state in the natural history of chlamydial infections. Women who harbor the organism may have few or no symptoms for months.

C trachomatis has become the most common cause of sexually transmitted disease in many countries.[17] The frequency of isolation from the cervix of women with acute salpingitis is between 5% and 40%. In a limited series, the organism was recovered from the fallopian tubes or peritoneal exudates of as many as 30% of patients with acute salpingitis. When one looks at the prevalence of *C trachomatis* infection among patients with prior salpingitis or infertility, the frequency of recovering the organism from patients with asymptomatic infection is alarming.

In contrast to gonococcal salpingitis, chlamydial tubal infection appears to be a true chronic, active infection. Intracellular organisms may persist in the genital tissue for extremely long periods and continue to produce silent, progressive tubal damage unless treatment with appropriate antibiotics is instituted.[19–24] When infertile patients with chlamydial antibodies undergo laparoscopic examination, frequently no history of an illness or procedure can be elicited to explain the presence of postinflammatory tubal damage.

In 1995, the World Health Organization Task Force on the prevention and management of infertility concluded a multicenter case-control study that compared women who had bilateral tubal occlusion with infertile women and age-matched pregnant controls.[25] Reproductive and sexual histories were evaluated and IgG antibodies to *C trachomatis* and *N gonorrhoeae* were measured. Women with past chlamydial or gonococcal infection or both were more likely to have bilateral tubal occlusion, a statistically significant finding; however, most of the women with bilateral occlusion reported no history of pelvic inflammatory disease systems. Women in the infertile group had a prevalence of *C trachomatis* antibodies (60%), which was similar to that of patients with bilateral tubal occlusion (71%).

According to the Centers for Disease Control and Prevention, chlamydial infections affect as many as 4 million men and women. More than 75% of cases of chlamydia among women are asymptomatic (which results in $2.1 billion being spent annually for chlamydia-related health costs). The tragedy of disease-related infertility will continue until eradication of chlamydial infection is made a global priority.[13,24]

The tubal disease associated with *C trachomatis* infection has been suggested to be medicated by an autoimmune cross reaction between the 60-kd chlamydial heat shock protein (HSP) and the 60-kd HSP found on human epithelial cells.[26] The cross reactivity is due to an almost 50% amino acid sequence shared between the two 60-kd proteins. Antibodies to *C trachomatis* were present in nearly 73% of women with tubal infertility compared with 32% of other causes of infertility. The chlamydial HSP 60 detected *Chlamydia* organisms associated infertility in infertile women with a sensitivity of 81.3% and a specificity of 97.5%. The reproductive consequences for women of serologic evidence of *C trachomatis* infection may be not only

pelvic inflammatory disease and tubal infertility but also reproductive loss due to ectopic pregnancy and spontaneous abortion.[27] Women previously infected with *C trachomatis* may also be at risk for preterm birth.[28] The positive predictive value of a seropositive result for preterm birth is 31%.

Additional studies performed on patients with tubal disease undergoing in vitro fertilization with and without serologic evidence of *C trachomatis* infection and chlamydial HSP 60 suggest another striking effect of certain chlamydial infections on reproductive potential. Although there were no differences in pregnancy rates or outcomes between *C trachomatis* seropositive versus seronegative groups, the *C trachomatis* positive group demonstrated a statistically significantly higher pregnancy rate than the chlamydial HSP 60 antibody negative patients (>40% versus 7%).[29] The reason for this finding has not yet been elucidated. Heat shock antibody is generally associated with inflammation. However, the putative trophoblast/lymphocyte cross-reactive (TLX) antigen necessary for the autoantiidiotypic antibodies to allow normal pregnancy is also likely to have a 60-kd molecular weight.[30] Whether the chlamydial HSP 60 antibody responds to this putative TLX antigen or works through other mechanisms remains to be determined.

M tuberculosis and *Coccidioides immitis,* among other organisms, are also fully capable of inducing permanent anatomic and functional sequelae, primarily by destroying the basement membrane. The frequency of genital tuberculosis among infertile women can range from 0.5% to 2.0% of all cases. A Mantoux intradermal skin test should be a standard part of every clinical evaluation of infertility, especially among patients who travel to and from countries where tuberculosis is prevalent. A positive reaction, which is induration more than 10 mm in diameter developing within 48 hours, should alert the physician to the possibility of genital tuberculosis. More important is a negative reaction, which for healthy patients effectively eliminates tuberculosis from diagnostic consideration.

ENDOMETRIAL-CERVICAL INFERTILITY OF INFECTIOUS CAUSATION

Gaps in our knowledge have been inferred by the high frequency of reproductive failure among patients without demonstrable evidence of endocrine dysfunction, hysterosalpingographic abnormalities, or any adverse finding in the postcoital test and with normal menstrual cycles and partners with no abnormalities in semen analysis. Our frustration has caused us to seek a possible causal relation between infertility and a specific organism functioning at the endocervical level. What has been the area of therapeutic controversy is whether a selected organism or flora exists eradication of which would restore the potential for a successful pregnancy. The principal two organisms incriminated in the hypothesis that are thought to function at the cervical level are *Mycoplasma hominis* and *Ureaplasma urealyticum.*

Women with secondary infertility tend to have an elevated vaginal pH and complex microbiologic flora in which the anaerobic component is increased both quantitatively and qualitatively. *Mycop hominis, U urealyticum,* or both can be isolated more frequently from such individuals than from matched controls. The fundamental question is whether either or both of these organisms can exert a negative cervical or endometrial influence on fertilization.[31,32]

The microbiologic hypothesis is based primarily on reports that initial isolation of mycoplasmata from the genital organs occurred more commonly among women with unexplained fertility than among matched controls and the observation that frequently after treatment of *Mycoplasma* infection conception occurred.[31,32] Indirect support for the hypothesis was furnished by the inference that infection of endometrial tissue by *Mycop hominis* may inhibit sperm migration by inducing changes in the ciliated cells that line the fallopian tubes in a manner similar to that described for *Mycop pneumoniae* infection.

A somewhat better case has been made for *U urealyticum* as a potentially correctable factor in secondary infertility.[31-36] At least one other study substantiated the report by Friberg[31] of a higher frequency of *U urealyticum* in a group of patients with unexplained infertility of at least 5 years' duration than among couples with proved fertility. A theoretic mechanism has been inferred from the observation that some strains of *U urealyticum* isolated from infertile couples have been shown to be able to produce neuraminidase-like substances.[19] Neuraminidase can interfere with implantation and blastocyst development in mice. This blastocystotoxic effect has been postulated as an explanation for infertility and spontaneous abortion among patients infected with *U urealyticum.*[27,34]

The problem with demographic studies has always been the appropriateness of the control group. The growth of *Mycop hominis* in the vagina is favored by pH shifts to the alkaline range. The organism achieves optimum growth at pH 7.4. *U urealyticum* prefers an environment somewhat acidic but relatively alkaline in comparison with normal vaginal pH. Both organisms grow best in microaerophilic environments. In studies that are carefully controlled and comparative, there is no difference in frequency of recovery of either *Mycop hominis* or *U urealyticum.* Any condition that elicits a local inflammatory response tends to enhance the probability of *Mycoplasma*

colonization. The prevalence of the organism increases with pregnancy, abortion, and the development of tubo-ovarian complexes.

In vitro studies have shown that *U urealyticum* does not alter the physiologic characteristics of vaginal fluid or cervical mucus, sperm penetration, or sperm viability in cervical mucus. In well-controlled studies, eradication of *Mycoplasma* with doxycycline therapy is not associated with an improved conception rate. It is the microbiologic environment that governs the presence or absence of these two organisms. A causal relation between subclinical infection with *Mycoplasma* and secondary infertility is not tenable according to existing data.

MICROBIOLOGIC EVALUATION

Exclusion of a tubal pathogen is the key to microbiologic evaluation for infertile patients.

Pathogens

Mycobacterium tuberculosis

The diagnosis of genital tuberculosis may be established on the basis of the histopathologic features of a *premenstrual* endometrial biopsy specimen or curettage fragments. One half of endometrial fragments are prepared for culture and guinea pig inoculation and the other half for histologic examination. Unfortunately, guinea pigs are not generally available, and conventional culture media may have to be used. The diagnosis is generally established by the presence of granulomas containing acid-fast bacilli. The failure to demonstrate the organism by the Ziehl–Neelsen technique does not invalidate the diagnosis except in the absence of evidence of delayed hypersensitivity (that is, a negative test with second-strength purified protein derivative [PPD]).

Occasionally, histologic examination of the endometrial tissue alone does not reveal disease because of sampling erors or noninvolvement of the endometrium when the fallopian tubes are the principal sites of infection. When a high index of suspicion exists, bacteriologic examination is important and should be performed. Menstrual blood collected in a Tassett cup provides additional material for culture. One variable usually not controlled is the point in the menstrual cycle at which the sample is taken. This variable influences the probability of organism recovery; for example, the progesterone phase is associated with diminished probability of recovery.

Hysterosalpingograms may reveal closed tubes with a tobacco-pouch deformity of the ampullary end or a rigid pipestem pattern. In contrast to the morphologic changes in chronic salpingitis the fimbriae are not involved. Some of the infected tubes demonstrate numerous fistulas. Because fallopian tubes infected with *M tuberculosis* are often segmentally obstructed, tubal operations seldom are successful in establishing patency or restoring function.

Chlamydia trachomatis

Tissue culture is the standard for laboratory diagnosis of *C trachomatis* infection. Although published methods are fairly standard, in practice many laboratories introduce variations that alter the sensitivity and specificity of the test.

Two components are needed to culture for *C trachomatis*: a cell-culture system and a method to identify inclusions growing in cell culture. The cell line of choice is McCoy. A particular strain of HeLa cells (HeLa 229) can be used, but this option is usually restricted to research laboratories. Specimen material is centrifuged into the cells for 1 hour and then incubated for 2 to 3 days in medium containing cycloheximide. Incubation can take place in individual vials with coverslips at the base or on flat-bottomed wells in plastic microtiter plates. The choice between methods is generally dictated by the number of specimens a laboratory has to process. The vial method is slightly more sensitive and less susceptible to cross contamination but is more time consuming and expensive.

Compared with other diagnostic tests for *C trachomatis,* the advantage of tissue culture is its specificity. With this method, the organism can be positively identified or saved for other marker studies such as immunotyping. It has been the method of choice for research studies. Determining the sensitivity and specificity has not been possible because it is the reference standard for other methods; however, it is estimated that culture has a sensitivity of 80% to 90% and a specificity of 100%.

Culture also has several disadvantages. The cost and complexity of laboratory requirements can be prohibitive. Specimens can be kept at 48°C only up to 24 hours (preferably 12 hours) before processing or must be frozen at –70°C if they cannot be inoculated within 24 hours. Specimens must be placed in specially prepared transport media. The cell monolayer may become contaminated with other bacteria or viruses, particularly in vaginal or rectal specimens.

In collecting any specimen for chlamydial culture, it is imperative to avoid sampling mucopurulent exudate. Because *C trachomatis* is an obligatory intracellular organism, the specimen must contain endocervical cells. Cotton swabs are best avoided because of the possible presence of cytotoxic material. Use of a Dacron or nylon swab with a plastic or wire shaft is advocated.

Compared with other diagnostic tests for *C trachomatis,* the advantage of tissue culture is its specificity. With this method, the organism can be positively identified or saved for other marker studies such as immunotyping. Thus culture is clearly the method of choice for research studies. It is estimated that culture has a sensitivity of 80%. Scrapings provided 102 (92.7%) of 110 diagnoses of cervical infection, the first scraping yielding 76 (69.0%), the second an additional 22 (20.0%), and the third another 4 (3.6%). These data are very similar to those documented for *N gonorrhoeae.* They clearly demonstrate that the use of a single swab underestimates the prevalence of chlamydial infection.

Techniques

Enzyme Immunoassay

An enzyme immunoassay (EIA) is used to measure antigen-antibody reactions through an enzyme-linked immunosorbent assay (ELISA) and requires a spectrophotometer. Processing time for specimens is approximately 4 hours. Questions continue to be raised about the reliability of EIA for *C trachomatis.* The sensitivity of the test has varied from 67% to 90%, the specificity from 92% to 97%, and the positive predictive value from 32% to 87% depending on the population studied. Much of the observed disparity has been attributed to variable sensitivity of the tissue culture systems with which the EIA has been compared. The advantages of ELISA are uncomplicated transport and storage of specimens, objective method of measurement in the laboratory, which involves standard equipment and does not depend on a specially trained observer, and the ability to test large numbers of specimens at one time.

DNA Probe

DNA probes has been introduced for the diagnosis of chlamydial infection. Nucleic acid hybridization tests are based on the ability of complementary nucleic acid strands specifically to align and associate to form stable double-stranded complexes. The probe is a chemoluminescent, labeled, single-stranded DNA probe that is complementary to the ribosomal RNA of the target organism. After the ribosomal RNA is released from the organism, the labeled DNA probe combines with the ribosomal RNA of the target organism to form a stable DNA:RNA hybrid. The labeled DNA:RNA hybrid is separated from the nonhybridized probe and measured. The principal advantage of DNA probes is the ability to screen concomitantly for *N gonorrhoeae.* The benefits derived from the detection of additional positive specimens for *N gonorrhoeae* outweigh the additional cost over more conventional diagnostic techniques. DNA probes for the detection of *C trachomatis* in the past have appeared to be just slightly less sensitive than culture or EIA. However, recent data suggest that molecular biologic techniques with polymerase chain reaction (PCR) are more reliable and specific than either ELISA or tissue culture in the detection of the presence of

Chlamydia infection in women without symptoms (P. Claman, personal communication, 1995).

Serologic Testing

Serologic diagnosis traditionally has relied on complement fixation (CF). Acute systemic infection produces a CF titer greater than 1:64, whereas infections limited to mucosal membranes produce a weak response. Microimmunofluorescence is more sensitive and is used preferentially. To be indicative of infection, serologic testing must demonstrate a fourfold or greater rise in IgG antibody titer or the presence of IgM antibodies for about 1 month.

INFECTIOUS COMPLICATIONS OF INTRAUTERINE INSEMINATION

Bacterial infection associated with intrauterine insemination (IUI) is a rare complication. A review of the literature identified only five cases of pelvic infection after IUI.[37] The prevalence of infectious complication is 1.83 per 1000 women undergoing IUI. To date there is little evidence to indicate that the prevalence is altered by administration of prophylactic antibiotics or washing semen samples with antibiotics. However, care must be taken to be certain that raw or unwashed semen is not injected into the uterus. Should that occur, severe cramping and even anaphylaxis have been reported. This situation is most likely to happen when donor sperm for IUI is obtained from a sperm bank and the person injecting the sample does not realize the semen was not shipped prepared for IUI. Extreme care is warranted whenever sperm is obtained or prepared at a source other than the physician's own facility.

VIRAL INFECTIONS AND THEIR CONTRIBUTION TO REPRODUCTION

Each year, approximately 75,000 women in the United States undergo artificial insemination with unrelated-donor semen.[38] Concern regarding transmission of viral infections by means of artificial insemination is warranted. Acquired immune deficiency syndrome (AIDS) is the most frequent killer of Americans 25 to 44 years of age. The spread of HIV is so rampant that AIDS is expected to be the second most frequent killer of women (behind heart disease) by the year 2000. The infectious potential of donor insemination is made painfully obvious by the fact that gonorrhea, hepatitis B, genital herpes infection, CMV infection, *Trichomonas vaginalis* infestation, *C trachomatis* infection, and HIV infection all have been transmitted by this route.[39–42] Most of these infections occurred

prior to 1986, when routine testing of all donors for these diseases was not performed and fresh semen samples typically were used. Today guidelines set forth by the American Society for Reproductive Medicine recommend testing both donors and recipients for a wide range of infectious diseases.[43] Donated semen samples are cryopreserved for 6 months, and the semen donor retested for diseases capable of seroconversion. Semen samples are not released for clinical use until the second test is negative.

Viral conditions may affect reproduction in another way. Couples in whom one spouse is seropositive for HIV are indirectly rendered infertile because of fear of transmission to the HIV-negative partner and to the fetus.[44] Although treatment by means of therapeutic insemination with husband's sperm for HIV-positive male and HIV-negative female couples has been reported,[45] it is extremely ill advised because not all HIV is contained within white blood cells, and the free virus cannot be washed away with certainty.[46] Such couples should be counseled to consider donor insemination if the man is infected and gestational surrogacy if the woman is infected. The ethical dilemma of counseling infertile couples infected with HIV is beyond the scope of this chapter.

CMV is another extremely important infection for both fertile and infertile couples of reproductive age. CMV infection is the most common congenital infection.[47] CMV infection manifests itself with flu-like symptoms in adults. Estimates suggest that 37,000 newborns in the United States annually have congenital CMV infection (1% of all live-born infants), and 10% of these infants manifest symptoms of infection. Approximately 85% of infants with symptoms experience some degree of mental retardation. Other symptoms of congenital CMV infection include deafness, blindness, intrauterine growth retardation, chorioretinitis, purpura, thrombocytopenia, microcephaly, hemolytic anemia, neonatal jaundice, hepatitis, and seizures. Transmission to the fetus is not limited to sexual exposure; it may occur by means of contact with blood products, urine, and saliva. After childbirth, transmission to the newborn may occur via breast milk.

Although congenital CMV infection may be transmitted to a newborn through reactivation of the latent virus, symptomatic disease is virtually always the result of a seronegative female's becoming infected during pregnancy.

Determination of infection is established by the presence of CMV IgG in serum. This test remains positive for life. Acute infection is detected with an initial rise in CMV IgM level, which remains elevated for about 1 month. Patients considering pregnancy should be tested initially for CMV IgM. If the test is positive, attempts at pregnancy should be delayed for 3 months, virtually eliminating congenital CMV infection as a problem.

PROCEDURAL SEQUENCE

The microbiologic evaluation for an infertile couple should include a PPD test and serologic testing for rubella and *Chlamydia*. Smears or swabs to detect *C trachomatis* should be obtained concomitantly. Once this information is received, an endometrial biopsy is performed for histologic analysis and possible culturing. If results of the PPD test are positive, a portion of the biopsy specimen or a second sample should be cultured for *M tuberculosis*.

If evidence of prior or current infection with *C trachomatis* is identified, we advocate treating the patient with doxycycline, 100 mg twice a day for 14 days. The patient's partner should be treated simultaneously. If the patient has no evidence of prior or current infection with *M tuberculosis* or *C trachomatis* but an endometrial biopsy shows evidence of a chronic inflammatory infiltrate, I perform a repeat biopsy of the endometrium to obtain cultures for microbiologic processing. Given totally negative cultures, I most infrequently offer a blind therapeutic challenge with a narrow-spectrum antibiotic and perform another biopsy 14 days after therapy. For such a patient, I explain that this approach is empirical. Patients who are seronegative for rubella are offered immunization, and treatment is delayed for 3 months. Infertile patients who need assisted reproductive technologies are screened in accordance with the guidelines recommended by the American Society for Reproductive Medicine.

REFERENCES

1. Schachter J: Chlamydial infection. *N Engl J Med* 298:428, 1978
2. Westrom L: Incidence: Effect of acute inflammatory disease on fertility. *Am J Obstet Gynecol* 121:707, 1975, 707–13
3. Monif GRG: Infection. In Seibel MM (ed), *Infertility: A Comprehensive Text.* Appleton & Lange, Norwalk, CT, 1990:235–240
4. Westrom L: Incidence, prevalence and trends of acute pelvic inflammatory disease and its consequences in industrialized countries. *Am J Obstet Gynecol* 138:880, 1980
5. Monif GRG: Choice of antibiotics and length of therapy in the treatment of acute salpingitis. *Am J Med* 78(Suppl 6B):188, 1985
6. Viberg L: Acute inflammatory conditions of the uterine adnexa. *Acta Obstet Gynecol Scand* 38(Suppl 4):1, 1964
7. Chow AW, Malkasian KL, Marshall JR, et al: The bacteriology of acute pelvic inflammatory disease. *N Engl J Med* 293:166, 1975
8. Eschenbach DA, Buchanan TM, Pollock HM, et al: Polymicrobial etiology of acute pelvic inflammatory disease: Value of cul-de-sac cultures and relative importance of gonococci and other aerobic or anaerobic bacteria. *Am J Obstet Gynecol* 122:876, 1975
9. Monif GRG, Welkos SL, Baer H, Thompson RLJ: Cul-de-sac isolates from patients with endometritis/salpingitis/peritonitis and gonococcal endocervicitis. *Am J Obstet Gynecol* 126:158, 1976
10. Monif GRG: Clinical staging of acute bacterial salpingitis and its therapeutic ramification. *Am J Obstet Gynecol* 143:489, 1982
11. March PA, Holmes KK, Oriel JD, Piot P, Schachter J (eds): *Chlamydial Infections.* Proceedings of the 5th International Symposium on Human Chlamydia Infections, June 15–19, 1982, Lund, Sweden. Amsterdam, Elsevier, 1982
12. Heynemann T: Entzuedung der adnexe. In: Seitzl, Amrelch AI, (eds), *Biologix unde Pathologic des Weibes,* ed 5. Munich, Urban & Schwarzenberg, 1953:19
13. Hedberg E, Anberg A: Gonorrheal salpingitis: Views on treatment and progress. *Fertil Steril* 16:125, 1965
14. Falk V: Treatment of acute non-tuberculosis salpingitis with antibiotics alone and in combination with glucocorticoids: Acute salpingitis with special reference to laparoscopy. *Acta Obstet Gynecol Scand* 44(Suppl 6):1, 1965
15. Hedberg E, Spetz SO: Acute salpingitis: Views on prognosis and treatment. *Acta Obstet Gynecol Scand* 37:131, 1958
16. Viberg L: Diagnosis of acute salpingitis: Interpretation of the pathogens with special reference to laparoscopy. *Acta Obstet Gynecol Scand* 54(Suppl 6): 1965
17. Monif GRG: Acute salpingitis. In: Monif GRG (ed), *Infectious Diseases in Obstetrics and Gynecology,* ed 3. Omaha, IDI, 1993:79–99
18. Aboulghar MA, Mansour RT, Serour GI: Ultrasonographically guided transvaginal aspiration of tubovarian abscesses and pyosalpinges: An optional treatment for acute pelvic inflammatory disease. *Am J Obstet Gynecol* 172:1501, 1995
19. Gump DW, Gibson M, Ashikawaga T: Infertile women and *Chlamydia trachomatis* infection. In: March PA, Holmes KK, Oriel JD, Piot P, Schachter J (eds), *Chlamydial Infections.* Proceedings of the 5th International Symposium on Hymen Chlamydial Infections, June 15–19, 1982, Lund, Sweden. Amsterdam, Elsevier, 1982
20. Washington AE, Gove S, Schachter J, Sweet RL: Oral contraceptives, *Chlamydia trachomatis* infection, and pelvic inflammatory disease: A word of caution about protection. *JAMA* 253:2246, 1985
21. Pummomen R, Terho P, Mikkanon V, et al: Chlamydia serology in infertile women by immunofluorescence. *Fertil Steril* 31:656, 1976
22. Sweet RL: Chlamydia salpingitis and infertility. *Fertil Steril* 38:530, 1982
23. Henry-Suchet J, Catalan F, Loffredo V, et al: *Chlamydia trachomatis* associated with chronic inflammation in abdominal specimens from women selected for tuboplasty. *Fertil Steril* 36:599, 1981
24. Henry-Suchet J, Catalan F, Loffredo V, et al: *Chlamydia trachomatis* and mycoplasma research by laparoscopy in cases of pelvic inflammatory disease and in cases of tubal obstruction. *Am J Obstet Gynecol* 138:1022, 1980
25. World Health Organization Task Force on the Prevention and Management of Infertility: Tubal infertility: Serologic relationship to past chlamydial and gonococcal infection. *Sex Transm Dis* 22:71, 1995

26. Toye B, Laferriere C, Claman P, Jessamine P, Peeling R: Association between antibody to chlamydial heat shock protein and tubal infertility. *J Infect Dis* 168:1236, 1993

27. Rae R, Smith IW, Liston WA, Kilpatrick DC: Chlamydial serologic studies and recurrent spontaneous abortion. *Am J Obstet Gynecol* 170:783, 1994

28. Claman P, Toye B, Peeling RW, Jessamine P, Belcher J: Serologic evidence of *Chlamydia trachomatis* infection and risk of preterm birth. *Can Med Assoc J* 153:259, 1995

29. Claman P, Amimi MN, Peeling R, Toye B, Jessamine P: Does serologic evidence of remote *Chlamydia trachomatis* infection and its heat shock protein (CHSP 60) affect in vitro fertilization–embryo transfer outcome? *Fertil Steril* 65:146, 1996

30. Stern PL, Beresford N, Thompson S, Johnson PM, Webb PD, Hole N: Characterization of the human trophoblast leukocyte common antigen molecules defined by monoclonal antibody. *J Immunol* 137:1604, 1986

31. Frieberg J: Mycoplasmas and ureaplasmas in infertility and abortion. *Fertil Steril* 33:351, 1980

32. Holmes KK: *Mycoplasma hominis*: A human pathogen. *Sex Transm Dis* 11:159, 1984

33. Stray-Pedersen B: Female genital colonization with *Ureaplasma urealyticum* and reproductive failure. *Obstet Gynecol Surv* 35:467, 1980

34. Seibel MM: Infection and infertility. In: De Cherney AH (ed), *Reproductive Failure*. New York, Churchill Livingstone, 1986: 203–218

35. Desai S, Cohen MS, Khatatmee M, Lenter E: *Ureaplasma urealyticum* (T-mycoplasma) infection: Does it have a role in male infertility: *J Urol* 124:469, 1980

36. Cassell GH, Brown MB, Younger JB, et al: Incidence of genital mycoplasmas in women at the time of diagnostic laparoscopy. *Yale J Biol Med* 56:557, 1983

37. Sacks PC, Simon JA: Infectious complications of intrauterine insemination: A case report and literature review. *Int J Fertil* 36:331, 1991

38. Centers for Disease Control and Prevention: Guidelines for preventing transmission of human immunodeficiency virus through transplantation of human tissue and organs. *MMWR Morb Mortal Wkly Rep* 43(Suppl RR-8):1, 1994

39. Arameta MRG, Mascola L, Eller A, et al: HIV transmission through donor artificial insemination. *JAMA* 273:854, 1995

40. Berry WR, Gottesfeld RL, Alter HJ, Vierling JM: Transmission of hepatitis B virus by artificial insemination. *JAMA* 257:1097, 1987

41. Moore DE, Ashley RL, Zarutskie PW, et al: Transmission of genital herpes by donor insemination. *JAMA* 261:3441, 1989

42. Nagel TC, Tagatz GE, Campbell BF: Transmission of *Chlamydia trachomatis* by artificial insemination. *Fertil Steril* 46:959, 1986

43. American Fertility Society: New guidelines for the use of semen donor insemination. *Fertil Steril* 53(Suppl 1):1, 1990

44. Peckham C, Gibb D: Mother-to-child transmission of the human immunodeficiency virus. *N Engl J Med* 333:298, 1995

45. Sempini AE, Levi-Setti P, Ravizza M, et al: Insemination of HIV-negative women with processed semen of HIV-positive partners. *Lancet* 340:1317, 1992

46. Ilaria G, Jacobs JL, Polsky B, et al: Detection of HIV-1 DNA sequences in preejaculatory fluid. *Lancet* 340:1469, 1992

47. Monif GRG: Cytomegaloviruses in infectious diseases in obstetrics and gynecology. Monif GRG (ed), 3rd edition, Omaha, IDT, 1993:2

CHAPTER 22

Molecular Genetics and Infertility

WILLIAM J. BUTLER · PAUL G. MCDONOUGH

Genetics and Molecular Biology

Genetics Control of Gametogenesis
  Oogenesis
  Spermatogenesis
  Pathophysiology of gametogenesis
  and fertilization
Other Known Genetic Causes of Infertility
  Multifactorial disorders
  Mendelian disorders
Molecular Genetics and Reproductive Biology

The burgeoning field of molecular biology has led to substantial advances in our understanding of clinical disease. In particular, the application of molecular biology in reproductive medicine has expanded our understanding of basic reproductive biology and provided new tools to investigate the causes of infertility and recurrent pregnancy loss. This chapter presents a brief basic review of molecular genetics, including the recombinant DNA techniques that are used in the diagnosis of genetic disorders. It then reviews how this technology has been applied to the problem of infertility. The review includes the genetic control of gametogenesis and sex determination, endocrine disorders that can lead to infertility, other genetic causes of infertility, and the genetics of recurrent pregnancy loss.

MOLECULAR GENETICS

Gene Structure

The molecular structure of deoxyribonucleic acid (DNA) was first described by Watson and Crick in 1953 (Fig 22–1).[1] DNA has a double helical structure composed of two chains of alternating deoxyribose and phosphate molecules linked by paired nitrogenous bases. The purine bases, adenine and guanine, pair specifically with the pyrimidine bases, thymine (replaced by uracil in RNA) and cytosine, respectively. This specific pairing results in the opposing chains' being both antiparallel and complementary. Denaturation or separation of the chains can allow

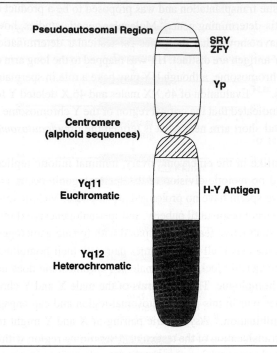

Figure 22–5. Human Y chromosome. Map of genes involved in sex determination.

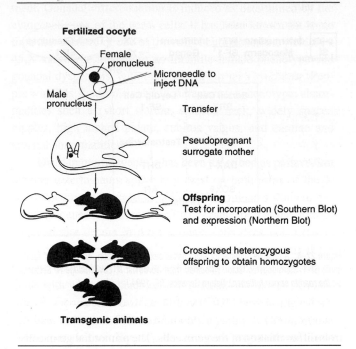

Figure 22–6. Insertional mutagenesis. Making transgenic animals.

One transgenic embryo that developed to maturity had a normal male phenotype with small testes but without spermatogenesis consistent with the findings in nontransgenic XX males. The direct evidence of germ-line sex reversal supports the hypothesis that *SRY* is the sex-determining region in mice and probably also in humans. There are still some unanswered questions, however. *SRY* sequences have been found in most but not all 46,XX males but not in 46,XX true hermaphrodites who also have testicular tissue.[48] Most 46,XY females have intact *SRY* genes, and approximately 10% exhibit mutations.[49,50] All mutations reported to date are located in a highly conserved 80–amino acid motif common to high-mobility group proteins, which are known to be DNA-binding transcription factors. Alternative mechanisms for sex reversal must be postulated to explain the exceptions.

SRY directs male gonadal differentiation. Differentiation of the Sertoli cell is an early male-specific change that, as previously noted, is important in inhibition of meiosis and direction of primordial germ-cell differentiation toward spermatogonia. Sertoli cells also produce MIS. The gene for MIS has been cloned and mapped to the short arm of chromosome 19.[51,52] MIS causes regression of the müllerian ducts during early male embryogenesis and has been noted to be expressed in granulosa cells in females where it may act to inhibit oocyte meiosis.[53] Experimental evidence is now accumulating demonstrating the role of *SRY* in the transcriptional regulation of

MIS.[54] The mechanism of action is not direct but appears to have intervening regulatory factors between *SRY* and the MIS promoter. *SRY* has also been shown to induce sexually dymorphic expression of SF-1 with early transcripts present in both sexes but subsequent levels declining in females during differentiation.[26,55] SF-1 binds to an upstream regulatory element of the MIS gene and may be one of the intervening regulatory factors between *SRY* and MIS expression (see Fig 22–4).

Two other genes have been implicated in the *SRY*-induced cascade leading to male sexual differentiation. The *SOX9* gene codes for a protein with a DNA-binding domain related to *SRY*. Mutation in one allele leads to a phenotype of severe dwarfism associated with XY female sex reversal.[56] Some XY females have a duplication in the short arm of the X chromosome that contains a gene encoding another member of the nuclear hormone receptor superfamily, *DAX 1*.[57] This gene is expressed in the genital ridge in mice of both sexes, and duplication may result in dose-sensitive sex reversal.

Another example of the dose effect is the presence of excess ovarian determinants in males with 47,XXY Klinefelter's syndrome leading to impaired spermatogenesis.[58] Approximately 12.5% of azospermic men (and 6.7% of oligospermic men) exhibit chromosomal anomalies, 70% of which are Klinefelter's syndrome. In men with oligospermia, robertsonian translocations are more frequent. The mechanism by which excess ovarian determinants on an extra X chromosome inhibit spermatogenesis is not clear. Balanced translocation carriers may be sterile secondary to the formation of long chromosome chains during meiosis I, inhibiting inactivation of the X chromosome and therefore causing a syndrome similar to the presence of an extra X.[59]

Other Genes That Affect Reproductive Function

Many patients may have abnormal gonadal development in the absence of a specific identifiable chromosomal or gene defect.[21,60] Reindollar et al[21] coined the term *chromosomally competent ovarian failure* (CCOF) to describe this condition. Females with 46,XX ovarian failure lack the phenotypic findings of patients with CIOF and may seek treatment either before puberty with sexual infantilism or after puberty with premature ovarian failure. Some retained reproductive function is more common among these patients than among those with privation of gonadal determinants.[22] Although the occurrence of CCOF is usually sporadic, some pedigrees exhibit autosomal recessive forms of inheritance.

Specific genetic syndromes have been identified that have gonadal failure as part of the phenotype. The gene for myotonia dystrophica has been identified and localized to the long arm of chromosome 19.[61] This is an autosomal dominant disorder characterized by progressive muscular dystrophy, myoclonus, cardiac involvement, and gonadal atrophy.[62] Mutations in the gene involve an increasing number of a three–base pair repeat sequence, which normally occurs in the 3′ untranslated region of the gene. When the number of repeats exceeds a threshold, the disease manifests itself.[61] Because the number of repeats can expand during meiosis, the severity of the disease can increase in subsequent generations, particularly when the abnormal gene is inherited from the mother.

Galactosemia is an autosomal recessive disease secondary to a deficiency of one of three different enzymes involved in galactose metabolism. The most common form of the disease involves the gene for galactose-1-phosphate uridyltransferase, which has been localized on the short arm of chromosome 9.[60] Patients homozygous for the mutated gene may have ovarian failure, possibly secondary to gonadal infiltration by abnormal metabolites.[63]

A particularly interesting syndrome associated with gonadal failure is Prader-Willi.[64] This is a sporadically occurring syndrome that affects males and females and is characterized by hypotonia, obesity, hyperphagia, mental retardation, and hypogonadotropic hypogonadism. Approximately one half of patients have a microdeletion on the long arm of chromosome 15 (15q11q13). The other half have uniparental isodisomy for the maternal chromosome 15 segment with loss of the paternally derived segment. Patients who have duplication of the paternally derived segment with loss of the maternally derived

segment have a phenotypically different syndrome, termed *Angelman syndrome*. The processes of genomic imprinting and uniparental isodisomy are discussed in the section on genetic causes of pregnancy loss.

REPRODUCTIVE ENDOCRINOLOGY

GnRH/GAP Gene

Molecular analysis of genes that encode hormones involved in the ovulatory process has given new insight into regulation of hypothalamic, pituitary, and gonadal function. Gonadotropin-releasing hormone (GnRH) is a decapeptide secreted from the hypothalamus that controls both synthesis and release of gonadotropins from the anterior pituitary gland. The gene for human GnRH has been cloned and localized to the short arm of chromosome 8. This single-copy gene contains 4 exons that encode a 92–amino acid precursor protein. This precursor molecule includes a 23–amino acid signal peptide, the GnRH decapeptide, three amino acids involved in processing, and a 56–amino acid protein termed *gonadotropin-associated peptide* (GnRH).[65] The existence of GAP had not been previously suspected, and studies have shown that it is both a potent gonadotropin secretagogue and a prolactin inhibitor.[66] The exact biologic function of GAP has yet to be determined, but studies have shown that the peptide is present in the hypothalamus and is present in the same cells as the messenger RNA for GnRH.

The *GnRH* gene is expressed in the hypothalamus and in the placenta. The mRNA in the placenta is approximately 1 kilobase (kb) longer than in the hypothalamus, because intron 1 is not spliced out during transcription. The promoter regions for placental and hypothalamic expression are different, implying differential transcriptional regulation.[67] Another interesting finding was the identification of a piece of mRNA derived from intron 1 that is transcribed from the opposite DNA strand (antisense) from that used to produce GnRH mRNA. Transcripts of this mRNA are present in cardiac muscle and in the hypothalamus and may be involved in GnRH transcriptional regulation.[68] The GnRH receptor gene has been identified. The gene codes for a 328–amino acid protein with seven transmembrane domains characteristic of G-protein–coupled receptors but lacking the carboxy-terminal intracytoplasmic domain. No mutations of this receptor gene have yet been described.

Much of the investigation of the *GnRH* gene was stimulated by the clinical condition of hypogonadotropic hypogonadism. One type of hypogonadotropic hypogonadism is Kallmann's syndrome, or isolated GnRH deficiency. It is characterized by hypogonadal function (anovulation in women and hypospermatogenesis in men) and may be inherited in an autosomal dominant, autosomal recessive or X-linked recessive manner.[69] There may also be anosmia secondary to absence of the olfactory bulbs and other associated anomalies. A hypogonadal mouse model was found to contain a large deletion that included exons III and IV of the *GnRH* gene.[70] The mRNA produces is truncated, resulting in absence of GnRH and GAP. An analogy was drawn to Kallmann's syndrome, but many patients in the study revealed normal GnRH gene architecture, although multiple polymorphisms have been identified.[71] One study has identified mutations in a gene on the short arm of the X chromosome in some male patients with Kallmann's syndrome, including multiple different deletions and point mutations. This gene (termed *KALIG 1*) appears to code for a neural cell adhesion molecule that plays an important part in the original migration of GnRH neurons.[72] The neurons that secrete GnRH originate in the olfactory placode and migrate into the brain with the olfactory apparatus. Failure in this migration results in anosmia and hypogonadotropic hypogonadism due to GnRH deficiency. Treatment with pulsatile GnRH or parenteral menopausal gonadotropins restores ovulation in women and spermatogenesis in men.[69]

Gonadotropin Genes

The gonadotropins, follicle-stimulating hormone (FSH) and luteinizing hormone (LH), are glycoprotein hormones that consist of a common α subunit linked to a unique β subunit.[73] The common α subunit is shared by both thyroid-stimulating hormone (TSH) and human chorionic gonadotropin (hCG) and differs at only a few of its 92 amino acids in each of these hormones. The unique β subunits confer specificity of action. Identification and analysis of the genes that code for both the α and β subunits has provided important information regarding the evolution and transcriptional regulation of these genes. They also have provided raw material for cloning by means of recombinant DNA technology to produce quantities of pure gonadotropin in the laboratory.

The gene for the α subunit was isolated, cloned, and sequenced from the human placenta, where the α subunit is present in great excess.[74] Southern blot analysis revealed a single fragment indicative of a single-copy gene. It was localized to the long arm of chromosome 6. The gene was found to be relatively large and to contain four exons. There is a cyclic adenosine monophosphate (cAMP) response element in the 5′ flanking region in the human gene. Glucocorticoids appear to inhibit α subunit expression by binding to this cAMP response element. Other transactivating factors also bind to this region and have been proposed as additional regulators.

The β subunits of LH and hCG are homologous.[73,75] Although both are glycosylated peptides, βhCG has a unique 24–amino acid carboxy-terminal extension with additional glycosylation. This increases the half-life of the βhCG molecule compared with the βLH subunit. Both βhCG and βLH are encoded by genes in a complex on the long arm of chromosome 19. This gene cluster consists of a single copy of the *βLH* gene and six genes of pseudogenes for *βhCG*. It has been proposed that the *βhCG* gene evolved from a common *βLH* ancestral gene and that duplications and rearrangements occurred after *βhCG* acquired its new function. Of these six genes, only *βhCG5* and *βhCG3* have been consistently shown to be expressed. The others are definitely inactive or possibly transcriptionally active at very low levels or under special circumstances. Different promoter regions allow for different physiologic regulation and tissue transcriptional specificity of the genes.[76] Alteration of the translational stop signal accounts for the carboxy-terminal extension of hCG. As noted, the peptides exhibit structural similarity that accounts for their immunologic cross reactivity and functional overlap, but the difference in the carboxy-terminal gives hCG a longer serum half-life. The different transcriptional regulation of these genes is shown by the expression of βLH in pituitary gonadotrophs and the exclusive expression of βhCG in the placenta.[77]

The gene for the β subunit of FSH is the most recently characterized of the gonadotropins.[78] It is a single-copy gene located on the short arm of chromosome 11 and containing three exons and two introns. Posttranscriptional processing results in differential splicing and polyadenylation, resulting in different lengths of mRNA. The gene is expressed in pituitary gonadotrophs in the same cells as βLH. The 3′ untranslated region is extremely long and may confer stability.

The regulation of gonadotropin subunit gene expression is complex. GnRH appears to increase both α and β subunit levels in the pituitary gland under most experimental conditions. Although sex steroids are generally considered to have their primary feedback effects at the level of the hypothalamus, estrogens have been shown to have both inhibitory and stimulatory effects on the transcription of gonadotropin genes. Both inhibin and activin exert their effects on FSH secretion at the pretranslational level of βFSH expression.[79] A mutation in the βLH gene has been found in a man with hypergonadotrophic hypogonadism; however, no women with mutated β-subunit gonadotropin genes have been identified.[73,80]

Recombinant DNA technology not only has provided insight into the normal structure, function, and regulation of hormones but also has provided potential for new therapeutic uses. Molecular cloning can be used to produce multiple copies of genes and with genetic engineering techniques used to attach appropriate DNA transcriptional control signals. These genes can be introduced into cells in a manner that allows gene expression and production of large quantities of pure hormone. Expression of glycoprotein hormones such as the gonadotropins is complex because of a requirement for posttranslational processing (glycosylation). Biologically active hCG, LH, and FSH are being produced in mammalian cell expression systems. This method should provide large quantities of pure hormones for clinical use and provide an in vitro system for the study of genetic mutations and the resultant functional derangements. It has the potential for applications in the diagnosis and management of clinical disease.

Inhibin and Activin

Although the existence of a substance termed *inhibin* has been postulated for many years secondary to the effects of testicular and ovarian follicle extracts on FSH secretion, the peptide responsible proved very difficult to isolate with standard biochemical techniques. A partial amino acid sequence was obtained that was used to predict a nucleotide sequence for screening a genomic library. This resulted in characterization and sequencing of the genes for inhibin and the related activin.[79] Inhibin is a heterodimer of a 133–amino acid α subunit linked to one of two β subunits. β A is a 115–amino acid peptide cleaved from a 426–amino acid precursor; β B is a 114–amino acid peptide cleaved from a 407–amino acid precursor. Activin is a dimer of two β subunits in any of three combinations: Activin A is a homodimer of β A; activin B is a homodimer of β B; and activin AB is a heterodimer. In contrast to the primary action of inhibin, which is to inhibit FSH secretion, activin stimulates FSH secretion and is therefore essentially a functional antagonist to the effect of inhibin on the pituitary gland.[81]

The formation of inhibin or activin is regulated by the relative levels of the α and β subunits.[82] There is a cAMP response element in the 5′ region of the α subunit gene, but this is absent in the β subunit genes, indicating differential regulation. An excess of α subunits results in inhibin formation, whereas a more equal ratio favors the formation of activin, because of the higher affinity of the β subunits for each other. Both α and β subunit genes are expressed in granulosa cells with complex regulation throughout folliculogenesis. FSH stimulation increases transcription of the β subunit genes.

In addition to their gonadal expression, both activin and inhibin subunit mRNA molecules are widely expressed in extragonadal tissues, including the adrenal glands, bone marrow, spleen, pituitary gland, kidneys, and brain.[82] There is extensive homology between the β subunit peptide and both tumor growth factor-β [TGFβ], a growth factor with pluralistic effects in multiple tissues, and MIS.[79] Activin may therefore be an autocrine/paracrine growth factor with widespread regulatory roles in numerous tissues.

Steroid Hormones

Application of contemporary molecular biologic techniques has altered the traditional view of steroidogenesis. It was previously believed that separate and distinct enzymes were involved in each intermediate conversion step of steroidogenesis. The elegant simplicity of the actual system was elaborated with molecular technology to identify and clone the genes for the enzymes involved. We now understand that multiple steps in steroidogenesis are catalyzed by a single enzyme.[83] The cytochrome P450 enzyme group is an important part of this process. The initial rate-limiting step in steroidogenesis is the conversion of cholesterol to pregnenolone in the mitochondria. This involves three distinct reactions: 20 α hydroxylation, 22 hydroxylation, and 20,22 lyase activity. Molecular analysis, however, revealed a single, unique gene that codes for a single identifiable enzyme. This was termed *cytochrome P450 side-chain cleavage* (P450scc). The gene was localized to chromosome 15 and was cloned and sequenced.[84] A single cap site and promoter region coordinates transcription of a single species of mRNA. This negates any possibility of serial isozymes, although posttranslational modification to effect enzyme specificity is still possible. Although a defect in P450scc once was thought to cause congenital lipoid adrenal hyperplasia, genetic analysis did not reveal any mutations. Point mutations causing premature stop codons have now been identified in the steroidogenic acute regulatory protein (*STAR*) gene in three patients.[85] STAR involved in cholesterol transport into mitochondria, and therefore is a mutation in the *STAR* gene is the probable cause of lipoid adrenal hyperplasia.

The next step in the steroid pathway is 3 βhydroxy-steroid dehydrogenase (3β-HSD)/Δ5 → Δ4 isomerase. This consists of two isozymes coded for by two contiguous genes on the short arm of chromosome 1.[86] This is a noncytochrome, P450-dependent enzyme in the endoplasmic reticulum. The genes are differentially regulated; type I is expressed in placenta and skin and type II is expressed in adrenal gland, ovary, and testis. A mutation in the type II gene has been identified in two families with congenital classic 3β-HSD deficiency.[87] The classic complete deficiency syndrome is present in infancy with a hypogonadal state, ambiguous genitalia, and complete absence of adrenal and gonadal steroids. It is fatal if not diagnosed early. A partial deficiency syndrome has been described with pubertal onset of hirsutism, acne, oligomenorrhea, and infertility in women, who often have had premature pubarche.[88,89]

Three other P450 enzymes are active in adrenal steroidogenesis. P450c17 catalyzes 17-hydroxylase and 17,20-lyase activity. The single-copy gene is on chromosome 10 and contains a possible steroid response element in the 5′ flanking region. A variety of mutations, including insertions and deletions, have been described.[90] Boys with P450c17 deficiency have ambiguous genitalia secondary to inability to synthesize testosterone. Girls often seek treatment because of delayed secondary sexual development and primary amenorrhea. Among girls, P450c17 deficiency can be misdiagnosed as gonadal dysgenesis.[91]

P450c21 (21-hydroxylase) is the most extensively studied

steroidogenic enzyme. The gene is located in the major histocompatibility complex on the short arm of chromosome 6.[92] There are two genes, *P450c21A,* which is a pseudogene, and *P450c21B,* which is the active gene. Because of its clinical importance, this enzyme is discussed in more detail later in this section.

The final P450 enzyme in adrenal steroidogenesis is P450c11. There are two isozymes encoded by separate but highly homologous genes on the long arm of chromosome 8.[93] One encodes the isozyme involved in synthesis of cortisol in both the zona glomerulosa and zona fasciculata of the adrenal gland. The second also catalyzes 18-hydroxylation and 18-oxidation in the zona glomerulosa for the synthesis of aldosterone. Several point mutations have been identified that lead to congenital 11-β hydroxylase deficiency.[94]

Congenital adrenal hyperplasia is a term that covers a variety of enzymatic defects that result in inadequate cortisol production and, in the classic case, masculinization of female external genitalia and adrenal insufficiency. More than two thirds of cases are secondary to a deficiency of P450c21. The more recently described late-onset adrenal hyperplasia results from a less severe defect in steroid synthesis. This is an autosomal recessive disease, which means the patient must inherit an abnormal gene from each parent. 21-hydroxylase P450c21 is duplicated and located in close proximity to the complement gene *C4* in the major histocompatibility complex on the short arm of chromosome 6.[83] The *B* gene is the actively transcribed gene, and the *A* gene is a pseudogene that is more than 95% homologous within the coding sequence but contains several mutated regions that cause defective gene expression.[95] Molecular analysis has identified numerous mutations that result in altered transcriptional regulation of the gene. In particular, gene duplications, deficiencies (deletions), and gene conversion of the active *B* gene to the inactive *A* gene have been documented.[96] Duplications and possibly gene conversions may result from mispairing with unequal crossing over of homologous chromosomes.

The highly variable phenotypes of patients with congenital adrenal hyperplasia are secondary to the diverse mutations found. Prenatal diagnostic testing and therapy are available for families in which there is an identifiable mutation. Duplications of either the *A* or *B* gene or both have been identified in patients with congenital adrenal hyperplasia and in unaffected healthy people. These duplications are most likely the result of unequal crossing over during meiosis. Mutations have been identified in a small percentage of patients with classic congenital adrenal hyperplasia. The most common mutations are gene conversions, which have been identified in both classic and adult-onset forms of the disease. In one large study, 76% of patients were presumed to have point mutations, 11% gene conversions, and 11% deletions.[97]

Classic congenital adrenal hyperplasia becomes apparent with adrenal insufficiency and ambiguous genitalia in girls and may be of the simple virilizing or salt-wasting form depending on the type of mutation and the degree of steroidogenic block. Nonclassic or adult-onset adrenal hyperplasia is found in 3% to 10% of women with hyperandrogenemia, oligoamenorrhea, and infertility.[98] These patients can be treated with low doses of steroids to suppress adrenocorticotropic hormone (ACTH) and reduce overproduction of adrenal androgens.

A discussion of steroid hormones would not be complete without mention of steroid hormone receptors. Of particular interest is the androgen receptor. Like other members of this steroid hormone receptor superfamily, the androgen receptor is considered to be a ligand-dependent transacting nuclear regulatory factor. It is located on the X chromosome, and the gene has been identified.[99] This receptor is of particular clinical interest because of its involvement in the androgen insensitivity syndromes (testicular feminization). These individuals have a genetic sex that is 46,XY, but because of resistance to the action of testosterone produced by the embryonic testis, the external genitalia do not masculinize. Because of the production of MIS, the müllerian system regresses, and the person has a blind-ending vaginal pouch. Both quantitative and qualitative defects in the androgen receptor have been associated with androgen insensitivity. These defects impair the actions of androgenic hormones and result in the heterogeneous phenotypic expression that occurs in this disorder.

The androgen receptor gene has been cloned and sequenced.[100] The coding region consists of eight exons and is similar to other steroid hormone receptors in that there is a highly conserved, central, cysteine-rich DNA-binding domain with two zinc fingers; a carboxy-terminal steroid-binding domain; and an amino-terminal region of variable length that may be involved in transcriptional activation of the target gene. A large deletion of the steroid-binding domain was reported in one family with complete androgen insensitivity syndrome.[101] Other mutations have involved new chain-termination codons leading to truncated transcripts and no translation and point mutations in both the steroid-binding and DNA-binding domains.[102] A possible gene rearrangement within the DNA-binding domain has been reported. A partial deletion of the androgen receptor gene was found in one phenotypically normal male patient with azoospermia (Fig 22–7).[103] Because the type of mutation appears to correlate with the degree of androgen resistance, molecular technology has expanded our understanding of sexual differentiation.

The estrogen receptor gene is another member of the steroid receptor superfamily. It has been localized to chromosome 6, but unlike the androgen receptor, until recently no mutations had been described. This absence of mutations was thought to be secondary to the presumed lethality of any muta-

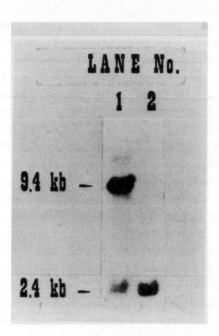

Figure 22–7. Deletion in exon 4 of the androgen receptor gene in a male patient with azoospermia. Lane 1, control; lane 2, patient. *(From Akin JW, et al: Evidence for partial deletion in the androgen receptor gene in a phenotypic male with azoospermia. Am J Obstet Gynecol 165:1981, 1991.)*

tion owing to the critical role of estrogen in embryo implantation. A man with an estrogen receptor gene mutation has now been identified.[104] He had normal sexual development but untested fertility. A mouse model using gene targeting to "knock out" the estrogen receptor gene resulted in infertile females with hypoplastic uteri and males with decreased fertility.[105]

GENETIC ASPECTS OF RECURRENT PREGNANCY LOSS

Although recurrent pregnancy loss is discussed in detail in Chapter 26, a brief review is appropriate in the context of genetic causes of infertility. Discussion of this subject requires a denominator, the basal pregnancy loss rate. This rate traditionally has been defined as the subsequent loss of a clinically recognized pregnancy. Various studies have placed this loss rate at 10% to 15%. Most of these losses were believed to occur within the first trimester, only 3% occurring from the second trimester on. Numerous studies have now shown that the actual loss rate for human pregnancies is much higher. Several workers have performed early pregnancy surveillance starting at or soon after the time of ovulation. These studies by means of very sensitive βhCG assays demonstrated a preclinical pregnancy loss rate of 22% to 60% before onset of the next menstrual period.[106] It appears that many human conceptions are lost after fertilization but before clinical diagnosis as a pregnancy (the first 2 gesta-

tional weeks). Some data show that a large percentage of these very early losses have a genetic cause. Hertig et al[107] examined a number of both preimplantation and early postimplantation embryos and showed severe morphologic disorganization that certainly may have been due to a severe genetic insult.

Studies using techniques to karyotype human gametes have shown a large number of cytogenetic abnormalities.[108] In men with normal semen analyses, 8% of sperm karyotypes using hamster egg penetration techniques were cytogenetically abnormal. Cytogenetic analysis of human oocytes revealed abnormalities in 15%. Limited studies on human preimplantation embryos have revealed a high percentage of karyotypic abnormalities. Thus it appears that many genetically determined pregnancy losses occur preclinically. This is consistent with what we know of most animal species and humans in whom abnormal gametes to appear to take part in fertilization and early embryonic development, but a process of zygote selection against genetically abnormal preimplantation embryos appears to take place.

After establishment of a viable intrauterine pregnancy as documented by means of early vaginal ultrasound scanning at 6 to 7 weeks of gestation, studies have shown that the actual clinical pregnancy loss rate is only 3.2%.[109] This rate varies depending on maternal age. The range is 1.5% for women younger than 25 years to 4.5% for women older than 35 years. Although clinical miscarriages are usually grouped by trimester, it does appear that most losses occur very early in the first trimester, before 8 weeks of gestation.

Studies of clinically recognized first-trimester pregnancy losses have consistently shown that 40% to 60% are cytogenetically abnormal aneuploid.[110] Hassold et al[111] showed a 46% incidence of chromosomal abnormalities, the most common being autosomal trisomy (44.5%) followed by monosomy (24%) and triploidy (15.1%). Autosomal monosomies rarely, if ever, occur. This finding may be consistent with findings of animal studies that show the severe lethality of this condition, which would be presumed to result in preclinical pregnancy loss.

Studies of cytogenetic abnormalities in trophoblasts obtained and cultured from first-trimester pregnancies have been criticized because of the known tendency for trophoblasts to be mosaic or to undergo artifactual chromosomal change in vitro. This would lead to overestimation of the percentage of pregnancy losses associated with cytogenetic abnormalities. Other studies, however, have shown that a cytogenetically abnormal trophoblast is less likely to grow, and therefore pregnancies successfully karyotyped may actually represent an excess of the cytogenetically normal pregnancies.

The incidence of cytogenetic abnormality decreases with increasing gestational age. Among second-trimester fetal losses, only 20% are found to be cytogenetically abnormal. In term stillbirths the incidence of chromosomal abnormalities was 5%.[112] This compares with a rate of 0.6% among liveborn term infants.

Warburton et al[113] studied recurrent pregnancy losses after one cytogenetically studied miscarriage. These researchers demonstrated that if the initial pregnancy loss is cytogenetically normal, there is an 80% likelihood that a subsequent loss will also be cytogenetically normal. The recurrence rate for cytogenetically abnormal losses, particularly trisomies, is not as high. If abortuses of couples with recurrent losses are cytogenetically abnormal, they are more likely to be abnormal because of structural chromosomal arrangements rather than recurrent trisomy or triploidy. Numerous studies of couples with two or more pregnancy losses have shown that between 2% and 5% have a major chromosomal rearrangement, either a balanced translocation or inversion.[114] The incidence is higher among couples with a mixed history of miscarriages and either healthy or ill liveborn infants.

Cytogenetic analysis of couples referred because of recurrent abortions has shown an excess of female partners who have low-level mosaicism for X-chromosome aneuploidy.[115] Studies have shown an increased risk of both spontaneous abortion and offspring with X chromosome aneuploidy among these patients. Studies with fluorescent in situ hybridization have confirmed a higher frequency of X-chromosome aneuploidy in peripheral white blood cells of patients with histories of recurrent abortions, further supporting the role of X-chromosome aneuploidy and mosaicism in the causation of recurrent abortion.

Embryonic aneuploidy is not the only genetic mechanism for early pregnancy loss. Recurrent euploidic abortions (normal chromosomes) may also be due to genetic problems caused by single-gene mutations.[112] The T locus in mice is a major histocompatibility complex–linked gene that is lethal when present in a homozygous state. Many studies have implicated parental human leukocyte antigen haplotypes in recurrent pregnancy loss. It is possible that genes linked to this immunologically important locus may be responsible for the apparent important role that immune function is now recognized to play in pregnancy loss. There are well-documented X-linked dominant genetic diseases that appear to be embryonically lethal in hemizygous males.[116] Disorders such as oral-facial-digital I syndrome and incontinentia pigmenti show only affected females with an excess of female births. Other lethal genes have been documented in animals. Insertional mutagenesis has even been used to induce a lethal recessive gene by means of insertion of a DNA sequence into a mouse α-1 collagen gene (see Fig 22–6).[117] When the heterozygous offspring were crossed, their homozygous progeny were unable to lay down a vascular system and could not develop beyond 13 days of embryonic life.

The genetic control of early embryonic development is poorly understood. Homeobox genes are DNA sequences first identified in *Drosophila melanogaster*. These genes appear to control expression of groups of other genes that control morphologic patterning of the embryo. The genes are highly conserved and have been identified in humans, where they are expressed in early embryonic development.[118] Mutations in *D melanogaster* have been shown to lead to severe embryonic disorganization with abnormal segmentation and development. Oncogenes are actually native human genes, many of which appear to code for growth factors or other substances important in early embryonic development. Abnormal activation can lead to neoplastic transformation and most probably to abnormal growth and embryonic development.[118] Leukemia inhibitory factor (LIF) is a polypeptide growth factor expressed in uterine endometrial glands during the window of receptivity for implantation of the blastocyst. A "gene knock out" experiment generated viable female mice homozygous for the mutant *LIF* gene with failure of implantation of blastocysts.[119] If the blastocysts were recovered and transferred to a pseudopregnant host mothers, they implanted and produced viable pups. It is certain that other genes are also critical in establishment and maintenance of pregnancy, but the precise role of single-gene mutation in human pregnancy loss remains to be defined.

A new concept of genetic regulations is that genes may be marked or imprinted as being of maternal or paternal origin.[64] This means that the somatic genes inherited from the mother or the father are not identical but may act in a separate way. This concept has been demonstrated in two well-described genetic syndromes—Prader-Willi and Angelman. Both syndromes result from the same microdeletion of chromosome 15 (q11-q13). However, the phenotypes of the syndromes are different. Not all people with either syndrome have the deletion. It has been shown that uniparental disomy, which means that the critical region on both chromosomes arises from a common parental source, either maternal or paternal, also results in the affected phenotype. Loss of the paternal region with duplication of the maternal region results in Prader-Willi syndrome; loss of the maternal region with duplication of the paternal region results in Angelman syndrome.[19]

The most extreme example of the effects of uniparental disomy is hydatidiform mole. This 46,XX tumor has a duplication of the entire paternal genome with loss of the entire maternal genome.[112] Solter[120] used highly inbred strains of mice to produce embryos in which both sets of chromosomes were either maternally or paternally derived. When both sets of chromosomes were maternally derived, the embryo exhibited normal embryonic development with poorly developed placental elements. When both sets of chromosomes were paternally derived, there was good placental development with poor embryonic development. This resulted in an animal model of a blighted ovum with the characteristic ultrasound finding of an empty sac. This certainly could explain the well-known phenomenon of empty sac and the diagnosis of a missed abortion with apparent severe embryonic disorganization but a normal karyotype at cytogenetic analysis of the products of conception. Studies are under way to examine genetic imprinting in both spontaneous and recurrent pregnancy loss.

REFERENCES

1. Watson JD, Crick FTC: Molecular structure of nucleic acids: A structure for deoxyribose nucleic acid. *Nature* 171:737, 1953

2. Gelehrter TD, Collins FS: *Principles of Medical Genetics.* Baltimore, Williams & Wilkins, 1990:9–23

3. Layman LC, McDonough PG: Molecular genetics in reproductive endocrinology. In: Wallach EE, Zacur HA (eds), *Reproductive Medicine and Surgery.* Baltimore, Mosby, 1995:3–38

4. Lanclos KD: Gene structure transcription and translation: *Infert Reprod Med Clin North Am* 5:1, 1994

5. Darnell JE: The processing of RNA. *Sci Am* 249:90, 1983

6. Wable E: The end of the message: 3′-end processing leading to polyadenylated messenger RNA. *Bioessays* 14:113, 1992

7. Smith HO, Wilcox KW: A restriction enzyme from *Hemophilus influenza.* I. Purification and general properties. *J Mol Biol* 51:379, 1970

8. Kelly TJ Jr, Smith HO: A restriction enzyme from *Hemophilus influenza.* II. Base sequence of the recognition site. *J Mol Biol* 51:393, 1970

9. Southern EM: Detection of specific sequences among DNA fragments separated by gel electrophoresis. *J Mol Biol* 98:503, 1975

10. Jeffreys AJ, Wilson V, Thein S: Hypervariable "minisatellite" regions in human DNA. *Nature* 314:67, 1985

11. Litt M, Luty J: A hypervariable microsatellite revealed by in vitro amplification of a dinucleotide repeat within the cardiac muscle action gene. *Am J Hum Genet* 44:397, 1989

12. Jeffreys AJ, Wilson V, Thein SL: Individual-specific "fingerprints" of human DNA. *Nature* 316:76, 1985

13. Fischer S, Lerman L: DNA fragments differing by single base-pair substitutions are separated in denaturing gradient gels: Correspondence with melting theory. *Proc Natl Acad Sci USA* 80:1579, 1983

14. Gray MR: Detection of DNA sequence polymorphisms in human genomic DNA by using denaturing gradient gel blots. *Am J Hum Genet* 50:331, 1992

15. Gray MR: Analyzing DNA sequence differences in clinical medicine. *Infert Reprod Med Clin North Am* 5:11, 1994

16. Saiki RK, Gelfand DH, Stoffel S, et al: Primer-directed enzymatic amplification of DNA with a thermostabile DNA polymerase. *Science* 239:487, 1988

17. Erlich HA, Gelfand DH, Srinsky JJ: Recent advances in the polymerase chain reaction. *Science* 252:1643, 1991

18. Cogan JD, Phillips JA: Polymerase chain reaction and DNA sequencing. *Infert Reprod Med Clin North Am* 5:29, 1994

19. Layman LC, Reindollar RH: The genetics of hypogonadism. *Infert Reprod Med Clin North Am* 5:53, 1994

20. Migeon BR, Kennedy JB: Evidence for the inactivation of an X chromosome early in the development of the human female. *Am J Hum Genet* 27:233, 1975

21. Reindollar RH, Byrd JR, McDonough PG: Delayed sexual development: A study of 252 patients. *Am J Obstet Gynecol* 140:371, 1981

22. Krauss CM, Turksoy RN, Atkins L, et al: Familial premature ovarian failure due to an interstitial deletion of the long arm of the X chromosome. *N Engl J Med* 317:125, 1987

23. Kaneko N, Kawagoe S, Hiroi M: Turner's syndrome: Review of the literature with reference to a successful pregnancy outcome. *Gynecol Obstet Invest* 29:81, 1990

24. Bedell MA, Brannan CI, Evans EP, et al: DNA rearrangements located over 100kb 5′ of the Steel (Sl)-coding region in the Steel-panda and Steel-contrasted mice deregulate: Sl expression can cause female sterility by disrupting ovarian follicle development. *Genes Dev* 9:455, 1995

25. Kriedberg JA, Sariola H, Loring JM, et al: *WT-1* is required for early kidney development. *Cell* 74:679, 1993

26. Luo X, Ikeda Y, Parker K: A cell-specific nuclear receptor is essential for adrenal and gonadal development and sexual differentiation. *Cell* 77:481, 1994

27. Eddy EM, Clark JM, Gong D, Fenderson BA: Origin and migration of primordial germ cells in mammals. *Gamete Res* 4:333, 1981

28. Motro B, van der Kooy D, Rossant J, et al: Contiguous patterns of c-*kit* and steel expression: Analysis of mutations in the W and SI loci. *Development* 113:1207, 1991

29. Resnick JL, Bixler LS, Cheng L, Donovan PJ: Long term proliferation of mouse primordial germ cells in culture. *Nature* 359:550, 1992

30. Jirasek JE: Principles of reproductive embryology. IV. Development of the ovary. In: Simpson JL (ed), *Disorders of Sexual Differentiation.* New York, Academic Press, 1976:75

31. Upadhyay S, Zamboni L: Ectopic germ cells: Natural model for the study of germ cell differentiation. *Proc Natl Acad Sci USA* 79:6584, 1982

32. Wachtell SS: The genetics of intersexuality: Clinical and theoretic perspectives. *Obstet Gynecol* 54:671, 1979

33. Goodfellow PJ, Darling SM, Thomas NS, Goodfellow PN: A pseudoautosomal gene in man. *Science* 234:740, 1986

34. Burgoyne PS, Levy ER, McLean A: Spermatogenic failure in male mice lacking HY antigen. *Nature* 320:170, 1986

35. Vergnaud G, Page DC, Simmler MC, et al: A deletion map of the human Y chromosome based on DNA hybridization. *Am J Hum Genet* 38:109, 1986

36. Muller U, Doulon T, Schmid M, et al: Deletion mapping of the testis determining locus with DNA probes in 46,XX males and 46,XY and 46,X,dic (Y) females. *Nucleic Acids Res* 14:6489, 1986

37. Disteche CM, Casanova M, Saal H, et al: Small deletions of the short arm of the Y chromosome in 46,XY females. *Proc Natl Acad Sci USA* 83:7841, 1986

38. Ashley T: A re-examination of the case for homology between the X and Y chromosomes of mouse and man. *Hum Genet* 67:372, 1984

39. Page DC, Mosher R, Simpson EM, et al: The sex determining re-

gion of the human Y chromosome encodes a zinc finger protein. *Cell* 51:1091, 1987

40. Tho SPT, Behzadian A: Detection and amplification of Y sequences. *Semin Reprod Endocrinol* 9:46, 1991

41. Palmer MS, Sinclair AH, Berta P, et al: Genetic evidence that *ZFY* is not the testis-determining factor. *Nature* 342:937, 1989

42. Sinclair AH, Foster JW, Spencer JA, et al: Sequences homologous to *ZFY,* a candidate human sex-determining gene, are autosomal in marsupials. *Nature* 336:780, 1988

43. Koopman P, Gubbay J, Collignon J, et al: *ZFY* gene expression patterns are not compatible with a primary role in mouse sex determination. *Nature* 342:940, 1989

44. Sinclair AH, Berta P, Palmer MS, et al: A gene from the human sex determining region encodes a protein with homology to a conserved DNA binding motif. *Nature* 346:240, 1990

45. Koopman P, Munsterberg A, Capel B, et al: Expression of a candidate sex-determining gene during mouse testis differentiation. *Nature* 348:450, 1990

46. Berta P, Hawkins JR, Sinclair AH et al: Genetic evidence equating SRY as the testis determining factor. *Nature* 348:448, 1990

47. Koopman T, Gubbay J, Vivian N, et al: Male development of chromosomally female mice transgenic for *Sry. Nature* 351:117, 1991

48. Tho SPT, Layman LC, Lanclos KD, et al: Absence of the testicular determining factor (TDF) gene *SRY* in XX true hermaphrodites (*n* = 5) and presence of this locus in most subjects (*n* = 22) with gonadal dysgenesis due to Y aneuploidy. *Am J Obstet Gynecol* 167:1794, 1992

49. Schmitt-Ney M, Thiele H, Kaltwaber P, et al: Two novel *SRY* missense mutations reducing DNA binding identified in XY females and their mosaic fathers. *Am J Hum Genet* 56:862, 1995

50. Hawkins JR, Taylor A, Berta P, et al: Mutational analysis of *SRY:* Nonsense and missense mutations in XY sex reversal. *Hum Genet* 88:471, 1992

51. Picard JY, Benarous R, Guerrier D, et al: Cloning and expression of cDNA for anti-müllerian hormone. *Proc Natl Acad Sci USA* 83:5464, 1986

52. Cohoen-Haguenauer O, Picard JY, Mattei MG, et al: Mapping of the gene for anti-müllerian hormone to the short arm of human chromosome 19. *Cytogenet Cell Genet* 44:2, 1987

53. Kim JH, Seibel MM, MacLaughlin DT, et al: The inhibitory effects of mullerian-inhibiting substance on epidermal growth factor induced proliferation and progesterone production of human granulosa-luteal cells. *J Clin Endocrinol Metab* 75:911, 1992

54. Hagg CM, King CY, Ukiyama E, et al: Molecular basis of sex determination: Activation of müllerian inhibiting substance gene expression by *SRY. Science* 266:1494, 1994

55. Shen W-H, Moore CCD, Ikeda Y, et al: Nuclear receptor steroidogenic factor 1 regulates the müllerian inhibiting substance gene: A link to the sex determination cascade. *Cell* 77:651, 1994

56. Wagner T, Wirth J, Meyer J, et al: Autosomal sex reversal and campomelic dysplasia are caused by mutations in and around the *Sry*-related gene SOX9. *Cell* 79:1111, 1994

57. Zanaria E, Muscatelli F, Bardoni B, et al: An unusual member of the nuclear hormone receptor superfamily responsible for X-linked adrenal hypoplasia congenita. *Nature* 372:635, 1994

58. Abyholm T, Stray-Pedersen S: Hypospermiogenesis and chromosomal aberrations: A clinical study of azospermic and oligospermic men with normal and abnormal karyotype. *Int J Androl* 4:546, 1981

59. Foreijt J: Meiotic studies of translocations causing male sterility in the mouse. II. Double heterozygotes for robertsonian translocations. *Cytogenet Cell Genet* 23:163, 1979

60. Layman LC: The genetics of ovarian failure. *Obstet Gynecol Report* 2:363, 1990

61. Caskey CT, Pizzuti A, Fu Y-H, et al: Triplet repeat mutations in human disease. *Science* 256:784, 1992

62. Clarke DG, Shapiro S, Monroe RG: Myotonia atrophica with testicular atrophy, urinary excretions of ICSH, androgens, and 17-ketosteroids. *J Clin Endocrinol* 16:1235, 1956

63. Kaufman FR, Kogut MD, Donnell GN, et al: Hypergonadotropic hypogonadism in female patients with galactosemia. *N Engl J Med* 304:994, 1981

64. Hall JG: Genomic imprinting: Review and relevance to human diseases. *Am J Hum Genet* 46:857, 1990

65. Seeburg PH, Adelman JP: Characterization of the cDNA for the precursor of human luteinizing hormone-releasing hormone. *Nature* 311:666, 1984

66. Nikolics K, Mason AJ, Szonyi E, et al: A prolactin-inhibiting factor within the precursor for human gonadotropin-releasing hormone. *Nature* 316:511, 1985

67. Radovick S, Wondisford FE, Nakayama Y, et al: Isolation and characterization of the human gonadotropin-releasing hormone gene in the hypothalamus and placenta. *Mol Endocrinol* 4:476, 1990

68. Adelman JP, Bond CT, Douglass J, Herbert E: Two mammalian genes transcribed from opposite strands of the same DNA locus. *Science* 235:1514, 1987

69. Layman LC: Idiopathic hypogonadotropic hypogonadism: Diagnosis, pathogenesis, genetics, and treatment. *Adolesc Pediatr Gynecol* 4:111, 1991

70. Mason AJ, Hayflick JS, Zoeller RT, et al: A deletion truncating the gonadotropin-releasing hormone gene is responsible for hypogonadism in the *hpg* mouse. *Science* 234:1366, 1986

71. Layman LC, Wilson JT, Huey LO, et al: Gonadotropin-releasing hormone, follicle stimulating hormone beta, and luteinizing hormone beta gene structure in idiopathic hypogonadotropic hypogonadism. *Fertil Steril* 57:42, 1992

72. Franco B, Guioli S, Pragliola A, et al: A gene deleted in Kallman's syndrome shares homology with neural cell adhesion and axonal path-finding molecules. *Nature* 353:529, 1991

73. Layman LC: Genetics of gonadotropin genes and the *GnRH/GAP* gene. *Semin Reprod Endocrinol* 9:22, 1991

74. Fiddes JC, Goodman HM: Isolation cloning and sequence analysis of the cDNA for the α-subunit of human chorionic gonadotropin. *Nature* 281:351, 1979

75. Talmadge K, Vamvakopoulos NC, Fiddes JC: Evolution of the genes for the subunits of human chorionic gonadotropin and luteinizing hormone. *Nature* 307:37, 1984

76. Jameson JL, Lindell CM, Haberner JF: Evolution of different transcriptional start sites in the human luteinizing hormone and chorionic gonadotropin beta subunit genes. *DNA* 5:277, 1986

77. Steger DJ, Altschmied J, Buscher M, Mellon P: Evolution of placenta-specific gene expression: Comparison of the equine and human gonadotropin α-subunit genes. *Mol Endocrinol* 5:243, 1991

78. Jameson JL, Becker CB, Lindell CM, Habener JF: Human follicle-stimulating hormone β-subunit gene encodes multiple messenger ribonucleic acids. *Mol Endocrinol* 2:806, 1988

79. Dye RB, Rabinovici J, Jaffe RB: Inhibin and activin in reproductive biology. *Obstet Gynecol Surv* 47:73, 1992

80. Weiss J, Axelrod L, Whitcomb RW, et al: Hypogonadism caused by a single amino acid substitution in the beta subunit of luteinizing hormone. *N Engl J Med* 326:1979, 1992

81. Ling N, Ying SY, Ueno N, et al: Pituitary FSH is released by a heterodimer of the beta-subunit from the two forms of inhibin. *Nature* 321:779, 1986

82. Meunier H, Rivier C, Evans RM, et al: Gonadal and extragonadal expression of inhibin alpha, beta A, and beta B subunits in various tissues predicts diverse functions. *Proc Natl Acad Sci USA* 85:247, 1988

83. Miller WL: Molecular biology of steroid hormone synthesis. *Endocr Rev* 9:295, 1988

84. Chung BC, Matteson KJ, Voutilainen R, et al: Human cholesterol side-chain cleavage enzyme, P450scc: CDNA cloning, assignment of the gene to chromosome 15 and expression in the placenta. *Proc Natl Acad Sci USA* 83:8962, 1986

85. Lin D, Sugawara T, Strauss JF III, et al: Role of steroidogenic acute regulatory protein in adrenal and gonadal steroidogenesis. *Science* 2167:1828, 1995

86. Lorence MC, Murray BA, Trant JM, et al: Human 3β-hydroxysteroid dehydrogenase/Δ5 → 4 Isomerase from placenta: Expression in non-steroidogenic cells of a protein that catalyzes the dehydrogenation/isomerization of C21 and C19 steroids. *Endocrinology* 126:2493, 1990

87. Rheaume E, Simard J, Morel Y, et al: Congenital adrenal hyperplasia due to point mutations in the type II 3β-hydroxysteroid dehydrogenase gene. *Nature Genet* 1:239, 1992

88. Temeck JW, Pang S, Nelson C, et al: Genetic defects of steroidogenesis in premature pubarche. *J Clin Endocrinol Metab* 64:609, 1987

89. Schram P, Zerah M, Mani P, et al: Nonclassical 3β-hydroxysteroid dehydrogenase deficiency: A review of our experience with 25 female patients. *Fertil Steril* 58:129, 1992

90. Yanase T, Simpson ER, Waterman MR: 17α-hydroxylase/17,20-lyase deficiency: From clinical investigation to molecular definition. *Endocr Rev* 12:91, 1991

91. Biglieri EG, Herron MA, Brust N: 17β-hydroxylase deficiency in men. *J Clin Invest* 45:1946, 1966

92. Levine LS, Zachmann M, New MI, et al: Genetic mapping of the 21-hydroxylase-deficiency gene within the HLA linkage group. *N Engl J Med* 299:911, 1978

93. White PC, Pascoe L: Disorders of steroid 11β-hydroxylase isoenzymes. *Trends Endocrinol Metab* 3:229, 1992

94. Carnow KM, Vitek J, White PC: Point mutations in *CYP11β1* causing steroid 11βhydroxylase deficiency (abstract). *Clin Res* 40:310, 1992

95. White PC, New MI, Dupont B: Structure of the human 21-hydroxylase genes. *Proc Natl Acad Sci USA* 83:5111, 1986

96. Reindollar RH, Gray MR: The molecular basis of 21-hydroxylase deficiency. *Semin Reprod Endocrinol* 9:334, 1991

97. White PC, Vitek A, Dupont B, New MI: Characterization of frequent deletions causing steroid 21-hydroxylase deficiency. *Proc Natl Acad Sci USA* 85:4436, 1988

98. Azziz R, Wells G, Zacur H, Acton RT: Abnormalities of 21-hydroxylase gene ratio and adrenal steroidogenesis in hyperandrogenic women with an exaggerated 17-hydroxyprogesterone response to acute adrenal stimulation. *J Clin Endocrinol Metab* 73:1327, 1991

99. Brown CJ, Goss SJ, Lubahn DB, et al: Androgen receptor locus on human X chromosome: Regional localization to Xq11-12 and description of a DNA polymorphism. *Am J Hum Genet* 44:264, 1989

100. Chang CS, Kokontis J, Liao ST: Molecular cloning of human and rat complementary DNA encoding androgen receptors. *Science* 240:324, 1988

101. Brown TR, Lubahn DB, Wilson EM, et al: Functional characterization of naturally occurring mutant androgen receptors from patients with complete androgen insensitivity. *Mol Endocrinol* 4:1759, 1990

102. Griffin JE: Androgen resistance: The clinical and molecular spectrum. *N Engl J Med* 326:611, 1992

103. Akin JW, Behzadian A, Tho SPT, McDonough PG: Evidence for partial deletion in the androgen receptor gene in a phenotypic male with azoospermia. *Am J Obstet Gynecol* 165:1891, 1991

104. Smith EP, Boyd J, Frank GR, et al: Estrogen resistance caused by a mutation in the estrogen-receptor gene in a man. *N Engl J Med* 331:1056, 1994

105. Lubahn DB, Moyer JS, Golding TS, et al: Alteration of reproductive function but not prenatal sexual development after insertional disruption of the mouse estrogen receptor gene. *Proc Natl Acad Sci USA* 90:11162, 1993

106. Edmonds DK, Lindsey KS, Miller JR, et al: Early embryonic mortality in women. *Fertil Steril* 38:447, 1982

107. Hertig AT, Rock J, Adams ED, Menkin MC: Thirty-four fertilized human ova, good, bad and indifferent, recovered from 210 women of known fertility: A study of biologic wastage in early human pregnancy. *Pediatrics* 25:202, 1959

108. Rudac E, Dor J, Mashiach S, et al: Chromosome analysis of multipronuclear human oocytes fertilized in vitro. *Fertil Steril* 41:538, 1984

109. Simpson JL, Mills SL, Holmes LB, et al: Low fetal loss rates after ultrasounds proved viability in early pregnancy. *JAMA* 258:2555, 1987

110. Boue J, Boue A, Lazar P: Retrospective and prospective epidemiological studies of 1500 karyotyped spontaneous human abortions. *Teratology* 12:11, 1975

111. Hassold TJ, Chen N, Funkhouser J, et al: A cytogenetic study of 1,000 spontaneous abortions. *Am J Hum Genet* 44:151, 1980

112. Tho SPT, McDonough PG: Genetics of fetal wastage, sporadic and recurrent abortion. *Infert Reprod Med Clin North Am* 5:157, 1994

113. Warburton D, Kline J, Stein A, et al: Does the karyotype of a spontaneous abortion predict the karyotype of a subsequent abortion? Evidence from 273 women with two karyotyped spontaneous abortions. *Am J Med Genet* 41:465, 1987

114. Tho SPT, Byrd JR, McDonough PG: Etiologies and subsequent reproductive performance of 100 couples with recurrent abortion. *Fertil Steril* 32:389, 1979

115. Singh DN, Hara S, Foster HW, et al: Reproductive performance in women with chromosome mosaicism. *Obstet Gynecol* 55:608, 1980

116. Wettke-Schafer R, Kantner G: X-linked dominant inherited diseases with lethality in hemizygous males. *Hum Genet* 64:123, 1983

117. Lohler J, Timpl R, Jaenisch R: Embryonic lethal mutation in mouse collagen I gene causes rupture of blood vessels and is associated with erythropoietic and mesenchymal cell death. *Cell* 38:597, 1984

118. Su BC, Strand D, McDonough PG, et al: Temporal and constitutive expression of homeobox-2 gene (*HU*-2), human-heat-shock gene (*HSP*-70) and oncogenes c-*sis* and n-*myc* in early human trophoblast. *Am J Obstet Gynecol* 150:1195, 1988

119. Stewart CL, Kaspar P, Brunet LJ, et al: Blastocyst implantation depends on maternal expression of leukemia inhibitory factor. *Nature* 359:75, 1992

120. Solter D: Differential imprinting and expression of maternal and paternal genomes. *Ann Rev Genet* 22:127, 1988

CHAPTER 23

Genetic Issues in Reproduction

MOSHE ZILBERSTEIN · MACHELLE M. SEIBEL

Patterns of Inheritance
Mendelian
Nonmendelian

Principles of Genetic Counseling
Conclusion

Medical genetics is the most rapidly evolving specialty in medicine. The Human Genome Project in the United States and similar endeavors in Europe diligently pursue the mapping and sequencing of the entire order of the human genetic composition (human genome). The goal is identification of all the human genes. The fallout of these ambitious projects has already had considerable impact on the practice of medicine because genes are discovered almost every week. Identification of genes confers better understanding of physiologic processes and elucidates the role of faulty genes in the pathogenesis and transmission of a wide array of disorders. The extraordinarily rapid pace of technologic and scientific advances poses a formidable burden on the practitioner to follow these developments and to apply them. It is important for every practitioner to understand basic processes and principles of medical genetics because the role that genetic factors play in pathologic processes are revealed. The knowledge has allowed precise diagnosis of genetic diseases, improved genetic counseling, and provided both more accurate prenatal diagnoses and novel opportunities for prevention. One must be familiar with the baseline risks (Table 23–1). The incidence of genetic diseases and other congenital anomalies apparent by the age of 25 is about 8%. Some genetic disorders are relatively common. Cystic fibrosis affects 1 in 2500 caucasians, sickle cell anemia affects 1 in 400 African Americans, and familial hypercholesterolemia affects 1 in 500 people (a disorder that is associated with increased risk of coronary heart disease).

Interestingly, advances in the mapping and isolation of new genes impact first and foremost on the practice of obstetrics and gynecology and reproduction. This is primarily because obstetricians and gynecologists traditionally are the purveyors of birth defect prevention. For example, prevention schemes include teratogen counseling and medication (folic acid). For their part, obstetricians and gynecologists contributed by developing sampling techniques for which the emerging molecular discoveries are complementary. Although the long-term objective of the Human Genome Project is to usher in new therapies (gene therapy), these are predicted to materialize in the far future. To devise new therapies, one must first elucidate the pathophysiologic process that brings about the disorder. It seems, however, that the advances in molecular genetics, that is, those that surround discoveries of genes, will first, and in the near future, allow new testing modalities rather than therapies. The nearest foreseen practical applications of the developments in medical genetics will be placed into the hands of obstetricians and gynecologists. These circumstances behoove practitioners to make rapid adjustments to emulate novel concepts, to learn new jargon, and

TABLE 23–1. BASELINE RISKS OF ABNORMAL OUTCOME OF PREGNANCY

Outcome	Risk
Congenital abnormality present at birth	1:30
Severe mental and physical handicap at birth	1:50
Spontaneous abortion	1:8
Couple infertile	1:10

Modified from Thompson et al: Thompson and Thompson's Genetics in Medicine, ed 5. Philadelphia, Saunders, 1991.

to become proficient in the implementation of genetic principles into practice.

A unique feature of genetic counseling is the tendency not only to focus on patients and their immediate families but also to include extended members of the family. This aspect is common ground to geneticists and reproduction specialists, who are used to extending their considerations to multiple patients, that is, the couple and their future offspring. In the setting of the infertility clinic, practitioners encounter genetic issues that require counseling in the following various circumstances: (1) as part of the evaluation of infertility, especially when the condition is intractable (severe oligospermia, recurrent abortion, premature menopause); (2) preconception counseling before treatment, including evaluation of family history, prevention of birth defects (folic acid treatment), and assessment of teratogenic exposure; (3) in pregnancy at about 9 weeks' gestation when options for prenatal testing and screening can still be used at the patient's request, as a result of specific testing (ultrasound finding), or after early miscarriage; (4) gamete donation when it is performed for genetic indications (about 3% of sperm donation) or when the discussion revolves around donor matching or donor recipient testing.

In the near future, preconception counseling will include routine discussion of preimplantation genetic diagnosis (PGD) for specific disorders in the family (chromosomal translocations or cystic fibrosis when a previous offspring is affected). It is also suggested that one discuss advanced maternal age or paternal age and inform patients of the age-related risk for miscarriage and possible options (risks and benefits) for prenatal testing.

This chapter is intended to provide basic understanding of the genetic issues that surround infertility and fertility management. Also delineated are principles of genetic counseling.

PATTERNS OF INHERITANCE

Mendelian

Mendelian Single-Gene Inheritance

Single-gene traits or disorders are transmitted through the expression of a single specific allele on one or both chromosomes of a chromosome pair. The pattern of inheritance of most single-gene traits has been inferred from the observed segregation of these traits within studied families. Single-gene traits are transmitted in a characteristic pattern in families. One can glean the pattern of inheritance of a given disorder from the family history. This pattern is determined by the location of the gene (either autosomal or X-linked). If the disease is expressed by heterozygotes (individuals who have one copy of the flawed gene and one normal copy), the pattern is dominant. If the person manifests the disorder only in the homozygous genotype (the person carries two copies of the flawed gene), the pattern is recessive. Genes are carried either on autosomal chromosomes or on sex chromosomes (mainly X chromosomes). Disorders therefore can be transmitted either as autosomal dominant or autosomal recessive or X-linked dominant or X-linked recessive.

Mendelian Single-Gene Disorders

Mendelian single-gene disorders result from defects (mutations) in a single gene. More than 12 million people in the United States are affected by single-gene disorders. These disorders account for 30% of pediatric hospitalizations, although individually the disorders are rare. Mendelian disorders are called *autosomal* if the mutated gene resides on one of the 22 pairs of autosomal chromosomes and X-linked if they are encoded by genes on the X chromosomes. The pattern of mendelian disorders follows the laws of segregation and independent assortment. Alleles (alternate forms of genes at a certain position or locus on the chromosome) at homologous loci segregate to different gametes during meiosis. Alleles at different loci sort independently (randomly) into the gametes during meiosis.

When a dominant disorder appears in a family for the first time as an isolated case, it can be caused by a new mutation. New mutations are occasionally associated with advanced paternal age. When a disorder arises by means of new mutation, the risk for recurrence in future pregnancies in the mother of the affected offspring is negligible. When such an assessment is given, one should carefully examine the parents to preclude the existence of a very mild form of the disorder in one of the parents. Most cases of achondroplasia can be accounted for by new mutations. If the condition exists in the parents, it can easily be recognized. On the other hand, in neurofibromatosis, individuals in the family who carry the mutated gene may present with a very mild phenotype. If one of the parents presents with unnoticed symptoms, the offspring's condition may erroneously be interpreted as a new mutation, and the risk to the child's future siblings is much higher than expected.

Some individuals who inherit autosomal dominant disorders may possess the abnormal gene but not have the disorder, a phenomenon referred to as *lack of penetrance*. People who belong to a family with such a disorder and are not affected carry up to a 10% risk they will transmit the disorder to their children. In some autosomal dominant disorders, parents may be carriers of germline mutations. Counseling for this condition is difficult because it may be associated with considerable risk depending on the proportion of gametes carrying the mutation. Counselors should be aware that a "new mutation" of an autosomal dominant disorder in the absence of a family history of the disease may be the result of nonpaternity, that is, the partner is not the father. The coincidental finding of nonpaternity raises ethical dilemmas because it alters the counseling for other family members.

The autosomal dominant pattern of inheritance is recognized on the basis of the following features: (1) consecutive generations in the family are affected in a pattern called *vertical transmission*; (2) males and females in the pedigree are equally affected and transmit the disease gene with equal frequency; (3) affected individuals have one affected parent (except for new mutations or those resulting from germ cell mutations); and (4) approximately 50% of affected parents of offspring also are affected. Examples of autosomal dominant disorders are listed in Table 23–2. To prevent fallacy in counseling, one should be aware of the difficulty in discerning the risks in some families because of late or variable onset, as in Huntington's disease, variable expressivity as in neurofibromatosis, and variable penetrance. Homozygosity for dominant genes is uncommon unless two people with the same disorder mate. In certain conditions, such as achondroplasia, this may happen quite frequently. Homozygous achondroplasia is a lethal condition, and the risk for homozygosity in a pregnancy that results from such mating is 25% homozygous lethal. The features of autosomal recessive inheritance are as follows:

1. The affected individuals are found within a single sibship, although the mutated gene is passed from one generation to another. This is called *horizontal transmission.*

2. Males and females are equally affected and transmit the mutant allele with equal probability.

TABLE 23–2. AUTOSOMAL DOMINANT DISORDERS

Achondroplasia
Acute intermittent porphyria
Adult polycystic kidney disease
Familial hypercholesterolemia
Huntington's disease
Myotonic dystrophy
Noonan's syndrome
Neurofibromatosis
Osteogenesis imperfecta (some forms)
Familial adenomatous polyposis of the colon
Tuberous sclerosis

TABLE 23–3. EXAMPLES OF AUTOSOMAL RECESSIVE DISORDERS

Cystic fibrosis
Congenital adrenal hyperplasia
Diastrophic dwarfism
Galactosemia
Homocystinuria
Oculocutaneous albinism
Phenylketonuria
Sickle cell anemia
Tay-Sachs disease
Thalassemia

3. Parents of the affected individual carry the mutant gene but they are clinically healthy (carriers).

4. Approximately 25% of the offspring of carrier parents are affected, 50% are phenotypically normal but are carriers, and 25% are normal and devoid of the mutation.

Autosomal recessive disorders (Table 23–3) usually are severe. Many of the inborn errors of metabolism have autosomal recessive patterns of inheritance. If the trait is rare, consanguinity between the parents of the affected individual is often observed. First cousins (this is the closest common consanguinity) share one eighth of these genes. Consanguinity in some cases is the sole reason for couples' seeking counseling. In some instances couples know the level of consanguinity, but in other instances the couple belongs to an ethnic group or religious isolate and questions consanguinity. Autosomal recessive conditions in a consanguinous family may appear to be dominant by virtue of a vertical pattern in the pedigree. It is usually helpful that one become familiar with the local population and ethnic composition.

X-Linked Recessive Disorders

The phenotype of an X-linked recessive condition (Table 23–4) is usually observed only in the man. Carrier females usually are unaffected. This is because although females have two X chro-

TABLE 23–4. X-LINKED RECESSIVE DISORDERS

Hemophilia A
Duchenne muscular dystrophy
Agammaglobulinemia
Lesch-Nyhan syndrome
Menkes' syndrome
Fabry's disease

mosomes, they are heterozygotes for the mutated gene, whereas because males are hemizygotes (have only one X chromosome), they express the abnormal phenotype. Special circumstances do exist in which carrier females express the disease phenotype of an X-linked recessive gene. Examples include Turner's syndrome (45X) if the mutation is carried on the only X chromosome, females with a translocation involving the X chromosome and an autosome with preferential inactivation of the normal chromosomes, and when nonrandom skewed inactivation of normal X chromosomes occur in most female cells.

The hallmarks of X-linked recessive transmission are (1) no male-to-male transmission; (2) gender differences (males are affected much more often than females; and (3) typical segregation (assuming male partner is unaffected and female partner is a noncarrier. Typical segregation is that all daughters of affected fathers are unaffected obligate carriers; none of the sons of affected fathers are affected; half of the sons of unaffected carrier mothers are affected; half of the daughters of unaffected carrier mothers are carriers; affected males in a family are related to each other through unaffected carrier females (uncle and nephew son of his sister).

X-Linked Dominant Inheritance

X-linked dominant inheritance is a rare mode of transmission in which a mutant gene gives rise to a disorder in both males and females. Examples include incontinentia pigmenti, orofaciodigital syndrome, and rickets resistant to vitamin D. In some disorders, the condition is lethal in hemizygous males. Many families with an X-linked dominant disorder have an excess of affected females. The characteristics of X-linked dominant inheritance are (1) no male-to-male transmission; (2) females are almost twice as likely to be affected as males (these conditions may be lethal among men; females who inherit the mutation are usually less severely affected); (3) if the partner is not affected and is not a carrier all daughters of affected fathers are affected; no sons of affected fathers are affected; half of the children of affected mothers are affected regardless of offspring sex; affected males in the family are related to each other through affected females.

Y-linked (Nolandric) Inheritance

Only a few examples of Y-linked inheritance exist, such as hairy ears. The hallmark of this mode of transmission is that only males are affected. An affected male passes the disease gene to all of his sons and none of his daughters.

Nonmendelian

More and more disorders are being discovered that are inherited in a nonmendelian pattern. It is beyond the scope of this chapter to discuss these patterns of inheritance in detail. It is, however, very important for every caregiver to be aware of their existence and to recognize these patterns because they play a role in the inheritance of some common conditions.

Unstable Mutations

The mechanism of disease in conditions that are inherited in a mendelian manner involves unstable trinucleotide repeats within or in the vicinity of the gene. The most common among this group of diseases are myotonic dystrophy, fragile X syndrome, and Huntington's disease. Although it basically demonstrates mendelian transmission, the pattern assumes unusual characteristics of inheritance. This pattern stems from instability of the mutation. The disorder becomes more severe in subsequent generations (anticipation), and sex biases exist in the inheritance of the more severe disorders (maternal in myotonic dystrophy and fragile X syndrome and paternal in Huntington's disease).

Imprinting

Imprinting is the term used to describe the now well-recognized phenomenon by which certain genes function differently depending on whether they are on a homologue chromosome that is inherited originally from the mother or from the father. Imprinting of the whole genome, specific chromosomes, chromosomal segments, and individual genes confers functional changes that occur during gametogenesis and generation of the eggs or the sperm cells. One of the best described examples is the deletion of the segment in the long arm of chromosome 15q11-13. When the deletion occurs in the paternally derived chromosome, the phenotype is Prader-Willi syndrome, which includes severe neonatal hypotonia and failure to thrive that later turns into obesity, behavioral problems, mental retardation, characteristic dysmorphic facial features, and small feet and hands. When the same deletion occurs in chromosome 15 derived from the mother, a distinctly different disorder appears. Angelman's syndrome is associated with severe mental retardation, microencephaly, ataxia, epilepsy, and lack of speech.

Mosaicism

Mosaicism refers to the existence of two or more cell lines of different chromosomal complement in the same person. Mosaicism may exist concurrently in both somatic and germ cells or be limited only to one of the cell groups. The effect of germline-gonadal mosaicism on inheritance, specifically of autosomal dominant and X-linked disorders, is discussed earlier in this chapter. Gonadal mosaicism is one explanation of the transmission of an autosomal dominant or X-linked disorder to more than one of the offspring when both parents are normal. In Duchenne muscular dystrophy, seemingly as many as 20% of mothers of isolated offspring with this disorder harbor gonadal mosaicism for the mutated gene.

Mitochondrial Inheritance

Mitochondria carry distinct DNA and mutation in this DNA can be the source of diseases as a result of mitochondrial dysfunction. Examples of diseases caused by mutation in mitochondrial DNA (mtDNA) include Leber's hereditary optic neuropathy (acute visual loss and neurologic symptoms) and myoclonic epilepsy with neurologic symptoms and ragged red fibers in skeletal muscle.

Mitochondria are the powerplant of the body. Disorders that compromise their function affect primary organs that are the principal consumers of aerobic oxidative energy—the kidneys, muscles, liver, and brain. Each mitochondrion contains several copies of mtDNA, and each cell contains a few hundred mitochondria. Each cell may contain normal and abnormal mitochondria (*heteroplasmy*). Mitochondria are maternally inherited through the cytoplasm of the egg. Sperm contribute no mitochondria to the zygote. The features of mitochondrial inheritance are (1) both males and females are equally affected and (2) transmission is only by affected females.

Complicating issues stem from the following facts: (1) Some mitochondrial dysfunction disorders are transmitted through nuclear mutations in nuclear genes that encode mitochondrial proteins that transmit in the mendelian manner. (2) It is difficult to predict the severity of mitochondrial disorders in offspring. Mitochondrial heteroplasmy in the eggs (the proportion of mutated mitochondria) determines the severity of the disease. (3) Many mitochondrial disorders appear sporadically in families. It is difficult to counsel relatives without symptoms who carry the mitochondrial mutation.

Chromosomal Abnormalities

Human somatic cells are diploid ($2n$) and contain 46 chromosomes. Gametes (egg or sperm) are haploid (n) and contain 23 chromosomes. After fertilization, the normally fertilized egg (zygote) contains 46 chromosomes, which is twice the haploid number. Of the 46 chromosomes 22 pairs are autosomes, and one pair is sex chromosomes. One should suspect chromosomal abnormalities in several situations, including many that are commonly encountered in the treatment of infertility. Approximately 15% of recognized pregnancies result in spontaneous abortion. More than half of these pregnancies are chromosomally abnormal. The frequency of chromosomal abnormalities among early fertilized zygotes and chemical pregnancies is higher. This information is being gained as early pregnancies in vitro become more accessible to observation in the laboratory. With pregnancies resulting in stillborns and neonatal fetal death, one can anticipate finding 5% chromosomal abnormalities. Chromosomal abnormalities occur in 0.6% of livebirths.

Chromosomal abnormalities may be *numerical*. *Polyploidy* means that a cell's chromosome number is a multiplication of the haploid set (n) and is higher than $2n$. Aneuploidy means the chromosome number is not a multiple of n but has either the addition of a chromosome ($2n + 1$ [trisomy]) or the loss of a chromosome ($2n - 1$ [monosomy]). Rarely aneuploidy is the result of more than one added or lost chromosome.

The second category of chromosomal abnormalities is *structural*. In these instances, the material on the chromosome is rearranged either on the same chromosome (inversion, deletion) or exchanged between chromosomes (translocation). Translocations can include almost a complete chromosome or segments of chromosomes. Structural abnormalities can either be functionally balanced whereby the amount of essential genetic material is preserved, or unbalanced, whereby there is a gain or loss of material. Balanced chromosomal structural abnormalities are usually compatible with a normal phenotype. These structural abnormalities, albeit balanced in somatic cells, are represented in germ cells. During meiosis, many of the gametes produced by an individual with a balanced translocation are unbalanced and give rise to zygotes that are incompatible with normal development. The frequency of translocations among parents with multiple spontaneous abortions is 2% to 5%. Similarly, 2% to 4% of infertile couples have an autosomal rearrangement. Chromosomal abnormalities can result in azoospermia and permature ovarian failure.

Approximately 0.5% of newborns have chromosomal abnormalities that are detected at birth or early in the neonatal period. Many other abnormalities, such as balanced translocations or sex chromosome abnormalities, are detected later in infancy, childhood, or adulthood. The most common autosomal abnormalities among newborns are trisomy 21, trisomy 18, and trisomy 13. The most common sex chromosomal abnormalities are Turner syndrome (45X), triple X (47XXX), and Kleinfelter's syndrome (XXY and XYY male). The most common indication for prenatal counseling and preconception counseling is advanced maternal age. The occurrence of chromosomal abnormalities among liveborn infants (especially trisomies) and of spontaneous abortions increases with age (see Table 23–1). This is a source of anxiety for many patients with infertility because they will be older than 35 years at term. Prenatal diagnosis is recommended to determine if the fetus is affected.

Indications for prenatal diagnosis include (1) maternal age 35 years or older at time of delivery; (2) a previous child with an autosomal trisomy such as Down syndrome, trisomy 18, or trisomy 13; (3) one parent is a carrier of a chromosomal rearrangement; (4) a previous child, the mother, or her partner has a neural tube defect; (5) pregnancy at risk for diagnosable genetic disorder; (6) parental anxiety (controversial).

There are noninvasive procedures designed to assess the status of the fetus. These include ultrasonography to identify birth defects and maternal serum α-fetoprotein (AFP) screening for open neural tube defects. Discussion of ultrasound for screening and diagnosis is beyond the scope of this chapter except to underscore that one needs to be familiar with ultrasound capabilities and limitations.

AFP is a glycoprotein produced by fetal liver, yolk sac, and in smaller quantities by the gastrointestinal tract of the fetus. Since the early 1970s, measurement of maternal serum AFP has been used to screen for open neural tube defects. Testing is preferred between 16 and 18 weeks' gestation but can be performed between 14 and 22 weeks' gestation. During pregnancy, maternal blood concentrations of AFP rise until about the 32nd week of pregnancy. Accurate dating of pregnancy and timing of conception are therefore very important for correct interpretation of the data. Because fertility clinics are likely to know the exact date of conception, clinic staff should convey this information to the prenatal caregiver for accurate interpretation of AFP results. Levels of AFP should be adjusted to maternal weight (levels inversely related to weight), race (maternal serum AFP is higher on average among African American population), and for insulin-dependent diabetes mellitus status (women with diabetes have lower level of maternal serum AFP), multiple pregnancies (twins, for example, produce twice the amount of maternal serum AFP). An elevated maternal serum AFP level can occasionally be explained by reasons other than a neural tube defect, especially when ultrasound examination does not show such an abnormality. Incorrect dating, multiple pregnancy, ventral wall defect, intrauterine fetal death, fetomaternal bleeding, fetal renal condition, or chromosomal abnormality (twice the prevalence among the general population if maternal serum AFP is above the cutoff) may indicate increased risk for fetal loss.

A multiple-marker screen has been introduced for the detection of trisomy 21 (Down syndrome). The use of this marker as a screening tool can be very instrumental in the general infertility population. The screen can be used in combination with an ultrasound examination for women close to the cutoff age for amniocentesis. One should, however, familiarize oneself with the risk of administrating a screening test to one's patient population. Appropriate counseling should be offered. The multiple-marker test has the following three components: (1) maternal serum AFP, (2) maternal serum human chorionic gonadotropin (hCG), and (3) maternal serum unconjugated estriol. The screening cutoff for this test is a risk cutoff. Some practitioners use 1:270 and others use 1:190. The overall detection rate is about 70% and is age dependent.

Almost all infertile couples undergoing treatment are attempting to conceive in the near future. Studies have shown that folic acid supplementation before conception provides up to a 72% protection against the risk of open neural tube defect. The recommended dose is 0.4 mg per day. Higher dosages are needed to prevent recurrences among patients with a family history of neural tube defects. All patients in our infertility clinic are advised to take 0.4 mg to 1 mg of folic acid daily.

Multifactorial Inheritance

Multifactorial inheritance describes traits and disorders that arise as a result of the combination and interaction of many genetic and nongenetic factors. They have familial characteristics but are also influenced by the environment. Some of the disorders are defined as *polygenic* to denote a primarily genetic causation that is brought about by interaction of several genes. In the context of gamete donation and donor-recipient matching, much consideration is given to quantitative traits like height, weight, and intelligence. It is usually believed that quantitative phenotypes are transmitted as multifactorial traits in healthy individuals. The traits usually present continuous variability, however, all possible variation can be seen between the extremes. General rules are that children resemble their parents with respect to normal traits, and usually the child's phenotype falls between that of the parents to resemble their average (regression to the mean).

Many common disorders are transmitted in a multifactorial polygenic pattern (hypertension, diabetes) and account for most of the morbidity and mortality among humans. Many times discerning that a certain disorder is multifactorial polygenic is achieved by exclusion, especially if the disorder is an isolated congenital abnormality. One should be aware that mendelian chromosomal or teratogenic causes can be identified for many syndromes of multiple congenital abnormalities. This can become a serious pitfall because multifactorial polygenic disorders carry an empiric risk far below to the recurrent risk of autosomal recessive or dominant disorders.

PRINCIPLES OF GENETIC COUNSELING

Practitioners of infertility treatment must familiarize themselves with the basic principles and ethics of genetic counseling. The principles of autonomy, privacy, confidentiality, and equity are fundamental to the process of counseling. Breaches of these principles may occur in rare circumstances when the breach is aimed at an extremely important goal, such as protection of others from severe and serious harm, and when there is no acceptable alternative to this action. There must be a high probability to prevent harm to others with the breach and the degree of infringement should be the minimum needed to achieve the goal. Any genetic counseling must adhere to the basic principles of ethics, which are beneficence (providing benefit to the patient), autonomy, justice (fair distribution of benefit and harm), utility (benefits and harm should be balanced), and nonmalfeasance (avoiding harm). In the context of a fertility clinic, imminent actions, namely treatment, are going to be taken to enhance the chance of conception.

The initial encounter with a couple seeking fertility treatment becomes the forefront of genetic consideration that may influence the patients' reproductive decision. The infertility specialist's role in conferring genetic counseling is not yet clearly defined, but it has become increasingly crucial. Every practitioner should be able to take an appropriate history and draw a pedigree and decide whether referral for further detailed genetic counseling is indicated. Common indications for genetic counseling are (1) planned conception or existing pregnancy in a woman 35 years or older or when the prospective father is older than 45 years; (2) one of the parents is known to harbor a chromosomal abnormality; (3) one of the prospective parents or both are known or believed to be carriers of a single-gene disorder, one is heterozygous for an autosomal dominant X-linked disorder, or both are heterozygous for a recessive disorder; (4) the finding of genetic or congenital abnormality or mental retardation in a close family member; (5) multiple spontaneous abortions, unexplained or anomalous pregnancy loss, or neonatal death; (6) exposure to potential teratogens; and (7) azoospermia or premature ovarian failure.

The purpose of genetic counseling is usually to provide couples sufficient information about their genetic circumstances without overwhelming them. The information given to couples may differ depending on the timing of the consultation, that is, preconception or postconception. Nondirectiveness is a core value of genetic counseling. The reproductive choices that are subsequently selected should reflect the couple's informed choice free from bias or coercion to the counselor's views or values. Although it might be difficult to implement, practitioners who undertake genetic counseling are prohibited from imposing their own preferences on patients. The counselor should be able to convey updated scientific and clinical information in a way that allows couples to understand and evaluate their options.

Various reproductive options are available to couples whose pregnancy carries high risk for disorders. Pregnancy can be pursued with or without prenatal diagnosis. Depending on the circumstances, the pregnancy can be terminated or maintained. In some instances, gamete donation should be discussed as an option during genetic counseling. Therapeutic insemination with donor sperm (TID) is an option when the father is affected with an autosomal dominant disorder or carries a chromosomal abnormality that leads to infertility, recurrent pregnancy or neonatal loss, or the birth of abnormal offspring. TID can also be offered when an existing child in the family is affected with an autosomal recessive disorder. Egg donation is an option for women who carry a chromosomal abnormality that leads to infertility, recurrent pregnancy loss, or the birth of

TABLE 23–5. PRENATAL DIAGNOSTIC TESTS

Test	Time	Risks	Purpose
Traditional amnio-centesis	15–18 weeks' gestation	0.5% commonly quoted for spontaneous abortion	Karyotype α-fetoprotein Potentially single-gene mutation
Early amnio-centesis	11–14 weeks' gestation (small experience mostly done at 14 weeks)	Failed sampling leakage of fluid 0.7%–4% Risk for spontaneous abortion 0.6% at 14 weeks but much higher earlier	Karyotype Potentially α-fetoprotein Single-gene mutation
Chorionic villus sampling	10–12 weeks' gestation (abdominal or transcervical)	Spontaneous abortion 0%–4.9% when compared with amniocentesis. Excess risk of birth defects is controversial Mosaicism 1%	Karyotype No α-fetoprotein testing Potential single-gene defects

abnormal offspring. Egg donation can also be offered to women with autosomal or X-linked disorders. Embryo donation (which could be considered early adoption) and traditional adoption are options. PGD emerges as an important, valid option of the future that must be explored before conception. Some couples may be interested in contraception, especially couples waiting for PGD or new medical developments. Sterilization may appeal to some couples, especially to those that have completed their families. Ultimately, the acceptability of any of these reproductive choices is the personal decision of the couple. Unfortunately, access to some possibilities may be limited because opportunity is not equal across society and definitely is not equal worldwide.

Counseling often requires making a clear distinction to the patient between direct testing and screening tests. The practitioner should be aware of and recognize the fundamental difference between direct diagnosis (Table 23–5) (for example, identification of the δF508 mutation of *CF* during amniocentesis when an affected sibling was identified) and screening tests such as measurement of AFP for screening for open neural tube defects. When many patients consent to testing, they do not fully understand the nature of a screening test and its primary objective to identify a population at risk.

The primary prerequisite for genetic counseling is an accurate and specific diagnosis of the condition for which the couple is seeking counseling. This prerequisite cannot be emphasized enough in the context of reproductive genetic counseling. One must remember that this counseling usually occurs at the final point of recourse, just before the couple is taking action to conceive, or when it might be strongly undesirable to terminate a pregnancy. Although counseling a couple for advanced maternal age is straightforward most of the time, when concern exists about the risk for a child with Down syndrome, information regarding a relative who is mentally retarded renders counseling futile without further information. Therefore it is sometimes necessary to postpone counseling until enough relevant information can be obtained regarding the disorder. Medical records should be perused to determine the exact diagnosis and how it was made. One should be aware of unprecedented rapid developments in the field of genetic diagnosis. As a result, many of the diagnoses made even in the recent past should be reevaluated with updated and more accurate testing and establishment of how other diagnoses were excluded. For example, birth defects such as clept lip and palate or open neural tube defect are mostly of the polygenic multifactorial pattern of inheritance with a recurrence risk among siblings of 2%–5% for clept lip and palate and 1%–2% for neural tube defects. However, in some cases clept lip and palate or neural tube defects are the result of syndromes that are inherited as autosomal recessive (encephalocele in Meckel's syndrome) with a 25% risk for recurrence. Open neural tube defects for example may be secondary to trisomy 8 and thus carry a lower recurrence risk. If a neural tube defect is secondary to teratogenic exposure such as to valproic acid or part of the amniotic band syndrome, counseling may be different.

Genetic history taking and the ability to draw a basic pedigree should be part of the initial encounter in the fertility clinic. A properly obtained and interpreted family history is the single most powerful instrument for genetic counseling in the context of the fertility clinic. It is an important tool for couples undertaking reproductive decisions and the single best tool for programs that offer gamete donation. Appropriate family history assists in reaching the correct diagnosis. Family history taking should have two inquiry styles: open-ended and close-ended questioning. After general information is recorded, one should make sure that information is collected regarding early-onset preventable disease, specific information regarding all first-degree relatives, other relatives, racial and ethnic background, and consanguinity. Information should be kept updated. One should pay attention to suspected hereditary disease in the family, severe as well as small birth defects, unexplained mental retardation, and possible teratogenic exposure. When an area of potential risk is revealed in the preconception encounter, the practitioner should review the history in further detail to clarify the actual risk. Ethnic origin must be discussed, because certain genetic disorders have a tendency to occur at higher frequency among certain ethnic groups. These disorders are amenable to carrier testing through population-based screening (Table 23–6). Consideration to ethnic background should be given

TABLE 23–6. SCREENING TESTS FOR GENETIC DISORDERS RELATED TO ETHNIC GROUP

Ethnic Group	Genetic Disorder	Test
Ashkenazi Jews (also French Canadians and Cajuns)	Tay-Sachs disease	Serum or leukocyte hexosaminidase A
African Americans	Sickle cell anemia, β-thalassemia	Hemoglobin electrophoresis
Mediterraneans (Greeks, Italians)	β-thalassemia	Mean corpuscular volume <80 Hemoglobin electrophoresis
Southeast Asians and Chinese	α-Thalassemia	Mean corpuscular volume <80 Hemoglobin electrophoresis
Northern European Caucasians	Cystic fibrosis	DNA analysis Population screening (still controversial)

when pregnancy is contemplated and when recipients and donors are matched for gamete donation.

Increasing numbers of autosomal recessive disorders are amenable to family-based carrier testing, such as α-antitrypsin deficiency, congenital adrenal hyperplasia, galactosemia, and phenylketonuria. Similar testing can be offered about some X-linked recessive disorders such as fragile X syndrome, muscular dystrophy, ornithine transcarbamylase deficiency, hemophilia A and B, and ocular albinism.

Most heterozygous individuals with autosomal dominant conditions are affected. Carrier testing for these conditions applies only to circumstances in which there is late onset of the symptoms, as in Huntington's disease, or when the manifestation is variable, as in neurofibromatosis. Some of the other autosomal dominant disorders that are currently amenable to carrier testing include familial hypercholesterolemia, myotonic dystrophy, and malignant hyperthermia. One should be aware that carrier testing, especially for presymptomatic autosomal dominant diseases, is a highly charged, controversial area among geneticists. Fertility specialists should be cautious before offering and certainly before performing such testing for their patients, especially in the context of gamete donation.

Estimation of genetic risk depends on the pattern of inheritance of the disorder. Practitioners who take it upon themselves to confer risk estimation for pre- and postconception couples should be familiar with the basic principles of inheritance. For example, mendelian (single-gene) disorders carry a high risk for recurrence. Chromosomal abnormalities typically carry low risk. Exceptions are the risk of recurrent pregnancy loss in specific reciprocal translocations or the 100% chromosomal abnormalities associated with certain translocations (for example, translocation 21:21), in which individuals never transmit a normal chromosome to their offspring. Practitioners should also be aware of their limitations and refer patients for formal genetic counseling when appropriate.

CONCLUSION

We have made an attempt to bridge two related medical fields: reproduction and genetics. This chapter is not a crash course in medical genetics or genetic counseling. It is intended to open a window for interested practitioners to the evolving issues in reproductive genetics. A list of basic texts for overview and for in-depth study is provided in the bibliography.

BIBLIOGRAPHY

Overview

Friedman JM, Dill FJ, Hayden MR, McGillivray BC: *Genetics,* ed 2. Baltimore, Williams & Wilkins, 1996

Gelehrter TD, Collins FS: *Principles of Medical Genetics.* Baltimore, Williams & Wilkins, 1990

Hall J (ed): *Medical Genetics I & II. Pediatr Clin North Am.* Philadelphia, Saunders, 1992

Kingston HM. ABC of Clinical Genetics. ed 2. BMJ Publishing Group. London, 1994

Thompson MW, McInnes RR, Willard HF: *Thompson and Thompson Genetics in Medicine,* ed 5. Philadelphia, Saunders, 1991

Prenatal Diagnosis and Genetic Testing

Filkins K, Russo JF: *Human Prenatal Diagnosis,* ed 2. New York, Dekker, 1990

Graham JM (ed): *I. Fetal Dysmorphology. II. Fetal Clinical Genetics. Clin Perinatol.* Philadelphia, Saunders, 1990

Gamete Donation

Seibel MM, Crockin S: *Family Building Through Egg and Sperm Donation: Medical, Legal and Ethical Issues.* Sudbury, Mass., Jones & Bartlett, 1996

In-depth Study

Baraitser M, Winter RM: *Color Atlas of Congenital Malformation Syndromes.* London, Mosby-Wolfe, 1996

Emery AEH, Rimoin DL: *Principles and Practice of Medical Genetics,* ed 2. New York, Churchill & Livingstone, 1990

Jones KL: *Smith's Recognizable Patterns of Human Malformations,* ed 4. Philadelphia, Saunders, 1988

Scriver CR, Beaudet AL, Sly WS, Valle D: *The Metabolic and Molecular Basis of Inherited Diseases,* ed 7. New York, McGraw-Hill, 1995

Vogel F, Motulsky AG: *Human Genetics: Problem and Approaches,* ed 2. Berlin, Springer Verlag, 1996 (in press)

CHAPTER 24

Neurologic Considerations

ANDREW G. HERZOG

Neurologic evaluation of infertility

Polycystic ovary disease   Skeletal asymmetry
Hypothalamic   Left handedness
 amenorrhea   Birth trauma
Functional   Febrile seizure
 hyperprolactinemia   Head injury
Unexplained infertility

EEG

Normal   Abnormal

Failure to conceive or ────────▶ Neurologic evaluation
respond to endocrine
therapy

Endocrine therapy

Responsive   Unresponsive

Continue   Trial of
treatment   antiseizure
                                  medication

Some common reproductive endocrine causes of infertility have been attributed to hypothalamic dysfunction. These include polycystic ovary (PCO) syndrome, hypothalamic amenorrhea (hypogonadotropic hypogonadism [HH]), and functional hyperprolactinemia. Considerable experimental and clinical investigative evidence suggests that each of these conditions may be the result of altered secretion of gonadotropin-releasing hormone (GnRH) or abnormal dopamine activity in the hypothalamus. The demonstration of a primary etiologic factor in the hypothal-

amus, however, is uncommon. It remains a possibility, therefore, that hypothalamic dysfunction may sometimes be secondary to extrahypothalamic influences. Indeed, the hypothalamus does not function in a vacuum in the brain. It is extensively and reciprocally interconnected with many cerebral and brainstem regions that modulate its activity. There is reason to consider in particular that the epileptic involvement of temporal lobe structures may contribute to hypothalamic dysfunction, the development of reproductive endocrine disorders, and infertility.

NEUROANATOMY AND EPILEPSY

Epilepsy affects approximately 1% of the population in the United States. It can be divided into two types, generalized and partial. Primary generalized seizures originate synchronously from the entire cerebral cortical mantle and result in loss of consciousness and generalized tonic-clonic seizures. Secondary generalized seizures result from the generalization of partial seizures. About three fourths of adults with seizures have partial epilepsy[1,2]; that is, seizures that originate from a small portion of cerebral cortex. This region is known as a *focus*.

Medial temporal lobe structures, especially the amygdala and hippocampus, are highly epileptogenic and are usually the sites of origin, or at least involvement, in partial epilepsy. These regions form part of the limbic system, where emotions are thought to be represented, and memory and learning take place. Activation of these regions with epileptic discharges can, therefore, lead to symptoms of heightened affect, including fear, anxiety, depression, and feelings of impending doom. Awareness may become intermittently impaired owing to the episodic interference of continuous memory formation by epileptic discharges. Learning may be disrupted intermittently or become persistently impaired.

Medial temporal lobe structures are heavily and reciprocally interconnected with other regions of the temporal lobe and with the insula. These areas of the brain elaborate perceptions of smell, taste, vision, and audition. Therefore, persons with epilepsy may experience auras of smell, taste, sight, or sound for which there are no environmental concomitants. Moreover, environmentally derived perceptions may be associated with exaggerated emotional and motivational significance by virtue of the heightened electrical activity in limbic structures. Deepened emotional state can lead to the development of persistently altered personality and behavior, commonly referred to as interictal features of temporal lobe epilepsy.[3] This syndrome is characterized by intense affect, depression, obsessions, paranoid ideation, circumstantiality, tangentiality, hyperreligiosity, hypergraphia, and altered sexuality or hyposexuality.

Medial temporal lobe structures are closely linked to the supplemental motor cortex and to the motor nucleus of the trigeminal nerve, which are regions of the brain that are responsible for motor activity such as deviation of the head and eyes and mouthing and chewing movements. Medial temporal structures are also extensively interconnected with the orbital frontal cortex, rostral hypothalamus, dorsal motor nucleus of the vagus, and solitary nucleus. These are sites of motor and sensory autonomic nervous system representation. Therefore, partial seizures are often associated with altered respiration, changes in cardiac rate, elevated blood pressure, enlargement of pupils, and even the occurrence of gooseflesh.

Finally, medial temporal lobe structures have extensive reciprocal, direct connections with hypothalamic regions involved in the regulation, production, and secretion of reproductive hormones. These medial temporal lobe structures have a critical role in the development and maintenance of the gonads, and they regulate the level of reproductive function and sexual behavior. These structures, moreover, manifest selective hormonal binding and show sensitive morphologic, physiologic, and biochemical changes in response to hormonal influence. The hormonal effects of human limbic stimulation, the reproductive and sexual effects of temporal lobectomy, and the sensitive relation of temporal lobe seizure frequency to reproductive endocrine levels all are consistent with the notion that limbic structures may have similar functions in humans.

REPRODUCTIVE DYSFUNCTION AND EPILEPSY

Reproductive dysfunction is unusually common among people who have epilepsy.[4–6] Some observations suggest that reproductive disorders are more common with partial seizures of temporal lobe origin (temporal lobe epilepsy [TLE]) than with generalized or focal motor seizure disorders.[4] Studies that deal exclusively or predominantly with women who have TLE reveal that 14% to 20% have amenorrhea and that more than 50% overall have some form of menstrual dysfunction.[5,7,8] Fertility is reduced to 69% to 80% of the expected number of offspring.[9,10] Investigations of men who have TLE show that 49% to 71% have diminished potency or altered sexual interest.[11–16]

Elevated prolactin levels,[17–19] elevated or decreased gonadotropin levels,[20–24] elevated or decreased gonadotropin response to stimulation,[23–25] decreased free testosterone levels,[26,27] and decreased 17-ketosteroid excretion[28] all have been shown to occur in the epileptic population. Two investigations in particular are noteworthy, because they demonstrated reproductive endocrine abnormalities that correlated significantly with sexual dysfunction. Decreased urinary excretion of 17-ketosteroids, specifically androsterone and dehydroepiandrosterone sulfate (DHEAS), was observed in men with epilepsy.[28] A positive correlation was found between the lowered excretion of androgens and reduced potency. It also was shown that men with epilepsy have reduced serum free testosterone levels.[27] These concentrations were associated with higher serum gonadotropin and prolactin levels and were related to diminished sex drive significantly.

Abnormalities in serum levels of gonadotropins, prolactin, and luteinizing hormone (LH) response to GnRH suggest altered function of the hypothalamic-pituitary axis. Primary structural lesions at the level of the hypothalamus or pituitary gland, however, have not been evident at computed tomography (CT) or clinical assessment and follow-up evaluation.[5,6,23] Similarly, clinical evaluations and imaging studies of peripheral endocrine organs have not demonstrated structural lesions that provide a cause of the findings.[5,6,23]

Abundant data suggest that altered function of temporal lobe structures, a factor common to all patients with TLE who have reproductive dysfunction, may contribute to reproductive and sexual changes. TLE generally originates from or involves limbic portions of the temporal lobe.[29] Some of these limbic structures comprise anatomically distinct functional divisions that exert opposing modulatory influences on the structure and function of reproductive organs.[30] A most notable example is the amygdala,[30] which can be divided into corticomedial and basolateral portions. Each has its largely separate outflow tract—the stria terminalis and ventral amygdalofugal pathway, respectively. Bilateral ablations of the basolateral portion of the amygdala in adult female deer mice can induce anovulatory cycles and PCO changes.[31] Stimulation of the corticomedial amygdala in a number of mammalian species can induce ovulation and uterine contractions.[32,33] Transection of the stria terminalis blocks the ovulatory response, whereas a lesion of the ventral amygdalofugal pathway has no such effect.[33]

Stimulation and ablation studies of rodents suggest that the corticomedial amygdala promotes sexual activity, whereas the basolateral amygdala inhibits it.[30,31] Bilateral amygdalectomy of adult male rats and cats results in marked degeneration of the testes.[34] Bilateral amygdalectomy of female monkeys induces amenorrhea and hypogonadal vaginal changes.[35] TLE in men is associated with a greater occurrence of decreased sexual interest, impotence, and abnormal semen analysis.[36] TLE in women is associated with a greater occurrence of menstrual disorders and anovulatory cycles.[37] Temporal lobectomy of men and women with TLE is commonly associated with improved reproductive and sexual function and less frequently with the development or exacerbation of reproductive and sexual dysfunction.[8,38–40]

Altered temporal lobe function may contribute to reproductive endocrine changes. With regard to gonadotropins, the amygdala has extensive, direct anatomic connections with the arcuate and preoptic hypothalamic nuclei, which are involved in the regulation, production, and secretion of GnRH[41] (Fig 24–1). Alterations in the physiologic frequency or concentration of pulsatile GnRH secretion can induce changes in serum LH and follicle-stimulating hormone (FSH) levels that resemble patterns in reproductive endocrine disorders such as PCO syndrome and HH.[42] Stimulation of the two main divisions of the amygdala or their outflow tracts can predictably and differentially affect the membrane potentials of the same ventromedial hypothalamic neurons.[43] Stimulation and ablation studies of the amygdala in conjunction with gonadotropin assays have shown that the two functional divisions of the amygdala can produce elevations or reductions in pituitary and serum LH levels.[31]

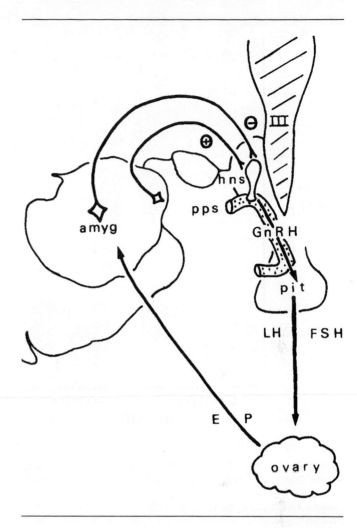

Figure 24–1. Cross section of the anterior temporal lobes and diencephalon depicts direct projections from the two anatomically distinct functional divisions of the amygdala (amyg) to the same ventromedial hypothalamic neurons. The different influences of these projections on hypothalamic neurosecretory cells (hns) modulate pulsatile gonadotropin-releasing hormone (GnRH) secretion. Releasing hormones enter the pituitary portal system (pps) and regulate the pattern of luteinizing hormone (LH) and follicle-stimulating hormone (FSH) secretion by the pituitary gland (pit). These gonadotropins induce ovulation and stimulate production of estradiol (E) and progesterone (P). Gonadal steroids bind to specific amygdaloid hormone receptors and influence neural activity, including epileptiform discharges.

Consistent with these data acquired in studies of animals is the finding that women with TLE have a range of early follicular phase serum LH levels that extend well above and below normal control values (Fig 24–2). This has led to the hypothesis that the involvement of temporal lobe limbic structures with seizure discharges may disrupt the normal limbic modulation of the hypothalamic regulation of pituitary secretion and promote the development of reproductive endocrine disorders (Fig 24–3).

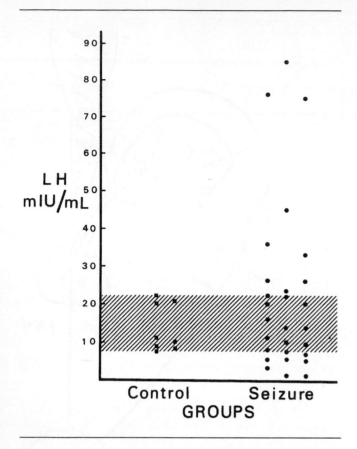

Figure 24-2. Graph shows the much broader range of baseline LH serum levels measured during the early follicular phase among 28 women with partial seizures of temporal lobe origin than among eight age-matched, healthy controls. This finding is consistent with the concept that involvement of the limbic system with epileptiform discharges may disrupt normal limbic modulation of hypothalamic regulation of pituitary gonadotropin secretion. *(From Herzog AG et al. Reproductive endocrine disorders in men with partial seizures of temporal lobe origin. Arch Neurol 43:347, 1986.)*

NEUROLOGIC CONSIDERATIONS OF MALE REPRODUCTIVE DYSFUNCTION

Androgens and Sexual Function in Men with Epilepsy

Reduced potency and hyposexuality occur in 38% to 71% of men with epilepsy.[4,11–16,44] The cause of these conditions is likely multifactorial, including psychosocial, epileptic, medicational, and hormonal factors.[13] Because androgens are considered to play an important role in the regulation of potency and libido,[45,46] measurement of serum levels of these hormones is a regular part of the medical evaluation. The most important androgen is testosterone. Testosterone exists in the serum in three forms: free, albumin bound, and sex hormone binding globulin (SHBG) bound.[47] Only about 2% of testosterone occurs in the free form, whereas 43% to 45% is bound to SHBG and 53% to 55% is bound to albumin.[47] There is general agreement that the SHBG-bound fraction of testosterone is not biologically active.[47–49] Considerable evidence exists, however, that the large pool of testosterone that is loosely bound to albumin is available to tissues.[48,49] Isojarvi et al[50] described three separate measures of serum testosterone in anticonvulsant-treated men with epilepsy. These investigators showed how the use of a particular medication or combination of medications can be associated with a low free androgen index (a measure of non–SHBG-bound testosterone) despite normal free testosterone and elevated serum levels of total testosterone. The data highlighted an important issue; that is, if androgen deficiency contributes to reproductive and sexual dysfunction among men with epilepsy,[6,22,27,28,51] which testosterone measurement is most relevant?

Several antiseizure medications induce the hepatic synthesis of increased amounts of SHBG that can result in normal or even elevated levels of total testosterone, yet they have been shown to reduce the concentrations of free or non–SHBG-bound testosterone.[26,27,50,52–54] Toone et al[27] found that reductions in free, but not total, testosterone were associated with decreased sexual interest. Fenwick et al[51] demonstrated a relation between decreased potency and low free testosterone levels. Isojarvi et al[50] showed that the free androgen index, one indicator of the non–SHBG-bound portion of testosterone, may be decreased despite normal free testosterone levels. The clinical significance of this finding is not known. My associates and I,[6] however, measured abnormally low non–SHBG-bound testosterone levels in five of eight treated epileptic men with diminished sexual interest or reduced potency. We[55] also observed in another study that among 13 men with epilepsy, those who were classified sexually healthy had an almost twofold higher average non–SHBG-bound testosterone value than those with reproductive or sexual dysfunction (2.4 vs 1.4 ng/mL [8.3 vs 4.8 nmol/L]). Nevertheless, only three of eight hyposexual men had levels below the normal control range, and the average values of both groups were normal. Only one total testosterone value was below the normal control range, and the average total testosterone values were not nearly as disparate (4.8 vs 4.0 ng/mL [16.6 vs 13.9 nmol/L]) between the sexually unaffected and affected groups. Free testosterone levels were not determined.

The demonstration by Isojarvi et al[50] that the free androgen index may be low when free testosterone levels are normal and our observations[6,55] that non–SHBG-bound testosterone may relate to the level of sexual activity suggest a need for an investigation that compares non–SHBG-bound and free testosterone in terms of their relation to reproductive and sexual dysfunction. Measures of non–SHBG-bound testosterone rather than free testosterone may potentially provide a more sensitive assessment of biologically and perhaps clinically significant androgen levels.

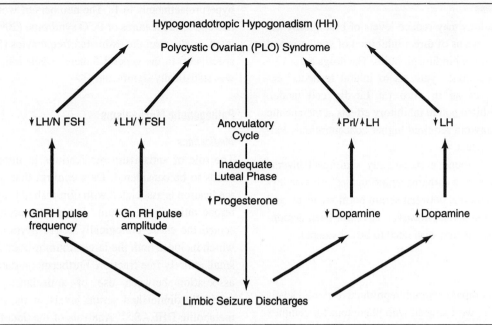

Figure 24–3. Possible mechanisms by which limbic seizure discharges may promote reproductive endocrine disorders and how abnormal reproductive hormone levels may influence epilepsy. Algorithm is based on a hypothesis that involvement of limbic structures with epileptiform discharges may disrupt normal limbic modulatory influences on hypothalamic secretion of GnRH. Altered frequency or amplitude of GnRH secretion may lead to patterns of pituitary secretion of LH and FSH, which are found in HH and PCO syndrome. Kindled limbic seizures alter brain dopamine levels. Hypothalamic dopamine exerts an inhibitory effect on pituitary LH and prolactin (Prl) secretion. Abnormal brain dopamine levels may alter pituitary gonadotropin and prolactin secretion, and promote the development of reproductive endocrine disorders. Reproductive endocrine disorders that are associated with partial seizures of temporal lobe origin are characterized by anovulatory cycles and diminished progesterone secretion. An elevated serum estrogen-to-progesterone ratio may promote the development of seizure discharges in the brain. *(Redrawn from Herzog AG et al: Reproductive endocrine disorders in men with partial seizures of temporal lobe origin.* Arch Neurol *43:347, 1986.)*

Neurologic Causes of Androgen Deficiency

Epilepsy

The disruption of normal temporolimbic modulation of hypothalamopituitary function by epileptiform discharges may promote the development of reproductive endocrine disorders.[56] Hypogonadism is unusually common among men with epilepsy. In our series of 20 men with partial seizures of temporal lobe origin, 11 (55%) had reproductive dysfunction or hyposexuality.[6] Nine of these 11 men (45% overall) had reproductive endocrine disorders, including HH in five (25%), hypergonadotropic hypogonadism in two (10%), and functional hyperprolactinemia in two (10%). Hypogonadism and abnormal semen analysis are as common among untreated as among treated men with epilepsy.[36] Lateralized cerebral and hypothalamic asymmetries moreover, may be responsible for the association of different patterns of reproductive endocrine secretion with left and right TLE.[55] The pulsatile secretion of LH over 8 hours during concomitant electroencephalographic (EEG) recording was evaluated among 12 men with unilateral paroxysmal temporal lobe epileptiform discharges and 11 healthy

men who acted as controls.[57] The LH pulse frequency was more variable among men with TLE than among controls, a finding that was statistically significant. Right temporal epileptiform activity was associated with greater LH pulse frequency than was left epileptiform activity, also a statistically significant finding. Paroxysmal unilateral slowing had opposite effects. The findings suggest that the laterality and nature of temporal lobe paroxysmal discharges may be important determinants of LH pulse frequency and the development of particular reproductive endocrine disorders.

Reproductive endocrine disorders may favor the development of TLE in men. Brain wave abnormalities, including temporal lobe epileptiform discharges, may occur with greater than expected frequency among men with these disorders.[58] Medial temporal lobe structures bind sex steroids, including testosterone.[59] Experimental data from studies with animals suggest that testosterone raises the electroshock seizure threshold and that orchiectomy lowers it.[60] Serum levels of free testosterone are usually decreased in the reproductive endocrine disorders associated with TLE in men[6,26,27] and may therefore favor the occurrence of epileptiform activity.

Antiseizure Medications

Antiseizure medications may reduce levels of biologically active testosterone by means of direct inhibition of synthesis and by means of induction of binding globulin. The drugs act at various levels of testosterone synthesis to inhibit testicular endocrine function.[61] In an in vitro rat Leydig cell model, carbamazepine exhibited potent inhibitory effects at therapeutic concentrations. Phenytoin required higher concentrations. Valproate had the least effect.

Macphee et al[54] found a statistically significant inverse correlation between serum carbamazepine and testosterone levels. Consistent correlations between serum hormone levels and antiseizure medication levels, however, have not been demonstrated.[22,27] Other factors may also need to be considered.

Estradiol

In an investigation comparing serum reproductive steroid levels between 20 men who were treated with phenytoin for complex partial seizures, 21 untreated men with complex partial seizures, and 20 age-matched healthy men who acted as controls, total and non–SHBG-bound estradiol levels were found to be significantly higher in the phenytoin group than in either the untreated or control groups,[62] a statistically significant finding. Barbiturates appear to have similar effects. These findings suggest that some antiseizure medications may lower free testosterone levels not only by means of induction of SHBG synthetase but also perhaps by means of induction of aromatase, which converts free testosterone to estradiol. Estradiol also increases SHBG synthesis. Moreover, it exerts a potent inhibitory influence on LH secretion and has been suggested to play an important role in negative feedback in men as well as in women.[63,64] Suppression of LH secretion results in HH. Chronically low free testosterone levels lead to testicular failure and hypergonadotropic hypogonadism. This may explain the frequent occurrence of both these reproductive endocrine disorders among men with epilepsy.[6] Finally, estradiol has been shown to produce premature aging of the hypothalamic arcuate nucleus, which secretes GnRH.[65,66]

NEUROLOGIC CONSIDERATIONS OF FEMALE REPRODUCTIVE DYSFUNCTION

In a study with a consecutive series of 50 women with clinical and EEG features of TLE, 28 (56%) had amenorrhea, oligomenorrhea, or abnormally long or short menstrual cycle intervals.[5] Nineteen (38%) of the 28 women with epilepsy and menstrual disorders had readily identifiable reproductive endocrine disorders: PCO syndrome in 10, HH (hypothalamic amenorrhea) in 6, premature menopause in 2, and functional hyperprolactinemia in 1.[5] The numbers of women with clinical and endocrine features of PCO syndrome (20%) and HH (12%) were greater than the estimated frequencies (5% and 1.5%, respectively) in the general female population, a difference that was statistically significant.

Pathogenetic Mechanisms

Medications

The role of antiseizure medications in infertility of women needs to be considered. Data confirm that use of antiseizure medication is associated with diminished free and total testosterone ratios in the serum.[5] Free testosterone actually represented the entire biologically active portion of testosterone, which includes both the large albumin-bound fraction and the small entirely free fraction. Furthermore, data demonstrate an association between use of antiseizure medication and markedly diminished serum levels of the adrenal androgen metabolite DHEAS.[5,67] Analysis of the data for women, however, did not show a statistically significant relation overall between the occurrence of menstrual disorders and the use of antiseizure medications (53% among users vs 60% among nonusers). Despite a demonstrated relationship between the use of valproate and PCO syndrome,[68] valproate was not yet in common use at the time of our investigation and was not one of the medications taken by any of the patients in the study. PCO syndrome was more common among the untreated (30%) than the treated (13%) women with epilepsy. PCO syndrome is characterized by abnormally high androgen levels. Antiseizure medications, such as barbiturates, phenytoin, and carbamazepine, induce hepatic enzymes and thereby lower biologically active androgen levels. Valproate does not. It is possible, therefore, that the higher occurrence of PCO syndrome among women who take valproate may be related to the failure of this medication to induce hepatic enzymes, which lower biologically active fractions of testosterone, although other potential mechanisms of action must be assessed. Therefore, although antiseizure medications alter reproductive hormone levels, it is unlikely that all the reproductive endocrine disorders among women with epilepsy can be attributed entirely to drug effects.

Neuroendocrine

Abnormal serum levels of gonadotropins and prolactin and an altered LH response to GnRH among these women suggest altered function of the hypothalamopituitary axis. Primary structural lesions at the level of the hypothalamus or pituitary gland, however, have not been evident at CT or clinical assessment and follow-up study.[5,23]

A role for altered temporolimbic EEG activity in the development of some reproductive endocrine disorders among women with epilepsy is supported by the finding of a statistically significant difference between the EEG laterality distributions associated with PCO syndrome and those associated with HH.[69] Among 30 women who had reproductive endocrine disorders and complex partial seizures with unilateral temporal lobe epileptiform discharges, there was a strong predominance of left-sided discharges (15 vs 1) with PCO syndrome and right-sided discharges (12 vs 2) with HH. Each distribution differed in a statistically significant way from that of 30 women with epilepsy who had no reproductive endocrine disorder (left/right = 17/13). Moreover, among women with PCO syndrome who had unilateral non–temporal lobe foci, six of seven had right-sided epileptiform discharges. This represented a statistically significant difference from the EEG laterality distribution among women with PCO syndrome who had temporal foci. These relations between altered patterns of reproductive hormonal secretion and the predominant laterality of EEG epileptiform discharges among women with epilepsy are consistent with a lateralized asymmetry in cerebral influences on reproductive endocrine function.

This hypothesis has been supported by investigations of the pulsatile secretion of LH by women with epilepsy. Untreated women with epilepsy have a higher LH pulse frequency than healthy controls,[70] whereas treated women have statistically significantly lower frequencies.[71] Left temporal epileptiform activity is associated with statistically significantly greater LH pulse frequency than right (left/right = 6/3; $P < .05$).[57] These findings suggest that the nature and laterality of temporal lobe EEG activity may be important determinants of LH pulse frequency and the development of particular reproductive endocrine disorders.

Neurotransmitter

Central dopaminergic mechanisms may contribute to the relation between TLE and reproductive endocrine disorders[56] (see Fig 24–3). Bromocriptine and dopamine lessen LH and prolactin secretion by the pituitary gland, and they are thought to act in the lateral palisade zone of the median eminence to inhibit GnRH secretion. Clinical studies of PCO syndrome reveal exaggerated suppression of LH levels with dopamine infusion and supranormal elevation of prolactin levels in response to haloperidol. These features and elevated baseline levels of LH and prolactin suggest a decreased level of dopamine activity in the hypothalamus of women with PCO syndrome.

The opposite has been proposed to explain HH. In the absence of hypothyroidism and structural lesions of the pituitary and peripheral endocrine glands, no organic origin is usually demonstrated to explain the low gonadotropin levels in HH. This amenorrhea is generally attributed to functional derangement of the hypothalamopituitary axis, especially excessive dopaminergic tone in the tuberoinfundibular region of the hypothalamus. Altered dopamine and homovanillic acid concentrations in the brains of animals with kindled amygdaloid seizures[72] and in the spinal fluid of patients with TLE[73] suggest a relation between TLE and brain dopamine metabolism. There is reason to consider, therefore, that epileptic discharges in medial temporal limbic structures may influence reproductive endocrine function by means of modulation of dopamine and GnRH levels in the hypothalamus.

Neural

Neural innervation of the gonads provides another potential mechanism by which altered brain function may induce reproductive and endocrine changes (Fig 24–4). This possibility has remained largely unexplored.[56] It has been demonstrated that bilateral ovariectomy is followed by a unilateral right-sided reduction in hypothalamic GnRH content, whereas unilateral ovariectomy on either side produces an ipsilateral increase in hypothalamic GnRH content.[74] These findings cannot readily be explained by endocrine factors alone.

The ovary is innervated both by sympathetic noradrenergic fibers that originate from neurons in the intermediolateral cell column of the spinal cord and by parasympathetic cholinergic fibers from the dorsal motor nucleus of the vagus. In rodent models, unilateral ovariectomy is generally associated with contralateral compensatory ovarian hypertrophy. Unilateral ovariectomy in association with 6-hydroxydopamine application to the remaining ovary results in decreased compensatory ovarian hypertrophy.[75] This has been attributed to blockage of noradrenergic neural transmission. Unilateral ovariectomy in association with bilateral vagotomy also results in diminished compensatory ovarian hypertrophy as well as in diminished elevations of serum LH and FSH levels and a prolonged estrus cycle.[76]

The amygdala has direct efferent projections to both the dorsal motor nucleus of the vagus and the dorsomedial and lateral regions of the hypothalamus.[56] The latter regulate the sympathetic response through direct projections to the neurons of the intermediolateral cell column of the spinal cord. Temporolimbic stimulation in adrenalectomized and hypophysectomized rats has been shown to increase or decrease estradiol and progesterone concentrations in the contralateral ovarian vein at 105 and 120 minutes, whereas ovarian blood flow remains unchanged.[77] Thus there is reason to investigate the possibility that involvement of medial temporal lobe structures with epileptiform discharges may disrupt normal limbic neural and neuroendocrine modulation of gonadal structure and function. The reverse may also be true. Sensory vagal fibers from the gonads terminate in the solitary nucleus of the medulla. The solitary nucleus is directly and extensively connected to the amygdala. The amygdala shows sensitive, short-latency, electrophysiologic responses to vagal stimulation. Therefore, sen-

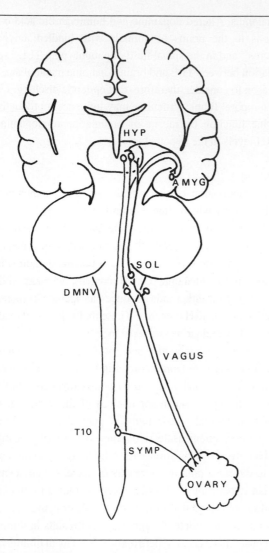

Figure 24–4. Neural pathways that may mediate limbic influences on gonadal structure and function. The amygdala (AMYG) has direct fiber projections to the dorsomedial and lateral regions of the hypothalamus (HYP). These regions are connected directly to the preganglionic sympathetic neurons in the intermediolateral cell column of the thoracolumbar spinal cord, from which originate sympathetic nerve fibers to the gonads. The amygdala also has direct and indirect projections to the dorsal motor nucleus of the vagus (DMNV), from which originate vagal fibers to the gonads. Afferent vagal fibers from the gonads project to the solitary nucleus in the medulla (SOL). The solitary nucleus has direct projections to the amygdala as well as to the hypothalamus.

sory input from pelvic reproductive structures may exert modulatory influences on limbic discharges.

Hormonal

Reproductive endocrine disorders may favor the development of TLE in women. Medial temporal lobe limbic structures bind hormones[59,78] and show sensitive electrophysiologic changes in response to hormonal influences.[79] Experimental and clinical data suggest that estrogen promotes interictal epileptiform brain wave activity and can precipitate clinical seizures. The antiestrogen clomiphene citrate has been shown to lessen both kainic acid–induced seizures in rats[80] and seizure frequency among epileptic women with reproductive endocrine disorders.[81] Progesterone also lessens the probability of interictal epileptiform activity and has benefitted some patients with epilepsy.[82–85] The anovulatory cycles in PCO syndrome and HH, therefore, may expose temporal lobe limbic structures to a constant estrogen effect without the normal progesterone elevation in the luteal phase and thereby heighten interictal epileptiform activity. In one study, 48 of 85 women (56%) with anovulatory cycles or amenorrhea were found to have EEG abnormalities, including some with focal paroxysmal epileptogenic discharges.[86] Treatment with clomiphene citrate restored EEG findings to normal in 26 women (54%). There was, moreover, an association between correction of the EEG and ovulation and pregnancy. Thus the hormonal changes associated with anovulatory cycles may favor the development of EEG abnormalities.

Prenatal Factors, Temporal Lobe Epilepsy, and Reproductive Endocrine Disorders

Another possibility to consider is that the association between TLE and some reproductive endocrine disorders may represent the parallel effects of prenatal factors common to the development of both the brain and the reproductive system. Both categories of disorder have a tendency to be familial. A genetically determined susceptibility to TLE was suggested by its greater than expected occurrence among first-order relatives.[87] Sex-linked dominant transmission[88] and autosomal dominant inheritance with variable expression[89] have been proposed to explain the high familial occurrence of PCO syndrome. Comparable studies of HH are not available. Premature menopause is reported to be familial.[90,91] It was attributed among four female members of one family to an interstitial deletion of the long arm of the X chromosome.[92] Autosomal dominant transmission with variable penetrance was proposed to explain the high familial frequency of HH among men.[93] Hypergonadotropic hypogonadism in disorders of gonadal differentiation is commonly associated with autosomal or sex chromosomal anomalies.[94] The possible contribution of hereditary traits or genetic linkage to the parallel development of both TLE and reproductive endocrine disorders warrants further investigation.

Data suggest that TLE and reproductive endocrine disorders may promote their mutual development. Specifically, involvement of limbic structures with epileptiform discharges may disrupt the normal modulation of reproductive endocrine function, and reproductive endocrine disorders may adversely affect neural activity in limbic structures and thereby enhance the development of TLE. Critical evaluation of these hypotheses with further research is required to obtain a better understanding of the interactions between reproductive endocrine disorders and epilepsy in the pathogenesis and management of both conditions.

Men and women with partial seizures may have a wide array of symptoms and findings. In the most obvious situations, seizures occur in clearly definable episodes and disrupt consciousness, memory, and continuing activities. In more subtle forms, symptoms blend with regular activities and perceptions. These forms are more difficult for patient and physician alike to diagnose. Many years may pass without recognition that the symptoms may be the manifestations of a potentially treatable, neuropathologic process that may also contribute to infertility. Therefore, the gynecologist and endocrinologist should obtain an EEG for patients who have reproductive or reproductive endocrine disorders that have neither a clearly definable primary cause in the reproductive or endocrine system nor an adequate response to therapy.

EEG studies are especially important if patients have emotional, behavioral, learning, perceptual, or autonomic manifestations consistent with a diagnosis of TLE. Suspicion should also be raised if there is evidence of left-handedness or skeletal asymmetry to suggest anomalous brain development or brain injury early in life. Other predisposing factors for brain wave abnormalities include a history of birth difficulty, febrile seizure, or head injury with loss of consciousness or memory. Most patients with partial seizures of temporal lobe origin have paroxysmal epileptiform activity or at least slowing of brain waves in temporal derivatives of an EEG. If results of a conventional EEG are normal, there is an additional 10% yield of positive findings of EEGs performed while the patient is asleep, especially with the use of nasopharyngeal or sphenoidal leads.

Some evidence exists that the return of brain wave function to normal may be associated with increased fertility. As noted earlier, results of EEGs were abnormal among most of one series of infertile women, and correction of the EEG was associated with ovulation and pregnancy.[86] The anticonvulsant phenytoin was used to treat 80 infertile women with an inadequate luteal phase and EEG abnormalities.[95] A 45% pregnancy rate was recorded within 4 months of the onset of therapy.

We used antiseizure medications to treat five women with newly diagnosed partial seizures and a 5- to 7-year history of unsuccessfully treated infertility in association with PCO syndrome. Three of the five women became pregnant within 3 months. Two of these women continued using antiseizure medication to term. The third patient tapered and discontinued the medication after learning of her pregnancy. All three women delivered apparently healthy, full-term babies. In several surgical series of unilateral temporal lobectomy for intractable epilepsy, improved seizure control was associated with normalization of reproductive function, restored fertility, and improved sexual behavior.[13–15,38,40]

Further investigations are required to establish the precise role of brain wave therapy in the treatment of infertility. Thorough neurologic and EEG evaluation of potential extrahypothalamic influences on reproductive and endocrine function should be considered for all infertile men and women who do not have a clearly definable primary cause identified in the reproductive or endocrine systems.

REFERENCES

1. Plan for Nationwide Action on Epilepsy. DHEW publication (NIH) 78-311. Washington, DC, Department of Health, Education, and Welfare, 1978, vol 2
2. Schomer DL: Current concepts in neurology: Partial epilepsy. *N Engl J Med* 309:356, 1983
3. Bear D, Fedio P: Quantitative analysis of interictal behavior in temporal lobe epilepsy. *Arch Neurol* 34:457, 1976
4. Gastaut H, Collomb H: Etude du comportement sexuel chez les epileptiques psychomoteurs. *Ann Med Psychol* 112:657, 1954
5. Herzog AG, Seibel MM, Schomer DL, et al: Reproductive endocrine disorders in women with partial seizures of temporal lobe origin. *Arch Neurol* 43:341, 1986
6. Herzog AG, Seibel MM, Schomer DL, et al: Reproductive endocrine disorders in men with partial seizures of temporal lobe origin. *Arch Neurol* 43:347, 1986
7. Jensen I, Vaernet K: Temporal lobe epilepsy: Follow-up investigation of 74 temporal lobe resected patients. *Acta Neurochir* 37:173, 1977
8. Trampuz V, Dimitrijevic M, Kryanovski J: Ulga epilepsije u patogenezi disfunkeije ovarija. *Neuropsihijatrija* 23:179, 1975
9. Dansky LV, Andermann E, Andermann F: Marriage and fertility in epileptic patients. *Epilepsia* 21:261, 1980
10. Webber MP, Hauser WA, Ottman R, Annegers JF: Fertility in persons with epilepsy: 1935–1974. *Epilepsia* 27:746, 1986
11. Hierons R, Saunders M: Impotence in patients with temporal lobe lesions. *Lancet* 2:761, 1966
12. Kolarsky A, Freund K, Machek J, et al: Association with early temporal lobe damage. *Arch Gen Psychiatry* 17:735, 1967
13. Taylor DC: Sexual behavior and temporal lobe epilepsy. *Arch Neurol* 21:510, 1969
14. Blumer D: Changes of sexual behavior related to temporal lobe disorders in man. *J Sex Res* 6:173, 1970
15. Jensen I, Larsen JK: Mental aspects of temporal lobe epilepsy. *J Neurol Neurosurg Psychiatry* 42:256, 1979
16. Shukla GD, Srivastava ON, Katiyar BC: Sexual disturbances in temporal lobe epilepsy: A controlled study. *Br J Psychiatry* 134:288, 1979
17. Abbott RJ, Browning MC, Davidson DL: Serum prolactin and cortisol concentrations after grand mal seizures. *J Neurol Neurosurg Psychiatry* 43:163, 1980

18. Pritchard PB III, Wannamaker BB, Sagel J, et al: Endocrine function following complex seizures. *Ann Neurol* 14:27, 1983

19. Dana-Haeri J, Trimble MR, Oxley J: Prolactin and gonadotropin change following generalized and partial seizures. *J Neurol Neurosurg Psychiatry* 46:331, 1983

20. Toone BK, Wheeler M, Fenwick PBC: Sex hormone changes in epileptics. *Clin Endocrinol (Oxf)* 12:391, 1980

21. Hoffman J, Kahlert T: Veraenderungen von sexual Hormonen bei maennlichen Epilepsie-Patienten unter Langzeittherapie. *Nervenarzt* 52:715, 1981

22. Rodin E, Subramanian MG, Gilroy J: Investigation of sex hormones in male epileptic patients. *Epilepsia* 25:690, 1984

23. Herzog AG, Russell V, Vaitukaitis JL, et al: Neuroendocrine dysfunction in temporal lobe epilepsy. *Arch Neurol* 39:133, 1982

24. Murialdo G, Manni R, DeMaria A, et al: Luteinizing hormone pulsatile secretion and pituitary response to gonadotropin-releasing hormone and to thyrotropin-releasing hormone in male epileptic subjects on chronic phenobarbital treatment. *J Endocrinol Invest* 10:27, 1987

25. Dana-Haeri J, Oxley J, Richens A: Pituitary responsiveness to gonadotropin-releasing and thyrotrophin-releasing hormones in epileptic patients receiving carbamazepine or phenytoin. *Clin Endocrinol (Oxf)* 20:163, 1984

26. Dana-Haeri J, Oxley J, Richens A: Reduction of free testosterone by antiepileptic drugs. *Br Med J (Clin Res Ed)* 284:85, 1982

27. Toone BK, Wheeler M, Nanjee M, et al: Sex hormones, sexual activity and plasma anticonvulsant levels in male epileptics. *J Neurol Neurosurg Psychiatry* 46:824, 1983

28. Christiansen P, Deigaard J, Lund M: Potens, fertilitet of konshormonudskillelse hos yngre manglige epilepsilidende. *Ugeskr Laeger* 137:2402, 1975

29. Falconer MA, Serafetinides EA, Corsellis JAN: Etiology and pathogenesis of temporal lobe epilepsy. *Arch Neurol* 10:233, 1964

30. Kaada B: Stimulation and regional ablation of the amygdaloid complex with reference to functional representations. In: Eleftheriou BE (ed), *The Neurobiology of the Amygdala.* New York, Plenum, 1972:205–281

31. Zolovick AJ: Effects of lesions and electrical stimulation of the amygdala on hypothalamic-hypophyseal regulation. In: Eleftheriou BE (ed), *The Neurobiology of the Amygdala.* New York, Plenum, 1972:745–762

32. Koikegami H, Yamada T, Usui K: Stimulation of the amygdaloid nuclei and periamygdaloid cortex with special reference to its effects on uterine movements and ovulation. *Folia Psychiatry Neurol Jpn* 8:7, 1954

33. Velasco ME, Taleisnik S: Release of gonadotropins induced by amygdaloid stimulation in the rat. *Endocrinology* 84:132, 1960

34. Yamada T, Greer MA: The effect of bilateral ablation of the amygdala on endocrine function in the rat. *Endocrinology* 66:565, 1960

35. Erickson LB, Wada JA: Effects of lesions in the temporal lobe and rhinencephalon on reproductive function in adult female rhesus monkeys. *Fertil Steril* 21:434, 1970

36. Taneja N, Kucheria K, Jain S, Maheshwari MC: Effect of phenytoin on semen. *Epilepsia* 35:136, 1994

37. Cummings LN, Giudice L, Morrell MJ: Ovulatory function in epilepsy. *Epilepsia* 36:353, 1995

38. Savard RJ, Walker E: Changes in social functioning after surgical treatment for temporal lobe epilepsy. *Social Work* 10:87, 1985

39. Taylor DC, Falconer MA: Clinical socioeconomic and psychological adjustment after temporal lobectomy for epilepsy. *Br J Psychiatry* 114:124, 1968

40. Cogen PH, Antunes JL, Correll JW: Reproductive function in temporal lobe epilepsy: The effect of temporal lobectomy. *Surg Neurol* 12:243, 1979

41. Renaud LP: Influence of amygdala stimulation on the activity of identified tuberoinfundibular neurons in the rat hypothalamus. *J Physiol* (Lond) 260:237, 1976

42. Knobil E: The neuroendocrine control of the menstrual cycle. *Recent Prog Horm Res* 36:53, 1980

43. Dreifuss JJ, Murphy JT, Gloor P: Contrasting effects of two identified amygdaloid efferent pathways on single hypothalamic neurons. *J Neurophysiol* 31:237, 1986

44. Fenwick PBC, Toone BK, Wheeler MJ, et al: Sexual behavior in a centre for epilepsy. *Acta Neurol Scand* 71:428, 1985

45. Davidson JM. Neurohormonal basis of sexual behavior. In: Greep RP (ed), *Reproductive Physiology II.* Baltimore, University Park Press, 13:225, 1977

46. Davidson JM, Camargo CA, Smith ER: Effects of androgen on sexual behavior in hypogonadal men. *J Clin Endocrinol Metab* 48:955, 1979

47. Sodergard R, Backstrom T, Shanbhag V, Carstensen H: Calculation of free and bound fractions of testosterone and estradiol-17 beta to plasma proteins at body temperature. *J Steroid Biochem* 16:801, 1982

48. Cummings DC, Wall SR: Non–sex hormone binding globulin and bound testosterone as a marker for hypogonadism. *J Clin Endocrinol Metab* 61:873, 1985

49. Manni A, Partridge WM, Cefalu W, et al: Bioavailability of albumin-bound testosterone. *J Clin Endocrinol Metab* 61:705, 1985

50. Isojarvi JIT, Pakarinen AJ, Ylipalosaari PJ, Myllyla VV: Serum hormones in male epileptic patients receiving anticonvulsant medication. *Arch Neurol* 47:670, 1990

51. Fenwick PBC, Mercer C, Grant R, et al: Nocturnal penile tumescence and serum testosterone levels. *Arch Sex Behav* 15:13, 1986

52. Barragry JM, Makin HLJ, Trafford DJH, et al: Effect of anticonvulsants on plasma testosterone and sex hormone binding globulin levels. *J Neurol Neurosurg Psychiatry* 41:913, 1978

53. Connell JM, Rapeport WG, Beastall GH, Brodie MJ: Changes in circulating androgens during short-term carbamazepine therapy. *Br J Clin Pharmacol* 17:347, 1984

54. Macphee GJA, Larkin JG, Butler E, et al: Circulating hormones and pituitary responsiveness in young epileptic men receiving long-term antiepileptic medication. *Epilepsia* 29:468, 1988

55. Herzog AG, Drislane FW, Schomer DL, et al: Abnormal pulsatile secretion of luteinizing hormone in men with epilepsy: Relation-

ship to laterality and nature of paroxysmal discharges. *Neurol* 40:1557, 1990

56. Herzog AG: A hypothesis to integrate partial seizures of temporal lobe origin and reproductive endocrine disorders. *Epilepsy Res* 3:151, 1989

57. Herzog AG, Coleman AE, Drislane FW, Schomer DS: Asymmetric temporal lobe modulation of luteinizing hormone secretion. *Neuroendocrinol* 60:35, 1994

58. Spark R, Wills C, Royal H: Hypogonadism, hyperprolactinemia, and temporal lobe epilepsy in hyposexual men. *Lancet* 1:413, 1984

59. Stumpf WE: Steroid-concentrating neurons in the amygdala. In: Eleftheriou BE (ed), *The Neurobiology of the Amygdala.* New York, Plenum, 1972:763–774

60. Longo LPS, Saldana LEG: Hormones and their influence in epilepsy. *Acta Neurol Latinoamer* 12:29, 1966

61. Kuhn-Velten WN, Herzog AG, Muller MR: Acute effects of anticonvulsant drugs on gonadotropin-stimulated and precursor-supported testicular androgen production. *Eur J Pharmacol* 181:151, 1990

62. Herzog AG, Levesque L, Drislane F, et al: Phenytoin-induced elevation of serum estradiol and reproductive dysfunction in men with epilepsy. *Epilepsia* 32:550, 1991

63. Loriaux D, Vigersky S, Marynick S, et al: Androgen and estrogen effects in the regulation of LH in man. In: Troen P, Nankin H (eds), *The Testis in Normal and Infertile Men.* New York, Raven, 1977:213

64. Winters S, Janick J, Loriaux L, Sherins R: Studies on the role of sex steroids in the feedback control of gonadotropin concentrations in men. II. Use of the estrogen antagonist clomiphene citrate. *J Clin Endocrinol Metab* 48:222, 1979

65. Brawer J, Schipper H, Robaire B: Effects of long-term androgen and estradiol exposure on the hypothalamus. *Endocrinology* 112:194, 1983

66. Finch CE, Felicio LS, Mobbs CV, Nelson JF: Ovarian and steroidal influences on neuroendocrine aging processes in female rodents. *Endocrinol Rev* 5:467, 1984

67. Levesque LA, Herzog AG, Seibel MM: The effect of phenytoin and carbamazepine on serum dehydroepiandrosterone sulfate in men and women who have partial seizures with temporal lobe involvement. *J Clin Endocrinol Metab* 63:243, 1986

68. Isojarvi JIT, Laatkainen TJ, Pakarinen AJ, et al: Polycystic ovaries and hyperandrogenism in women taking valproate for epilepsy. *N Engl J Med* 329:1383, 1993

69. Herzog AG: A relationship between particular reproductive endocrine disorders and the laterality of epileptiform discharges in women with epilepsy. *Neurol* 43:1907, 1993

70. Bilo L, Meo R, Valentino R, et al: Abnormal patterns of luteinizing hormone pulsatility in women with epilepsy. *Fertil Steril* 55:705, 1991

71. Drislane FW, Coleman AE, Schomer DL, et al: Altered pulsatile secretion of luteinizing hormone in women with epilepsy. *Neurol* 44:306, 1994

72. Sato M, Nakashima T: Kindling: Secondary epileptogenesis, sleep and catecholamines. *Can J Neurol Sci* 2:439, 1975

73. Papeschi R, Molina-Negro P, Sourkes TL, et al: The concentration of homovanillic and 5-hydroxyindoleacetic acid in ventricular and lumbar CSF. *Neurol* 22:1151, 1972

74. Gerandai I, Rotstejn WH, Marchetti B, et al: Unilateral ovariectomy induced luteinizing hormone-releasing hormone content changes in the two halves of the mediobasal hypothalamus. *Neurosci Lett* 9:333, 1978

75. Gerandai I, Marchetti B, Maugeri S, et al: Prevention of compensatory ovarian hypertrophy by local treatment of the ovary with 6-OHDA. *Neuroendocrinology* 27:272, 1978

76. Burden HW, Lawrence IE: The effect of denervation on compensatory ovarian hypertrophy. *Neuroendocrinology* 23:368, 1977

77. Kawakami M, Kubo K, Vemura T, et al: Involvement of ovarian innervation in steriod secretion. *Endocrinology* 109:136, 1981

78. Pfaff DW, Keiner M: Estradiol-concentrating cells in the rat amygdala as part of a limbic-hypothalamic hormone-sensitive system. In: Eleftheriou BE (ed), *The Neurobiology of the Amygdala.* New York, Plenum, 1972:775–792

79. Sawyer CH: Functions of the amygdala related to the feedback actions of gonadal steroid hormones. In: Eleftheriou BE (ed), *The Neurobiology of the Amygdala.* New York, Plenum, 1972: 745–762

80. Nicoletti F, Speciale C, Sortino MA, et al: Comparative effects of estradiol benzoate, the antiestrogen clomiphene citrate, and the progestin medroxyprogesterone acetate on kainic acid–induced seizures in male and female rats. *Epilepsia* 26:252, 1985

81. Herzog AG: Clomiphene therapy in epileptic women with menstrual disorders. *Neurology* 38:432, 1988

82. Herzog AG: Intermittent progesterone therapy and frequency of complex partial seizures in women with menstrual disorders. *Neurology* 36:1607, 1986

83. Herzog AG: Progesterone therapy in women with complex partial and secondary generalized seizures. *Neurol* 45:1660–1662, 1995

84. Mattson RH, Cramer JA, Caldwell BV, et al: Treatment of seizures with medroxyprogesterone acetate: Preliminary report. *Neurology* 34:1255, 1984

85. Zimmerman AW, Holden KR, Reiter EO, et al: Medroxyprogesterone acetate in the treatment of seizures associated with menstruation. *J Pediatr* 83:959, 1973

86. Sharf M, Sharf B, Bental E, et al: The electroencephalogram in the investigation of anovulation and its treatment by clomiphene. *Lancet* 1:750, 1969

87. Andermann E: Multifactorial inheritance of generalized and focal epilepsy. In: Anderson VE, Hauser WA, Penry JK, et al (eds), *Genetic Basis of the Epilepsies.* New York, Raven, 1982: 355–374

88. Givens JR: Hirsutism and hyperandrogenism. *Adv Intern Med* 21:221, 1976

89. Jaffee WL, Vaitukaitis JL: Polycystic ovarian syndrome. In: Vaitukaitis JL (ed), *Clinical Reproductive Neuroendocrinology.* New York, Elsevier, 1982:207–230

90. Coulam CB, Stringfellow S, Hoefnagel D: Evidence for a genetic factor in the etiology of premature ovarian failure. *Fertil Steril* 40:693, 1983

91. Mattison DR, Evans MI, Schwimmer WB, et al: Familial premature ovarian failure. *Am J Hum Genet* 36:134, 1984

92. Krauss CM, Turksoy RN, Atkins L, et al: Familial premature ovarian failure due to an interstitial deletion of the long arm of the X chromosome. *N Engl J Med* 317:125, 1987

93. Santen RJ, Paulsen CA: Hypogonadotropic eunuchoidism. I. Clinical study of the mode of inheritance. *J Clin Endocrinol Metab* 36:47, 1973

94. Grumbach MD, Conte FA: Disorders of sex differentiation. In: Williams RH (ed), *Textbook of Endocrinology.* Philadelphia, Saunders, 1981:423–514

95. Gautray JP, Jolivet A, Goldenberg F, et al: Clinical investigation of the menstrual cycle. II. Neuroendocrine investigation and therapy of the inadequate luteal phase. *Fertil Steril* 29:275, 1978

CHAPTER 25

Body Weight and Reproduction

G. WILLIAM BATES

Effects of Body Fat on Hormone
Secretion and Metabolism
Treatment of Underweight Women

Treatment of Overweight Women
Summary

Fascination with thinness and dietary control pervades a large segment of U.S. society.[1,2] One need only witness the number of men and women jogging or running along the streets of U.S. cities, towns, and villages, or notice the prolific number of books and articles written on diet and weight control. Health centers abound. Many are associated with health care institutions. Recent research[3] linked excessive body weight with early mortality among women, and the authors of the study recommended that women lose weight to levels *below* recommended levels in current United States guidelines.

Body weight, specifically body fat, plays an essential role in the initiation and maintenance of reproductive function of men and women.[4,5] Moreover, once pregnancy occurs, the existing amount of body fat at conception and the weight gain during pregnancy appear to influence pregnancy outcome.[6] A high proportion of well-trained athletes, ballet dancers, gymnasts, and women who control their weight excessively experience amenorrhea.[7-10] Women who are obese also have a high incidence of amenorrhea and infertility.[11] Thus there must be an optimal body weight for successful reproductive function.

Six percent of cases of primary infertility in which ovulatory dysfunction is present result from being excessively underweight, and another 6% from being excessively overweight.[12] Therefore, 12% of infertility is caused by female body weight disorders. (The impact of body weight disorders on male repro-

duction is unknown.) More than 70% of these women conceive spontaneously if their weight disorder is corrected through a weight-gaining or a weight-reduction diet as appropriate.[13,14] Yet body weight is often considered last in an infertility evaluation. It may be ignored entirely until other diagnostic studies and therapeutic interventions have proved normal or futile. In my opinion, the body weight *of both partners* of the infertile couple should be considered first when there is an obviously slender or obese body habitus. Appropriate counseling about the effects of body weight on reproductive function can save a couple time and money in achieving pregnancy.

EFFECTS OF BODY FAT ON HORMONE SECRETION AND METABOLISM

Body fat affects gonadotropin secretion at the time of puberty and in association with weight loss. In prepubertal children, there is little secretion of the gonadotropins—follicle-stimulating hormone (FSH) and luteinizing hormone (LH). With the onset of puberty, there is increased secretion of both FSH and LH, but secretion of LH is greater. With the establishment of ovulatory cycles (and spermatogenesis in boys) the gonadotropin secretory pattern seen in sexually mature adults develops.[15] These dynamic changes are presented in Fig 25–1.

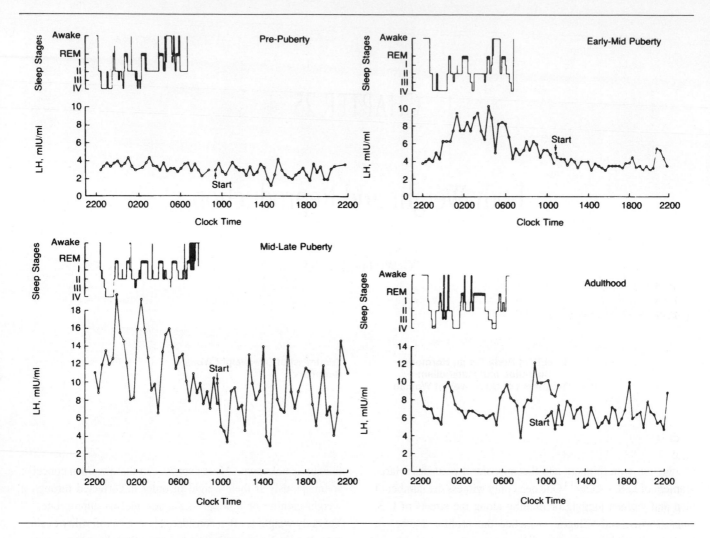

Figure 25–1. 24-hour luteinizing hormone (LH) secretory pattern in stages of puberty. *(From Katz J, et al: Weight and circadian luteinizing hormone secretory pattern in anorexia nervosa.* Psychosom Med *4:549, 1978.)*

With loss of body fat, the gonadotropin secretory pattern reverts to an intrapubertal pattern and then a prepubertal pattern if the weight loss is so severe as to constitute anorexia nervosa.[16] Thus we see dynamic changes in gonadotropin secretory pattern with downward changes in body weight.

Virgersky et al[17] described the changes in gonadotropin secretion in secondary amenorrhea associated with simple weight loss. In simple weight loss, there is first an increase in the secretion of LH similar to the pattern seen in polycystic ovarian (PCO) disease. With additional weight loss, there is suppression of both FSH and LH to levels seen among prepubertal children. Genazzani et al[18] found decreased LH pulse frequency and pulse amplitude among women with hypothalamic amenorrhea associated with weight loss. Reichman et al[19] found lengthening of the follicular phase of the cycle in women who ate a controlled diet. Therefore, if the gonadotropin secretory pattern of a slender woman mimics that found in PCO disease, *weight loss*

is considered the cause of hypothalamic dysfunction and infertility. If the gonadotropin secretory pattern is similar to that of a child, there is usually a profound loss (or deficiency) of body fat that necessitates dietary therapy to restore normal ovulatory cycles. When body weight is restored to within 5% of predicted ideal body weight (IBW), gonadotropin secretory patterns return to normal and ovulatory cycles resume.[20] An example of the LH-to-FSH ratios among a group of women with deviations from ideal body weight is presented in Fig 25–2.

In addition to the effects of body weight changes on gonadotropin secretion, there is an alteration in the metabolism of estradiol-17β among slender and obese women. Fishman et al[21] were the first to demonstrate deviations from expected pathways of estradiol-17β metabolism in association with anorexia nervosa and obesity. By infusing radiolabeled estradiol-17β and measuring the urinary products, they found that underweight women had a preferential metabolism of estradiol-17β to the 2-

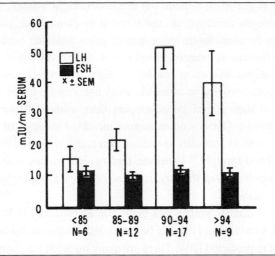

Figure 25-2. Serum gonadotropin levels among 44 women at various percentages of ideal body weight. *(From Bates GW, et al: Reproductive failure in women who practice weight control. Fertil Steril 1982;37:373.)*

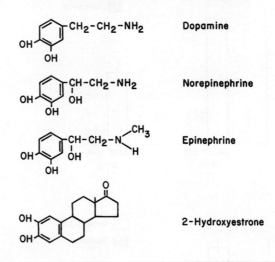

Figure 25-3. Structural similarity between the catecholamine neurotransmitters and catechol estrone. The catechol ring is the site of metabolic inactivation by catechol-O-methyltransferase. *(From Bates GW: On the nature of the hot flash. Clin Obstet Gynecol 1981;24:231.)*

hydroxylated estrogens 2-hydroxyestrone and 2-hydroxyestradiol. These estrogens—designated catechol estrogens because of their structural similarity to the catecholamines—act as antiestrogens and downregulate estradiol receptors and hypothalamic gonadotropin-releasing hormone (GnRH) secretion. The structural similarities of catecholamines and catechol estrogens is presented in Fig 25-3.

In obese women the preferential route of estradiol metabolism is to estriol, a weak, but nevertheless, active estrogen. Thus in obese women, estradiol is not completely cleared to a metabolically inactive estrogen but to a metabolite that has estrogenic action. The differential metabolic pathways of estradiol in thin and obese women were confirmed by Hershcopf et al.[22]

Sitteri and Macdonald,[23] by infusing radiolabeled androstenedione and estrone into obese women, found that obese women have increased conversion of androstenedione to estrone in adipose tissue. Not only do obese women (and men) have increased metabolism of estradiol to estriol, but also obese people have increased extraglandular production of estrone in adipose tissue. Obese people are hyperestrogenic.

Because PCO syndrome is more common among obese than thin women, Yen[24] postulated that the increased estrone level associated with obesity could increase pituitary secretion of LH, which would increase ovarian secretion of androstenedione. This theory holds in practice. Obese, anovulatory women have elevated androstenedione, estrone, and LH levels. When they take oral contraceptives to suppress LH secretion, there is

decrease in the plasma concentrations of androstenedione and estrone. Moreover, when obese women lose weight, their reproductive cycles and levels of ovarian hormones return to normal.[14,25] The effects of weight loss on gonadotropin secretion and plasma androgen concentrations are shown in Figs 25-4 and 25-5.

Underweight and overweight conditions alter gonadotropin secretion and sex steroid hormone metabolism. These metabolic alterations lead to decreased reproductive function

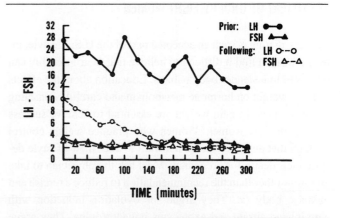

Figure 25-4. Serum gonadotropin secretion of an obese, infertile woman before (136% ideal body weight) and after (122% ideal body weight) weight loss.

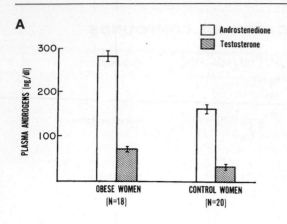

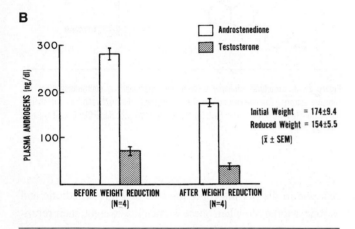

Figure 25–5. A. Serum androstenedione and testosterone levels of obese and normal-weight women. **B.** Changes in serum androstenedione and testosterone levels after weight loss by four women.

It is important to point out that underweight women, who are estrogen deficient, do not respond to clomiphene citrate therapy because clomiphene citrate requires adequate estradiol to be effective. Hypoestrogenism is part of the condition of low body weight. Women of low body weight who receive exogenous gonadotropins to stimulate ovulation require fewer ampules of menopausal gonadotropins than women of normal body weight. Obese women require increased ampules of gonadotropins to stimulate ovulation compared with women of normal body weight.[26] However, *underweight women with hypoestrogenism need the largest amount of gonadotropins to induce ovulation.*[27]

If a woman weighs less than 95% of predicted IBW for height, I recommend that she be counseled to increase her body weight to predicted IBW. There are many methods for computing IBW. It can be calculated from underwater weighing, from radiolabeled clearance studies, or from calculation of the Quetelet index. I calculate IBW by using the median weight for a medium frame of the Metropolitan Life Insurance Table.[28] The 1983 Metropolitan Life Insurance table for body weight is presented in Table 25–1. The median weight for a medium frame is the base IBW. The deviation of the patient's weight from IBW is calculated to derive the patient's percentage of IBW. If the percentage of deviation from IBW is more than 5% below IBW, I recommend that the patient gain to that weight.

A diet high in fat and calories is recommended. Foods such as ice cream, french fries, butter, and cheese facilitate weight gain. Weight gain at the rate of ½ pound (0.2 kg) per week is

and may be the cause of infertility for as many as 15% of infertile couples.

TREATMENT OF UNDERWEIGHT WOMEN

Because dieting is such an accepted part of the U.S. lifestyle, infertile women find it difficult to believe that their infertility can be linked to a slender body habitus. Education about the effects of body weight on hormone metabolism and careful counseling about the need to gain weight are essential to achieve success by underweight women. Women who practice weight control through diet and exercise do not want to alter their lifestyle despite their desire for pregnancy. Most ask the physician to take any steps other than the recommendation to reduce exercise and increase body fat. They argue for ovulation induction with clomiphene citrate and exogenous gonadotropins. They argue for one of the assisted reproductive technologies instead of recommendations to gain weight.

TABLE 25–1. 1983 METROPOLITAN INSURANCE COMPANY HEIGHT AND WEIGHT TABLE FOR WOMEN

Height		Weight (lb)		
Feet	**Inches**	**Small Frame**	**Medium Frame**	**Large Frame**
4	10	102–111	109–121	118–131
4	11	103–113	111–123	120–134
5	0	104–115	113–126	122–137
5	1	106–118	115–129	125–140
5	2	108–121	118–132	128–143
5	3	111–124	121–135	131–147
5	4	114–127	124–138	134–151
5	5	117–130	127–141	137–155
5	6	120–133	130–144	140–159
5	7	123–136	133–147	143–163
5	8	126–139	136–150	146–167
5	9	129–142	139–153	149–170
5	10	132–145	142–156	152–173
5	11	135–148	145–159	155–176
6	0	138–151	148–162	158–179

advised. Some women want to reach IBW as quickly as possible. I discourage rapid weight gain. Infertile, underweight women can expect conception within 6 to 8 months *after* restoration of body weight.

Another way to help women identify their low body weight is to ask them to sketch themselves at the present weight and at the recommended IBW. Distortions of body image sometimes are present in these sketches. The greater the distortion of body image, the more difficult it is for that particular woman to achieve weight gain. Examples of sketches made by underweight women are presented in Figs 25–6 and 25–7.

Encouragement is beneficial. Praise should be lavish when women are able to gain weight. Negative criticism is withheld if weight gain does not occur as rapidly as expected. One should ask how family members (husband and parents) react to the idea of weight gain. Often, family members have already made the suggestion that the infertile woman is underweight and could benefit from weight gain. The support of family members should be enlisted to encourage weight gain.

With weight gain, the woman can be expected to become euestrogenic. Therefore, she should expect increased breast size and increased cervical mucous secretion. Because these are positive changes, they should be emphasized.

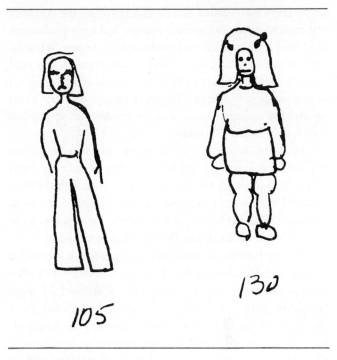

Figure 25–7. Self-sketch of a severely underweight woman at present body weight and at predicted ideal body weight. Note the distorted body image.

TREATMENT OF OVERWEIGHT WOMEN

Obese women are more apt to acknowledge the impact of obesity on reproductive function than are slender women. However, the challenge of weight loss is just as daunting for obese women as is the challenge of weight gain for slender women. Most obese people (men and women) have tried diets, exercise programs, and other methods to lose weight, but have not been successful. When a physician recommends a weight reduction program for obese people trying to conceive, this recommendation is viewed as another wasted effort.

The approach the physician takes to weight reduction shapes the outcome. Like underweight women, obese women need education and counseling. Moreover, they need encouragement and understanding with praise for accomplishments in weight reduction.

Because androgens are anabolic steroids, and because many obese women have androgen excess, evaluation of infertility for an obese woman begins with measurement of gonadotropins (FSH and LH), prolactin, androstenedione, total testosterone, and dehydroepiandrosterone sulfate (DHEAS). If androstenedione or testosterone level is elevated, oral contraceptive therapy is recommended to downregulate pituitary gonadotropin secretion with the effect of reducing ovarian androgen production.[29] This step facilitates weight reduction.

Obese, infertile women find it paradoxic to take oral contraceptives when the objective is pregnancy. Yet when they are

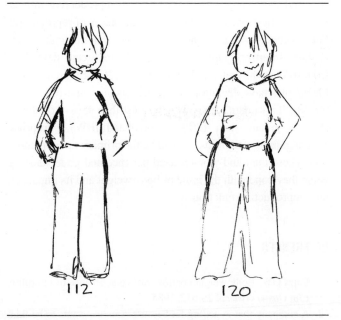

Figure 25–6. Self-sketch of an underweight, infertile woman at present body weight and at predicted ideal body weight. Note the healthy self-image.

taught about the anabolic role of androgens and the effects of oral contraceptives in lowering ovarian androgen production, they often readily accept oral contraceptive therapy. When infertile women begin therapy with oral contraceptives, they must be given a realistic time period to take the oral contraceptives. I usually suggest 6 months. Weight reduction does not occur rapidly; the realistic expectations for reaching an appropriate body weight is 6 to 12 months.

Next, the patient is given a weight reduction diet of less than 1200 calories a day and less than 20 g of fat a day. Most people lose about 1 pound (0.45 kg) per week with this diet. Men and women are counseled that they can eat many foods and stay within the caloric and fat limits. Patients should be given examples of foods that fit within these guidelines.

Finally, patients are given an exercise program to coincide with the weight reduction diet. They are encouraged to walk 3 miles a day. A suggestion is to measure a distance 1.5 miles from home and to walk that distance and back every day. Some patients prefer a treadmill or a track. However, these methods make it easy to stop early, become bored, and lose interest. Walking long distances allows one to do other things, such as listen to music, learn new languages, listen to books on tape, or share time with family and friends. Exercise time can be used for productive thinking time or social time. As people become comfortable with walking, they begin to jog part of the distance. This is encouraged. Patients should be advised to purchase *good* running shoes for the daily walking program. This provides a measure of protection from joint and muscle fatigue and injury.

Most women are able to lose 1 pound (0.45 kg) a week with this program of oral contraceptive suppression (if androgens are elevated), diet, and exercise. Patients should return for follow-up visits at 4- to 6-week intervals to measure their progress and receive encouragement. Praise is part of the therapy.

Many obese women request ovulation induction with clomiphene citrate or menopausal gonadotropins; many have previously received clomiphene citrate. Clomiphene citrate is a lipid-soluble compound that is sequestered in adipose tissue. Clomiphene citrate also competes with estrogens for estrogen receptors. Because obese women are hyperestrogenic, more clomiphene citrate is required to induce ovulation than for women of normal body weight. Shepard et al[30] reported that body weight affects the amount of clomiphene citrate required to induce ovulation. Among women who weigh more than 175 pounds (78.6 kg), 200 mg of clomiphene citrate a day was required to induce ovulation in the study by Shepard et al. These data are presented in Fig 25–8. Similarly, large amounts of menopausal gonadotropins are required to induce ovulation for obese women.[27]

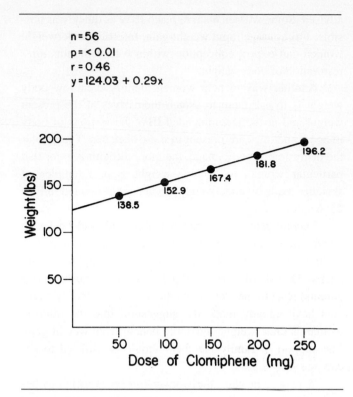

Figure 25–8. Relation of ovulatory dose of clomiphene citrate to body weight. *(From Shepard MK, et al: Relationship of weight to successful induction of ovulation with clomiphene citrate. Fertil Steril 1979;32:641. Reprinted with permission of the publisher, the American Fertility Society.)*

SUMMARY

Body fat plays a critical role in human reproduction. Both excess and deficiency of body fat lead to reproductive failure. Body weight is one of the first potential causes of reproductive failure among both men and women who seek treatment of infertility. Infertile couples are not likely to accept deviations from IBW as the cause of infertility. Yet 12% or more of infertile couples have deviations from IBW as the cause of their infertility. If a woman's body weight is less than 95% of predicted IBW or greater than 120% of predicted IBW, appropriate weight gain or weight loss should be the primary recommendation. These men and women need patience and understanding while they cope with the issue of body weight and its impact on their reproductive function.

REFERENCES

1. Bates GW: Body weight control practice as a cause of infertility. *Clin Obstet Gynecol* 28:632, 1985
2. A company that is getting fat because America wants to be thin. *Business Week* November 19:70, 1984

3. Manson JE, Willett WC, Stampfer MJ, et al: Body weight and mortality among women. *N Engl J Med* 333:677, 1995

4. Frisch RE, Ravelle R: Height and weight at menarche and a hypothesis of critical body weights and adolescent events. *Science* 169:397, 1970

5. Frisch RE, McArthur J: Menstrual cycles: Fatness as a determinant of minimum weight for height necessary for their maintenance or onset. *Science* 185:949, 1974

6. Kulpa PJ, White BM, Visscher R: Aerobic exercise in pregnancy. *Am J Obstet Gynecol* 156:139, 1987

7. Warren MP: The effects of exercise on pubertal progression and reproductive function in girls. *J Clin Endocrinol Metab* 51:1150, 1980

8. Schwartz B, Cumming DC, Riordan E, Selye M, Yen SSC: Exercise-associated amenorrhea: A distinct entity? *Am J Obstet Gynecol* 141:662, 1981

9. Frisch RE, Wyshak G, Vincet L: Delayed menarche in and amenorrhea of ballet dancers. *N Engl J Med* 303:17, 1980

10. Constantini NW, Warren MP: Menstrual dysfunction in swimmers: A distinct entity. *J Clin Endocrinol Metab* 80:2740, 1995

11. Rogers J, Mitchell GW: The relation of obesity to menstrual disturbances. *N Engl J Med* 247:53, 1952

12. Green BB, Weiss NS, Daling JR: Risk of ovulatory infertility in relation to body weight. *Fertil Steril* 50:721, 1988

13. Bates GW, Bates SR, Whitworth NS: Reproductive failure in women who practice weight control. *Fertil Steril* 37:373, 1982

14. Bates GW, Whitworth NS: Effect of body weight reduction on plasma androgens in obese, infertile women. *Fertil Steril* 38:406, 1982

15. Boyar RM, Finkelstein JW, Roffwarg H, et al: Synchronization of augmented luteinizing hormone secretion with sleep during puberty. *N Engl J Med* 287:582, 1972

16. Boyar RM, Katz J, Finkelstein JW, et al: Anorexia nervosa: Immaturity of the 24-hour luteinizing hormone secretory pattern. *N Engl J Med* 291:861, 1974

17. Virgersky RA, Anderson AE, Thompson RH, et al: Hypothalamic dysfunction in secondary amenorrhea associated with simple weight loss. *N Engl J Med* 297:1141, 1977

18. Genazzani AD, Petraglia F, Gabbri G, et al: Evidence of luteinizing hormone secretion in hypothalamic amenorrhea associated with weight loss. *Fertil Steril* 54:222, 1990

19. Reichman ME, Judd JT, Taylor PR, et al: Effect of dietary fat on length of the follicular phase of the menstrual cycle in a controlled diet setting. *J Clin Endocrinol Metab* 74:1171, 1992

20. Sherman BM, Halmi KA, Zamudio R: LH and FSH response to gonadotropin-releasing hormone in anorexia nervosa: Effect of nutritional rehabilitation. *J Clin Endocrinol Metab* 49:601, 1975

21. Fishman JA, Boyar RM, Hellman L: Influence of body weight on estradiol metabolism in young women. *J Clin Endocrinol Metab* 41:989, 1975

22. Hershcopf RJ, Bradlow HL, Fishman J: Differential hydroxylations of estrone and estradiol in man. *J Clin Endocrinol Metab* 62:170, 1986

23. Sitteri PK, Macdonald PC: Role of extraglandular estrogen in human endocrinology. In: Green PO, Eastwood EB (eds), *Handbook of Physiology.* Vol 2. Washington, DC, American Physiological Society, 1973:615

24. Yen SSC: The polycystic ovary syndrome. *Clin Endocrinol (Oxf)* 12:177, 1980

25. Mitchell GW, Rogers J: The influence of weight reduction on amenorrhea in obese women. *N Engl J Med* 249:835, 1953

26. Halme J, Hammond MG, Bailey L, Talbert LM: Lower doses of human menopausal gonadotropin are associated with improved success with in vitro fertilization in women with low body weight. *Am J Obstet Gynecol* 158:64, 1988

27. Chong AP, Rafael RW, Forte CC: Influence of weight in the induction of ovulation with menopausal gonadotropin and human chorionic gonadotropin. *Fertil Steril* 46:599, 1986

28. Metropolitan Life Insurance Company Health and Safety Education Division. Metropolitan Life Insurance Company, New York, NY, 1983

29. Givins JR, Anderson RN, Wiser WL, Fish SA: Dynamics of suppression of FSH, LH, androstenedione, and testosterone in PCO using an oral contraceptive. *J Clin Endocrinol Metab* 38:727, 1974

30. Shepard MK, Balmaceda JP, Leija CG: Relationship of weight to successful induction of ovulation with clomiphene citrate. *Fertil Steril* 32:641, 1979

CHAPTER 26

Recurrent Pregnancy Loss

CAROLYN B. COULAM

Evaluation of Recurrent Pregnancy Loss
Three or more consecutive spontaneous abortions

Establish if previous
liveborn or stillborn
Verify recurrent pregnancy
losses are with same
partner

Obtain genetic history
Assess for autoimmune disease
Exclude genetic disorders
Review gestational ages of
pregnancy losses

Determine need for psychologic support
Discuss possible causes

Chromosomal analysis

Abnormal | Normal

Genetic counseling   Hysterosalpingogram,
Normal child, 30%   hysteroscopy, hysterosonogram
Consider donor
gametes   Normal   Abnormal

Endometrial studies   Surgical treatment
Serum progesterone

Abnormal | Normal

?Progesterone treatment   Autoantibodies
?Clomiphene treatment   Reproductive immunophenotyping
                          Embryotoxicity assay (ETA)

Positive | Negative

Immunotherapy   Psychologic support
Autoantibodies   ?Empiric treatment

Heparin, ASA   + CD56+   Leukocyte antibody detection assay
Prednisone, ASA +ETA
IVIg   IVIg

                      Positive   Negative
                      IVIg   IVIg
                                  WBC
                                  Immunization

Spontaneous abortion is the expression of products of conception before 20 weeks' gestation. According to the World Health Organization (1992), 150,000 spontaneous abortions occur each day. Spontaneous abortion is the most common complication of pregnancy; it occurs among at least 75% of all women trying to become pregnant.[1] Most of these losses are unrecognized and occur before or with the expected menses.[2] The remaining 15% to 20% are spontaneous abortions or ectopic pregnancies diagnosed after clinical recognition of pregnancy. As many as 5% of all couples conceiving experience two consecutive abortions, and 2% have three or more consecutive losses.[3] These recurrent spontaneous abortions have been described as a syndrome.[4] All of these losses result in substantial physical and emotional pain and medical expense.

Until recently, little attention had been focused on the problem of recurrent abortion. Recommendations for the care of couples experiencing recurrent abortion have been conflicting. To treat this disorder effectively, a proper diagnosis must be made. Although genetic, anatomic, infectious, hormonal, and immunologic factors have been implicated in the causation of recurrent spontaneous abortion, the roles of anatomic defects[5] and hormonal deficiencies[6] have been questioned and the role of infection seriously doubted.[7] Thus the principal causes of recurrent spontaneous abortion are left to chromosomal abnormalities and immunologic factors. The frequency with which each of these factors contributes to recurrent spontaneous abortion has been the subject of recent studies.

PROPOSED MECHANISMS OF RECURRENT SPONTANEOUS ABORTION

Early pregnancy loss can result from abnormalities within the conceptus or the endometrium.

Abnormal Conceptus

It has been recognized for some time that products of at least 50% of early spontaneous abortions are cytogenetically abnormal.[8] This figure contrasts markedly with the prevalence of chromosomal abnormalities observed among stillbirths (5%) and livebirths (0.5%).[1] The most plausible explanation for the large number of chromosomal abnormalities among lost pregnancies is that most chromosomal abnormalities result in disordered development incompatible with prolonged intrauterine survival. The extent to which chromosomal abnormalities contribute to recurrent abortion was previously thought to be relatively low (5%).[7] Current data indicate that 60% of all abortuses from women experiencing recurrent abortion are chromosomally abnormal (Table 26–1).

TABLE 26–1. RESULTS OF CHROMOSOMAL ANALYSIS FROM 100 PRODUCTS OF CONCEPTION OBTAINED AFTER SPONTANEOUS ABORTION AMONG WOMEN WITH A HISTORY OF RECURRENT SPONTANEOUS ABORTION

Karyotype	n	%
Normal	41	41
Abnormal	59	59
Total	100	100

Risk factors for a chromosomally abnormal conceptus include advanced maternal age[9,10] and history of subfertility.[11,12]

Maternal Age

The association of advanced maternal age and risk of spontaneous abortion is well known and has been shown to be related to increasing odds for fetal chromosomal trisomy.[13] Therefore, the increased risk of first-trimester loss with advanced maternal age is attributable to embryonic chromosomal abnormalities in sporadic abortions. Maternal age as a risk factor for recurrent spontaneous abortion has been both reported[14,15] and refuted.[16–18] Authors who report an association between maternal age and recurrent spontaneous abortion found the rate of spontaneous abortion rises with maternal age only after 35 years of age.[19] However, when multiple logistic regression analysis was performed to compare the relative importance of maternal age and obstetric history for prediction of fetal chromosomal abnormalities, maternal age was the most significant predictor of fetal trisomy.[9]

Evidence exists that some couples are at risk for conceptions complicated by recurrent aneuploidy.[11–20] The birth of a trisomic infant places a woman at increased risk for a subsequent trisomic conceptus.[21] Analysis of data from women who have had two or more karyotyped abortions, when adjusted for maternal age, suggests an increased risk for women who have had a trisomic abortion to have a subsequent trisomic abortion.[13]

History of Subfertility

Women who are infertile have a threefold higher frequency of spontaneous abortion than the fertile population.[12] Women experiencing recurrent spontaneous abortion have a twofold increase in the frequency of infertility compared with the general population.[11] It has been estimated that 50% of fertilized oocytes actually implant in the endometrium, and 43% of those that do implant are lost before clinical pregnancy is recognized.[2,12,22] Women who experience recurrent pregnancy loss before the time of clinically perceived pregnancy seek treatment of unexplained infertility. The associations between spontaneous abortion and infertility suggest a common mechanism in a subset of couples experiencing both. To gain further insight into the mechanisms that might be involved, clinical and preclinical pregnancy losses occurring after various assisted reproductive technologies were studied.

Clinical Versus Preclinical Pregnancy Loss

Pregnancy losses after clinical recognition of implantation by means of visualization of a gestational sac with transvaginal ultrasonography and preclinical pregnancy losses diagnosed by means of documentation of elevations in serum human chorionic gonadotropin (hCG) concentrations before demonstration of implantation by means of visualization of a gestational sac with transvaginal ultrasonography in 500 pregnancies after in vitro fertilization/embryo transfers (IVF/ET) were studied. The frequency of clinical and preclinical losses was compared with maternal age and type of endometrial stimulation before embryo transfer.[23] The frequency of clinical pregnancy loss increased with increasing maternal age ($r = .971$, $R^2 = .95$, $P = .005$). No significant differences in rates of clinical pregnancy losses were observed when gonadotropin-stimulated and nonstimulated cycles were compared.[23] When the rate of preclinical loss was compared with the age of the woman from whom the oocytes were retrieved, linear regression analysis revealed no significant association between preclinical loss and age of the woman contributing the oocyte ($r = .8$, $R^2 = .65$, $P = .1$).[23] A significant difference in the frequency of preclinical loss was observed when gonadotropin-stimulated cycles were compared with nonstimulated cycles. Preclinical pregnancy losses were more frequent when IVT/ET cycles were compared with donor oocyte recipient cycles and frozen-thawed embryo transfers (FET) ($P = .0001$). That the decreased frequency of preclinical losses in the nonstimulated cycles was not related to hormonal supplementation was evident when pregnancy loss rates after ET in natural and hormonally controlled endometrial cycles were compared. That the decreased frequency of preclinical losses observed after FET was not due to embryo selection from survival after freezing and thawing was evident in a comparison of pregnancy loss rates after fresh and frozen-thawed ETs among donor oocyte recipients. Thus clinical pregnancy loss results largely from abnormalities of the conceptus, and preclinical pregnancy loss appears to be largely related to abnormalities in the endometrium.

Abnormal Endometrium

The endometrium consists of glandular epithelium, stroma, and lymphomyeloid cells. To support successful pregnancy, the endometrium must differentiate into decidua. In humans, the endometrium develops into decidua under the influence of hormones and lymphoid and trophoblastic cells. Any event that would interfere with the activities of hormones and lymphoid or trophoblastic cells can inhibit normal development of decidua. Events thought to be able to interfere with decidual function have been categorized as anatomic, hormonal, and immunologic.[7] Anatomic defects proposed to interfere with decidual function include endometrial polyps, submucous fibroids, and uterine synechiae. Müllerian duct defects do not appear to cause first-trimester pregnancy loss.[5] Hormonal deficiencies associated with first-trimester pregnancy loss have involved progesterone.[6] Data are accumulating supporting a role of the lymphoid cells and immune system in first-trimester pregnancy loss.[24–27]

At the time of implantation, trophoblastic cells communicate with endometrial and lymphoid cells. Communication is mediated by cytokines and cell surface proteins. Human leukocyte antigen G (HLA-G), a protein expressed on the cell surface of the trophoblast,[28] is recognized by a CD8[+] lymphocyte. The CD8[+] lymphocyte secretes cytokines that promote trophoblastic cell growth and differentiation.[29] As the trophoblastic cells proliferate and invade the endometrium, they differentiate into an inner cytoblastic and an outer syncytiocytoblastic layer. Any agent that interferes with differentiation of cytotrophoblast to syncytiotrophoblast can inhibit the normal development of a pregnancy. Antiphospholipid antibodies (APA) have been shown to inhibit differentiation of cytotrophoblast to syncytiotrophoblast,[30] and their presence in sera of women have been associated with adverse pregnancy outcome.[31]

Trophoblastic cells are resistant to lysis by cytotoxic T lymphocytes and natural killer (NK) cells, but they are susceptible to activated NK cells or lymphokine-activated killer (LAK) cells.[32–34] Suppression of activation of NK to LAK cells is necessary for successful pregnancy to occur. A number of cytokines have been shown to prevent LAK cell activation and abortion in mice. These cytokines include interleukin-3 (IL-3), granulocyte-macrophage colony-stimulating factor (GM-CSF), transforming growth factor β_2 (TGFβ_2),[29,34,35] and a 34-kd protein produced by CD8[+] cells with progesterone receptors.[36] Local production of these cytokines at the fetodecidual interface has been studied, but there is also evidence of systemic activity.[34] These factors can be measured systemically as circulating embryotoxins in an embryotoxicity assay.[37,38] Circulating NK (CD56[+]) cells can be measured, and identification of elevated percentages of circulating CD56[+] cells has been associated with early loss of karyotypically normal pregnancies.[39] Thus identification of circulating elevated concentrations of antiphospholipids (and other autoantibodies including antithyroid and antinuclear antibodies) and elevated percentages of CD56[+] cells and embryotoxins have been used to identify women at risk for immunologic components contributing to pregnancy wastage.

DIAGNOSIS

An important component in treating couples with recurrent pregnancy loss is establishing the correct diagnosis. Causes of recurrent pregnancy loss have included chromosomal defects, abnormalities of the uterus, hormonal deficiencies, and immunologic factors.[7] Therefore, the term *recurrent spontaneous abortion* is neither a diagnosis nor a disease but rather a description of an event that occurs as a result of a disease or diseases. Understanding the mechanisms involved in recurrent spontaneous abortion allows a more focused approach to identifying risk factors associated with recurrent spontaneous abortion that aid in the diagnosis. Tools available to facilitate the diagnosis of recurrent pregnancy loss include chromosomal analysis, examination of the uterine cavity, evaluation of endometrial receptivity, and immunologic tests (Table 26–2).

Chromosomal Analysis

Chromosomal analysis can be performed on products of conception originating from couples experiencing recurrent spontaneous abortion or on peripheral leukocytes from the parents. Chromosomal abnormalities can be identified in 60% of karyotyped fetuses before the 12th week of gestation.[40] Parental chromosomal structural abnormalities (usually balanced translocations) can be found in 6% of couples experiencing recurrent spontaneous abortion.[7]

The results of a chromosomal analysis performed on the products of conception of a lost pregnancy can help predict subsequent pregnancy outcome. A history of a previous trisomy is a risk factor for another trisomy.[10,41] The risk of spontaneous abortion in a subsequent pregnancy is increased when a normal embryonic karyotype is found in abortus material.[41] Boué et al[8]

TABLE 26–2. EVALUATION FOR RECURRENT PREGNANCY LOSS

Chromosomal Analysis
  Parents
  Products of conception

Examination of Uterine Cavity
  Hysteroscopy
  Hysterosalpingography
  Hysterosonography

Evaluation of Endometrial Receptivity
  Serum progesterone
  Endometrial biopsy
  Integrins
  Ultrasonography

Immunologic Tests
  Autoantibodies
  CD56+ cells
  Embryotoxicity assay
  Leukocyte antibody detection assay

---

found the risk for subsequent spontaneous abortion to be 16% to 17% when an embryonic chromosomal abnormality was diagnosed in a single spontaneous abortion compared with 23% when the embryonic karyotype was normal. Morton et al[42] reported an abortion rate of 23% when the embryonic karyotype was normal compared with rates of 15% to 17% after losses with chromosomal errors. Most important, the subsequent losses after loss of a karyotypically normal conceptus had a high probability of also being chromosomally normal.[8,10,18,41,42] Thus with a history of recurrent spontaneous abortion, demonstration of normal embryonic karyotype may be the most important indication for diagnostic evaluation and possible treatment of women experiencing recurrent spontaneous abortion. At the present time, the only way to identify such women is to have the results of chromosomal analysis of previous pregnancy losses available.

Examination of the Uterine Cavity

Examination of the uterus is considered part of the complete examination of women experiencing recurrent spontaneous abortion. Techniques used to evaluate the uterine cavity include hysteroscopy,[43] hysterosalpingography,[44] and hysterosonography.[45,46] When the results of these methods have been compared, hysterosonography has been shown to be the most accurate method of detection and evaluation of size, intracavitary growth, and location of intrauterine lesions.[47] In a study of 600 women undergoing hysterosonography for evaluation of recurrent pregnancy loss and infertility, 499 (83.7%) had normal findings and 101 (16.8%) had abnormal findings.[46] The abnormalities were müllerian duct anomalies (11%), endometrial polyps (40%), uterine synechiae (31%), submucous fibroid (17%), T-shaped uterus (1%), and retained intrauterine device (IUD) (1%). The role of müllerian duct defects as a cause of recurrent spontaneous abortion has been questioned.[5] The roles of endometrial polyps and submucous fibroids have not been clearly defined. Uterine synechiae have been reported to be the result of abortion rather than the cause.[48] Until the contributions of anatomic lesions within the uterine cavity to the causation of recurrent spontaneous abortion are determined, evaluation of the uterine cavity might be best obtained with an accurate, simple office procedure that does not require an anesthetic agent or contrast material. Such a procedure would decrease risk for allergic reactions and decrease cost. Hysterosonography is such a simple and safe method for evaluation of the uterine cavity.

Evaluation of Endometrial Receptivity

Successful implantation and normal early embryonic growth require a receptive endometrium. A receptive endometrium can be produced by means of administration of estrogen and progesterone, as has been shown by studies using a human donor oocyte as a model.[49] Many investigations have focused on the mechanisms by which estrogen and progesterone ensure successful pregnancy. Although estrogen is necessary for normal folliculogenesis and oocyte maturation, progesterone does not affect oocyte quality or fertilizability.[50] With the human donor egg recipient as a model, the role of progesterone appears to involve preparation of the endometrium to ensure uterine receptivity that allows the fertilized egg to implant.[51] Lack of progesterone-induced uterine receptivity results in preimplantation failure and infertility. Postimplantation failure associated with decreased progesterone production is believed to result from nonviable pregnancies, because serum progesterone concentrations are high at 4 weeks of gestation in women who have spontaneous abortions and decrease by 5 to 6 weeks of gestation.[52] Although the role of hormonal factors has been implicated as a cause of infertility, the role of hormones in recurrent spontaneous abortion is less obvious. Nonetheless, luteal-phase defects, characterized by inadequate endometrial maturation resulting from insufficient progesterone production, have been reported to cause recurrent spontaneous abortion. Methods used to diagnose luteal-phase defects include histologic dating of endometrial biopsy specimens, determination of serum progesterone concentration, endometrial expression of integrins, and ultrasonography.

Endometrial Biopsy

Endometrial biopsy has been the standard for the diagnosis of luteal-phase defects.[53] Development of the endometrium has been theorized to reflect the end-organ response to progesterone and provide a bioassay that is independent of fluctuations in serum hormone levels.[54] Endometrial maturation is assessed by means of correlating histologic dating of the biopsy specimen; as defined by the criteria of Noyes et al,[55] with chronologic dating. Chronologic dating is traditionally assigned retrospectively by counting backward from the onset of the next menstrual period and assuming that ovulation occurs on day 14 of that cycle. The diagnosis of luteal-phase defect has been made by means of showing a discrepancy between histologic and chronologic dating of more than 2 days.[56] This technique has an accuracy rate of 25% to 35%.[54,57] Because of the low accuracy rate, several investigators believe that the chronologic date should be calculated prospectively by counting forward from the day of luteinizing hormone (LH) surge or the day of follicle rupture as documented with ultrasound.[58,59] When ultrasonic confirmation of follicular rupture was used as a reference for chronologic dating of the endometrium, the prevalence of the diagnosis of out-of-phase biopsy specimen was 1% compared with 32% when the onset of the next menstrual period was used[59] (Fig 26–1). More important, when the frequency of out-of-phase endometrial biopsy specimens was compared for women having recurrent spontaneous abortion and fertile women, the diagnosis of

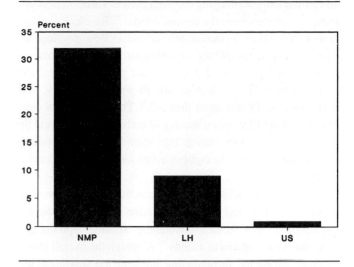

Figure 26–1. Prevalence of diagnosis of luteal-phase defect based on onset of next menstrual period (NMP), urinary luteinizing hormone (LH) surge, and ultrasonic confirmation of follicle rupture (US).

luteal-phase defect was higher among fertile controls.[59] The diagnosis of luteal-phase defect based on an out-of-phase endometrial biopsy does not predict pregnancy outcome. Its utility in the evaluation of reproductive disorders, therefore, has been questioned.[60]

Serum Progesterone Concentrations

To evaluate the function of the corpus luteum, researchers have advocated measurement of one luteal product, progesterone, during the secretory phase. Secretory phase progesterone concentration in saliva,[61] plasma,[62] and serum[63] have been described. An important criticism of a single value of progesterone concentration to diagnose luteal-phase defect is the pulsatility of its secretion, with as much as 10-fold variations.[62] To reduce this variability, some investigators have suggested multiple sampling frequency as a means to assess luteal-phase adequacy.[53] The ready availability of serum progesterone assays has made this a theoretically attractive approach.

Ultrasonography of the Endometrium

Transvaginal ultrasound probes with high frequency and high definition allow a close view of the changes observed in the pattern and thickness of the endometrium. Studies have correlated ultrasonic patterns with the menstrual phase of the cycle[64] and with subsequent pregnancy rate.[65] The sonographic finding of an endometrial thickness of 6 mm or more and a triple-line pattern in the late follicular phase can be used to predict successful implantation.[66]

Transvaginal ultrasonography with color-flow imaging

and pulsed Doppler imaging has been used to visualize flow velocity waveforms from the uterine arteries.[67] Results have suggested impedance to uterine arterial blood flow provides an index of uterine receptivity for implantation.[65–67] Implantation rates per embryo were 15.3% when the pulsatility index (PI) was 1.00 to 1.99, 22.2% when the PI was 2.00 to 2.99, and zero when the PI was more than 3.0.[67] The investigators concluded that the PI value on the day of embryo transfer could be used to increase implantation rate after IVF by determining when embryos should be cryopreserved until the uterus is more receptive.

To assess the utility of endometrial thickness, endometrial echogenic pattern, and mean PI of uterine arteries in predicting implantation, 400 women undergoing assisted reproductive procedures participated in a study.[65] Although the overall sensitivity of ultrasound in predicting implantation was high, the specificity was low (25%), suggesting that many embryos do not implant for reasons other than uterine receptivity (Table 26–3). The results obtained with these data suggest that ultrasonographic findings, echogenic pattern, and uterine arterial impedance can be used to predict as many as 28% of failures to become pregnant after use of assisted reproductive techniques (see Table 26–3). No other published method can be used to predict the failure of embryos to implant this accurately.

Thus, ultrasonography provides a noninvasive and immediate marker of uterine receptivity reflecting an adequate luteal phase.

Integrins

β3 is a marker protein that is consistently present during implantation in healthy, fertile women but not in women with maturational delay of the endometrium (luteal-phase defect).[67,68] This protein is a member of the integrin family and is a subunit of the αV/β3 vitronectin receptor. When the expression of αV, β3, and their ligand, osteopontin, was studied in endometrium throughout the menstrual cycle, all were absent during the proliferative phase.[67,68] The expression of αV increases soon after ovulation, and epithelial β3 expression abruptly increases starting on day 20 of the menstrual cycle.[67] Osteopontin showed an increase in the early secretory phase that reached a plateau on day 20 of the cycle. After day 25, epithelial cell expression of osteopontin disappeared, whereas a marked increase in its expression by stromal decidual cells occurred late in the secretory phase.[68] αV/β3 is expressed by invading human trophoblasts. The investigators concluded that epithelial cell expression of the β3 integrin subunit after day 20 of the endometrial cycle may define the onset of uterine receptivity and that coexpression of the functional αV/β3 integrin and its ligand, osteopontin, on the endometrial glandular cells are markers of uterine receptivity and define the window of trophoblastic cell attachment to the endometrial epithelium on days 20 to 25 of the cycle.[67] Furthermore, the authors hypothesized that osteopontin may be the extracellular ligand that provides the molecular bridge that mediates adhesion of the trophoblastic cells to the endometrial cells, indicating a continued role for αV/β3 ligand in the process of trophoblastic invasion during implantation. Results from studies with infertile women showed that these observations and conclusions have clinical applications.[69] Although all fertile women who acted as controls had normal β3 expression on endometrial biopsy specimens, only 16 of 42 women (38%) with unexplained infertility had β3 expression.[69] These results suggest that uterine receptivity may be an important factor in the decreased cycle fecundity of women with unexplained infertility. The role of integrins in the diagnosis of recurrent pregnancy loss has not been defined.

Immunologic Tests

Medical attention has focused on immunologic factors involved in recurrent spontaneous abortion. It is estimated that more than 80% of heretofore unexplained recurrent pregnancy losses can be explained on the basis of immunologic factors. Since the fetus develops from genetic contributions from both the mother and the father, it has been customary to divide immunologic factors into inappropriate responses directed toward the mother's contribution to the pregnancy (autoimmune) or the father's contribution (alloimmune). Autoimmune and alloimmune factors can be identified with blood tests.

Autoimmune Factors

Autoimmune risk factors contributing to recurrent pregnancy loss can be manifested as elevated concentrations of circulating autoantibodies or an increase in the ratio of circulating CD4 to CD8 cells.

Autoantibodies. Increased concentrations of circulating autoantibodies associated with recurrent pregnancy loss include APA,[70,71] lupuslike anticoagulant,[72–75] antinuclear antibodies,[76–79] and antithyroid antibodies.[80–82]

TABLE 26–3. FREQUENCY AND ACCURACY OF ULTRASONOGRAPHIC FINDINGS IN PREDICTING IMPLANTATION AMONG 400 CYCLES OF ASSISTED REPRODUCTIVE TECHNOLOGIES

Measurement	Percentage		
	Lack of Multilayer Pattern	*PI > 3.3*	*Either*
Frequency	14	15	28
Sensitivity	95	71	89
Specificity	20	25	21
Negative predictive value	86	46	75

PI, pulsatility index.

Approximately 20% of women who experience recurrent miscarriages have positive tests for ALA.[70] Anticardiolipin antibody is one APA that is commonly used as an indicator of the presence of APA. Although anticardiolipins can be found in many women who experience recurrent spontaneous abortion, the correlation is not universal. The role of anticardiolipin antibodies as a cause of pregnancy loss has been questioned, and other APA such as phosphatidylserine antibodies have been accepted as more accurate markers of pregnancy loss.[83] Analyzing six or seven antiphospholipids gives a more representative idea of the underlying process associated with pregnancy failure and provides a more sensitive test.[70] Since APA syndrome is characterized by polyclonal activation, people with APA syndrome would be expected to display more than one APA on the panel. Because a false-positive test can result from other stimulation, it is important to reconfirm the presence of APA by repeating the test in 6 to 8 weeks.[84]

About 3% of women who experience recurrent miscarriages have positive tests for lupuslike anticoagulant.[74] Only 9% of people with systemic lupus erythematosus (SLE) have a positive lupus anticoagulant test.[85] Thus not every woman with a positive lupuslike anticoagulant test has a positive test for SLE. The tests used to detect lupus anticoagulants include partial thromboplastin time, kaolin clotting time, and dilute Russel viper venom time.[86]

Antinuclear antibodies have been reported to be associated with recurrent spontaneous abortion.[76–79] The mechanisms by which antinuclear antibodies cause pregnancy loss are not known. The association between antinuclear antibodies and recurrent pregnancy loss may be causal, but antinuclear antibodies probably represent a marker of polyclonal activation of an underlying process.

The presence of thyroid antibodies has been shown to be a risk factor for miscarriage[80,81] and recurrent spontaneous abortion.[82] Women who have thyroid antibodies miscarry at appropriately twice the rate of women without them. Both thyroglobulin antibodies and thyroid microsomal (thyroid peroxidase) antibodies are related to an increased miscarriage rate. When sensitive assays are used, 31% of women who experience recurrent miscarriage have been shown to have positive tests for one or both antithyroid antibodies. When only the hemagglutination blood test is used, one of five women with thyroid antibodies does not receive a correct diagnosis.

Lymphocytes. Autoimmune disease can be diagnosed by means of determining the ratio of types of white blood cells (WBCs) to each other. The ratio of helper T lymphocytes (CD4) to suppressor T lymphocytes (CD8) is elevated when some autoimmune disorders or autoimmune components contributing to recurrent spontaneous abortions are present.

Alloimmune Factors

In the past, tests used to assess alloimmune problems included HLA testing for antigen sharing between partners, a test to detect the presence of maternal antipaternal lymphocytotoxic antibodies, and a test to identify the presence of blocking factors through lymphocyte culture reaction. More recent studies, however, have shown that these laboratory tests cannot be used to predict miscarriage or any other pregnancy outcome.[87] Tests currently available to identify an alloimmune cause of recurrent miscarriage include measurement of the circulating percentage of WBCs known as NK or CD56[+] cells[29] and the embryotoxicity assay.[37,38,88] In addition, leukocyte antibody detection tests can be used to identify people who will not likely benefit from treatment with leukocyte immunization. Leukocyte antibody detection tests therefore should be performed before a husband's leukocyte immunization therapy is considered.

CD56[+] Cells. Monocytes present within the decidua at the site of implantation that express CD56[+] have been associated with successful pregnancy outcome.[24,89–92] NK cells within the CD56 phenotype were found to be more abundant in normal human term placentas than in cord and maternal blood in a study in which expression of progesterone receptors was suggested to be responsible for such an abundance of CD56[+] NK cells.[93] A deficiency of these cells has been observed in biopsy specimens of the placental bed from women with incipient miscarriage.[24] Studies with animals have demonstrated a role of CD56[+] cells in abortion.[91,92,94,95] In this model, the success of the fetal allograft was, in part, the result of local suppression at the level of the decidua by factors secreted by the CD56[+] cells.[24–27,94,96] Other studies suggested the systemic regulation of antitrophoblast killer cells in reproductive success.[97–99] In a study by Clark et al,[94] peripheral NK cells from women who experienced recurrent abortion participated in cytotoxic responses to placental cells from each woman's own conceptus.

The concentration of circulating CD56[+] cells has been shown to correlate with pregnancy outcome among women carrying a singleton gestation and in women with an obstetric history of recurrent pregnancy loss.[39] Percentages of CD56[+] cells greater than 12% predicted loss of karyotypically normal pregnancy.[39]

When peripheral NK cell activities were studied in women experiencing recurrent spontaneous abortion before and after immunotherapy by means of husband leukocyte immunization, a correlation was found between NK cell activity and conception and pregnancy outcome.[98] All women in whom NK activity decreased after immunotherapy became pregnant and had healthy babies. In contrast, women in whom NK activity greatly increased after immunotherapy did not become pregnant more than 12 months after treatment.[99]

Intravenous immunoglobulin (IVIg) therapy has been shown to modulate NK (CD56[+]) cell activity.[100] When women with a history of recurrent spontaneous abortion with elevated levels of circulating CD56[+] cells were treated with IVIg, all had healthy infants.[39]

Embryotoxicity Assay. A variety of cytokines and soluble mediators that promote implantation and early embryo growth have been identified in decidual tissue. Certain cytokines can be directly or indirectly cytotoxic to a conceptus.[101] Activated lymphocytes and macrophages from women with a history of recurrent spontaneous abortion when stimulated with trophoblast produced soluble factors that were toxic to mouse embryos and human placental cell lines.[102] A number of investigators have identified these embryotoxic factors in sera of women experiencing reproductive failure.[37,38,101–105] Circulating embryotoxic factors have been suggested as a basis for a new classification of idiopathic recurrent spontaneous abortion.[104] The prevalence of embryotoxic factors among women experiencing recurrent spontaneous abortion is 24%.[38] These embryotoxic factors can be produced by activated lymphocytes stimulated with trophoblasts.[103] Since IVIg therapy has been shown to regulate both T-cell and B-cell function,[106,107] a rationale is provided for the management of recurrent spontaneous abortion associated with circulating embryotoxins. IVIg therapy administered to such patients has resulted in livebirths.[39]

Leukocyte Antibody Detection Assay. This test indicates a woman's physiologic response to pregnancy.[87] Induction of antibodies directed against leukocyte antigens by the mother in response to allostimulation through reproductive processes is a well-known phenomenon among mammals.[108] In the past, maternal antibody recognition of parental lymphocytes has been evaluated with bioassays such as lymphocytotoxicity testing and mixed lymphocyte culture reactions. Serologic studies indicate that these antibodies often are cytotoxic in vitro. It had been speculated that these lymphocytotoxic antibodies might be detrimental to pregnancy,[109] but no evidence exists to support this theory. In fact, most data suggest that the presence of lymphocytotoxic antibodies is a predictor of successful pregnancy outcome.[110,111] Fertile women have antipaternal lymphocytotoxic antibodies more frequently than infertile women and those who have recurrent abortions ($P < .0001$).[87] This observation suggested an association between maternal exposure to pregnancy and the presence of such antibodies. To test this suggestion, total exposure to pregnancy (number of pregnancies multiplied by the duration of each pregnancy) was calculated from 449 obstetric histories.[87] As the time of exposure to pregnancy increased, so did maternal production of lymphocytotoxic antibodies. The association between gravidity and duration of pregnancy with the presence of lymphocytotoxic antibodies supports the concept

that lymphocytotoxic antibodies are the result of successful pregnancy rather than the cause of unsuccessful pregnancy.

Blockade of antibodies in potentially deleterious maternal immune responses has been postulated as a mechanism for successful pregnancy.[112] The blocking antibody hypothesis is based on the presumption that an antiembryonal cell–mediated immune response would cause all pregnancies to abort if the response were not intercepted. It has been suggested that this interception is accomplished by anti-idiotypic antibodies. However, blocking activity is not always detected in the sera of women with normal pregnancies.[112] In addition, normal pregnancy can occur in B-cell–deficient agammaglobulinemic women and mice.[113] Like the presence of maternal antipaternal lymphocytotoxic antibodies, mixed lymphocyte culture inhibitors are more frequent in sera of fertile than infertile women ($P < .001$) and are associated with the number and duration of pregnancies.[87] Thus it appears that the presence of mixed lymphocyte culture inhibitors and antipaternal lymphocytotoxic antibodies represents a response to pregnancy rather than a cause of failed pregnancy.

A more sensitive assay for the measurement of antibodies to paternal leukocytes than lymphocytotoxicity testing and mixed lymphocyte culture reactions is the leukocyte antibody detection assay by means of fluorescence-activated cytometry.[114] The absence of detection of maternal recognition of paternal cells in the assay would be useful in selecting women for various treatment regimens. If immunotherapy with immunization is going to be considered as a treatment option, a woman already showing an allogeneic response to the husband's WBCs in the leukocyte antibody detection assay would not be expected to respond and could be considered for alternative forms of treatment such as IVIg therapy. Treatment with IVIg would provide passive immunization of anti-idiotypic antibodies[115] as well as modulation of B-cell,[107] T-cell,[106] and NK-cell function.[100]

Prevalence of Diagnosis

Whereas in the past, most couples experiencing recurrent pregnancy loss were believed to have an immunologic factor as the cause, recent data suggest more than half of the pregnancies lost by couples experiencing recurrent abortions have chromosomal abnormalities evident in the products of conception (Table 26–4).

TREATMENT

Therapy should be directed at the cause of recurrent pregnancy loss. Tests available to help direct the approach to treatment include chromosomal analyses for both partners to diagnose chromosomal abnormalities; evaluation of the uterine cavity

TABLE 26–4. PREVALENCE OF DIAGNOSIS AMONG COUPLES WITH RECURRENT PREGNANCY LOSS

Diagnosis	Previous (%) (*n* = 225)	Current (%) (*n* = 224)
Genetic causes	6	60
Anatomic defects	1	1
Hormonal deficiency	1	1
Immunologic causes	67	30
Unexplained	25	10

TABLE 26–5. REPRODUCTIVE PERFORMANCE BEFORE AND AFTER METROPLASTY

Patients	Before	After
Total	21	20
Pregnant	20 (95%)	17 (85%)
With living children	0 (0%)	14 (70%)

(hysteroscopy, hysterosalpingography, or hysterosonography) to diagnose anatomic defects; luteal-phase evaluation of the endometrium with measurement of serum progesterone concentration to diagnose hormonal deficiencies; and immunologic tests, including autoantibody testing; quantitation of circulating CD56+ cells; and assays for detection of embryotoxicity and leukocyte antibodies to diagnose immunologic factors (see Table 26–2).

Chromosomal Abnormalities

Chromosomal abnormalities are found in 60% of karyotyped products of conception and 6% of parental leukocytes among women who experience recurrent spontaneous abortion.[7,8,40] Trisomies and monosomy for the X chromosome are the most frequent chromosomal abnormalities in first-trimester abortions,[18] and robertsonian translocations usually are seen in members of couples who experience recurrent abortions.[116]

At the time of initial visit, pedigree analysis and chromosomal studies of peripheral blood from both members of the couple are used to identify known genetic factors. No treatment is available either for detected parental chromosomal translocation or for a multifactorial genetic disorder that is operative in the production of abortions, with or without fetal malformations. Therapeutically, the chance of delivering a full-term living child is 20% to 30% depending on the specific translocation or genetic disorder. Cytogenetic studies of chorionic villi and amniotic fluid, ultrasonography, and α-fetoprotein levels are indicated in future pregnancies for these patients. Use of donor gametes is a treatment option, and high successful pregnancy rates have been reported.

Anatomic Defects

Müllerian duct anomalies have been thought to be causal in recurrent spontaneous abortion. Studies show a marked improvement in fetal salvage rates after metroplasty (Table 26–5). However, when the outcome among patients who underwent metroplasty was compared with that among women with the same uterine abnormality who did not undergo surgical treatment, the livebirth rates were the same[5] (Table 26–6). The in-

vestigators analyzed the reproductive outcome of 140 patients with uterine anomalies. Twenty-one patients underwent metroplasty, and 119 did not. Seventeen of the nonsurgical patients were matched with the surgical patients by age, chief symptom at the time of diagnosis, gravidity, and type of anomaly, and these women served as matched controls. The remaining 102 nonsurgical patients did not have clinically significant problems and served as additional controls.

Follow-up data were available after the diagnosis of uterine anomaly for 20 of the surgical patients, 17 of the nonsurgical matched controls, and 52 of the other controls. The percentages of patients with living children after the diagnosis of uterine anomaly were 71% and 80% for each of the nonsurgical groups compared with 70% for those who underwent metroplasty. Although fetal salvage rates improved markedly after metroplasty, outcome was similar to that of controls who deferred surgical repair.

Observations at hysteroscopy have provided evidence that uterine adhesions represent an effect rather than a cause of multiple pregnancy losses.[48] Just as the efficacy of metroplasty in the treatment of multiple pregnancy loss is being questioned, so too is the role of these anatomic defects as a cause.

Two additional anatomic defects deserve mention. A small, T-shaped uterus identified at hysterosalpingography suggests in utero exposure to diethylstilbestrol. The hypoplastic uterine corpus is associated with recurrent spontaneous abortions and premature labor. No treatment of this problem exists. A history of recurrent second-trimester pregnancy losses preceded by painless cervical effacement and dilatation is a typical history of incompetent cervix. Treatment involves placing a

TABLE 26–6. OBSTETRIC OUTCOME WITH AND WITHOUT METROPLASTY AFTER THE DIAGNOSIS OF UTERINE ANOMALY

Patients	Surgical	Nonsurgical Matched	Controls Other
Total	20	17	52
Pregnant	17 (85%)	17 (100%)	49 (94%)
With living children	14 (70%)	12 (71%)	42 (81%)

McDonald or Shirodkar cervical cerclage during the second trimester of the next pregnancy.

Hormonal Deficiencies

The role of progesterone deficiency in recurrent spontaneous abortion has been investigated in two areas. The first was an attempt to implicate low pregnanediol levels in pregnancy. Results among women who were treated with exogenous progesterone were no different from those among patients who received a placebo.[117,118] The second approach was to diagnose the insufficient effect of progesterone on the endometrium during the luteal phase of the menstrual cycle and to initiate treatment with exogenous hormones a few days after ovulation. The effect of treatment on pregnancy rates with luteal-phase deficiency has been reviewed.[119] One randomized controlled trial found a statistically significant benefit of treatment with progesterone suppositories or oral dehydrogesterone compared with no treatment (relative risk, 1.9; 95% confidence interval 0.4 to 8.1). Three other comparative studies showed no statistically significant benefit. Case-series reports (before-after studies) claiming benefit failed to account for the effect of regression to that mean. The reviewers concluded that the benefit of treatment of luteal-phase deficiency is not known. Both the diagnosis and treatment of luteal-phase defect have been the subject of considerable debate. The published data call into question the existence of luteal-phase defect as a clinically significant entity. If luteal-phase defect emerges as a clinical entity, its importance will most likely be in implantation defects that become clinically apparent as unexplained infertility and not recurrent spontaneous abortion.

Immunologic Factors

Understanding the mechanisms involved in recurrent spontaneous abortion allows a focused approach to specific treatment. Tests useful in directing an approach to immunotherapy include autoantibody testing, quantitation of circulating CD56[+] cells, and performance of assays for the detection of embryotoxicity and leukocyte antibodies.

Immunotherapy for Recurrent Spontaneous Abortion Associated with Autoantibodies

Autoantibodies associated with recurrent pregnancy loss include antiphospholipid and antinuclear and antithyroid antibodies. The patients in most of the clinical trials of immunotherapy for autoantibody-associated recurrent spontaneous abortion have been women expressing APA. Treatment options for APA syndrome have included low-dose aspirin, prednisone and aspirin, heparin and aspirin, and IVIg. Table 26–7 summarizes the treatment options for recurrent pregnancy loss associated with APA and the associated livebirth rates.

TABLE 26–7. SUMMARY OF RESULTS REPORTED IN THE LITERATURE USING VARIOUS TYPES OF TREATMENT OF RECURRENT SPONTANEOUS ABORTION ASSOCIATED WITH ANTIPHOSPHOLIPID ANTIBODIES

Treatment	References	Total No. of Patients	No. of Successful Pregnancies	% Successful Pregnancies
Aspirin, prednisone, heparin	Kwak et al, 1992[70]	50	38	76
Aspirin, prednisone	Cowchock, 1991[31]	134	95	71
	Hasegawa et al, 1992[120]			
Aspirin, heparin	Lubbe and Liggins, 1985[72]	37	29	78
	Cowchock et al, 1988[121]			
	Cowchock, 1991[31]			
IVIg (in combination with the above drugs)	Lubbe and Liggins, 1985[72]	14	10	71
	Carreras et al, 1988[122]			
	Francois et al, 1988[123]			
	Scott et al, 1988[124]			
	Parke et al, 1989[125]			
	MacLachlan et al, 1990[126]			
IVIg alone	MacLachlan et al, 1990[126]	3	3	100
	Christiansen et al, 1992[127]			
Aspirin	Cowchock, 1991[31]	42	19	45
	Kutteh and Webster, 1996[128]			
No treatment	Cowchock et al, 1988[121]	30	3	10

IVIg, intravenous immunoglobulin.

Aspirin. Low-dose aspirin (80 mg/day) alone has been advocated in the treatment of recurrent spontaneous abortion associated with APA. However, results of clinical trials have shown it to be half as effective as treatment that includes prednisone or heparin.[31,128] In a prospective, controlled trial of aspirin alone versus heparin with aspirin for the treatment of recurrent spontaneous abortion associated with APA, heparin with aspirin provided a significantly better outcome than aspirin alone (livebirth rate 83% versus 46%, $P < .05$).[128]

Prednisone and Aspirin. Most patients with reported recurrent spontaneous abortion have been treated with combinations of prednisone and aspirin. Prednisone is usually given as a daily dose of 40 to 60 mg beginning at the diagnosis of pregnancy. A daily dose of 80 mg of aspirin is usually started before conception. The goal of or rationale for this type of therapy is suppression of APA before conception.

Early reports from noncontrolled studies have been summarized by Cowchock.[31] The average livebirth rate among women with at least two pregnancy losses associated with APA after treatment with prednisone and aspirin was 70%. A randomized, controlled trial subsequently confirmed the efficacy of prednisone and aspirin for the treatment of recurrent spontaneous abortion associated with APA.[120] In that study, women treated with prednisone and aspirin had a livebirth rate of 77% compared with untreated women serving as controls who had a livebirth rate of 8%. However, risks associated with the dosage of prednisone used to treat recurrent spontaneous abortion associated with APA include signs of iatrogenic Cushing's syndrome, severe acne, increased risk for gestational diabetes, osteopenia, posterior capsular cataract, listeriosis, pneumonia, and even maternal death of miliary tuberculosis.[129–132] Early preeclampsia is more common in pregnancy among women receiving prednisone, and premature rupture of membranes and associated preterm birth almost always occur after prednisone therapy.[131,132]

Heparin and Aspirin. Because of the side effects connected with prednisone treatment of recurrent spontaneous abortion associated with APA, alternative treatments were sought. Because most of the clinical conditions associated with APA have a vascular or thrombotic origin, heparin has been investigated for the treatment of recurrent spontaneous abortion associated with APA. Treatment regimens using heparin for the treatment of recurrent spontaneous abortion associated with APA are summarized in Table 26–7. Even though heparin has been used with and without prednisone, the livebirth rate in all studies ranges from 74% to 88% compared with control values of 11% (no treatment)[121] and with 45% (aspirin alone).[31,128] When a controlled clinical trial compared heparin and aspirin with prednisone and aspirin for the treatment of recurrent spontaneous

abortion associated with APA, livebirth rates of 75% were the same in both groups. However, both maternal morbidity and the frequency of preterm delivery were higher among pregnant women treated with prednisone, a statistically significant difference. Therefore, the current recommendations for first-attempt treatment of recurrent spontaneous abortion associated with APA is heparin and aspirin. Heparin is usually administered at a dose of 5000 to 10,000 units subcutaneously twice a day along with aspirin 80 mg a day. Side effects of heparin therapy include prolonged coagulation times, thrombocytopenia, and osteoporosis.[133,134]

Intravenous Immunoglobulin Therapy. IVIg therapy has been used as treatment of recurrent spontaneous abortion associated with APA. Originally, IVIg therapy was used to treat women who had not been successful in pregnancy and previously treated with aspirin and prednisone or aspirin alone. The rationale for the use of IVIg therapy in the original studies was the suppression of lupus anticoagulant in a woman being treated for severe thrombocytopenia.[135] IVIg was nearly always given with prednisone or heparin plus aspirin.[72,122–126,132] The estimated total success rate of 71% for women at very high risk for pregnancy failure with a history of previous treatment failures suggested IVIg treatment was effective.[132] More recently, IVIg therapy alone has been used successfully to treat women with APA.[127] This report along with a previous report of successful treatment with IVIg for a woman who had lost 12 previous pregnancies while being treated with aspirin and heparin or prednisone[136] suggest IVIg therapy alone is successful in treating women with recurrent spontaneous abortion associated with APA.

Immunotherapy for Recurrent Spontaneous Abortion Associated with Elevated Concentrations of Circulating CD56⁺ Cells

Recent data suggest that IVIg therapy is useful in maintaining pregnancies in women with a history of recurrent spontaneous abortion who lose karyotypically normal embryos after detection of embryonic cardiac activity on ultrasonographic examination and who demonstrate elevated levels of NK (CD56⁺) cells in maternal blood.[39] In this study, 13 women received IVIg and none experienced a pregnancy loss. The frequency of elevated levels of circulating CD56⁺ cells associated with viable outcome were compared between women receiving and women not receiving IVIg (Table 26–8). A significantly higher proportion of women with CD56⁺ cell levels raised more than 12% had viable pregnancies when they received IVIg ($P = .0002$).

Immunotherapy for Recurrent Spontaneous Abortion Associated with Circulating Embryotoxins

Embryotoxic factors have been identified in 24% to 60% of women experiencing recurrent spontaneous abortion.[37,38,101–105] These women had successful pregnancies after IVIg therapy or

TABLE 26–8. COMPARISONS IN FREQUENCY OF CD56+ CELLS >12% AND ≤12% BETWEEN SINGLETON GESTATIONS TREATED AND NOT TREATED INTRAVENOUS IMMUNOGLOBULIN (IVIg) AMONG WOMEN WITH VIABLE PREGNANCIES

IVIg	Viable Pregnancy	CD56+ >12%	CD56+ ≤12%	P Value
Yes	13	10 (77)	3 (23)	.0002
No	27	3 (11)	24 (89)	

Numbers in parentheses are percentages of the total number of viable pregnancies.

progesterone supplementation.[37,39] However, none of these studies reported control results. Although it makes sense that immunotherapy that modulates cytokine production should be effective in modulating cytokine production that results in embryotoxic activity, further studies of immunotherapy for the treatment of recurrent spontaneous abortion associated with circulating embryotoxins are required to determine efficacy.

Immunotherapy for Recurrent Spontaneous Abortion Associated with None of the Aforementioned Immunologic Markers and Low Levels of Leukocyte Antibody Detection

Since the first reports of immunotherapy resulting in successful treatment of recurrent spontaneous abortion,[137,138] the treatment most commonly used has been leukocyte immunization.[139–143] However, therapeutic tests of the hypothesis in clinical trials evaluating leukocyte immunization for the treatment of recurrent spontaneous abortion and alternative treatments were sought. IVIg therapy is an alternative treatment reported to result in successful pregnancies.[144]

Allogenic Leukocyte Immunotherapy for Recurrent Spontaneous Abortion. Clinical trials evaluating allogenic leukocyte immunization have both supported[139,140] and refuted[141,142] this method of immunotherapy for the treatment of recurrent spontaneous abortion. Explanations for the conflicting results reported in these trials included small sample sizes, heterogeneity of populations from trial to trial, baseline differences within trials even after randomization (a problem associated with small sample sizes), and the uncontrolled use of cointerventions that confound the treatment effect.[145–147]

To address the uncertainties caused by conflicting results with respect to the effectiveness of immunotherapy by means of leukocyte immunization, a worldwide collaborative observational study and meta-analysis were performed.[143] Fifteen centers participated in the study. Nine randomized trials (seven double-blinded) were evaluated independently by two data analysis teams to assure conclusions were robust. Although the independent analyses used different definitions and statistical methods, the results were similar (Table 26–9). The percentages of livebirth ratios (ratio of livebirth in treatment and control

groups) with 95% confidence intervals were 1.16 (range, 1.01 to 1.34; $P = .03$) and 1.21 (range, 1.04 to 1.37; $P = .02$). The absolute differences in livebirth rates between treatment and control groups were 8% and 10%, respectively, in the respective analyses. Results in the randomized clinical trials and nonrandomized clinical trials were similar and consistent with those of noncontrolled trials previously reviewed and summarized.[140]

Immunotherapy Using Intravenous Immunoglobulin as Treatment of Recurrent Spontaneous Abortion. Since the Worldwide Collaborative Observational Study and Meta-Analysis on Allogenic Leukocyte Immunotherapy for Recurrent Spontaneous Abortion showed a low treatment effect with an absolute reduction of risk of further abortion between 8% and 10% (the number of patients one needs to treat to achieve one additional livebirth is between 9 and 13),[143] alternative treatments of recurrent spontaneous abortion have been sought. Among the alternative treatments reported to result in successful pregnancies is IVIg therapy.[127,144,148–150] Immunomodulation with IVIg has been postulated to result from passively transferred blocking or anti-idiotypic antibodies,[115] blockade of the Fc receptor,[151] enhancement of suppressor T-cell function,[106] downregulation of B-cell function,[107] reduction of activation of complement components,[152,153] NK cell activity, and cytokine production.[100]

A recent prospective, randomized double-blind, placebo-controlled trial of IVIg in the treatment of women with recurrent spontaneous abortion showed that the difference in livebirth rates between women receiving IVIg (62%) and placebo (34%) was significant ($P = .04$)[144] (Table 26–10). According to the magnitude of effect, one needs to treat four women to achieve one additional livebirth, making IVIg therapy three times more effective than leukocyte immunization.

SUMMARY

Recurrent pregnancy loss is a health care concern. Safe and effective treatments are necessary. Because women who experi-

TABLE 26–9. RESULTS OF WORLDWIDE COLLABORATIVE OBSERVATIONAL STUDY AND META-ANALYSIS ON ALLOGENIC LEUKOCYTE IMMUNOTHERAPY FOR RECURRENT SPONTANEOUS ABORTION: COMPARISON OF RESULTS OF TWO INDEPENDENT ANALYSES

	Analysis No. 1	Analysis No. 2
Number of patients	430	449
Relative treatment effect	1.16 (1.01–1.34)	1.21 (1.04–1.37)
Additional number of livebirths per 100 treated women	7.6 (4.6–11.7)	10 (6.5–14.5)
Number needed to treat for one additional livebirth	13 (8.5–21.7)	10 (6.9–15.4)

Numbers in parentheses are 95% confidence intervals.

TABLE 26–10. RESULTS OF RANDOMIZED PLACEBO-CONTROLLED TRIAL USING INTRAVENOUS IMMUNOGLOBULIN (IVIg) FOR THE TREATMENT OF RECURRENT SPONTANEOUS ABORTION: OUTCOME AMONG 61 PREGNANT WOMEN RANDOMIZED TO RECEIVE IVIg OR PLACEBO (ALBUMIN)

Pregnancy Outcome	n	IVIg		Placebo		P Value
		No.	%	No.	%	
Delivery	29	18	62	11	38	.04
Abortion	32	11	34	21	66	.04
Blighted ovum	15	8	53	7	47	NS
Intrauterine death	17	3	18	14	82	.004
Total	61	29	48	32	52	NS

NS, nonsignificant.
Numbers in % columns are percentages of the total (*n*).

ence recurrent pregnancy loss are a heterogeneous population, specific markers are necessary to identify those who will respond to various treatments. The presence of APA helps identify women with recurrent pregnancy loss who are most likely to respond to heparin and aspirin treatment. An elevated concentration of NK cells in maternal blood and a loss of karyotypically normal embryos after detection of cardiac activity at ultrasonographic examination helps identify women who are most likely to respond to IVIg treatment. An obstetric history of recurrent primary abortion with an absence of maternal antipaternal lymphocytotoxic antibodies and APA is used to predict which women are most likely to respond to allogeneic leukocyte immunization. However, the treatment effect is low, with a livebirth rate of 60%, which represents an enhancement over no treatment in the range of 8% to 10%. The difference in livebirth rates between women receiving IVIg therapy and women receiving placebo was 28%. Women experiencing recurrent spontaneous abortion who have high, as opposed to low, levels of leukocyte antibody do not respond to leukocyte immunization therapy. They do, however, respond to treatment with IVIg, the overall success rate of IVIg being 70%.

It is important to be able to identify women likely to respond to various forms of immunotherapy. Chromosomal abnormalities are evident in 60% of recurrent abortions. Women who experience recurrent aneuploidy in their abortuses would not be expected to respond to immunotherapy. At present, the only way to identify such women is to have the results of chromosome analysis of previous pregnancy losses available. Having access to this information will require a change in current obstetric practice to obtaining karyotyping of all pregnancy losses. The cost-effectiveness of chromosomal studies of abortuses is apparent when costs of evaluation and treatment are considered.

Although it is beyond the scope of this chapter to discuss in detail the emotional component of recurrent pregnancy loss,[154] it must be remembered that this event takes an enormous emotional toll on couples, and in some ways it is even more devastating and anxiety provoking than not conceiving at all. Psychological consultation should be offered to all couples experiencing this situation. It is hoped that specific therapy based on pathogenesis rather than empiricism will lead to successful treatment of this frustrating clinical problem.

REFERENCES

1. Boklage CE: Survival probability of human conceptions from fertilization to term. *Int J Fertil* 35:189, 1990
2. Wilcox AJ, Weinberg CR, O'Connor JF, et al: Incidence of early loss of pregnancy. *N Engl J Med* 319:189, 1988
3. Coulam CB: Epidemiology of recurrent spontaneous abortion. *Am J Reprod Immunol* 26:23, 1991
4. Strobino BR, Kline J, Shrout P, et al: Recurrent spontaneous abortion: Definition of a syndrome. In: Porter IH, Hook EB (eds), *Embryonic and Fetal Death.* New York, Academic Press, 1980:315
5. Kirk EP, Chuong CJ, Coulam CB, Williams TJ: Pregnancy after metroplasty for uterine anomalies. *Fertil Steril* 59:1164, 1993
6. Lloyd R, Coulam CB: Recurrent spontaneous abortion: Frequency of diagnosis of luteal phase defect. *Am J Reprod Immunol Microbiol* 16:103, 1988
7. Coulam CB: Unexplained recurrent pregnancy loss: Epilogue. *Clin Obstet Gynecol* 29:999, 1986
8. Boué J, Boué A, Lazar P: Retrospective and prospective epidemiological studies of 1,500 karyotyped spontaneous human abortions. *Teratology* 12:11, 1975
9. Cowchock FS, Gibas Z, Jackson LG: Chromosome errors as a cause of spontaneous abortion: The relative importance of maternal age and obstetric history. *Fertil Steril* 59:1011, 1993
10. Warburton D, Kline J, Stein Z, Hutzler M, Chin A, Hassold T. Does the karyotype of a spontaneous abortion predict the karyotype of a subsequent abortion? Evidence from 273 women with two karyotyped spontaneous abortions. *Am J Hum Genet* 41:465, 1987
11. Coulam CB: Association between infertility and spontaneous abortion. *Am J Reprod Immunol* 27:128, 1992
12. Jansen RPS: Spontaneous abortion incidence in the treatment of infertility. *Am J Obstet Gynecol* 143:451, 1982
13. Warburton D: Chromosomal causes of fetal death. *Clin Obstet Gynecol* 30:268, 1987
14. Risch HA, Weiss NS, Clarke EA, Miller AB: Risk factors for spontaneous abortion and its recurrence. *Am J Epidemiol* 128:420, 1988
15. Regan L: A prospective study of spontaneous abortion. In: Beard RW, Sharp F (eds), *Early Pregnancy Loss: Mechanisms and Treatment.* London, Royal College of Obstetrics and Gynaecology, 1988:23
16. Parazzini F, Acaia B, Ricciardeiello O, Fedele L, Liata P, Candiani GB: Short-term reproductive prognosis when no cause can be found for recurrent miscarriage. *Br J Obstet Gynaecol* 95:654, 1988

17. Cowchock FS, Smith JB, David S, Scher J, Batzer F, Carson S: Paternal mononuclear cell immunization therapy for repeated miscarriage: Predictive variables for pregnancy success. *Am J Reprod Immunol* 22:12, 1990

18. Strobino B, Fox HE, Kline J, Stein Z, Susser M, Warburton D: Characteristics of women with recurrent spontaneous abortions and women with favorable reproductive histories. *Am J Public Health* 76:986, 1986

19. Alberman E: The epidemiology of repeated abortion. In: Beard RW, Sharp F (eds), *Early Pregnancy Loss: Mechanisms and Treatment.* New York, Springer-Verlag, 1988:9

20. Lippman A, Ayme S: Fetal death rates in mothers of children with trisomy 21 (Down syndrome). *Ann Hum Genet* 48;303, 1984

21. Stene J, Stene E, Mikkelsen M: Risk for chromosome abnormality at amniocentesis following a child with a non-inherited chromosome aberration. *Prenat Diagn* 4:81, 1984

22. Leridan H: *Human Fertility: The Basic Components.* Chicago, University of Chicago Press, 1977:1–9

23. Coulam CB: Implantation failure. *Hum Reprod* 10:1338–1340, 1995

24. Michel M, Underwood J, Clark DA, Mowbray J, Beard RW: Histologic and immunologic study of uterine biopsy tissue of incipiently aborting women. *Am J Obstet Gynecol* 161:409, 1989

25. Clark DA, Lea RG, Underwood J, et al: A subset of recurrent first trimester abortion women show subnormal TGFβ2 suppressor activity at the implantation site associated with miscarriage. *J Immunol Immunopharmacol* 12:83, 1992

26. Clark DA, Lea RG, Denburg J, et al: Transforming growth factor beta related suppressor factor in mammalian pregnancy decidual: Homologies between the mouse and human in successful pregnancy and in recurrent unexplained abortion. In: Chaouat G, Mowbray J (eds), *Cellular and Molecular Biology of the Materno-Fetal Relationship,* 1991:171–179.

27. Lea RG, Underwood J, Flanders KC, et al: A subset of patients with recurrent spontaneous abortion is deficient in transforming growth factor beta-2-producing suppressor cells in decidua near the placental attachment site. *Am J Reprod Immunol* 34:52–57, 1995

28. Wei X, Orr HT: Differential expression of HLAE, HLAF and HLAG transcripts in human tissue. *Hum Immunol* 29:131, 1990

29. Chaouat G, Menu E, Athanassakis I, Wegmann TG: Maternal T cells regulate placental size and fetal survival. *Reg Immunol* 1:143, 1988

30. Rote NS: Antiphospholipid antibodies: Lobsters or red herrings? *Am J Reprod Immunol* 28:31, 1992

31. Cowchock S: The role of antiphospholipid antibodies in obstetric medicine. *Curr Obstet Med* 1:229, 1991

32. Drake BL, Head JR: Murine trophoblast can be killed by lymphokine-activated killer cells. *J Immunol* 143:9, 1989

33. King A, Loke YW: Human trophoblast and JEG choriocarcinoma cells are sensitive to lysis by IL-2–stimulated decidual NK cells. *Cell Immunol* 129:435, 1990

34. Clark DA, Flanders KC, Banwatt D, et al: Murine pregnancy decidual produces a unique immunosuppressive molecule related to transforming growth factor β-2. *J Immunol* 144:3008, 1990

35. Chaouat G, Menu E, Clark DA, Menisci M, Do M, Wegmann TG: Control of fetal survival in CBA X DBA/2 mice by lymphokine therapy. *J Reprod Fertil* 89:447, 1990

36. Szekeres-Bartho J, Autran B, Debre P, Andreu G, Denver L, Chaouat G: Immunoregulatory effects of a suppressor factor from healthy pregnancy women's lymphocytes after progesterone induction. *Cell Immunol* 122:281, 1989

37. Ecker JL, Laufer MR, Hill JA: Measurement of embryotoxic factors is predictive of pregnancy outcome in women with a history of recurrent abortion. *Obstet Gynecol* 81:84, 1993

38. Roussev RG, Stern JJ, Thorsell L, Thomason EJ, Coulam CB: Validation of an embryotoxicity assay. *Am J Reprod Immunol* 34:1, 1994

39. Coulam CB, Goodman C, Roussev RG, Thomason EJ, Beaman KG: Systemic CD56$^+$ cells can predict pregnancy outcome. *Am J Reprod Immunol* 33:40, 1995

40. Stern JJ, Dorfmann A, Gutierrez-Najan AJ, Cerrillo M, Coulam CB: Frequency of abnormal karyotypes among abortuses from women with and without a history of recurrent spontaneous abortion. *Fertil Steril* 65:220–254, 1995

41. Hassold T: A cytogenetic study of repeated spontaneous abortion. *Am J Hum Genet* 32:723, 1980

42. Morton NE, Chiu D, Holland C, Jacobs PA, Pettay D: Chromosome anomalies as predictors of recurrence risk for spontaneous abortion. *Am J Med Genet* 28:353, 1987

43. Shamma FN, Lee G, Gutmann JN, Lavy G: The role of office hysteroscopy in *in vitro* fertilization. *Fertil Steril* 58:1237, 1992

44. Prevedourakis C, Loutradis D, Kalianidis C, Markis N, Aravantinos D: Hysterosalpingography and hysteroscopy in female infertility. 9:2353, 1994

45. Parsons AK, Lense JJ: Sonohysterography for endometrial abnormalities: Preliminary results. *J Clin Ultrasound* 21:87, 1993

46. Coulam CB, Stern JJ, Soenksen DM, Britten S, Bustillo M: Hysterosonogram: A simple method of assessing the uterine cavity. Presented at Gynecoradiology Special Interest Group, 20th Annual Meeting of the American Fertility Society, November 5–10, 1994, San Antonio, Texas

47. Cicinelli E, Romano F, Anastasio PS, Blasi N, Parisi C, Galantino P: Transabdominal sonohysterography, transvaginal sonography and hysteroscopy in the evaluation of submucous myomas. *Obstet Gynecol* 85:42, 1995

48. Shaffer W: Role of uterine adhesions in the cause of multiple pregnancy losses. *Clin Obstet Gynecol* 29:912, 1986

49. Sauer MV, Paulson RJ, Lobo RA: Reversing the natural decline in human fertility: An extended clinical trial of oocyte donation to women of advanced reproductive age. *JAMA* 268:1275, 1992

50. Silverburg KM, Burns WN, Olive DL, Riehl RM, Schenken RS: Serum progesterone levels predict success of in vitro fertilization/embryo transfer in patients stimulated with leuprolide acetate and human menopausal gonadotropins. *J Clin Endocrinol Metab* 73:797, 1991

51. Meldrum DR: Female reproductive aging: Ovarian and uterine factors. *Fertil Steril* 59:1, 1993

52. Stern JJ, Voss F, Coulam CB: Early diagnosis of ectopic pregnancy

using receiver-operator characteristic curves of serum progesterone concentrations. *Hum Reprod* 8:775, 1993

53. Rosenfeld DL, Garcia CR: A comparison of endometrial histology with simultaneous plasma progesterone determinations in infertile women. *Fertil Steril* 26:1256, 1976

54. McNeely MJ, Soules MR: The diagnosis of luteal phase deficiency: A critical review. *Fertil Steril* 51:582, 1989

55. Noyes RW, Hertig AT, Rock J: Dating the endometrial biopsy. *Fertil Steril* 1:3, 1950

56. Jones GES: Some newer aspects of the management of infertility. *JAMA* 147:1123, 1949

57. Coulam CB, Stern JJ: Endocrine factors associated with recurrent spontaneous abortion. *Clin Obstet Gynecol* 37:730, 1994

58. Shoupe D, Mishell DR Jr, Lacarra M, et al: Correlation of endometrial maturation with four methods of estimating day of ovulation. *Obstet Gynecol* 72:88, 1986

59. Peters AJ, Lloyd RP, Coulam CB: Prevalence of out-of-phase endometrial biopsy specimens. *Am J Obstet Gynecol* 166:1738, 1992

60. Batista MC, Cartledge TP, Merino MJ, et al: Mid-luteal phase endometrial biopsy does not accurately predict luteal function. *Fertil Steril* 59:294, 1993

61. Tulppala M, Björses U-M, Stenman U-H, Wahlström OJ, Ylikorkala O: Luteal phase defect in habitual abortion: Progesterone in saliva. *Fertil Steril* 56:41,1991

62. Abraham GE, Maroulis GB, Marshall JR: Evaluation of ovulation and corpus luteum function using measurements of plasma progesterone. *Obstet Gynecol* 44:522, 1974

63. Pillet MC, Wu TF, Adamson GD, Subak LL, Lamb EJ: Improved prediction of post-ovulatory day using temperature recording, endometrial biopsy, and serum progesterone. *Fertil Steril* 53:614, 1990

64. Hamilton MPR, Fleming R, Coutts JRT, MacNaughton MC, Whitfield CR: Luteal phase deficiency: Ultrasonic and biochemical insights into pathogenesis. *Br J Obstet Gynaecol* 97:569, 1990

65. Coulam CB, Bustillo M, Soenksen DM, Britten S: Ultrasonographic predictors of implantation after assisted reproduction. *Fertil Steril* 62:1004, 1994

66. Bustillo M, Krysa LW, Coulam CB: Uterine receptivity in an oocyte donation program. *Human Reprod* 10:442–446, 1995

67. Lessey BA, Damjanovich L, Courtifaris C, Castlebaum A, Albelda SM, Buck CA: Integrin adhesion molecules in the human endometrium: Correlation with the normal and abnormal menstrual cycle. *J Clin Invest* 90:188, 1992

68. Courtifaris C, Lessey BA: Coexpression of endometrial osteopontin and its receptor, the αV/β3 integrin, define the window of human uterine receptivity to embryo implantation. Presented at the 40th Annual Meeting of the Society for Gynecologic Investigation, March 31–April 3, 1993, Toronto, Ontario, Canada

69. Lessey BA, Castlebaum A: Characterization of the αV/β3 integrin in endometrium of patients with unexplained infertility: A prospective controlled study. Presented at the 40th Annual Meeting of the Society for Gynecologic Investigation, March 31–April 3, 1993, Toronto, Ontario, Canada

70. Kwak JYH, Gilman-Sachs A, Beaman KD, Beer AE: Autoanti-

bodies in women with primary recurrent spontaneous abortion of unknown etiology. *J Reprod Immunol* 22:15, 1992

71. Silver RM, Branch DW: Recurrent miscarriage: autoimmune considerations. *Clin Obstet Gynecol* 37:745, 1994

72. Lubbe WF, Liggins GC: Lupus anticoagulant and pregnancy. *Am J Obstet Gynecol* 153:322, 1985

73. Howard MA, Firkin BG, Healy DL, et al: Lupus anticoagulant in women with multiple spontaneous miscarriage. *Am J Hematol* 26:175, 1987

74. Petri M, Golbus M, Anderson R, Whiting-O'Keefe Q, Corash L, Hellmann D: Antinuclear antibody, lupus anticoagulant, and anticardiolipin antibody in women with idiopathic habitual abortion. *Arthritis Rheum* 30:601, 1987

75. Harris EN, Chan JKH, Asherson RA, et al: Thrombosis, recurrent fetal loss, and thrombocytopenia. *Arch Intern Med* 146:2153, 1986

76. Cowchock S, Dehoratius RJ, Wapner RJ, Jackson LG: Subclinical autoimmune disease and unexplained abortion. *Am J Obstet Gynecol* 152:367, 1984

77. Garcia-De la Torre I, Hernandez-Vasquez L, Angulo-Vasquez J, Romero-Ornelas A: Prevalence of antinuclear antibodies in patients with habitual abortion and in normal and toxemic pregnancies. *Rheumatol Int* 4:87, 1984

78. Harger JH, Rabin BS, Marchese SG: The prognostic value of antinuclear antibodies in women with recurrent pregnancy losses: A prospective controlled study. *Obstet Gynecol* 73:419, 1989

79. Xu L, Chang V, Murphy A, et al: Antinuclear antibodies in sera of patients with recurrent pregnancy wastage. *Am J Obstet Gynecol* 163:1493, 1990

80. Stagnaro-Green A, Roman SH, Cobin RH, El-Harazy E, Alvarez-Marfany M, Davies TF: Detection of at-risk pregnancy by means of highly sensitive assays for thyroid autoantibodies. *JAMA* 264:1422, 1990

81. Glinoer D, Fernandez Soto M, Bourdoux P: Pregnancy in patients with mild thyroid abnormalities: Maternal and fetal repercussions. *J Clin Endocrinol Metab* 73:421, 1991

82. Pratt D, Novotny M, Kaberlein G, Dudkiewicz A, Gleicher N: Antithyroid antibodies and the association with non-organ-specific antibodies in recurrent pregnancy loss. *Am J Obstet Gynecol* 168:837, 1993

83. Rote NS, Lyden TW, Vogt E, Ng AK: Antiphospholipid antibodies and placental development. In: Hunt JS (ed), *Immunology of Reproduction*. New York, Springer-Verlag, 1994:285–302

84. Harris EN: The second international anticardiolipin standardization workshop: The Kingston anti-phospholipid antibody study (KAPS) group. *Am J Clin Pathol* 94:476, 1990

85. Petri M, Rheinschmidt M, Whiting-Okeefe Q, Hellman D, Corash L: The frequency of lupus anticoagulant in systemic lupus erythematosus. *Ann Intern Med* 106:524, 1987

86. Triplett DA: Antiphospholipid antibodies and recurrent pregnancy loss. *Am J Reprod Immunol* 20:52, 1989

87. Coulam CB: Immunologic tests in the evaluation of reproductive disorders: A critical review. *Am J Obstet Gynecol* 167:1844, 1992

88. Thomason EJ, Roussev RG, Stern JJ, Coulam CB: Prevalence of

embryotoxic factor in sera from women with unexplained recurrent abortion. *Am J Reprod Immunol* 33:333, 1995

89. Croy BA, Gambel P, Rossant J, Wegmann TG: Characterization of murine decidual natural killer (NK) cells and their relevance to the success of pregnancy. *Cell Immunol* 93:315, 1985

90. Starkey PM, Sargent LL, Redman CWG: Cell populations in human early pregnancy decidua: Characterization and isolation of large granular lymphocytes by flow cytometry. *Immunology* 65:129, 1988

91. Clark DA, Drake B, Head JR, Stedronska-Clark J, Banwatt D: Decidua-associated suppressor activity and viability of individual implantation sites of allopregnant mice. *J Reprod Immunol* 17:253, 1990

92. Clark DA, Chaouat G, Mogil R, Wegmann TG: Prevention of spontaneous abortion in DBA/2-mated CBA/J mice by GM-CSF involves CD8+ T cell-dependent suppression of natural effector cell cytotoxicity against trophoblast target cells. *Cell Immunol* 154:143, 1994

93. Roussev RG, Higgins NG, McIntyre JA: Phenotypic characterization of normal human placental cells. *J Reprod Immunol* 25:15, 1993

94. Clark DA, Lea RG, Podor T, Daya S, Banwatt D, Harley CB: Cytokines determining the success or failure of pregnancy. *Ann N Y Acad Sci* 626:524, 1991

95. Clark DA, Blair C: NICHD conference on materno-feto placental interactions. *J Reprod Fertil* 92:231, 1991

96. Croy BA, Guilbert LJ, Browne MA, et al: Characterization of cytokine production by the metrial gland and granulated metrial gland cells. *J Reprod Immunol* 19:149, 1991

97. Clark DA: Host immunoregulatory mechanisms and the success of the conceptus fertilised in vivo and in vitro. In: Beard RW, Sharp F (eds), *Early Pregnancy Failure: Mechanisms and Treatment,* Aston-Under-Lyme, UK, Peacock Press, 1988:215–232

98. Makida R, Minami M, Takamizawa M, Juji T, Fujii T, Mizuno M: Natural killer cell activity and immunotherapy for recurrent spontaneous abortion. *Lancet* 2:579, 1991

99. Yokoyama M, Sano M, Sonoda K, Nozaki M, Nakamura GI, Nakano H: Cytotoxic cells directed against placental cells detected in human habitual abortions by an in vitro terminal labelling assay. *Am J Reprod Immunol* 31:197, 1994

100. Newland AC: The use and mechanisms of action of intravenous immunoglobulin: An update. *Br J Haematol* 72:301, 1989

101. Hill JA, Polgar K, Harlow BL, Anderson DJ: Evidence of embryo- and trophoblast-toxic cellular immune response(s) in women with recurrent spontaneous abortion. *Am J Obstet Gynecol* 166:1044, 1992

102. Hill JA, Haimovici F, Anderson DJ: Products of activated lymphocytes and macrophages inhibit mouse embryo development in vitro. *J Immunol* 139:2250, 1987

103. Chavez DJ, McIntyre JA: Sera from women with histories of repeated pregnancy losses cause abnormalities in mouse peri-implantation blastocyst. *J Reprod Immunol* 6:273, 1984

104. Oksenberg JR, Brautbar C: In vitro suppression of murine blastocysts growth by sera from women with reproductive disorders. *Am J Reprod Immunol* 11:118, 1986

105. Zigril M, Fein A, Carp H, Toder V: Immuno-potentiation reverses the embryotoxic effect a serum from women with pregnancy loss. *Fertil Steril* 56:653, 1991

106. Delfraissy JF, Tchernia G, Laurian Y: Suppressor cell function after intravenous gammaglobulin treatment in adult chronic idiopathic thrombocytopenic purpura. *Br J Haematol* 60:315, 1985

107. Nydegger UE: Hypothetic and established action mechanisms of therapy with immunoglobulin G. In: Imbach P (ed), *Immunotherapy with Intravenous Immunoglobulins.* London, Academic Press, 1991:27–36

108. Newman MJ, Hines HC: Production of fetally stimulated lymphocytotoxic antibodies by primiparous cows. *Anim Blood Groups Biochem Genet* 10:87, 1979

109. McIntrye JA, Faulk WP, Nichols-Johnson VR, Taylor CG: Immunological testing and immunotherapy in recurrent spontaneous abortion. *Obstet Gynecol* 67:169, 1986

110. Mowbray JF: Autoantibodies, alloantibodies and reproductive success. *Cur Opin Immunol* 1982:1:741–743

111. Toder V, Strassburger D, Carp H, et al: Immunopotentiation and pregnancy loss. *J Reprod Fertil* 37:79, 1989

112. Rocklin RF, Kitzmiller JL, Garvey MR: Maternal-fetal relations. II. Further characterization of an immunologic blocking factor that develops during pregnancy. *Clin Immunol Immunopathol* 22:305, 1982

113. Roger JC: Lack of a requirement for a maternal humoral immune response to establish or maintain successful allogeneic pregnancy. *Transplantation* 40:372, 1985

114. Gilman-Sach A, Luo SP, Beer AE, Beaman KD: Analysis of anti-lymphocyte antibodies by flow cytometry or microlymphocytotoxicity in women with recurrent spontaneous abortions immunized with paternal leukocytes. *J Clin Lab Immunol* 30:53, 1989

115. Brand A, Witvliet M, Class FHJ: Beneficial effect of intravenous gammaglobulin in a patient with complement-mediated autoimmune thrombocytopenia due to IgM-antiplatelet antibodies. *Br J Haematol* 69:507, 1988

116. Dewald GW, Michels VV: Recurrent miscarriages: cytogenetic causes and genetic counseling of affected families. *Clin Obstet Gynecol* 29:865, 1986

117. Goldzieher JW: Double-blinded trial for a progestin in habitual abortion. *JAMA* 188:651, 1964

118. Klopper A, Macnaughton MC: Hormones in recurrent abortion. *Br J Obstet Gynaecol* 72:1022, 1965

119. Karamardian LM, Grimes PA: Luteal phase deficiency: Effect of treatment of pregnancy rates. *Am J Obstet Gynecol* 167:1391, 1992

120. Hasegawa I, Takakuwa K, Goto S, et al: Effectiveness of prednisone/aspirin therapy for recurrent aborters with antiphospholipid antibody. *Hum Reprod* 7:203, 1992

121. Cowchock FS, Wapner RJ, Needleman L, Filer R: A comparison of pregnancy outcome after two treatments for antibodies to cardiolipin (ACA). *Clin Exp Rheumatol* 6:200, 1988

122. Carreras LO, Perez GN, Vega HR, Maclouf J: Lupus anticoagulant and recurrent fetal loss: Successful treatment with gammaglobulin. *Lancet* 2:393, 1988

123. Francois A, Freund M, Reym P: Repeated fetal losses and the lupus anticoagulant. *Ann Intern Med* 109:933, 1988

124. Scott JR, Branch W, Kochenour NK, Ward K: Intravenous immunoglobulin treatment of pregnancy patients with recurrent pregnancy loss caused by antiphospholipid antibodies and Rh immunization. *Am J Obstet Gynecol* 159:1055, 1988

125. Parke A, Maier D, Wilson D, Andreoli J, Ballow M: Intravenous gammaglobulin, antiphospholipid antibodies, and pregnancy. *Ann Intern Med* 110:495, 1989

126. MacLachlan NA, Letsky E, DeSwiet M, et al: The use of intravenous immunoglobulin therapy in the management of antiphospholipid antibody associated pregnancies. *Clin Exp Rheumatol* 8:221, 1990

127. Christiansen OB, Mathiesen O, Lauristen JG, Grunnet N: Intravenous immunoglobulin treatment of women with multiple miscarriages. *Hum Reprod* 7:718, 1992

128. Kutteh WH: Antiphospholipid antibody associated recurrent pregnancy loss: Treatment with heparin and low-dose aspirin alone. *Am J Obstet Gynecol* 174:1, 1996

129. Branch DW, Scott JR, Kochenour NK, Hershgold E: Obstetric complications associated with the lupus anticoagulant. *N Engl J Med* 313:1322, 1985

130. Alarcon-Segovia D, Deleze M, Oria CV, et al: Antiphospholipid antibodies and the antiphospholipid antibody syndrome in systemic lupus erythematosus. *Medicine* 68:353, 1989

131. Ramsdon CF, Farquharson RG: A woman with twelve first trimester losses in whom lupus anticoagulant was detected and treated with steroids, sandoglobulin, and heparin. *Clin Exp Rheumatol* 8:221, 1990

132. Cowchock FS, Resse EA, Balaban D, Branch DW, Plouffe L: Repeated fetal losses associated with antiphospholipid antibodies: A collaborative trial comparing treatment with prednisone to low dose heparin. *Am J Obstet Gynecol* 166:1318, 1992

133. Babcock RB, Dumper CW, Scharfman WB: Heparin-induced immunothrombocytopenia. *N Engl J Med* 295:237, 1976

134. McVerry B, Spearing R, Smith A: SLE anticoagulant: Transient inhibition by high dose immunoglobulin infusions. *Br J Haematol* 61:579, 1985

135. Wapner RJ, Cowchock FS, Shapiro SS: Successful treatment in two women with antiphospholipid antibodies and refractory pregnancy losses with intravenous immunoglobulin infusions. *Am J Obstet Gynecol* 161:1271, 1989

136. Bernstein RM, Crawford RJ: Intravenous IgG therapy for anticardiolipin syndrome: A case report. *Clin Exp Rheumatol* 6:198, 1988

137. Beer AE, Quebbeman JF, Ayers JW, Haines RF: Major histocompatibility complex antigens, maternal and paternal immune responses and chronic habitual abortions in humans. *Am J Obstet Gynecol* 141:987, 1981

138. Taylor C, Faulk WP: Prevention of recurrent abortions with leukocyte transfusions. *Lancet* 2:68, 1981

139. Mowbray JF, Lidlee H, Underwood JL, Gibbings C, Reginald PW, Beard RW: Controlled trial of treatment of recurrent spontaneous abortion by immunization with paternal cells. *Lancet* 1:941, 1985

140. Gatenby PA, Cameron K, Simes RJ, et al: Treatment of recurrent spontaneous abortion by immunization with paternal lymphocytes: Results of a controlled trial. *Am J Reprod Immunol* 29:88, 1993

141. Cauchi MN, Lemi D, Young DE, Klosa M, Pepperell RJ: Treatment of recurrent spontaneous aborters by immunization with paternal cells: Controlled trial. *Am J Reprod Immunol* 25:16, 1991

142. Ho H, Gill TJ III, Hsuish HJ, Jiang JJ, Lee TY, Hsish CY: Immunotherapy for recurrent spontaneous abortion in a Chinese population. *Am J Reprod Immunol* 25:10, 1991

143. Recurrent Miscarriage Immunotherapy Trialists Group: Worldwide collaborative observational study and meta-analysis on allogenic leukocyte immunotherapy for recurrent spontaneous abortion. *Am J Reprod Immunol* 32:55, 1994

144. Coulam CB, Krysa L, Stern JJ, Bustillo M: Intravenous immunoglobulin for treatment of recurrent pregnancy loss. *Am J Reprod Immunol* 34:333–337, 1995

145. Coulam CB, Clark DA: Report from the Ethics Committee on Immunotherapy, American Society of Immunology of Reproduction. *Am J Reprod Immunol* 26:93, 1991

146. Coulam CB, Clark DA, Beer AE: Report from the Ethics Committee on Immunotherapy. *Am J Reprod Immunol* 28:3, 1992

147. Coulam CB: Report from the Ethics Committee on Immunotherapy. *Am J Reprod Immunol* 30:45, 1993

148. Mueller-Eckhardt G, Heine O, Neppert J, Kunzel W, Mueller-Eckhardt C: Prevention of recurrent spontaneous abortion by intravenous immunoglobulin. *Vox Sang* 56:151, 1989

149. Mueller-Eckhardt G, Huni O, Poltrin B: IVIg to prevent recurrent spontaneous abortion. *Lancet* 1:424, 1991

150. Maruyama T, Makino T, Iwasaki K, et al: The influence of intravenous immunoglobulin treatment on maternal immunity in women with unexplained recurrent miscarriage. *Am J Reprod Immunol* 31:7, 1994

151. Kimberly RP, Salmon JE, Bussell JB, et al: Modulation of mononuclear phagocyte function by intravenous gammaglobulin. *J Immunol* 132:745, 1987

152. Kulics J, Rajnavolgye E, Fust G, Gergely J: Interaction of C3 and C3b with immunoglobulin. *J Mol Immunol* 20:805, 1983

153. Zielinski CC, Pries P, Eibl MM: Effect of immunoglobulin substitution of serum immunoglobulin and complement concentration. *Nephron* 40:253, 1985

154. Seibel MM, Taymor ML: Emotional aspects of infertility. *Fertil Steril* 37:127, 1982

CHAPTER 27

Aging and Reproduction

GEORGE B. MAROULIS

The Effect of Age on Fertility Rates in
    Different Populations
Effect of Age on the Components of
    the Female Reproductive System
    Ovary
    Uterus

Hypothalamus
Cervix
Fallopian tubes
Effect of Age on Male Fertility
Abortion Rate in Relation to Age
Conclusion

The process of aging affects all biologic systems. These changes become apparent at different ages in different systems of the human body and become more obvious when the system is required to function at its maximum potential. For the reproductive system, which for women has a finite life, the maximum potential, that is, fertility, begins declining in the mid thirties, about 10 years before menstrual irregularities appear. Besides fertility, aging is associated with decreases in hormonal production of estrogen in the reproductive system, which influences the skeletal and cardiovascular systems. This chapter focuses on the age-related decrease in reproductive potential, which is due to: (1) intrinsic aging of the reproductive system; (2) weathering, which refers to the increase with age of certain conditions that influence the reproductive system; and (3) socioeconomic factors that influence the reproductive system.[1]

Intrinsic aging refers to the changes expected and anticipated with time in the components of the reproductive system, such as the hypothalamic-pituitary axis, ovary, uterus, fallopian tubes, and cervix. *Weathering* refers to events that occur with advancing age that affect the reproductive system directly or indirectly, such as endometriosis, pelvic infection,

smoking, diabetes and obesity. In men, an example of such a problem is impotence, which can be influenced by diabetes, therapy for hypertension, and impaired cardiac function. Many *socioeconomic* factors can influence the fertility potential of women, such as poor nutrition, poor health, promiscuity, and pelvic infection. An additional social factor that may influence an age-specific decrease in fertility in modern society is the delay in marriage and the desire for childbearing, because women and men may pursue their careers first and want to have a family later. By the time such couples want to have children, age becomes a factor. It is interesting that during the 1990s, there is a projected 22% decrease in the number of women who want to conceive before the age of 35 years. Since 1970, there has been a 50% increase in the number of women who have their first child after the age of 35 years.[2,3] In addition, in years past when women delayed their childbearing, they were not necessarily sexually active. In today's world, sexual practices have changed. Contraception is widely used, women have more sexual partners, and the risk for pelvic inflammatory disease and tubal damage increase with advancing age.[4]

THE EFFECT OF AGE ON FERTILITY RATES IN DIFFERENT POPULATIONS

In evaluating fertility potential, two terms are frequently used: *fecundability* and *fertility rate*.[5] *Fecundability rate* is the probability of conceiving during one menstrual cycle. It is estimated by counting the observed conceptions during a number of cycles and dividing it by the total number of menstrual cycles of women who engage in sexual intercourse and do not practice contraception. *Fertility rate* is the probability of conceiving within 1 year within a given population. It is estimated by counting the number of livebirths in 1 year and dividing it by the total population of women in the reproductive age group. These rates usually underestimate the fertility potential for the following reasons: (1) early pregnancy and subclinical losses are often ignored and not estimated, and (2) the assumption that all women under observation have sexual intercourse, ovulate, or have timed intercourse with ovulation to maximize the fertility potential may not be correct. Many women may, for example, have irregular anovulatory cycles, use contraception, and not be sexually active. Such facts are not known by the investigators. The results from natural populations are depicted in Fig 27–1.

Natural fertility rates are estimated from populations such as the Hutterites in North America and other populations in Europe, such as in Geneva in the 16th century and 17th century.[6] The fertility rate remains relatively stable until the ages of 30 to 32 years, after which they decline. Comparing fertility rates with those of women 20 to 24 years of age, there is a drop of 4% to 8% among women 25 to 29 years of age, 15% to 19% among women 30 to 34 years of age, 26% to 46% among women 35 to 39 years of age, and up to 92% among women 45 to 49 years of age. In such natural populations, the fecundability and fertility rates usually underestimate the fertility potential of older women for reasons already pointed out. Data from the United States (1981) do not reflect the natural fertility rate, since the population is practicing contraception. However, it is of interest to see the effect of the various social influences on fertility rate. The maximum potential for the fertility and fecundability rates among older women is best estimated among women who are trying to become pregnant using treatments such as gamete intrafallopian transfer (GIFT),[7] in vitro fertilization (IVF),[8] therapeutic insemination with donor sperm (TID)[9] or in natural populations from late 1700s and early 1800s, such as those of Ireland, Belgium, and Sweden. In these populations women purposely delayed childbearing and tried to become pregnant at older ages.[7–9] In such populations, the mean age of marriage was more than 27 years and even close to 30 years. The statistics show that women 40 years of age and older can have fertility rates near 40% and are not hopelessly infertile.[10] Fig 27–2 shows the fertility potential from studies of women undergoing artificial insemination or other therapeutic procedures such as IVF or GIFT. Fertility potential is presumed to be maximal among women undergoing TID because the reproductive system of these women is presumed to be normal. In one study, all women had documented good progesterone levels, normal hysterosalpingograms, normal menses, and no history of endometriosis. To ensure proper timing, inseminations were based on detection of the luteinizing hormone (LH) surge.[11] The highest pregnancy rate (30% per cycle) was observed among women 20 to 24 years of age, followed by a plateau (16% to 19% per cycle) until the age of 42 to 44 years, when the rate dropped to less than 5% per cycle.[9,11]

Reversal of tubal ligation for women older than 40 years can be successful, although the success rate is less than that among women younger than 40 years (45% vs 66%).[13] Simi-

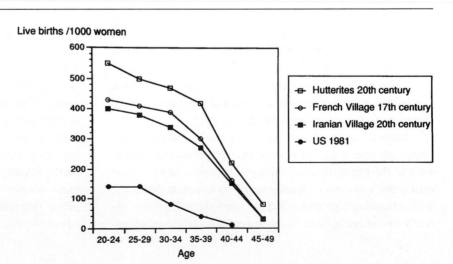

Figure 27–1. Fertility rate among natural populations and a U.S. population.

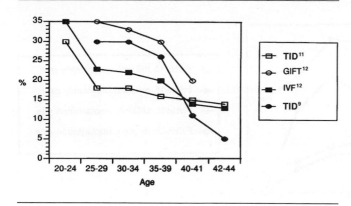

Figure 27–2. Pregnancy rate per cycle among infertile patients undergoing various treatments.

larly, women undergoing induction of ovulation also notice a decrease in pregnancy rates with increased age. Pregnancy rate among anovulatory women younger than 36 years receiving human menopausal gonadotropin (hMG) was reported to be 35% compared with 10% per cycle among women older than 36 years, whereas the abortion rate increased from 15.5% to 29%.[14]

EFFECT OF AGE ON THE COMPONENTS OF THE FEMALE REPRODUCTIVE SYSTEM

From data already presented, there is evidently a decrease in fertility rate with age. In women, the main reason for decreased fertility appears to be decreased ovarian function and oocyte quality. There is still a controversy about the possible importance of aging of the uterus, hypothalamus-pituitary axis, cervix, and fallopian tube to fertility .

Ovary

Ovarian function is characterized by: (1) the quality and quantity of oocytes released and (2) the hormonal milieu of the preovulatory follicle and postovulatory corpus luteum and its progesterone production.

The oocyte reservoir, oocyte quality, and ovarian responsiveness to gonadotropic stimulation may decline with advancing age. The age-related changes in ovarian function effect menstrual cyclicity, particularly after 40 years of age. The menstrual cycles become shorter and irregular 3 to 9 years before the onset of menopause. The shortening of the follicular phase is associated with a decrease in serum estradiol level throughout the cycle and a shortening of the length of the menstrual cycle. Serum follicle-stimulating hormone (FSH) level increases slightly with advancing age while LH level usually remains unchanged.[15] After the LH surge, both the serum progesterone level and the length of the luteal phase remain unchanged. In

one study, however, the incidence of a short luteal phase increased among women between 45 and 50 years of age. In another study, progesterone levels decreased, suggesting inadequate function of the corpus luteum.[16,17] In support of this finding, luteal cells from older women displayed a decreased ability to secrete progesterone and inhibin compared with cells from younger women.[18]

This decline in ovarian function and its reserve with age is progressive and subtle. A marker of this decline is a rising level of early follicular (cycle day 2 to 3) serum FSH level.[19] Another marker of ovarian function is inhibin, a polypeptide hormone secreted by the granulosa cells.[20] Serum FSH stimulates the increase in inhibin and estradiol levels, reflecting the growing number of follicles. A decrease in follicular inhibin is the earliest sign of ovarian aging. It precedes the decrease of follicular estradiol production and is probably the factor that allows the increase in serum FSH level.[21] Actually, a rise in cycle day 3 serum FSH level greater than 15 IU/L in women of any age has a predictive value for poor reproductive potential and a decrease in the number of oocytes.[22] The quality of the oocytes correlates negatively with age, particularly for women older than 38 years. In these women, a rising serum FSH level is associated with a further decrease in implantation rate within similar age groups.[21] If cycle day 3 serum FSH level exceeds 15 IU/L, fertility rates decrease (Fig 27–3). Levels greater than 25 IU/L are usually associated with a zero pregnancy rate.[22]

Other efforts to screen women older than 35 years for diminished ovarian reserve have been described. They include the clomiphene citrate challenge test (CCCT) and the gonadotropin-releasing hormone (GnRH) analog stimulation test.[23,24] The CCCT is based on the premise that in response to a clomiphene-induced increase in serum FSH levels, women with normal ovarian reserve produce enough estrogen and inhibin to keep serum FSH levels within normal range, whereas among those with poor follicular development FSH levels rise. After an intake of 100 mg of clomiphene citrate from cycle day 5 to cycle day 9, serum FSH level is measured on day 10. A normal CCCT response on day 10 shows an FSH level less than 20 IU/L. An FSH level greater than 20 IU/L (Leeco assay) is indicative of decreasing ovarian reserve. The decrease correlates with age so that 3% of patients had such a response before the age of 30 years, 7% at 30 to 34 years of age, 10% at 35 to 39 years of age, and 26% at 40 years of age and after.[23] An abnormal test is a prognostic factor for decreased fertility potential within all age groups.[23]

A GnRH agonist stimulation test designed to stimulate ovarian function has been described. According to this test, on cycle day 2, leuprolide acetate (1.0 mg/mL) is given, and estradiol is measured 24 hours later. An increase in estradiol production after administration of GnRH is associated with an increasing pregnancy rate. A change in estradiol level of less than 15 pg/mL (55 pmol/L) is associated with a pregnancy rate less than

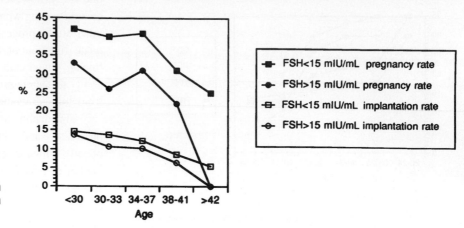

Figure 27–3. Influence of age and FSH level on implantation and pregnancy rates. *(From Toner JR, Scott RT:* Semin Reprod Endocrinol *13:1, 1995.)*

5%. A change of 100 pg/mL (367 pmol/L) or more is associated with a pregnancy rate of 35%.[24]

These two tests seem to enhance the predictability of ovarian response. Age, however, even in the presence of a normal test, is a determining factor, so these tests of ovarian responsiveness should be evaluated within the framework of each age group.

Oocyte depletion is an ongoing process from birth until menopause and beyond. Because the actual decrease in the number of oocytes may contribute to the decrease in fecundability rate and an increase in the rate of chromosomal abnormalities and abortion, finding a way to decrease the rate of depletion of oocytes in women who plan and want to prolong their childbearing age would be important. Today, there is no method by which oocyte depletion can be delayed, although data for women taking oral contraceptives suggest that menopause may be slightly delayed.[25] Factors that may be used to predict faster oocyte depletion are early menarche, age at last pregnancy, poor nutrition, smoking, and a family history of early menopause.[26,27] Premature menopause is most frequently attributed to defects in ovarian differentiation, such as gonadal dysgenesis, mumps oophoritis, autoimmune diseases, or the consequence of the treatment of certain diseases with irradiation or chemotherapy with alkylating agents.[28]

It is estimated that during fetal life as many as 7 million oogonia are present in a woman's ovaries; at birth the number is reduced to 2 million; and by menarche, to 300,000. Between menarche and menopause, approximately 1000 oocytes are consumed every month, but only a few oocytes are released. It is hypothesized that the total number of the population of human ovarian follicles is composed of two populations: (1) the nongrowing follicles and (2) the early growing follicles. It is theorized that in younger women, there is depletion of the nongrowing follicles, mainly by atresia, but in older women, nongrowing follicles enter the growing pool at an accelerated rate.

The mechanisms that accelerate the entrance of nongrowing follicles into a growth phase may depend on the increase in FSH levels that occurs with increasing age.[29]

The change in the quality of the oocytes with advancing age is the reason for the observed increase in the number of chromosomal anomalies that occurs with increasing age. Down syndrome and certain chromosomal anomalies, which increase with maternal age, however, may be the consequence of the decrease in the oocyte pool rather than the effect of age per se.[30] The possible relation of fetal aneuploidy to dwindling oocyte pool is suggested on the basis of data from studies of animals. The data show that unilateral ovariectomy of mice led to an increase in the rate of fetal aneuploidy with maternal age.[31] The increase with age in the rate of congenital defects due to oocyte disturbances could be even more terrible than thought up to now because of the relationship of Down syndrome to the Alzheimer type of neuropathology.[32] This relationship between Alzheimer's disease and Down syndrome is observed only among children who have the chromosomal defect. There is no evidence that Alzheimer's disease is more prevalent in the normal offspring of older women.[32,33]

In older women, oocytes are fertilized, but the resulting conceptus has a decreased implantation rate. The reason for this decreased implantation rate is not clear, but it may be related to decreased embryo quality and not to the quality of the uterine environment. Existing data also suggest that oocyte aging may affect the nucleus, leading to defective nuclear development or chromosomal aberrations.[32] There is an increasing rate of aneuploidy among oocytes that are not fertilized, and advanced maternal age increases the rate of aneuploidy among oocytes.[34,35] That oocyte aging is most probably the key to the decreased implantation rate among older women is clearly shown by the increase in implantation rates when embryos developing from oocytes obtained from younger women are implanted in older women. Another possible reason was proposed by Cohen et al,[36] who postulated that in older women hatching of embryos is impaired.

All these changes in ovarian function due to age are not clearly understood. It is not clear whether it is the decreasing number of follicles or the follicular milieu or age that is responsible for the change of the menstrual cycle pattern and the ovarian function. Possible changes in the vascularity of the ovaries may play a role in ovarian aging. In a study by Gonzalez et al,[37] ovaries from postmenopausal women were compared with those of women in their earlier reproductive years. The investigators found that in postmenopausal ovaries the arteries, veins, and arterioles had a lumen diminution as much as 88.5%; 94.2% of specimens had a thickened wall, which may support the hypothesis that vascular aging, including thickening of the blood vessels and diminished lumen, may lead to a decreased blood supply and a change in the function of the ovaries.[37] Further studies of ovarian blood supply are needed to confirm these findings. A recent study[38] using Doppler ultrasound found that the impedance (resistance index) of the ovarian artery in postmenopausal women progressively increase from 5 to 15 years after menopause, suggesting a progressive decrease in ovarian blood flow with age that was not reversed by estrogen replacement therapy. Uterine flow also decreased with age but improved with estrogen therapy.[38]

Uterus

Studies with animals such as rabbits, mice, and hamsters have implied that the aging uterus is responsible for much of the decreased implantation rate and increased pregnancy wastage observed with aging. For women, available data on the effect of aging on uterine receptivity are controversial in that some studies suggest a decrease in uterine receptivity with age, but most studies do not. The studies in which endometrial receptivity appeared to decrease with age showed that when oocytes obtained from women younger than 30 years were given to two groups of recipients of different ages, the implantation rates were much higher among recipients 35 years of age or younger compared with those older than 35 years.[8,39] Endometrial histologic findings are frequently reported to be abnormal among women who undergo hyperstimulation. The frequency is higher among women older than 35 years than among women younger than 35 years.[40,78] It has also been reported that a decrease in endometrial receptivity among women older than 40 years may be reversed with additional progesterone supplementation, such as an increase from 50 mg to 100 mg intramuscularly daily before embryo transfer.[40]

Most studies have failed to show a statistically significant effect of age on endometrial receptivity. Endometrial thickness during the pre- and postovulatory state has been correlated with implantation; however, age does not seem to affect the thickness of the endometrium.[41] The appearance of the endometrium of women without ovarian function, after estrogen replacement therapy is similar to that of women 26 to 60 years of age.[42] Sauer et al[43] found that there was no difference in endometrial receptivity among age groups ranging from 30 to 59 years. Abortion rates were also equal among all these age groups, with the exception that prior exposure to chemotherapy may alter endometrial integrity and lead to greater pregnancy wastage among women receiving donated embryos.[43] Another study[44] showed that when oocytes obtained from young donors were distributed among younger and older recipients, the implantation rates were the same, again suggesting no effect of age on endometrial receptivity.

The question of the effect of aging on the endometrium is not settled. More studies are needed to evaluate possible changes on the molecular level, which may be revealing. One such study showed that epidermal growth factor (EGF) and insulin-like growth factor 1 (IGF-1) expression in perimenopausal and premenopausal women is higher than that of postmenopausal women.[45] These changes, however, are probably due to estrogen levels and may be reversible.

Another age-related factor which may influence implantation is the presence of leiomyomas, endometrial hyperplasia, and polyps, the frequency of which increases with age.[46]

Hypothalamus

Aging may cause hypothalamic changes that lead to a decrease in certain body functions in animals.[47] The observed changes in hypothalamic norepinephrine and dopamine are important because they reduce secretion of gonadotropic hormones and stop the estrous cycle in female rats.[47] Decreases in hypothalamic norepinephrine and dopamine levels have been reported in older humans, but it is not clear whether these are related to changes in body functions.[47] Indeed, among humans, the effect of age on the hypothalamus and pituitary gland has not been adequately studied. In addition, most of the available data on the effects of aging on the hypothalamus that refer to rodents may not be applicable to primates. Among women, advancing age, according to one study, did not affect gonadotropic production or LH pulse frequencies or amplitude.[48] However, another study[49] found that aging resulted in a decrease in the secretion of gonadotropins among postmenopausal women. When two groups of postmenopausal women (average age of 80.3 versus 53.8 years) were stimulated with GnRH, the older postmenopausal women achieved a lower mean LH level composed of attenuated LH pulse amplitudes and pulse frequencies, whereas the FSH secretion of older women was also characterized by lower mean FSH levels with lower FSH pulse amplitudes but not pulse frequencies.[49] It seems that there are changes in gonadotropin production in the later postmenopausal years, probably after 60 years of age. It is interesting that the positive and negative feedback mechanism seems to remain intact with advancing age.[50] The biologic activity of the secreted gonadotropins, however, may change with age. A study by Wide and Hobson[51] showed that the biologic activity of gonadotropins among older women is less than that of younger women.

The consistency of the pituitary gland has been studied in relation to advancing age. One study[52] found increasing fibrosis of the pituitary gland after the fourth decade of life. However, the gland appears to have great reserves of gonadotropins, so secretion of these hormones is not influenced substantially until extreme losses of tissue or functional capacity have occurred. Some additional information may be supportive of this view; it is reported that the neurons of the suprachiasmatic nucleus decrease during normal aging.[53]

Cervix

The endocervix changes in appearance at different ages. During childhood and puberty, the cells of the endocervical mucosa are low columnar. After the onset of menstrual cycles, they are ciliated mucus columnar cells. These cells have two functions: (1) synthesis of mucins and (2) accumulation within the endocervical canal of mucus, water, and soluble proteins, which provide, under the influence of estrogens, the proper environment for good sperm transfer. In postmenopausal women, the height of the endocervical cells decreases in size and the stroma of the cervix changes from reticular connective tissue to collagen connective tissue. With increasing age the endocervix changes from an organ that responds cyclicly to estrogen to an organ that produces noncyclic secretions, the role of which is probably to defend against bacteria and infections.[54] The decrease in functional ability of the cervix is a result of decreasing estrogens; to what extent this decrease affects sperm transfer is not clear. No studies have investigated the role of aging in the postcoital test or mucous production and how these may relate to fertility.

Fallopian Tubes

The main function of the fallopian tubes in reproduction is to transport ova and provide the appropriate environment for fertilization. The transportation of an ovum is influenced by (1) the contractility of the muscular wall of the fallopian tube, (2) the ciliary activity of the oviduct, (3) the secretion of the oviduct, and (4) the diameter of the lumen. Some of these factors are influenced by estrogen and progesterone because the smooth muscle and secretory cells of the human oviduct contain estrogen and progesterone receptors, whereas the ciliary cells do not.[55] Tubal mobility is influenced by age and menopause because of decreasing estrogen levels. However, this oviductal ciliary activity can be restored in women who receive estrogens. The secretions of the oviduct are at a maximum in the late follicular phase, but after menopause there is a decrease in the secretory cell height and activity. These functions are restored by the administration of estrogen.[56] Whether these age-related changes in the oviduct, which appear to be secondary to steroid secretion by the ovary, can delay oocyte transport and play a role in the increased incidence of ectopic pregnancy or decreased fertility is not known. Ectopic pregnancy rate increases with age and smoking, but whether this change is the direct effect of aging or other factors such as smoking, pelvic infection, or endometriosis is not clear.[57]

EFFECT OF AGE ON MALE FERTILITY

The role of the age of the male partner in fertility is not known. In one study, the data for women and men born in the mid 19th century were evaluated as to the effect of the age of the wife, the age of the husband, and the duration of the marriage on the pregnancy rate. The wife's age contributed to a decrease in fertility after the age of 35 years, whereas among men the decline started at the age of 40. By the age of 65 years the fertility rate of men had dropped to 36% of that among men between the ages of 20 and 24 years.[58]

Among men, advancing age is associated with a decrease in plasma levels of free testosterone. It is generally believed that this decrease is primarily due to decreased testicular function. Indeed, the observation of increasing levels of LH supports the idea of primary testicular dysfunction.[59] However, in one study[60] hypothalamic aging was implicated more than testicular dysfunction as the cause of decreased testosterone. In this study the LH pulse frequency and duration increased with age, the amplitude decreased, and the mean serum LH and FSH concentrations increased. It was then theorized that the main event in the aging of the hypothalamus-testicular axis is the decrease in LH amplitude. This decrease leads to lower serum testosterone levels, causing an increase in LH pulse frequency and duration. The increase leads to an increase in basal gonadotropin release and an increase in LH levels.[60] Further investigation as to the mechanism of aging in the hypothalamic-pituitary-gonadal axis is needed for men. The physiologic significance of LH pulses remains unclear as far as Leydig cell function is concerned. Whereas pulsatile GnRH secretion is required for LH release, the Leydig cells do not require pulsatile LH release, since they can be stimulated by human chorionic gonadotropin (hCG), which has a long half life.[61]

Studies that focus on testicular function suggest that there is an age-related decrease in spermatogenesis, total sperm count, and sperm motility and morphology in older men.[62-64] McLeod and Gold[65] reported a decreased conception rate among older men, and Ducot et al[66] have made similar observations. However, none of these studies answered definitively the question of "men's fertility change with age" because: (1) they did

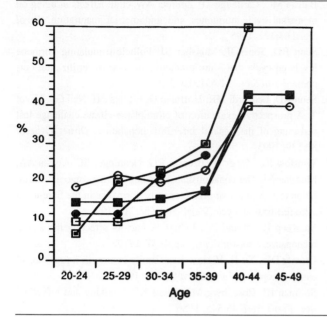

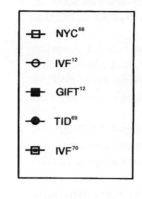

Figure 27–4. Abortion rate at different maternal ages. NYC, New York.

not evaluate the effect of maternal age and (2) they did not account for the possibility that decreases in spermatogenesis may not be important unless the sperm count is less than what is considered normal.

ABORTION RATE IN RELATION TO AGE

The abortion rate increases with advancing age, which decreases the overall potential for fertility among older women[67] (Fig 27–4). Studies from healthy populations have shown that the incidence of spontaneous abortion among women older than 40 years is approximately 30%. It is likely, however, that this rate is an underestimate of the actual rate, since many early abortions are not recognized. In longitudinal studies, as many as 60% of conceptions detected by means of a rise in βhCG level usually abort within the first 12 weeks of pregnancy.[71] Studies with public and private patients in New York City[68] and pregnant physicians[72] show a progressive increase in abortion rate with age. Results of IVF, GIFT, and TID show that compared with an abortion rate of 7% to 15% among women between the ages of 20 and 29 years, women 40 years of age or older have an abortion rate that exceeds 40%.[12,69,70]

The age-related increase in abortion rate occurs among both chromosomally normal and abnormal conceptuses. The increase in chromosomal abnormalities is primarily due to trisomies, which suggests a loss of oocyte integrity with advancing age. The age-related increase in the number of chromosomally normal conceptuses suggests a possible decline in uterine receptivity or a decline in normal growth of the conceptus. Cytogenetic studies of abortuses show that more than 50% of abortuses are chromosomally abnormal.[73] Most are aneuploid, 17%

are triploid, and some are structural rearrangements, mosaics, sex chromosome trisomies, and autosomal monosomies. Advancing age increases aneuploidy and the number of abnormal-appearing embryos. Older women have a higher incidence of hypodiploidy or hyperdiploidy.[35]

Few data exist regarding the effect of paternal age on spontaneous abortion. One study suggested that there may be an increased rate of Down syndrome due to paternal age.[74] Other chromosomal disorders that are possibly related to the increasing paternal age are the Iso-X syndrome and trisomy-16.[68,75] One study suggested that the source of the chromosomes contributing to trisomy-21 may be the father about 25% of the time.[76] In another study, however, no paternal effect on the Down syndrome was found.[77]

CONCLUSION

Although aging is a natural process that cannot be prevented, an understanding of its contribution to infertility is useful in treating and counseling patients. This is particularly true in light of the increasing numbers of patients of advanced reproductive age seeking treatment of infertility.

REFERENCES

1. Susser M: *Community Psychiatry: Epidemiologic and Social Themes.* New York: Random House, 1968
2. Fonteyn VJ, Isadanb A: Nongenetic implications of childbearing after the age of thirty-five. *Obstet Gynecol Surv* 43:709, 1988

3. Advance report of final natality studies 1982: NCHS Monthly Vital Statistics, Repro 33 (Suppl):1984

4. Mosher WE, Pratt WF: Reproductive impairments among married couples in the United States. Vital and Health Statistics, Series 23, No. 11, National Center for Health Studies. Washington, DC, U.S. Government Printing Office, 1982

5. Kline J, Stein Z, Susser M: Aging and reproduction. I. Fecundity, fertility and gestation. In: Kline J, Stein Z, Susser M (eds), *Conception to Birth.* New York: Oxford University Press, 1989:259

6. Henry L: Some data on natural fertility. *Eugenics Quar Rev* 8:81, 1961

7. Penzias AS, Thompson IE, Alper MM, Oskowitz SP, Berger MJ: Successful use of gamete intrafallopian transfer does not reverse the decline in fertility in women over 40 years of age. *Obstet Gynecol* 77:37, 1991

8. Rotsztejn DA, Asch RH: Effect of aging on assistive reproductive technologies (ART): Experience from egg donation. *Semin Reprod Endocrinol* 9:272, 1991

9. Byrd W, Bradshaw K, Carr B, Edman C, Odom J, Ackerman G: A prospective randomized study of pregnancy rates following intrauterine and intracervical insemination using frozen donor sperm. *Fertil Steril* 52:521, 1990

10. Menken J, Larsen U: Fertility rates and aging: In: Mastroianni L, Paulsen CA (eds), *Aging, Reproduction and the Climacteric.* New York, Plenum, 1986:147

11. Stovall DW, Toma SK, Hammoud MG, Talbert LM: The effect of age on female fecundity. *Obstet Gynecol* 77:33, 1991

12. Medical Research International: The American Fertility Society Special Interest Group: In-vitro fertilization/embryo transfer in the United States—1989 results from IVF-ET registry. *Fertil Steril* 55:14, 1991

13. Trimbos-Kemper TCM: Reversal of sterilization in women over 40 years of age: A multicenter study in the Netherlands. *Fertil Steril* 53:575, 1990

14. Dor J, Itzkowic DJ, Mashiach S, Lunenfeld B, Serr DM: Cumulative conception rates following gonadotropin therapy. *Am J Obstet Gynecol* 136:102, 1980

15. Sherman BM, Koreman SG: Hormonal characteristics of the human menstrual cycle throughout reproductive life. *J Clin Invest* 55:699, 1975

16. Lenton EA, Landgren BM: The normal menstrual cycle. In: Shearman RP (ed), *Clinical Reproductive Endocrinology.* Edinburgh, Churchill Livingstone, 1985:92–93

17. Reyes F, Winter J, Faiman L: Pituitary-ovarian relationships preceding the menopause. *Am J Obstet Gynecol* 129:557, 1977

18. Pellicer A, Mari M, De Los Santos M, et al: Effect of aging on the human ovary: The secretion of immunoreactive L-inhibin and progesterone. *Fertil Steril* 61:663, 1994

19. Lenton EA, Sexton L, Lee S, Cooke ID: Progressive changes in LH/FSH ratio in women throughout reproductive life. *Maturitas* 10:35, 1988

20. McLachlan RI, Robertson D, Dekretcher DM, Burger HG: Plasma inhibin levels during gonadotropin induced ovarian hyperstimulation for IVF: A new index of follicular function. *Lancet* 1:1233, 1986

21. Batista MC, Cartledge TP, Zellmer AW, et al: Effects of aging on menstrual cycle hormones and endometrial maturation. *Fertil Steril* 64:492, 1995

22. Scott RD, Toner JP, Muasher SJ: Follicle-stimulating hormone levels on cycle day 3 are predictive of in-vitro fertilization outcome. *Fertil Steril* 51:651, 1989

23. Scott RD, Leonardi MR, Hoffman G, Ellions EH, Neil GS, Navot T: A prospective evaluation of clomiphene citrate challenge test screening of the general infertility population. *Obstet Gynecol* 82:539, 1993

24. Winslow KL, Toner JP, Brezski RG, Oehninger SC, Acosta AA, Muasher SJ: The gonadotropin-releasing hormone agonist stimulation test: A sensitive predictor of performance in the flare-up in vitro fertilization cycle. *Fertil Steril* 56:711, 1991

25. VanKeep PA, Brand PC, Lehert P: Factors affecting the age at menopause. *J Biosoc Sci* 6(Suppl):37, 1979

26. Cramer DW, Xu H, Harlow BL: Family history as a predictor of early menopause. *Fertil Steril* 64:740, 1995

27. Stillman RJ, Rosenberg MT, Sachs BP: Smoking and reproduction. *Fertil Steril* 46:545, 1986

28. Vermeulen A: Environment, human reproduction, menopause and andropause. *Environ Health Perspect* 101(Suppl 2):91, 1993

29. Gougon A, Echohard R, Phalabard JC: Age related changes of the population of human ovarian follicles: Increase in the disappearance rate of non-growing and early growing follicles in aging women. *Biol Reprod* 50:653, 1994

30. Kline J, Levin B: Trisomy and age at menopause predicted association given a link with rate of oocyte atresia. *Pediatr Perinat Epidemiol* 6:225, 1992

31. Brook J, Gosden G, Chandley AC: Maternal aging and aneuploid embryos: Evidence for the mouse that biological and not chronological age is the important influence. *Hum Genet* 66:41, 1984

32. Finch CE: The evolution of ovarian oocyte decline with aging and possible relationships to Down syndrome and Alzheimer's disease. *Exp Gerontol* 29:299, 1994

33. Farrer LA, Cupples IA, Conner L, Wolf PA, Growdon JH: Association of decreased paternal age and late onset of Alzheimer's disease: An example of genetic imprinting. *Arch Neurol* 48:599, 1993

34. Macas E, Floersheim, Hotz E, et al: Abnormal chromosomal arrangements in human oocytes. *Hum Reprod* 5:703, 1990

35. Munne S, Alikani M, Tonkin G, Grifo J, Cohen J: Embryo morphology, developmental rates, and maternal age are correlated with chromosome abnormalities. *Fertil Steril* 64:382, 1995

36. Cohen J, Alikani M, Trowbridge J, Rosenwaks Z: Implantation enhancement by selective assisted hatching using zona drilling of human embryos with poor prognosis. *Hum Reprod* 5:685, 1992

37. Gonzalez OV, Martinez NL, Rodriguez G, Ancer J: Pattern of vascular aging of the postmenopausal ovary. *Ginecol Obstet Mex* 60:1, 1992

38. Kurjak A, Kupesic S: Ovarian senescence and its significance on uterine and ovarian perfusion. *Fertil Steril* 64:532, 1995

39. Levran D, Ben-Schloo I, Dor J, et al: Aging of the endometrium and oocytes: Observations on conception and abortion rate in an egg donation model. *Fertil Steril* 56:1091, 1991

40. Meldrum DR: Female reproductive aging: Ovarian and uterine factors. *Fertil Steril* 59:1, 1990

41. Feichtinger W, Kemeter P: Uterine ultrasound. In: Edward RG, Purdy JM, Steptor PC (eds), *Implantation of the Human Embryo.* London, Academic Press, 1985:335

42. Sauer MV, Miles A: Evaluating the effects of age and the endometrial responsiveness to hormone replacement therapy: Histologic and tissue receptive analysis. *J Assist Reprod Genet* 10:47, 1993

43. Sauer MV, Paulson RJ, Ary BA, Lobo A: Three hundred cycles of oocyte donation at the University of Southern California: Assessing the effect of age and infertility diagnosis on pregnancy and implantation rates. *J Assist Reprod Genet* 11:92, 1994

44. Navot D, Drews MR, Bergh TA: Age-related decline in female fertility is not due to diminished capacity of the uterus to sustain embryo implantation. *Fertil Steril* 61:97, 1994

45. Leone M, Constantini C, Gallo G, et al: Role of growth factors in the human endometrium during aging. *Maturitas* 16:31, 1993

46. Dicker D, Goldman JA, Ashkenazi J, Feldberg D, Dekel A: The value of hysteroscopy in elderly women prior to in-vitro fertilization-embryo transfer (IVF-ET): A comparative study. *J In Vitro Fertil Embryo Transf* 7:267, 1990

47. Meites J: Role of hypothalamic catecholamines in aging processes. *Acta Endocrinol* 125(Suppl 1):98, 1991

48. Alexander SE, Aksel S, Hazelton JM, Yeoman RR, Gilmore SM: The effect of aging on hypothalamic function in oophorectomized women. *Am J Obstet Gynecol* 162:446, 1990

49. Rossmanith WG, Scherbaum WA, Lauritzen: Gonadotropin secretion during aging in postmenopausal women. *Neuroendocrinology* 54:211, 1991

50. Odell WD, Swerdloff RS: Progesterone induced luteinizing and follicle stimulating hormone surge in post-menopausal women: A stimulated ovulatory peak. *Proc Natl Acad Sci USA* 61:529, 1968

51. Wide L, Hobson BM: Qualitative difference in follicle stimulating hormone activity in the pituitaries of young women compared to that of men and elderly women. *J Clin Endocrinol Metab* 56:371, 1983

52. Greenberg SR: The pathogenesis of hypophyseal fibrosis in aging: Its relationship to tissue iron deposition. *J Gerontol* 30:531, 1975

53. Swaab DF, Hofman MA, Lucassen PJ, Purba JS, Raadsheer FC, Van de Nes JA: Functional neuroanatomy and neuropathology of the human hypothalamus. *Anat Embryol* 187:317, 1993

54. Nicosia SV: Aging of the human endocervix. *Semin Reprod Endocrinol* 9:206, 1991

55. Yeko TR, Handler A: Effect of aging on tubal function and ectopic pregnancy. *Semin Reprod Endocrinol* 9:215, 1991

56. Donnez J, Casanas-Roux F, Ferin J, Thomas K: Changes in ciliation and cell height in human tubal epithelium in the fertile and post fertile years. *Maturitas* 5:39, 1983

57. Centers for Disease Control: Ectopic pregnancy in the United States, 1979–1985. *Morb Mortal Wkly Rep.* 37:9, 1988

58. Mineau G, Trussell J: A specification of marital fertility by parents' age at marriage and marital duration. *Demography* 19:335, 1982

59. Vermeulen A: Clinical review 24: Androgenes in the aging male. *J Clin Endocrinol Metab* 73:221, 1991

60. Veldhuist JD, Urban RJ, Lizarralde G, Johnson ML, Iranmanesh A: Attenuation of luteinizing hormone secretory burst amplitude as approximate basis for the hypoandrogenism of healthy aging men. *J Clin Endocrinol Metab* 75:707, 1992

61. Vermeulen A, Kaufman JN: Editorial: Role of the hypothalamic-pituitary function in the hypoandrogenism of healthy aging. *J Clin Endocrinol Metab* 75:704, 1992

62. Werner AM, Barnhard J, Gordon JW: The effects of aging on sperm and oocytes. *Semin Reprod Endocrinol* 9:231, 1991

63. Schwartz D, Mayoux MJ, Spira A, et al: Semen characteristics as a function of age in 833 fertile men. *Fertil Steril* 39:530, 1983

64. Nieschlag E, Lammers U, Freischem CW, Langer K, Wickings EJ: Reproductive functions in young fathers and grandfathers. *J Clin Endocrinol Metab* 55:676, 1982

65. MacLeod J, Gold RZ: The male factor in fertility and infertility. VII. Semen quality in relation to age and sexual activity. *Fertil Steril* 4:10–33, 1953

66. Ducot B, Spira A, Feneux D, Jouannet P: Male factors and the likelihood of pregnancy in infertile couples. II. Study of clinical characteristics—Practical consequences. *Int J Androl* 11:395, 1988

67. Maroulis G: Effect of aging on fertility and pregnancy. *Semin Reprod Endocrinol* 9:165, 1991

68. Stein ZA: A woman's age: Childbearing and childrearing. *Am J Epidemiol* 121:327, 1985

69. Virro MR, Shewchuck AB: Pregnancy outcome in 242 conceptions after artificial insemination with donor sperm and effects of maternal age on the prognosis for successful pregnancy. *Am J Obstet Gynecol* 148:518, 1984

70. Edwards RG: In vitro fertilization and embryo replacement. *Ann N Y Acad Sci* 442:1, 1985

71. Gosden RG: Maternal age: A major factor affecting the prospects and outcome of pregnancy. *Ann N Y Acad Sci* 142:45, 1984

72. Roman E: Maternal age, pregnancy interval and spontaneous abortion. In: *Spontaneous Abortion and Its Relationship to Various Maternal and Obstetric Factors.* London, University of London, 1982. Thesis.

73. Eiben B, Borgmann S, Schubbe I, Hansmann I: Cytogenetic study directly from chorionic villi of 140 spontaneous abortions. *Hum Genet* 77:137, 1987

74. Magenis RE, Chamberlain J: Paternal origin of non dysjunction. In: de la Cruz F, Gerald PS (eds), *Trisomy 21 Down's syndrome.* NICHD-Mental Retardation Research Center Series. Baltimore, University Park Press, 1981

75. Lenz W: Epidemiology of congenital malformations. *Ann N Y Acad Sci* 123:228, 1965

76. Wagenbichler P, Killian W, Reth, et al: Origin of the extra chromosome No. 21 in Down's syndrome. *Hum Genet* 32:13, 1976

77. Erickson JD: Down's syndrome, paternal age, maternal age and birth order. *Ann Hum Genet* 41:289, 1978

78. Maroulis GB: unpublished data.

PART VI

Ultrasound

tubal patency.[60-64] While normal saline solution is injected into the uterine cavity through an endocervical catheter, TVS is used to assess the flow of the saline solution through the tubes, the presence of hydrosalpinx before and after injection, and the presence of free fluid in the cul-de-sac. Results have been satisfactory; complete consistency with laparoscopic findings was in the range of 50%[63] to 76%.[62] It should be remembered that agreement in the observations at HSG and laparoscopic chromopertubation have been reported to be on the order of 55% to 75%.[65,66]

Imaging of flow within the fallopian tubes with color Doppler sonography has been described to have promising results. Peters and Coulam[65] showed an 81% sensitivity and 94% specificity for this technique when they compare the results with those of chromopertubation at laparoscopy. Overall agreement of sonographic results with observations at laparoscopy and results of HSG with those of chromopertubation at laparoscopy were 86% and 71%, respectively. This difference, however, was not statistically significant. In a subsequent study by the same group,[67] results of color Doppler HSG correlated significantly better with laparoscopic chromopertubation findings when compared with x-ray HSG (82% versus 57%, respectively, $P = .015$). Yarali et al[68] also found color Doppler HSG highly sensitive (93%) and specific (83%) when laparoscopic chromopertubation was used as the standard.

The recent development of hysterosalpingo-contrast-sonography (HyCoSy) with an echo-enhancing agent (Ecovist, Schering AG, Germany) may improve the diagnostic efficacy of ultrasonography. This agent is superior to saline solution as a contrast medium, because direct observation of flow in the tube, indicative of tubal patency, is possible.[69] With B-mode scanning only, Schlief and Deichert[66] found a sensitivity of 88% to 90% and specificity of 100% for both tubes. The addition of color Doppler sonography further improved the diagnostic accuracy, with a sensitivity of approximately 92% and a specificity of 100%, when compared with HSG and laparoscopy for detecting tubal patency. The same group subsequently showed that accuracy can be improved to 100% if contrast flow in a short segment of the fallopian tube can be depicted by means of color Doppler scanning.[70]

The foregoing data suggest that color Doppler HSG after injection of saline solution or an echocontrast agent compares favorably with HSG in the evaluation of the patency of the fallopian tubes and correlates highly with laparoscopic findings. Although the risk of infection still exists, the absence of ionizing radiation and avoidance of potential allergic reactions to iodinated contrast agents, both inherent in HSG, without sacrificing diagnostic accuracy, make HyCoSy a valuable clinical tool. Because it is a safe, well-tolerated and relatively inexpensive process that can be performed in a short time as an outpatient procedure,[71] use of HyCoSy has the potential to become established policy in the evaluation of infertility. Further clinical experience is needed before the role of HyCoSy can be defined.

Ultrasound-Guided Tubal Catheterization

Fine catheters can be introduced through the uterine cavity into the tubal ostium under sonographic guidance.[72,73] For patients with promixal tubal occlusion suggested by findings at HSG, the diagnosis can be excluded or confirmed, and definitive treatment with the use of a guide wire[72] or balloon tuboplasty can be attempted.[73] The catheter may be viewed at ultrasonography by means of injection of micro-bubble emulsion or fine highly echogenic bubbles of air to confirm tubal recanalization. The same ultrasound-guided catheterization techniques can be used during assisted-conception treatment cycles for intratubal insemination and for gamete intrafallopian transfer (GIFT) and zygote intrafallopian transfer (ZIFT).

Endometrial Changes During Spontaneous and Induced Cycles

During the menstrual cycle, the endometrium undergoes typical morphologic changes according to the stage of the cycle, that is, menstrual, proliferative, and secretory. These serial changes can be monitored by means of sonography. It was shown in 1979 that the sonographic appearance of the endometrium during the spontaneous ovulatory cycle correlates well with cycle stage.[74] Many investigators have subsequently shown a similar correlation among patients undergoing ovarian stimulation for ovulation induction or for IVF.

The two aspects of the endometrium that can be recognized by means of sonography and appear to change throughout the menstrual cycle are (1) thickness and (2) reflectivity or echogenicity. Both aspects have been found to represent the circulating levels of ovarian steroids. Because of its higher resolution, TVS is particularly suited for delineation of the aforementioned endometrial changes and has greater precision than TAS.[46]

The uterus and endometrium should always be scanned in both the longitudinal and transverse planes. Endometrial thickness is measured on both sides of the midline, through the central longitudinal axis of the uterine body. The measurement is performed from the echogenic interface of the junction between endometrium and myometrium and actually represents the doubling of two layers of endometrium.

The endometrium progressively thickens during the cycle. The stratum functionalis, composed of the spongiosum and compactum layers, is the layer that undergoes the cyclical changes of proliferation, degeneration, and menstrual loss. The stratum basalis, which provides the regenerative endometrium after menses, remains intact throughout the cycle. Sonographic measurements of double endometrial thickness represent the stratum functionalis. At ultrasonographic examination, a thin, hypoechoic halo is seen surrounding the functionalis; this halo probably corresponds to the basalis layer and the inner layer of the myometrium.[75,76] This hypoechoic band is not included in the measurement of endometrial thickness.

During menstruation, while the functionalis layer of the endometrium is being shed, the endometrium appears sonographically as a thin, slightly irregular continuous single line of echogenic interface (Fig 28–16). Some hypoechoic areas related to extravasated blood and sloughing tissue may be depicted as well. An endometrial thickness less than 5 mm is usually seen during menses and at the early to midfollicular phase. The largest increase in endometrial thickness occurs between the early and late proliferative phase (Fig 28–17). As the follicular phase continues and serum estrogen concentrations rise, the endometrium gradually thickens, reaching a total anterior-posterior width of up to 8 to 14 mm at the time of ovulation. This increase in thickness is accompanied by changes in endometrial reflectivity. The functional endometrial layer of enlarging glands and stroma appears hypoechoic relative to the outer myometrium (Fig 28–18). This hypoechoic area develops around a prominent midline echo. Because the innermost layer of a compact endometrium may be edematous, a multilayered triple-line pattern is seen at the late proliferative or periovulatory period.[77,78]

During the luteal phase, usually within 48 hours after ovulation, a hyperechoic endometrium can be identified that represents secretory transformation. It is similar in appearance to the decidua seen in early pregnancy. The increase in echogenicity is probably related to storage of mucus and glycogen in the hypertrophied and tortuous endometrial glands. Compared with the follicular phase, endometrial thickness may plateau, or

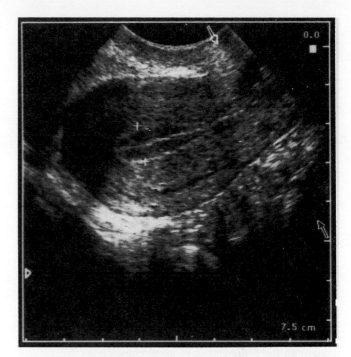

Figure 28–17. Transvaginal scan of the endometrium at midfollicular phase showing a triple-layer endometrium. *(Courtesy of M. Seibel, MD.)*

thicken further, peaking around the midsecretory phase of a spontaneous cycle (Fig 28–19). This transformation in endometrial reflectivity is considered strong evidence that ovulation has occurred. In anovulatory patients, lack of change in endometrial appearance or hyperplastic linings with exaggerated endometrial thickness may be suggested by sonographic findings and confirmed by hormonal assays and endometrial biopsies. Ultrasonography alone, however, cannot fully replace endometrial

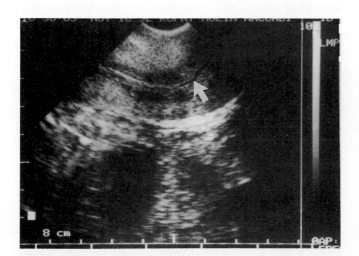

Figure 28–16. Transvaginal scan of the uterus showing the endometrial canal during menstruation. The hypoechogenic rim represents blood within the uterine cavity (arrow).

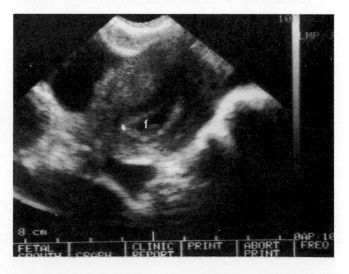

Figure 28–18. Transvaginal scan of the uterus showing the endometrial cavity after ovulation with fluid (*f*) and an echogenic endometrial rim.

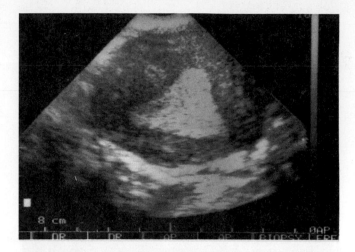

Figure 28–19. Transvaginal scan of the uterus. The hyperechogenic, shiny endometrium is typical of the luteal phase.

biopsy for assessment of the adequacy of the luteal phase endometrium and for diagnosis of luteal-phase defect.[79,80]

A marked increase in uterine volume, as estimated by means of sonography, occurs during the follicular phase of the cycle. This increase has been shown to be maximal during the periovulatory period and to correlate positively with serum estradiol concentrations.[81–83] Strohmer et al[84] demonstrated a strong correlation between individual uterine size and endometrial thickness in the midfollicular and early luteal phase of stimulated cycles. They suggested that endometrial thickness is determined by the individual uterine architecture and therefore cannot be used to predict the likelihood of implantation. The relevance of myometrial changes is poorly understood and has not been well studied, partially because of difficulty obtaining myometrial tissue for morphologic analysis.

Estimation of endometrial volumes can be sought by measurement of the long axis, anteroposterior, and transverse dimensions of the endometrium. Fleischer et al[76] showed that during spontaneous ovulatory cycles, endometrial volumes demonstrate a statistically significant increase between proliferative (1.6 ± 0.4 mL) and secretory phase endometrium (3.6 ± 0.8 mL).

Endometrial thickness as seen at sonography reliably reflects a patient's hormonal status. The cyclic changes of the endometrium may serve as a useful clinical tool in the evaluation of infertility for patients with amenorrhea. Both the transabdominal[85] and the transvaginal[86] routes can be used to measure endometrial thickness, which can serve as a reliable marker of estrogenic status and be used to predict the usefulness and results of the progesterone challenge test. By means of TVS, Morcos et al[86] selected an endometrial thickness of 1.5 mm or less to predict absence of bleeding after administration of progesterone. They reported a sensitivity and specificity of 94% and

93%, respectively. By using this method, patients with a thin endometrium can save time and the extra visit necessary to document a negative progesterone challenge test. Similarly, for patients with dysfunctional uterine bleeding, endometrial thickness may guide the physician to the desired treatment. A thick endometrium may indicate the use of progesterone, whereas a thin endometrium may indicate the need for combined estrogen and progesterone therapy.[87]

Different ovulation induction regimens do not seem to influence endometrial thickness, as was shown by Imoedemhe et al,[88] in a study in which endometrial thickness was compared among three groups of patients undergoing IVF on three different ovulation induction regimens. The authors found that endometrial thickness for all three groups was similar and comparable to that observed among a group of spontaneously ovulating fertile controls despite supraphysiologic estradiol levels in stimulated cycles. Furthermore, no correlation between endometrial thickness and peripheral ovarian steroid levels was found during the periovulatory period,[88] as was shown by other groups as well.[74,89–91] A possible explanation to this phenomenon is that there is a threshold of serum estradiol concentration necessary for normal endometrial growth and above which no further increase in thickness occurs. In a spontaneous ovulatory cycle, the maximal effect of circulating estrogens on endometrial thickness is virtually achieved. When exogenous estrogens are administered, the favorable endometrial pattern in terms of thickness and relectivity is achieved sooner in women taking higher doses of estrogen, and this is reflected in higher estradiol levels.[92]

One exception is, perhaps, the effect of clomiphene citrate on the endometrium. Several investigators have shown an adverse effect of clomiphene citrate on endometrial thickness when used alone[77,93–95] or in combination with human menopausal gonadotropin (hMG)[88,90,96,97] for ovulation induction, although in some of the studies measurements remained within the range of normal control values.[88,95] The morphometric correlate of this finding was demonstrated by Rogers et al,[97] who found reduced endometrial glandular volume after a clomiphene citrate and hMG protocol compared with buserelin acetate and hMG. This deleterious effect can be reversed by the addition of ethinyl estradiol to the treatment regimen.[98]

Endometrial Thickness and Reflectivity as Predictors of Implantation

Investigators of assisted reproductive technologies have added the entity endometrial receptivity to their vocabulary as part of the effort to explain the disappointingly low pregnancy rates achieved after "successful" treament cycles in terms of high oocyte retrieval rates and satisfactory embryo quality and transfer rates.[99] Although still poorly defined, endometrial receptiv-

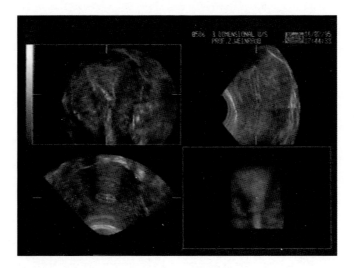

Figure 28–5. Three-dimensional ultrasound scan of the uterus. Three perpendicular planar re-formation sections are shown. Conventional longitudinal and transverse sections through the uterus appear in the left lower and upper right areas. The third plane (upper left and lower right) is a coronal section rarely displayed on a routine two-dimensional ultrasound scan.

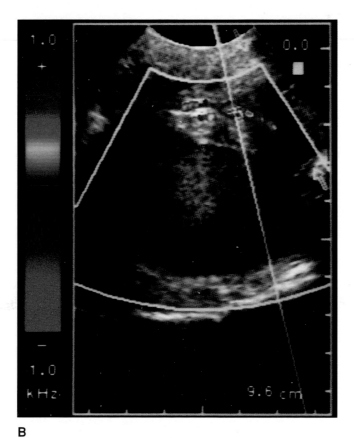

B

Figure 28–11. B. Color Doppler appearance of chocolate cyst. *(Courtesy of M. Seibel, MD.)*

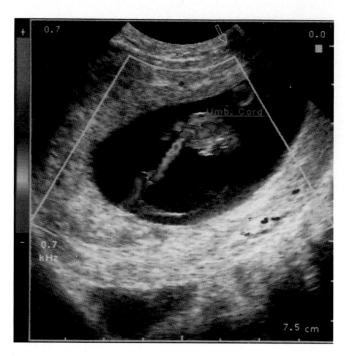

Figure 28–32. Doppler flow ultrasound scan demonstrating the fetus and the umbilical cord. The yolk sac is above the fetus, and the amnionic sac surrounds it. *(Courtesy of M. Seibel, MD.)*

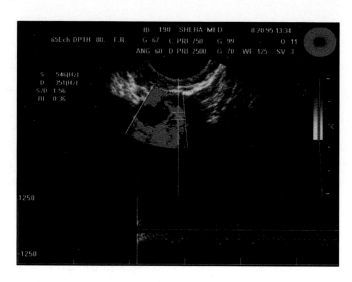

Figure 28–34. Intraovarian energy color Doppler flow velocity waveforms during the luteal phase showing low impedance to flow (resistance index 0.36) typical of corpus luteum formation with neovascularization.

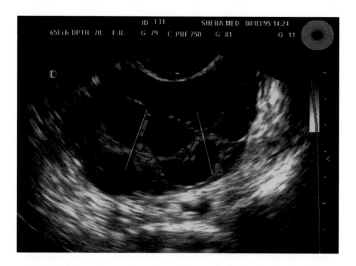

Figure 28–35. Energy Doppler flow in a hyperstimulated ovary. Note dispersal of color in the septa.

ity has been the subject of intense investigation during the last decade, and much effort has been directed toward the sonographic depiction of endometrial thickness and reflectivity. Doppler velocimetry of uterine and ovarian vessels also is commonly used in this context.

Researchers are in almost general accord that an endometrial thickness of at least 6 to 7 mm and a triple-line reflectivity pattern at the periovulatory period reflect normal endometrial development during the follicular phase of spontaneous and stimulated cycles. However, whether endometrial thickness and reflectivity correlate well with implantation remains controversial.

Pregnancy with an endometrial thickness less than 6 or 7 mm is a rare event. Presence of a hyperechoic endometrium less than 6 mm thick at the periovulatory period is associated with a negative predictive value for conception of 100%.[83,100–102] It has been suggested that the underdeveloped, thin endometrium may be a result of inability of the endometrium to respond to estradiol, rather than inadequate estradiol levels, since serum estradiol concentrations are not markedly different from concentrations in cycles in which an adequate endometrium develops.[83]

No agreement exists among investigators on whether fertilization and implantation can be predicted when a thicker endometrium is present. Gonen et al[100] and Gonen and Casper[101] found a markedly thicker endometrium on the day before oocyte recovery in women who conceived after IVF-ET compared with those who did not. Similarly, Check et al[103] and Shoham et al[83] found that endometrial thickness on the day of administration of human chorionic gonadotropin (hCG) was significantly greater in pregnant than in nonpregnant women undergoing IVF-ET or ovulation induction, a difference that was statistically significant. The authors suggested that endometrial thickness may be used to predict the likelihood of implantation. Glissant et al[89] also reported that endometrial thickness was greater in conception than in nonconception IVF-ET cycles but concluded that it was not possible to predict the probability of pregnancy with endometrial thickness alone. Guirgis et al[104] conducted a study with 350 patients who underwent GIFT. The investigators compared the results of TVS examinations on the day of hCG administration with the findings on scans performed on the day of the operation. They found more frequent and more marked increases in endometrial thickness and reflectivity among women who subsequently conceived, as compared to those who did not, a statistically significant difference. Dickey et al[105] showed improved fecundity and less biochemical pregnancies after cycles of assisted reproductive techniques if, on the day of hCG administration, endometrial thickness was 9 mm or greater but also 14 mm or less. In contrast to the foregoing studies, other investigators demonstrated no statistically significant difference in mean en-

dometrial thickness during the periovulatory period when conception and nonconception cycles were compared.[102,106–108]

Opinions also vary regarding the predictive value of endometrial thickness during the luteal phase. Shoham et al[83] showed that after ovulation induction, midluteal phase endometrial thickness of 11 mm or more was a good predictor of conception. Rabinowitz et al[107] showed that an endometrial thickness of 13 mm was a prerequisite for pregnancy in an IVF-ET program. Other investigators, however, reported no detectable sonographic endometrial changes during the luteal phase, which would allow prediction of pregnancy.[88,89,106]

Conclusive evidence on the predictive value of the endometrial reflectivity pattern has not been presented. Gonen et al[101] found a correlation between successful pregnancy and a triple-line endometrial echo pattern, as opposed to an intermediate isoechogenic pattern with an absent, central echogenic line or an entirely homogeneous hyperechogenic endometrium. Similar observations were also made by some investigators[102,103,108–110] but not by others.[111] It has been suggested that a multilayered endometrial pattern may also be used to predict the likelihood of fertilization in vitro.[101,112] Furthermore, it has been shown that this favorable pattern at TVS examination is an accurate predictor of successful donor-egg cycles prepared with exogenous hormones[92] and of successful donor artificial insemination during natural cycles.[91] It has therefore been suggested that administration of progesterone to women receiving exogenous estrogen in preparation for a donor oocyte transfer should be deferred until a multilayered endometrium is evident at sonography.[92,102] In contrast, Check et al[113] found no correlation between an endometrial echo pattern and pregnancy rate in donor-oocyte–ET cycles.

In summary, whether or not sonographic evaluation of endometrial thickness and reflectivity can be used to predict the likelihood of implantation has not been clearly defined. Most investigators agree that the positive predictive value of endometrial thickness alone is low,[89,100,101,103,108] but a threshold value of less than 6 mm has a great negative predictive value for the subsequent occurrence of pregnancy.[83,100,101] Also unknown are whether unfavorable endometrial patterns tend to recur in successive cycles and whether hormonal manipulations (introduction of or changes in stimulation protocols) can be used to modify the endometrium.

At present, there are considerable difficulties in interpreting the contradictory results of studies on endometrial thickness and reflectivity patterns as predictors of pregnancy. Partial explanations may be found in the small size of most of the study groups, the impact of different stimulation protocols on the sonographic image of the endometrium, the use of different scanning routes (transvaginal versus transabdominal) and measurement techniques, and the variability in timing of scans and therapeutic procedures (eg, IVF-ET, GIFT, or artificial insemination). Future studies of endometrial characteristics, conducted with more uniform methods, will help to define the value of sonographic evaluation of endometrial development for the prediction of implantation.

Subendometrial Myometrial Contractions

The observation that a nonpregnant uterus has inherent contractility dates back to the last century. Initial studies of myometrial contractility incorporated pressure-wave catheter-based transducers placed within the uterine cavity. The main disadvantage of these methods was their invasiveness, which, in addition to the considerable discomfort and risk of infection, restricted the size of study groups and could potentially induce artificial changes in contractility. The noninvasive nature of ultrasound renders it well suited for detection and analysis of subendometrial myometrial contractility. Birnholz[114] used TAS to describe endometrial movements that were not associated with visible myometrial contractions, as was later demonstrated by Abramowicz and Archer by means of TVS.[115] Transabdominal studies in this context have virtually been replaced by TVS, and the origin of contraction has been attributed to the innermost layer of the myometrium.[116-119] Appreciation of subendometrial myometrial contractions is enhanced by review of taped real-time images in a fast-forward mode on a videocassette recorder with dynamic tracking. In this way, the direction, symmetry, frequency, and amplitude of uterine contractions can be evaluated. The technique, however, has not been standardized.

Two main types of myometrial contractions have been described. The first type consists of random contractions of the entire myometrium, similar to the contractions described with dysmenorrhea or during pregnancy (Braxton-Hicks contractions). These contractions may be described by the women as painful, and their frequency is markedly diminished in the periovulatory period. The second type consists of subtle, wave-like subendometrial myometrial contractions, which are not perceived by the women. Because of the potential relevance to the process of human reproduction, it is this type of contraction that currently draws attention and interest.

The direction of contraction is determined as antegrade if it starts at the uterine fundus and moves toward the cervix. A contraction is retrograde if it starts at the cervix and moves toward the fundus. Subendometrial myometrial contractions display a coherent pattern that is closely related to the phase of the menstrual cycle. Antegrade contractions are almost solely confined to menstruation. Throughout the follicular phase to the periovulatory period, retrograde contractions become progressively consistent and increase in frequency, amplitude, and percentage, attaining their maximum on the day of ovulation.[117] During the periovulatory period, subendometrial myometrial contractions can be seen in 85% of normal, fertile ovulatory pa-

tients,[118] and more than 80% of contractions are retrograde.[117,118] The reported frequencies of contraction waves range between about 3 cycles/min[117] and up to 10 cycles/min[118] during the periovulatory period. The pattern of subendometrial myometrial contractions is essentially reversed in the luteal phase, and contractions progressively decline until menstruation.

The regulatory mechanisms that control subendometrial myometrial contractions are unkown. However, the biphasic pattern of follicular rise and luteal fall in contractility seems to be correlated with serum concentration of ovarian steroids, with a stimulatory effect of estrogen during the follicular phase, culminating at midcycle, and an inhibitory effect of estrogen plus progesterone during the luteal phase. This hypothesis is supported by the observation that compared with spontaneously ovulatory women, women undergoing controlled ovarian hyperstimulation (COH) for IVF-ET have enhanced subendometrial myometrial contractions during midcycle, and women taking oral contraceptives have less prominent contractions.[115] It has therefore been speculated that the purpose of the contractions is to enhance the fertility of women, perhaps through involvement in active transport of spermatozoa toward the tubal ostia by means of symmetric, high-frequency, retrograde contractions, which are typical for midcycle.[115,117,118] Another possible mechanism for fertility enhancement was suggested by de Vries et al,[116] who found that all contractions in the luteal phase are retrograde, but short and asymmetric, and may therefore help maintain the blastocyst in the uterine cavity until implantation. This theory was not supported by Narayan and Goswamy,[119] who found no statistically significant differences in subendometrial myometrial contractility on the day of ET in conception and nonconception IVF-ET cycles.

Many questions regarding subendometrial myometrial contractility remain unanswered: Is contractility involved in the pathophysiology of unexplained infertility, or habitual abortions as has been suggested?[114,116] Can it be used to predict implantation after spontaneous and induced cycles? Is myometrial contractility affected by uterine or adnexal abnormalities or by different treatment protocols? What can be said at the moment is that this phenomenon deserves further investigation as another possible factor involved in endometrial receptivity.

Ovarian Changes During the Natural Cycle

Normal follicular development, ovulation, and formation of a functional corpus luteum are the prerequisites of adequate reproductive function. The sequence of these events has been elegantly demonstrated at serial ultrasound examinations over the course of the spontaneous ovulatory cycle.[3,120,121] The morphologic changes in the walls of preovulatory follicles[122] and the characteristics of actual follicular evacuation have been observed at TVS.[123] Both clinical and sonographic findings can be used to evaluate ovulatory function and dysfunction. The hormonal changes that occur during the cycle determine the sequence of events that can be observed in both the ovaries and the uterus. Without a thorough understanding of the hormonal changes during the menstrual cycle, interpretation of any ultrasonographic findings will be incomplete and often inadequate.

In the early follicular phase of the menstrual cycle, a cohort of developing follicles is recruited from the pool of nonproliferating primordial follicles present within the ovaries.[124] The initiation of follicular development is a continuous process. Most of these primordial follicles never develop beyond the early preantral phase and undergo spontaneous regression. Some, however, develop under the influence of follicle-stimulating hormone (FSH), and the granulosa cells contained within these antral follicles start to produce estrogen. When they have reached a diameter of 2 to 3 mm, the follicles may be detected by means of TVS. On approximately cycle day 8, when it is 8 to 10 mm in diameter, a single dominant follicle is selected from this group.[125,126] Some of the nondominant follicles are detectable with ultrasound, and it has been shown that they continue to grow until the time of selection. Thereafter there is a decrease in their mean growth slopes in the dominant ovary only. The final diameter of the follicles, however, always remains less than 11 mm.[126]

While the nondominant follicles undergo atresia or developmental arrest, the dominant follicle continues to grow at a linear rate of 2 to 3 mm per day. In 5% to 11% of normal cycles, two dominant follicles develop, but always on opposite ovaries.[124] The diameter of the dominant follicle increases from 12 mm to 23 mm over the 5 days preceding ovulation. During the 24 hours before ovulation the dominant follicle undergoes a rapid exponential growth, and ovulation generally occurs when the mean diameter of the follicle is between 18 and 24 mm[127] (Figs 28–20 and 28–21). It has been shown that the amount of estrogen produced by a single follicle increases as the follicle matures. A linear correlation exists between the follicular diameter and serum estradiol level,[3,128] but the variation within and between these two measurements is too large to allow prediction of ovulation within less than 1.4 ± 1.2 days.[128] Similarly, as a single measurement, the variation in maximum preovulatory diameter has not proved a particularly useful index for prediction of ovulation.[5,127] Transvaginal ultrasonography considerably improves the sensitivity of ultrasonography for ovulation detection. This was demonstrated by Vermesh et al,[129] who were able to detect ovulation, defined as disappearance of the dominant follicle in all 31 cycles studied. During the later stages of development, the cumulus oophorus may be seen as an eccentrically located mural protrusion consisting of low-level echoes, approximately 1 to 3.6 mm in diameter, and this may be regarded as a sign of follicular maturity and that ovulation will occur within 18 to 36 hours.[3,46,130–132] Visualization of the cumu-

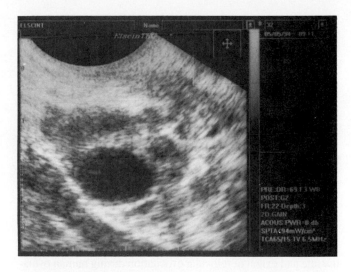

Figure 28–20. Transvaginal scan showing a preovulatory follicle about 20 mm in diameter.

lus oophorus by means of TVS and TAS has been reported in 60% to 65% and more than 80% of preovulatory follicles, respectively.[46,133]

Different signs of follicular maturity and impending ovulation have been documented.[130,134] Decreased follicular wall reflectivity and crenellation or a double contour indicates that ovulation will occur within 6 to 10 hours. By means of TVS, the site of stigma formation can be depicted as well.[122,123] These indications reflect the changes in and around the follicle that occur after the luteinizing hormone (LH) surge has begun. These signs are probably not seen frequently enough, and they are too operator dependent to be useful on a routine basis. No reproducible sonographic signs have been definitely shown to reliably predict imminent ovulation.[131]

Ovulation occurs about 36 to 38 hours after the serum LH surge begins.[130] Because detection of the LH surge in urine is somewhat delayed, ovulation occurs approximately 24 hours after a positive urine assay is found. The process of ovulation was observed ultrasonically by means of documentation of the disappearance of a large preovulatory follicle and the subsequent formation of a corpus luteum.[5,127] There was some variation among patients, but all showed a decrease in the size of the follicle either rapidly or over a period of 30 min followed by the development of a corpus hemorrhagicum soon after.[5] Evidence of ovulation can be seen in about 90% of normal cycles.[127] These changes are described as the follicle's disappearing completely, collapsing, and becoming irregular in shape and filled with mixed high- and low-level echoes as the corpus hemorrhagicum forms.[127,131] In addition, up to 50 mL of fluid not previously seen may be present in the cul-de-sac, although some free fluid may be detected before follicular rupture as a result of transudation from the dominant follicle.

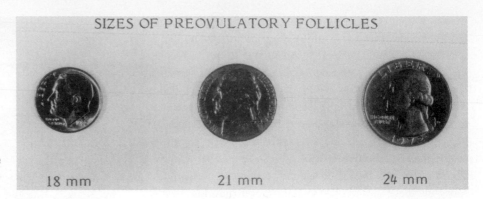

SIZES OF PREOVULATORY FOLLICLES

18 mm   21 mm   24 mm

Figure 28–21. Coins used as references to illustrate the sizes of preovulatory follicles. *(Courtesy of M. Seibel, MD.)*

One group of investigators found considerable variation in the rate and extent of follicular evacuation during human ovulation, as evidenced by means of TVS.[123] All follicles displayed an initial burst of fluid; more than 50% of the follicles lost the first half of their fluid within 15 seconds. The rest of the fluid drained from the follicle at more variable rates. The time required to reach complete follicular evacuation ranged from 6 seconds to more than 18 minutes (mean 6.1 ± 1.1 minutes), but some follicles did not empty entirely. It was therefore speculated that the variability during follicular evacuation may influence successful expulsion of the oocyte from the follicle.[123] A substantial number of women, however, especially those with induced multiple ovulations, do not demonstrate sonographic evidence of ovulation until the second morning after detection of the urine LH surge.[135] This temporal relation may adversely affect pregnancy rates in timed insemination cycles.

Within days the corpus luteum becomes round and closer to uniformly echogenic. In the absence of pregnancy, the corpus luteum lasts for 14 days, at which time it rapidly regresses in size and becomes less well demarcated and blends with surrounding ovarian tissue to become a corpus albicans around the time of menstruation. At ultrasonography a corpus luteum typically appears as a cyst with well-defined walls and low-level internal echoes, reflecting its hemorrhagic contents. Through most of the normal cycle, from development of the follicle to the disappearance of the corpus luteum at menstruation, a cystic structure is present on one or the other ovary. This structure may vary in size depending on the degree of development and hemorrhage. For this reason, care should be taken not to interpret a cyst seen at ultrasound examination erroneously as evidence of a pathologic condition, because frequently it is a normal finding in most premenopausal women.

Both TAS and TVS can be used for evaluation of ovulatory dynamics. The transvaginal approach is currently preferred because of the improved resolution with the high-frequency transducers. Follicular diameter is usually determined from the mean of maximal longitudinal and transverse diameter measurements, or three dimensions may be used for this purpose, al-

lowing improvement of accuracy and reproducibility.[136] Variations in measurements of mean follicular diameter exist; the measurements tend to be smaller for the same observer than for several observers.[137] The 95% confidence interval for a follicle measured to be 15 mm by a single observer is 13 to 17 mm, whereas for multiple observers it is 12 to 18 mm. The greatest measurement errors are associated with larger follicles.[138] This finding may be of clinical significance, since therapeutic decisions are commonly based on the ultrasonographic estimation of the size of the dominant follicle. Follicular volume can be calculated by use of the formula for ovoid structures: $\pi/6 \cdot a \cdot b \cdot c$ (where a, b, and c are the largest diameters measured on three planes).[136] It has been suggested that the 2D image of the follicle depicted with ultrasonography corresponds well with the 3D structure and, hence, its total volume.[6,138] The mean diameter of round and polygonal follicles accurately predicts total follicular volume as measured during follicular aspiration. However, the volume of ellipsoid follicles cannot be predicted with measurement of the longest, shortest, or mean diameter, and this fact should be taken into consideration during clinical decision making.[139]

Ovulatory Factors

Ultrasound plays an important role in the evaluation and management of anovulation. With three exceptions, however, it is far less useful in determining the causative factors of anovulation or oligo-ovulation. The three areas in which ultrasound may assist in the diagnosis are PCO syndrome, luteinized unruptured follicle (LUF), and the empty follicle syndrome.

Polycystic Ovary Syndrome

The diagnosis of PCO disease can be established with the characteristic hormonal profile (raised serum levels of LH, or high ratios of LH to FSH, or high androgen and insulin concentrations), coupled with obesity, hirsutism, and menstrual disorders. The diagnosis is confirmed with ovarian biopsy. It may also be suggested by certain ultrasonographic features. Because of the noninvasive nature of the modality, ultrasonography has virtually replaced visualization and biopsy of the ovaries at laparoscopy or laparotomy. There is, however, no agreement regarding the ultrasonographic definition of PCO syndrome, just as there is continuous debate over the clinical and biochemical definitions of the syndrome. Furthermore, the sonographic findings typical of PCO syndrome may be seen among women who do not show the characteristic clinical and biochemical changes, and it also is not always seen when the clinical and biochemical features do exist. The classic ultrasonographic picture of PCO (Fig 28–22) may be seen in patients with various clinical conditions such as hypothalamic amenorrhea, adrenal and thyroid disorders, and in perimenarchal girls. Thus the ultrasonographic findings of polycystic or multifollicular ovaries are not pathognomonic for PCO disease.

With the advent of ultrasonography, it has been shown that PCO are more common than was previously realized. The prevalence of PCO diagnosed at TAS among healthy women was 21% to 23%,[140–142] and TVS yielded similar results.[142] When PCO are seen incidently in women during an ultrasonographic examination, about 50% of the patients have the classic signs and symptoms associated with PCO syndrome.[143,144] Among 25% a variant of the syndrome is seen, and among another 25%, no clinical abnormality is detected.[143] Adams et al[145] reported that PCO were found among 26% of women with amenorrhea, 87% with oligomenorrhea, and 92% with idiopathic hirsutism. Pache et al[146] showed that patients with oligomenorrhea or amenorrhea who suffered from infertility, ovarian polycystic changes evidenced at TVS correlate well with the clinical and endocrine findings associated with the PCO disease.

The sonographic features of PCO syndrome reflect the morphologic changes that occur in ovaries with multiple, poorly

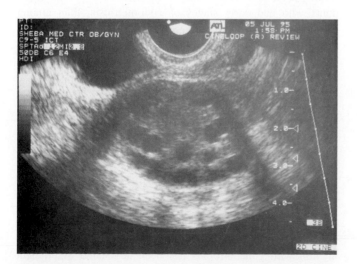

Figure 28–22. Transvaginal scan of an enlarged ovary containing multiple peripheral small follicles with hypertrophied stroma in a patient with PCO syndrome.

developed, atretic follicles situated at the periphery of the ovaries, which are enlarged and demonstrate stromal hypertrophy.[143,147] Until now, however, no definite criteria for sonographic diagnosis had been established.

Ovarian enlargement (>6 cm^3) is seen in about 71% of patients with hormonally defined PCO disease,[148] and the ovaries are usually twice the normal size. Ovarian volumes have been inconsistently calculated by use of one of several formulas for ovoid structures,[149,150] or by use of ovarian cross section (with two diameters only).[151] Ovarian enlargement becomes more apparent with increased duration of disease. Nevertheless, approximately 29% of patients have no ovarian enlargement. The ovary may become spherically enlarged, rather than ellipsoid. Several sonographic measurements are used to detect this spheroidal enlargement: the ovarian diameter exceeds the anteroposterior diameter of the fundus of the uterus,[143] the uterine width–to–ovarian length ratio is less than 1,[151] and the ovarian roundness ratio (ovarian width/ovarian length) is greater than 0.7.[150,151]

PCO contain several immature, atretic follicles, less than 10 mm in diameter and crowded at the surface around hyperechoic stromal tissue. The number of these follicles can be determined by means of scanning the ovary from the inner to the outer margins in longitudinal cross sections[152] or by counting the follicles in a single ovarian plane.[151,153] Hence, considerable differences can be expected soley on the basis of the method chosen for counting the follicles. With TVS, the number of follicles necessary to establish the diagnosis of PCO has been reported to vary from more than 5[150] or 10[144,153] to at least 15.[154] In a study conducted with TVS,[152] the maximum number of developing follicles found in women who acted as controls was 11. Although most patients with PCO had more than 11 follicles, a statistically significant number had fewer than 11 follicles, reducing the sensitivity of follicular number alone as a predictor of PCO. Increased stromal echogenicity is considered an important sonographic sign of PCO,[144,153,154] but this appraisal has the important disadvantage of being purely subjective. Several authors have found increased stromal echogenicity to be the most accurate single sonographic sign of PCO.[151,152] The reported sensitivity and specificity are 94% and 90%, respectively.[152]

With conventional TAS, the detection and counting of follicles less than 5 mm in diameter is not always possible, especially in obese women. The ovaries may appear relatively sonolucent, making the appreciation of stromal echogenicity difficult and inaccurate. The enhanced resolution and visualization of TVS are expected to simplify and improve the accuracy of diagnosis of PCO. Until now, however, the results of studies comparing TAS and TVS have been conflicting.[142,151] Ardaens et al[151] compared ultrasound findings collected with TAS and TVS for a population of patients believed to have PCO. The sonographic features of PCO were seen with both modalities in less than one third of the patients. Whereas the internal ovarian features of PCO were more frequently identified with TVS than with TAS, external features, such as increased ovarian area, uterine-to-ovarian size ratio, and excessive ovarian roundness, were equally delineated with both modalities. Regarding internal ovarian features, the most important difference was noted in the appreciation of ovarian stroma. With use of TVS 57% of patients were judged to have increased ovarian stroma, but this finding was found with TAS in only 4.8% of the patients. Similarly, Fox et al[154] found that TAS did not allow detection of 30% of PCO, compared with an almost 100% detection rate with TVS. In contrast, Farquhar et al[142] evaluated the use of TAS versus TVS in the diagnosis of PCO in a population of randomly selected women. There was no difference, however, in the prevalence of PCO found with both techniques. There also was no difference between TVS and TAS in number of follicles or the size of follicles detected. Some women had PCO detected with TVS but not with TAS, and vice versa. The agreement between the two methods of screening was 78% for PCO, 97% for normal ovaries, and 92% overall.

In summary, the ultrasonographic definition of PCO should be further refined. The broad spectrum of clinical and sonographic features typical of the disease does not allow establishment of strict criteria for single sonographic criteria that would provide an accurate means of diagnosis. One possible solution for this problem would be to use combinations of criteria. Pache et al[152] by means of TVS showed that combining measurements of follicular size and ovarian volume increases the power of discrimination between normal and polycystic ovaries with a sensitivity of 92% and a specificity of 97%. In the near future, as 3D ultrasonography is being introduced into clinical practice, another improvement in diagnostic accuracy might be achieved. In the interim, the cardinal features of multiple small follicles in an enlarged ovary, especially when associated with increased stromal echogenicity, should strongly raise the possibility of PCO.

The Luteinized Unruptured Follicle Syndrome

LUF is a condition in which the follicle fails to rupture and expel the oocyte within the ovulatory interval of 38 hours after the LH surge. The diagnosis of LUF syndrome once consisted of laparoscopic demonstration of lack of ovarian stigma in the early luteal phase in a patient with an apparently normal LH surge. The diagnosis was confirmed at recovery of an oocyte from the unruptured follicle. With the advent of ultrasound, the LUF can be easily demonstrated at serial examinations after the LH surge.[155–158] Therefore, any dominant follicle that persists 48 hours after the LH peak is abnormal and may be taken as evidence of LUF. The LUF retains its echo-free cystic appearance with no signs of collapse. Beginning at the early

luteal phase, and during several days of temperature rise or elevation of serum progesterone concentration, the follicular wall demonstrates gradual thickening, representing hypertrophy of the luteinized granulosa cells. With the use of sonography, Check et al[159] identified two distinct types of LUF syndrome: (1) mature follicle LUF, in which release of an ovum was not demonstrated after the follicle attained maturity, and (2) luteinization LUF, in which luteinization, evidenced by an increase in serum progesterone concentration, occurs before follicular maturation. The patterns of endogenous gonadotropin and ovarian steroid secretion appear normal, as does the length of the luteal phase, leading to the conclusion that the endocrine function of the corpus luteum is preserved. However, without follicular rupture, the amount of peritoneal fluid and concentration of ovarian steroids are decreased compared with normal ovulation.[160,161]

The frequency of LUF syndrome and its contribution to infertility is not known. It has been reported to occur in approximately 11% of cycles of normal women[156] and in 11.5% to more than 50% of cycles of patients with unexplained infertility.[157,162] It is still unknown whether the syndrome occurs occasionally or in a repetitive manner. Among a population of 60 women with infertility of mixed causes, LUF was diagnosed in 52 (13.5%) of apparently ovulatory cycles.[163] A high incidence of LUF was observed in patients with PCO (37.5%), endometriosis (24.7%), and a history of pelvic operations (26.2%). At aspiration of the 384 follicles during the luteal phase, the presence of an entrapped postmature oocyte, a direct evidence of LUF, was demonstrated in 6 of 19 cases (31.5%) in which the hormonal profiles for the aspirated follicular fluid coincided with the preoperative diagnosis. It has been suggested that periovarian abnormality may interfere with follicular rupture. Among patients with unexplained infertility who underwent diagnostic laparoscopy, the incidence of LUF was higher (35%) among patients who had early stages of endometriosis, than among patients who did not have endometriosis (11%).[164] Aspiration of follicles yielded degenerated oocyte cumuli in 43% of LUFs, which appear to be more common among patients with unexplained infertility, occurring in more than 50% of cycles.[157] It is not known whether this syndrome occurs continuously in all cycles or occurs only occasionally. The results of the foregoing studies suggest that LUF syndrome might be observed more frequently among patients with pelvic or periovarian abnormalities that interfere with follicular rupture. This syndrome may be an etiologic factor in unexplained infertility. Because it is believed to be more common among patients who have mild or minimal endometriosis, LUF syndrome may be one cause of endometriosis-related infertility. Finally, although ovulation induction with gonadotropins has been advocated as efficient therapy for LUF syndrome,[159] LUF may occur after administration of hCG in hMG-stimulated cycles.[165]

The Empty Follicle Syndrome

The empty follicle syndrome represents another type of ovulatory dysfunction. It was described after the observation that some follicular aspirates contained no oocytes.[166,167] Hilgers et al[168] defined the empty follicle syndrome sonographically as absence of the cumulus oophorus in a mature follicle. By means of TVS, the prevalence of this syndrome among a population of infertile patients was found to be 66/152 (43.4%).[133] The frequency increased with age and was independent of gravidity.

The existence of the empty follicle syndrome as a separate entity in spontaneous and induced cycles is still being questioned. First, although the sonographic demonstration of the cumulus oophorus has been reported in more than 80% of mature follicles,[133] it is a rather difficult, time-consuming, and operator-dependent task, with variable degrees of success. Furthermore, it has been claimed that the structure identified as the cumulus may represent artifactual echoes or a small follicle projecting into the dominant follicle.[131] Absence of the cumulus oophorus may simply result from failure to detect this tiny structure during an ultrasonographic examination. Another viable explanation of this phenomenon is that some cases of failed oocyte retrieval might have been caused by premature ovulation. Premature ovulation has been shown to occur in 2% of GIFT cycles.[104] Aspiration of the follicle to seek the presence or absence of an oocyte may aid in the diagnosis but would be possible only during cycles of an assisted reproductive technique. Even this could not be considered absolutely accurate. Moreover, stimulated cycles are different from spontaneous cycles in the effects of therapeutic drugs. Recently it was suggested that occurrence of the empty follicle syndrome during induction of ovulation may be a "pharmaceutical industry syndrome," resulting from lack of exposure to biologically active hCG.[169] Further studies are needed before the existence and importance of the empty follicle syndrome can be validated.

MONITORING THERAPY

Safety Considerations

Although concern has been expressed regarding the safety of exposure of preovulatory oocytes to ultrasound,[170] until now both experimental work and clinical experience have not identified any harmful effects.[171,172] The use of vaginal transmission gel during TVS, however, has been associated with an adverse effect on sperm motility and viability,[173] which could interfere with fertilization. Therefore, the use of ultrasound transmission gel should be avoided during the periovulatory period among patients who practice timed natural intercourse or cervical insemination. Alternatives are use of normal saline solution or incubation media.

Artificial Insemination

For patients with irregular cycles, monitoring follicular development and endometrial thickness may be of considerable help in timing of insemination.[91] Once the dominant follicle achieves a diameter of 18 mm, ultrasound examinations may be performed daily. Insemination should be performed on the day ultrasound criteria of ovulation are demonstrated. As an alternative, the final stage of ovulation may be triggered by hCG when the dominant follicle has reached sufficient size, and insemination is performed the next morning. Not all authors, however, agree on the ability of ultrasound monitoring to enhance the success rate of therapeutic insemination with therapeutic donor insemination (TID), and this subject may still be regarded as controversial.[174]

Ovulation Induction

Oligo-ovulation or anovulation is present among approximately 20% of infertile couples. Except for those with ovarian failure, ovulation can be induced successfully for most patients. The aim is to induce development of one or more follicles and continue their growth to maturity and ovulation. Typically, the drugs used are clomiphene citrate and preparations of hMG and purified urinary FSH. Pulsatile administration of GnRH also has been successfully used for induction of ovulation in patients with hypothalamic amenorrhea or PCO disease. Synthetic preparations of GnRH agonists are commonly used for pituitary downregulation during ovulation induction in treatment cycles of assisted reproductive techniques. The same principles of ultrasound monitoring generally apply to the different regimens of ovulation induction therapy.

After the initiation of ovulation induction therapy, under the influence of high levels of circulating gonadotropins, the ovaries undergo enhanced follicular response, and the process of selection is overridden, allowing smaller, codominant follicles to escape from atresia. If adequate FSH support is given, development of multiple follicles commonly occurs, and this kind of therapy is therefore often called controlled ovarian hyperstimulation. Ultrasound monitoring allows the number and size of developing follicles to be observed easily. The likelihood of complications of ovulation induction, such as ovarian hyperstimulation and multiple gestations, can be predicted and reduced with careful monitoring. Because repeated ultrasound examinations are both expensive and time consuming for patients, follicular development is not monitored in all instances, as, for example, when clomiphene citrate is administered. The likelihood that large numbers of follicles will develop when this drug is used is small, because the development of more than two dominant follicles is uncommon.[120]

The Baseline Ultrasonographic Scan

When gonadotropins are used for induction of ovulation, ultrasound monitoring is advised.[175] An initial scan of the pelvis is obtained before therapy is initiated to establish the presence of any ovarian or uterine abnormalities. If, for example, there have been recent stimulated cycles, ultrasonography may confirm the resolution of hyperstimulated ovaries and exclude the presence of residual ovarian cysts. Even if all subsequent monitoring is to be performed with a transvaginal transducer, it is recommended that conventional, full-bladder TAS be performed initially. This technique allows the whole pelvis to be well visualized. The transvaginal transducer has only a limited field of view, and any abnormality that lies more than 6 or 7 cm from the transducer may not be depicted. During therapy, monitoring with TVS is generally preferred because of better patient compliance, combined with enhanced resolution and greater precision in the measurement of follicular diameter.

The baseline ultrasonographic examination is important during cycles of assisted reproductive techniques. The presence of an ovarian cyst in the early follicular phase is frequently encountered. Although ovarian cysts may occur spontaneously, they are more often noted after COH in a previous cycle and after pituitary downregulation with GnRH agonists. Despite their common occurrence, the impact of the presence of ovarian cysts on the outcome of cycles of assisted reproductive techniques and hence the management of these cysts, remains controversial. The presence of ovarian cysts has been shown to compromise the success of IVF.[176,177] Ovarian cysts not only interfere with stimulation but also can impair monitoring of follicular growth and interfere with ovarian accessibility during oocyte retrieval. Ovarian cysts may obscure and distort the growing follicles. Cysts also may lead to errors in evaluation of follicular growth, because they tend to grow during COH and may therefore be misinterpreted as growing follicles. This is especially true when more than one cyst is present or when the cyst is multilocular. In addition, if it is functional (steroid-secreting), the cyst may adversely affect the hormonal milieu in which the other follicles will develop.

Goldberg et al[176] showed that patients with ovarian cysts before ovulation induction had a lower estradiol level and a higher cancellation rate than those without ovarian cysts. Thatcher et al[177] demonstrated that the outcome for these patients worsens if one attempts to proceed with ovarian stimulation despite the presence of a cyst. In another study,[178] in which hMG and hCG were administered without IVF, patients undergoing stimulation in the presence of a baseline cyst required significantly more hMG than did those without. Other groups report that cysts have no adverse effect on IVF outcome and advise proceeding with COH despite the presence of cysts. Hornstein et al[179] found no statistically significant difference in maximum serum estradiol level, cycle cancellation rate, number of oocytes recovered, number of embryos transferred, and pregnancy rate per cycle between patients with a cyst and those without a cyst. Similarly, Karande et al[180] showed that small ovarian cysts detected at the baseline ultrasonographic examination do not have a negative impact on ovarian stimulation or pregnancy rates in an IVF program.

Options for management of ovarian cysts in the early follicular phase of an assisted reproductive technique cycle include cancellation of ovarian stimulation, initiation of stimulation despite the presence of a cyst, or TVS-guided aspiration of the cyst. The presence of baseline ovarian cysts has been a frequent cause of cancellation or postponement of a cycle because of concern that the cyst may grow further, undergo torsion, rupture, or compromise the potential for follicular development. Although poorer outcomes for induced cycles with baseline ovarian cysts have not been invariably demonstrated, several assisted reproductive technology programs perform TVS-guided aspiration of these cysts before ovulation induction rather than canceling or postponing the cycle.[176] Rizk et al[181] addressed this problem by differentiating patients with ovarian cysts present before exogenous gonadotropin stimulation from those with cysts that developed after pituitary downregulation with a GnRH agonist. For each group, the outcome of IVF cycles was compared between patients with and patients without cyst aspiration. Among the group with baseline spontaneous ovarian cysts that were aspirated, the number of follicles on the side of aspirated cysts was significantly higher than the number of follicles among the group who did not undergo aspiration. There were, however, no differences between the two subgroups in the total number of follicles or oocytes in both ovaries or in fertilization and pregnancy rates. Aspiration of ovarian cysts that developed after pituitary downregulation with a GnRH agonist did not show a beneficial effect on the outcome of IVF in any respect.

The presence of endometriotic cysts at the baseline ultrasonographic examination should be generally ignored, and aspiration of endometriomas is not recommended. However, controversy exists on this issue as well. Dicker et al[182] showed that aspiration of an endometriotic cyst before ovulation induction for IVF had a beneficial effect on cycle outcome.

Diagnosis of PCO at the baseline ultrasonographic scan is important, mainly because these patients are prone to ovarian hyperstimulation syndrome (OHSS). A reduced dose of gonadotropins, combined with meticulous monitoring, is recommended for these patients to decrease the risk of this complication. In addition, the diagnosis of PCO may be of prognostic value with regard to the outcome of assisted reproductive techniques, since although considerably more oocytes were recovered from patients with PCO, low fertilization rates were demonstrated for this group as compared with women with normal ovulation and with tubal-factor infertility.[183]

Monitoring Follicular Growth

Ultrasound monitoring of the ovaries is normally started on the 5th day after the start of gonadotropin administration, usually on cycle days 7 to 10 (Fig 28–23). By this time the developing follicles are approximately 10 mm in diameter, and the extent of ovarian response may be appreciated. The timing and frequency of subsequent scans can thus be determined. This early scan may be of prognostic value for the outcome of IVF. It has been shown that the pattern of early growth of the follicles is more important than the absolute measurements on the day of hCG administration.[184] If several follicles lie side to side they may be compressed and lose their singular spherical shape, giving a cartwheel appearance. Although many gynecologists advocate measuring the follicles in all three dimensions, in practice this often proves to be painstaking and the results frequently are confusing to interpret, particularly when large numbers of follicles are present. A single mean diameter for each follicle averaged from only two dimensions is usually all that is necessary. This measurement may be obtained with the ovary in either the longitudinal or transverse projection, but the same projection must be used in all subsequent scans. Most important, however, is careful assessment of the size of the dominant or leading follicle.

Follicles grow approximately 2 mm per day. Between 18 and 23 mm is regarded as an optimal size for mature follicles; however, they may vary considerably in size, particularly in cy-cles induced with gonadotropins. For this reason, in patients with oligo-ovulation or anovulation, the diameter of the largest follicle is commonly used as a guide for oocyte maturity. If the largest follicle has reached a diameter of at least 18 mm, ovulation may be triggered with administration of hCG. In contrast to clomiphene-stimulated cycles, a spontaneous LH surge is not frequent in stimulation protocols in which gonadotropins are used. Nevertheless, withholding hCG while awaiting growth of other follicles may result in either a premature LH surge or in spontaneous luteinization of an unruptured follicle. In both instances, the planned therapeutic interventions must be canceled. With the wide use of GnRH agonists, premature ovulation and luteinization have become rare and confined mainly to women who do not comply with the administration schedule.

For patients undergoing IVF, it is necessary to develop a larger number of follicles so that more than one or two ova can be harvested (Fig 28–24). Various protocols may be used, but all are designed to develop many more follicles than would be desirable for women with oligo-ovulation or anovulation.[186] Again, the optimum size is between 18 and 23 mm, but it is unlikely that all follicles develop at the same rate. Mature ova may be obtained from follicles between 12 and 34 mm, although 15 and 23 mm are more typical diameters. Within this range no statistically significant differences in fertilization rates have been noticed. The gynecologist must therefore attempt to develop many follicles in this range while avoiding a spontaneous LH surge. When oocytes are harvested with ultrasound guidance, it should be remembered that puncturing a follicle larger than 20 mm is considerably easier than puncturing one of 12 mm.

Accurate prediction of an LH surge is not possible with ultrasound. Similarly, when multiple follicles develop, the sono-

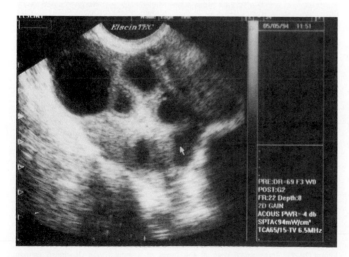

Figure 28–23. Transvaginal scan of the ovary showing a dominant follicle during treatment with clomiphene citrate.

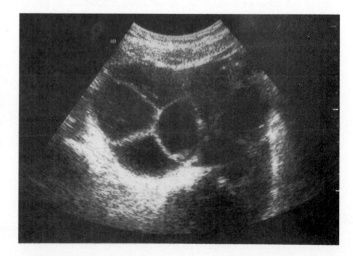

Figure 28–24. Transvaginal scan of stimulated ovaries in a patient undergoing IVF before oocyte retrieval.

graphic signs of imminent ovulation are extremely difficult to recognize. Thus, when one times oocyte retrieval, the ultrasound findings should not be used in isolation. Other clues, such as serum estradiol and LH or progesterone levels, should also be monitored. If the patient has had previous induced cycles, these should also be reviewed, because cyclic patterns frequently emerge and can assist in the timing of oocyte retrieval.

Combining Other Monitoring Techniques

The timing of hCG administration is critical. Too early and the oocytes might undergo atresia or fail to provide mature eggs; too late and the oocytes may be overmature. In addition, in many patients, a spontaneous LH surge may occur, causing considerable difficulty in correct timing of oocyte retrieval. Because the size of the follicle does not always correlate with maturity, it is not surprising that ultrasonographic findings alone have not been completely successful for estimating maturity.[186] For this reason, in most programs estradiol levels are monitored when ultrasound examinations are performed.[128] In a normal cycle there is reasonable correlation between the mean diameter of the dominant follicle and the estradiol level, which is usually about 400 pg/mL (1470 pmol/L).[3,187] In the presence of numerous follicles of variable sizes, correlation is poor.[6] Claims of statistically significant correlation between estradiol level and mean follicular volume in these patients[188] do not appear to be valid. Generally, when estradiol level is between 1000 and 2000 pg/mL (3670 and 7340 pmol/L) the follicles are mature. Because a satisfactory estradiol level may be produced by a few mature follicles or a larger number of small immature follicles, the combination of ultrasound findings and measurement of estradiol level allows better patient care. Observation of endometrial thickness may be of value under these circumstances, since thickness tends to increase maximally around the time of ovulation. In addition, endometrial thickness may allow prediction of failure of implantation. In the presence of an endometrial thickness of less than 7 mm, withholding the administration of hCG to allow further thickening should be strongly considered, if it is still possible.[83,100,101] As estradiol level rises, there is an increasing frequency of OHSS.[189] The gynecologist should therefore attempt to balance the need for many mature follicles with the likelihood of OHSS if estradiol level rises too high.

Although ultrasonography is commonly used during gonadotropin therapy in conjunction with hormonal assays to monitor patients undergoing COH, it has been shown that it is possible to run a successful ovulation induction program solely on the basis of ultrasound monitoring.[83] If a low-dose, stepwise regimen is used, this approach has been found safe in terms of preventing multiple pregnancies and diminishing the incidence and severity of OHSS. Similarly, a large series of GIFT cycles

has been reported in which monitoring was carried out solely with the use of ultrasound scans with excellent results.[190]

In most circumstances follicular development does not require further monitoring after hCG administration. The follicles usually grow between 2 and 4 mm in the 36 hours before ovulation. If evidence of ovulation is required, another ultrasound scan 2 days after hCG administration is recommended to search for signs such as a decrease in size or the disappearance of a number of follicles and fluid in the cul-de-sac. In addition, cystic enlargement of the ovaries indicates development of OHSS and also may be taken as evidence of ovulation. This rarely occurs in any but induced cycles. Conversely, in the absence of ultrasound evidence of ovulation, a second dose of hCG may be administered.

COMPLICATIONS OF OVULATION INDUCTION

Ovarian Hyperstimulation Syndrome

OHSS is the most serious complication associated with ovulation induction. Some degree of ovarian hyperstimulation occurs in all women who respond to ovulation induction therapy. This syndrome is characterized by varying degrees of cystic enlargement of the ovaries after ovulation (Fig 28–25). In its mild and moderate forms, OHSS is usually self-limited and requires no active therapy other than observation and plasma volume and electrolyte replacement. In the severe form of OHSS, massive cystic enlargement of the ovaries occurs accompanied by hemoconcentration and third space accumulation of fluid in the form of ascites, pleural, and pericardial effusions (Fig 28–26).

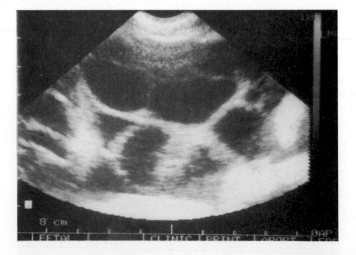

Figure 28–25. Transvaginal scan of the ovary of a patient who developed ovarian hyperstimulation syndrome after induction of ovulation with gonadotropins. Note the enlarged ovary with multiple ovarian cysts.

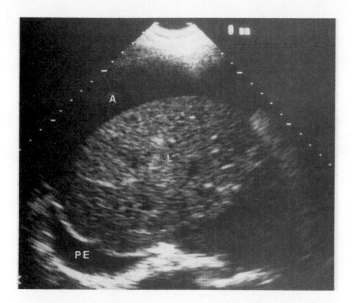

Figure 28–26. Ultrasound findings in ovarian hyperstimulation. *L,* liver; *A,* ascites; *PE,* pleural effusion. The white line between *PE* and *L* is the diaphragm. *(Courtesy of M. Seibel, MD.)*

The full clinical syndrome may be further complicated by renal failure and oliguria, hypovolemic shock, thromboembolic phenomena, adult respiratory distress syndrome, and even death.[191] This is of great importance because about 0.5% of otherwise healthy young women who participate in assisted reproduction programs may experience severe OHSS[192] and suffer severe morbidity and even mortality from this purely iatrogenic condition. Fortunately, this degree of severity is uncommon. Other forms of OHSS characterized by ovarian enlargement without evidence of ascites, effusion, or hemoconcentration are common, being demonstrated in 44% of ovulation inductions.[193]

Ultrasound plays an important role in prediction, detection, monitoring, and even therapy for OHSS. In fact, OHSS is an entity in which prevention, diagnosis, and management currently rely mainly on ultrasonographic findings.

Prevention of severe OHSS is important because once full OHSS has developed, there is no definitive treatment. Apart from supportive therapy, hardly any benefit can be derived from the different medical treatments that have been suggested.[192] Because the key to prevention of severe OHSS is early identification of patients at risk, there have been many attempts to define this population. Sonographic markers of high risk include evidence of PCO during the baseline examination, the necklace sign (small, early antral follicles 2 to 8 mm in diameter arranged around the periphery of the ovary, during the early follicular phase), and development of multiple follicles during the mid to late follicular phase.[192] A definite correlation exists between the development of OHSS and the number of follicles present at ovulation[194] and estradiol level. The larger the number of folli-

cles and the higher the estradiol level, the more likely it is OHSS that will occur. Ovarian hyperstimulation syndrome tends to occur among women whose ovaries contain multiple small or intermediate-sized follicles. Thus, a specific preovulatory follicular configuration characterizes patients at risk for development of OHSS.[194] The value of ovarian ultrasonography in the prediction of OHSS is emphasized. Further risk factors include young age (less than 35 years) and lean habitus.[192] The risk is further increased if a protocol that includes a GnRH agonist is used.[192]

OHSS is almost exclusively related to the presence of either exogenous or endogenous hCG (that is, when hCG is used for luteal support and in the presence of pregnancy, respectively).[192] Withholding hCG does not necessarily prevent ovulation and subsequent development of OHSS because spontaneous LH surges occasionally occur. The symptoms and signs of OHSS start developing soon after ovulation and are worse after 8 to 10 days. In the absence of pregnancy, the symptoms diminish over a period of 10 days. If the patient becomes pregnant, ovarian enlargement may persist for many weeks.[193]

Once OHSS has developed, ultrasonography serves an important role in monitoring the extent of ovarian enlargement and degrees of production of ascitic fluid. In fact, these two sonographic findings are the more important criteria for classification of stages of OHSS.[191,192] The sonographic appearance of a hyperstimulated ovary is almost distinctive. It consists of the presence of multiple, large, thin-walled cysts on the periphery of the enlarged ovaries. Free fluid in the abdomen can be easily demonstrated at both TAS and TVS. Because ovarian hyperstimulation usually is deliberate and a larger number of follicles and higher estradiol levels are present in patients undergoing assisted reproductive techniques, some degree of OHSS is present in almost all patients. Indeed, the term *controlled ovarian hyperstimulation* often is used to describe ovulation induction for assisted reproduction. It should be stated that during cycles of assisted reproductive techniques, the content of the follicles is usually thoroughly aspirated. Thus the ovaries are not as markedly enlarged as after ovulation induction. Therefore, it has been suggested that for such patients the classification of OHSS should rely more on the general clinical features and laboratory values than on ovarian enlargement.[192] Whether follicular aspiration during assisted reproductive treatments reduces the risk for OHSS is still debatable.[192]

Ultrasonography is well suited to evaluation of the extent of OHSS and whether the condition is in progression or under resolution. In severe and life-threatening OHSS unresponsive to medical therapy, paracentesis becomes an important modality. Paracentesis should be performed transabdominally with ultrasound guidance. Transvaginal, ultrasound-guided aspiration of ascitic fluid has been described as an effective and safe method.[195]

Multiple Gestations

Although it is ideal if only one or two follicles develop in patients who need ovulation induction, numerous follicles develop in most women. This does increase the probability of multiple gestations, but these actually occur in only about 10% to 20% of patients. Therefore, the presence of many follicles should not preclude the administration of hCG. When three or more preovulatory follicles are detected, however, careful discussion with the couple before administration of hCG is essential.

Attempts to correlate the incidence of multiple gestations with the amount of estrogen secreted by the developing follicles have not met with success.[196] Because ultrasound provides accurate information concerning the number and size of growing follicles, it was hoped that it would also help to predict, and thus to reduce, the risk for multiple gestations. Navot et al[197] compared the findings of the preovulatory scan in singleton and multiple gestations resulting from ovulation induction with gonadotropins. They were able to show that in the presence of intermediate-sized follicles 15 to 17 mm in diameter, in addition to a single dominant follicle of 18 mm or more in diameter, the risk for multiple gestation increases in a statistically significant way. The retrospective study, however, was biased, because the investigators tended to withold hCG in an effort to reduce the risk for multiple gestations when two or more dominant follicles were detected. In a prospective study, Ben-Nun et al[198] reported that the number and size of follicles visualized on the day of hCG administration had no predictive value for the occurrence of multiple gestations. Incorporation of low-dose, stepwise gonadotropin treatment regimens has been found to be efficient for reduction in the number of leading follicles and thus for the prevention of multiple gestations.[199] In assisted reproduction programs, the multiple pregnancy rates can be reduced by limiting the number of replaced embryos to two or possibly three, and cryopreserving the others.[200]

Sonography plays an essential role in the early recognition and management of multiple gestation. It can also provide accurate determination of the locations, number of gestational sacs, placentas, and amniotic compartments (Fig 28–27). Ultrasound-guided selective reduction of multiple gestations has been reported as an efficient method by which the number of developing embryos can be controlled. Although not without risk, this procedure can be successfully accomplished with either TAS[201] or TVS.[202]

ULTRASOUND-GUIDED PROCEDURES

Oocyte Retrieval with Ultrasound Guidance

Ultrasound has almost exclusively replaced laparoscopy in guiding oocyte retrieval in assisted reproduction programs.

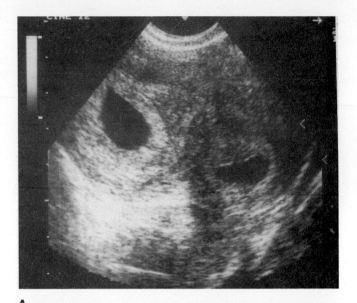

Figure 28–27. Twin gestation. **A.** In a septated uterus. **B.** In a tube, representing twin tubal pregnancy. *U*, uterus.

All ultrasound-directed methods for oocyte retrieval avoid the trauma, morbidity, and anesthetic risks of laparoscopy. Three methods of ultrasound-guided oocyte retrieval have been reported: transabdominal-transvesical, transurethral-transvesical, and transvaginal. The first studies used a transabdominal-transvesical approach.[203,204] Although a satisfactory rate of oocyte recovery has been achieved with this technique, it is not widely used because of the considerable discomfort to the patient. A periurethral-transvesical approach has had wider application.[205] This technique can be performed without considerable discomfort for a sedated patient. The oocyte recovery rate is comparable with that of laparoscopic retrieval. In the first report of transvaginal ultrasound-guided follicle puncture, the needle was guided with a standard transabdominal technique; the vagina and ovaries were scanned through a full bladder.[9] Subsequently, the advent of the transvaginal probe with biopsy attachment made it possible to harvest oocytes with the transvaginal approach.[206,207]

Of the ultrasound-guided methods for oocyte retrieval, the transvaginal approach has distinct advantages, similar to those that apply to use of a vaginal transducer in scanning to evaluate follicular growth (Fig 28–28). Because the transducer is close to the ovaries, a high-frequency, high-definition transducer can be used, ensuring excellent visualization of the follicles and avoiding injury to the bladder, intestine, or blood vessels. Because the patient's pain and discomfort are minimal and recovery is quick, oocyte retrieval can be performed in an outpatient setting. Better control of all aspects of oocyte retrieval is possible compared with other ultrasound guidance methods. Furthermore, the procedure can be performed by a single operator, instead of requiring both a sonographer and a gynecologist. It has been demonstrated that the use of laparoscopy has no advantage over the transvaginal technique of oocyte retrieval.[208]

Transvaginal, ultrasound-guided oocyte retrieval is not risk-free.[209] The introduction of a sharp aspiration needle through the vaginal wall and into the ovary may injure the adjacent intestinal, uterine, and adnexal organs and blood vessels. Minor vaginal hemorrhage is quite common, with a reported incidence of 8.6% to 24%.[210] Such bleeding usually responds to application of local pressure and is therefore of minimal clinical significance. Although much rarer, but of greater clinical significance, hemoperitoneum may be caused by direct damage to pelvic organs or to pelvic blood vessels misinterpreted as ovar-

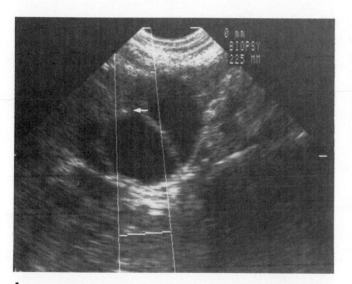

A

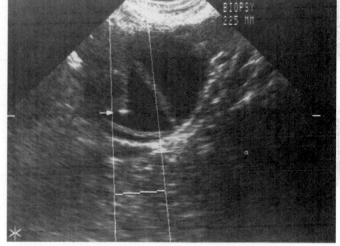

B

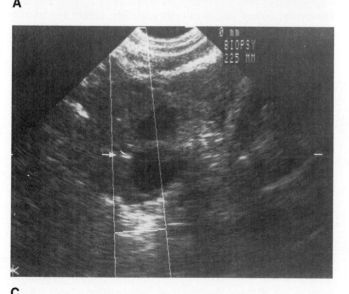

C

Figure 28–28. Transvaginal oocyte retrieval. **A.** The tip of the needle (arrow) before follicle aspiration. **B.** The needle (arrow) advanced into the follicle. **C.** The follicle has been aspirated. The needle tip is depicted (arrow).

ian follicles. The second, most common, complication is pelvic infection, caused by microorganisms introduced to the peritoneal cavity by the collecting needle. Infection also may result from exacerbation of PID or from trauma to a loop of intestine. A history of PID may imply a higher risk for pelvic reinfection. Follicle puncture–related complications were reported among 0.5% of cycles, and postoperative infections were reported among 0.3% of embryo transfers.[211] Bleeding and infections introduced by the needle may be serious and sometimes are fatal.[212] Overall, transvaginal ultrasound-guided oocyte retrieval is considered a safe procedure, complications of which are relatively rare. Therefore, this technique is now regarded as the method of choice for harvesting oocytes in most assisted reproduction programs.

In many patients with extensive tubal disease and adhesions, the ovaries may not be equally accessible with all approaches. An ovary that lies high within the pelvis is more likely to be accessible with the transabdominal than with the transvaginal approach. Similarly, an ovary behind the uterus or low within the cul-de-sac can be approached only through the vagina. Competency in more than one method of oocyte retrieval is therefore recommended to accommodate all patients.

Ultrasound-Guided Gamete Transfer

In cycles in which GIFT was used, ultrasound was initially used only to assist ovulation induction, and laparoscopy was used to retrieve oocytes and place them into the fallopian tubes. The feasibility of catheterization of the distal portion of the fallopian tube with TVS guidance, by means of a specially designed catheter, has been reported. The technique enables successful transfer of oocytes, sperm, zygotes, and embryos.[213–215] However, transvaginal GIFT seems to be less effective. In a retrospective comparison between laparoscopic and ultrasound-guided GIFT, higher pregnancy rates were achieved with laparoscopy.[216] Some gynecologists have used TVS to perform oocyte retrieval followed by the transfer of oocytes and sperm into the uterus.[217] Gamete uterine transfer (GUT) has the advantage of not requiring patency of the fallopian tubes (Fig 28–29).

Ultrasound-Guided Embryo Transfer

ET after IVF treatment is considered a relatively simple procedure. However, in an attempt to improve pregnancy rates, especially when difficult transfers are encountered, or when uterine anomalies are present, performing this procedure with TAS or TVS has been suggested.[218,219] Transvaginal-transmyometrial ultrasound-guided ET also has been suggested as a means to improve implantation and pregnancy rates.[220] The value of ultrasound-guided ET has yet to be evaluated.

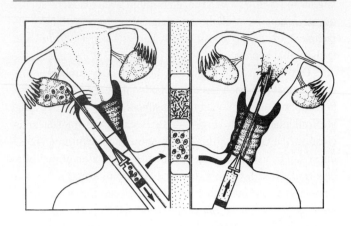

Figure 28–29. Schematic of gamete uterine transfer. *(Courtesy M. Seibel, M.D.)*

Other Ultrasound-Guided Procedures

Ultrasound guidance has been shown to allow effective aspiration of ovarian cysts, assessment of tubal patency, and selective reduction in multiple gestations. In addition, TVS is an important tool in the investigation of early gestation and early recognition of ectopic pregnancy. Successful TVS-guided aspiration of the contents of an unruptured tubal gestational sac[221] and injection of lethal substances such as methotrexate[222,223] or potassium chloride[224] into the sac have been reported and are currently being used in some centers.

MONITORING PREGNANCY

Early Pregnancy

During the earliest phases of embryonic life, before a chorionic cavity has formed, the embryo is not detectable with ultrasound. This chorionic cavity forms 30 to 34 days after the last menstruation, when it rapidly becomes detectable with ultrasound. If a a vaginal transducer is used, a clearly defined gestational sac usually can be detected by 32 days. No yolk sac or fetal parts can be seen, and a gestational sac may be confused with a decidual cast. By 35 days, by means of a vaginal transducer, a yolk sac can be seen within the gestational sac. This proves conclusively the presence of an intrauterine pregnancy. The gestational sac grows about 1 mm a day; if the standard sector scanner is used, the sac is usually not easily visible until day 35, and the yolk sac generally is not seen until day 40 (Fig 28–30). By this time or soon after, a fetal pole may be detected with the vaginal probe. From these data, it can be seen that an intrauterine pregnancy cannot be detected for at least 16 days from conception, or 30 days after the last menstruation (Table 28–1).

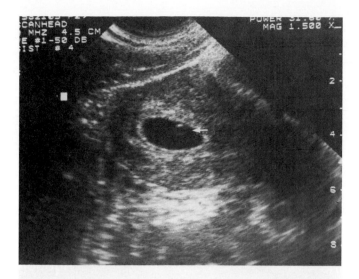

Figure 28–30. Longitudinal scan of the uterus reveals a yolk sac (arrow) within a gestational sac. This is absolute proof that the sac represents an intrauterine pregnancy. A double decidual sign is depicted on the fundal and posterior aspects of the gestational sac.

Unless a yolk sac can be detected, the presence of an intrauterine pregnancy cannot be determined absolutely. A gestational sac without a detectable yolk sac or fetal pole may be confused with a decidual cast, a point of confusion when an ectopic pregnancy is suspected.

Attempts have been made to differentiate a gestational sac from a decidual cast, often referred to as a pseudogestational sac or pseudosac of pregnancy.[225] When implantation of the blastocyst occurs at around the 6th day after conception, it does so into one or another wall of the endometrium. As the embryo develops and the chorionic sac appears, the embryo tends to lie in an eccentric position within the uterine cavity, surrounded by markedly thickened endometrium. This position forms the basis of what is termed the *intradecidual sign* (Fig 28–31A,B), which is claimed to be both highly sensitive and specific for the diagnosis of intrauterine pregnancy. Conversely, a decidual cast or pseudosac is a centrally located, sac-shaped anechoic area in which the endometrium of the uterine wall is of similar thickness on both sides of the sac (Fig 28–31C,D). These are the findings whether a transvaginal or transabdominal transducer is used.

Another sign that may be helpful in confirming the presence of pregnancy when neither yolk sac nor fetal pole is detectable is the ultrasonographic demonstration of line of separation beween the decidua parietalis and the decidua capsularis (Fig 28–31E,F). This is represented as a lucent line between the two echogenic lines caused by the two decidual layers. This sandwich is what is called the *double decidual sac sign,* which is good evidence of an intrauterine rather than an ectopic pregnancy.

TABLE 28–1. AFFIRMATION OF INTRAUTERINE PREGNANCY

Day After Last Menstrual Period	β-hCG 2nd IS (mIU/mL)	Ultrasound Findings
23	—	Positive
32	±500	Gestational sac
35	±1,800	Yolk sac, gestational sac
40	>5,000	Fetal pole, yolk sac
45	>10,000	Embryo, fetal pole

Even when one or another of these signs is present, if ectopic gestation is suspected, it is prudent to repeat the ultrasound examination in 5 to 7 days to confirm the presence of a yolk sac or fetal pole within the gestational sac, proving beyond doubt the existence of an intrauterine pregnancy (Fig 28–32; see color plate facing page 460).

DOPPLER VELOCIMETRY OF THE UTERINE AND OVARIAN CIRCULATION

The introduction of Doppler ultrasound technology has opened a new era in reproductive medicine, allowing noninvasive assessment of uterine and ovarian blood flow, thereby shifting and extending the role of ultrasound studies from purely morphologic to a more physiologic aspect. Advances and refinements of Doppler ultrasound technology have made it possible to study flow velocity waveforms (FVWs) as an accurate indicator of uterine and ovarian perfusion. In the uterine circulation, the main-stem uterine arteries and their branches, the arcuate and radial arteries, and even the spiral arteries which traverse the endometrium, can all be studied (Fig 28–33). Blood flow in the ovary can be assessed at Doppler examination of the ovarian artery, vessels in the ovarian stroma, intra-ovarian structures such as the periovulatory follicle, and the corpus luteum.

The technical aspects of Doppler velocimetry are beyond the scope of this chapter, and the reader is referred elsewhere for a more thorough discussion.[226–227] Briefly, Doppler indices of FVWs reflect blood flow impedance distal to the point of sampling, in other words, downstream resistance to blood flow. Three indices are commonly used to express FVWs. The systolic-to-diastolic (S/D) ratio and the Pourcelot resistance index (RI) are the simplest to measure. However, the pulsatility index (PI) is the only one that can be used when there is no end-diastolic flow or reversed flow. According to the formula used to calculate the PI, the value of the index increases if proximal blood flow remains constant while the distal vascular bed constricts. Conversely, a low PI indicates decreased impedance to blood flow in the distal vasculature. The PI is the least convenient index because it necessitates digitizing the entire wave-

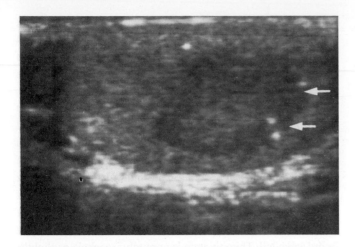

Figure 28–37. Longitudinal scan shows a well-defined, hyperechoic mass in the testis representing a seminoma (arrows).

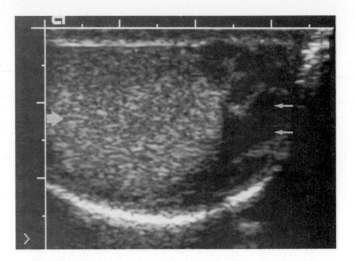

Figure 28–38. Adjacent to the normal testis (thick arrow) is a serpiginous hypoechoic area representing a varicocele (thin arrows).

nologist should be able routinely to diagnose these tumors (Fig 28–37).

Varicoceles are a frequent and treatable cause of infertility.[265] In this condition, the veins of the pampiniform plexus that accompany the epididymis become elongated, distorted, and distended. The veins of the pampiniform plexus usually measure 0.5 to 1.5 mm in diameter and are readily seen. Care must be taken not to overdiagnose this condition. Most (98%) of varicoceles occur on the left side, attributable to the venous drainage into the left renal vein rather than directly into the inferior vena cava, which drains the right spermatic vein. This arrangement increases pressure in the left spermatic vein, leading to valvular incompetence. For this reason, varicoceles tend to enlarge when the man stands or during a Valsalva maneuver. Ultrasound examination with a high-frequency, high-resolution linear probe reveals serpiginous dilated veins within and around the epididymis (Fig 28–38). These dilated veins should be greater than 2 mm in diameter. Color Doppler imaging often does not show flow even at the appropriate settings, but movement of the blood may be readily visualized at gray-scale imaging.

Absence or partial absence of the epididymis occasionally may occur. For this reason, it is necessary to demonstrate both the head and tail of the epididymis. Enlargement of the epididymis may indicate chronic or old infection, which may be associated with blockage of the vas. A careful clinical history for infection is probably more accurate and certainly less expensive than ultrasonography. Frequently, other abnormalities such as epididymal cysts, spermatoceles, hydroceles, calcifications or cysts of the tunica albuginea may be seen around the epididymis. These are not generally associated with infertility.

Transport System Failure

Abnormalities of the distal sperm transport system are commonly the cause of a low-volume ejaculate.[266] Transrectal ultrasonography allows good visualization of the seminal vesicles, vas deferentia, and the ejaculatory ducts as they pass through the prostate.

In the axial plane, the paired seminal vesicles give a characteristic bow tie appearance (Fig 28–39). Medially the ampullae of the vasa represent the normal dilatation of these structures. Bilateral or unilteral agenesis of the seminal vesicles or vasa deferentia either separately or in combination is a common cause of low ejaculatory volumes and may be readily detected at transrectal ultrasonography.[266] Hypoplasia or cysts of the seminal vesicles, although less common, also may be detected. Blockage of the ejaculatory duct may be caused by the presence of stones or cysts. The course of the ejaculatory ducts through the prostate to the verumontanum can usually be followed with careful scanning technique. Therefore, stones or

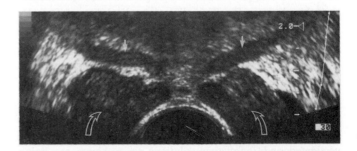

Figure 28–39. Transrectal ultrasound scan showing normal paired seminal vesicles (open arrows) and paired vasa deferentia (closed arrows).

cysts may be demonstrated. In these instances, if no other abnormality is found, curative surgical treatment is a possibility.

It must be remembered that in a large number of men undergoing examinations for infertility for any cause, no abnormality is found. It is also important to recognize that a demonstrated abnormality may not always be the cause of infertility and that complete evaluation is still necessary. Proper ultrasound examination of the prostate and seminal vesicles necessitates meticulous technique, superior equipment, and a thorough knowledge of both the anatomy and the potential pathologic condition. Anything less will inevitably result in an inadequate or inaccurate diagnosis.

ACKNOWLEDGMENTS

Our thanks to Dr. B. Caspi, Dr. Y. Zalel, and Prof. Z. Weinraub for providing some of the figures.

REFERENCES

1. Kratochwil A, Urban GU, Friedrich F: Ultrasonic tomography of the ovaries. *Ann Chir Gynecol* 61:211, 1972
2. Hackeloer B, Nitschke S, Daume E, Sturm G, Buchholz R: Ultrasonics of ovarian changes under gonadotropin stimulation. *Geburtshilfe Frauenheilkd* 38:185, 1977
3. Hackeloer BJ, Fleming R, Robinson HP, Adam AH, Coutts JRT: Correlation of ultrasonic and endocrinologic assessment of human follicular development. *Am J Obstet Gynecol* 135:122, 1979
4. Kerin JF, Warnes GM, Crocker J, et al: 3-Hour urinary radioimmunoassay for luteinizing hormone to detect onset of preovulatory LH surge. *Lancet* 1:430, 1980
5. O'Herlihy C, de Crespigny L, Robinson HP: Monitoring ovarian follicular development with real-time ultrasound. *Br J Obstet Gynaecol* 87:613, 1980
6. Montzavinos T, Garcia JE, Jones HW Jr: Ultrasound measurement of ovarian follicles stimulated by human gonadotropins for oocyte recovery and in vitro fertilization. *Fertil Steril* 40:461, 1983
7. Seibel MM, McArdle CR, Thompson IE, Berger MJ, Taymor ML: The role of ultrasound in ovulation induction: A critical appraisal. *Fertil Steril* 36:573, 1981
8. Gleicher N, Friberg J, Fullan N, et al: Egg retrieval for in vitro fertilization sonographically controlled vaginal culdocentesis. *Lancet* 2:508, 1983
9. Dellenbach P, Nisand I, Moreau L, et al: Transvaginal sonographically controlled ovarian follicle puncture for egg retrieval. *Lancet* 2:1467, 1984
10. Schwimer SR, Lebovic J: Transvaginal pelvic ultrasonography. *J Ultrasound Med* 3:381, 1984
11. Frederick J, Paulson RJ, Sauer MV: Routine use of vaginal ultrasonography in the preoperative evaluation of gynecologic patients: An adjunct to resident education. *J Reprod Med* 36:779, 1991
12. Yee B, Barnes RB, Vargyas JM, Marrs RP: Correlation of transabdominal and transvaginal ultrasound measurements of follicle size and number with laparoscopic findings for in vitro fertilization. *Fertil Steril* 47:828, 1987
13. Andreotti RE, Thompson GH, Janowitz W, Shapiro AG, Zusmer NR: Endovaginal and transabdominal sonography of ovarian follicles. *J Ultrasound Med* 8:555, 1989
14. Timor-Tritsch IE: Is office use of vaginal ultrasonography feasible? *Am J Obstet Gynecol* 162:983, 1990
15. Hill LM, Coulam CB, Kislak SL, Peterson CS, Runco CJ: Sonographic evaluation of the cervix during ovulation induction. *Am J Obstet Gynecol* 157:1170, 1987
16. Hall DA: Sonographic appearance of normal ovary, of polycystic disease, and of functional ovarian cysts. *Semin Ultrasound* 4:149, 1983
17. Cohen HL, Tice HM, Mandel FS: Ovarian volumes measured by US: Bigger than we think. *Radiology* 177:189, 1990
18. Sauer MV, Agnew C, Worthen N, et al: Reliability of ultrasound in predicting leiomyoma volume. *J Reprod Med* 33:612, 1988
19. Narayan R, Goswamy RK. Transvaginal sonography of the uterine cavity with hysteroscopic correlation in the investigation of infertility. *Ultrasound Obstet Gynecol* 3:129, 1993
20. Nakamura Y, Yoshimura Y: Treatment of uterine leiomyomas in perimenopausal women with gonadotropin-releasing hormone agonists. *Clin Obstet Gynecol* 36:660, 1993
21. Fedele L, Bianchi S, Dorta M, Brioschi D, Zanotti F, Vercellini P: Transvaginal ultrasonography versus hysteroscopy in the diagnosis of uterine submucous myomas. *Obstet Gynecol* 77:745, 1991
22. Goldberg BB, Liu JB, Kuhlman K, Merton DA, Curtz AB: Endoluminal gynecologic ultrasound: Preliminary results. *J Ultrasound Med* 10:583, 1991
23. Huang RT, Chou CY, Chang CH, Yu SC, Yao BL: Differentiation between adenomyoma and leiomyoma with transvaginal ultrasonography. *Ultrasound Obstet Gynecol* 5:47, 1995
24. Balen FG, Allen CM, Gardener JE, Siddle NC, Lees WR: 3-dimensional reconstruction of ultrasound images of the uterine cavity. *Br J Radiol* 66:588, 1993
25. Shalev E, Shimoni Y, Peleg D: Ultrasound controlled operative hysteroscopy. *J Am Coll Surg* 179:70, 1994
26. Buttram VC: Müllerian anomalies and their management. *Fertil Steril* 40:159, 1983
27. Reuter KL, Daly DC, Cohen SM: Septate versus bicornuate uteri: Errors in imaging diagnosis. *Radiology* 172:749, 1989
28. Malini S, Valdes C, Malinak R: Sonographic diagnosis and classification of anomalies of the female genital tract. *J Ultrasound Med* 3:397, 1984
29. Pennes DR, Bowerman RA, Silver TM: Congenital uterine anomalies and associated pregnancies: Findings and pitfalls in the sonographic diagnosis. *J Ultrasound Med* 4:531, 1985
30. Ohl J, Nisand I, Dellenbach P: Resection under echographic con-

trol of septate uteri. *J Gynecol Obstet Biol Reprod (Paris)* 20:538, 1991

31. McArdle CR, Berezin A: Ultrasound demonstration of uterus subseptus. *J Clin Ultrasound* 8:139, 1980

32. Scanlan KA, Pozniak MA, Fagerholm M, Shapiro S: Value of transperineal sonography in the assessment of vaginal atresia. *Am J Roentgenol* 154:545, 1990

33. Boulot P, Deschamps F, Hedon B, Laffargue F, Viali JL: Prenatal diagnosis of an abdomino-pelvic hydrometrocolpos: A case report. *Eur J Obstet Gynecol Reprod Biol* 40:233, 1991

34. Petit P, Thomas D, Moerman P, Fryns JP: Abdominal distention as the first echographic sign of hydrometrocolpos in a female fetus. *Eur J Obstet Gynecol Reprod Biol* 39:99, 1991

35. Viscomi G, Gonzales R, Taylor K: Ultrasound detection of uterine anomalies after diethylstilbestrol (DES) exposure. *Radiology* 136:733, 1980

36. Sample W, Lippe B, Gyepes M: Gray scale ultrasonography of the normal female pelvis. *Radiology* 125:477, 1977

37. Pellerito JS, McCarthy SM, Doyle MB, Glickman MG, DeCherney AH: Diagnosis of uterine anomalies: Relative accuracy of MR imaging, endovaginal sonography, and hysterosalpingography. *Radiology* 183:795, 1992

38. Jurkovic D, Geipel A, Gruboeck K, Jauniaux E, Natucci M, Campbell S: Three-dimensional ultrasound for the assessment of uterine anatomy and detection of congenital anomalies: A comparison with hysterosalpingography and two-dimensional sonography. *Ultrasound Obstet Gynecol* 5:233, 1995

39. Confino E, Friberg J, Giglia RV, Gleicher N: Sonographic imaging of intrauterine adhesions. *Obstet Gynecol* 66:596, 1985

40. Mendelson EB, Bohm-Velez M, Joseph N, Neiman HL: Endometrial abnormalities: Evaluation with transvaginal sonography. *Am J Roentgenol* 150:139, 1988

41. Zighelboim I, Szczedrin W, Zambrano O: Management of IUD users with non-visible threads. *Adv Contracept* 6:91, 1990

42. Knudsen HJ, Rasmussen K: The "forgotten" intrauterine device: A cause of infertility. *Arch Gynecol Obstet* 253:143, 1993

43. Caspi B, Weissman A, Elchalal U: Lost IUD thread as a possible cause of infertility. *Int J Gynaecol Obstet* 43:65, 1993

44. Marcus SF, Bhattacharya J, Williams G, Brinsden P, Hamou J: Endometrial ossification: A cause of secondary infertility—Report of two cases. *Am J Obstet Gynecol* 170:1381, 1994

45. Fried AM, Rhodes RA, Morehouse IR: Endometrioma: Analysis and sonographic classification of 51 documented cases. *South Med J* 86:297, 1993

46. Blumenfeld Z, Yoffe N, Bronshtein M: Transvaginal sonography in infertility and assisted reproduction. *Obstet Gynecol Surv* 46:36, 1990

47. Friedman H, Vogelzang RL, Mendelson EB, Neiman HL, Cohen M: Endometriosis detection by ultrasound with laparoscopic correlation. *Radiology* 157:217, 1985

48. Athey PA, Diment DD: The spectrum of sonographic findings in endometriosis. *J Ultrasound Med* 8:487, 1989

49. Sandler MA, Karo JJ: The spectrum of ultrasonic findings in endometriosis. *Radiology* 127:229, 1978

50. Kupesic S, Kurjak A: Normal and abnormal ovarian circulation. In: Kurjak A (ed), *Ultrasound and the Ovary.* London, Parthenon, 1994:201–202

51. Arrive L, Hriack H, Martin MC: Pelvic endometriosis: MR imaging. *Radiology* 171:687, 1989

52. Togashi K, Nishimura K, Kimura I, et al: Endometrial cysts: Diagnosis with MR imaging. *Radiology* 180:73, 1991

53. Tessler FN, Perrella RR, Fleischer AC, Grant EG: Endovaginal sonographic diagnosis of dilated fallopian tubes. *Am J Roentgenol* 153:523, 1989

54. Reuter K, Cohen S, Daly D: Ultrasonic presentation of giant hydrosalpinges in asymptomatic patients. *J Clin Ultrasound* 15:45, 1987

55. Karasick S, Goldfarb AF: Peritubal adhesions in infertile women: Diagnosis with hysterosalpingography. *Am J Roentgenol* 152:777, 1989

56. Hoffer FA, Kozakewich H, Colodny A, Goldstein DP: Peritoneal inclusion cysts: Ovarian fluid in peritoneal adhesions. *Radiology* 169:189, 1988

57. Lande IM, Hill MC, Cosco E, et al: Adnexal and cul-de-sac abnormalities: Transvaginal sonography. *Radiology* 166:325, 1988

58. Timor-Tritsch IE, Rottem S, Levron Y: The fallopian tubes. In: Timor-Tritsch IE, Rottem S (eds), *Transvaginal Sonography.* New York, Elsevier, 1988:45

59. Rasmussen F, Larsen C, Justesen P: Fallopian tube patency demonstrated at ultrasonography. *Acta Radiol* 27:61, 1986

60. Allahbadia GN: Fallopian tubes and ultrasonography: The Sion experience. *Fertil Steril* 58:901, 1992

61. Mitri FF, Andronikou AD, Perpinyal S, Hofmeyer GJ, Sonnendecker EW: Clinical comparison of sonographic hydrotubation and hysterosalpingography. *Br J Obstet Gynaecol* 98:1031, 1991

62. Tufekci EC, Girit S, Bayirili E, Durmusoglu F, Yalti S: Evaluation of tubal patency by transvaginal sonosalpingography. *Fertil Steril* 57:336, 1992

63. Friberg B, Joergensen C: Tubal patency studied by ultrasonography: A pilot study. *Acta Obstet Gynecol Scand* 73:53, 1994

64. Bonilla-Musoles F, Simon C, Serra V, Sampaio M, Pellicer A: An assessment of hysterosalpingosonography (HSSG) as a diagnostic tool for uterine cavity defects and tubal patency. *J Clin Ultrasound* 20:175, 1992

65. Peters AJ, Coulam CB: Hysterosalpingography with color Doppler ultrasonography. *Am J Obstet Gynecol* 164:1530, 1990

66. Schlief R, Deichert U: Hysterosalpingo-contrast-sonography of the uterus and fallopian tubes: Results of a clinical trial of a new contrast medium in 120 patients. *Radiology* 178:213, 1991

67. Stern J, Peters AJ, Coulam CB: Color Doppler ultrasonography assessment of tubal patency: A comparison study with traditional techniques. *Fertil Steril* 58:897, 1992

68. Yarali H, Gurgan T, Erden A, Kisnisci HA: Colour Doppler hysterosalpingography: A simple and potentially useful method to evaluate fallopian tube patency. *Hum Reprod* 9:64, 1994

69. Deichert U, Schlief R, van de Sandt M, Juhnke I: Transvaginal hysterosalpingo-contrast-sonography (Hy-Co-Sy) compared with conventional tubal diagnostics. *Hum Reprod* 4:418, 1989

70. Deichert U, Schlief R, van de Sandt M, Daume E: Transvaginal

hysterosalpingo-contrast-sonography for the assessment of tubal patency with gray scale imaging and the additional use of pulsed wave Doppler. *Fertil Steril* 57:62, 1992

71. Balen FG, Allen CM, Siddle NC, Lees WR: Ultrasound contrast hysterosalpingography: Evaluation as an outpatient procedure. *Br J Radiol* 66:592, 1993

72. Lisse K, Sydow P: Fallopian tube catheterization and recanalization under ultrasonic observation: A simplified technique to evaluate tubal patency and open proximally obstructed tubes. *Fertil Steril* 56:198, 1991

73. Confino E, Tur-Kaspa I, Gleicher N: Sonographic transcervical balloon tuboplasty. *Hum Reprod* 7:1271, 1992

74. Hall DA, Hann LE, Ferrucci JT, et al: Sonographic morphology of the normal menstrual cycle. *Radiology* 133:185, 1979

75. Fleischer AC, Kalemeris CG, Machin JE, et al: Sonographic depiction of the normal and abnormal endometrium with histopathologic correlation. *J Ultrasound Med* 8:445, 1986

76. Fleischer AC, Gordon AN, Entman SS, Kepple DM: Transvaginal scanning of the endometrium. *J Clin Ultrasound* 18:337, 1990

77. Fleischer AC, Pittaway DE, Beard LA: Sonographic depiction of endometrial changes occurring with ovulation induction. *J Ultrasound Med* 3:341, 1984

78. Forrest TS, Elyaderani MK, Muilenburg MI, Bewtra C, Kable WT, Sullivan P: Cyclic endometrial changes: US measurements with histologic correlation. *Radiology* 167:233, 1988

79. Doherty CM, Silver B, Binor Z, Molo MW, Radwanska E: Transvaginal ultrasonography and the assessment of luteal phase endometrium. *Am J Obstet Gynecol* 168:1702, 1993

80. Li TC, Nuttall L, Klentzeris L, Cooke ID: How well does ultrasonographic measurement of endometrial thickness predict the results of histological dating. *Hum Reprod* 7:1, 1992

81. Adams JM, Tan SL, Wheeler MJ, Morris DV, Jacobs HS, Franks S: Uterine growth in the follicular phase of spontaneous ovulatory cycles and during luteinizing hormone-releasing hormone-induced cycles in women with normal or polycystic ovaries. *Fertil Steril* 49:52, 1988

82. Eden JA, Place J, Carter GD, Jones J, Alaghband-Zadeh J, Pawson ME: What are the ultrasound and biochemical features of impending ovulation? *Aust N Z J Obstet Gynaecol* 28:225, 1988

83. Shoham Z, Di Carlo C, Patel A, Conway GS, Jacobs HS: Is it possible to run a successful ovulation induction program based solely on ultrasound monitoring? The importance of endometrial measurements. *Fertil Steril* 56:836, 1991

84. Strohmer H, Obruca A, Rander KM, Feichtinger W: Relationship of the individual uterine size and the endometrial thickness in stimulated cycles. *Fertil Steril* 61:972, 1994

85. Shulman A, Shulman N, Weissenglass L, Bahary C: Ultrasonic assessment of the endometrium as a predictor of oestrogen status in amenorrheic patients. *Hum Reprod* 4:616, 1989

86. Morcos RN, Leonard MD, Smith M, Bourguet C, Makii M, Khawli O: Vaginosonographic measurement of endometrial thickness in the evaluation of amenorrhea. *Fertil Steril* 55:543, 1991

87. Lewit N, Thaler I, Rottem S: The uterus: A new look with transvaginal sonography. *J Clin Ultrasound* 18:331, 1990

88. Imoedemhe DAG, Shaw RW, Kirkland A, Chan R: Ultrasound measurement of endometrial thickness on different ovarian stimulation regimens during in vitro fertilization. *Hum Reprod* 2:545, 1987

89. Glissant A, de Mouzon J, Frydman R: Ultrasound study of the endometrium during in vitro fertilization cycles. *Fertil Steril* 44:786, 1985

90. Lenz S, Lindenberg S: Ultrasonic evaluation of endometrial growth in women with normal cycles during spontaneous and stimulated cycles. *Hum Reprod* 5:377, 1990

91. Gonen Y, Calderon I, Dirnfeld M, Abramovici H: The impact of sonographic assessment of the endometrium and meticulous hormonal monitoring during natural cycles in patients with failed donor artificial insemination. *Ultrasound Obstet Gynecol* 1:122, 1991

92. Shapiro H, Cowell C, Casper RF: The use of vaginal ultrasound for monitoring endometrial preparation in a donor oocyte program. *Fertil Steril* 59:1055, 1993

93. Wolman I, Sagi J, Pauzner D, Yovel I, Seidman DS, David MP: Transabdominal ultrasonographic evaluation of endometrial thickness in clomiphene citrate-stimulated cycles in relation to conception. *J Clin Ultrasound* 22:109, 1994

94. Eden JA, Place J, Carter GD, Jones J, Alaghband-Zadeh J, Pawson ME: The effect of clomiphene citrate on follicular phase increase in endometrial thickness and uterine volume. *Obstet Gynecol* 73:187, 1989

95. Randall JM, Templeton A: Transvaginal sonographic assessment of follicular and endometrial growth in spontaneous and clomiphene citrate cycles. *Fertil Steril* 56:208, 1991

96. Gonen Y, Casper RF: Sonographic determination of a possible adverse effect of clomiphene citrate on endometrial growth. *Hum Reprod* 5:670, 1990

97. Rogers PAW, Polson D, Murphy CR, Hosie M, Susil B, Leoni M: Correlation of endometrial histology, morphometry, and ultrasound appearance after different stimulation protocols for in vitro fertilization. *Fertil Steril* 55:583, 1991

98. Yagel S, Ben-Chetrit A, Anteby E, Zacut D, Hochner-Celnikier D, Ron M: The effect of ethinyl estradiol on endometrial thickness and uterine volume during ovulation induction by clomiphene citrate. *Fertil Steril* 57:33, 1992

99. Yaron Y, Botchan A, Amit A, Peyser R, David MP, Lessing JB: Endometrial receptivity in the light of modern assisted reproductive technologies. *Fertil Steril* 62:225, 1994

100. Gonen Y, Casper RF, Jacobson W, Blankier J: Endometrial thickness and growth during ovarian stimulation: A possible predictor of implantation in in vitro fertilization. *Fertil Steril* 52:446, 1989

101. Gonen Y, Casper RF: Prediction of implantation by the sonographic appearance of the endometrium during controlled ovarian stimulation for in vitro fertilization (IVF). *J In Vitro Fertil Embryo Transf* 7:146, 1990

102. Coulam CB, Bustillo M, Soenksen DM, Britten S: Ultrasonographic predictors of implantation after assisted reproduction. *Fertil Steril* 62:1004, 1994

103. Check JH, Nowroozi K, Choe J, Dietterich C: Influence of en-

dometrial thickness and echogenic patterns on pregnancy rates during in vitro fertilization. *Fertil Steril* 56:1173, 1991

104. Guirgis RR, Alshawaf T, Craft IL: Preoperative ultrasonic assessment of women undergoing gamete intrafallopian transfer: A prospective study of 350 cases. *Ultrasound Obstet Gynecol* 3:124, 1993

105. Dickey RP, Olar TT, Curole DN, Taylor SN, Rye PH: Endometrial pattern and thickness associated with pregnancy outcome after assisted reproduction technologies. *Hum Reprod* 7:418, 1992

106. Fleischer AC, Herbert CM, Sacks GA, Wenz AC, Entman SS, James AE Jr: Sonography of the endometrium during conception and nonconception cycles of in vitro fertilization and embryo transfer. *Fertil Steril* 46:442, 1986

107. Rabinowitz R, Laufer N, Lewin A, et al: The value of ultrasonographic endometrial measurement in the prediction of pregnancy following in vitro fertilization. *Fertil Steril* 45:824, 1986

108. Welker BG, Gembruch U, Diedrich K, Al-Hasani S, Krebs D: Transvaginal sonography of the endometrium during ovum pickup in stimulated cycles for in vitro fertilization. *J Ultrasound Med* 8:549, 1989

109. Serafini P, Batzofin J, Nelson J, Olive D: Sonographic uterine predictors of pregnancy in women undergoing ovulation induction for assisted reproductive treatments. *Fertil Steril* 62:815, 1994

110. Fleischer AC, Herbert CM, Hill GA, et al: Transvaginal sonography of the endometrium during induced cycles. *J Ultrasound Med* 10:93, 1991

111. Khalifa E, Brzyski RG, Oehninger S, Acosta AA, Muasher SJ: Sonographic appearance of endometrium: The predictive value for the outcome of in vitro fertilization in stimulated cycles. *Hum Reprod* 6:677, 1992

112. Smith B, Porter R, Ahuja K, Craft I: Ultrasonic assessment of endometrial changes in stimulated cycles and in vitro fertilization and embryo transfer program. *J In Vitro Fertil Embryo Transf* 1:233, 1984

113. Check JH, Nowroozi K, Choe J, Lurie D, Dietterich C: The effect of endometrial thickness and echo pattern on in vitro fertilization outcome in donor oocyte-embryo transfer cycle. *Fertil Steril* 59:72, 1993

114. Birnholz JC: Ultrasonic visualization of endometrial movements. *Fertil Steril* 41:157, 1984

115. Abramowicz JS, Archer DF: Uterine endometrial peristalsis: A transvaginal ultrasound study. *Fertil Steril* 54:451, 1990

116. de Vries K, Lyons EA, Ballard G, Levi CS, Lindsay DJ: Contractions of the inner third of the myometrium. *Am J Obstet Gynecol* 162:679, 1990

117. Lyons EA, Taylor PJ, Zheng XH, Ballard G, Levi CS, Kredentser JV: Characterization of subendometrial myometrial contractions throughout the menstrual cycle in normal fertile women. *Fertil Steril* 55:771, 1991

118. Chalubinski K, Deutinger J, Bernaschek G: Vaginosonography for recording of cycle-related myometrial contractions. *Fertil Steril* 59:225, 1993

119. Narayan R, Goswamy R: Subendometrial-myometrial contractil-

ity in conception and non-conception embryo transfer cycles. *Ultrasound Obstet Gynecol* 4:499, 1994

120. Ritchie WGM: Sonographic evaluation of normal and induced ovulation. *Radiology* 161:1, 1986

121. Luciano AA, Peluso J, Koch EI, Maier D, Kuslis S, Davison E: Temporal relationship and the reliability of the clinical, hormonal, and ultrasonographic indices of ovulation in infertile women. *Obstet Gynecol* 75:412, 1990

122. Martinuk SD, Chizen DR, Pierson RA: Ultrasonographic morphology of the human preovulatory follicle wall prior to ovulation. *Clin Anat* 5:339, 1992

123. Hanna MD, Chizen DR, Pierson RA: Characteristics of follicular evacuation during human ovulation. *Ultrasound Obstet Gynecol* 4:488, 1994

124. Ritchie WGM: Ultrasound in the evaluation of normal and induced ovulation. *Fertil Steril* 43:167, 1985

125. Hodgen GD: The dominant ovarian follicle. *Fertil Steril* 38:281, 1982

126. Pache TD, Wladimiroff JW, de Jong FH, Hop WC, Fauser BCJM: Growth patterns of nondominant ovarian follicles during the normal menstrual cycle. *Fertil Steril* 54:638, 1990

127. Queenan JT, O'Brien GD, Bains LM, Simpson J, Collins WP, Campbell S: Ultrasound scanning of ovaries to detect ovulation in women. *Fertil Steril* 34:99, 1980

128. Bryce RL, Shutter B, Sinosich MI, Stiel JN, Picker RH, Saunders DM: The value of ultrasound, gonadotropin and estradiol measurements for precise ovulation prediction. *Fertil Steril* 37:42, 1982

129. Vermesh M, Kletzky OA, Davajan V, Israel R: Monitoring technique to predict and detect ovulation. *Fertil Steril* 47:259, 1987

130. Seibel MM, Smith DM, Levesque L, et al: The temporal relationship between the luteinizing hormone surge and human oocyte maturation. *Am J Obstet Gynecol* 142:568, 1982

131. Zandt-Stastny D, Thorsen MK, Middleton WD, et al: Inability of sonography to detect imminent ovulation. *Am J Roentgenol* 152:91, 1989

132. Hilgers TW, Kimball CR, Keck SJ, Dvorak AD, Tamisiea DF, Yaksich PJ: Assessment of the empty follicle syndrome by transvaginal sonography. *J Ultrasound Med* 11:313, 1992

133. Lenz S: Ultrasonic study of follicular maturation, ovulation and development of corpus luteum during normal menstrual cycles. *Acta Obstet Gynecol Scand* 64:15, 1985

134. Jaffe R, Abramowicz J, Ben Aderet N: Correlation between the endocrine profile of ovulation and the ultrasonically detected "double contour" of the preovulatory follicle. *Gynecol Obstet Invest* 24:119, 1987

135. Pearlstone AC, Surrey ES: The temporal relation between the urine LH surge and sonographic evidence of ovulation: Determinants and clinical significance. *Obstet Gynecol* 83:184, 1994

136. DeCherney AH, Laufer N: The monitoring of ovulation induction using ultrasound and estrogen. *Clin Obstet Gynecol* 27:993, 1984

137. Forman RG, Robinson J, Yudkin P, Egan D, Reynolds K, Barlow DH: What is true follicular diameter: An assessment of the repro-

ducibility of transvaginal ultrasound monitoring in stimulated cycles. *Fertil Steril* 56:989, 1991

138. Simonetti S, Veeck LL, Jones HW Jr: Correlation of follicular fluid volume with oocyte morphology from follicles stimulated by human menopausal gonadotropin. *Fertil Steril* 44:177, 1985

139. Penzias AS, Emmi AM, Dubey AK, Layman LC, De Cherney AH, Reindollar RH: Ultrasound prediction of follicle volume: Is the mean diameter reflective? *Fertil Steril* 62:1274, 1994

140. Polson DW, Adams J, Wadsworth J, Franks S: Polycystic ovaries: A common finding in normal women. *Lancet* 1:870, 1988

141. Clayton RN, Ogden V, Hodgkinson J, et al: How common are polycystic ovaries in normal women and what is their significance for the fertility of the population. *Clin Endocrinol* 37:127, 1992

142. Farquhar CM, Birdsall M, Manning P, Mitchell JM: Transabdominal versus transvaginal ultrasound in the diagnosis of polycystic ovaries in a population of randomly selected women. *Ultrasound Obstet Gynecol* 4:54, 1994

143. Swanson M, Sauerbrei EE, Cooperberg PL: Medical implications of ultrasonically detected polycystic ovaries. *J Clin Ultrasound* 9:219, 1981

144. Conway GS, Honour JW, Jacobs HS: Heterogeneity of the polycystic ovary syndrome: Clinical endocrine and ultrasound features in 556 patients. *Clin Endocrinol (Oxf)* 30:459, 1989

145. Adams J, Polson DW, Franks S: Prevalence of polycystic ovaries in women with anovulation and idiopathic hirsutism. *Br Med J* 293:355, 1986

146. Pache TD, de Jong FH, Hop WC, Fauser BCJM: Association between ovarian changes assessed by transvaginal sonography and clinical and endocrine signs of the polycystic ovary syndrome. *Fertil Steril* 59:544, 1993

147. Parisi L, Tramonti M, Derchi LE, Casciano S, Zurli A, Rocchi P: Polycystic ovarian disease: Ultrasonic evaluation and correlations with clinical and hormonal data. *J Clin Ultrasound* 12:21, 1984

148. Hann LE, Hall DA, McArdle CR, Seibel MM: Polycystic ovarian disease: Sonographic spectrum. *Radiology* 150:531, 1984

149. Orsini LF, Venturoli S, Lorusso R, Plochinotta V, Paradisi R, Bovicelli L: Ultrasonic findings in polycystic ovarian disease. *Fertil Steril* 43:709, 1985

150. Yeh HC, Futterweit W, Thornton JC: Polycystic ovarian disease: US features in 104 patients. *Radiology* 163:111, 1987

151. Ardaens Y, Robert Y, Lemaitre L, Fossati P, Dewailly D: Polycystic ovarian disease: Contribution of vaginal endosonography and reassessment of ultrasonic diagnosis. *Fertil Steril* 55:1062, 1991

152. Pache TD, Wladimiroff JW, Hop WCJ, Fauser BCJM: How to discriminate between normal and polycystic ovaries: Transvaginal US study. *Radiology* 183:421, 1992

153. Adams J, Franks S, Polson DW, et al: Multifollicular ovaries: Clinical and endocrine features and response to pulsatile gonadotropin releasing hormone. *Lancet* 2:1375, 1985

154. Fox R, Corrigan E, Thomas PA, Hull MGR: The diagnosis of polycystic ovaries in women with oligo-amenorrhea: Predictive power of endocrine tests. *Clin Endocrinol (Oxf)* 34:1271, 1991

155. Coulam CB, Hill LM, Breckle R: Ultrasonic evidence for luteinization of unruptured preovulatory follicles. *Fertil Steril* 37:524, 1982

156. Kerin JF, Kirby C, Morris D, et al: Incidence of luteinized unruptured follicle phenomenon in cycling women. *Fertil Steril* 40:620, 1983

157. Liukkonen S, Koskimies AI, Tenhunen A, Ylostalo P: Diagnosis of luteinized unruptured follicle (LUF) syndrome by ultrasound. *Fertil Steril* 41:26, 1984

158. Killick S, Elstein M: Pharmacologic production of luteinized unruptured follicles by prostaglandin synthetase inhibitors. *Fertil Steril* 47:773, 1987

159. Check JH, Dietterich C, Nowroozi K, Wu CH: Comparison of various therapies for the luteinized unruptured follicle. *Int J Fertil* 37:33, 1992

160. Koninckx PR, Renaer M, Brosens IA: Origin of peritoneal fluid in women: An ovarian exudation product. *Br J Obstet Gynaecol* 87:177, 1980

161. Janssen-Caspers HAB, Kruitwagen RFPM, Wladimiroff JW, deJong FH, Drogendijk AC: Diagnosis of luteinized unruptured follicles by ultrasound and steroid hormone assays in peritoneal fluid: A comparative study. *Fertil Steril* 46:823, 1986

162. Hamilton MP, Fleming R, Coutts JR, Macnaughton MC, Whitfield CR: Luteal cysts and unexplained infertility: biochemical and ultrasonic evaluation. *Fertil Steril* 54:32, 1990

163. Toda T: Ultrasonographical study on luteinized unruptured follicle. *Nippon Sanka Fujinka Gakkai Zasshi* 42:1195, 1990

164. Mio Y, Toda T, Harada T, Terakawa N: Luteinized unruptured follicle in the early stages of endometriosis as a cause of unexplained infertility. *Am J Obstet Gynecol* 167:271, 1992

165. Bateman BG, Kolp LA, Nunley WC, et al: Oocyte retention after follicle luteinization. *Fertil Steril* 54:793, 1990

166. Coulam CB, Bustillo M, Schulman JD: Empty follicle syndrome. *Fertil Steril* 46:1153, 1986

167. Ben Shlomo I, Schiff E, Levran D, Ben-Rafael Z, Mashiach S, Dor S: Failure of oocyte retrieval during in vitro fertilization: A sporadic event rather than a syndrome. *Fertil Steril* 55:324, 1991

168. Hilgers TA, Dvorak AD, Tamisiea DF, Ellis RL, Yaksich PJ: Sonographic definition of the empty follicle syndrome. *J Ultrasound Med* 8:411, 1989

169. Hochschild FZ, Fernandez E, Mackenna A, Fabres C, Altieri E, Lopez T: The empty follicle syndrome (EFS): A pharmaceutical industry syndrome (abstract). Presented at the 50th Annual Meeting of the American Fertility Society, November 5–10, 1994, San Antonio, Texas

170. Demoulin A, Bologne R, Hustin J, Lambotte R: Is ultrasound monitoring of follicular growth harmless? *Ann N Y Acad Sci* 442:146, 1985

171. Williams SR, Rotchild R, Wesolowski D, Austin C, Speroff L: Does exposure of preovulatory oocytes to ultrasound radiation affect reproductive performance? *J In Vitro Fertil Embryo Transf* 5:18, 1988

172. Stewart HD, Stewart HF, Morre RM, Garry J: Compilation of reported biologic effects data and ultrasound exposure level. *J Clin Ultrasound* 13:167, 1985

173. Shimonovitz S, Yagel S, Zacut D, et al: Ultrasound transmission gel in the vagina can impair sperm motility. *Hum Reprod* 9:482, 1994

174. Depypere HT, Gordts S, Campo R, Comhaire F: Methods to increase the success rate of artificial insemination with donor semen. *Hum Reprod* 9:661, 1994

175. McArdle CR, Seibel MM, Weinstein F, Hann LE, Nickerson C, Taymor ML: Induction of ovulation monitored by ultrasound. *Radiology* 148:809, 1983

176. Goldberg MJ, Miller FM, Friedman CI, Dodds WG, Kim MH: Effect of baseline ovarian cysts on in vitro fertilization and gamete intrafallopian transfer cycles. *Fertil Steril* 55:319, 1991

177. Thatcher SS, Jones E, DeCherney AH: Ovarian cysts decrease the success of controlled ovarian stimulation in in vitro fertilization cycles. *Fertil Steril* 52:812, 1989

178. Tummon IS, Henig I, Radwanska E, Binor Z, Rawlins R, Dmowski WP: Persistent ovarian cysts following administration of human menopausal and chorionic gonadotropins: An attenuated form of ovarian hyperstimulation syndrome. *Fertil Steril* 49:244, 1988

179. Hornstein MD, Barbieri RL, Ravnikar VA, McShane PM: The effects of baseline ovarian cysts on the clinical response to controlled ovarian hyperstimulation in an in vitro fertilization program. *Fertil Steril* 52:437, 1989

180. Karande VC, Scott RT, Jones GS, Muasher SJ: Non-functional ovarian cysts do not affect ipsilateral or contralateral ovarian performance during in vitro fertilization. *Hum Reprod* 5:431, 1990

181. Rizk B, Tan SL, Kingsland C, Steer C, Mason BA, Campbell S: Ovarian cyst aspiration and the outcome of in vitro fertilization. *Fertil Steril* 54:661, 1990

182. Dicker D, Goldman JA, Feldberg D, Ashkenazi J, Levy T: Transvaginal ultrasonic needle-guided aspiration of endometriotic cysts before ovulation induction for in vitro fertilization. *J In Vitro Fertil Embryo Transf* 8:286, 1991

183. Dor J, Shulman A, Levran D, Ben-Rafael Z, Radak E, Mashiach S: The treatment of patients with polycystic ovarian syndrome by in vitro fertilization and embryo transfer: A comparison of results with those of patients with tubal infertility. *Hum Reprod* 5:816, 1990

184. Nayudu PL: Relationship of constructed follicular growth pattern in stimulated cycles to outcome after IVF. *Hum Reprod* 6:465, 1992

185. Seibel MM: A new era in reproductive technology: In vitro fertilization, gamete intrafallopian transfer and donated gametes and embryos. *N Engl J Med* 318:828, 1988

186. Buttery B, Trouson A, McMater R, Wood C: Evaluation of diagnostic ultrasound as a parameter of follicular development in an in vitro fertilization program. *Fertil Steril* 39:458, 1983

187. Kerin JF, Edmonds DK, Warnes GM, et al: Morphological and functional relationships of graafian follicle growth to ovulation in women using ultrasonic, laparoscopic and biochemical measurements. *Br J Obstet Gynaecol* 88:81, 1981

188. Marrs RP, Vargyas JM, March CM: Correlation of ultrasonic and endocrinologic measurements in human menopausal gonadotropin therapy. *Am J Obstet Gynecol* 145:417, 1983

189. Schenker JG, Weinstein D: Ovarian hyperstimulation syndrome: A current survey. *Fertil Steril* 30:255, 1978

190. Craft I, Ah-Moye M, Al-Shawaf T, et al: Analysis of 1071 GIFT procedures: The case for a flexible approach to treatment. *Lancet* 2:1094, 1988

191. Golan A, Ron-El R, Herman A, Soffer Y, Weinraub Z, Caspi E: Ovarian hyperstimulation syndrome: An update review. *Obstet Gynecol Surv* 44:430, 1989

192. Navot D, Bergh PA, Laufer N: Ovarian hyperstimulation syndrome in novel reproductive technologies: Prevention and treatment. *Fertil Steril* 58:249, 1992

193. McArdle CR, Seibel MM, Hann LE, Weinstein F, Taymor ML: The diagnosis of ovarian hyperstimulation (OHS): The impact of ultrasound. *Fertil Steril* 39:464, 1983

194. Blankstein J, Shalev J, Saadon T, et al: Ovarian hyperstimulation syndrome: Prediction by number and size of preovulatory follicles. *Fertil Steril* 47:597, 1987

195. Aboulghar MA, Mansour RT, Serour GI, Amin Y: Ultrasonically guided vaginal aspiration of ascites in the treatment of severe ovarian hyperstimulation syndrome. *Fertil Steril* 53:933, 1990

196. Schwartz M, Jewelewicz R: The use of gonadotropins for induction of ovulation. *Fertil Steril* 35:3, 1981

197. Navot D, Goldstein N, Mor Yosef S, Simon A, Relon A, Birkenfeld A: Multiple pregnancies: Risk and prognostic variables during induction of ovulation with human menopausal gonadotropins. *Hum Reprod* 6:1152, 1991

198. Ben-Nun I, Cohen I, Shulman A, Fejgin M, Goldberger S, Beyth Y: The inability of preovulatory ovarian scan to predict multifetal pregnancy occurrence in a follow-up of induction of ovulation with menotropins. *Fertil Steril* 60:781, 1993

199. Shoham Z, Patel A, Jacobs HS: Polycystic ovarian syndrome: Safety and effectiveness of stepwise and low-dose administration of purified follicle-stimulating hormone. *Fertil Steril* 55:1051, 1991

200. Staessen C, Janssenswillens C, van den Abbeel E, Devroey P, van Steirtegem AC: Avoidance of triplet pregnancies by elective transfer of two good quality embryos. *Hum Reprod* 8:1650, 1993

201. Evans MI, Dommergues M, Wapner RJ, et al: Efficacy of transabdominal multifetal pregnancy reduction: Collaborative experience of the world's largest centers. *Obstet Gynecol* 82:61, 1993

202. Timor-Tritsch IE, Peisner DB, Monteagudo A, Lerner JP, Sharma S: Multifetal pregnancy reduction by transvaginal puncture: Evaluation of the technique used in 134 cases. *Am J Obstet Gynecol* 168:799, 1993

203. Lenz S, Lauritsen JG: Ultrasonically guided percutaneous aspiration of human follicles under local anesthesia: A new method of collecting oocytes for in vitro fertilization. *Fertil Steril* 38:673, 1982

204. Lewin A, Laufer N, Rabinowitz R, Margalioth EJ, Bar I, Schenker JG: Ultrasonically guided oocyte collection under local anesthesia: The first choice method for in vitro fertilization—A comparative study with laparoscopy. *Fertil Steril* 46:257, 1986

205. Parsons J, Riddle A, Booker M, et al: Oocyte retrieval for in vitro

fertilization by ultrasonically guided needle aspiration via the urethra. *Lancet* 1:1076, 1985

206. Russel JB, DeCherney AH, Hobbins JC: A new transvaginal probe and biopsy guide for oocyte retrieval. *Fertil Steril* 47:350, 1987

207. Kemeter P, Feichtinger W: Transvaginal oocyte retrieval using a transvaginal sector scan probe combined with an automated puncture device. *Hum Reprod* 1:21, 1986

208. Gonen Y, Blanker J, Casper RF: Transvaginal ultrasonically guided follicular aspiration: A comparative study with laparoscopically guided follicular aspiration. *J Clin Ultrasound* 18:257, 1990

209. Schenker JG, Ezra Y: Complications of assisted reproductive techniques. *Fertil Steril* 61:411, 1994

210. Bennet SJ, Waterstone JJ, Cheng WC, Parsons J: Complications of transvaginal ultrasound-directed follicle aspiration: A review of 2670 consecutive procedures. *J In Vitro Fertil Embryo Transf* 10:72, 1993

211. Bergh T, Lundkvist O: Clinical complications during in vitro fertilization treatment. *Hum Reprod* 7:625, 1992

212. Dicker D, Ashkenazi J, Feldberg D, Levy T, Dekel A, Ben-Rafael Z: Severe abdominal complications after transvaginal ultrasonically guided retrieval of oocytes for in vitro fertilization and embryo transfer. *Fertil Steril* 59:1313, 1993

213. Jansen RP, Anderson JC: Catheterisation of the fallopian tubes from the vagina. *Lancet* 2:309, 1987

214. Jansen RP, Anderson JC, Sutherland PD: Non-operative embryo transfer to the fallopian tube. *N Engl J Med* 319:288, 1988

215. Bustillo M, Munabi AK, Schulman JD: Pregnancy after nonsurgical ultrasound guided gamete intrafallopian transfer. *N Engl J Med* 319:313, 1988

216. Jansen RP, Anderson JC: Transvaginal versus laparoscopic gamete intrafallopian transfer: A case controlled retrospective comparison. *Fertil Steril* 59:836, 1993

217. Seibel MM: The role of ultrasound in infertility. In: Seibel MM, Blackwell RE (eds), *Ovulation Induction*. New York, Raven, 1994:171–190

218. Hureley VA, Osborn JC, Leoni MA, Leeton J: Ultrasound-guided embryo transfer: A controlled trial. *Fertil Steril* 55:559, 1991

219. Al Whawaf T, Dave R, Harper J, Linehan D, Riley P, Craft I: Transfer of embryos into the uterus: How much do technical factors affect pregnancy rates. *J Assist Reprod Genet* 10:31, 1993

220. Kato O, Takatsuka R, Asch RH: Transvaginal-transmyometrial embryo transfer: The Towako method—Experiences of 104 cases. *Fertil Steril* 59:51, 1993

221. Davidson G, Leeton J: Management of unruptured tubal pregnancy by aspiration of sac under ultrasound control. *Lancet* 2:276, 1988

222. Feichtinger W, Memeter P: Conservative treatment of ectopic pregnancy by transvaginal aspiration under sonographic control and methotrexate injection. *Lancet* 1:381, 1987

223. Leeton J, Davidson G: Nonsurgical management of unruptured tubal pregnancy with intra-amniotic methotrexate: Preliminary report of two cases. *Fertil Steril* 50:167, 1988

224. Timor-Tritsch I, Baxi L, Peisner DB: Transvaginal salpingocentesis: A new technique for treating ectopic pregnancy. *Am J Obstet Gynecol* 160:459, 1989

225. McArdle CR: Ultrasound in infertility. In: Seibel MM (ed), *Infertility: A Comprehensive Text*. Norwalk, CT, Appleton & Lange, 1990:285–310

226. Thaler I, Manor D, Brandes J, Rottem S, Itskovitz J: Basic principles and clinical applications of the transvaginal Doppler duplex system in reproductive medicine. *J In Vitro Fertil Embryo Transf* 7:74, 1990

227. Fleischer AC: Ultrasound imaging 2000: Assessment of uteroovarian blood flow with transvaginal color Doppler sonography—Potential clinical applications in infertility. *Fertil Steril* 55:684, 1991

228. Taylor KJ, Burns PN, Wells PN, Conway DI, Hull MG: Ultrasound Doppler flow studies of the ovarian and uterine arteries. *Br J Obstet Gynaecol* 92:240, 1985

229. Feichtinger W, Putz M, Kemeter P: Transvaginal Doppler sonography for measuring blood flow in the pelvis. *Ultraschall Med* 9:30, 1988

230. Deutinger J, Reinthaller A, Bernaschek G: Transvaginal pulsed Doppler measurement of blood flow velocity in the ovarian arteries during cycle stimulation and after follicle puncture. *Fertil Steril* 51:466, 1989

231. Scholtes MCW, Wladimiroff JW, van Rijen HJM, Hop VCJ: Uterine and ovarian flow velocity waveforms in the normal menstrual cycle: A transvaginal Doppler study. *Fertil Steril* 52:981, 1989

232. Steer CV, Campbell S, Pampiglione JS, Kingsland CR, Mason BA, Collins WP: Transvaginal colour flow imaging of the uterine arteries during the ovarian and menstrual cycles. *Hum Reprod* 5:391, 1990

233. Long MG, Boultbee JE, Hanson ME, Begent RH: Doppler time velocity waveform studies of the uterine artery and uterus. *Br J Obstet Gynaecol* 96:588, 1989

234. Goswamy RK, Steptoe PC: Doppler ultrasound studies of the uterine artery in spontaneous ovarian cycles. *Hum Reprod* 3:721, 1988

235. Kupesic S, Kurjak A: Uterine and ovarian perfusion during the periovulatory period assessed by transvaginal color Doppler. *Fertil Steril* 60:439, 1993

236. Steer CV, Campbell S, Tan SL, et al: The use of transvaginal color flow imaging after in vitro fertilization to identify optimum uterine conditions before embryo transfer. *Fertil Steril* 57:372, 1992

237. Santolaya-Forgas J: Physiology of the menstrual cycle by ultrasonography. *J Ultrasound Med* 11:139, 1992

238. Sladkevicius P, Valentin L, Marsal K: Blood flow velocity in the uterine and ovarian arteries during the normal menstrual cycles. *Ultrasound Obstet Gynecol* 3:199, 1993

239. Fugino Y, Ito F, Matuoka I, Kojima T, Koh B, Ogita S: Pulsatility index of uterine artery in pregnant and non-pregnant women. *Hum Reprod* 8:1126, 1993

240. Zaidi J, Jurkovic D, Campbell S, Okokon E, Tan SL: Circadian variation in uterine artery blood flow indices during the follicular phase of the menstrual cycle. *Ultrasound Obstet Gynecol* 5:406, 1995

241. Steer CV, Tan SL, Mason BA, Campbell S: Midluteal-phase vaginal color Doppler assessment of uterine artery impedance in a subfertile population. *Fertil Steril* 61:53, 1994

242. Kurjak A, Kupesic-Urek S, Schulman H, Zalud I: Transvaginal color flow Doppler in the assessment of ovarian and uterine blood flow in infertile women. *Fertil Steril* 56:870, 1991

243. Goswamy RK, Williams G, Steptoe PC: Decreased uterine perfusion: A cause of infertility. *Hum Reprod* 3:955, 1988

244. Strezik K, Grab D, Vasse V, Hutter W, Roesenbusch B, Terinde R: Doppler sonographic findings and their correlation with implantation in an in vitro fertilization program. *Fertil Steril* 52:825, 1989

245. Strohmer J, Herczeg H, Plockinger B, Kemeter P, Feichtinger W: Prognostic appraisal of success and failure of an in vitro fertilization program by transvaginal Doppler ultrasound at the time of ovulation induction. *Ultrasound Obstet Gynecol* 1:272, 1991

246. Favre R, Bettahar K, Grange G, et al: Predictive value of transvaginal uterine Doppler assessment in an in vitro fertilization program. *Ultrasound Obstet Gynecol* 3:350, 1993

247. de Ziegler D, Bessis R, Frydman R: Vascular resistance of uterine arteries: Physiological effects of estradiol and progesterone. *Fertil Steril* 55:775, 1991

248. Achiron R, Levran D, Sivan E, Lipitz S, Dor J, Mashiach S: Endometrial blood flow response to hormone replacement therapy in women with premature ovarian failure: A transvaginal Doppler study. *Fertil Steril* 63:550, 1995

249. Applebaum M: The uterine biophysical profile. *Ultrasound Obstet Gynecol* 5:67, 1995

250. Merce LT, Garces D, Barco MJ, de la Fuente F: Intraovarian Doppler velocimetry in ovulatory, disovulatory and anovulatory cycles. *Ultrasound Obstet Gynecol* 2:197, 1992

251. Hata K, Hata T, Senoh D, et al: Change in ovarian arterial compliance during the human menstrual cycle assessed by Doppler ultrasound. *Br J Obstet Gynaecol* 97:163, 1990

252. Weiner Z, Thaler I, Levron J, Lewit N, Itskovitz-Eldor J: Assessment of ovarian and uterine blood flow by transvaginal color Doppler in ovarian-stimulated women: Correlation with the number of follicles and steroid hormone levels. *Fertil Steril* 59:743, 1993

253. Bourne TH, Jurkovic D, Waterstone J, Campbell S, Collins WP: Intrafollicular blood flow during human ovulation. *Ultrasound Obstet Gynecol* 1:53, 1991

254. Collins W, Jurkovic D, Bourne T, Kurjak A, Campbell S: Ovarian morphology, endocrine function and intra-follicular blood flow during the peri-ovulatory period. *Hum Reprod* 6:319, 1991

255. Campbell S, Bourne TH, Waterstone J, et al: Transvaginal color blood flow imaging of the periovulatory follicle. *Fertil Steril* 60:433, 1993

256. Zalud I, Kurjak A: The assessment of luteal blood flow in pregnant and non-pregnant women by transvaginal color Doppler. *J Perinat Med* 18:215, 1990

257. Baber RJ, McSweeney MB, Gill RW, et al: Transvaginal pulsed Doppler assessment of blood flow to the corpus luteum in IVF patients following embryo transfer. *Br J Obstet Gynaecol* 95:1226, 1988

258. Tikanen H: The role of vascularization of the corpus luteum in the short luteal phase studied by Doppler ultrasound. *Acta Obstet Gynecol Scand* 73:321, 1994

259. Bourne TH, Reynolds K, Waterstone J, et al: Paracetamol-associated luteinized unruptured follicle syndrome: Effect on intrafollicular blood flow. *Ultrasound Obstet Gynecol* 1:420, 1991

260. Battalgia C, Artini PG, D'Ambrogio G, Genazzani AD, Genazzani AR: The role of color Doppler imaging in the diagnosis of polycystic ovary syndrome. *Am J Obstet Gynecol* 172:108, 1995

261. Tekay A, Martikainen, Jouppila P: Doppler parameters of the ovarian and uterine blood circulation in ovarian hyperstimulation syndrome. *Ultrasound Obstet Gynecol* 6:50, 1995

262. Pellicer A, Ballester MJ, Serrano MD, et al: Aetiological factors involved in the low response to gonadotropins in infertile women with normal basal serum follicle stimulating hormone levels. *Hum Reprod* 9:806, 1994

263. Balakier H, Stronell RD: Color Doppler assessment of folliculogenesis in in vitro fertilization patients. *Fertil Steril* 62:1211, 1994

264. Rumack CM, Wilson SR, Charboneau JW: *Diagnostic Ultrasound.* St. Louis, Mosby Year Book, 1991

265. Wolverson MK, Houltoun E, Heiberg E, et al: High resolution real time sonography of scrotal varicocele. *Am J Roentgenol* 141:775, 1983

266. Kuligowska E, Baker CE, Oates BD: Male infertility: Role of transrectal ultrasound in diagnosis and management. *Radiology* 185:353, 1992

PART VII

Hormonal Treatment of Infertility of Women

CHAPTER 29

Ovulation Initiation with Clomiphene Citrate

DIRAN CHAMOUN · HOWARD D. McCLAMROCK · ELI Y. ADASHI

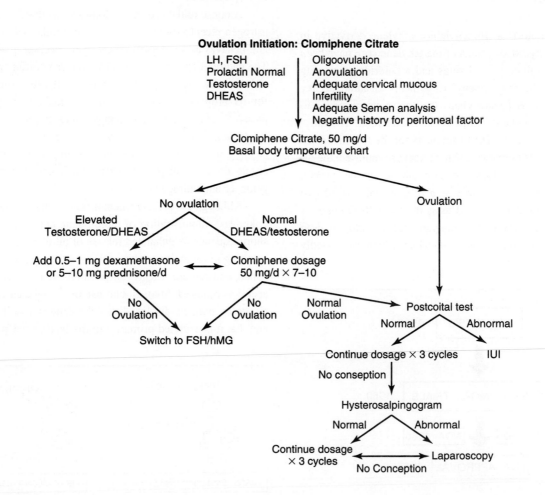

Ovulation Initiation: Clomiphene Citrate

LH, FSH   Oligoovulation
Prolactin Normal   Anovulation
Testosterone   Adequate cervical mucous
DHEAS   Infertility
     Adequate Semen analysis
     Negative history for peritoneal factor

Clomiphene Citrate, 50 mg/d
Basal body temperature chart

No ovulation   Ovulation

Elevated Testosterone/DHEAS   Normal DHEAS/testosterone

Add 0.5–1 mg dexamethasone or 5–10 mg prednisone/d   Clomiphene dosage 50 mg/d × 7–10

No Ovulation   No Ovulation   Normal Ovulation   Postcoital test

Switch to FSH/hMG

Normal   Abnormal

Continue dosage × 3 cycles   IUI

No conseption

Hysterosalpingogram

Normal   Abnormal

Continue dosage × 3 cycles   Laparoscopy

No Conception

Synthesized in 1956, clomiphene citrate was first used in clinical trials as early as 1960[1] (Fig 29–1). These efforts were followed in short sequence by the appearance of the first published report describing the successful use of the drug to induce ovulation in humans.[2] Specifically, clomiphene citrate (still known as MRL-41) was shown to effect ovulation in 28 of 36 women with chronic anovulation; confirmatory reports followed.[3–11] An investigational new drug application having been filed in 1962, approval for widespread clinical use of clomiphene citrate was ultimately granted by the U.S. Food and Drug Administration (FDA) in 1967 with the stipulation that the total dosage consumed per treatment cycle not exceed 750 mg. The original William S. Merrell Company patent rights[12] have expired, leading to the introduction of preparations listed under brand names other than Clomid, such as Serophene, a product of Serono Laboratories (Randolph, MA). By most accounts, the efficacy of the various brands of clomiphene citrate appears comparable.

PHARMACOLOGY

Clomiphene citrate is a triphenylchloroethylene derivative in which the four hydrogen atoms of the ethylene core have been substituted with three phenyl rings and a chloride anion (Fig 29–2). One of the three phenyl rings bears an aminoalkoxy (OCH_2–CH_2–$N[C_2K_5]_2$) side chain, the importance of which to the action of clomiphene citrate remains uncertain. The dihydrogen citrate moiety ($C_6H_8O_7$) accounts for the fact that commercially available preparations in clinical use represent the dihydrogen citrate salt form of clomiphene citrate proper. Clomiphene citrate is available as a racemic mixture of two stereochemical isomers referred to as the *trans* (62%) and *cis* (38%) isomers (Fig 29–3). In some parts of the world, the drug is available in its *cis* form as a 10-mg tablet, which is reportedly

OCH_2—CH_2—$N(C_2H_5)_2$

$\cdot C_6 H_8 O_7$

Cl

2-[p-(2-chloro-1,2-diphenylvinyl) phenoxy] triethylamine dihydrogen citrate

Figure 29–2. Structural formula of clomiphene citrate.

equipotent with the 50-mg tablet sold in the United States. Limited experience suggests that the clinical utility of clomiphene citrate may indeed be due to its *cis* isomer.[13,14] It remains uncertain, however, whether *cis*-clomiphene citrate is more effective than clomiphene citrate proper in terms of ovulation and conception rates.[15–18]

A nonsteroidal estrogen, clomiphene citrate interacts with estrogen receptor-binding proteins not unlike native estrogens and behaves as a competitive estrogen receptor antagonist.[19,20] The nature of the interaction, however, may differ from that of the naturally occurring ligand. Specifically, the drug is known for its propensity toward prolonged nuclear receptor occupancy.[20–22] Indeed, it may occupy nuclear receptor sites for weeks at a time, as compared with native estrogens capable of clearing the cell within 24 hours. Of importance, clomiphene citrate does not display progestational, corticotropic, androgenic, or antiandrogenic properties.

Although the precise mechanism of action remains largely unknown, administration of clomiphene citrate is followed in short sequence by enhanced release of pituitary gonadotropins, resulting in follicular recruitment, selection, assertion of dominance, and rupture. Clearly then otherwise intact reproductive access is required. Studies with use of ^{14}C-labeled clomiphene citrate by humans disclosed that the drug is readily absorbed and that it is excreted primarily in the feces.[23–25] Up to 50% of

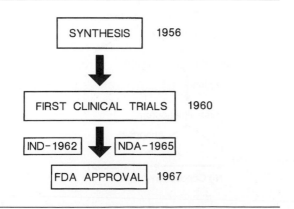

| SYNTHESIS | 1956 |

FIRST CLINICAL TRIALS | 1960

IND-1962 | NDA-1965

FDA APPROVAL | 1967

Figure 29–1. Developmental landmarks of clomiphene citrate. IND, investigational new drug application; NDA, new drug application; FDA, U.S. Food and Drug Administration.

OCH_2-CH_2-$N(C_2H_5)_2$

$\cdot C_6H_8O_7$

Cl

TRANS = ENCLOMIPHENE CITRATE

OCH_2-CH_2-$N(C_2H_5)_2$

Cl

$\cdot C_6H_8O_7$

CIS = ZUCLOMIPHENE CITRATE

Figure 29–3. Stereochemical isomers of clomiphene citrate.

the compound is excreted within 5 days. Computations based on a half-life estimate of 5 days suggest finite residual drug concentrations until and possibly beyond midcycle. The role of the residual at midcycle in the ovulatory agenda remains uncertain.[26]

ADMINISTRATION

Indications

The primary indication for the use of clomiphene citrate is normogonadotropic, normoprolactinemic, anovulatory infertility.[27–29] Patients with inappropriate gonadotropin release (an increased luteinizing hormone–to–follicle-stimulating hormone [LH/FSH] ratio), as occurs in the polycystic ovary (PCO) syndrome, are also excellent candidates for clomiphene citrate therapy.[27–29] Eligible patients are likely to have a chronic anovulatory disorder that often dates back to puberty. They are also likely to be well estrogenized as assessed by progestin-induced withdrawal bleeding, normal to high circulating levels of estrone and estradiol-17β, and the occasional finding of abnormal endometrial growth such as cystic hyperplasia. Of importance, it is the adequate estrogen milieu of eligible patients that resulted in the suggestion that clomiphene citrate may initiate ovulation because of its antiestrogenic property. In contrast, initiation of ovulation with this compound is generally unsuccessful in hypogonadotropic (estrogen-poor) women, although an empirical trial may be in order.[30–32] Although hyperprolactinemic chronic anovulation may respond to clomiphene citrate[33] such patients should be treated with a dopamine receptor agonist such as bromocriptine.

The empiric use of clomiphene citrate in conjunction with intrauterine insemination (IVI) to treat normally ovulating women with unexplained infertility has gained some popularity.[34–38] The rationale behind the use of clomiphene citrate by these patients has been to overcome any subtle, unpredictable ovulatory dysfunction and possibly to enhance fertilization by increasing the number of oocytes available.[38,39] Finally, in this age of cost containment, attention has again been focused on natural[40–43] and clomiphene citrate–stimulated[45–47] in vitro fertilization (IVF) cycles in an attempt not only to control cost but also to minimize the risks associated with assisted reproductive technologies. Nevertheless, the precise role of clomiphene citrate in the treatment of unexplained infertility and in assisted reproductive cycles remains to be established.

Contraindications

Pregnancy

The unintentional administration of clomiphene citrate during pregnancy might occur under unmonitored circumstances in which absence of a period after a clomiphene citrate cycle may be taken to mean apparent treatment failure. Thus the old clinical dictum of no period, no clomiphene citrate appears to be just as timely as it was when the drug was originally formulated. Increased physician awareness, basal body temperature charting, and pregnancy testing should minimize, if not eliminate, the use of the drug during early pregnancy.

Liver Dysfunction

Liver disease or a history of liver dysfunction is generally viewed as a contraindication to the use of clomiphene citrate. Because the drug is metabolized, if only in part at the level of the liver, when administered in the setting of suboptimal liver function, its effects may prove to be unmanageable and even harmful.

Ovarian Cysts

Because clomiphene citrate is capable of stimulating follicular growth, further enlargement of a preexisting ovarian cyst or of a residual (posttreatment) enlarged ovary may prove to be potentially harmful,[48,49] such as in the rare occurrence of massive ovarian enlargement.[50] Thus patients should be examined for possible ovarian enlargement as clinically indicated after clomiphene citrate therapy. Allowances must be made for the ovary to return to normal size either spontaneously over time or with the use of combination oral contraceptives.

Visual Symptoms

Withholding clomiphene citrate on the basis of its causing visual symptoms is a precautionary measure for which little scientific support exists. Discontinuation of the drug appears warranted if such symptoms (night blindness, scotomata) do occur, because use of the agent is elective and because unforeseen and potentially irreversible (optic neuropathy)[51,52] ophthalmologic sequelae may be avoided.

Monitoring

The use of clomiphene citrate generally does not require intense monitoring. Basal body temperature charting is recommended as an adjunctive measure, however, because of its low cost, simplicity, and harmlessness. Other monitoring options might also be considered as dictated by clinical course.

Steroidogenic Monitoring

The so-called triple 7 regimen is based on the anticipation that the successful initiation of ovulation with clomiphene citrate is marked by unique alterations in serum levels of estradiol-17β and progesterone.[53] Specifically, documentation is sought for a preovulatory increase in estradiol-17β level and a subsequent rise in luteal progesterone level.[54,55] If the various hormonal determinations are timed relative to the last oral dose of clo-

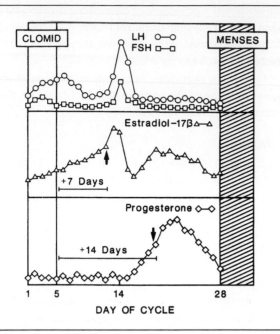

Figure 29–4. Hormonal monitoring of clomiphene (Clomid)–initiated ovulation.

miphene citrate, the triple 7 regimen can be used whether clomiphene citrate is administered for 5, 7, or 10 days.

The protocol used at the University of Maryland calls for determination of the circulating levels of estradiol-17β 7 days after the patient takes the last clomiphene citrate tablet (Fig 29–4). Accordingly, monitoring for estradiol-17β occurs well within the projected window of ovulation; that is, 5 to 10 days after the last oral dose. Using this approach, a preovulatory increase in estradiol-17β level is commonly detected if it is assumed that successful follicular recruitment, selection, and assertion of dominance have occurred. Progesterone sampling is generally performed 7 days after the estradiol determination; that is, 14 days after the last oral dose of clomiphene citrate. This system optimizes the detection of a possible luteal rise. A follow-up office visit is scheduled 7 days after progesterone sampling, which is 21 days after the patient takes the last clomiphene citrate tablet.

Although this regimen involves two hormonal determinations in the course of a cycle, useful information may be derived under circumstances characterized by an apparent lack of response, for example, when basal body temperature charting remains inconclusive or in the face of an apparent treatment failure. Under these circumstances, hormonal monitoring yields indispensable information relative to the occurrence of ovulation or the lack thereof.

Sonographic Monitoring of Follicular Development

Now widely available, ultrasonography may be used independently of or concurrently with hormonal monitoring.[56,57] In fact,

ultrasound monitoring is particularly useful for women who prove to be eligible for human chorionic gonadotropin (hCG) treatment. Follicular monitoring with hCG administration to trigger ovulation affords better cycle control and predictability of ovulation and thus better timing of intercourse or IUI. Best results may therefore be anticipated with the combination of several monitoring modalities.

Establishment of Dosage

The recommended starting dosage for clomiphene citrate is 50 mg daily for a total of 5 days. Although an unequivocal relation between dose level and multiple gestation has not been demonstrated, it is likely that such correlation does exist. It is suggested that use be made of the lowest dose of clomiphene citrate consistent with successful outcome. Therapy may be initiated at any time in the absence of recent uterine bleeding. Patients with chronic anovulation may start treatment at any time. Indeed, uterine bleeding, either spontaneous or induced, is not imperative before the initiation of ovulation. More commonly, treatment is started on or about the fifth day of the cycle after progestin-induced bleeding or spontaneous dysfunctional uterine bleeding, although an earlier or later starting date (up to day 8) is acceptable.

The simplest protocols call for graded incremental therapy when the subsequent cycle dosage proves to be ineffective in inducing ovulation.[58,59] Such decisions can and should be made immediately after the treatment cycle in question. In the absence of ovulation, new treatment courses may begin as early as 30 days after initiation of the previous cycle. Lack of response to 200 or 250 mg daily for 5 days suggests that a change of course is in order. Most pregnancies, however, occur at dosages of 150 mg daily or less (Table 29–1).

Once an ovulatory dosage is obtained, additional modification is neither advantageous nor required. Instead, a 4- to 6-month effort at conception is indicated before any further intervention. This is because of the finding that most clomiphene citrate–associated conceptions[60] are anticipated within the first six ovulatory cycles (Table 29–2). Intercourse every other day

TABLE 29–1. DOSE EFFECTS OF CLOMIPHENE CITRATE

Dose (mg)	Ovulatory Rate (%)	Conception Rate (%)
50	52.1	52.8
100	21.9	20.7
150	12.3	9.8
200	6.9	8.8
250	4.9	6.2

From Gysler M, et al: A decade's experience with an individualized clomiphene treatment regimen including the effect on the postcoital test. Fertil Steril 37:161, 1982.

TABLE 29–2. CLOMIPHENE CITRATE–RELATED CONCEPTIONS: EFFECT OF DURATION OF TREATMENT

Ovulatory Cycle	Cumulative Conceptions (%)
1	51.8
2	76.7
3	84.5
5	91.2
≥6	100.0

From Gysler M, et al: A decade's experience with an individualized clomiphene treatment regimen including the effect on the postcoital test. Fertil Steril 37:161, 1982.

for 1 week beginning 4 days after the last day of clomiphene citrate administration ensures optimal timing for conception.

OVULATION FAILURE

Total Lack of Response

Total lack of response refers to the absence of follicular development and the consequent lack of ovulation after treatment with clomiphene citrate (Fig 29–5). Under these circumstances, consideration might be given to increasing the duration of clomiphene citrate therapy.[61–63] It has long been recognized that prolonged administration of relatively low doses of the drug may succeed when shorter-term high-dose regimens have failed. Although the mechanisms underlying this phenomenon

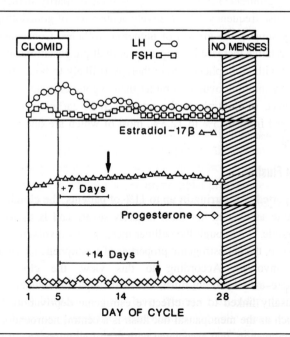

Figure 29–5. Anovulatory response to clomiphene citrate (Clomid).

remain uncertain, it is tempting to speculate that this form of therapy results in more persistent and seemingly more efficient increments in the release of pituitary gonadotropin with consequent ovarian stimulation.

In addition, consideration may be given to dexamethasone supplementation.[64–72] The mechanisms underlying the ability of dexamethasone to synergize with clomiphene citrate are unknown, but it is abundantly clear that these two agents may promote ovulation initiation, particularly in the presence of elevated dehydroepiandosterone sulfate. It remains unknown whether dexamethasone lowers the circulating levels of adrenal androgens (which might otherwise inhibit folliculogenesis or aromatase activity), or whether glucocorticoids may synergize with clomiphene citrate at the level of the hypothalamus—that is, participate in the release of hypothalamic gonadotropin-releasing hormone (GnRH).[73]

Partial Lack of Response

Clomiphene citrate–associated ovulation failure need not be complete. The drug may bring about follicular maturation and progressive increments in serum estradiol-17β level (Fig 29–6). Despite a seemingly adequate preovulatory rise in estradiol-17β level, however, ovulation may not occur for reasons that remain largely unknown. Although ovulation and conception do not occur, the apparent lack of a midcycle gonadotropin surge can be bypassed by the exogenous administration of hCG.

It is anticipated that hormonal monitoring and ultrasonographic follicular measurements will precisely identify patients for whom clomiphene citrate results in follicular maturation but not ovulation and who are candidates for hCG administration. Failure to use these adjunctive modalities may result in the administration of hCG either unnecessarily or at a suboptimal time. It has been estimated that 10% to 20% of women do not conceive with peak clomiphene citrate doses even when supplemented with hCG.

CONCEPTION FAILURE

Failure to conceive refers to the lack of conception in the face of an apparent ovulatory pattern. This requires that clomiphene citrate–associated reproductive tract dysfunction be ruled out.[6,9,74–77] In addition, other possible concurrent infertility factors (for example, male or tuboperitoneal) must be evaluated if not properly assessed before this point.

Clomiphene citrate has been shown to have an antiestrogenic effect on the vaginal epithelium,[6,9,74] uterine cervix,[6,9,74,75,77] and endometrium.[6,74–77] The literature on the effect of clomiphene citrate on cervical mucus has been controversial. Some investigators have reported an adverse effect,[77–86] and others

long-term, prospective, multicenter trial to help resolve these issues.

SUMMARY

Clomiphene citrate remains one of the most widely prescribed medications in the treatment of infertility. It is the medication of choice for a wide range of ovulatory dysfunctions. Women with hyperprolactinemia should not receive the drug, and despite some preliminary reports on the use of clomiphene citrate in regularly ovulating women, its utility for an empiric treatment is still controversial. These two relative contraindications notwithstanding, clomiphene citrate remains a safe, effective, reasonably inexpensive method of therapy for infertility due to disorders of ovulation.

APPENDIX. FAULKNER CENTRE FOR REPRODUCTIVE MEDICINE PATIENT CONSENT FOR THE USE OF CLOMIPHENE CITRATE (CLOMID OR SEROPHENE)

Clomiphene Citrate is an orally administered medication to induce (bring on) ovulation. It can also be used to test the ovaries' responsiveness. Approximately 10% of women taking clomiphene experience some side effects or adverse reactions. Common side effects you may have include:

1. *Multiple births* occur in 6% to 10% of women who conceive on clomiphene. The vast majority of these deliveries are twins, with less than 1% of reported deliveries being triplets or more. If a multiple pregnancy occurs, complications of the pregnancy include: an increased risk of premature labor and/or delivery, fetal injury or death due to prematurity, miscarriage, and toxemia of pregnancy.

2. *Miscarriage* rates in women taking clomiphene vary from 10% to 25%. The miscarriage rate in the general population is 10% to 20%. The reason for a possible increased miscarriage rate is unknown.

3. *Ovarian hyperstimulation* may occur causing the formation of benign ovarian cysts. These cysts may occasionally cause abdominal pain, discomfort, and swelling and very rarely cause the ovary to twist or bleed, which may require abdominal surgery. The cysts usually go away over two to four weeks, but may persist longer. Although an increased incidence of ovarian tumors has been suggested with more than six months of clomiphene treatment, a cause and effect has not been proven. Promptly call your physician if you experience pain or an increase in discomfort.

4. *Breast tenderness* and/or soreness.

5. *Hot flashes* may occur while taking clomiphene. They stop with no consequences.

6. *Transient hair loss* may rarely happen, especially if repeated cycles of clomiphene are required. This stops once treatment is discontinued and is not permanent.

7. *Visual blurring* stops once treatment is discontinued, but requires that you report the reaction promptly to your physician.

8. *The risk of congenital malformations* (birth defects) in children conceived by clomiphene is no different from the incidence of congenital malformations in the general population. However, patients taking clomiphene can have an abnormal baby. To be safe, never take clomiphene if you may be pregnant or once pregnancy is confirmed.

9. *Other* minor reactions include: mood swings, headache, nausea, vomiting, fatigue, insomnia, dizziness, and nervousness. These are limited to the cycle of treatment with clomiphene.

If you experience other adverse reactions, or have any questions concerning your treatment with clomiphene, please contact the office at (617) 983-7300.

I have read the above information and have had all questions answered to my satisfaction. I consent to the use of clomiphene citrate.

Patient Signature   Date

The undersigned has gone over this consent form with the patient and answered any questions and explained any terms that were unfamiliar to the patient.

Signature   Date

Revised 10/31/96

REFERENCES

1. Palopoli FP, Feil VJ, Allen RE, Holtkamp DE, Richardson A Jr: Substituted aminoalkoxytriarylhaloethylenes. *J Med Chem* 10:84, 1967

2. Greenblatt RB, Barfield WE, Jungck EC, Ray AW: Induction of ovulation with MRL/41. *JAMA* 178:101, 1961

3. Charles D: M.R.L. 41 in the treatment of secondary amenorrhea and endometrial hyperplasia. *Lancet* 2:278, 1962

4. Greenblatt BR, Roy S, Mahesh VB, Barfield WE, Jungck EC: Induction of ovulation. *Am J Obstet Gynecol* 84:900, 1962

5. Roy S, Greenblatt RB, Mahesh VB, Jungck EC: Clomiphene citrate: Further observations on its use in induction of ovulation in the human and on its mode of action. *Fertil Steril* 14:575, 1963

6. Whitelaw MJ, Grams LR, Stamm WJ: Clomiphene citrate: Its uses and observations on its probable action. *Am J Obstet Gynecol* 90:355, 1964

7. Puebla RA, Greenblatt RB: Clomiphene citrate in the management of anovulatory uterine bleeding. *J Clin Endocrinol* 24:863, 1964

8. Kistner R: Further observations on the effects of clomiphene citrate in anovulatory females. *Am J Obstet Gynecol* 92:380, 1965

9. Lamb EJ, Guderian AM: Clinical effects of clomiphene in anovulation. *Obstet Gynecol* 28:505, 1966

10. Jones GS, Moraes-Ruehsen MD: Clomiphene citrate for improvement for ovarian function. *Am J Obstet Gynecol* 99:814, 1967

11. MacGregor AH, Johnson JE, Bunde CA: Further clinical experience with clomiphene citrate. *Fertil Steril* 19:616, 1968

12. Allen RE, Palopoli FP, Schumann EL, Vancampan MG Jr: U.S. Patent Office 2:914, 561, 1959

13. Charles D, Klein T, Lunn SF, Loraine JA: Clinical and endocrinological studies with the isomeric components of clomiphene citrate. *J Obstet Gynaecol Br Commonw* 76:1100, 1969

14. Pandya G, Cohen MR: The effect of cis-isomer of clomiphene ci-

trate (cisclomiphene) on cervical mucus and vaginal cytology. *J Reprod Med* 8:133, 1972

15. MacLeod SC, Mitton DM, Parker AS, Tupper WRC: Experience with induction of ovulation. *Am J Obstet Gynecol* 108:814, 1970

16. Murthy YS, Parekh MC, Arronet GH: Experience with clomiphene and cisclomiphene. *Int J Fertil* 16:66, 1971

17. Van Campenhout J, Borreman E, Hyman A, et al: Induction of ovulation with cis clomiphene. *Am J Obstet Gynecol* 115:321, 1973

18. Connaughton JF Jr, Garcia CR, Wallach EE: Induction of ovulation with cisclomiphene and a placebo. *Obstet Gynecol* 43:697, 1974

19. Clark JH, Markaverich BM: The agonistic-antagonistic properties of clomiphene: Review. *Pharmacol Ther* 15:467, 1982

20. Clark JH, Peck EJ Jr: Oestrogen receptors and antagonism of steroid hormone action. *Nature* 251:446, 1974

21. Clark JH, Peck EJ Jr: Estrogen-receptor binding: Relationship to estrogen-induced responses. *J Toxicol Environ Health* 1:561, 1976

22. Adashi EY, Hsueh AJW, Yen SSC: Alterations induced by clomiphene in the concentrations of oestrogen receptors in the uterus, pituitary gland and hypothalamus of female rats. *J Endocrinol* 87:383, 1980

23. Schreiber E, Johnson JE, Plotz EJ, Wiener M: Studies with 14C labeled clomiphene citrate. *Clin Res* 14:287, 1966

24. Holtkamp DE, Staples RE, Greslin JG, Davis RH: Pharmacodynamics of clomiphene in animals. *Excerpt Med Int Congr Ser* 133:68, 1966

25. Clomiphene citrate (Clomid). William S. Merrell Company. *Clin Pharmacol Ther* 8:891, 1967

26. Terakawa N. Shimizu I, Tsutsumi H, Aono T, Matsumoto K: A possible role of clomiphene citrate in the control of pre-ovulatory LH surge during induction of ovulation. *Acta Endocrinol* 190:58, 1985

27. Goldfarb AF, Crawford R: Polycystic ovarian disease, clomiphene and multiple pregnancies. *Obstet Gynecol* 34:307, 1969

28. Yen SSC, Vela P, Ryan KJ: Effect of clomiphene citrate in polycystic ovary syndrome: Relationship between serum gonadotropin and corpus luteum function. *J Clin Endocrinol* 31:7, 1970

29. Lunenfeld B, Insler V: Classification of amenorrhoeic states and their treatment by ovulation induction. *Clin Endocrinol* 3:223, 1974

30. Spellacy WN, Cohen WD: Clomiphene treatment of prolonged secondary amenorrhea associated with pituitary gonadotropin deficiency. *Am J Obstet Gynecol* 97:943, 1967

31. Marshall JC, Fraser TR: Amenorrhea in anorexia nervosa: Assessment and treatment with clomiphene citrate. *Br Med J* 4:590, 1971

32. Garcia-Flores RF, Vazquez-Mendez J: Progressive dosages of clomiphene in hypothalamic anovulation. *Fertil Steril* 42:543, 1984

33. Greenblatt RB, Faucher G, Mahesh VB, et al: Ovulation and pregnancy in the Chiari-Frommel syndrome: Report of 10 cases. *Fertil Steril* 17:742, 1966

34. Glazener CM, Coulson C, Lambert PA, et al: Clomiphene treatment for women with unexplained infertility: Placebo-controlled study of hormonal responses and conception rates. *Gynecol Endocrinol* 4:75, 1990

35. Collins JA: Superovulation in the treatment of unexplained infertility. *Semin Reprod Endocrinol* 8:165, 1990

36. Deaton JL, Gibson M, Blackmer KM, Nakajima ST, Badger GJ, Brumsted JR: A randomized, controlled trial of clomiphene citrate and intrauterine insemination in couples with unexplained infertility or surgically corrected endometriosis. *Fertil Steril* 54:1083, 1990

37. Arici A, Byrd W, Bradshaw K, Kutteh HW, Marshburn P, Carr BR: Evaluation of clomiphene citrate and human chorionic gonadotropin treatment: A prospective, randomized, crossover study during intrauterine insemination cycles. *Fertil Steril* 61:314, 1994

38. Rodin DA, Fisher AM, Clayton RN: Cycle abnormalities in infertile women with regular menstrual cycles: Effects of clomiphene citrate treatment. *Fertil Steril* 62:42, 1994

39. Coutts JRT, Fleming R, Carswell W, et al: The defective luteal phase. In: Jacobs HS (ed), *Advances in Gynecological Endocrinology*. London, Royal College of Obstetrics and Gynecology, 1978:65–91

40. Foulot H, Ranoux C, Dubuisson JB, Rambaud D, Aubriot FX, Poirot C: In vitro fertilization without ovarian stimulation: A simplified protocol applied in 80 cycles. *Fertil Steril* 52:617, 1989

41. Lenton EA, Cooke ID, Hooper M, et al: In vitro fertilization in a natural cycle. *Clin Obstet Gynecol* 6:229, 1992

42. Claman P, Domingo M, Garner P, Leader A, Spence JEH: Natural cycle in vitro fertilization-embryo transfer at the University of Ottowa: An inefficient therapy for tubal infertility. *Fertil Steril* 60:298, 1993

43. Paulson RJ, Sauer MV, Francis MM, Macaso TM, Lobo RA: In vitro fertilization in unstimulated cycles: The University of California experience. *Fertil Steril* 57:290, 1992

44. MacDougall MJ, Tan SL, Hall V, Balen A, Mason BA, Jacobs HS: Comparison of natural with clomiphene citrate–stimulated cycles in in vitro fertilization: A prospective, randomized trial. *Fertil Steril* 61:1052, 1994

45. Seibel MM: Toward reducing risks and costs of egg donation: A preliminary report. *Fertil Steril* 64:199, 1995

46. Corfman RS, Milad MP, Bellavance TL, Ory SJ, Erickson LD, Ball GD: A novel ovarian stimulation protocol for use with the assisted reproductive technologies. *Fertil Steril* 60:864, 1993

47. Steinkampf MP, Kretzer PA, McElroy E, Conway-Myers BA: A simplified approach to in vitro fertilization. *J Reprod Med* 37:199, 1992

48. Roland M: Problems of ovulation induction with clomiphene citrate with report of a case of ovarian hyperstimulation. *Obstet Gynecol* 33:55, 1970

49. Scommegna A, Lash SR: Ovarian overstimulation, massive ascites and singleton pregnancy after clomiphene. *JAMA* 207:753, 1969

50. Southam AL, Janovski NA: Massive ovarian hyperstimulation with clomiphene citrate. *JAMA* 181:443, 1962

51. Lawton AW: Optic neuropathy associated with clomiphene citrate therapy. *Fertil Steril* 61:390, 1994

52. Rock T, Dinar Y, Romem M: Retinal periphlebitis after hormonal treatment. *Ann Ophthalmol* 21:75, 1989

53. Swyer GIM, Radwanska E, McGarrigle HHG: Plasma oestradiol and progesterone estimation for the monitoring of induction of

ovulation with clomiphene and chorionic gonadotropin. *Br J Obstet Gynaecol* 82:794, 1975

54. Fritz MA, Speroff L: The endocrinology of the menstrual cycle: The interaction of folliculogenesis and neuroendocrine mechanisms. *Fertil Steril* 38:509, 1982

55. Fritz MA, Speroff L: Current concepts of the endocrine characteristics of normal menstrual function: The key to diagnosis and management of menstrual disorders. *Clin Obstet Gynecol* 26:647, 1983

56. Seibel MM, Blackwell RE: *Ovulation Induction.* New York, Raven Press, 1994

57. O'Herlihy C, Pepperell RJ, Robinson HP: Ultrasound timing of human chorionic gonadotropin administration in clomiphene stimulated cycles. *Obstet Gynecol* 59:40, 1982

58. Rust LA, Israel R, Mishell DR Jr: An individualized graduated therapeutic regimen for clomiphene citrate. *Am J Obstet Gynecol* 120:785, 1974

59. Drake TS, Tredway DR, Buchanan GC: Continued clinical experience with an increasing dosage regimen of clomiphene citrate administration. *Fertil Steril* 30:274, 1978

60. Gysler M, March CM, Mishell DR Jr, Bailey EJ: A decade's experience with an individualized clomiphene treatment regimen including its effect on the postcoital test. *Fertil Steril* 37:161, 1982

61. Adams R, Mishell DR Jr, Israel R: Treatment of refractory anovulation with increased dosage and prolonged duration of cyclic clomiphene citrate. *Obstet Gynecol* 39:562, 1972

62. Lobo RA, Granger LR, Davajan V, Mishell DR Jr: An extended regimen of clomiphene citrate in women unresponsive to standard therapy. *Fertil Steril* 27:762, 1982

63. O'Herlihy C, Pepperell RJ, Brown JB, et al: Incremental clomiphene therapy: A new method for treating persistent anovulation. *Obstet Gynecol* 58:535, 1981

64. Chang RJ, Abraham GE: Effect of dexamethasone and clomiphene citrate on peripheral steroid levels and ovarian function in a hirsute amenorrheic patient. *Fertil Steril* 27:640, 1972

65. Lobo RA, Paul W, March CM, Granger L, Kletzky OA: Clomiphene and dexamethasone in women unresponsive to clomiphene alone. *Obstet Gynecol* 60:497, 1982

66. Check JH, Rakoff AE, Roy BK: Induction of ovulation with combined glucocorticoid and clomiphene citrate therapy in a minimally hirsute woman. *J Reprod Med* 19:159, 1977

67. Lisse K: Combined and clomiphene-dexamethasone therapy in cases with resistance to clomiphene. *Zentrabl Gynakol* 102:645, 1980

68. Higashiyama S, Yasuda J, Otubo K, Ikada H: Ovulation induction with prednisolone-clomiphene therapy in clomiphene failure. *Jpn J Fertil Steril* 26:1, 1981

69. Diamant YZ, Evron S: Induction of ovulation by combined clomiphene citrate and dexamethasone treatment in clomiphene citrate nonresponders. *Eur J Obstet Gynaecol Reprod Biol* 11:335, 1981

70. Daly DC, Walters CA, Soto-Albors CE, Tohan N, Riddick DH: A randomized study of dexamethasone in ovulation induction with clomiphene citrate. *Fertil Steril* 41:844, 1984

71. Hoffman D, Lobo RA: Serum dehydroepiandrosterone sulfate and the use of clomiphene citrate in anovulatory women. *Fertil Steril* 43:196, 1985

72. Singh KB, Dunnihoo DR, Mahajan DK, Bairnsfather LE: Clomiphene-dexamethasone treatment of clomiphene-resistant women with and without the polycystic ovary syndrome. *J Reprod Med* 37:215, 1992

73. Miyake A, Tasaka K, Sakumoto T, Nagahara Y, Aono T: Hydrocortisone elicits the effect of clomiphene citrate on luteinizing hormone-releasing hormone in vitro. *Acta Endocrinol* 107:145, 1984

74. Van Campenhout J, Simard R, LeDuc B: The antiestrogenic effect of clomiphene in the human being. *Fertil Steril* 19:700, 1968

75. Wall JA, Franklin RR, Kaufmann RH, Kaplan A: The effects of clomiphene citrate on the endometrium. *Am J Obstet Gynecol* 93:842, 1965

76. Kistner RW, Lewis JL, Steiner GJ: Effects of clomiphene citrate on endometrial hyperplasia in the premenopausal female. *Cancer* 19:115, 1966

77. Graff G: Suppression of cervical mucus during clomiphene therapy. *Fertil Steril* 22:209, 1971

78. Van der Merwe JV: The effect of clomiphene and conjugated estrogens on cervical mucus. *S Afr Med J* 60:347, 1981

79. Maxson WS, Pittaway DE, Herbert CM, Garner CH, Wentz AC: Antiestrogenic effect of clomiphene citrate: Correlation with serum estradiol concentrations. *Fertil Steril* 42:356, 1984

80. Tepper R, Lunenfeld B, Shalev J, Oradia J, Blankenstein J: The effect of clomiphene citrate and tamoxifen on the cervical mucus. *Acta Obstet Gynecol Scand* 67:311, 1988

81. Kokia E, Bider D, Lunenfeld B, Blankstein J, Mashiach S, Ben-Raphael Z: Additional exogenous estrogens to improve cervical mucus following clomiphene citrate medication. *Acta Obstet Gynecol Scand* 69:139, 1990

82. Langer R, Golan A, Ron-El R, Pansky M, Newman M, Caspi E: Hormonal changes related to impairment of cervical mucus in cycles stimulated by clomiphene citrate. *Aust N Z J Obstet Gynaecol* 30:254, 1990

83. Randall JM, Templeton A: Cervical mucus score and in vitro sperm-mucus interaction in spontaneous and clomiphene citrate cycles. *Fertil Steril* 56:465, 1991

84. Gelety TJ, Buyalos RP: The effect of clomiphene citrate and menopausal gonadotropins on cervical mucus in ovulatory cycles. *Fertil Steril* 60:471, 1993

85. Acharya U, Irvine DS, Hamilton MP, Templeton AA: The effect of three anti-oestrogen drugs on cervical mucus quality and in vitro sperm-cervical mucus interaction in ovulatory women. *Hum Reprod* 8:437, 1993

86. Massai MR, De Ziegler D, Lesobre V, Bergeron C, Frydman R, Bouchard P: Clomiphene citrate affects cervical mucus and endometrium morphology independently of the changes in plasma hormone levels induced by multiple follicular recruitment. *Fertil Steril* 59:1179, 1993

87. Van Hall EV, Mastboom JL: Luteal phase insufficiency in patients treated with clomiphene. *Am J Obstet Gynecol* 103:165, 1969

88. Jones GS, Maffezzoli RD, Strott CA, et al: Pathophysiology of reproductive failure after clomiphene-induced ovulation. *Am J Obstet Gynecol* 108:847, 1970

89. Garcia J, Jones SG, Wentz AC: The use of clomiphene citrate. *Fertil Steril* 28:707, 1977

90. Gonen Y, Casper RF: Sonographic determination of a possible adverse effect of clomiphene citrate on endometrium growth. *Hum Reprod* 5:670, 1990

91. Dickey RP, Olar TT, Taylor SN, Curole DN, Matulick EM: Relationship of endometrial thickness and pattern to fecundity in ovulation induction cycles: Effect of clomiphene citrate alone and with human menopausal gonadotropins. *Fertil Steril* 59:756, 1993

92. Rogers PA, Paulson D, Murphy CR, Hosie M, Susil B, Leoni M: Correlation of endometrial histology, morphometry, and ultrasound appearance after different stimulation protocols for in vitro fertilization. *Fertil Steril* 55:583, 1991

93. Fleischer AC, Pittaway DE, Beard LA, et al: Sonographic depiction of endometrial changes occuring with ovulation induction. *J Ultrasound Med* 3:341, 1984

94. Imoedemhe DA, Shaw RW, Kirkland A, Chan R: Ultrasound measurement of endometrial thickness on different ovarian stimulation regimens during in vitro fertilization. *Hum Reprod* 2:545, 1987

95. Eden JA, Place J, Carter GD, Jones J, Alagband-Zadeh J, Pawson ME: The effect of clomiphene citrate on follicular phase increase in endometrial thickness and uterine volume. *Obstet Gynecol* 73:187, 1989

96. Whitelaw MJ, Kalman CG, Grams LR: The significance of the high ovulation rate versus the low pregnancy rate with Clomid. *Am J Obstet Gynecol* 107:865, 1970

97. Hancock KW, Oakey RE: The low incidence of pregnancy following clomiphene therapy. *Int J Fertil* 18:49, 1973

98. Lamb EJ, Colliflower WW, Williams JW: Endometrial histology and conception rates after clomiphene. *Obstet Gynecol* 39:389 1972

99. Gorlitsky GA, Kase NG, Speroff L: Ovulation and pregnancy rates with clomiphene citrate. *Obstet Gynecol* 51:265, 1978

100. Hammond MG, Halme JK, Talbert LM: Factors affecting the pregnancy rate in clomiphene citrate induction of ovulation. *Obstet Gynecol* 62:196, 1983

101. Kistner RW: The infertile woman. *J Nurs* 73:1937, 1973

102. Asch RH, Greenblatt RB: Update on the safety and efficacy of clomiphene citrate as a therapeutic agent. *J Reprod Med* 17:175 1976

103. Ross GT, Cargille CM, Lipsett MB, et al: Pituitary and gonadal hormones in women during spontaneous and induced ovulatory cycles. *Recent Prog Horm Res* 26:1, 1970

104. Atlay RD, Pennington GW: The use of clomiphene citrate and pituitary gonadotropin in successive pregnancies: The Sheffield quadruplets. *Am J Obstet Gynecol* 109:402, 1971

105. Aiken RA: An account of the "Birmingham sextuplets." *J Obstet Gynaecol Br Commonw* 76:684, 1969

106. Jones GS, De Moraes-Ruehsen M: Induction of ovulation with human gonadotropins and with clomiphene. *Fertil Steril* 16:461, 1965

107. Laufer N, Pratt BM, DeCherney AH, et al: The in vivo–in vitro effects of clomiphene citrate on ovulation, fertilization and development of cultured mouse oocytes. *Am J Obstet Gynecol* 147:633, 1983

108. Wramsby H, Fredga K, Liedholm P: Chromosome analysis of human oocytes recovered from preovulatory follicles in stimulated cycles. *N Engl J Med* 316:121, 1987

109. Seibel MM, Smith DM: The effect of clomiphene citrate on human preovulatory oocyte maturation in vivo. *J In Vitro Fertil Embryo Transf* 6:3, 1989

110. Boue JG, Boue A: Increased frequency of chromosomal anomalies in abortions after induced ovulation. *Lancet* 1:679, 1973

111. Mor-Joseph S, Anteby SO, Granat M, Brzezinski A, Evron S: Recurrent molar pregnancies associated with clomiphene citrate and human menopausal gonadotropins. *Am J Obstet Gynecol* 151:1095, 1985

112. Harlap S: Ovulation induction and congenital malformations. *Lancet* 2:961, 1976

113. Shoham Z: Epidemiology, etiology, and fertility drugs in ovarian epithelial carcinoma: Where are we today? *Fertil Steril* 62:433, 1994

114. Bamford TM, Steele SJ: Uterine and ovarian carcinoma in a patient receiving gonadotropin therapy: Case report. *Br J Obstet Gynaecol* 89:962, 1982

115. Atlas M, Menczer J: Massive hyperstimulation in borderline carcinoma of the ovary. *Acta Obstet Gynecol Scand* 61:261, 1982

116. Ben-Hur H, Dgani R, Lancet M, Katz Z, Nissim F, Rosenman D: Ovarian carcinoma masquerading as ovarian hyperstimulation syndrome. *Acta Obstet Gynecol Scand* 65:813, 1986

117. Carter ME, Joyce DN: Ovarian carcinoma in a patient hyperstimulated by gonadotropin therapy for in vitro fertilization: A case report. *J In Vitro Fertil Embryo Transf* 4:126, 1987

118. Kulkarni R, McGarry JM: Follicular stimulation and ovarian cancer (letter). *Br Med J* 299:740, 1989

119. Dietle J: Ovulation and ovarian cancer (letter). *Lancet* 2:445, 1991

120. Goldberg GL, Rundowitz CD: Ovarian carcinoma of low malignant potential, infertility, and induction of ovulation: Is there a link? *Am J Obstet Gynecol* 166:853, 1992

121. Nijman HW, Burger CW, Baak JPA, Schats R, Vermorken JB, Kenemans P: Borderline malignancy of the ovary and controlled hyperstimulation, a report of two cases. *Eur J Cancer* 28A:1971, 1992

122. Whittemore AS, Harris R, Itnyre J, et al: Characteristics relating to ovarian cancer risk: Collabortive analysis of 12 U.S. case-control studies. I. Methods. *Am J Epidemiol* 136:1175, 1992

123. Whittemore AS, Harris R, Itnyre J, et al: Characteristics relating to ovarian cancer risk: Collaborative analysis of 12 U.S. case-control studies. II. Invasive epithelial ovarian cancer in white women. *Am J Epidemiol* 136:1184, 1992

124. Harris R, Whittemore AS, Itnyre J, et al: Characteristics relating to ovarian cancer risk: Collaborative analysis of 12 U.S. case-control studies. III. Epithelial tumors of low malignant potential in white women. *Am J Epidemiol* 136:1204, 1992

125. Whittemore AS, Harris R, Itnyre J, et al: Characteristics relating to ovarian cancer risk: Collaborative analysis of 12 U.S. case-control studies. IV. The pathogenesis of epithelial ovarian cancer. *Am J Epidemiol* 136:1212, 1992

126. Horn-Ross PL, Whittemore AS, Harris R, et al: Characteristics relating to ovarian cancer risk: Collaborative analysis of 12 U.S. case-control studies. VI. Non-epithelial cancers among adults. *Epidemiology* 3:490, 1992

127. Hartge P, Schiffman MH, Hoover R, McGowan L, Lesher L, Norris HJ: A case-control study of epithelial ovarian cancer. *Am J Obstet Gynecol* 161:10, 1989

128. Cramer DW, Hutchison GB, Welsh WR, Scully RE, Ryan KJ: Determinants of ovarian cancer risk. I. Reproductive experiences and family history. *J Natl Cancer Inst* 71:711, 1983

129. Nasca PC, Greenwald P, Chorost S, Richart R, Caputo T: An epi-demological case-control study of ovarian cancer and reproductive factors. *Am J Epidemiol* 119:705, 1984

130. Whittemore AS. Fertility drugs and risk of ovarian cancer. *Hum Reprod* 8:999, 1993

131. Cohen J, Forman R, Harlap S, et al: IFFS experts group report on the Whittemore study related to the risk of ovarian cancer associated with the use of infertility agents. *Hum Reprod* 8:996, 1993

132. Rossing MA, Daling JR, Weiss NS, Moore DE, Self SG. Ovarian tumors in a cohort of infertile women. *N Engl J Med* 331:771, 1994

133. Ron E, Lunenfeld B, Menczer J, et al: Cancer incidence in a co-hort of infertile women. *Am J Epidemiol* 125:780, 1987

CHAPTER 30

Ovulation Induction with Human Menopausal Gonadotropin

BRUNO LUNENFELD · EITAN LUNENFELD

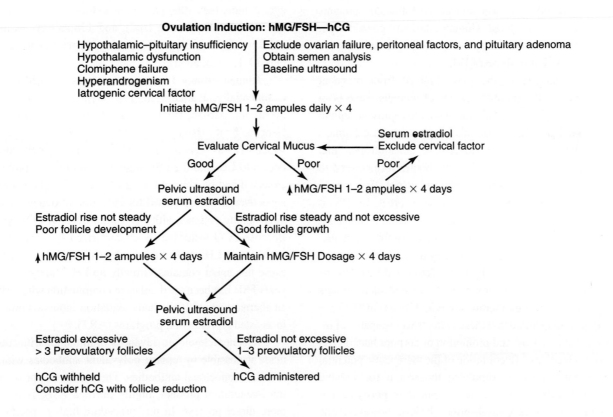

HISTORICAL PERSPECTIVES

One of the most far-reaching discoveries ever made in reproductive biology was that the male and female reproductive systems are under the functional control of the anterior hypophysis. Crowe et al demonstrated in 1909 that partial hypophysectomy of adult dogs provoked atrophy of the reproductive organs and prevented sexual development in juvenile animals.[1] It took nearly 20 years before investigators obtained firm evidence that the male and female reproductive systems were under the functional control of the pituitary gland. This evidence was based on the demonstration that implantation of anterior pituitary glands evoked rapid development of sexual puberty in immature animals[2]; hypophysectomized immature male and female animals failed to mature sexually[3]; and in adult hypophysectomized animals, sexual characteristics regressed rapidly.

Soon afterward, the three gonadotropic factors were discovered. Follicle-stimulating hormone (FSH), as its name indicates, is primarily responsible for follicular recruitment, selection, growth, and ripening. Luteinizing hormone (LH) is responsible for the final maturation of the FSH-stimulated follicles, ovulation, and transformation of the follicular remnants into functional corpora lutea. Human chorionic gonadotropin (hCG), the hormone secreted by the trophoblastic cells, has biologic actions similar to those of LH.

These hormones, in the past obtained from pregnant mares' serum and the pituitary glands of animals, have been used clinically to induce ovulation. Gonadotropins of animal origin are no longer used for this purpose because humans rapidly produce antibodies to nonprimate gonadotropins that neutralize their clinical effects. The antibodies formed tend to be specific for the preparations injected and do not affect the action of gonadotropins obtained from other sources. In 1954 it was demonstrated that kaolin extracts from pooled menopausal urine contained FSH and LH activity in comparable amounts.[4] These extracts prevented atrophy of Leydig cells and retained complete spermatogenesis in hypophysectomized rats. On the basis of these findings the authors predicted that such extracts could open up interesting therapeutic possibilities. In 1957 the same group demonstrated that these extracts were capable of inducing follicular growth and promotion of corpora lutea in hypophysectomized rats.[5] Recognition of the therapeutic potential of human gonadotropins stimulated the search for suitable sources for extraction. Most investigators were purifying gonadotropins from menopausal urine (hMG); however, one group obtained them by processing human pituitary glands (human pituitary gonadotropin [hPG]).

One pituitary gland contains as much FSH as 2 to 5 liters of postmenopausal urine. A suitable product was obtained by means of single-fraction purification with ammonium sulfate or ethanol. Ovulation was induced successfully with hPG followed by hCG.[6]

The scarcity of the postmortem pituitary glands needed for the production of hPG eliminates the possibility of their widescale use. However, hPG continued to be used in Australia and other parts of the world. When Creuzfeld-Jakob disease was identified in patients who received hPG, it was banned from clinical use.[7,8] Pharmaceutical companies such as Ares-Serono (Rome, Italy) and Organon International (Akso Nobel N.V. of the Netherlands) directed their attention to the preparation of extracts from urine. The initial urinary extract was prepared by means of the kaolin-acetone method, purified first with ammonium acetate ethanol and then by permutit chromatography. This preparation is a potent ovarian stimulant in humans.[9] Although these postmenopausal urinary preparations were of only 3% to 4% purity and contained more than 97% copurified urinary proteins, the scientific community and regulatory agencies accepted these materials for clinical use, because no alternatives were available. During 1962 three pregnancies resulted after 16 courses of treatment of 10 women.[10] Since that time it is estimated that more than one million women have been treated with hMG. Published results exist on more than 8000 anovulatory patients who received hMG for more than 22,000 cycles; more than 1000 patients who took hMG and underwent intrauterine insemination (IUI), and 138,238 cycles in which hMG was used in assisted reproductive treatment (ART) (Tables 30–1, 30–2, 30–3).

Human urinary FSH as an alternative to hMG became commercially available in 1987. The production of FSH (Metrodin, Serono, Rome, Italy, and the Ares-Serono Group, Geneva, Switzerland) was essentially a "passive" process in which LH was separated from bulk material by polyvalent antibodies to LH, and the FSH together with urinary proteins was collected and lyophylized for use. FSH offers theoretic advantages over hMG when used for induction of ovulation, particularly among patients with polycystic ovary (PCO) syndrome. Because PCO syndrome is characterized by abnormally elevated serum LH levels, the use of purified FSH is attractive because this agent contains virtually no LH. During the last few years FSH has been used either in combination with hMG or as an alternative to hMG in many ovulation-induction protocols or in assisted reproduction programs (ART).

Recent technologic advances in immunopurification have made it possible to replace polyvalent antibodies with highly specific monoclonal antibodies. The production process of the third-generation product, highly purified FSH, is therefore a more direct process. In this procedure highly specific monoclonal antibodies to FSH selectively bind the FSH molecules in the hMG bulk material as they pass through the affinity column. The unbound urinary protein and the LH pass through the column and are removed. The column then contains pure FSH. This is extracted from the column as a highly purified product devoid of both LH and contaminating urinary proteins. As a re-

TABLE 30–1. CONCEPTION RATES FOLLOWING GONADOTROPIN THERAPY IN ANOVULATORY PATIENTS

Author	No. of Patients	No. of Cycles	Pregnancies		
			Number	Per Cycle (%)	Per Patient (%)
Australian Department of Health[11] (1981)	1056	4008	552	13.8	52.3
Bettendorf et al[12] (1981)	756	1585	224	14.1	29.6
Butler et al[13] (1970)	134	438	31	7.1	23.1
Caspi et al[14] (1974)	101	343	62	18.1	61.4
Ellis & Williamson[15] (1975)	77	332	43	13.0	55.8
Gemzell[16] (1970)	228	463	101	21.8	44.3
Goldfarb[17] (1982)	442	1098	118	10.7	26.7
Healy et al[18] (1980)	40	159	33	20.8	82.5
Kurachi et al[19] (1983)	2166	6096	523	8.6	24.1
Lunenfeld et al[20] (1985)	1107	3646	424	11.6	38.3
Potashnik et al[a] (1986)	262	580	85	14.6	32.4
Spadoni et al[21] (1974)	62	225	26	11.6	41.9
Thompson & Hansen[22] (1970)	1190	2798	334	11.9	28.1
Tsapoulis et al[23] (1974)	320	320	163	—	50.9
Total	7941	21,771[b]	2719	11.7[b]	34.2

[a]Potashnik G, Glassner M, Holzbert G, Insler V (unpublished data).
[b]Excludes Tsapoulis et al data.

sult of this improved processing, Metrodin HP (Fertinex, Serono Laboratories, Norwell, MA) contains less than 0.1 IU of LH activity and less than 5% of unidentified urinary proteins. The specific activity of the FSH in this preparation has been increased, from approximately 100 to 150 IU/mg of protein for Metrodin to about 9000 IU/mg of protein for Metrodin HP.

The purity is also increased from 1% to 2% in Metrodin to 95% in Metrodin HP. Because of the enhanced purity of Metrodin HP, the total amount of injected protein is very small. Therefore, Metrodin HP is suitable for subcutaneous administration. Batch-to-batch variability is practically eliminated and the product lends itself to detailed analysis by means of physicochemical methods in addition to classic in vivo bioassay. This purified preparation also allows better assessment of the pharmacodynamics and pharmacokinetics of FSH.

The technical developments have made it possible to redesign ovulation-induction protocols (for example, low-dose regimens, low-dose increments, subcutaneous injection). These new protocols may prove to be more efficient and may result in fewer multiple pregnancies, a lower abortion rate, and an even lower risk of hyperstimulation. With the use of highly purified FSH preparations, a reevaluation of the role of estrogen as a marker of ovulation induction may be necessary. The accessibility of Metrodin HP brings into question whether it is ethical to continue using earlier FSH preparations that possess only 100 to 200 IU of FSH per milligram of protein and contain 95% copurified urinary proteins. The highly purified urinary preparations will likely replace all commercially available hMG and Metrodin preparations within the next 2 years.

TABLE 30–2. CONCEPTION RATES FOLLOWING hMG SUPEROVULATION IN OVULATORY WOMEN TREATED FOR UNEXPLAINED OR MALE-FACTOR INFERTILITY WITH GONADOTROPIN THERAPY (COH) COMBINED WITH TIMED INTERCOURSE OR INTRAUTERINE INSEMINATION

Author	No. of Patients	Total No. of Cycles	Pregnancies		
			Number	Per Cycle (%)	Per Patient (%)
Serhal et al[24] (1988)	48	77	5	6.5	15.6
Wellner et al[25] (1988)	97	388	12	3.1	12.4
Chaffkin et al[26] (1991)	266	695	85	12.2	32.0
Chang et al[27] (1993)	343	467	72	15.4	—
Aboulghar et al[28] (1993)	268	463	93	20.1	34.7
Total	1022	2090	267	12.8	26.1

COH, controlled ovarian hyperstimulation.

TABLE 30–3. CONCEPTION RATES FOLLOWING SUPEROVULATION GONADOTROPIN THERAPY (COH) COMBINED WITH ART

Author	No. of Oocyte Retrievals	No. of Transfer Cycles	Pregnancies		
			Number	Per Cycle (%)	Per Patient (%)
Cohen et al[29] (1993)	138,238	116,201	26,411	19.1	22.7

ART, assisted reproductive treatments such as IVF-ET, GIFT, ZIFT, and TET. The numbers are based on reports from 760 centers in 33 countries and cover the year 1991.

CHEMISTRY, CLEARANCE, AND PHYSIOLOGY

Since the 1960s the principal elements of the mechanisms of action, control, and regulation of secretion of gonadotropins have been elucidated,[30] and the structure of the hormones has been determined. Gonadotropins are glycoproteins with a molecular weight of about 30,000 daltons and consisting of about 20% carbohydrate. The carbohydrate moieties in the molecules are fucose, mannose, galactose, acetyl glucosamine, and N-acetyl neuraminic acid.[31] The sialic acid content varies widely among the glycoprotein hormones, from 20 residues in hCG and five in FSH to only one or two in LH. These differences are largely responsible for the variations in the isoelectric points of gonadotropins. The carbohydrate moieties are complex. They may be branched or straight chains, and they contain sialic acid as an important constituent, particularly at the ends of the chains.

Different sialic acid content also accounts for both the variation in molecular weight of the hormone isolated from various sources and the differences in biologic activity determined by means of in vivo assays (Table 30–4). The higher the sialic acid content, the longer is the biologic half-life. Thus the increased amount of carbohydrate in hCG is responsible for the fact that its half-life is significantly longer than that of LH or FSH. Whereas the β subunit of LH contains only one carbohydrate group, the β subunit of hCG contains six. The function of these carbohydrate groups is not fully known, except that removing the terminal neuraminic acid (sialic acid) residues drastically shortens the half-lives of the circulating hormones in blood. For this reason, desialylated preparations of human LH, hCG, and FSH show considerably reduced biologic activity in vivo but retain activity in either specific in vitro biologic assays, in which membrane receptors or isolated target cells are used. Therefore, attempts to measure these hormones by means of immunoassay or in vitro bioassay do not express the actual bioactivity in vivo. Deglycosylated hormones in vitro can act as competitive antagonists of the actions of the intact hormone on cyclic adenosine monophosphate (cAMP) production and to a lesser extent on steroid hormone biosynthesis.

The gonadotropic hormones consist of two hydrophobic, noncovalently associated α and β subunits. The three-dimensional structure of each subunit is maintained by internally cross-linked disulfide bonds. Gonadotropic hormones can be disassociated into individual subunits with denaturing agents (10 M urea at pH 4.5 or 1 M propionic acid).[32] The pure subunits possess limited biologic activity, but the activity is regenerated when the two subunits are allowed to recombine. All of the gonadotropins as well as thyroid-stimulating hormone (TSH) share a common α subunit of 92 amino acid residues in the same sequence, containing five disulfide bonds as well as two carbohydrate moieties at positions 52 and 78. The β subunits of FSH, LH, and hCG are unique to each hormone and confer their biologic specificity; they have amino acid chains of variable lengths (116 to 147 amino acid residues) and contain six disulfide bonds. In the β subunits of hCG, two branched-chain moieties are attached to asparagine at positions 13 and 30. Smaller, linear sugar groups are attached by means of o-serine linkage to serines within the unique hCG COOH-terminal peptide at residues 121, 127, 132, and 138. Highly purified FSH isolated from human pituitary glands has a specific activity of 10,000 IU/mg. Highly purified hCG has a specific activity of 11,000 to 13,500 IU/mg. Studies with methods that allowed analysis of the genes and gene products showed that the two subunits of the gonadotropic hormones are translated from separate messenger RNAs,[33] and both are synthesized as precursors. This is followed by cleavage of the signal peptide leader sequence by the signal peptidase. The nascent polypeptide α and β subunits are

TABLE 30–4. MICROHETEROGENEITY OF FSH: CHARACTERISTICS OF THE ACIDIC AND BASIC ISOFORMS

Characteristic	Estradiol	
	Basic Isoform	Acidic Isoform
Activity		
In vitro	High	Low
In vivo	Low	High
Sialic acid content	Low	High
Clearance	Rapid	Slow
Half-life	Short	Long
Receptor binding	High	Low
Signal transduction	High	Low

The overall in vivo bioactivity is higher because of its longer half-life and lower clearance.

Gonadal steroids and GnRH influence pituitary neuraminidase and sialyltransferase activity to generate changes in isoforms.

Follicula

As follic
apparen
gonadot
to assure
most exc
granulos
chemical
lates the
aromatas
ulosa cel
duces sy
leading t
nadotrop
ovary, bu
and ovul

The
latory me
action in
FSH stin
secretes
preferent
drostene
leading t
probably
largest nu
tration o
size, inhi
FSH sec
growing
becomes
nadotrop
other pa
factor (IC
to fulfill t

Stud
that each
1 respons
lular tran
IGFs can
cells. IGI
kinase me
ligand to
of tyrosin
lation/de
IGF-1. H
ducing IC
bind to a
producin;
pete for f

then glycosylated by means of en bloc attachment of high-mannose-complex–type oligosaccharides to two asparagine residues of each subunit. Excess mannose and glucose residues are trimmed from the intermediates (Fig 30–1). Thereafter, peripheral monosaccharides *N*-acetyl glucosamine, galactose, and *N*-acetyl neuraminic acid are attached sequentially to complete the oligosaccharide structures. The α and β subunits then combine noncovalently in a two-step reaction to form the biologically active glycoproteins.[34]

The task of producing recombinant gonadotropin molecules has, however, proved to be difficult. Whereas bacteria efficiently produce nonglycosylated peptides such as insulin, and yeast has been cloned for the production of certain vaccines, prokaryotic cells are incapable of correctly glycosylating the peptide subunits to produce biologically active gonadotropins. The complex sugars are important for proper folding of the polypeptide backbone. The sites and extent of glycosylation determine tertiary structure, length of degradation time, the regions of the molecule exposed to target cell receptors, and exposure of the molecule to mechanisms that regulate metabolism in vivo. Recombinant glycosylated peptides may be synthesized by certain mammalian cell lines. The ovary cells of Chinese hamsters are known to be suitable host cells for the production of glycosylated recombinant proteins. Such cell lines were chosen for the expression of recombinant human FSH and LH. The expression of human FSH dimer was achieved by means of transfection of Chinese hamster ovary cells with a genomic clone that contained the complete FSH β coding sequence together with the α subunit minigene. Stable cell lines expressing FSH dimer in relatively abundant amounts were selected. The resulting recombinant FSH was more homogenous than the most purified pituitary FSH preparations, providing a basis for clinical use. Specific cell clones have now been selected for large-scale production of recombinant FSH.

The resultant preparations are very pure and have a high biologic potency (>10,000 IU/mg protein).

With such recombinant FSH, ovulation induction followed by pregnancies has been reported.[35–39] Furthermore, these preparations have proved as efficient as the urinary preparations. With recombinant DNA technology and highly defined cell culture techniques, recombinant DNA gonadotropins are now being prepared on an industrial scale. What would currently require 30 million liters of urine per year will ultimately be produced by genetically engineered cells in defined chemical culture medium comprising only a small fraction of that volume. It is our hope that in the not too distant future DNA technology will provide an almost endless supply of human gonadotropins. Moreover, recombinant DNA technology allows the design of potential therapeutically active gonadotropin agonists and antagonists by altering key proteins and carbohydrate regions in the α and β subunits of FSH and LH.[40]

Information regarding metabolism of gonadotropic hormones is scarce. It has been shown that purified preparations of human FSH, LH, and hCG injected intravenously into humans have serum half-lives (as determined with bioassays) of 180 to 240 minutes, 42 to 60 minutes, and 6 to 8 hours, respectively. The half-lives of the α and β subunits of LH were found to be only 16 minutes. The higher carbohydrate content of hCG (10%) is responsible for its longer half-life than that of human FSH (5%) and LH (2%). Because of rapid hepatic clearance, removal of sialic acid from hCG reduces the half-life to minutes and results in correspondingly low biologic activity in vivo.

The mean metabolic clearance rate (MCR) of FSH in women has been determined to be 14 mL/min; the MCR in men has not been determined. The MCR of LH is 25 to 30 mL/min in women regardless of ovulatory state and is almost 50% higher in healthy men. The disappearance curves for both hormones are multiexponential, indicating distribution in more than three mathematical compartments. Among premenopausal women, daily production rates of LH are 500 to 1000 IU with a marked preovulatory rise, whereas rates among postmenopausal women are 3000 to 4000 IU daily. These values indicate that the pituitary content of LH (and probably of FSH) is turned over once or twice daily and that rapid biosynthesis of gonadotropins must be necessary to maintain the normal levels of pituitary storage and secretion. Only 3% to 10% of the daily production of FSH and LH is excreted in the urine in a biologically active form; however, the rate of urinary gonadotropin secretion may be used to reflect both physiologic and pathologic conditions. The recovery of exogenous gonadotropins among the urine of fertile and infertile people is 10% to 20% of the administered hormone. Urinary excretion of gonadotropins accounts for only 5% of the MCR. The MCR of hMG among people with hypogonadotropism is 0.4 to 1.7 mL/min.

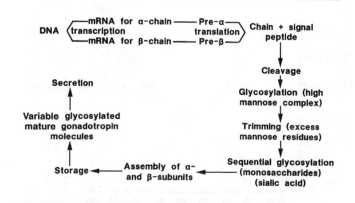

Figure 30–1. Schematic of the main steps of gonadotropin production in the gonadotrope.

FOLLICULAR▌

Early studies▌
licular devel▌
independent.▌
follicular dev▌
tered and ret▌
10 weeks for▌
gle layer of▌
capable of g▌
ration, and c▌
stimulation c▌
30–2). Whei▌
growth, no n▌
sent at the be▌
licles degen▌
remain, and▌
from atresia▌
Only one ma▌
undergo atre▌
estrogenic n▌
velopment. /▌
with follicul▌

In the ▌
genesis is pr▌

atresia. Exogenous gonadotropin stimulation, specifically FSH, can save follicles from degeneration and allow multiple ovulation.[49] Disturbances in the pulsatile pattern of GnRH secretion or improper gonadotropin stimulation derange follicular development, which may result in anovulation. The severity of this derangement may range from hypoestrogenic amenorrhea to regular cycles with only subtle abnormalities in follicular development and hormonal profiles in women with unexplained infertility.[50]

Follicular Dominance

With use of the threshold principle advocated initially in the mid 1960s,[51,52] it is somewhat possible to regulate the number of follicles that reach dominance and ovulate. Low-dose FSH step-up protocols could therefore decrease the occurrence of hyperstimulation and multiple pregnancies. Estrogen production by the dominant follicle initiates the midcycle LH surge, ovulation, and luteinization. Excessive LH at this stage can cause premature luteinization of the dominant follicle expressed by an untimely progesterone increase.[53]

Diagnosis and treatment of specific abnormalities in an infertile woman depend to a large extent on an understanding of the structural and functional components of the elaborate system that governs the ovarian cycle. The technical developments that have led to the production of highly purified urinary and recombinant FSH and a deeper understanding of the pharmacodynamics and pharmacokinetics of these preparations have made it possible to redesign ovulation-inducing protocols that may prove to be more efficient and result in fewer multiple pregnancies, a lower abortion rate, and a lower risk of hyperstimulation than seen with earlier treatment protocols.

SELECTION OF PATIENTS FOR FIRST- AND SECOND-LINE GONADOTROPIN THERAPY

The possibilities for classification of anovulatory patients are virtually unlimited, depending on the clinical laboratory facilities available and the purpose to be served. Every classification may be valuable as long as acceptable, measurable, and well-defined variables are used and a reasonable compromise is achieved among accuracy, effort, and cost. The guidelines are based on up-to-date scientific information and technical advances. They are therapeutically oriented to gonadotropins as first- or second-line therapy.

Hypothalamic–Pituitary Insufficiency

The cause of amenorrhea among women who do not have withdrawal vaginal bleeding after progesterone challenge may be target unresponsiveness or hypothalamic–pituitary insufficiency.

Bleeding after cyclic estrogen–progesterone administration eliminates the diagnosis of uterine causes such as congenital abnormalities or a severe uterine adhesion such as Asherman's syndrome. Low or normal FSH and LH levels rule out ovarian failure and point to pituitary insufficiency.

All women with pituitary insufficiency need both exogenous FSH and LH for follicular development and therefore benefit from hMG–hCG or FSH/LH–hCG therapy. When pulsatile GnRH is used, it is necessary to differentiate hypothalamic insufficiency and pituitary failure. Patients with pituitary failure cannot respond to pulsatile GnRH (Fig 30–3).

Hypothalamic Dysfunction with Normal Prolactin and Androgen Levels

Lack of ovulation among nonandrogenized, normoprolactinemic women secondary to chronic hypothalamic dysfunction is probably the most common cause of menstrual disorders. Patients in this category also have a variety of symptoms that may range from luteal-phase defects to amenorrhea. This form of amenorrhea usually responds to progesterone challenge with vaginal bleeding.

Stress, alterations in body weight, and excessive athletic activity can cause chronic hypothalamic anovulation. If change in lifestyle does not restore ovulation, clomiphene citrate should be considered first. Only for women who do not ovulate with doses of up to 150 mg/day for 5 days or who do not conceive despite suggestive ovulation for three to six cycles should FSH/hCG therapy be initiated. In the rare situation in which follicular development occurs without sufficient estrogen production, as demonstrated at ultrasonography with lack of endometrial development, FSH should be supplemented with LH or substituted with hMG.

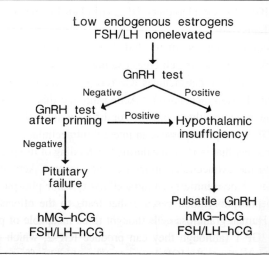

Figure 30–3. Algorithm for the differential diagnosis of amenorrhea in patients with low endogenous estrogens.

Figure 30–2. F▌
primordial follicle▌

Iatrogenically Induced Cervical Factor

When a patient with hypothalamic dysfunction with normal prolactin and androgen levels appears to respond well to treatment with clomiphene citrate but does not conceive, a postcoital test should be repeated. Should serial determinations of the cervical score[54] and well-timed postcoital tests reveal persistently poor cervical mucus with predominantly immotile spermatozoa, a deleterious effect of clomiphene citrate on the cervical mucus should be taken into consideration (Fig 30–4).

Clomiphene citrate, acting as an antiestrogen, may severely depress the vaginal epithelium and, to a lesser degree, the endocervical crypts. Because clomiphene therapy results in multifollicular development, the elevated estrogen levels usually override this effect. In some cases, however, the antiestrogenic effect results in thick, tenacious mucus, which may prevent conception by hindering sperm migration through the cervical canal. The discrepancy between the ovulation rate and the conception rate after clomiphene therapy may in some cases be due to the suppressive effect of the drug on the uterine cervix. The use of estrogens in combination with clomiphene citrate as a means of improving the quality of the cervical mucus remains a controversial issue. Low dosages of synthetic estrogens such as ethinyl estradiol, 20 μg, or conjugated estrogens such as Premarin (Wyeth-Ayerst Laboratories, New York, NY), 0.3 mg daily on cycle days 10 to 17, are typical.

If penetration of the cervical mucus by spermatozoa does not improve after treatment with estrogens in combination with clomiphene citrate, IUI with the partner's sperm may be attempted. Therapy with FSH-hCG or hMG-hCG may also serve as second-line therapy among such patients, because it induces ovulation without deleterious effect on the cervical mucus.

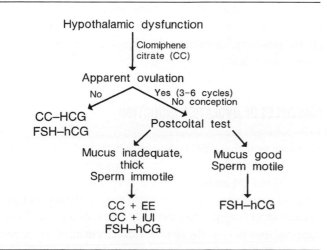

Figure 30–4. Iatrogenic cervical factor in patients with hypothalamic dysfunction treated with clomiphene citrate (CC).

Premature Luteinization

Premature luteinization is a specific category of anovulation. It is frequently unrecognized or is misdiagnosed as unexplained infertility, luteal-phase defect, or luteinized unruptured follicle (LUF) syndrome. It occurs if there is an untimely LH surge in response to rising estrogen at a time when the follicle is still immature. It can only be diagnosed if an LH peak is detected in the presence of immature follicles as seen during ultrasonography. It can be speculated that this entity represents an exaggerated sensitivity of the pituitary gland to the rising levels of estrogen, resulting in an LH surge. This assumption may explain the failure of clomiphene citrate or hMG to restore ovulation in these women. Because both of these agents cause multiple follicular development with exaggerated estrogen responses, a premature LH peak is even more likely to occur. A rational therapeutic approach is to abolish the estrogen-evoked positive feedback mechanism. This can be effectively accomplished by use of a potent GnRH agonist.[55]

Anovulation due to recurrent premature luteinization necessitates a triphasic therapeutic approach. A GnRH agonist is administered until the positive feedback is abolished (2 to 7 weeks). Thereafter, hMG or FSH is given in conjunction with the agonist until at least one follicle reaches maturation as judged during ultrasonography and with estrogen levels. Then hCG is administered to induce ovulation (Fig 30–5).

Hypothalamic–Pituitary Dysfunction Associated with Hyperandrogenism

An androgenized anovulatory patient typically has a history of acne, seborrhea, and hirsutism that may or may not be associated with obesity. Elevated androgen production may arise from the ovaries, the adrenal cortex, or both. Accurate determination of the predominant source assists the clinician in choosing the correct treatment to restore ovulation. Figure 30–6 illustrates such an approach.

An androgenized patient with normal or elevated testosterone levels who also has normal levels of DHEAS should be considered to have PCO syndrome. An elevated LH-to-FSH ratio (greater than 3) is an additional characteristic of this entity. High-resolution ultrasound imaging of the pelvis provides anatomic confirmation of this diagnosis. Peripheral cysts of 4 to 6 mm average diameter and an echo-dense central stroma are typically observed. This corresponds well with the macroscopic appearance of the cut surface of the PCO. In patients with PCO syndrome, chronic increased LH secretion continuously stimulates the proliferation of stromal and thecal cells and increases production of intraovarian and intrafollicular androgens. Intrafollicular androgens are associated with follicular atresia, probably through inhibition of both FSH and LH receptors. This

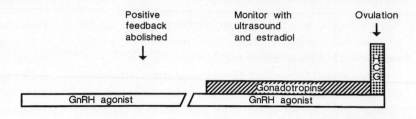

Figure 30–5. Triphasic treatment scheme. (*From Shadmi AL, et al. Abolishment of the positive feedback mechanism: A criterion for temporary medical hypophysectomy by LH-RH agonist. Gynecol Endocrinol 1:1, 1987.*[59])

mechanism fits the hormonal pattern and morphologic appearance described earlier.

Chronically elevated LH secretion may have manifold causes. It may be initiated through increased androstenedione–testosterone production from either an ovarian or adrenal source. The peripheral conversion of androstenedione-testosterone to estrone-estradiol, primarily in adipose tissue, enhances LH secretion. The relation of obesity to this disease is unequivocal and its impact on the clinical expression of the syndrome most important; however, a hypothalamic–pituitary disorder cannot be excluded as the origin. The first-line treatment, regardless of cause, is clomiphene citrate. This agent increases gonadotropin secretion and, despite an even further increase in LH levels in some women, allows selection, growth, and maturation of a single follicle. In other patients clomiphene citrate causes many follicles to grow and results in hyperstimulation. For patients with an inappropriate response to clomiphene, gonadotropin therapy, preferably an FSH preparation, should be used to attempt to override the FSH–LH imbalance. For some patients FSH is capable of interrupting the self-perpetuating biochemical cycle of PCO syndrome.[56–58]

For women in whom both of these types of therapy fail, a more rational approach may be indicated. Long-term administration of GnRH analogs has been shown to be effective in downregulating pituitary gonadotropin secretion.[59] These agents

were used successfully in conjunction with gonadotropins for women with the PCO syndrome who previously had not conceived with exogenous gonadotropin therapy alone.[60] During GnRH analog therapy, gonadotropin secretion diminishes and the FSH–LH imbalance is corrected within 3 to 4 weeks.[9,59] When this stage has been reached, treatment is initiated. Figure 30–7 illustrates this approach in a patient whom other therapeutic regimens had failed and who conceived after this kind of triphasic therapy.

Use of hMG in Presumably Ovulating Women

Although the use of hMG-hCG by anovulatory women is widely accepted and of definite value, the applicability of these agents by presumably ovulatory women, is not without controversy. Such patients include those with unexplained infertility or luteal-phase defect, those undergoing therapeutic insemination, and those with cervical-factor infertility who take the hormones for mucus production. The potential exists for OHSS and multiple gestation. In contrast to these risks is the realization that among these women, empiric use of hMG is associated with a pregnancy rate of approximately 12%.[61] Although still low, this rate was significantly higher than those among corresponding control groups and not dissimilar from rates achieved with in vitro fertilization (IVF). Some authors, however, found pregnancy rates of 14% among untreated women with unexplained infertility.[62] Therefore, the empiric use of hMG remains of uncertain value.

PRINCIPLES OF OVULATION INDUCTION

To induce ovulation, FSH is necessary in the early phase of the cycle to recruit and select follicles. For growth and maturation, both FSH and LH are necessary. For IVF, in which the aim is to obtain many oocytes, increased gonadotropin stimulation theoretically should begin during the early recruitment phase. To induce ovulation in vivo, the aim is the development of one or two mature follicles, and gonadotropin stimulation should be delayed until the selection phase (see Fig 30–2).

Most gonadotropin preparations used for therapeutic purposes contain both FSH and LH in various proportions. It has

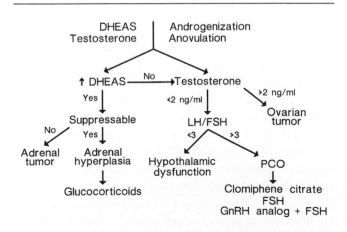

Figure 30–6. Algorithm for the differential diagnosis of androgenization of women.

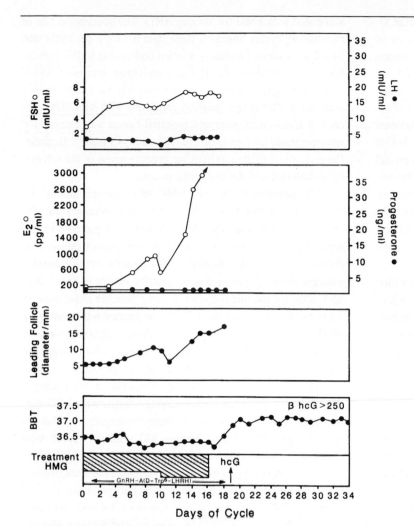

Figure 30–7. Profile of women who conceived after triphasic therapy. (*From Shadmi AL, et al. Abolishment of the positive feedback mechanism: A criterion for temporary medical hypophysectomy by LH-RH agonist. Gynecol Endocrinol 1:1, 1987.*)

been shown that administration of hMG or purified FSH can override the normal mechanism of ovarian follicular selection. It was demonstrated that among normogonadotropic patients administration of hMG on cycle day 2 produced considerably more follicles than administration from day 9.[63] Apparently, the earlier FSH administration is started during the cycle (before the selection phase), the more follicles are recruited.

Although the timing and FSH content of hMG preparations determine the number of follicles rescued and selected, the LH content determines the steroidogenic pattern. Final maturation of the follicles is brought about by the combination of FSH and LH. This stage takes between 4 and 6 days and is expressed by a steady geometric increment of estrogens and a daily increase in follicular diameter of about 1.5 to 2 mm/day. Ovulation is induced by means of administration of LH or LH-like material (hCG) when one or two follicles have reached a diameter of 16 mm or more, a classic endometrial pattern with a thickness on ultrasound scans of more than 8 mm, serum progesterone levels less than 1 ng/mL (3 nmol/L), and serum estradiol levels ideally between 450 and 900 pg/mL (1650 and 3300

pmol/L). When estradiol levels are greater than 2000 pg/mL (7340 pmol/L) or three or more preovulatory follicles are present, hCG should be withheld, or if circumstances allow, the patient should be referred for follicular reduction. This technique involves aspiration of excessive follicles after hCG administration. The excessive eggs are fertilized and cryopreserved, and the remaining follicles allowed to ovulate in vivo. Should the patient not conceive in this specific cycle, the cryopreserved embryos are transferred in subsequent cycles. The use of this technique should reduce multiple gestations and hyperstimulation to a minimum. The absolute estradiol value deemed unsafe may vary from center to center depending on the type of estradiol assay used.

MONITORING OF GONADOTROPIN THERAPY

By monitoring ovulation induction, one can assess the daily gonadotropin dose that is effective in evoking an ovarian response (threshold dose), the length of time required for follicular maturation, and the appropriate time to trigger ovulation with hCG. Furthermore, it should help to prevent hyperstimulation, or at least to detect it as early as possible. Ideally, for these purposes a combination of ultrasonography to assess the number and size of growing follicles and measurement of estrogen level to indicate functional integrity should be used.[64] Because levels of estrogens reflect the total estrogen secretion of all functional follicular structures, however, a baseline ultrasonogram before gonadotropin administration is useful in all instances and crucial for women who received ovulation-induction therapy in the previous cycle. Endogenous estrogen production affects several cervical values, which can be assessed by a point scoring system (the cervical score).[54] The score shows a reasonably good correlation with rising estrogen levels and is a particularly useful guide in establishing the effective daily dosage of gonadotropins.

The initial dosage of FSH is usually 75 to 150 IU/day (one to two ampules of Pergonal [Serono], Humagon [Organon], or Metrodin [Serono], Metrodin HP [Ares-Serono, Switzerland], Gonal-F [Ares-Serono, Switzerland], Puregon [Organon International, Akso Nobel, The Netherlands]). If no rise in estrogen occurs within 5 days (as determined by means of cervical score or measuring the level) and no alarming clinical signs are noted, the daily dosage is increased by half (½) to two ampules. Treatment is continued at the higher dosage for 4 to 6 days, the growth and maturation phase. This phase is monitored with ultrasonography to determine the number and size of follicles, and by means of estrogen level measurement to determine their functional capacity.[64,65] The effective dosage is one that causes a clinically significant and steady estrogen rise. With this method of monitoring ovulation induction, two ultrasonograms and estrogen determinations usually are sufficient. Increases in estrogen levels greater than 100% a day are excessive. If this occurs, the dosage should be reduced by one ampule. If the estrogen level does not rise steadily, the daily dosage is again increased by half (½) to two ampules for 4 to 6 days. If the estrogen rise is steady and not excessive, the same dosage is continued until the level is between 450 and 900 pg/mL (1650 and 3300 pmol/L) and one or two follicles have reached a diameter of 16 mm or greater, endometrial thickness is 8 mm or more, and serum progesterone levels are less than 1 ng/mL (3 nmol/L). At that point ovulation is triggered with the administration of 5000 to 10,000 IU of hCG.

RESULTS OF TREATMENT

Tables 30–1 through 30–3 show published results on nearly 8000 anovulatory patients who received hMG for more than 22,000 cycles, more than 1000 ovulatory patients for whom hMG was used in combination with IUI, and in 138,238 cycles stimulated with hMG for various ARTs. The conception rate in anovulatory cycles based on these data is 11.7% per cycle and 34.2% per patient. Ovulatory women undergoing hMG stimulation in conjunction with IUI can anticipate success rates of 12.8% per cycle and 26.1% per patient. Similar results can be anticipated after superovulation combined with ART. The efficacy of hMG–hCG treatment reported herein was determined retrospectively by means of life-table analysis from a database. Pregnancy was related to both the primary cause of the infertility disturbance and the age of the patient.

The pregnancy rate with hMG–hCG therapy among patients with amenorrhea with hypothalamic–pituitary insufficiency or failure was very high. Among 279 patients in our series, 82% conceived.[30] The cumulative pregnancy rate was affected by age in a statistically significant way. Among patients younger than 35 years, the pregnancy rate was more than 95% after six treatment cycles. Among patients older than 35 years the rate was only 60%.[30] The pregnancy rates following hMG–hCG therapy among amenorrheic, oligoovulatory, or anovulatory patients who underwent unsuccessful clomiphene citrate therapy was 55%. Patients older than 35 years have much less likelihood of becoming pregnant than women younger than 35 years. Pregnancy rates among women with PCO syndrome are difficult to estimate because the diagnosis of this entity has been ill defined. Among 827 patients treated with clomiphene citrate, 76% ovulated but only 33% conceived within 6 months.[67] Among patients with clomiphene-resistant disease, treatment with hMG resulted in a 58% conception rate after an average of 2.4 treatment cycles.[68] A multicenter study was conducted with purified FSH (Metrodin) to treat patients who did not conceive after various therapies. This clinical trial achieved a pregnancy rate of 30%. The average length of therapy was 2.4 cycles per patient. Since the introduction of long-term administration of GnRH analogs, a number of reports with a triphasic treatment regimen have appeared in the literature. Results appear promising among well-selected patients, but it is clearly not the first line of therapy.

Results in the treatment of LUF syndrome, infertility due to untimely LH surges, and unexplained infertility have been disappointing. The introduction of purified FSH and GnRH analogs may change the poor prognosis for these patients. These medications alone or combined with IVF and embryo transfer (IVF-ET) or with gamete intrafallopian transfer (GIFT), seem theoretically promising. It is too early to quantify results because the number of patients treated is small.

True success rates are concealed in the number of livebirths. A review of 1346 miscarriages after hMG therapy showed an abortion rate of 21.5%.[30] There was no significant difference in abortion rate with respect to diagnostic groups; however, it was higher in the first conception cycle than in the second or third. This was independent of whether the second

TABLE 30–5. CLASSIFICATION OF HYPERSTIMULATION

Laboratory and Clinical Findings	Adverse Reaction					
	Mild				Severe	
	1		2		3	
	1	2	3	4	5	6
Excessive steroid production	+	+	+	+	+	+
Ovarian enlargement		+	+	+	+	+
Abdominal discomfort		+	+	+	+	+
Palpable ovarian cysts		?	+	+	+	+
Abdominal distention			+	+	+	+
Nausea			+	+	+	+
Vomiting				+	+	+
Diarrhea				?	+	+
Ascites					+	+
Hydrothorax						+
Severe hemoconcentration						+
Thromembolic phenomena						?

From Lunenfeld B, et al: Short and long term survey of patients treated with hMG/hCG and follow-up of offspring. In: Genanziani AR, et al (eds), Proceedings of the First International Congress on Gynecological Endocrinology. Lancashire, England, Parthenon, 1987:459–468.

conception occurred spontaneously (13%) or followed induction of ovulation with hMG–hCG (12.8%).

Short-term Safety

No consistent drug-related adverse effects have been reported with gonadotropin therapy. Most of the adverse reactions noted with hMG–hCG are due to ovarian responsiveness and sensitivity to the amount administered. Because most of the treatment protocols aim to induce multifollicular development, the main complications are hyperstimulation, multiple pregnancy, and obstetric and postnatal complications due to multiple gestation.

Hyperstimulation

The prevalence of mild hyperstimulation (Table 30–5 ranges between 31% and 60% in different large series. The prevalence of severe hyperstimulation ranges between 0.25% and 1.8% and has been declining with the use of serum estradiol and pelvic ultrasonography. With correct monitoring, the rate of severe hyperstimulation should not surpass 0.25%.

Multiple Gestations

The overall multiple pregnancy rate is about 26%. Of these, 74% are twins. With ultrasonic monitoring, it is possible to prevent or at least decrease the occurrence of multiple pregnancies; however, every such attempt has reduced the overall pregnancy rate. The increased conception rate with multifollicular development and transfer of more than one embryo has been well demonstrated in IVF programs.

The course of gestation appears to be normal. Analysis of the mode of delivery showed a high frequency of interventions, breech extractions, vacuum extractions, forceps deliveries, and cesarean sections. The high prevalence of obstetric interventions may be explained by a high rate of multiple pregnancies, primiparity ratios, and psychologic factors involved in patients' with long-standing infertility delivering a "premium child."

Sex Ratios

The sex ratio (M:F) of single births is 1.06 (54% boys) and of twins is 0.72 (42% boys).[30] The number of triplets was too small to analyze. One group reported 32 boys and 50 girls among the single births (39%) with a twin M:F ratio of 0.78.[14a] In another series, the rate of male children in single pregnancies was 51.8%,[12] but in twin and triplet pregnancies it was 53.8% and 66.7%, respectively. The typical secondary sex ratio at 28 weeks' gestation is considered to be 106 boys to 100 girls.[69,70] This higher number of boys probably reflects the interplay between the primary sex ratio and sex differences in early prenatal mortality. It is known that the number of boys decreases with an increasing number of children at birth. This is regarded as being due to the better survival of female offspring rather than a relative loss of boys.[71,72]

The sex ratios were 1.043 for twins, 1.007 for triplets, and 0.940 for quadruplets.[72] The high frequencies of girls in our twin series and of male twins and triplets in two other series,[12] were probably due to the rather small numbers involved. By combining all three series, one approaches the expected sex ratios, indicating clearly the importance of sufficiently large numbers to estimate similarity or divergence in the figures.

Congenital Malformations

Until 1970 serious malformations were reported among 4 of 122 infants born.[73] During the years 1970 to 1972 no serious malformations occurred among the 87 infants examined in the neonatal period. Another report on 157 infants after gonadotropin therapy revealed four infants classified as having serious malformations and 11 with various slight malformations.[14] Preliminary data on 66 infants born as a result of hMG–hCG treatment after 28 weeks' gestation revealed two with a serious malformation and five with slight malformations (15.21 and 75.8/1000 livebirths, respectively).[74] This prevalence did not differ significantly from the 10.3 serious and 72.4 slight malformations per 1000 livebirths reported for the population as a whole. The prevalence of congenital malformations in healthy populations has been reported to be 12.7 per 1000 livebirths after 28 weeks' gestation, with a range of 3.1 to 22.5.[75,76] This increases to 23.1 per 1000, which is manifested at the age of 5. A congenital malformation rate of 3% was observed in the neonatal period, with twice as many occurring in twin births, most of which were monozygotic.[77] The clinical evidence does not indicate that babies born after hMG–hCG ovulation induction are at any greater risk of malformation than the population as a whole.

The postnatal development of the children born did not deviate from acceptable norms. Of 26 daughters,[78] including five pairs of twins, of amenorrheic women who conceived before 1969, 22 (84.6%) reported regular menses, usually associated with pelvic pain (95%). One girl had oligomenorrhea (interval 35 to 45 days), and two had experienced menarche 2 and 4 months before the interview for the study. Only one girl had not yet experienced menarche. The mean age at menarche was 12.3 years (range 10 to 14 years), which was slightly lower than the mean age of 12.6 years among general female populations of children born in Israel[79] and the United States.[80] The mean weight and height of the girls was similar to the 50th percentile values of the healthy population of the same ages born in Israel.[77] Examination of medical histories did not disclose any special data except the usual childhood diseases. All girls had normal psychomotor and mental development.

It can be concluded that the girls examined are developing normally, both physically and mentally, and have normal secondary sex characteristics. A functional hypothalamic-pituitary–ovarian-uterine axis is evidenced by the appearance of menarche followed by normal regular cycles. This observation is of special importance among the girls whose mothers had pituitary failure or insufficiency, indicating that the disease is not necessarily hereditary. Although the number of postpubertal girls examined so far is too small to allow final conclusions, we believe that the group in the study was of sufficient size to reassure clinicians, the treated mothers, and their offspring that no serious defect in pubertal development is expected to occur as the result of treatment.

Long-term Safety

Nulliparity has been a consistently reported risk factor for carcinoma of the breast and endometrium.[81–85] Among the 1438 functionally infertile patients in our series,[30] the rate of hormone-associated tumors was 1.5 times the expected rate. For carcinoma of the breast it was 1.4 times higher and for endometrial cancers 8.0 times higher. In an attempt to assess whether risk factors could be linked to different causes in this heterogeneous group, these infertile patients were analyzed according to three types: (1) amenorrheic patients with low endogenous estrogen and gonadotropin levels (141 patients); (2) infertile women displaying both estrogens and postovulatory progesterone whose infertility was due to mechanical infertility, male-factor infertility, or unexplained infertility (712 patients); and (3) amenorrheic or anovulatory women displaying endogenous

estrogens but lacking or having less than normal postovulatory progesterone levels (992 patients).

In the first group, the observed hormone-associated cancer rate was lower than expected for all sites. Not a single case of breast, endometrial, or other hormone-associated cancer was detected (although 1.68 were expected) in patients of this group independent of whether hMG–hCG therapy was followed by pregnancy. Among the women in the second group, no increased risk for hormone-associated cancer was observed. In the third group the observed rates of uterine and breast cancer were 10.3 and 1.8 times greater than expected, respectively.

For 187 women with functional infertility who were treated with hMG-hCG, no record of conception exists. In this group, three breast cancers were observed and 1.1 were expected. This figure is 2.83 times greater than the expected rate in a matched population. Furthermore, two cases of endometrial cancer were found, whereas only 0.07 were expected. This figure is 28.6 times the expected rate. In contrast, among the 198 women who conceived between 1965 and 1975 after induction of ovulation with hMG-hCG, not a single case of breast or endometrial cancer was observed. Our investigation indicates that women treated with hMG-hCG are not at increased risk for cancer.

Because the number of women who underwent each specific treatment was small, the statistical power to detect minor effects of treatment was low; however, a large cancer risk would certainly have been detected. It seems from the results presented that among the infertile patients, only anovulatory women with unopposed estrogens are at increased risk for uterine and breast cancer. Induction of ovulation with hMG-hCG followed by conception seems to reduce the risk. The interpretation of these results must be tempered by the fact that most of these women have not yet entered the natural cancer age. In one publication, Whitemore et al[86] used a large combined data set derived from case control studies in the United States. They interpreted their findings to show that an increased risk for ovarian cancer associated with infertility in part may be due to the use of fertility drugs.

The global study population of the three studies used by Whitemore et al[86] in this analysis was 2278 women, of whom only 1723 were included in the analysis. The data related to infertility drugs were calculated from 20 ever-married patients with invasive epithelial ovarian cancer treated with infertility drugs and 11 controls. This very small number of subjects is responsible for the extremely wide 95% confidence interval of 2.3–315.6 with a mean risk of 27.0 for women who despite receiving fertility drugs did not conceive. Conception reduced this risk to levels of fertile controls.

The data of Whitemore et al[86] contrast with our results,[30,87] which indicate that hMG–hCG therapy does not increase risk for cancer. Because the number of women receiving each specific treatment was small, and most of the patients in our study had not yet reached the age of the maximal cancer risk, the statistical power to detect minor effects of treatment was low. We therefore reinvestigated our data again 10 years later. Preliminary results representing more than 56,000 woman years identified no indication that treatment of anovulatory patients with hMG–hCG increases their risk for cancer, even though the mean age of the women reached 50.6 years and the follow-up period was lengthened to 21.9 years. An increasing number of studies strongly suggest that an association between gonadotropin therapy and ovarian or other cancer is highly unlikely.[89-91]

Gonadotropins as ovulation-inducing drugs, if administered to properly selected patients in correct dosages and with effective monitoring of treatment, are relatively safe for both patients and offspring. It can be concluded that anovulatory patients have a 60% to 80% chance of delivering a healthy baby. For infertility due to mechanical factors, microsurgical and IVF procedures have changed the once-grim prognosis. The likelihood of conception varies from 60% to 70% for tubal anastomosis or adhesiolysis to 20% to 30% for neosalpingostomy[92] and 10% to 20% for IVF.[93] These rates are still much smaller than for infertility due to endocrine factors.

REFERENCES

1. Lunenfeld B, Donini P: Historic aspects of gonadotropins. In: Greenblat RB (ed), *Ovulation.* Toronto, Lippincott, 1966: 105–115

2. Zondek B, Ascheim S: Das Hormon des Hypophysenvorderlappens: Testobject zum Nachweis des Hormons. *Klin Wochenschr* 6:248, 1927

3. Smith PE, Engle ET: Experimental evidence regarding role of anterior pituitary in development and regulation of genital system. *Am J Anat* 40:159, 1927

4. Borth R, Lunenfeld B, de Watteville H: Activité gonadotrope d'un extrait d'urines de femmes en ménopause. *Experientia* 10:266, 1954

5. Borth R, Lunenfeld B, Riotton G, et al: Activité gonadotrope d'un extrait de femmes en ménopause (2nd communication). *Experientia* 13:115, 1957

6. Gemzell CA, Diczfalusy E, Tillinger G: Clinical effect of human pituitary follicle-stimulating hormone (FSH). *J Clin Endocrinol Metab* 18:1333, 1958

7. Cochius JI, Mack K, Burns RJ: Creuzfeld-Jakob disease in a recipient human pituitary derived gonadotrophin. *Aust N Z J Med* 20:592, 1990

8. Dumble LD, Klein RD: Creuzfel-Jakob disease legacy for Australian women treated with human pituitary gonadotropins. *Lancet* 340:848, 1992

9. Borth R, Lunenfeld B, Menzi A: Pharmacologic and clinical effects of a gonadotropin preparation from human postmenopausal urine. In: Albert A, Thomas MC (eds), *Human Pituitary Gonadotropins.* Springfield, IL, Thomas, 1961:255

10. Lunenfeld B, Sulimovici S, Rabau E, et al: L'induction de l'ovulation dans les amenorrhees hypophysaires par un traitement combiné de gonadotrophines urinaires ménopausiques et de gonadotrophines chorioniques. *Compt Rend Soc Fr Gynecol* 5:287, 1962

11. Australian Department of Health, Results of hMG therapy. Personal communication, 1981

12. Bettendorf G, Braendle W, Sprotte CH, Weise CH, Zimmerman: Overall results of gonadotropin therapy. In: Insler V, Bettendorf G (eds), *Advances in Diagnosis and Treatment of Infertility.* New York, Elsevier-North Holland, 1981:21–26

13. Butler JK: Oestrone response patterns and clincal results following various pergonal dosage schedules. In: Butler JK (ed), *Developments in the Pharmacology and Clinical Uses of Human Gonadotrophins.* High Wycombe England, G. D. Searle, 1970:42

14. Caspi E, Levin S, Bukovsky J, Weintraub Z: Induction pregnancy with human gonadotropins after clomiphene failures in menstruating ovulatory infertility patients. *Isr J Med Sci* 10:249, 1974

14a. Caspi E, Ronen J, Schreyer P, et al: Pregnancy and infant outcome after gonadotropin therapy. *Br J Obstet Gynaecol* 83:967, 1976

15. Ellis JD, Williamson JG: Factors influencing pregnancy and complication rates with human menopausal gonadotropin therapy. *British J Obstet Gynaec* 82:52, 1975

16. Gemzell CA: Recent results of human gonadotropin therapy. In: Bettendorf G, Insler V (eds), *Clinical Application of Human Gonadotropins.* Stuttgart, Thieme Verlag, 1970:6

17. Goldfarb AF, Schlaff S, Mansi ML: A life-table analysis of pregnancy yield in fixed low-dose menotropin therapy for patients in whom clomiphene citrate failed to induce ovulation. *Fertil Steril* 37:629, 1982

18. Healy DL, Kovacs GT, Pepperell RJ, Burger HG: A normal cumulative conception rate after human pituitary gonadotropin. *Fertil Steril* 34:341, 1980

19. Kurachi K: Problems concerning ovulation induction. *Nippon Sanka Fujinka Gakkai Zashi* 35:1127, 1983

20. Lunenfeld B, Mashiah S, Blankstein J: Induction ovulation with gonadotropins. In: Shearman R (ed), *Clinical Reproductive Endocrinology.* New York, Churchill Livingstone, 1985:523

21. Spadoni LR, Cox DW, Smith DC: Use of human menopausal gonadotropin for the induction of ovulation. *Amer J Obstet Gynecol* 120:988, 1974

22. Thompson LR, Hansen LM: Pergonal (menotropin): A summary of clinical experience in the induction of ovulation and pregnancy. *Fertil Steril* 21:844, 1970

23. Tsapoulis AD, Zourlaz PA, Comninos AC: Observations on 320 infertile patients treated with human gonadotropins (human menopausal gonadotropin/human chorionic gonadotropin. *Fertil Steril* 29:492, 1978

24. Serhal PF, Katz M, Little V, Woronowski H: Unexplained infertility—the value of Pergonal superovulation combined with intrauterine insemination. *Fertil Steril* 49:602–606, 1988

25. Welner S, DeCherney AH, Polan ML: Human menopausal gonadotropins: A justifiable therapy in ovulatory women with long-standing idiopathic infertility. *Fertil Steril* 158:111–117, 1988

sufficient but follicle diameter is 15 or 16 mm, FSH may be withheld and the patient "coasts" for 24 hours. A serum estradiol measurement and pelvic ultrasound examination are repeated the next day, and hCG is administered that afternoon. Patients who need more than 14 days of treatment or more than three ampules (225 IU) of FSH a day are unlikely to respond to this form of treatment. With this protocol 94% of pregnancies occurred within two treatment cycles.[60] Pregnancy and nonpregnancy cycles were compared for characteristics associated with a successful outcome. Success was most likely among patients with more "classic" PCO syndrome, that is, those with obesity, high body surface area (>1.78 m²), LH/FSH ratio greater than 2.5, and testosterone level greater than 80 ng/dL (27.7 nmol/L). Ovarian hyperstimulation is more likely to occur in nonconception cycles. These data are helpful in counseling patients with PCO syndrome who need ovulation induction with FSH.

Another group of authors administered a relatively low dose of FSH to a group of patients with PCO syndrome diagnosed at ultrasound examination who has at least one endocrine abnormality, that is, an elevated LH or testosterone level or both. FSH was initiated 2 or 3 days after menses at a dosage of one ampule (75 IU) a day for 14 days. If no response was seen, the dose was increased by half an ampule (37.5 IU) per day. The dose was increased by one half ampule every 7 days until a follicle 12 mm or more in diameter was found, after which the dose remained constant until ovulation.[64] Ovulation was induced with 5000 IU of hCG when the dominant follicle was 18 mm or more in diameter. Ovulation occurred in 75% of patients and 77% of cycles induced, and a single dominant follicle developed in 70% of cycles. Similar results were obtained when hMG was administered according to the same protocol. The results of the study suggested that low doses and longer duration of treatment both are important aspects of gonadotropin treatment of PCO syndrome.

In a separate protocol, we compared administration of a short course of uFSH (5±1 days), which is of similar duration to clomiphene, to the aforedescribed protocol (11±4 days). In spite of comparable estradiol levels (short, 887 pg/mL [3260 pmol/L]; long, 856 pg/mL [3140 pmol/L]) and numbers of preovulatory follicles (short, 2.0; long, 1.7), no pregnancies occurred in the short protocol group. These data suggest that effective folliculogenesis in PCO syndrome necessitates more than 6 days of uFSH administration to simulate the normal physiologic requirements for maturation.

One group of authors used a pulsatile infusion pump to administer FSH intravenously to patients with PCO syndrome.[71] Eight patients received 75 to 112.5 IU a day. A pulse interval of 120 minutes was used to infuse 6.7 IU per pulse. hCG was used to trigger ovulation. All patients had four or more follicles, and four patients had between seven and 15. Five of eight patients experienced ovarian overstimulation; per one woman it was se-

vere with ascites and altered coagulation values. There was one triplet and one quadruplet pregnancy. Although it is innovative, in my opinion intravenous administration of FSH must be used with great caution in the treatment of ovulatory disorders associated with PCO syndrome. It is possible, however, that this modality may prove useful to women who respond poorly to ovulation-induction protocols for in vitro fertilization (IVF).

In another treatment approach, FSH was used in sequence with intravenous pulsatile administration of GnRH. GnRH administration was initiated on cycle day 2 after a progestin-induced bleed at a dosage of 20 μg per pulse every 59 minutes. On cycle days 5, 7, and 9 patients received two ampules of FSH (75 IU per ampule) per day. If an ultrasound examination performed on day 10 revealed at least one follicle 12 mm or more in diameter GnRH was continued and FSH discontinued. If the desired stage was not reached, two ampules of FSH were given daily until at least one follicle 18 mm or more in diameter formed; 5000 IU hCG then was administered. Ovulation occurred in 13 to 15 days in all patients, and only one follicle developed in each patient.

Other authors have used a step-down dosage regimen for induction of ovulation in PCO syndrome.[65] Patients with PCO syndrome initially were given a GnRH agonist for 3 weeks. Either hMG or FSH was added at a dosage of 150 IU a day intramuscularly and was continued until at least one follicle attained a diameter of 9 mm. The gonadotropin dosage was then decreased to 1.5 ampules (112.5 IU) for 2 days and then further reduced to one ampule (75 IU) a day until one to three follicles achieved a diameter of 18 mm or more. On that day the GnRH agonist and the gonadotropins were discontinued, and 10,000 IU of hCG was given intramuscularly. Twenty-two of 28 patients ovulated. Pregnancy rates were not stated.

Controlled, prospective studies comparing uFSH and hMG for ovulation induction in PCO syndrome suggest that ovulation and pregnancy rates are comparable.[61–65,68,72] Use of uFSH, however, appears to result in fewer complications if prospective monitoring of cycles is conducted with estrogen measurements and pelvic ultrasound examinations. Multiple protocols are available. Further refinement of dosage and duration of treatment will no doubt enhance the effectiveness and safety of use of uFSH for the treatment of anovulation in patients with PCO disease.

Urinary Follicle-Stimulating Hormone for In Vitro Fertilization

Successful IVF and embryo transfer (ET) is positively correlated with the number of oocytes retrieved and the number of embryos transferred.[73] For this reason, many IVF centers have begun incorporating uFSH into their treatment protocols for controlled ovarian hyperstimulation (COH). Studies with intact monkeys have shown uFSH capable of recruiting several follicles with infrequent spontaneous LH surges.[69] Although this is a potentially undesirable outcome for ovulation induction in PCO syndrome, lack of an LH surge is highly desirable at IVF centers. Workers must precisely document the onset of the LH surge or time of hCG administration to plan oocyte retrieval.

Administering uFSH for IVF also poses a theoretic concern. Unlike patients with hypothalamic amenorrhea, who respond poorly to purified FSH, patients undergoing IVF have normal levels of circulating endogenous LH. Therefore, the addition of exogenous LH could result in enhanced androgen production and follicular atresia. To address this concern, 28 ovulatory cycles were studied prospectively and randomly treated with clomiphene citrate, 50 to 100 mg/day for 5 days, and hMG, 225 IU/day for 3 days; clomiphene citrate and uFSH; or uFSH alone. Peripheral levels of androstenedione decreased in a statistically significant way with use of uFSH alone or in sequence with clomiphene citrate.[74] Mean serum estradiol levels were not statistically different (Table 31–4). The results of this study suggested that uFSH is less androgenic than hMG for ovulation induction in IVF cycles. Furthermore, ovulation induction with hMG compared with uFSH results in a statistically significant increase in follicular fluid androgen levels.[75] Both these findings suggest that use of uFSH may improve oocyte quality and, indirectly, pregnancy rates achieved by means of IVF.

Clinical trials with uFSH alone have resulted in a tendency to larger number of oocytes retrieved, embryos transferred, and pregnancies achieved compared with hMG regimens.[76–81] One group used FSH therapy alone after pituitary desensitization and found FSH alone fully effective and highly successful.[82] When uFSH is compared with extra hMG for augmenting treatment during follicular recruitment (cycle days 3, 4, and possibly 5), more mature oocytes are retrieved, higher numbers of embryos are transferred, and pregnancy rates are increased considerably.[77,83] Other groups have not found an advantage with uFSH alone over hMG. In fact a higher frequency of short luteal phases in uFSH-stimulated cycles was reported. One report suggested that uFSH may be associated with an increased prevalence of empty follicle syndrome.[84] All the empty follicles occurred in patients with unexplained infertility, however, and may represent an entity that existed before the IVF program was begun. Use of rFSH has also been evaluated in a multicenter, prospective, randomized study in conjunction with use of a GnRH agonist.[85,86] The rFSH was found to be as safe and effective as uFSH for stimulation of ovarian follicular development. If FSH and hMG are equally effective medications for IVF, the increasing availability of rFSH with its lack of immunogenicity and improved batch-to-batch consistency (because the isoform profile is controlled) may make rFSH the drug of choice for assisted reproductive technology, especially since it appears that rFSH can be used safely and successfully even following an IgE-mediated allergic reaction to uFSH. This will certainly be the case if manufacturers market rFSH less expensively than the currently available urinary extracts.

TABLE 31–4. PERIPHERAL SEX STEROID VALUES IN OVULATORY MENSTRUAL CYCLES AUGMENTED WITH REGIMENS OF PURE URINARY FOLLICLE-STIMULATING HORMONE AND HUMAN MENOPAUSAL GONADOTROPIN

Treatment	$E_2 \bar{x} \Delta$	$P \bar{x} \Delta$	$T \bar{x} \Delta$	$\Delta_4 \bar{x} \Delta$
CI–hMG ($n = 7$)	698.2 (NS)	0.14 (NS)	0.24 (NS)	2.25 (< .05)
CI–uFSH ($n = 13$)	638.5 (NS)	0.43 (NS)	0.07 (NS)	0.45
uFSH ($n = 8$)	55.8	0.19 (NS)	0.11 (NS)	0.17

E_2, estradiol; P, progesterone; T, testosterone; CI, clomiphene.
From Oskowitz SP, Seibel MM, Taymor ML: Comparative effects on sex steroids of pure urinary follicle-stimulating hormone and human menopausal gonadotropins in clomiphene-primed ovulatory cycles. Presented at the 41st Annual Meeting of the American Fertility Society, September 27–October 5, 1985, Chicago. Reprinted with permission of the publisher, The American Fertility Society.

REFERENCES

1. Zondek B, Aschheim S: Des Hormon des Hypophysenvorderlappens. *Klin Wochenschr* 6:248, 1927
2. Smith PE, Engle ET: Experimental evidence regarding the role of anterior pituitary in the development and regulation of the genital system. *Am J Anat* 40:159, 1927
3. Cole HH, Hart GH: The potency of blood serum of mares in progressive stages of pregnancy in effecting the sexual maturation of immature rats. *Am J Physiol* 93:57, 1930
4. Hamblem EC, David CD: Treatment of hypoovarianism by the sequential and cyclic administration of equine and chorionic gonadotropins. *Am J Obstet Gynecol* 50:137, 1945
5. Buxton CL: The pitfalls of clinical research. *J Clin Endocrinol Metab* 13:231, 1953
6. Gemzell CA, Diczfalusy E, Tillinger KG: Clinical effect of human pituitary follicle-stimulating hormone. *J Clin Endocrinol Metab* 18:1333, 1958
7. Donini P, Puzzuoli D, Montezeniola R: Purification of gonadotropins from human menopause urine. *Acta Endocrinol (Copenh)* 45:321, 1964
8. Lunenfeld B, Sulimovici S, Rabau E, Eshkol A: L'induction de l'ovulation dans les amenorrhoea hypophysaires par un traitement combiné de gonadotrophines urinaires ménopausiques et de gonadotrophines chorionique. *C R Soc Fr Gynecol* 35:346, 1962
9. Taymor ML, Sturgis SH, Lieberman BL, Goldstein DP: Induction of ovulation with human postmenopausal gonadotropin. I. Case selection and results of therapy. *Fertil Steril* 17:731, 1966
10. Taymor ML, Sturgis SH: Induction of ovulation with human postmenopausal gonadotropin. II. Probable causes of overstimulation. *Fertil Steril* 17:736, 1966
11. Karam K, Taymor ML, Berger KJ: Estrogen monitoring and the prevention of ovarian overstimulation during gonadotropin therapy. *Am J Obstet Gynecol* 115:L972, 1973

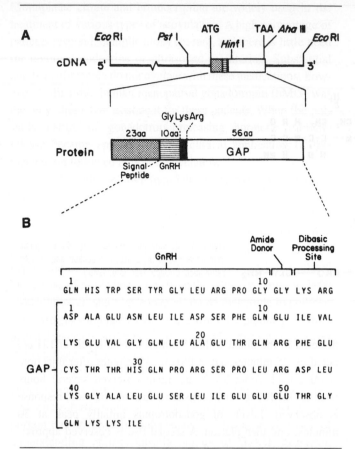

Figure 32–4. Structure and encoded amino acid sequence of human placental cDNA for prepro-GnRH. **A.** Partial-restriction endonuclease map. The coding region is located between the initiation codon for protein synthesis ATG and the termination codon TAA. Schematic representation of the encoded protein identifies the three domains of signal peptide, GnRH, and GAP with the respective sizes in amino acid (aa) residues. **B.** Amino acid sequences of GnRH and GAP with an enzymatic processing site separating the two moieties. Numbers refer to the respective positions within GnRH (1–10) or GAP (1–56). *(From Seeberg PH, Adelman JP: Characterization of cDNA for precursor luteinizing hormone–releasing hormone. Nature 311:666, 1984.)*

priming, or so-called upregulation. Constant infusions of GnRH downregulate by depleting receptors (or desensitize postreceptor response).

Analogs of GnRH with higher potency and longer half-lives than the parent peptide have been developed by means of substitution or omission of certain amino acids from the decapeptide. When administered intermittently, these agonists/antagonists (Fig 32–6) act as if a constant GnRH infusion were being given. Downregulation ensues, with a profound reduction in gonadotropin secretion. Iatrogenic induction of a hypogonadal state with GnRH analogs appears useful in the management of steroid-hormone–dependent disorders such as precocious puberty, endometriosis, uterine fibroids, prostate disease, and hyperandrogenic states. Furthermore, by blocking endogenous gonadotropin secretion, especially the LH surge,

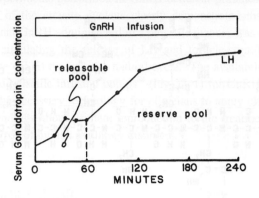

Figure 32–5. Gonadotropin responses to continuous intravenous infusion of GnRH. *(From Keye WR Jr: Regulation of pituitary response to gonadotropin-releasing hormone. In: Sciarra JJ (ed), Gynecology and Obstetrics. New York, Harper & Row, 1987, vol. 5.)*

these analogs appear helpful in improving the predictability of ovarian response to hMG therapy, especially among clomiphene-resistant patients with polycystic ovary (PCO) syndrome and in superovulation regimens for in vitro fertilization (IVF).[55,56]

Secretion

GnRH is cleaved from its precursor and secreted primarily by cells located within the arcuate nucleus. These cells share characteristics of both neuronal and endocrine gland cells. They respond to steroid hormones as well as to neurotransmitters such as catecholamines and endogenous opiates. The releasing hormone and its precursor are synthesized on ribosomes, packaged into granules by the Golgi apparatus, and transported down the axon for storage and secretion primarily into the portal vessels of the pituitary stalk. It is these GnRH fibers of the tuberoinfundibular tract that govern gonadotropin secretion.

Physiologic studies have shown that gonadotropin response to GnRH is strikingly dependent on the mode of administration and the surrounding hormonal milieu. In monkeys, intermittent pulsed administration of this peptide results in a sustained release of FSH and LH, whereas continuous infusion results in inhibition of both gonadotropins (Fig 32–7).[57] In addition, ovarian products (steroids and protein hormones) can modulate gonadotropin secretion, resulting in the cyclic hormonal changes observed during a normal menstrual cycle even if GnRH is administered at a set pulse frequency.[1]

GnRH Physiology in a Normal Menstrual Cycle

Endogenous GnRH is difficult to measure directly because of its very short half-life, the fact that it is secreted into the pituitary portal circulation, and the possibility that peripheral lev-

	AGONISTS				GNRH		ANTAGONISTS	
	D-Trp[6]	Leuprolide	Buserelin	Nafarelin				
1	—	—	—	—	pyro-Glu	N-Ac-D-Na(2)	Ac-Δ^2-Pro	NAc-D-p-Cl-Phe
2					His	D-pCl-Phe	p-F-D-Phe	NAc-D-p-Cl-Phe
3					Trp	D-trp	D-Trp	D-Trp
4					Ser			
5					Tyr			
6	D-Trp	D-Leu	D-Ser(tBu)	D-Nal(2)	Gly	D-hArg(Et$_2$)	D-Trp	D-Phe
7					Leu			
8					Arg			
9					Pro			
10		NHEt	NHEt		Gly-NH$_2$	D-Ala		D-Ala

Figure 32–6. Structure of GnRH decapeptide and sites of substitutions in some of its agonistic and antagonistic analogs. *(From Andreyko JL, et al: Therapeutic uses of gonadotropin-releasing hormone analogs.* Obstet Gynecol Surv *42:1, 1987.)*

els do not reflect portal values. Therefore our understanding of its physiologic role has been facilitated by animal experiments demonstrating that observed peripheral blood LH pulses accurately reflect a preceding bolus of hypothalamic GnRH secreted into the portal circulation (Fig 32–8).[58] These data support the notion that hypothalmic GnRH activity may be in-

ferred by the study of pituitary LH pulses in peripheral blood.[59]

Studies of normal menstrual cycles conducted in this manner have shown that GnRH is regulated by neurotransmitters such as catecholamines and endogenous opiates. Norepinephrine appears to stimulate hypothalamic GnRH secretion by way

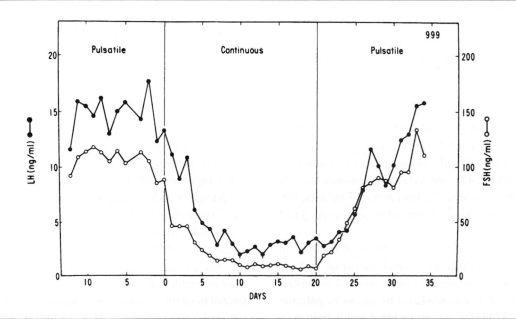

Figure 32–7. When GnRH is administered by means of continuous infusion to a hypothalamic-lesioned rhesus monkey, desensitization and downregulation of the GnRH receptor take place. This leads to marked reduction of both LH and FSH levels. *(From Belchetz PE, et al: Hypophyseal responses to continuous and intermittent delivery of hypothalamic godadotropin-releasing hormone.* Science *202:631, 1978.)*

control of premature LH release, and of disordered luteal-phase function, becomes potentially remediable by means of elimination of pathologic conditions related to disordered pituitary responsiveness.

Luteal Phase Support After Ovulation with Pulsatile GnRH

After follicles mature with GnRH, an endogenous LH surge occurs that initiates ovulation. The quality of the LH surge, however, is often not sufficient to provide adequate luteal-phase support. Therefore, after ovulation, medication must be continued.[93] This can be accomplished with either continuation of the pulsatile GnRH or discontinuation of the pulsatile GnRH and administration of progesterone or human chorionic gonadotropin (hCG). We have found it most convenient and cost-effective to administer hCG, 2500 IU intramuscularly, beginning the day after ovulation and every third day thereafter for a total of three doses.

GNRH AGONISTS AND ENDOMETRIOSIS ASSOCIATED WITH INFERTILITY

The effectiveness of LHRH agonists on symptomatic endometriosis has been well established.[94–97] In a randomized, placebo-controlled study,[95] it was found that treatment with the GnRH agonist leuprolide acetate improved pelvic pain, pelvic tenderness, dysmenorrhea, and dyspareunia. Treatment with GnRH agonists led to improvement in endometriosis as evaluated at laparoscopy. In another randomized study,[96] it was found that the percentage of women with severe symptoms of endometriosis decreased from 40% to 5% to 10% after treatment with nafarelin. When they compared their results to those with use of danazol, the authors found that nafarelin was as effective as danazol. However, danazol treatment was associated with weight gain, edema, myalgia, and increased liver enzyme levels. Danazol also impaired lipid profiles by decreasing serum cholesterol and high-density lipoprotein levels and increasing low-density lipoprotein levels. Nafarelin had no negative effects on blood lipids and only a minimal effect on serum alkaline phosphatase level. (Similar findings related to lipid profiles were obtained in a study in which buserelin and danazol were compared.[98]) In the nafarelin study,[96] the pregnancy rate among women who attempted to conceive was 39% according to 1-year follow-up findings. No statistically significant difference was found in pregnancy rate after danazol and after nafarelin treatment.

The relation between endometriosis and infertility remains unclear. There is little doubt that fertility decreases when endometriosis involves the ovaries and when the adhesions involve the fallopian tubes and ovaries. The association between minimal and mild endometriosis and infertility is less clear.

Some studies suggest that minimal and mild endometriosis decrease fertility.[99–101] Other studies showed no association,[102] and the authors suggested that the pregnancy rate among women with minimal and mild endometriosis is not improved by therapy with GnRH agonists.[103] A large multicenter study is being conducted in Canada to evaluate the association between minimal and mild endometriosis and infertility.

Although medical treatment of pain-related endometriosis is effective, its efficacy in the management of infertility-related endometriosis is questionable. Adhesions associated with endometriosis and large endometriomas are best treated surgically by means of laparoscopy. Laparoscopic treatment of endometriosis is associated with a high fecundity rate even in the presence of advanced disease, and there is a trend suggesting increased pregnancy rates.[104] The treatment is lysis of adhesions, excision of endometriotic implants, and excision of endometriomas. The incidence of pregnancy is independent of the stage of endometriosis (pregnancy rate, 70%), but is directly related to the duration of infertility.[100,105] Some surgeons believe that preoperative treatment with hormones facilitates surgical therapy by softening the endometriotic implants. Others do not share this view. Most pregnancies occur within a year of the operation, and pre- or postoperative treatment with hormones unnecessarily delays conception. Hughes et al[103] reported that hormonal suppression is ineffective therapy for endometriosis-related infertility.

It appears that surgical therapy may be superior to therapy with GnRH agonists in the treatment of endometriosis-related infertility. There is also no clear evidence that medical treatment is of any benefit to future fertility.

GnRH AGONISTS AND MYOMA ASSOCIATED WITH INFERTILITY

The association between myomas and infertility or repeated pregnancy wastage is not fully understood. Several authors[106,107] demonstrated that more than 50% of infertile women with leiomyomata uteri conceived within 1 year after myomectomy. Myomectomy may also be associated with a decrease in the risk of subsequent miscarriage. The precise reason is not clear. Reduction of the implantation space, mechanical compression of the fallopian tube, delay in sperm transport due to increased uterine surface, and interference with uterine vascularization causing endometrial impairment and implantation are the possible explanations. Nevertheless, the finding of a myoma in an infertile woman does not necessarily indicate myomectomy is necessary.

For women with infertility or repeated pregnancy wastage, myomectomy is indicated if the uterus is 16 weeks' gestational size or larger, especially if the myoma impinges on the uterine cavity, or if the uterine cavity is markedly distorted by multiple myomas. Other indications are menorrhagia or pressure symptoms due to the enlarging uterus. It is imperative to exclude other causes of infertility before considering myomectomy. Submucous myomas can be removed at hysteroscopy, although some risk of uterine perforation and subsequent damage to the intestine exists.[108]

Preoperative treatment with GnRH agonists has been advocated by several authors. In a randomized, placebo-controlled study, 77% of women treated with leuprolide acetate had at least a 26% reduction in uterine volume, and 38% experienced more than 50% shrinkage.[109] Treatment is given for 3 months, because a longer duration rarely results in marked additional shrinkage. Leuprolide acetate is usually given in a depot form (3.75 mg intramuscularly every 4 weeks). Although it is not always necessary, women with uterine leiomyoma of larger than 16 weeks' gestational size generally benefit from this preoperative treatment. The main advantage is to allow time to improve the patients' hematologic status. Other advantages are reduction in the amount of blood loss due to the decrease in the vascularity and size of the myoma and easier removal of a smaller myoma. Reduction in the size of the myoma also facilitates performance of myomectomy at laparoscopy. Some surgeons have suggested that pretreatment with GnRH agonists is associated with loss of tissue planes, leading to more difficult dissection of the tumor. We do not share this view. Because bleeding is a potential complication, autologous blood donation or preoperative treatment with ferrous sulfate is recommended for women undergoing myomectomy.

Laparoscopic myomectomy is associated with several advantages, including reduced blood loss, short hospital stay, and rapid recovery. However, laparoscopic myomectomy can lead to inadequate multilayered closure, which may lead to uterine fistula, dehiscence, and rupture. The uterine defect also can be closed extracorporeally with a minilaparotomy incision.[110] The incision is large enough to accommodate the myoma (laparoscopy-assisted myomectomy). The advantages of this approach over laparotomy are reduced length of hospital stay, more rapid postoperative recovery, and possibly less adhesion formation. Periadnexal adhesions are an important cause of reduced fertility after myomectomy.

Estrogen has been reported to be associated with increased adhesion formation in animal models.[112–114] In a rabbit model, animals on which ovariectomy had been performed had a lower total adhesion score than animals with ovaries.[112] In a rat model, fat necrosis and fibrotic changes were found less often in the absence of estrogen.[114] In monkeys, adhesion formation in animals treated with the GnRH agonist leuprolide acetate occurred less often than in intact animals.[113] These findings suggest the possible role of estrogen in encouraging adhe-

sion formation. Whether the hypoestrogenic state leads to less postmyomectomy adhesion formation in humans remains unknown. In any event, other advantages of use of GnRH agonists make it a useful treatment for women undergoing myomectomy.

GnRH AGONISTS FOR OVARIAN STIMULATION IN ASSISTED REPRODUCTION

IVF is a successful procedure the results of which compare favorably with those of spontaneous conception in a natural menstrual cycle of a fertile woman.[115] IVF has helped thousands of infertile women conceive.[116] Although the methods of oocyte recovery and embryo transfer are now uniform at most IVF centers,[117] there is still no consensus about the ideal method of ovarian stimulation. Regimens involving the use of gonadotropins, either alone or combined with clomiphene citrate, necessitate close monitoring of follicular growth and are associated with a high incidence of premature LH surges. In 1984, the use of the GnRH agonist buserelin together with hMG was first reported for ovarian stimulation for IVF.[118] Since that publication, a number of studies have suggested that the use of GnRH agonists prevents spontaneous LH surges and improves follicular response, fertilization, and implantation rates leading to a net increase in pregnancy rate per cycle.[119]

Although the use of GnRH agonists together with gonadotropins has gained widespread popularity and is the sole method of ovarian stimulation in many programs, a number of issues concerning use of these agents remain unresolved. Some of these issues are examined in light of recent developments.

Routine Use of GnRH Agonists for All Patients Undergoing IVF

Most studies describing the superiority of GnRH agonists over conventional stimulation regimens have been conducted with patients who had a poor or abnormal response in previous cycles.[120] There have been relatively few prospective, randomized studies comparing the use of GnRH agonists with conventional stimulation regimens among patients who do not have a specific indication for the use of GnRH agonists. Neveu et al[119] and Antoine et al[121] reported statistically significantly better results among women who received GnRH agonists, but other authors[122] have found no statistically significant differences.

A meta-analysis by Hughes et al[123] of randomized and quasirandomized studies showed that GnRH agonists reduced cancellation rates, increased the number of oocytes recovered, and improved clinical pregnancy rates per cycle begun and per embryo transfer.

Our group[124] studied the results for almost 2900 women who underwent one of five stimulation regimens exclusively

GnRH agonists on the ovary to inhibit steroidogenesis and gonadotropin receptor formation.[151] Unfortunately, the use of GnRH agonists does not reduce the incidence of OHSS. In fact, several studies have suggested that there may be an increased incidence of OHSS when GnRH agonists are used.[152,153] MacDougall et al[85,86] studied the association of OHSS with IVF. They found that pretreatment with GnRH agonists significantly increased the prevalence of severe OHSS (1.1% compared with 0.2%, $P<.05$) compared with ovarian stimulation with clomiphene citrate and hMG[85] and that patients with a pretreatment ultrasound diagnosis of PCO are also at increased risk.[86] Wada et al[154] also reported an increased incidence of OHSS among patients with PCO.

Because there is no definitive treatment of OHSS and management is symptomatic rather than curative, prevention is important. There are a few strategies for preventing OHSS among patients considered to be at increased risk during monitoring, that is, patients with a large number of ovarian follicles and who have a high serum estradiol concentration on the day of hCG administration.

First, hCG can be withheld, the cycle abandoned, and a new cycle begun 1 or 2 months later. This is the safest option, but many patients and clinicians are reluctant to embark on this course of action because of the difficulties of treatment and the emotional and financial commitment invested by the patient. Moreover, this policy results in cancellation of a high proportion of cycles that will not progress to clinical hyperstimulation. Second, hCG could be withheld and the GnRH agonist continued until pituitary desensitization is achieved, at which point hMG is re-commenced at a lower dose. However, discontinuing hMG and re-commencing follicular stimulation with a lower dose of gonadotropin may take anywhere from 24 to 56 days,[152] and repeat stimulation with a lower dose of hMG may still lead to excessive stimulation or, conversely, inadequate response of the ovaries. Third, one may proceed with oocyte collection but freeze all pre-embryos for transfer in a subsequent cycle.[155] A study by Wada et al.[156] showed that elective cryopreservation of all embryos from women with high estradiol levels reduced the severity but not the incidence of symptomatic OHSS. If cryopreservation is used, there is no advantage in continuing administration of GnRH agonists.[157] Fourth, glucocorticoids can be administered after oocyte recovery and slowly tapered off over a 10-day period. However, the only prospective, randomized study that addressed this issue showed no benefit for glucocorticoid administration.[158] The use of intravenous albumin in patients at high risk for OHSS has been suggested,[159] but some recent studies have questioned the usefulness of this approach.[160]

It would therefore appear that there is no ideal method of preventing OHSS. Because PCO is a definite high-risk factor, it would be prudent to assess ovarian morphology by means of ul-

trasound scan at the beginning of treatment. If PCOs are identified, then the dose of gonadotropins used should initially be low and be cautiously increased if necessary. If, despite these precautions, there are many preovulatory follicles and high serum estradiol levels on the day of presumed hCG administration, then the choice of which of the aforementioned must be carefully considered for the individual patient. In practice, the decision is influenced to some extent by the results of cryopreservation in the particular IVF program. If a decision is made to proceed with oocyte recovery, then every follicle, including small and medium-sized ones, should be emptied[161] because the presence of these follicles contributes to the risk for OHSS.

GnRH Agonists and Miscarriage Rates

Two studies have suggested that the use of GnRH agonists may reduce miscarriage rates among some patients. Homburg et al[162] conducted a study with 239 women with PCO in whom clomiphene therapy had failed, who underwent GnRH agonist and hMG therapy ($n = 110$) or hMG therapy only ($n = 128$) for ovulation induction ($n = 138$) or IVF ($n = 101$). The miscarriage rate among women undergoing induction of ovulation who took GnRH agonists and hMG was 16.7% compared with 39.4% among women who took hMG alone. For patients undergoing IVF, the comparable figures were 18.2% and 38.5%. Balen et al[163] studied the risk of miscarriage among 1060 IVF pregnancies related to age, cause of infertility, ovarian morphology, and treatment regimen. The miscarriage rate was 23.6% among women with normal ovaries compared with 35.8% among those with PCO ($P = .0038$). Women whose ovaries were normal at ultrasound examinations were just as likely to miscarry if they were treated with gonadotropins and clomiphene citrate or with the long buserelin protocol. Those with PCO, however, had a statistically significant reduction in the rate of miscarriage when treated with the long buserelin protocol (20.3%) compared with gonadotropins and clomiphene citrate (47.2%).

CONCLUSIONS

The introduction of GnRH and its agonists into infertility treatment has been an important advance in reproductive medicine. Pulsatile GnRH has an important, albeit somewhat limited, role at the moment for induction of ovulation in patients with clomiphene-resistant anovulation. It is the preferred treatment of patients with HH. Data suggest GnRH may have a greater role in the treatment of patients with PCO syndrome than hitherto believed. GnRH agonists offer another option for induction of ovulation, and there are some preliminary data that use of these drugs may reduce miscarriage rates. GnRH agonists are useful in pretreatment of fibroids before myomectomy and are widely used in the treatment of endometriosis.

In the context of assisted reproduction, the use of GnRH agonists increases pregnancy rate, decreases miscarriage rate, and increases livebirth rate after IVF. It allows flexible timing of hCG administration. The long protocol of GnRH agonist administration should, in general, be the ovarian stimulation regimen of choice for use in IVF today.

REFERENCES

1. Knobil E: The neuroendocrine control of the menstrual cycle. *Recent Prog Horm Res* 36:53, 1980
2. Harris GW: The pituitary stalk and ovulation. In: Vilee CA (ed), *Control of Ovulation.* New York, Pergamon, 1961: 56
3. Campbell HJ, Feuer G, Garcia J, Harris GW: The infusion of brain extracts into the anterior pituitary gland and the secretion of gonadotrophic hormones. *J Physiol* 157:30P, 1961
4. McCann SM, Talesnik S, Friedman H: LH-releasing activity in hypothalamic extracts. *Proc Soc Exp Biol Med* 104:432, 1960
5. Matsuo H, Baba Y, Nair RMG, Arimura A, Schally AV: Structure of the porcine LH and FSH releasing factor. I. The proposed amino acid sequence. *Biochem Biophys Res Commun* 43:1334, 1971
6. Burgus R, Butcher M, Ling N, Guillemin R: Structure moleculaire du facteur hypothalamique (LRF) d'origina ovine controlant la secretion de l'hormone gonadotrope hypophysaire de luteinisation (LH). *Seances Acad Sci* (III) 273:1611, 1971
7. Schally AV: Aspects of hypothalamic regulation of the pituitary gland: Its implications for the control of reproductive processes. *Science* 202:18, 1978
8. Guillemin R: Peptides in the brain: The new endocrinology of the neuron. *Science* 202:390, 1978
9. Taymor ML: The use of luteinizing hormone-releasing hormone in gynecologic endocrinology. *Fertil Steril* 25:992, 1974
10. Grimes EM, Thompson IE, Taymore ML: The sequence of pituitary responses to synthetic luteinizing hormone-releasing hormone (LH-RH) throughout the normal menstrual cycle. *Acta Endocrinol* 79:625, 1975
11. Feore JC, Taymore ML: The relationship between the pituitary response to luteinizing hormone-releasing hormone and the ovulatory response to clomiphene citrate. *Fertil Steril* 27:1240, 1976
12. Mortimer RH, Fleischer N, Lev-Gur M, et al: Correlation between integrated LH and FSH levels and the response to luteinizing hormone-releasing factor (LRF). *J Clin Endocrinol Metab* 43:1240, 1976
13. Reiter EO, Root AW, Duckett GE: The response of pituitary gonadotrope to a constant infusion of luteinizing hormone-releasing hormone (LHRH) in normal prepubertal and pubertal children and in children with abnormalities of sexual development. *J Clin Endocrinol Metab* 43:400, 1976
14. Wentz AC, Andersen RN: Response to repetitive luteinizing hormone-releasing hormone stimulation in hypothalamic and pituitary disease. *Am J Obstet Gynecol* 138:364, 1980
15. Kastin AJ, Zarate A, Midgley AR, et al: Ovulation confirmed by pregnancy after infusion of porcine LHRH. *J Clin Endocrinol Metab* 33:980, 1971
16. Grimes EM, Taymor ML, Thompson IE: Induction of timed ovulation with synthetic luteinizing hormone-releasing hormone in women undergoing insemination therapy. I. Effect of a single parenteral administration at mid-cycle. *Fertil Steril* 26:277, 1975
17. Acosta AA, Buttram VC, Malinak LR, et al: The use of synthetic luteinizing hormone-releasing hormone in induction of ovulation. *Fertil Steril* 26:1173, 1975
18. Huang KE: The induction of ovulation in amenorrheic patients with synthetic luteinizing hormone-releasing hormone: The significance of pituitary responsiveness. *Fertil Steril* 27:65, 1976
19. Huang KE: Use of synthetic luteinizing hormone-releasing hormone in induction of ovulation in amenorrheic patients. *Fertil Steril* 26:796, 1975
20. Keller PJ: Induction of ovulation by synthetic luteinizing hormone-releasing factor in infertile women. *Lancet* 2:570, 1972
21. Breckwoldt M, Czygan PJ, Lehman F, Bettendorf G: Synthetic LH-RH as a therapeutic agent. *Acta Endocrinol* 75:209, 1974
22. Crosignani PG, Trojsi L, Attansio A, et al: Hormonal profiles in anovulatory patients treated with gonadotropins and synthetic luteinizing hormone-releasing hormone. *Obstet Gynecol* 46:15, 1975
23. Maia H Jr, Barbosa I, Maia H, et al: Induction of ovulation with clomiphene citrate followed by LH-RH in women. *Int J Gynaecol Obstet* 21:1, 1983
24. Nakano R, Katayama K, Mizuno T, Tojo S: Induction of ovulation with synthetic luteinizing hormone-releasing hormone. *Fertil Steril* 24:471, 1974
25. Phansey SA, Barnes MA, Williamson HO, et al: Combined use of clomiphene and intranasal luteinizing hormone-releasing hormone for induction of ovulation in chronically anovulatory women. *Fertil Steril* 34:446, 1980
26. Kotsuji F, Kitaguchi M, Okamura Y, Tojo S: Luteinizing hormone-releasing hormone (LH-RH) treatment for inducing clomiphene response in anovulatory patients with hypogonadotropic hypogonadism. *Asia Oceania J Obstet Gynaecol* 8:139, 1982
27. Akande EO, Carr PJ, Dutton A, et al: Effect of synthetic gonadotropin-releasing hormone in secondary amenorrhea. *Lancet* 2:112, 1972
28. Casas PRF, Badano AR, Aparicio N, et al: Luteinizing hormone-releasing hormone in the treatment of anovulatory infertility. *Fertil Steril* 26:549, 1975
29. Hammond CB, Wiebe RH, Haney A, Yancy SG: Ovulation induction with luteinizing hormone-releasing hormone in amenorrheic infertile women. *Am J Obstet Gynecol* 135:924, 1979
30. Hanker JP, Bohnet HG, Leyendecker G, Schneider HPG: LH-RH therapy in functional amenorrhea based on clinical subclassification. *Int J Fertil* 25:222, 1980
31. Henderson SR, Bonnar J, Moore A, MacKinnon PCB: Luteinizing hormone-releasing hormone for induction of follicular maturation and ovulation in women with infertility and amenorrhea. *Fertil Steril* 27:621, 1976

95. Dlugi AM, Miller JD, Knittle J: Lupron depot (leuprolide acetate) for depot suspension in the treatment of endometriosis: A randomized placebo-controlled, double blind study. *Fertil Steril* 54:419, 1990

96. The Nafarelin European Endometriosis Trial Group: Nafarelin for endometriosis: A large scale, danazol-controlled trial efficacy and safety, with 1 year follow-up. *Fertil Steril* 57:514, 1992

97. Wheeler JM, Knittle JD, Miller JD: Depot leuprolide acetate versus danazol in the treatment of women with symptomatic endometriosis: A multicenter, double blind randomized clinical trial. II. Assessment of safety. *Am J Obstet Gynecol* 169:26, 1993

98. Dlugi AM, Rufo S, D'Amico JF, Seibel MM: A comparison of the effect of buserelin versus danazol on plasma lipoproteins during treatment of pelvic endometriosis. *Fertil Steril* 49:913, 1988

99. Nowroozi K, Chase JS, Check JH, Wu CH: The importance of laparoscopic coagulation of mild endometriosis in infertile women. *Int J Fertil* 32:442, 1987

100. Nezhat C, Crowgey S, Nezhat F: Videolaseroscopy for the treatment of endometriosis associated infertility. *Fertil Steril* 51:237, 1989

101. Tulandi T, Mouchawar M: Treatment-dependent and treatment-independent pregnancy among women with minimal and mild endometriosis. *Fertil Steril* 56:790, 1991

102. Seibel MM: Does minimal endometriosis always require treatment? *Contemp Obstet Gynecol* 34:84, 1989

103. Hughes EG, Fedorkow DM, Collins JA: A quantitative overview of controlled trials in endometriosis-associated infertility. *Fertil Steril* 59:963, 1993

104. Adamson GD, Lu J, Subak LL: Laparoscopic CO_2 laser vaporization of endometriosis compared with traditional treatments. *Fertil Steril* 50:704, 1988

105. Olive DL, Martin DC: Treatment of endometriosis-associated infertility with CO_2 laser laparoscopy: The use of one and two-parameter exponential models. *Fertil Steril* 48:18, 1987

106. Buttram VC Jr, Reiter RC: Uterine leiomyomata: Etiology, symptomatology and management. *Fertil Steril* 36:433, 1981

107. Tulandi T, Murray C, Guralnick M: Adhesion formation and reproductive outcome after myomectomy and second-look laparoscopy. *Obstet Gynecol* 82:213, 1993

108. Sullivan B, Kenney P, Seibel MM: Hysteroscopic resection of fibroid with thermal injury to sigmoid closed by primary repair. *Obstet Gynecol* 80:546, 1992

109. Friedman AJ, Hoffman DI, Browneller RW, Miller JD: Treatment of leiomyomata uteri with leuprolide acetate depot: A double-blind, placebo-controlled, multicenter study. *Obstet Gynecol* 77:720, 1991

110. Nezhat C, Nezhat F, Bess O, Nezhat CH: Laparoscopically assisted myomectomy: A report of a new technique in 57 cases. *Int J Fertil* 39:39, 1994

111. Tulandi T, Collins JA, Burrows E, et al: Treatment-dependent and treatment-independent pregnancy among women with periadnexal adhesions. *Am J Obstet Gynecol* 162:354, 1990

112. Metzger DA, Breault DT, Chaffkin L, et al: The role of estrogen suppression versus oophorectomy in adhesion formation (abstract P347). In: Abstracts of the Scientific Sessions of the 40th Annual Meeting of The Society for Gynecologic Investigations, Toronto, Ontario, 1993: 356

113. Grow DR, Coddington CC, Seltman H, et al: Role of hypoestrogens in adhesion formation after myometrial surgery in primates (abstract O-002). In: Abstracts of the Scientific Oral and Poster Sessions of the 50th Annual Meeting of The American Fertility Society, San Antonio, Texas, 1994: S1

114. Wright JA, Sharpe KL: Gonadotrophin releasing hormone agonist (GnRHa) therapy reduces postoperative adhesion formation and reformation following adhesiolysis in rat models for adhesion formation and endometriosis (abstract O-119). In: Abstracts of Scientific Oral and Poster Sessions of the 50th Annual Meeting of The American Fertility Society, San Antonio, Texas, 1994: S58

115. Tan SL, Steer C, Royston P, Rizk P, Mason BA, Campbell S: Conception rates and in vitro fertilization. *Lancet* 335:299, 1990

116. Tan SL, Royston P, Campbell S, et al: Cumulative conception and live birth rates after in vitro fertilization. *Lancet* 339:1390, 1992

117. Tan SL, Bennett S, Parson J: Surgical techniques for oocyte recovery and embryo transfer. *Br Med Bull* 628, 1990

118. Porter RN, Smith W, Craft IL, et al: Induction of ovulation for in vitro ferilization using buserelin and gonadotrophins. *Lancet* 2:1284, 1984

119. Neveu S, Hedon B, Bringer J, et al: Ovarian stimulation by a combination of a gonadotropin-releasing hormone agonist and gonadotrophins for in-vitro fertilization. *Fertil Steril* 47:639, 1987

120. Cummins JM, Yovich JM, Edinsinghe WR, Yovich JL: Pituitary down-regulation using leuprolide for the intensive ovulation management of poor prognosis patients having in vitro fertilization (IVF) related treatments. *J In Vitro Fertil Embryo Transf* 6:345, 1989

121. Antoine JM, Salat-Baroux J, Alvarez S, et al: Ovarian stimulation using human menopausal gonadotrophins with or without LHRH analogues in a long protocol for in vitro fertilization: A prospective randomized comparison. *Hum Reprod* 5:565, 1990

122. Dor J, Ben-Shlomo I, Levran D, Rudak E, Yunish M, Mashiach S: The relative success of gonadotropin-releasing hormone analogue, clomiphene citrate and gonadotropin in 1099 cycles of in vitro fertilization. *Fertil Steril* 58:986, 1992

123. Hughes EG, Federkow DM, Daya S, Sagle M, de Koppel P, Collins J: The routine use of gonadotropin-releasing hormone agonists prior to in vitro fertilization and gamete intrafallopian transfer: A meta-analysis of randomized controlled trials. *Fertil Steril* 58:888, 1992

124. Tan SL, Maconochie N, Doyle P, et al: Cumulative conception and livebirth rates after in-vitro fertilization with, and without, the use of the long, short and ultrashort regimens of the luteinizing hormone releasing hormone agonist, buserelin. *Am J Obstet Gynecol* 171:513, 1994

125. Penzias AS, Shamma FN, Gutmann JN, Jones EE, DeCherney A, Lavy G: Nafarelin versus leuprolide in ovulation induction for in vitro fertilization: A randomized clinical trial. *Obstet Gynecol* 79:739, 1992

126. Parinaud J, Oustry P, Perineau M, Reme J-M, Monrozies X, Pon-

tonnier G: Randomized trial of three luteinizing hormone-releasing hormone analogues used for ovarian stimulation in an in vitro fertilization program. *Fertil Steril* 57:1265, 1992

127. Filicori M, Flamigni C, Cognigni G, et al: Comparison of the suppressive capacity of different depot gonadotropin-releasing hormone analogs in women. *J Clin Endocrinol Metab* 77:130, 1993

128. Tan SL, Kingsland C, Campbell S, et al: The long protocol of administration of gonadotrophin-releasing hormone agonist is superior to the short protocol for ovarian stimulation for in vitro fertilization. *Fertil Steril* 57:810, 1992

129. Macnamee M, Howles CM, Edwards RG, Taylor PJ, Elder KT: Short term luteinizing hormone releasing hormone treatment: Prospective trial of a novel ovarian stimulation regimen for in vitro fertilization. *Fertil Steril* 52:264, 1989

130. Dirnfeld M, Gonen Y, Lissak A, et al: A randomized prospective study on the effect of short and long buserelin treatment in women with repeated unsuccessful in vitro fertilization (IVF) cycles due to inadequate response. *J In Vitro Fertil Embryo Transf* 8:339, 1991

131. Stanger J, Yovich JL: Reduced in-vitro fertilization of human oocytes from patients with raised basal luteinizing hormone levels during the follicular phase. *Br J Obstet Gynaecol* 92:385, 1985

132. Howles C, Macnamee MC, Edwards RG, Goswamy R, Steptoe PC: Effect of high tonic levels of luteinizing hormone on outcome of in-vitro fertilization. *Lancet* 2:521, 1986

133. Wren M, Tan SL, Waterstone J, Parsons J: A comparative study of the optimum dose and route of administration of buserelin for pituitary downregulation in vitro fertilization. *Hum Reprod* 6:1370, 1991

134. Salat-Baroux J, Alvarez S, Marie Antoine J, et al: Comparison between long and short protocols of LHRH agonist in the treatment of polycystic ovary disease by in-vitro fertilization. *Hum Reprod* 3:535, 1988

135. Rizk B, Tan SL, Kingsland C, Steer C, Mason BA, Campbell S: Ovarian cyst aspiration and outcome of in-vitro fertilization. *Fertil Steril* 54:661, 1990

136. Loumaye E, Vankrieken L, Depreester S, Psalti I, de Cooman S, Thomas K: Hormonal changes induced by short-term administration of a gonadotropin-releasing hormone agonist during ovarian hyperstimulation for in vitro fertilization and their consequences for embryo development. *Fertil Steril* 51:105, 1989

137. Fleming R, Jamieson ME, Coutts JRT: The use of GnRH-analogs in assisted reproduction. In: Matson PL, Lieberman BA (eds), *Clinical IVF Forum: Current Views in Assisted Reproduction*. Manchester, England, Manchester University Press, 1990:1–19

138. Ho PC, Chan YF, So WK, Yeung WSB, Chan STH: Luteinizing hormone (LH) surge in patients using buserelin spray during ovarian stimulation for assisted reproduction. *Gynecol Endocrinol* 4(suppl 2):112, 1990

139. Balen A, Tan SL, Jacobs HS: Hypersecretion of luteinizing hormone: A significant cause of infertility and miscarriage. *Br J Obstet Gynaecol* 100:1082, 1993

140. Daya S: Short versus long protocol using gonadotropin releasing hormone agonists (GnRHa) for in vitro fertilization cycles: A meta-analysis (abstract P-058). Abstracts of the Scientific Oral and Poster Sessions of the 49th Annual Meeting of the American Fertility Society, Montreal, Quebec, Canada. 1993: P058

141. Pellicer A, Simon C, Miro F, et al: Ovarian response and outcome of in-vitro fertilization in patients treated with gondatrophin releasing hormone analogues in different phases of the menstrual cycle. *Hum Reprod* 4:285, 1989

142. Williams RF, Hodgen GD: Disparate effects of human chorionic gonadotropin during the late follicular phase in monkeys: Normal ovulation, follicular atresia, ovarian acyclicity, and hypersecretion of follicle-stimulating hormone. *Fertil Steril* 33:64, 1980

143. Tamada T, Matsumoto S: Suppression of ovulation with human chorionic gonadotropin. *Fertil Steril* 20:840, 1969

144. Punnonen R, Ashorn R, Vilja R, Heinonen PK, Kujansuu E, Tuohimaa P: Spontaneous luteinizing hormone surge and cleavage of in vitro fertilized embryos. *Fertil Steril* 49:479, 1988

145. Zorn JR, Boyer P, Guichard A: Never on a Sunday: Programming for IVF-ET and GIFT. *Lancet* 1:385, 1987

146. Vauthier D, Lefebvre G: The use of gonadotropin-releasing hormone analogs for in vitro fertilization: Comparison between the standard form and long-acting formulation of D-Trp-6-luteinizing hormone-releasing hormone. *Fertil Steril* 51:100, 1989

147. Dimitry ES, Bates SA, Oskarsson T, Margara R, Winston RML: Programming in vitro fertilization for a 5- or 3-day week. *Fertil Steril* 55:934, 1991

148. Clark L, Stanger J, Brinsmead M: Prolonged follicle stimulation decreases pregnancy rates after in vitro fertilization. *Fertil Steril* 55:1192, 1991

149. Tan SL, Balen A, Hussein El, et al: A prospective randomized study of the optimum timing of human chorionic gonadotropin administration after pituitary desensitization in in vitro fertilization. *Fertil Steril* 57:1259, 1992

150. Golan A, Ron-El, Herman A, Weinraub Z, Soffer Y, Caspi E: Ovarian hyperstimulation following D-Trp-6 luteinizing hormone releasing hormone microcapsules and menotropin for in vitro fertilization. *Fertil Steril* 50:912, 1988

151. Hsueh AJW, Jones PBC: Extrapituitary actions of gonadotropin-releasing hormone. *Endocr Rev* 2:437, 1981

152. Forman RG, Frydman R, Egan D, Ross C, Barlow DH: Severe ovarian hyperstimulation syndrome using agonists of gonadotropin-releasing hormone for in vitro fertilization: A European series and a proposal for prevention. *Fertil Steril* 53:502, 1990

153. Tanbo T, Dale PO, Kjekshus E, Abyholm T: Stimulation with human menopausal gonadotropin versus follicle-stimulating hormone after pituitary suppression in polycystic ovarian syndrome. *Fertil Steril* 53:798, 1990

154. Wada I, Matson PL, Troup SA, Lieberman BA: Assisted conception using buserelin and human menopausal gonadotrophins in women with polycystic ovary syndrome. *Br J Obstet Gynaecol* 100:365, 1993

155. Amso NN, Ahuja KK, Morris N, Shaw RW: The management of predicted ovarian hyperstimulation involving gonadotropin-releasing hormone analog with effective cryopreservation of all pre-embryos. *Fertil Steril* 53:1087, 1990

156. Wada I, Matson PL, Troup SA, Morroll DR, Hunt L, Lieberman BA: Does elective cryopreservation of all embryos from women at risk of ovarian hyperstimulation syndrome reduce the incidence of the condition. *Br J Obstet Gynaecol* 100:265, 1993

157. Wada I, Matson PL, Horne G, Buck P, Lieberman BA: Is continuation of a gonadotrophin releasing hormone agonist (GnRHa) necessary for women at risk of developing the ovarian hyperstimulation syndrome? *Hum Reprod* 7:1090, 1992

158. Tan SL, Balen A, Hussein El, Campbell S, Jacobs HS: The administration of glucocorticoids for the prevention of ovarian hyperstimulation syndrome in in vitro fertilization: A prospective randomized study. *Fertil Steril* 57:378, 1992

159. Asch RH, Ivery G, Goldsman M, Frederick JL, Stone SC, Balmaceda JP: The use of intravenous albumin in patients at high risk for severe ovarian hyperstimulation syndrome. *Hum Reprod* 8:1015, 1993

160. Shaker A, Zosmer A, Dean N, Bekir J, Jacobs HS, Tan SL: A randomized study comparing intravenous albumin and transfer of fresh embryos with cyropreservation of all embryos for subsequent transfer in patients at high risk of developing ovarian hyperstimulation syndrome. *Fertil Steril* 65:992, 1996

161. Tan SL, Waterstone J, Wren M, Parsons J: A prospective randomized study comparing aspiration only with aspiration and flushing for transvaginal ultrasound directed oocyte recovery. *Fertil Steril* 57:356, 1992

162. Homburg R, Levy T, Berkovitz D, et al: Gonadotropin-releasing hormone agonist reduces the miscarriage rate for pregnancies achieved in women with polycystic ovarian syndrome. *Fertil Steril* 59:527, 1993

163. Balen A, Tan SL, MacDougall MJ, Jacobs HS: Miscarriage rates following in-vitro fertilization are increased in women with polycystic ovaries and reduced by pituitary desensitisation with buserelin. *Hum Reprod* 8:959, 1992

CHAPTER 33

Treatment of Infertility
with Dopamine Agonists

SCOT M. HUTCHISON · HOWARD A. ZACUR

Comparison of ergot and non-ergot dopamine agonists in the treatment of hyperprolactinemia

Drug	Recommended Dosage	Route of Administration	Duration of Action	Response	Common Side Effects
Ergot					
Parlodel	2.5–10 mg/day (divided)	PO	8 to 12 hrs.	Resolution of symptoms Lowers prolactin Shrinks adenomas	CNS Dizziness, headache, syncope, Nasal stuffiness GI vomiting, nausea Cardiovascular Orthostatic hypotension
Parlodel SRO (Sandoz, Basle, Switzerland)	2.5-15 mg once-a-day	PO	24 hrs.	Similar	Similar
Parlodel LA	50–100mg q-monthly	IM	~28d	Similar	Similar, milder transient
Parlodel, vaginal route	2.5 mg once-a-day	Vaginal	24 hrs.	Similar	Less GI
Mesulergine	0.25–2.0 mg/day (divided)	PO	~ 10 hrs.	Similar	Similar more prevalent
Lisuride (Dopergin, Schering AG Germany)	0.2–0.5 mg/day (divided)	PO	8–12 hrs.	Similar	Similar nausea, dizziness drowsiness more prevalent
Teguride	0.25–1.5 mg/day (divided)	PO	<24 hrs.	Similar	Similar transient central more prevalent
Hydergine	6–12 mg/day (divided)	PO	<24 hrs.	Lower	None reported
Pergolide	0.025–0.1 mg once-a-day	PO	24–48 hrs.	Similar	Similar fever, nasal congestion hypotension more common
Dihydroergocriptine (POLI Industria Chimica S.P.A. Milan, Italy)	20–30 mg/day (divided)	PO	<12 hrs.	Similar	Similar, less frequent, less severe
Carbergoline Farmitalia Carlo Erba, Milan, Italy	0.25–1 mg q weekly or twice weekly	PO	7–14 days	Similar	Similar hypotension more common
Non-ergot					
CV-205-502 Norprolac or quinagolide (Sandoz, Basle, Switzerland)	0.075–0.15 mg once-a-day	PO	24 hrs.	Similar to better	Similar, milder transient, less common

Inability of the pituitary gland to stimulate normal ovarian follicular development and trigger oocyte release results in a lost chance at conception. Repetition of this dysfunctional process results in infertility. Normal ovarian follicular development and oocyte release require appropriate pituitary secretion of the gonadotropins luteinizing hormone (LH) and follicle-stimulating hormone (FSH) as well as appropriate secretion of the lactogenic hormone prolactin. Abnormal pituitary LH secretion is discussed in detail in Chapter 7. Abnormal pituitary secretion of prolactin and its role in infertility are discussed in Chapter 9.

The catecholamine dopamine regulates secretion of LH at the level of the hypothalamus and prolactin at the level of the pituitary gland. As a consequence of the interrelationships between dopamine, prolactin, and gonadotropin secretion, dopamine agonists have been successfully used in therapy for infertility. This review focuses on this treatment method.

PROLACTIN PHYSIOLOGY AND PATHOPHYSIOLOGY

Prolactin is a 199–amino acid protein of approximately 23 kd in its nonglycosylated form.[1] The secretion of this hormone by the pituitary gland is largely controlled by means of tonic inhibition via dopaminergic input from the hypothalamus. This inhibition is mediated by the D_2 receptor subtype on the lactotrope membrane with activation of an inhibitory G protein, which causes a decrease in adenylate cyclase activity.[2] Functional receptors for dopamine vary from lactotrope to lactotrope,[3] and this may be the explanation for failure of dopamine agonists to lower serum prolactin levels uniformly in all people with hyperprolactinemia.

Hyperprolactinemia can markedly diminish reproductive function. Overproduced prolactin stimulates hypothalamic dopamine secretion, which decreases release of gonadotropin-releasing hormone (GnRH).[4] A deficiency in hypothalamic dopamine activity has been suggested as the cause of abnormal LH secretion in women with polycystic ovary (PCO) syndrome.[5,6] Mildly altered GnRH pulsatility in hyperprolactinemia may lead first to poor granulosa cell luteinization and then to luteal-phase defects[7] as prolactin level rises. A sustained rise in prolactin level is followed by anovulation and amenorrhea.[8] Women with PCO syndrome often have mildly elevated serum prolactin levels, but these may not be higher than those of the general population.[9]

Hyperprolactinemia may be identified in 0.17% of the male population and 1.20% of the female population.[10] Approximately 5% of women with menstrual irregularity, infertility, hirsutism, or galactorrhea are found to have hyperprolactinemia (serum prolactin levels exceeding 20 ng/mL [20 μg/L]). In approximately 50% of women with hyperprolactinemia a pituitary abnormality such as microadenoma is identified if imaging studies of the gland are performed.[11]

Prolactin as a hormone was discovered in a rabbit by Stricker and Grueter in 1928.[12] The existence of a distinct human prolactin molecule remained in doubt for many years thereafter because it was believed that growth hormone (GH) acted as the prolactin molecule in humans. This belief was challenged after the discovery of a human prolactin molecule distinct from human GH in the laboratories of Frantz and Kleinberg[13] and Huang et al[14] in the early 1970s. This discovery was soon followed by the identification of endocrine conditions associated with elevated prolactin levels.

BROMOCRIPTINE AND PROLACTIN

During an investigation of reproduction, Shelesnyak found in 1954 that ergot alkaloids inhibited the process of implantation in rats. Shelesnyak later showed that this effect could be reversed either by progesterone[15] or by prolactin.[16] Zeilmaker and Carlsen[17] then showed that the abortifacient action of one of the ergot alkaloids, ergocornine, worked specifically at the pituitary gland by means of an unknown mechanism. As a result, work soon began to develop an ergot alkaloid drug capable of inhibiting pituitary prolactin release. This work resulted in the development of 2-Br-α ergocryptine mesylate, also known as CB154, bromocriptine mesylate, or by its trade name Parlodel[18,19] (Sandoz Pharmaceuticals, East Hanover, NJ) (Fig 33–1).

Dopamine inhibition of prolactin secretion was suspected from many animal experiments performed in the early 1970s.[20] Because inhibition of prolactin release in rats by use of bromocriptine was prevented by use of the receptor blocker chlorpromazine,[21] it was suspected that bromocriptine prevented secretion of pituitary prolactin by acting via dopamine receptors.[22] The ability of bromocriptine to affect prolactin release in humans was soon reported[23] followed by its use in clinical studies to treat galactorrhea.[24] In retrospect it was fortuitous

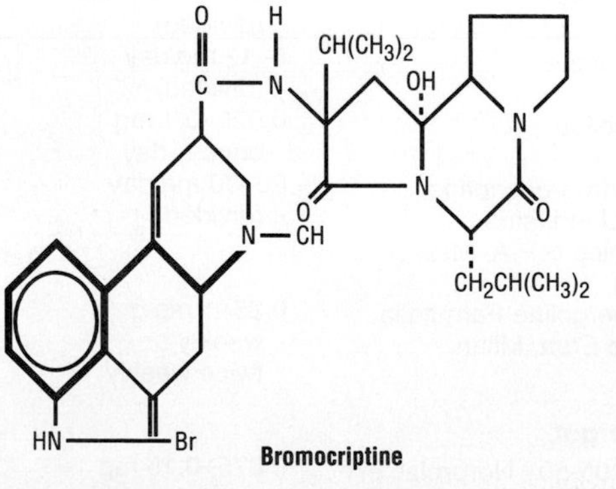

Figure 33–1. Structural formula of bromocriptine.

that the discovery of a human prolactin molecule and a radioimmunoassay to measure it occurred almost simultaneously with the discovery of a drug capable of treating patients with elevated levels of prolactin.

EVALUATION FOR HYPERPROLACTINEMIA

Before any treatment is administered to a patient believed to have hyperprolactinemia, it is essential to confirm the diagnosis. Prolactin is best measured under ideal circumstances to avoid misinterpretation of results. To minimize artifactual elevations in serum prolactin level, blood drawing should occur when the patient is awake, nonstressed emotionally or physically, and in the follicular phase of the cycle if menses occurs.[25] If this initial serum value is elevated, another sample should be collected for verification.

Before treatment it is essential to exclude other explainable causes of hyperprolactinemia, such as primary hypothyroidism. Medications may contribute to hyperprolactinemia, and these should be identified. Phenothiazines such as chlorpromazine[26] and fluphenazine,[27] which block dopamine receptors, and opiates,[28] which alter dopamine turnover, cause increased serum levels of prolactin. Women treated with metoclopramide,[29] tricyclic antidepressants,[30] and monamine oxidase (MAO) inhibitors[31] may also exhibit hyperprolactinemia. Lithium can prevent thyroxine release from the thyroid gland, causing primary hypothyroidism and hyperprolactinemia.[32]

Patients with certain diseases are expected to have hyperprolactinemia as a consequence of the underlying disease. For example, patients with chronic renal disease who need dialysis do not adequately filter a pituitary prolactin-releasing factor.[33] Patients with cirrhosis of the liver, regardless of current alcohol use, may have hyperprolactinemia resulting from altered hypothalamic dopamine secretion due to encephalopathy and not hepatic injury.[34]

Regardless of the cause of hyperprolactinemia, unless it can be unequivocally demonstrated that the cause is a continuing problem such as concomitant drug therapy, it is reasonable to request imaging of the pituitary gland by means of magnetic resonance (MR) with gadolinium enhancement or by means of computed tomography (CT). This recommendation is made to determine if pituitary masses, stalk compression, or hypothalamic masses exist before the beginning of treatment. Although most pituitary masses are prolactin-secreting prolactinomas, some of these masses may secrete hormones other than prolactin. Lactotrope and non–hormone-producing pituitary tumors account for 30% to 40% of all pituitary lesions.[35] Gonadotropic cell adenomas are responsible for 10% to 20%,[36] and adrenocorticotropic hormone (ACTH)– and GH-secreting tumors each account for 10% to 20% of the total.[37] Non-

prolactin-secreting pituitary tumors disrupt the inhibitory influence of the hypothalamus on the normal prolactin-secreting lactotropes, causing "sympathetic" hyperprolactinemia. Appropriate treatment of a patient whose pituitary lesion is a prolactinoma may be different than that of a patient whose pituitary lesion is not a prolactinoma.

MEDICAL MANAGEMENT OF INFERTILITY ASSOCIATED WITH HYPERPROLACTINEMIA

At present, several dopamine agonists can be used to decrease serum prolactin levels and bring about the return of normal reproductive function to most patients. Of these agents, bromocriptine is perhaps the best studied and the most widely used. In the U.S. market, bromocriptine constitutes the only drug approved specifically for the management of reproductive dysfunction related to hyperprolactinemia. It is also indicated for acromegaly and Parkinson's disease. The indication of bromocriptine for the suppression of postpartum lactation has been voluntarily withdrawn in the United States because of unproven allegations of thromboembolic events and myocardial infarction.[38] Bromocriptine is an ergot alkaloid–derived dopamine receptor agonist that appears to bind both D_1 and D_2 dopamine receptors. The side effects appear to be mediated through the D_1 receptor, because more specific D_2 agonists are better tolerated.[39] Approximately 50% of patients who take the drug experience some adverse effect (such as nausea, orthostatic hypertension, nasal stuffiness, or fatigue). Most of these effects are mild and resolve with time, but 5% to 10% of patients discontinue bromocriptine use because of severe nausea and vomiting.[40] Other, more severe adverse reactions such as gastrointestinal bleeding, alcohol intolerance, cold-induced vasospasm, pulmonary fibrosis, and psychosis may occur, especially with the higher doses used for treatment of Parkinson's disease.[41] Rare and uncommon side effects of bromocriptine include alopecia, reported by two patients,[42] and acute induced elevation in aspartate and alanine aminotransferase levels in another patient.[43]

BROMOCRIPTINE PHARMACOLOGY

After oral administration of bromocriptine, 28% of the drug is absorbed from the gastrointestinal tract resulting in peak blood levels within 1 to 3 hours. Almost all of the absorbed drug reaches the liver initially and is eventually excreted in the feces (98%). Very little drug is found in the circulation 14 hours after oral administration.[44] Bromocriptine is metabolized to at least 30 excretory products,[45] but only intact drug is believed active in inhibiting prolactin secretion.[46] The effectiveness of

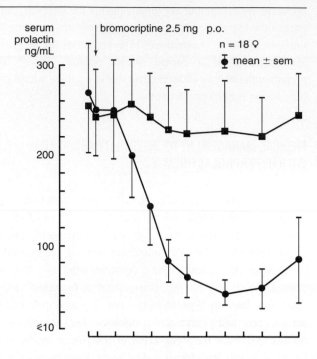

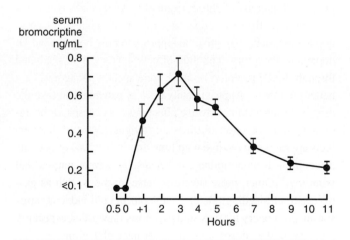

Figure 33–2. Prolactin and bromocriptine concentrations (mean ± SE) of hyperprolactinemic women (*n* = 18) before (——■——) and after (——●——) taking 2.5 mg of bromocriptine at 0 hours.

than oral administration of the same dose[50] (Fig 33–4), a circumstance believed to be due to decreased enterohepatic metabolism. Vaginal bromocriptine may even be considered for infertile couples with hyperprolactinemia. Although a decrease in sperm motility following bromocriptine exposure in vitro has been noted, women have conceived after its vaginal administration.[51]

Bromocriptine therapy typically requires multiple doses throughout the day, because its half-life is 3.3 hours.[46] This multiple dose requirement has been thought to decrease patient compliance. If bromocriptine is taken as directed and is well tolerated, as many as 95% of patients with amenorrhea or oligomenorrhea ovulate and resume normal menses.[52,53]

Oral bromocriptine is best started after a negative serum pregnancy test (if the patient has amenorrhea or oligomenorrhea) and at the lowest possible dose with dosage titrated to the prolactin response. Normalization of the serum/plasma prolactin concentration is the desired goal of therapy. To decrease the severity of adverse reactions, the medication is taken with food at bedtime, and the initial dose is 1.25 mg (one-half of a 2.5-mg tablet). It is often helpful to begin taking the drug on a Friday night to have the weekend to adjust the dosage. Precau-

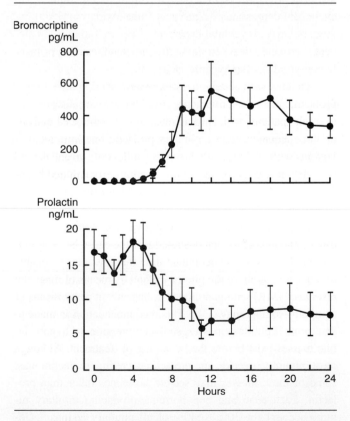

Figure 33–3. Plasma levels of bromocriptine and prolactin (mean ± SE) of five women after vaginal administration of 2.5 mg of bromocriptine. (*From Vermesh M, et al: Vaginal bromocriptine: Pharmacology and effect on serum prolactin in normal women. Obstet Gynecol 72:693, 1988.*)

bromocriptine in inhibiting pituitary prolactin secretion is sustained with an effect observed for at least 9 hours after oral administration of a single 2.5-mg tablet[46] (Fig 33–2). Bromocriptine also may be administered vaginally, resulting in a maximal decline in serum prolactin 11 hours after vaginal administration of a standard 2.5-mg tablet of bromocriptine placed in the posterior fornix of the vagina in healthy women[47] (Fig 33–3). Use of vaginally administered bromocriptine also has been successful in decreasing the serum prolactin concentration of women with hyperprolactinemia.[48,49] After 7 hours circulating serum bromocriptine concentrations are higher after vaginal

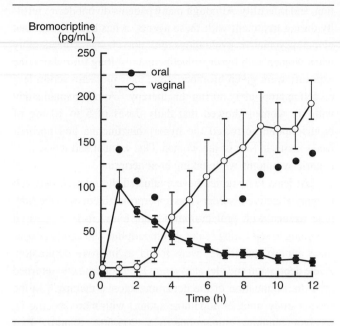

Bromocriptine (pg/mL)

Figure 33–4. Serum levels of bromocriptine after oral (*n* = 7) and vaginal (*n* = 8) administration of a 2.5-mg dose. (*From Katz E, et al: Increased circulating levels of bromocriptine after vaginal compared with oral administration. Fertil Steril 55:882, 1991.*)

tions regarding operation of machinery or automobiles are in order. Prolactin levels can be checked a few days after the patient begins taking the medication and after each dose adjustment. The initial increase in dose (if required) should be from 1.25 mg to 2.5 mg at bedtime. Additional stepwise increases of 1.25 mg may be taken first in the morning and then in the afternoon; the usual maximum dose is 2.5 mg three times per day.

For patients who cannot tolerate oral bromocriptine because of severe nausea and vomiting, vaginal administration may be tried, which usually decreases symptoms related to oral bromocriptine therapy. The percentage of maximum decline in serum prolactin level is statistically similar with either route of administration.[54] Many patients report no adverse effects after up to 2 years of continuous vaginal administration, causing some authors to advocate vaginal administration as first-line treatment of patients who require bromocriptine therapy.[55]

To decrease cost and increase compliance, several studies have evaluated the administration of oral bromocriptine in an intermittent manner. Bromocriptine was only given to infertile women during the follicular phase of the menstrual cycle.[56–58] A recurrence of hyperprolactinemia in the luteal phase was noted, but apparently normal luteal function (as measured by means of normal serum progesterone levels) and a high rate of pregnancy followed. A recent randomized, prospective study of low-income infertile women with hyperprolactinemia confirmed the effectiveness and decreased expense of intermittent bromocriptine therapy. The investigators found that intermittent therapy was tolerated better than continuous bromocriptine therapy.[59]

They also found that the rebounding high prolactin levels in the luteal phase decreased with further cycles of therapy.

Alternative methods of delivery of bromocriptine have been investigated to overcome the adverse reactions and short half-life of conventional oral therapy. Both a long-acting injectable form and a slow-release oral form of bromocriptine exist, but are available only to patients outside the United States. Injectable forms of bromocriptine are made by means of administration of the drug with a carrier material. Polylactic acid initially was used for this purpose, but this carrier material has a very long half-life. Bromocriptine is now embedded in glucose-initiated poly (dl-lactide-co-gycolide) microspherules with a maximal degradation time of 3 months and is marketed as a long-acting repetitive (LAR) bromocriptine.[60] The long-acting oral preparation of bromocriptine, known as slow oral release (SRO), is administered in a capsule that possesses defined osmotic properties.[61] In a double blind, randomized study of oral as opposed to injectable bromocriptine, similar side-effect profiles were seen, but a single monthly injection of 50 mg of bromocriptine given intramuscularly decreased prolactin levels just as well as 7.5 mg of oral bromocriptine given daily.[62] SRO bromocriptine (5 and 10 mg/day) was compared with one 2.5- or 5-mg tablet of bromocriptine given twice daily in randomized double-blind trials. The once-daily SRO form was shown to be equally efficacious in decreasing hyperprolactinemia as a twice-a-day regimen with conventional bromocriptine.[61] A similar incidence of adverse effects between the two regimens was reported in another study.[63] A third study found fewer side effects with the SRO form of the drug.[64]

Longer acting forms of bromocriptine have proved to be effective in the treatment of infertile patients with pituitary micro- and macroadenomas. Several studies of the injectable form of bromocriptine used from 1 to more than 4 years demonstrated an average reduction in adenoma size of 50% after 1 year of therapy.[65–68] Successful use of injectable bromocriptine by patients with pituitary microadenomas intolerant of oral bromocriptine has been reported.[60] Bromocriptine is effective in shrinking pituitary adenomas because it inhibits not only the synthesis and release of prolactin from the pituitary lactotrope but also mitosis of these cells.[69] Because of presumed variations in lactotroph response to dopamine, there remains a 20% chance that an adenoma will not shrink after bromocriptine therapy is instituted.[69] When pituitary prolactin-producing adenomas are shrunk with bromocriptine an increase in fibrous or connective tissue at the tumor site is found, which may make future operations, if contemplated, more difficult to perform.[70] Longer-acting forms of bromocriptine may or may not reduce the incidence of adverse effects when given to patients with pituitary adenomas but will likely improve compliance.

Because bromocriptine often is used to treat patients with infertility associated with hyperprolactinemia, a common question is what to do when pregnancy occurs. It is best to advise the use of barrier contraception until the first menses (usually about 8 weeks after therapy is initiated) to minimize drug exposure in early pregnancy. There does not seem to be an increased risk for spontaneous abortion,[71] nor does there appear to be a teratogenic effect of bromocriptine on the fetus[72,73] despite the fact that bromocriptine crosses the placenta and has been shown to lower fetal serum levels of prolactin.[74] However, most authors believe it is best to stop bromocriptine therapy once pregnancy is diagnosed, because dopamine agonists may have unknown effects on fetal neural development. If symptomatic enlargement of a pituitary adenoma should occur during pregnancy, bromocriptine therapy may be restarted. Continuous administration of bromocriptine to prevent neurologic complications in pregnant women with prolactinomas[75] and in one woman with empty sella syndrome has been reported.[76] No adverse reactions were documented in these studies. Use of bromocriptine throughout pregnancy to prevent adenoma enlargement has been suggested, but use of prophylactic dopamine agonist therapy may be questioned in view of eight uneventful pregnancies reported among four women with pituitary macroadenomas and suprasellar extension who all stopped bromocriptine therapy after the diagnosis of pregnancy.[77] Pregnancy itself does not seem to aggravate hyperprolactinemia or cause adenoma recurrence in women successfully treated with surgical therapy.[78] The results of one study have suggested that term pregnancy and multiparity may cause spontaneous improvement in hyperprolactinemia.[79] This may result from spontaneous infarction of the adenoma within the pituitary gland postpartum.

As mentioned previously, a variety of medications given for psychiatric indications cause hyperprolactinemia, anovula-

tion, and infertility. Although many patients do not desire fertility during treatment with these agents, it has been shown that global psychiatric evaluations did not change considerably when women with hyperprolactinemia resulting from thorazine exposure were given bromocriptine; their prolactin serum levels fell appropriately during this therapy.[80] Another small study with six women showed that daily doses of 5 to 10 mg of bromocriptine corrected the hyperprolactinemia and normalized menses in four of the women. One woman had worse psychiatric symptoms while taking bromocriptine.[81]

At least two studies have evaluated the relation between primary affective disorders and hyperprolactinemia. In the first, nine women with prolactinomas were found to be depressed according to self-rating scales. Bromocriptine and another dopamine agonist, pergolide, were found to improve depression. Acute depression and elevated serum levels of prolactin returned after discontinuation of the dopamine agonist therapy.[82] In the second study, another dopamine agonist with more specific D_2 receptor binding, quinagolide (CV 205-502, Sandoz, East Hanover, NJ) was found to improve psychometric test results among depressed patients better than bromocriptine. However, both drugs improved depressive symptoms over baseline.[83]

OTHER DOPAMINE AGONISTS

Several other compounds have been shown reliably to decrease serum prolactin levels, and all bind dopamine D_2 receptors, some with much greater affinity than bromocriptine. Among these are pergolide, quinagolide (CV 205-502), metergoline, cabergoline, and terguride (Fig 33–5). With drug half-lives greater than that of bromocriptine, these dopamine agonists

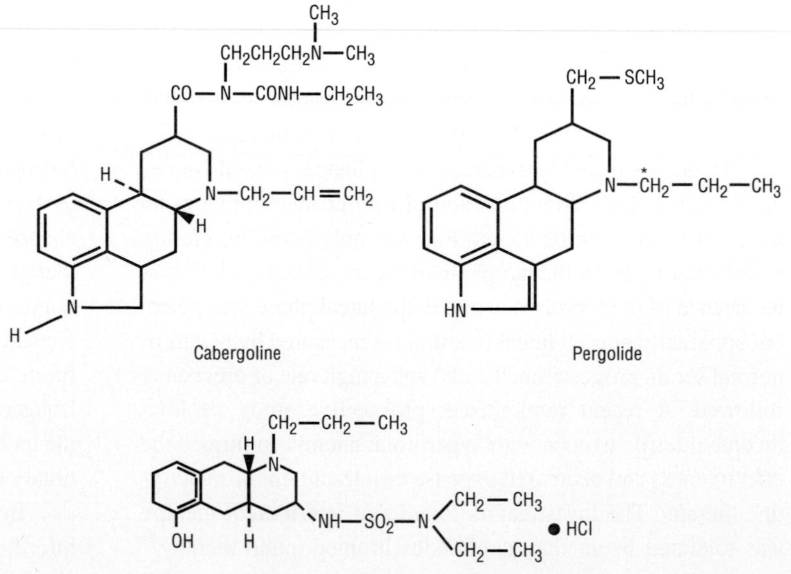

Figure 33–5. Structural formulae of pergolide, cabergoline, and quinagolide.

may require only once-daily dosing. Unfortunately, these long half-lives mean that detectable quantities of drug are found in the maternal serum for long periods of time. This complicates use of these agents for infertility, because discontinuation of the drug with confirmation of pregnancy likely results in substantial early fetal exposure.

There have been no recent reports of pregnancies complicated by the use of these drugs or fetal malformations with use, but there is not the body of data that exists with bromocriptine to declare these agents as safe in pregnancy. However, for the 5% to 18% of patients who are resistant to bromocriptine, these agents may be the only choice other than a transsphenoidal operation to manage hyperprolactinemia.[84–86] Interestingly, resistance to one or more dopamine agonists appears to be mediated either by a reduction in the affinity or density of D_2 receptor sites[86,87] or by a postreceptor defect that renders the guanine nucleotide-binding protein G_o deficient.[88]

Pergolide (Permax, Eli Lilly, Indianapolis, IN) is a synthetic ergolide that lacks the peptide side chain of bromocriptine.[89] It is approved in the United States for the treatment of patients with Parkinson's disease. Although not approved for the treatment of hyperprolactinemia, it has been shown in several clinical studies to decrease prolactin secretion in vivo[90–92] while effectively decreasing the size of pituitary adenomas.[93,94] Pergolide is about 100 times more potent than bromocriptine on a weight-to-weight basis, which is reflected in its much-reduced dosage compared with bromocriptine. Pergolide is administered at least once a day, because its effect can be observed 72 hours after the last dose. In one randomized, controlled, multicenter trial,[44] pergolide was found to be as efficacious as bromocriptine in decreasing prolactin secretion, reducing galactorrhea and breast tenderness, and causing resumption of normal menses. With both drugs similar numbers of patients reported adverse effects, but the patients taking pergolide more commonly reported a flu-like syndrome and vasodilatation than patients taking bromocriptine. Dosage of pergolide in the study was 25 μg per day orally with the evening meal for the first 3 days. If no adverse effect was noted, the dose was increased to 50 μg per day. Subsequent dose escalations were in steps of 25 to 50 μg. Total daily dose did not exceed 500 μg. Other studies have also shown pergolide to be as effective as bromocriptine in the management of hyperprolactinemia.[95,96] One of these studies demonstrated that once-a-day pergolide administration was as effective in the treatment of patients with hyperprolactinemia as multiday dosage of bromocriptine.[96]

Pergolide was shown in a study to be effective in reducing the size of pituitary microadenomas and to decrease prolactin concentrations in a proportion of patients resistant to bromocriptine therapy.[97] The side effects reported were similar to those of bromocriptine therapy, and the maximum dose in the study was 200 μg per day. Treatment duration of up to 5 years was not accompanied by complications.

Cabergoline (Farmitalia, Milan, Italy) is a dopamine agonist with high selectivity and affinity for the dopamine D_2 receptor. It is indicated for the treatment of patients with hyperprolactinemia but is not currently available in the United States. Cabergoline may receive Food and Drug Administration (FDA) approval to be prescribed for hyperprolactinemia in the near future. It requires only twice per week dosing, does not seem to affect other endocrinologic values, and appears to be safe for use in suppression of puerperal lactation.[98] Tolerability of cabergoline appears to be somewhat better than that of bromocriptine (perhaps because of the decreased frequency of dosage), and long-term use appears to be safe.[99] Compared with bromocriptine, cabergoline decreased serum prolactin level more rapidly among puerperal women after a single dose of 1.0 mg than did twice daily bromocriptine, 2.5 mg, taken for 14 days; it also suppressed lactation.[100] Athough a single 300-μg dose of cabergoline was slightly less effective in lowering prolactin levels 6 hours after single administration than 2.5 mg bromocriptine taken orally (55% decline versus 64%), its effect persisted for 7 days whereas that of bromocriptine lasted only 1 day.[101] In a large, double-blind study comparing cabergoline with bromocriptine in the treatment of women with hyperprolactinemic amenorrhea,[102] a maximum dose of cabergoline of 1.0 mg twice weekly was more effective in restoring normal ovulatory cycles than was a maximum of 5.0 mg of bromocriptine taken twice a day. The number of women who had stable normoprolactinemia also was higher in the cabergoline group. The prevalence of severe adverse reactions was lower among the cabergoline-treated group; 3% discontinued the study compared with 12% in the bromocriptine-treated group. Compliance with the cabergoline regimen was found to be better than with the bromocriptine regimen. Cabergoline has been used successfully to treat a patient with pituitary macroadenoma.[103] The drug may be administered vaginally with good results among patients with hyperprolactinemia intolerance of oral dopaminergic agents.[104]

Because of the limited clinical experience with cabergoline in pregnancy, it is currently recommended that the drug be stopped 1 month before conception is attempted. This recommendation seems reasonable. One study[105] found that 23 of 28 previously amenorrheic women continued to have ovulatory cycles for at least 6 months after cabergoline withdrawal, although only five remained normoprolactinemic. The manufacturer of cabergoline reports that among 222 pregnancies of 201 women exposed to cabergoline, the spontaneous abortion rate for 170 pregnancies with known outcome was 13%. This is well within the normal rate of pregnancy loss. The fetal malformation rate was within normal limits, and no malformation occurred more than once.[106]

Another dopamine agonist, although not derived from ergot, is *quinagolide* (CV 205-502, Norprolac, Sandoz, Basel, Switzerland). This drug is an octohydrobenzo-(g)-quinolone which has a structure similar to that of apomorphine and ergoline. Quinagolide is available in Europe and on a special-needs basis to patients in the United States through a few investigators in tertiary care institutions. Unfortunately, the process of obtaining FDA approval for this drug has not been completed. It is, however, another drug that may be successfully used to treat hyperprolactinemic bromocriptine-intolerant or bromocriptine-resistant patients who have or do not have a pituitary adenoma.[107–110] Quinagolide has better dopamine D_2 receptor affinity than bromocriptine,[111] and this may afford it greater tolerability over bromocriptine. In contrast to quinagolide, bromocriptine may act as a D_1 receptor antagonist as well as an antagonist at α-1-adenoreceptors and serotonin receptors, which may be responsible for many of the side effects reported by bromocriptine users.[112] In four studies, patients with bromocriptine intolerance were better able to tolerate quinagolide therapy.[39,113–115] In a large double-blind, randomized study, once-daily quinagolide (50 μg) was compared with once-daily bromocriptine (2.5 mg). No differences were seen in efficacy of suppression of prolactin or side effects.[116] No difference has been shown between bromocriptine and quinagolide in ability to shrink pituitary adenomas,[117] but comparison studies are compromised by the inability to establish a dose-response relation. That is, there is a lack of correlation between pretreatment prolactin concentration, final drug dose, and time required to normalize prolactin concentration.[118]

Quinagolide has been compared with cabergoline for treatment of patients with hyperprolactinemia.[119] In an open, randomized, cross-over trial, quinagolide 75 μg daily was compared with cabergoline 0.5 mg twice a week. Cabergoline was found to cause fewer adverse effects and to normalize prolactin levels more frequently. In addition, cabergoline was found to suppress prolactin levels for a longer period of time after cessation of therapy. Some patients intolerant of cabergoline tolerated quinagolide. Most patients had resolution of symptoms (generally nausea) within the first week of therapy.[120]

Hydergine (Sandoz, Basel, Switzerland) has also been shown to inhibit prolactin secretion and induce ovulation in patients with hyperprolactinemic amenorrhea. Hydergine is a mixed ergot alkaloid compound that has been shown to increase cognitive function in selected patients. It currently is indicated only for this purpose in the United States. In one study[121] hydergine was shown to be especially useful in induction of ovulation in women whose baseline serum prolactin levels were less than 100 ng/mL (100 μg/L). The drug did not induce normoprolactinemia in women with high baseline prolactin levels, nor did it induce ovulation in these women. However, the six women who returned to normal ovulatory function had seven pregnancies, and four healthy infants were delivered. In addition, no patient experienced any adverse effects during the study. It appears that for women who cannot tolerate bromocriptine and have lower serum prolactin concentrations, hydergine may be considered a second-line drug.

Other ergot-derived dopamine agonists have been developed to treat hyperprolactinemic states. These include metergoline, terguride, and lisuride. These drugs have been shown to be as effective as bromocriptine with similar side effects.[122–125] Of interest is the observation from these studies that some patients appear to tolerate one ergot preparation better than another. None of these preparations is available in the United States.

LONG-TERM USE OF DOPAMINE AGONISTS

Lack of adverse effects of long-term bromocriptine therapy has been reported in one study in which 75 hyperprolactinemic women with and without pituitary adenomas (micro or macro) were treated for 5 to 9 years.[126] Necrotic changes in prolactinomas after long-term administration were reported,[127] perhaps explaining why some patients exhibit a sustained lowering of prolactin levels after cessation of bromocriptine use.[128,129] Caution must be advised, however; one study with 12 women with macroadenomas successfully treated with bromocriptine for as long as 7 years showed that 11 patients had recurrence of hyperprolactinemia after stopping treatment. One of these patients had tumor reexpansion.[130]

ALTERNATIVES TO DOPAMINE AGONISTS

In the treatment of hyperprolactinemic women with ovulatory dysfunction who cannot tolerate any medical therapy and desire to conceive, it is important to know that induction of ovulation and conception can be accomplished without dopamine agonists. Clomiphene citrate in combination with human chorionic gonadotropin (hCG) has been shown to induce ovulation in many of these women.[131] Menotropins also have been used successfully by hyperprolactinemic patients with ovulatory dysfunction.[132]

DOPAMINE AGONIST THERAPY FOR NORMOPROLACTINEMIC INFERTILITY

Dopamine agonists have been used to manage infertility in women with normal prolactin levels who were either menstruating or amenorrheic. One rationale for this treatment is that "occult" hyperprolactinemia may be responsible for the observed infertility. Use of a dopamine receptor blocker[133] or thyrotropin-releasing hormone (TRH)[134] to enhance prolactin secretion has been suggested as methods to identify patients with "occult" hyperprolactinemia. In one study involving 305 women with a normal basal prolactin level, administration of TRH resulted in an exaggerated prolactin response (exceeding 86 ng/mL [86 μg/L]) in 48.[135] This response was interpreted as being indicative of occult or subclinical hyperprolactinemia. A transient increase in prolactin level during the midportion of the menstrual cycle in women with unexplained infertility has been reported. These women were treated with bromocriptine, and 18 of 45 couples conceived within 3 months of the start of therapy.[136] Normoprolactinemic women with unexplained infertility and galactorrhea also have been treated with bromocriptine and have become pregnant.[137] Bromocriptine has also been reported to be efficacious in therapy for ovulatory dysfunction associated with normoprolactinemic galactorrhea.[138] Bromocriptine has not, however, proved more successful than placebo in the treatment of women with unexplained infertility with normal prolactin levels.[139]

The diagnostic category of "unexplained infertility" as it currently exists may be too broad to allow detection of specific subgroups of infertile couples with normoprolactinemia who may benefit from dopamine agonist therapy. For example, prolactin plays a role in regulating the immune system.[140] Various immunologic disorders have been proposed as causes of infertility. In a 1994 study bromocriptine was shown to reverse the inhibitory effect of macrophages on human sperm motility.[141] Thus the beneficial effects of bromocriptine in the treatment of some women with unexplained infertility and normal prolactin levels may be mediated by the immune system rather than the hypothalamic-pituitary-ovarian axis.

DOPAMINE AGONIST THERAPY AND POLYCYSTIC OVARY SYNDROME

Bromocriptine has been used to treat infertility in ovulatory women with PCO syndrome.[142] The rationale for providing this treatment is that exogenous administration of a dopamine agonist may correct a dopamine deficiency state within the hypothalamus, initially causing inappropriate release of GnRH followed by inappropriate pituitary LH secretion. Only a few studies have investigated the use of bromocriptine to treat women with PCO syndrome. One of the earliest of these suggested a beneficial effect of dopamine agonist therapy for PCO syndrome by showing that ovulation occurred in four cycles of nine among seven treated women.[143] In one double-blind, crossover study involving 20 women with PCO syndrome, each was given placebo or bromocriptine. Three patients ovulated when given bromocriptine, but two of these three were hyperprolactinemic. All women experienced some type of side effect.[144] In another double-blind, controlled study of bromocriptine and placebo involving 55 patients with PCO syndrome, it was shown that the endocrine profile was not different between

groups before treatment. After treatment clinical results were no different between groups. An ovulatory cycle was recorded for 12 of 28 patients taking bromocriptine versus 8 of 27 taking placebo.[145] Among patients with PCO syndrome with normal prolactin levels, gonadotropin levels were unaltered by bromocriptine therapy in one study performed in the United States.[146] This result was later corroborated by a similar study performed in Brazil.[147]

SUMMARY

Most patients with hyperprolactinemia and infertility respond well to bromocriptine, the first-line therapy for this indication. Bromocriptine dosages can be quickly titrated with patient tolerance and serum prolactin levels as a guide. A somewhat flexible maximum dose of 2.5 mg three times a day is the upper limit for therapy. For patients who are intolerant of bromocriptine given orally, vaginal administration can be considered (as can SRO or injectable bromocriptine for patients outside the United States). For patients who are still intolerant (or resistant) to bromocriptine, other dopamine agonists can be used. Two thirds of bromocriptine-intolerant and one third of bromocriptine-resistant patients tolerate and respond to another agent. With the use of longer-acting agents such as pergolide, cabergoline, or quinagolide, the dose of drug must be titrated carefully to prolactin level, because these agents tend to cause a slow, progressive decrease in serum prolactin level that may take weeks or longer to observe. If severe adverse experiences are encountered with dopamine agonists, discontinuation of the drug usually causes a rapid resolution of symptoms. Women who conceive while using bromocriptine should discontinue the drug when pregnancy is confirmed. Women who desire pregnancy and are taking a long-acting dopamine agonist should discontinue therapy about 1 month before attempting conception. At present, there does not seem to be an indication for dopamine agonist treatment of infertile women with normoprolactinemia and normal ovulatory function, although this may change as an understanding of the function of prolactin is gained.

REFERENCES

1. Nicoll CS, Mayer GL, Russel SM: Structural features of prolactins and growth hormones that can be related to their biologic properties. *Endocr Rev* 7:169, 1986
2. Wood DF, Johnston JM, Johnston DG: Dopamine, the dopamine D$_2$ receptor and pituitary tumors. *Clin Endocrinol* 35:455, 1991
3. Lyque EH, Munoz de Toro M, Smith PI, et al: Subpopulations of lactotropes detected with reverse hemolytic plaque assay show differential responsiveness to dopamine. *Endocrinology* 118:2120, 1986

4. LeBlanc H, Lachelin GCL, Abu-Fadil S, et al: Effects of dopamine on pituitary secretion in humans. *J Clin Endocrinol Metab* 43:668, 1976

5. Yen SSC: The polycystic ovary syndrome. *Clin Endocrinol* 12:177, 1980

6. Quigley ME, Rakoff JS, Yen SSC: Increased luteinizing hormone sensitivity to dopamine inhibition in polycystic ovary syndrome. *J Clin Endocrinol Metab* 52:231, 1981

7. Adashi EY, Resnick CE: Prolactin as an inhibitor of granulosa cell luteinization: Implications for hyperprolactinemia-associated luteal phase dysfunction. *Fertil Steril* 48:131, 1987

8. Franks S, Murray MF, Jequier AM: Incidence and significance of hyperprolactinemia in women with amenorrhea. *Clin Endocrinol* 4:597, 1975

9. Zacur HA, Foster GV: Hyperprolactinemia and polycystic ovarian syndrome. *Semin Reprod Endocrinol* 10:236, 1992

10. Miyai K, Ichihara K, Kondo, Mon S: Asymptomatic hyperprolactinemia and prolactinoma in the general population: Mass screening by paired assays of serum prolactin. *Clin Endocrinol (Oxf)* 25:549, 1986

11. Batrinos ML, Panitsa-Faflia CH, Tsinganou E, et al: Incidence and characteristics of microprolactinomas (3–5 mm) in 4199 women assayed for prolactin. *Horm Metab Res* 24:384, 1992

12. Stricker P, Grueter F: Action du lobe anterieur de l'hypophyse sur la montee laiteuse. *Compt Rend Soc Biol* 99:1978, 1928

13. Frantz AG, Kleinberg DL: Prolactin: Evidence that it is separate from growth hormone in human blood. *Science* 170:745, 1970

14. Hwang P, Guyda H, Friesen H: A radioimmunoassay for human prolactin. *Proc Natl Acad Sci USA* 68:1902, 1971

15. Shelesnyak MC: Ergotoxine inhibition of deciduomata formation and its reversal by progesterone. *Am J Physiol* 179:301, 1954

16. Shelesnyak MC: Maintenance of gestation in ergotoxine treated pregnant rats by exogenous prolactin. *Acta Endocrinol (Kbh)* 27:99, 1958

17. Zeilmaker GH, Carlsen RA: Experimental studies on the effect of ergocornine methane sulfonate on the luteotrophic function of the rat pituitary gland. *Acta Endocrinol (Kbh)* 41:321, 1962

18. Fluckiger E, Wagner H: 2-Br-α-ergocryptine: Beeinflussung von fertilitat und laktation bei der ratte. *Experientia* 24:1130, 1968

19. Yanai R, Nagasawa H: Suppression of mammary hyperplastic nodule formation and pituitary prolactin secretion in mice induced by ergocornine and 2-Br-α ergocryptine. *J Natl Cancer Inst* 45:1105, 1970

20. Zacur HA, Foster GV, Tyson JE: Multifactorial regulation of prolactin secretion. *Lancet* 1:410, 1976

21. Fluckiger E: The pharmacology of bromocriptine. In: Bayliss RIS, Turner P, Maclay WP (eds), *Pharmacological and Clinical Aspects of Bromocriptine (Parlodel)*. Tunbridge Wells, Kent, England, MCS Consultants, 1976:12

22. Fuxe K, Corrodi H, Hokfelt T, et al: Evidence for prolonged dopamine receptor stimulation. *Med Biol* 52:121, 1974

23. Del Pozo E, Brun Del Re R, Varga L, et al: The inhibition of prolactin secretion in man by CB154 (2-Br-α-ergocryptine). *J Clin Endocrinol* 35:768, 1972

24. Besser GM, Parke L, Edwards CRW, et al: Galactorrhea: Successful treatment with reduction of plasma prolactin levels by bromoergocryptine. *Br Med J* 3:669, 1972

25. Zacur HA, Hutchison SM: Evaluation and therapy of hyperprolactinemia. In: Wallach EE, Zacur HA (eds), *Reproductive Medicine and Surgery*. St. Louis, Mosby–Year Book, 1995:196

26. Kleinberg DL, Noll GL, Franz AG: Chlorpromazine stimulation and l-dopa suppression of plasma prolactin in man. *J Clin Endocrinol Metab* 33:873, 1971

27. Langer G, Sachav EJ, Gruen PH, et al: Human prolactin responses to neuroleptic drugs correlate with antischizophrenic potency. *Nature* 266:639, 1977

28. Wardlaw SL, Wehrneberg WB, Ferin M, et al: Failure of beta endorphin to stimulate prolactin release in the pituitary stalk sectioned monkey. *Endocrinology* 107:1663, 1980

29. Sowers JR, McCallum RW, Hershman JM, et al: Comparison of metoclopramide with other dynamic tests of prolactin secretion. *J Clin Endocrinol Metab* 43:679, 1976

30. Turkington RW: Prolaction secretion in patients treated with various drugs. *Arch Intern Med* 130:349, 1972

31. Slater SL, Lipper S, Shiling DJ, et al: Elevation of plasma-prolactin by monamine oxidase inhibitors. *Lancet* 2:275, 1977

32. Kable WT: Drug-induced primary hypothyroidism and hyperprolactinemia (letter). *Fertil Steril* 35:483, 1981

33. Sievertson GD, Lim VS, Nakawatase C, et al: Metabolic clearance and secretion of human prolactin in normal subjects and inpatients with chronic renal failure. *J Clin Endocrinol Metab* 50:846, 1980

34. Corenblum B, Shaffer EA: Hyperprolactinemia in hepatic encephalopathy may result from impaired central dopaminergic transmission. *Hum Metab Res* 21:675, 1989

35. Kovacs K: Pathology of pituitary tumors. *Endocrinol Metab Clin N Am* 16:529, 1987

36. Snyder PJ: Gonadotroph cell pituitary adenoma. *Endocrinol Metab Clin N Am* 16:755, 1987

37. Molitch ME, Russel EJ: The pituitary incidentaloma. *Ann Intern Med* 112:925, 1990

38. Letter to pharmacists dated August 18, 1994, advising voluntary withdrawal of the indication of post-partum lactation for Parloael®, Sandoz Pharmaceuticals, East Hanover, New Jersey

39. Vilar L, Burke CW: Quinagolide efficacy and tolerability in hyperprolactinemic patients who are resistant to or intolerant of bromocriptine. *Clin Endocrinol* 41:821, 1994

40. Friesen H, Tolis G: The use of bromocriptine in the galactorrhea-amenorrhea syndromes: The Canadian Cooperative study. *Clin Endocrinol* 6:91, 1977

41. Weil C: The safety of bromocriptine in long-term use: A review of the literature. *Curr Med Res Opin* 10:25, 1986

42. Fabre N, Montastruc JL, Rascol O: Alopecia: An adverse effect of bromocriptine. *Clin Neuropharmacol* 16:266, 1993

43. Liberato NL, Poli M, Bollati P, et al: Bromocriptine-induced acute hepatitis. *Lancet* 340:969, 1992

44. Schran HF, Bhuta SI, Schwratz HJ, et al: The pharmacokinetics of bromocriptine in man. In: Goldstein M, Calne DB, Liberman A,

Thorner MO (eds), *Ergot Compounds and Brain Function: Neuroscience and Neuropsychiatric Aspects.* New York, Raven, 1980:125

45. Parkes D: Bromocriptine. *N Engl J Med* 301:873, 1979

46. Thorner MO, Schran HF, Evans WS, et al: A broad spectrum of prolactin suppression by bromocriptine in hyperprolactinemic women: A study of serum prolactin and bromocriptine levels after acute and chronic administration of bromocriptine. *J Clin Endocrinol Metab* 50:1026, 1980

47. Vermesh M, Fossum GT, Kletzky OA: Vaginal bromocriptine: Pharmacology and effect on serum prolactin in normal women. *Obstet Gynecol* 72:693, 1988

48. Kletzky OA, Vermesh M: Effectiveness of vaginal bromocriptine in treating women with hyperprolactinemia. *Fertil Steril* 51:269, 1989

49. Katz E, Schran H, Adashi EY: Successful treatment of a prolactin producing pituitary macroadenoma with intravaginal bromocriptine mesylate: A novel approach to intolerance of oral therapy. *Obstet Gynecol* 73:517, 1989

50. Katz E, Weiss BE, Hassell A, et al: Increased circulating levels of bromocriptine after vaginal compared with oral administration. *Fertil Steril* 55:882, 1991

51. Chenette PE, Siegel MS, Vermesh M, et al: Effect of bromocriptine on sperm function in vitro and in vivo. *Obstet Gynecol* 77:935, 1991

52. Del Pozo E, Varga L, Wyss H, et al: Clinical and hormonal response to bromocriptine (CB154) in the galactorrhea syndrome. *J Clin Endocrinol Metab* 39:18, 1974

53. Vance ML, Evans WS, Thorner MO: Bromocriptine. *Ann Intern Med* 100:78, 1984

54. Dash RJ, Ajmani AK, Sialy R: Prolactin (PRL) response to oral or vaginal bromoergocriptine in hyperprolactinemic women. *Horm Metab Res* 26:164, 1993

55. Ginsburg J, Hardiman P, Thomas M: Vaginal bromocriptine: Clinical and biochemical effects. *Gynecol Endocrinol* 6:119, 1992

56. Coelingh Bennink HJT, van der Steeg HJ: Ovulation induction by bromocriptine (abstract). *Fertil Steril* 28:347, 1977

57. Polatti F, Bolis PF, Ravagni-Probizer MF, et al: Treatment of hyperprolactinemic amenorrhea by intermittent administration of bromocryptine (CB154). *Am J Obstet Gynecol* 131:792, 1978

58. Coelingh Bennink HJT: Intermittent bromocriptine treatment for the induction of ovulation in hyperprolactinemic patients. *Fertil Steril* 31:267, 1979

59. Parra A, Crespo G, Coria I, et al: Clinical and hormonal response to short-term intermittent versus continuous oral bromocriptine therapy in hyperprolactinemic women. *Int J Fertil* 40:96, 1995

60. Espinos JJ, Rodriquez-Espinosa J, Webb SM, et al: Long acting repeatable bromocriptine in the treatment of patients with microprolactinoma intolerant or resistant to oral dopaminergics. *Fertil Steril* 62:926, 1994

61. Weingrill CO, Mussio W, Moraes CRS, et al: Long-acting oral bromocriptine (Parlodel SRO) in the treatment of hyperprolactinemia. *Fertil Steril* 57:331, 1992

62. Ciccarelli E, Grottoli S, Minola C, et al: Double blind randomized study using oral or injectable bromocriptine in patients with hyperprolactinemia. *Clin Endocrinol* 40:193, 1994

63. Biberoglu K, Atasu T, Shabgahi B, et al: Tolerability, safety, and efficacy of two formulations of Parlodel: a slow release oral form (SRO) versus registered Parlodel capsules. *Gynecol Obstet Invest* 37:6, 1994

64. Moro M, Maraschini C, Toja P, et al: Comparison between a slow-release oral prepration of bromocriptine and regular bromocriptine in patients with hyperprolactinemia: A double blind, double dummy study. *Horm Res* 35:137, 1991

65. Beckers A, Petrossians P, Abs R, et al: Treatment of macroprolactinomas with the long-acting and repeatable form of bromocriptine: A report on 29 cases. *J Clin Endocrinol Metab* 75:275, 1992

66. Brue T, Lancranjan I, Louvet JP, et al: A long-acting repeatable form of bromocriptine as long term treatment of prolactin secreting macroadenomas: A multi center study. *Fertil Steril* 57:74, 1992

67. Lengyel AM, Mussio W, Imamura P, et al: Long acting injectable bromocriptine (Parlodel LAR) in the chronic treatment of prolactin-secreting macroadenomas. *Fertil Steril* 59:980, 1993

68. Ciccarelli E, Mioler C, Grottoli S, et al: Long term therapy of patients with microprolactinoma using repeatable injectable bromocriptine. *J Clin Endocrinol Metab* 76:484, 1993

69. Bevan JS, Webster J, Burke CW, et al: Dopamine agonists and pituitary tumor shrinkage. *Endocr Rev* 13:220, 1992

70. Esiri MM, Bevan JS, Burke CW, et al: Effect of bromocriptine treatment on the fibrous tissue content of prolactin secreting and nonfunctioning macroadenomas of the pituitary gland. *J Clin Endocrinol* 63:383, 1986

71. Turkalj I, Bran P, Krupp P: Surveillance of bromocriptine in pregnancy. *JAMA* 247:1589, 1982

72. Czeizel A, Kiss R, Racz K, et al: Case-control cytogenetic study in offspring of mothers treated with bromocriptine early in pregnancy. *Mutat Res* 210:23, 1989

73. Raymond JP, Goldstein E, Konopka P, et al: Follow-up of children born of bromocriptine-treated mothers. *Horm Res* 22:239, 1985

74. Bigazzi M, Ronga R, Lancranjan I, et al: A pregnancy in an acromegalic woman during bromocriptine treatment: Effects on growth hormone and prolactin in the maternal, fetal, and amniotic fluid compartments. *J Clin Endocrinol Metab* 48:9, 1979

75. Konopka P, Raymond JP, Merceron RE, et al: Continuous administration of bromocriptine in the prevention of neurological complications in pregnant women with prolactinomas. *Am J Obstet Gynecol* 146:935, 1983

76. Georgiev DB, Dokumov SI: Continuous bromocriptine treatment of empty sella syndrome aggravating pregnancy: A case report. *Gynecol Obstet Invest* 32:243, 1991

77. Ahmed M, Al-Dossary E, Woodhouse NJ: Macroprolactinomas with suprasellar extension: Effect of bromocriptine withdrawal during one or more pregnancies. *Fertil Steril* 58:492, 1992

78. Hirohata T, Uozumi T, Mukada K, et al: Influence of pregnancy on the serum prolactin level following prolactinoma surgery. *Acta Endocrinol (Copenh)* 125:259, 1991

79. Ampudia X, Puig-Domingo M, Schwarzstein D, et al: Outcome

and long-term effects of pregnancy in women with hyperprolactinemia. *Eur J Obstet Gynecol Reprod Biol* 46:101, 1992

80. Cohn JB, Brust J, DeSerio F, et al: Effect of bromocriptine mesylate on induced hyperprolactinemia in stabilized psychiatric outpatients undergoing neuroleptic treatment. *Neuropsychobiology* 13:173, 1985

81. Smith S: Neuroleptic-associated hyperprolactinemia: Can it be treated with bromocriptine? *J Reprod Med* 37:737, 1992

82. Mattox JH, Buckman MT, Bernstein J, et al: Dopamine agonists for reducing depression associated with hyperprolactinemia. *J Reprod Med* 31:694, 1986

83. Lappohn RE, van de Weil HB, Brownell J: The effect of two dopaminergic drugs on menstrual function and psychologic state in hyperprolactinemia. *Fertil Steril* 58:321, 1992

84. Franks S, Horrocks PM, Lynch SS, et al: Effectiveness of pergolide mesylate in long term treatment of hyperprolactinemia. *Br Med J* 286:1177, 1983

85. Ahmed SR, Shalet SM: Discordant responses of prolactinoma to two different dopamine agonists. *Clin Endocrinol (Oxf)* 24:421, 1986

86. Pellegrini I, Costa R, Grisoli F, et al: Abnormal dopamine sensitivity in some human prolactinomas. *Horm Res* 31:19, 1989

87. Pellegrini I, Rasolonjanahary R, Gunz G, et al: Resistance to bromocriptine in prolactinomas. *J Clin Endocrinol Metab* 69:500, 1989

88. Collu R, Bouvier C, Lagace G, et al: Selective deficiency of guanine nucleotide-binding protein G_O in two dopamine-resistant pituitary tumors. *Endocrinology* 122:1176, 1988

89. Kleinberg DL, Lieberman A, Todd J, et al: Pergolide mesylate: A potent day-long inhibitor of prolactin in rhesus monkeys and patients with Parkinson's disease. *J Clin Endocrinol Metab* 51:152, 1980

90. L'Hermite M, Debusschere P: Potent 48 hours inhibition of prolactin secretion by pergolide in hyperprolactinemic women. *Acta Endocrinol (Copenh)* 101:481, 1982

91. Bergh T, Nillius SJ, Wide L: The long-acting dopamine agonist pergolide mesylate for treatment of hyperprolactinemia. *Acta Eur Fertil* 15:421, 1984

92. Blackwell RE, Bradley EL, Kline LB, et al: Comparison of dopamine agonists in the treatment of hyperprolactinemic syndromes: A multicenter study. *Fertil Steril* 39:744, 1983

93. Kleinberg DL, Boyd AE, Wardlaw S, et al: Pergolide for the treatment of pituitary tumors secreting prolactin or growth hormone. *N Engl J Med* 309:704, 1983

94. Kendall-Taylor P, Hall K, Johnston DG, et al: Reduction in size of prolactin-secreting tumors in men treated with pergolide. *Br Med J* 285:465, 1982

95. Kletzky OA, Borenstein R, Mileikowsky GN: Pergolide and bromocriptine for the treatment of patients with hyperprolactinemia. *Am J Obstet Gynecol* 154:431, 1986

96. Lamberts SWJ, Quik RFP: A comparison of the efficacy and safety of pergolide and bromocriptine in the treatment of hyperprolactinemia. *J Clin Endocrinol Metab* 72:635, 1991

97. Berezin M, Avidan D, Baron E: Long-term pergolide treatment of

hyperprolactinemic patients previously unsuccessfully treated with dopaminergic drugs. *Isr J Med Sci* 27:375, 1991

98. Rains CP, Bryson HM, Filton A: Cabergoline: A review of its pharmacological properties and therapeutic potential in the treatment of hyperprolactinemia and inhibition of lactation. *Drugs* 49:255, 1995

99. Ciccarelli E, Giusti M, Miola C, et al: Effectiveness and tolerability of long term treatment with cabergoline, a new long-lasting ergoline derivative, in hyperprolactinemic patients. *J Clin Endocrinol Metab* 69:725, 1989

100. European Multicenter Study Group for Cabergoline in Lactation Inhibition: Single dose cabergoline versus bromocriptine in inhibition of puerperal lactation: Randomized, double-blind, multicentre study. *BMJ* 302:1367, 1991

101. Ferrari C, Barbieri C, Caldara R, et al: Long-lasting prolactin lowering effect of cabergoline, a new dopamine agonist, in hyperprolactinemic patients. *J Clin Endocrinol Metab* 63:941, 1986

102. Webster J, Piscitelli G, Polli A, et al: A comparison of cabergoline and bromocriptine in the treatment of hyperprolactinemic amenorrhea. *N Engl J Med* 331:904, 1994

103. Paoletti AM, Depau GF, Mais V, et al: Effectiveness of cabergoline in reducing follicle-stimulating hormone and prolactin hypersecretion from pituitary macroadenoma in an infertile woman. *Fertil Steril* 62:882, 1994

104. Motta T, de Vincentiis S, Marchini M, et al: Vaginal cabergoline in the treatment of hyperprolactinemic patients intolerant to oral dopamineigas. *Fertil Steril* 65:440, 1996

105. Ferrari C, Paracchi A, Mattei AM, et al: Cabergoline in the long-term therapy of hyperprolactinemic disorders. *Acta Endocrinol (Copenh)* 126:489, 1992

106. Bevan JS, Davis JRE: Cabergoline: An advance in dopaminergic therapy. *Clin Endocrinol* 41:709, 1994

107. Razzaq R, O'Halloran DJ, Beardwell CG, et al: The effects of CV 205-502 in patients with hyperprolactinemia intolerant and/ or resistant to bromocriptine. *Horm Res* 39:318, 1993

108. Merola B, Sarnacchiaro F, Colao A, et al: Positive response to compound CV 205-502 in hyperprolactinemic patients resistant or intolerant of bromocriptine. *Gynecol Endocrinol* 8:175, 1994

109. Vance ML, Lipper M, Klibanski A, et al: Treatment of prolactin secreting macroadenomas with the long-acting non-ergot dopamine agonist CV 205-502. *Ann Intern Med* 112:668, 1990

110. Khalfallah Y, Claustrat B, Grochowicki M, et al: Effects of a new prolactin inhibitor, CV 205-502, in the treatment of human macroprolactinomas. *J Clin Endocrinol Metab* 71:354, 1990

111. Brue T, Pellegrini I, Gunz G, et al: Effects of the dopamine agonist CV 205-502 in human prolactinomas resistant to bromocriptine. *J Clin Endocrinol Metab* 74:577, 1992

112. Nordmann R, Fluckiger EW, Petcher TJ, et al: Endocrine actions of the potent dopamine D2-agonist CV 205-502 and related octahydrobenzo [g] quinolones. *Drugs of the Future* 13:951, 1988

113. Van der Heijden PFM, de Wit W, Brownell J, et al: CV 205-502, a new dopamine agonist, versus bromocriptine in the treatment of hyperprolactinemia. *Eur J Obstet Reprod Biol* 40:111, 1991

114. Glaser B, Nesher Y, Barziliai S: Long term treatment of

bromocriptine intolerant prolactinoma patients with CV 205-502. *J Reprod Med* 39:449, 1994

115. Van der Lely AJ, Brownell J, Lamberts SWJ: The efficacy and tolerability of CV 205-502 (a nonergot dopaminergic drug) in macroprolactinoma patients and in prolactinoma patients intolerant to bromocriptine. *J Clin Endocrinol Metab* 72:1136, 1991

116. Verhelst JA, Froud AL, Touzel R, et al: Acute and long-term effects of once-daily oral bromocriptine and a new long-acting non-ergot dopamine agonist, quinagolide, in the treatment of hyperprolactinemia: A double-blind study. *Acta Endocrinol (Copenh)* 125:385, 1991

117. Durantean L, Chanson P, Lavoine A, et al: Effect of the new dopaminergic agonist CV 205-502 on plasma prolactin levels and tumor size in bromocriptine-resistant prolactin. *Clin Endocrinol* 34:25, 1991

118. Shoham Z, Homburg R, Jacobs HS: CV 205-502: Effectiveness, tolerability, and safety over 24-month study. *Fertil Steril* 55:501, 1991

119. Giusti M, Porcella E, Carraro A, et al: A cross-over study with the two novel dopaminergic drugs cabergoline and quinagolide in hyperprolactinemic patients. *J Endocrinol Invest* 17:51, 1994

120. Vance ML, Cragun JR, Reimnitz C, et al: CV 205-502 treatment of hyperprolactinemia. *J Clin Endocrinol Metab* 68:336, 1989

121. Tamura T, Satoh T, Minakami H, et al: Effect of hydergine in hyperprolactinemia. *J Clin Endocrinol Metab* 69:470, 1989

122. Crosignani PG, Ferrari C, Liuzzi A, et al: Treatment of hyperprolactinemic states with different drugs: A study with bromocriptine, metergoline and lisuride. *Fertil Steril* 37:61, 1982

123. Bohnet HG, Kato K, Wolf AS: Treatment of hyperprolactinemic amenorrhea with metergoline. *Obstet Gynecol* 67:249, 1986

124. Dallabonzana D, Liuzzi A, Oppizzi G, et al: Chronic treatment of pathological hyperprolactinemia and acromegaly with the new ergot derivative terguride. *J Clin Endocrinol Metab* 63:1002, 1986

125. Ciccarelli E, Touzel R, Besser M, et al: Terguride: A new dopamine agonist drug—A comparison of its neuroendocrine and side effect profile with bromocriptine. *Fertil Steril* 49:589, 1988

126. Corenblum B, Taylor PJ: Long term follow-up of hyperprolactinemic women treated with bromocriptine. *Fertil Steril* 40:596, 1983

127. Gen M, Uozumi T, Ohta M, et al: Necrotic changes in prolactinomas after long term administration of bromocriptine. *J Clin Endocrinol Metab* 59:463, 1984

128. Moriondo P, Travaglini P, Nissim M, et al: Bromocriptine treatment of microprolactinomas: Evidence of stable prolactin decrease after drug withdrawal. *J Clin Endocrinol Metab* 60:764, 1985

129. Rasmussen C, Bergh T, Wide L: Prolactin secretion and menstrual function after long term bromocriptine treatment. *Fertil Steril* 48:550, 1987

130. Van't Verlaat J, Croughs RJM: Withdrawal of bromocriptine after long term therapy for cacroprolactinomas: Effect on plasma prolactin and tumor size. *Clin Endocrinol* 34:175, 1991

131. Radwanska E, McGarrigle HH, Little V, et al: Induction of ovulation in women with hyperprolactinemic amenorrhea using clomiphene and human chorionic gonadotropin or bromocriptine. *Fertil Steril* 32:187, 1979

132. Farine D, Dor J, Lupovici N, et al: Conception rate after gonadotropin therapy in hyperprolactinemia and normoprolactinemia. *Obstet Gynecol* 65:658, 1985

133. Suginami H, Hamada K, Kohji Y: Ovulation induction with bromocriptine in normoprolactinemic anovulatory women. *J Clin Endocrinol Metab* 62:899, 1986

134. Steinberger E, Nader S, Rodrigez-Riqau L, et al: Prolactin response to thyrotropin-releasing hormone with ovulatory dysfunction and its use for selection of candidates for bromocriptine therapy. *J Endocrinol Invest* 13:637, 1990

135. Asukai K, Uemura T, Minaguchi H: Occult hyperprolactinemia in infertile women. *Fertil Steril* 60:423, 1993

136. Ben-David M, Schenker JG: Transient hyperprolactinemia: A correctable cause of idiopathic female infertility. *J Clin Endocrinol Metab* 57:442, 1983

137. DeVane GW, Guzick DS: Bromocriptine therapy in normoprolactinic women with unexplained infertility and galactorrhea. *Fertil Steril* 46:1026, 1986

138. Padilla SL, Person GK, McDonough PG, et al: The efficacy of bromocriptine in patients with ovulatory dysfunction and normoprolactinemic galactorrhea. *Fertil Steril* 44:695, 1985

139. Peperell RJ: Prolactin and reproduction. *Fertil Steril* 35:267, 1980

140. Gala RR: Prolactin and growth hormone in the regulation of the immune system. *Proc Soc Exp Biol Med* 198:513, 1991

141. Scommegna A, Ye SH, Prins GS: Bromocriptine reverses the inhibitory effect of macrophages on human sperm motility. *Fertil Steril* 61:331, 1994

142. Goldzieher JW, Young RL: Selected aspects of polycystic ovarian disease. *Endocrinol Metab Clin North Am* 21:141, 1992

143. Seibel MM, Oskowitz S, Kamrava M, et al: Bromocriptine response in normoprolactinemic patients with polycystic ovary disease: A preliminary report. *Obstet Gynecol* 64:213, 1984

144. Tabbakh GH, Loutfi IA, Azab I, et al: Bromocriptine in polycystic ovarian disease: A controlled clinical trial. *Obstet Gynecol* 71:301, 1988

145. Buvat J, Buvat-Herbaut M, Marcolin G, et al: A double-blind controlled study of the hormonal and clinical effects of bromocriptine in the polycystic ovary syndrome. *J Clin Endocrinol Metab* 63:119, 1986

146. Steingold KA, Lobo RA, Judd HL, et al: The effect of bromocriptine on gonadotropin and steroid secretion in polycystic ovarian disease. *J Clin Endocrinol Metab* 62:1048, 1986

147. Ferriani RA, Silva de Sa MF, Moura MD, et al: Dopamine might not be involved in the pathogenesis of polycystic ovary syndrome. *Gynecol Endocrinol* 3:317, 1989

PART VIII

Surgical Treatment of Female-Factor Infertility

CHAPTER 34

Diagnostic and Operative Hysteroscopy

PATRICK J. TAYLOR · VICTOR GOMEL

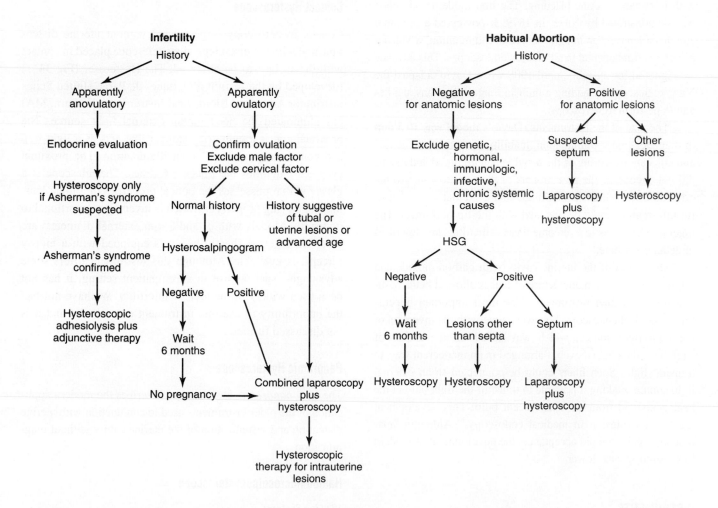

A vaginal speculum recovered from the ashes of Pompeii and now exhibited in the archeological museum in Naples is the first example of an instrument used to visualize the interior of the female genital tract. In 1805, Admiral Nelson won his great victory off Cape Trafalgar. In the same year, Bozzini (cited by Lindemann)[1] was reprimanded by the medical faculty of Vienna for "undue curiosity" in attempting to visualize the interior of the urethra of a living human being. He also observed the cervix using a tubular speculum, with light from a candle being reflected with a mirror.

Aubinais (cited by Lyon)[2] is credited incorrectly with the first hysteroscopy in 1864. In fact, he observed the emergence of a fetal head from a cervix.

A 12-mm device with which the urethra could be investigated was introduced by Desormeaux.[3] The first true hysteroscopy was performed in 1869 by Pantaleoni using Desormeaux's device.[4] Pantaleoni inspected and cauterized with silver nitrate polyps the uterine cavity of a 60-year-old woman with intractable uterine bleeding. The first modern endoscope was demonstrated by Nitze[5] in 1879. It possessed a proximal and distal lens and an integral source of illumination, which are principles fundamental to all modern endoscopes. This advance was ignored for 29 years, until 1908 when David[6] adapted the Nitze endoscope by adding a built-in magnifying lens and began to perform hysteroscopy.

The size of the instruments (David's model was 10.5 mm in diameter), poor illumination, inability to distend the uterus, and constant obscuring of the distal lens with blood and mucus did not encourage the practitioners of the time to embrace the procedure with enthusiasm. Munde[7] believed that as much useful information could be obtained with the tip of a finger. The ingenious attempts to overcome these difficulties are described in detail elsewhere.[1,8,9]

Distention of the uterine cavity with carbon dioxide and improvement in the manufacture of lenses allowed better visualization with finer instruments. The most important impetus for all medical endoscopy, however, came with the invention of the cold light source, which was based on the ability of stretched silica fibers, even if arranged in an incoherent way, to transmit light. Such fibers could be connected to an external light source, making it possible to transmit the light but not the heat generated from an incandescent bulb. This development led to an explosion in medical endoscopy.[10] Although laparoscopy[11] gained rapid acceptance, the development of modern hysteroscopy was slower.

INSTRUMENTS

Along with the evolution of hysteroscopy as an important diagnostic and therapeutic tool has come an awareness that proper training, credentialing, and monitoring are essential for optimal clinical outcomes. As a result, various organizations and societies have established guidelines for training and credentialing operative endoscopists.[12–14] In general, diagnostic hysteroscopy is considered a level I procedure not requiring further training. More advanced procedures such as endometrial resection or ablation, division or resection of a uterine septum, endoscopic surgical therapy for Asherman's syndrome, resection of uterine myomas, and fallopian tube cannulation are considered level II procedures necessitating additional training.

Since the early 1960s, hysteroscopic technology has advanced in three parallel directions, and several techniques have evolved. The three types of hysteroscopes in current use are contact, panoramic, and the Hamou microcolpohysteroscope (MCH). Accessory equipment includes a viewing system, a gaseous liquid distention medium if indicated, and ancillary instruments.

Contact Hysteroscope

Contact hysteroscopy is performed without uterine distention, and with the distal lens of the telescope placed in contact with the surface to be observed. The Hysteroser (Fig 34–1) (developed by the Institut d'Optiques de Paris, United States distributor Advanced Biomedical Instruments, Woburn, MA) has eliminated the need for an external light source. The proximal end is a cylindric chamber that acts as a light trap and concentrates ambient room illumination. The proximal eyepiece magnifies the image 1.6 times. The telescope is a glass rod that possesses the optical properties of a thick lens, the magnifying property of which is inversely proportional to its length. Models with 6- and 8-mm external diameters are used. An external sheath, which is equipped with a biopsy forceps, is available. Although this instrument offers some advantages, such as use in an outpatient setting, it has not been used widely in the area of infertility. We have not had the opportunity to use this instrument extensively, and it is not discussed further.

Panoramic Hysteroscope

The term *panoramic hysteroscopy* describes the modern application of the older instruments used in conjunction with uterine distention and visualization of the uterine cavity without magnification.

Hamou Microcolpohysteroscope

Viewing Systems

A 150-watt cold light source connected with either a fiberoptic or alcohol-filled cable is adequate for all purposes with the exception of photography, which requires a xenon light source for

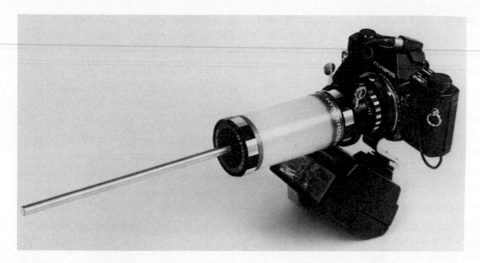

Figure 34–1. The contact hysteroscope (Hysteroser) with camera and flash attachments.

optimum results. The telescopes are adapted cystoscopes and have external diameters that range from 4 to 6 mm. Both 180° and foroblique viewing systems are available. The range of models produced by various instrument makers has been reviewed extensively.[15]

Hysteroscopes come equipped with a diagnostic sheath and a larger operative sheath through which ancillary instruments can be introduced. In some small-bore models, the external sheath has been adapted to accept miniature flexible biopsy forceps, electroprobes, and scissors. An external sheath into which dissecting scissors are incorporated is also available. Our experience has been that the flexible instruments are too fragile for performing many operative procedures.

The Hamou MCH[16] (Karl Storz Endoscopy America, Culver City, CA) is a compound instrument that can be used as a panoramic hysteroscope, a contact hysteroscope, or a microscope. The microscopic properties are made possible by a lens system that allows magnification of 1, 20, 60, and 150 times. Although the higher magnifications are of value in investigating premalignant disease of the cervix and endometrium, they have little role in procedures for infertility. A second model, the Hamou II that dispenses with the turret lens and the higher magnifications has been introduced (Fig 34–2). Both models can be focused by use of a knurled wheel.

Distention Media

The distention media used in hysteroscopy have been reviewed extensively.[17] Because the uterine cavity is a potential space, for effective panoramic viewing, the walls must be separated with a distention medium. Distention media must be easy to handle

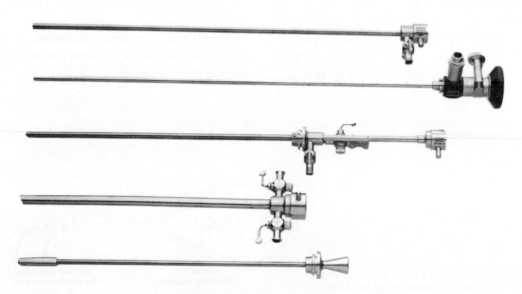

Figure 34–2. The Hamou II microhysteroscope.

and immiscible with blood, and they must pose no risk for local or systemic effects. If electrosurgical instruments are to be used, the medium must not be capable of conducting electrical current. Each of the currently available media meets the specifications to a greater or lesser degree.

Carbon Dioxide. We have largely abandoned the use of carbon dioxide for conventional panoramic hysteroscopy. A gas-tight seal is required at the cervix, and the specially designed suction cups tend to be somewhat cumbersome. If this approach is to be used, only insufflation equipment specifically designed for hysteroscopy is safe. Insufflators designed for laparoscopy must never be used to perform hysteroscopy. Whereas hysteroscopic insufflators deliver 100 mL of carbon dioxide per minute, the minimum flow rate of the laparoscopic insufflator is 1 L per minute. Such volumes of carbon dioxide carry a substantial risk for causing a lethal gas embolism.

Although the standard constant-pressure–variable-flow or constant-flow–variable-pressure insufflators are adequate, Hamou perfected an electronic variable-pressure–variable-flow insufflator (Fig 34–3). This device uses an electronic molecular counter that allows for programmable control of both the flow and the pressure of carbon dioxide.

Intrauterine pressure should not exceed 100 mm Hg. At these pressures, flow rates of 40 to 60 mL/minute are safe.[18] The view is clear, sharp, and excellent for photography if carbon dioxide is used. Troublesome gas bubbles can form and obscure the view if there is fluid or mucus within the uterine cavity. Bleeding also becomes a hindrance, making surgical manipulations difficult.

Dextrose 5% in Water. Dextrose 5% in water (D5W) is particularly useful for outpatient hysteroscopy. The large volumes required as it flows freely from the cervix are offset by the fact that D5W is inexpensive. Dissection is difficult, however, because of the ease with which D5W mixes with blood. Therefore, mucus and blood must be flushed from the uterine cavity. This can be achieved by means of introduction of a fine polyethylene catheter through the operating channel. Injection of D5W through this catheter results in pressures greater than can be achieved with the flow from the hysteroscopic sheath itself (see Fig 34–3). One instills D5W by connecting one inflow channel of the sheath to a 500-mL plastic bag wrapped in a blood pressure cuff that is inflated to a pressure of 80 to 120 mm Hg. Approximately 150 mL will be used in 10 minutes. With this system, the usual intrauterine pressure is 40 mm Hg, but pressures of 100 to 110 mm Hg are required to visualize the tubal ostia.[19] These higher intrauterine pressures may be achieved with additional inflation of the blood pressure cuff.

Normal Saline Solution. Normal saline solution is readily available and inexpensive. It is isotonic and thus poses no risk for causing hemolysis if intravasation occurs. Saline solution is miscible with blood and is not satisfactory if bleeding is anticipated. Lasers can be safely used in this environment, but saline solution conducts electricity, precluding its use with electrosurgical instruments.

High-Viscosity Fluids. Polyvinyl prolidene (4% Luviskol K-90), a mixture of different polymers, was originally proposed as a uterine distention medium. It proved to be unsuitable.

Hyskon. Hyskon (Pharmacia, Piscataway, NJ) is a dextran with an average molecular weight of 70,000 made to 32% in 10% dextrose.[20] Hyskon is electrolyte free, nonconductive, and biodegradable. No special instruments are required, and the medium can be instilled through a 20-mL syringe connected either directly or by means of a short piece of polyethylene tubing to one of the inflow taps of the sheath. Hyskon is particularly valuable in short operative procedures, because it does not mix with blood. The principal disadvantage, aside from expense, is that Hyskon becomes sticky as it dries. Immediately after use of Hyskon, the instruments and their moving parts must be rinsed thoroughly to prevent them from jamming. If jamming occurs, the stopcock should not be forced but should be soaked for a few minutes in hot water.

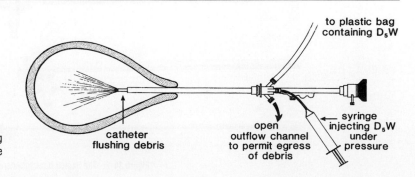

Figure 34–3. Catheter used to flush debris from the uterus; D5W is flowing in through one channel. The catheter is introduced through the operative stopcock, and the outflow channel is left open to allow egress of the debris.

Glycine. Glycine is an amino acid in 1.5% solution. It is suitable for use in electrosurgical procedures. Glycine is nonhemolytic, but intravasation may cause nausea and vertigo. If large volumes are retained, fluid overload and high-output cardiac failure may occur. The metabolites of glycine can cause encephalopathy.

Sorbitol. d-Glucitol is made up in a 3% solution. It is miscible with blood and is slightly hypotonic. Sorbitol is safe to use with electrosurgical equipment but if absorbed can cause hemolysis. Patients with diabetes are at some risk for hyperglycemia.

Although the pressure cuff delivery system for fluid media is satisfactory for both diagnostic and operative procedures, many surgeons prefer to use a pump that automatically controls the pressure and flow rate. It is imperative during all operative procedures that fluid balance be monitored accurately.

Ancillary Instruments

Minimum equipment for routine diagnostic hysteroscopy includes a calibrated probe, fine suction irrigation catheters, soft tubal probes, scissors, and biopsy forceps. These instruments may be flexible, semiflexible, or rigid. For diagnostic work, flexible instruments are adequate and can be introduced through a somewhat smaller external sheath. If operative work is to be undertaken, rigid instruments are required and must be introduced directly along the axis of the operating sheath, necessitating use of a hysteroscope with an offset eyepiece. The external sheath, by necessity, must be larger.

Both the shaft and handle of electrosurgical instruments should be insulated. Neuwirth and Amin[21] described a modification of a urologic resectoscope that accommodates a standard hysteroscope. A cutting loop is powered by a transistorized unit set to 60 to 80 W of cutting current. The depth of burn with this instrument is not greater than 2 mm.

Fine laser probes have become available. Although we find a modification of an MCH to be the instrument of choice for diagnostic work, if operative procedures are to be undertaken, a resectoscope or a surgical operating panoramic hysteroscope equipped with rigid instruments is preferable.

HYSTEROSCOPIC TECHNIQUE

Preoperative Investigation

Before hysteroscopy is performed, a complete history is taken and a physical examination performed. For a patient seeking treatment of infertility or habitual abortion, endoscopy should be one of the last procedures after other causes of the symptoms have been excluded with less invasive means.

Preliminary investigations include the blood group and hemoglobin level of both partners. The woman's degree of immunity to rubella should be ascertained. We have abandoned Venereal Disease Research Laboratory (VDRL) testing, because we did not encounter a positive result in 1700 examinations.[22] Cervical, vaginal, and seminal cultures should be performed for both the common infective organisms and for *Chlamydia* and *Mycoplasma* species. If an infective agent is detected, appropriate antibiotic therapy should be administered and the infection eradicated before hysteroscopy. If general anesthesia is planned, the patient's fitness for anesthesia must be evaluated. Informed consent for the procedure must be obtained.

Timing

Optimum evaluation of the uterine cavity of a patient reporting infertility or habitual abortion can be achieved during the follicular phase of the menstrual cycle. If hysteroscopy is to be combined with laparoscopy, there are advantages to performing the latter procedure in the immediately postovulatory phase, when, for example, evidence of ovulation can be sought. There is no contraindication to performing hysteroscopy at this time.

Positioning the Patient

Hysteroscopy is performed with the patient in the dorsal lithotomy position with her feet in stirrups. Although every attempt should be made to achieve asepsis, no antiseptic solution should be introduced into the vagina if carbon dioxide is to be used as the distention medium. All antiseptic solutions are soapy and dirty the distal lens of the instrument, and they usually are carried into the uterine cavity. Although the bubbles produced by antiseptic solutions are quite spectacular, they hinder adequate visualization. Because the patient is instructed to void before the procedure, catheterization is rarely necessary.

A bimanual examination is performed to determine the position and mobility of the uterus. This elementary precaution protects against perforation of a retroverted uterus. The cervix is exposed with a speculum, and the anterior part of the cervix is grasped with a single-toothed tenaculum. The tenaculum is placed in the vertical plane when the Hamou MCH is used.

Anesthesia

Most diagnostic hysteroscopies can be performed without anesthesia.[23] For selected patients, paracervical blockade with 1% bupivacaine, 10 mL injected on each side of the cervix, provides adequate analgesia provided that 10 minutes are allowed to elapse from the time of injection. Patients who undergo general anesthesia include those who are extremely apprehensive, the few patients for whom attempted procedures have proved to be too uncomfortable in the office or outpatient setting, and patients undergoing hysteroscopy combined with laparoscopy either as a diagnostic procedure or when laparoscopic monitoring of intrauterine surgical procedures is indicated.[24]

Technique

With modern small-caliber diagnostic hysteroscopes, no prior cervical dilation is required. Occasionally, however, it is necessary to dilate the cervix. The uterus should be sounded and the cervix dilated to a size of dilator just smaller than the external diameter of the hysteroscope sheath.

The hysteroscope is inserted through the sheath and connected to the light source (see Fig 34–3), and the distention medium and the sheath are filled with either carbon dioxide or fluid medium. With the distention medium flowing, the hysteroscope is inserted through the external ostium, and the speculum is removed.

When carbon dioxide is used as the distention medium, the insufflator (Fig 34–4) is preset at a flow rate of 30 mL/minute and at a pressure of 90 mm Hg. Once the gas is flowing, the tip of the telescope is inserted to the external ostium. The flow of carbon dioxide produces a microcavity in the cervical canal immediately distal to the tip of the hysteroscope. As the cervical canal is distended, the instrument is gradually advanced into the microcavity. With this method of introduction under direct vision, atraumatic advancement is possible, which is usually pain free and bloodless. The length, morphology, and any pathologic features of the cervical canal can be evaluated. As the instrument enters the uterine cavity, an excellent, clear panoramic view is obtained.

Uterine viewing begins as the cavity is entered and should not proceed if the lens is obscured by mucus or blood. A red appearance over the end of the lens suggests that the telescope is in contact with the uterine wall and should immediately be withdrawn a few centimeters. If the examination is difficult and the pressure very low despite a high flow rate, a leak in the system or uterine perforation should be suspected.

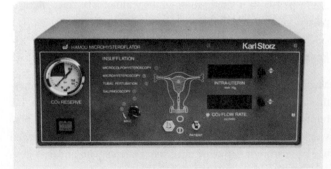

Figure 34–4. The Microhysteroflator.

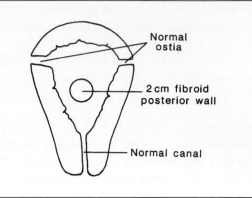

Figure 34–5. Sketch documents hysteroscopic findings.

An excellent view is obtained as the uterine cavity distends. A systematic inspection should be made beginning with the fundus. Each tubal ostium and the anterior, posterior, and lateral uterine walls are identified. Inspection of the cervical canal is repeated as the instrument is withdrawn.

It is important to document all findings.[25] Both still and videophotography provide elegant records. Nevertheless, the dictated operative report and a free hand sketch of the uterine cavity and any associated lesions are simple and inexpensive and may be of inestimable value (Fig 34–5).

CONTRAINDICATIONS

Hysteroscopy should not be performed during menstruation. Not only does the blood make visualization more difficult, but also at least a theoretic risk exists that the passage of endometrial fragments through the fallopian tubes may predispose the patient to subsequent endometriosis. A history of recent or present acute pelvic infection[23] and any suggestion of early pregnancy constitute absolute contraindications. Great care must be taken in the treatment of patients suffering from Asherman's syndrome,[26] because the uteri in these patients are unusually friable and easily perforated.

COMPLICATIONS

It is clear that diagnostic hysteroscopy for infertile patients or women with habitual abortion is a low-risk procedure. Complications may arise from the anesthetic agent or distention medium, during cervical dilation, and during the performance of diagnostic and especially operative hysteroscopy. Failure to complete the procedure must also be considered a complication. Complications of specific operative procedures are described later in this chapter.

Anesthesia

The risks of anesthesia, either general or local, are no different for hysteroscopy than for any other surgical procedure. Any risk of general anesthesia can be avoided if the procedure is performed without general anesthesia. Hypersensitivity may occasionally occur even with use of local anesthetic agents, however. If a local anesthetic has been augmented with administration of parenteral hypnotics, hallucinations may occur. This is particularly likely with the use of ketamine, diazepam, and droperidol.

Distention Medium

The use of DA5W is essentially risk free. Rare cases of anaphylaxis to dextran have been reported.[27] This usually occurs if the uterine cavity has been traumatized, allowing high volumes of dextran (Hyskon) to enter the systemic circulation. Although use of carbon dioxide may be associated with postoperative shoulder tip pain, hypercardia, and cardiac arrhythmias do not occur unless the method of insufflation is inappropriate.[28] The most feared complication of use of carbon dioxide is venous gas embolism. The risk is low when appropriate insufflators are used.

Risks of Cervical Dilation

During cervical dilation, it is possible to form a false passage or perforate the uterus (Fig 34–6; see color plate facing page 580). Fortunately, these events are rare. More frequently, the tenaculum tears free. Such an event occurred in 4 of 836 women who underwent hysteroscopy as part of an infertility investigation.[30] Although in this series, we recorded only cases that necessitated suturing to control bleeding, dislodgment of the tenaculum is frequent but usually trivial.

Uterine Perforation

Uterine perforation may be caused by the sound, the dilator, or the hysteroscope, or it may occur during operative procedures. Uterine perforation should be suspected when the instrument has passed to a great depth, and it should be considered probable if large volumes of distention medium instilled at low pressures result in no uterine distention. Perforation occurred in 2 of 1014 patients undergoing diagnostic hysteroscopy. In both cases, the instrument was used by a learner under instruction.[31] Lindemann[32] reported 6 perforations in a total of 5200 carbon dioxide hysteroscopies. Perforation is unlikely to occur when the hysteroscope is advanced under constant visual control. Perforation is more likely to occur during an operative procedure such as division of uterine synechiae or septa and myomectomy. Simple uterine perforation does not appear to be a serious complication. Previously, we recommended that assessment lap-

aroscopy be performed if uterine perforation occurred.[25] We now recommend watchful waiting unless there is reason to believe the perforation results from use of an energy source such as electricity or laser. In such instances, laparoscopy may be insufficient to evaluate fully the possible sequelae. Fortunately, penetrating thermal injury to the colon often can be managed successfully with primary repair.[33]

The rare instances in which obvious hemorrhage is seen, require immediate attention. Otherwise, the patient is observed for 2 to 3 hours, a baseline hematocrit is obtained, and vital signs are monitored. If her condition is stable, the patient is discharged and asked to return for a follow-up visit in the office the next day. At that time, the patient is reexamined, her temperature and pulse are recorded, and the hematocrit is repeated. Signs of peritonitis or intraperitoneal hematoma formation necessitate readmission and treatment. It is wise to explain to the patient the nature of such complications and instruct her to contact the office immediately should she experience pain, bleeding, or fever.

Infection

Acute infection after diagnostic hysteroscopy appears to be a rare complication. In a series of 1000 Hamou MCH hysteroscopies, only 1 severe and 7 mild pelvic infections were identified.[34] The severe infection occurred during removal of a tubal stent after a tuboplasty. These same investigators did not record a single instance of infection among 3000 subsequent evaluations. Infection is more likely to occur after prolonged operative procedures, especially when repeated insertion and removal of the hysteroscope has been necessary. Infection is manifested 48 to 72 hours after the procedure with pelvic pain, vaginal discharge, and fever. The use of prophylactic antibiotics is recommended with operative procedures.

Uterine Synechiae

Blind diagnostic curettage in the treatment of infertile patients is correlated with subsequent formation of intrauterine adhesions.[35] Diagnostic hysteroscopy does not appear to pose a similar risk. We performed 112 second-look hysteroscopies among patients undergoing laparoscopy and hysteroscopy before tubal reconstructive operations followed by second-look laparoscopy and hysteroscopy 6 weeks after the original procedure. No patients were determined to have intrauterine adhesions preoperatively, and none showed fresh adhesion formation at the time of the second-look procedure.

Other Complications

Other minimal complications of hysteroscopy have been reported, including perforation of a thin-walled hydrosalpinx at the time of carbon dioxide hysteroscopy. A similar occurrence was reported when dextran was used.[23] We reported a total complication rate among 2014 combined laparoscopies and diagnostic hysteroscopies of less than 1%.[31]

Failure to complete hysteroscopy has been reported to occur among zero to 8% of patients.[24] Such failure occurred among 21 (2.08%) of 1010 patients.[31] Reasons included an inability to dilate the cervix in 11 instances, blood obscuring the view in 4 instances, and air bubbles hindering visualization in 6 instances. The disastrous visualization of an early pregnancy in one patient was described elsewhere.[36] The most common cause of failure is inability to dilate the cervix. This almost never occurs when a small-bore instrument and carbon dioxide are used.

ROLE OF DIAGNOSTIC HYSTEROSCOPY IN INFERTILITY AND HABITUAL ABORTION

The role of hysteroscopy in the treatment of patients reporting infertility or habitual abortion is to detect the presence and confirm the exact nature of any intrauterine lesions that may be contributing to the condition.

Timing

Infertility

The investigation for an infertile couple should be concluded as rapidly, accurately, inexpensively, and noninvasively as possible. According to these criteria, in most instances, endoscopic evaluation should be one of the later investigations. At the first visit, a simple examination of the woman's menstrual pattern allows triage into two large groups, those in which the woman is (1) apparently ovulatory and (2) apparently anovulatory.

Ovulatory Women. When a woman apparently is ovulatory, ovulation should be confirmed with a basal body temperature (BBT) graph and measurement of serum progesterone levels. Two properly collected semen samples should be analyzed, and the sperm–cervical mucus interaction determined with a postcoital test. If a male factor or cervical factor is detected and there is no history of tubal or uterine disease, these factors should be treated for 6 months before further investigation of the uterine cavity and fallopian tubes. Only if such treatment is unsuccessful should evaluation of the lower genital tract of the woman be undertaken. If the women's history is suggestive of tubal or uterine disease or if she is of advanced reproductive age (older than 35 years), the lower genital tract should be evaluated before any additional therapy is undertaken.

If the preliminary evaluation demonstrates normal ovulation, normal male factors, and normal sperm–cervical mucus interaction, the lower genital tract should be evaluated. The initial procedure should be hysterosalpingography (HSG).[37]

Anovulatory Women. The detailed work-up for an anovulatory woman with amenorrhea is described in Chap 6. The role of hysteroscopy is largely restricted to patients for whom a diagnosis of Asherman's syndrome is suspected. Because of disturbed menstrual function, the patients may initially be believed to be anovulatory. These patients may have amenorrhea, normal levels of gonadotropin and prolactin, and negative withdrawal bleeding when challenged with an estrogen-progestin combination. For such patients, diagnosis and treatment can be carried out during one procedure.

Habitual Abortion

Strictly speaking, the diagnosis of habitual abortion should be made only when three consecutive pregnancy losses of less than 20 weeks' gestation have occurred with a fetus weighing less than 500 g. A theoretic study of Malpas in 1938[39] predicted a 75% risk for subsequent spontaneous abortion among such patients. More likely, however, these women probably have a 70% likelihood of carrying any subsequent pregnancy to term.[39] Nevertheless, these patients have an increased likelihood of a specific cause for abortion, such as genetic, hormonal, anatomic, immunologic, infective, or chronic systemic disease.

The role of hysteroscopy is to detect anatomic uterine lesions. The uterine cavity should be investigated with both HSG and hysteroscopy. If the history suggests an anatomic lesion, as may be the case when a surgeon who performed curettage during a previous abortion noted the probable presence of an intrauterine septum, HSG and hysteroscopy should be performed early. If no such history exists, investigation of the uterine cavity should be delayed until the karyotype of both partners has been determined and the woman has undergone appropriate evaluation, including assessment of her thyroid status and luteal phase adequacy, cervical and endometrial cultures for *Chlamydia* and *Mycoplasma* species, and assessment of her toxoplasmosis titer.[40] The possible role of the shared human leukocyte (HLA) antigens between partners and embryo toxic factor (see Chap 26) is beyond the scope of this chapter.

Complementary Role of Hysterosalpingography and Hysteroscopy

In most instances, the preliminary investigation of the lower genital tract should be with HSG. Advantages of initial HSG include (1) identification of uterine anomalies and intrauterine lesions; (2) identification of cornual occlusion or lesions even in the presence of cornual patency; (3) immediate identification of distal tubal occlusion and assessment of intratubal architecture; and (4) planning of a laparoscopic reparative operation if distal tubal occlusion is found.[41]

Just as wide discrepancy has been reported between HSG and laparoscopic findings,[42] a similar incongruence between

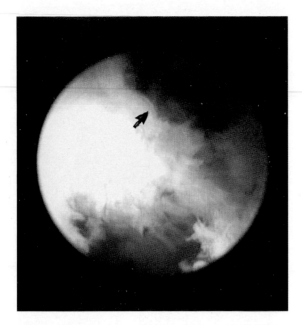

Figure 34–6. Hysteroscopic view of endometrial cavity (arrows) and false passage caused by introduction of the hysteroscope (bottom).

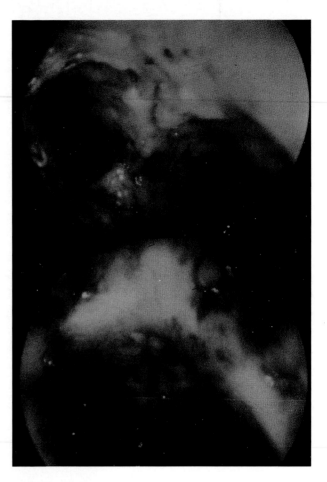

Figure 34–9. Dense intrauterine adhesions (top) before and (bottom) after removal. *(Courtesy of Dr. J. Hamou.)*

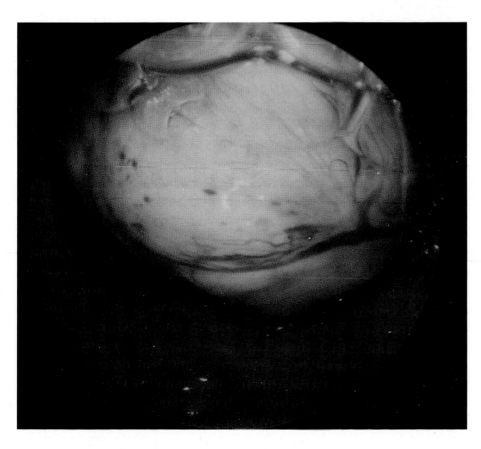

Figure 34–10. A large submucous fibroid. *(Courtesy of Dr. J. Hamou.)*

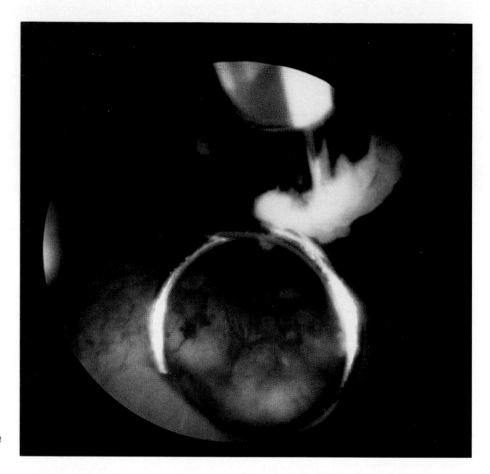

Figure 34–11. Electrosurgical snare is used to remove submucous fibroids. *(Courtesy of Dr. J. Hamou.)*

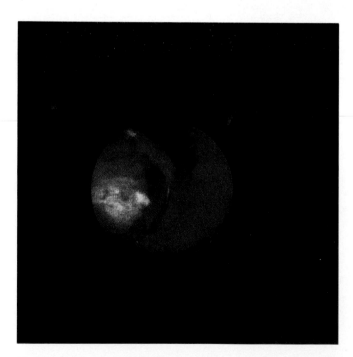

Figure 34–12. The resectoscope loop in use to divide a septum. *(Courtesy of Dr. A. H. DeCherney.)*

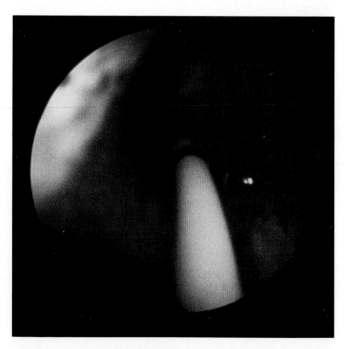

Figure 34–13. Cannulation of the tubal ostium.

HSG and hysteroscopic findings has been noted. Siegler[43] compared the results among 104 patients seeking treatment of infertility on whom both HSG and hysteroscopy were performed. Hysteroscopy failed in eight patients. Uterine abnormalities were suggested at HSG for 19 patients; 2 of these patients were found to have an entirely normal uterus at the time of hysteroscopy. Septa were confirmed at HSG in six patients, adhesions in five, and submucous fibroids in two. An unsuspected uterine lesion was found in 30 (39%) of 77 hysteroscopic examinations. One hundred forty-two patients were examined with hysteroscopy, in 63 of whom results of previous HSG had been reported as abnormal. Hysteroscopic evaluation was normal for 20 patients (32%).[44]

Comparison of HSG and hysteroscopy in the treatment of 91 infertile patients resulted in a divergence of opinion about the findings for 40% of the patients.[45] In a study by Snowden et al,[46] HSG indicated an abnormality in 16 (21%) of 77 women. At hysteroscopy, findings were confirmed for 11 and refuted for 5 of 61 patients who had normal HSG findings, and hysteroscopy allowed detection of an unsuspected lesion in only 1 patient (1%). The discrepancy between the findings of Snowden et al and those of other investigators may be accounted for by the fact that most lesions apparently missed at HSG are small, and the ability to detect such lesions depends on the care with which the HSG is performed. In the study by Snowden et al,[46] 21% of patients had radiologic evidence of intrauterine abnormalities, a frequency considerably higher than that reported elsewhere.[47]

We compared HSG and hysteroscopic findings for 254 women[31] (Table 34–1). Correlation between the findings was good when results of HSG were abnormal. Hysteroscopy is of particular value in identification of the exact nature of a lesion when the radiologic report notes a filling defect. Although hysteroscopy may be more accurate in identification of small polyps and filmy adhesions, congruence between HSG and endoscopic findings is excellent with respect to uterine malformations.[48]

TABLE 34–1. COMPARISON OF HYSTEROSALPINGOGRAPHIC AND HYSTEROSCOPIC FINDINGS

| Hysteroscopic Findings | Normal (n = 232) | Hysterosalpingographic Findings Abnormal (n = 22) | | | |
		Filling Defect (n = 16)	Adhesions (n = 2)	Polyps (n = 1)	Septa (n = 3)
Normal	166	3	—	—	—
Adhesions	45	4	2	—	—
Polyps	18	9	—	1	—
Myomata	3	—	—	—	—
Septa	0	—	—	—	3

Combined Laparoscopy and Hysteroscopy

For infertile patients, it has been our practice to combine hysteroscopy with laparoscopy. Both procedures can be performed safely under the same general anesthesia. Among 677 infertile women in whom both procedures were performed successfully, the results with both modalities were considered normal for 156 patients (23.0%), and the findings of one or both procedures were abnormal for 521 patients (77.0%). We believe the combination of laparoscopy and hysteroscopy offers the most complete evaluation of the lower reproductive tract.[49]

The most frequently detected intrauterine lesion among patients seeking treatment because of habitual abortion is a uterine septum. Hysteroscopy does not allow differentiation between a septate and a bicornuate uterus. For evaluation of a malformed uterus, combined laparoscopy and hysteroscopy can be of inestimable value, although advances in magnetic resonance imaging (MRI) and to some extent ultrasonography[50] can assist in provision of such refined differentiation.

Findings

Table 34–2 demonstrates the hysteroscopic findings for five series of infertile patients. In the past, we performed all diagnostic hysteroscopies using dextran 70 as the distention medium. We had the opportunity to compare the specific findings for 992 women examined with this method with the findings for 335 women who underwent hysteroscopy with a Hamou 1 instrument and carbon dioxide as the distention medium[52] (Table 34–3). In all instances, the apparent detection rate was considerably higher when dextran was used. We were forced to conclude from these data that many of the findings in our preliminary studies were artifactual and that although fibroids and septa were detected with roughly the same prevalence, adhesions and polyps were noted much less frequently when carbon dioxide was used. On the basis of these findings, we now use carbon dioxide exclusively when performing hysteroscopy for diagnostic purposes. Despite these somewhat unsettling findings, the most frequently noted lesions among patients seeking treatment because of infertility are polyps, adhesions, fibroids, and septa.

Polyps

The following discussion is illustrated by Figs 34–7 through 34–13 (Figs 34–9 to 34–13; see color plate facing page 580). Mucous polyps (Fig 34–7) occur within the uterine cavity and must be differentiated from dislodged strips of endometrium and myomata. In contrast to myomata, which are fixed, polyps undulate gently with the flow of the distention medium. The final histologic diagnosis may be difficult to substantiate and may reflect the fact that after removal, the typical histologic charac-

TABLE 34–2. HYSTEROSCOPIC FINDINGS FOR FIVE SERIES OF INFERTILE WOMEN

Findings	1977[axx]	1977[a43]	1980[44]	Taylor et al[b]	1984[c51]
Number of patients	34	167	142	701	128
Failed procedure	2	0	0	24	0
Normal cavities	20	68	54	419	45
Polyps or polyposis	2	60	34	89	6
Adhesions	4	19	28	155	27
Uterine malformations	2	9	9	9	2
Fibroids	2	11	–	5	4
Scarred cavity	4	–	–	–	–
Cervical stenosis	–	–	3	–	6
Cesarean section	–	–	3	–	–
Scar defect	–	–			–
Vascular abnormalities	–	–	–	–	6
Endometritis	–	–	–	–	10
Bone metaplasia	–	–	–	–	1
Abnormalities (%)	44	59.3	62.0	41.6	64.8

[a]Panoramic hysteroscopy.
[b]Unpublished data.
[c]Contact microhysteroscopy.
Adapted form Hamou J, and Taylor PJ: Panoramic, contract, and microcolpohysteroscopy in gynecologic practice. Curr Probl Obstet Gynecol 2:1, 1982.

teristics of polyps may be lost. A Hamou MCH, if used at high magnification, allows in situ histologic diagnosis. Polyps may also be noted at the tubal ostia (see Fig 34–8).

Adhesions

Although patients with the classic amenorrhea traumaticum of Asherman[26] describe amenorrhea, adhesions (see Fig 34–9) may occur with no disturbance of menstrual function. Among 69 patients in whom intrauterine adhesions were detected, 23 had normal cyclic menses.[53] The formation of these adhesions is usually preceded either by pregnancy, particularly missed abortion, or intrauterine manipulation. Vascularization and fibrosis probably have a role in placental fragments after either spontaneous abortion or delivery.[53] Among 192 women, the probable

TABLE 34–3. SPECIFIC HYSTEROSCOPIC FINDINGS FOR TWO GROUPS OF WOMEN WHO UNDERWENT SUCCESSFUL HYSTEROSCOPY

Distention Medium Group and Findings	Primary Infertility (n = 493) (%)	Secondary Infertility (n = 344) (%)	Reversal (n = 155) (%)
Dextran 70			
Normal	350 (71.0)	188 (54.6)	104 (67.0)
Adhesions	74 (15.0)	103 (29.9)	28 (18.1)
Polyps	59 (12.0)	40 (11.6)	19 (12.2)
Fibroids	6 (1.2)	7 (2.0)	2 (1.3)
Septa	4 (0.8)	6 (1.7)	2 (1.3)
Total abnormalities	**143 (29.0)**	**156 (45.3)**	**51 (32.9)**
Carbon dioxide	(n = 160)	(n = 118)	(n = 57)
Normal	153 (95.6)	105 (89.0)	54 (94.5)
Adhesions	4 (2.5)	5 (4.2)	1 (2.0)
Polyps	2 (1.2)	0	0
Fibroids	1 (0.6)	0	1 (2.0)
Septa	0	8 (6.8)	1 (2.0)
Total abnormalities	**7 (4.4)**	**13 (11.0)**	**3 (5.0)**

Some percentages do not equal 100 because of rounding.
From Taylor PJ, et al: A comparison of dextran 70 with carbon dioxide as a distention medium for hysteroscopy in patients with infertility or requesting reversal of a prior tubal sterilization. Fertil Steril 47:861, 1987.
Reproduced with permission of the publisher, The American Fertility Society.

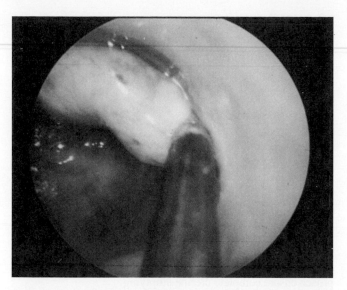

Figure 34–7. A large mucous polyp. The miniaturized electrode has been placed preparatory to electrocoagulation of the base. *(Courtesy of Dr. J. Hamou.)*

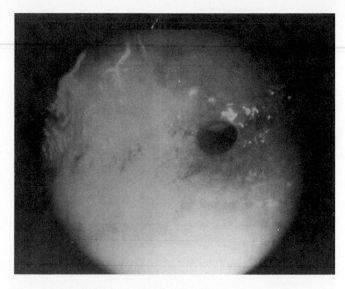

Figure 34–8. Intratubal polyp. *(Courtesy of Dr. J. Hamou.)*

etiologic event was puerperal curettage for 39, spontaneous abortion for 72, therapeutic abortion for 59, molar abortion for 9, diagnostic curettage for 1, myomectomy for 5, and cesarean section for 7. The use of intrauterine contraceptive devices (IUDs) has been implicated in the formation of adhesions.[44] We have also remarked on the role of diagnostic curettage in adhesion development.[34]

At histologic examination, these adhesions may be composed of endometrial, myofibrous, or connective tissue,[54] and they may be noted as lying centrally within the uterine cavity or projecting laterally as shelves from the uterine walls.[55] They can be differentiated at hysteroscopy by their surface appearance and the force required to divide them. The exact histologic nature of adhesions can be determined in vivo at 60 times magnification with a Hamou MCH. Most adhesions are either endometrial or myofibrous and can be seen lying centrally within the uterine cavity. This subject has been reviewed extensively.[56]

Fibroids

Fibroids (see Fig 34–10) bulge into the uterine cavity. The endometrium over them is thin, and they are frequently covered with obvious vessels. Fibroids are smooth, firm, pale, and rounded, and they may be pedunculated or sessile. Many fibroids may be removed with an electrosurgical snare (see Fig 34–11). The technique is described later.

Septa

The appearance of a septum at hysteroscopic examination is characteristic (see Fig 34–12). The dark uterine cornua are obviously separated by a central fibrous band. The surface appearance of the septum depends on the effect of reproductive steroids on the endometrium and varies throughout the menstrual cycle.

Endometritis

If it is suspected that there is acute infection, hysteroscopy is contraindicated. It is interesting how many cases of both acute and chronic endometritis are identified in patients with no symptoms. The endometrium has an appearance similar to that observed at colposcopy when the cervix is infected. The mucosa is congested and the orifices of the glands are white. The overall appearance is one of speckling akin to that of chronic cervicitis.

Relevance of Lesions Detected at Hysteroscopy

Polyps

Large polyps are uncommon, but it is reasonable to postulate that they may hinder implantation. It is probable that the finding of small mucous polyps in patients with infertility and habitual abortion is simply incidental. We are unable to demonstrate any statistically significant difference in the prevalence of hysteroscopically detected polyps among women with primary or secondary infertility or in those requesting reversal of tubal sterilization. This last group, although not a perfect control group, has served in all our studies as potentially fertile controls.[31,42,52]

Adhesions

Undoubtedly the adhesions of Asherman's syndrome are a recognizable cause of infertility. The exact relevance of less dense adhesions seen in women with regular cycles has yet to be ascertained. Although in our earlier studies[35] we demonstrated a statistically significantly higher prevalence of adhesions among patients with secondary infertility, our most recent observations have caused some doubts about the validity of these studies. This is an intriguing problem that remains to be resolved.

It may well be that adhesions play a role in habitual abortion. An improved live delivery rate was demonstrated in a group of women among whom such adhesions were diagnosed at HSG.[57] Adhesions were identified in 51 women with a history of habitual abortion.[55] Subsequently, 18 women remained infertile, 12 conceived and aborted, and 19 delivered at term. Although these studies do not allow the conclusion that intrauterine adhesions are a cause of habitual abortion, they certainly raise the suspicion.

Fibroids

It is probable that most uterine leiomyomata are not causative of infertility.[58] This statement must be made with reservation in the case of submucous lesions. Fibroids, however, do predispose to habitual abortion. A review by Buttram and Reiter[58] of Hicks's data demonstrated that among 441 women with uterine leiomyomata, 181 (41%) experienced spontaneous abortion.

Uterine Malformations

It is unlikely that anomalies of the reproductive tract are a cause of infertility, but they have been implicated in the causation of habitual abortion. In one study, the abortion rate was 33.8% among women with a bicornuate uterus, 22% among those with a septate uterus, and 34.6% among women with a single uterine horn.[59] Such malformations occur in 1 of every 700 women.[60]

OPERATIVE HYSTEROSCOPY

Hysteroscopy not only allows accurate diagnosis of intrauterine lesions but also in many instances provides an avenue by which therapeutic maneuvers can be performed. Polyps, fibroids, adhesions, and septa all can be managed by hysteroscopic means. In addition, it is possible to cannulate the fallopian tubes under hysteroscopic guidance to unblock proximal occlusion or inject gametes in embryos to assist in conception.

Polyps

Large polyps should be removed. Although removal of small intrauterine polyps may not influence the outcome for patients with infertility or habitual abortion, it seems appropriate that polyps be removed when detected. The procedure is simple and essentially risk free. It must be acknowledged that such removals are probably performed more to relieve anxiety than to manage infertility. Some infertile women who are aware of the presence of uterine polyps may continue to believe that these lesions are the cause of the infertility until something is done to remove them.

Single polyps can be removed simply by means of simple transection of the base with a hysteroscopic electrosurgical probe or a resectoscope with 50-W current. Because of its softness, the excised polyp can be pulled and extracted intact through the cervix with a polyp forceps (see Fig 34–7). Multiple polyps are best managed by means of removal of the hysteroscope, curettage, and immediately revisualization of the uterine cavity. If residual lesions are identified, they can be removed with a snare or by means of a second curettage. This approach ensure complete uterine emptying.

When the base of a large polyp cannot be clearly visualized, the polyp can be morcellated with a resectoscope until the base is visible, at which point the base is transected. Among 164 women who had undergone curettage for abnormal uterine bleeding, hysteroscopic examination revealed residual lesions in 101.[61] Of these 101 patients, 51 had not obtained relief from bleeding. After hysteroscopic evaluation and repeated curettage controlled with hysteroscopy, only two of these patients returned with bleeding within 1 year.

Adhesions

Intrauterine adhesions have been classified on the basis of their extent and nature as (1) mild (filmy and composed of endometrial tissue producing partial or complete uterine cavity occlusion); (2) moderate (fibromuscular and usually thick but covered with endometrium occluding the uterine cavity partially or totally); and (3) severe (composed of connective tissue only and partially or totally occluding the uterine cavity).[62]

Filmy adhesions frequently rupture under the pressure of the distension medium, or they may be dislodged with the tip of the hysteroscope. Another technique is target abrasion.[53] The distal tips of foroblique hysteroscopes are angled and somewhat sharp. In target abrasion, the tip is brought under direct visual control against one pole of the adhesion and is used to abrade progressively the attachment of the adhesion to the uterine wall. This procedure is repeated at the opposite pole for long adhesions (see Fig 34–9). This technique was successful for 59 of 69 patients as an office procedure. The other 10 patients required general anesthesia, because the procedure was too painful or the adhesions were remarkably dense.

Although it can indeed be performed in the office, it has been our practice to perform target abrasion with general anesthesia and laparoscopic monitoring. Undoubtedly patients with adhesions have a very friable uterus that is prone to perforation.[19] Other authors[63] have recommended a similar approach. Moderate and severe adhesions must be excised with a scissors, neodymium:ytterium-aluminum-garnet (Nd:YAG) laser, or electrical knife.

Hysteroscopic observation begins within the cervical canal. When adhesions are present in the cervical canal or in the internal ostium, they are divided first and the hysteroscope is gradually advanced. As adhesions are divided, the uterine cavity expands and to facilitate visualization and division of further adhesions. Once the hysteroscope reaches the fundal region, an attempt is made to visualize the tubal ostia. Valle and Sciarra[62] suggest injection of methylene blue into the uterine cavity (through the inflow channel of the hysteroscope) when difficulty is encountered differentiating between adhesions and the endometrial lining. Endometrium usually stains well with methylene blue, whereas connective tissue and myometrium do not.

The use of concomitant transabdominal ultrasonographic monitoring recently has been recommended to facilitate dissection and to identify any pockets of adenomyosis that can be associated with the adhesions.[64]

Once the adhesions have been removed in all but the most minor cases, particularly if there has been any diminution in menstrual flow, an IUD may be placed within the uterine cavity and the patient may be given conjugated estrogens (Premarin), 2.5 mg daily for 60 days, during the last 10 days of which she also takes medroxyprogesterone (Provera), 5 mg twice daily. Once these medications are discontinued and withdrawal bleeding occurs, the IUD should be removed.

In very severe cases, an intrauterine hemostasis balloon (Mentor Corporation, Goleta, CA) may be used. This silicone elastomer balloon has the size and shape of the uterine cavity. The device is connected to a two-way ball control valve via silicone tubing and thus can be inflated with sterile saline solution.

An alternative approach to this regimen, made necessary by the fact that use of IUDs has been virtually discontinued in North America, is to administer Premarin and medroxyprogesterone acetate and to perform a second-look hysteroscopy 6 weeks after the initial procedure. Any residual adhesions can be removed at this time.

It must be remembered that removal of intrauterine adhesions predisposes the patient to a number of potential difficulties in any ensuing pregnancy. In a series of 192 patients in whom adhesions were treated by means of hysteroscopic lysis, 79 (41.1%) became pregnant; of these, 29 patients (36.7%) experienced spontaneous abortions, 2 had premature deliveries, and 45 experienced at least one term delivery.[55] Eight patients who delivered required manual removal of the placenta or postpartum curettage. There is a distinct risk of placenta accreta af-

ter lysis of intrauterine adhesions. Among three women with this condition, two needed treatment by means of cesarean hysterectomy.[65]

In the series reported by Valle and Sciarra[62] there were 187 patients. Among the 43 patients with adhesions classified as mild, 35 (81%) achieved pregnancy. Among the 97 patients with moderate adhesions, 64 (66%) had term pregnancies. Of the 47 patients with severe adhesions, 15 (32%) had term pregnancies.

Fibroids

Small submucous fibroids can be managed by means of hysteroscopic excision with a resectoscope.[21] Pedunculated tumors are easily managed by means of electrosurgical division of the pedicle. Sessile lesions can be shaved until flush with the surrounding endometrium. When hysteroscopic excision of fibroids is performed with a resectoscope, glycine or sorbitol is the distention medium of choice, because they are relatively nonconductive substances.

The approach to be taken depends on the size of the lesion, position of the lesion, and the number of tumors. Lesions 5 cm or less in diameter, protrude for 75% or more of their volume into the uterine cavity, and are single can be resected without preparation in a one-step procedure.

Single lesions that are predominantly within the cavity but are larger than 5 cm, those that are 74% to 50% in the cavity, and those smaller than 2.5 cm in diameter but more than 50% intramural can be managed after suppression by means of administration of a gonadotropin-releasing hormone (GnRH) agonist in a single-step procedure.[66] Larger lesions that are predominantly intramural or multiple tumors necessitate excision at two or more sessions.

Hysteroscopic myomectomy avoids the need for an abdominal incision and a hysterotomy and reduces postoperative discomfort, hospital stay, and recovery period. The procedure commences with a thorough hysteroscopic evaluation of the uterine cavity to identify the location and size of the fibroids and to ensure that hysteroscopic resection is possible. The cervix is dilated and the resectoscope introduced. The myoma is then shaved with the resectoscopic loop and 50 to 90 W of cutting current. Small arterial bleeders are controlled with 50 W of pure coagulation current. The loop of the resectoscope is placed at the most distant part of the tumor, the generator is activated immediately before the resection loop makes contact with the tissue, and the resectoscope is drawn toward the cervix.

With repeated strokes of the loop, small slices of the tumor are excised. These tumor slices float in the distention medium. When chips of tissue interfere with visualization, they are trapped against the outer sheath of the resectoscope by means of the loop and are removed from the uterine cavity together with resectoscope. A polyp forceps also can be used to retrieve the fragments of tumor from the uterine cavity. The procedure is continued until excision of the whole fibroid when the fibroid is totally submucous and until flush with the endometrium if the fibroid is partly intramural. With the latter type of partially resected fibroids, the remaining portion of the tumor is extruded in time toward the cavity, facilitating resection at a second procedure performed several weeks later.

Some surgeons have attempted to devascularize the remaining portion of the myoma.[67] To achieve this, a Nd:YAG laser fiber is introduced perpendicularly into the body of the myoma as far as possible and the laser is activated as the fiber is slowly removed. The procedure is repeated by means of introduction of the laser fiber through various sites of the myoma until distinct craters with brown borders are visible throughout the remaining portion of the fibroid. The same result can also be obtained electrosurgically. This procedure induces necrobiosis, which is called *myolysis*. The residual largely shrunk and devascularized myoma, which usually protrudes into the cavity in time, may be removed easily at a second-stage procedure 2 months later.

Several studies of hysteroscopic myomectomy[21,68–75] were summarized by Robert and Farrell.[76] Among 1040 women, 114 had infertility and 926 abnormal uterine bleeding. Postoperative hemorrhage was by far the most common complication, occurring in 44 women (4.3%). This can usually be controlled by means of insertion of a Foley catheter or an intrauterine hemostasis balloon. While the catheter is in place, the patient should receive systemic antibiotics. Only four patients needed emergency hysterectomies.

Preoperative hysteroscopy also plays a role in the treatment of patients with multiple fibroids who need abdominal myomectomy. If no intrauterine lesions are identified, an opening into the uterine cavity can be avoided. If there are submucous lesions that are amenable to hysteroscopic resection, such an approach obviates an opening into the cavity.

Pregnancy rates as high as 66% have been reported after hysteroscopic myomectomy.[71] Others investigators also had encouraging results.[69,73,75] Corson and Brooks[69] and Robert and Farrell[76] remarked that the outlook for subsequent fertility is better among women with secondary rather than primary infertility, suggesting that for the latter, a factor or factors other than fibroids may be operant.

Unfortunately, none of the aforecited studies had a no-treatment arm, making it impossible to determine with certainty whether removing the lesions was responsible for the patients' fertility. Although it is recognized that only a randomized, prospective study of treatment versus observation would answer this question, it is highly unlikely that such a study can be mounted. Until it is, it will be difficult, if not impossible, not to accede to the request of any informed infertile woman or one who suffers from habitual abortion that a myomectomy be performed. Hysteroscopy is the route of choice for submucous lesions.

Uterine Septa

When a uterine septum is detected at HSG, particularly in patients with habitual abortion, the next step should be to perform either MRI or combined laparoscopy and hysteroscopy. It is only by these means that the exact configuration of the uterus can be determined. Hysteroscopy is of no value in the surgical treatment of a patient with a bicornuate uterine deformity.

A septum with a base less than 1 cm thick can be managed effectively with hysteroscopy. Once it has been visualized, the lesion is divided with hysteroscopic scissors. This is a remarkably bloodless procedure. Although both argon and YAG lasers have been used to divide uterine septa, performing the procedure with rigid scissors or a resectoscope[77] is simpler, quicker, and requires less expensive equipment (Fig 34–12). In addition, unlike lasers and a resectoscope, a rigid scissors causes no thermal tissue damage beyond the line of section.

Many workers recommend the preoperative use of GnRH agonists, which cause marked endometrial thinning, avoidance of mucous debris, and a decrease in uterine blood flow. Others prefer to perform the procedure without preoperative preparation but in the proliferative phase of the cycle.

The uterine cavity is first inspected with a hysteroscope. The cervix is dilated to introduce the operative sheath through which the rigid scissors and hysteroscope are introduced. The septum is divided in the center with progressive horizontal incisions starting from the inferior margin and gradually moving toward the fundus. The incision is continued until the hysteroscope can be moved freely between the two tubal ostia, at which point the cavity assumes a normal appearance.

Querleu et al[77] described an ultrasound-guided technique to divide septa. They performed the procedure with general anesthesia or neuroleptanalgesia. The bladder was filled with 250 mL of normal saline solution through a Foley catheter. An assistant placed the transducer of a real-time scanner in a longitudinal or transverse position according to the surgeon's needs. The uterus was assessed and the septum was measured in width and length. Laparoscopic scissors of 4.5 mm diameter were used to divide the septum under ultrasonographic control. The scissors were introduced transcervically into the uterine cavity without cervical dilation. The scissors were opened and one of the blades was placed on the left and the other on the right side of the lower extremity of the septum. The septum was divided at an equal distance from the anterior and posterior surfaces of the uterus. The procedure was considered complete when the upper limit of the transection and the serosal surface of the fundus was 10 mm. After the operation the patients were given cyclic hormonal therapy for 3 months, although the investigators acknowledged the controversial nature of such treatment.

Querleu et al[77] reported on a series of 24 patients, 7 of whom had complete uterine and cervical septa, 11 had complete uterine septa, and 6 had partial uterine septa. There were no complications. Fifteen of the 24 patients had third-trimester deliveries or ongoing pregnancies at the time of publication of the results. Among 12 women who had experienced recurrent pregnancy losses, 10 achieved pregnancies that went beyond the second trimester. Nine of these women delivered at term or had an ongoing third-trimester pregnancy. A similar technique has been described in which the procedure is performed under fluoroscopic control with the use of HSG control media.[78] These investigators reported on a series of 34 patients, of whom 31 had prior pregnancy losses. At the time that the report was published, 12 of 34 patients had delivered live infants and 13 were pregnant, 10 of whom were beyond 20 weeks of gestation.

DeCherney et al[79] treated 103 patients with the resectoscopic method. All patients were treated during the proliferative phase of the menstrual cycle. Dextran 70 was the distention medium, and all patients were monitored with laparoscopy. The septum was incised with a cutting current of 30 W/second. The operating time varied between 20 and 40 minutes. Resection was performed successfully on 72 patients; 31 had lesions that were considered inoperable. Only one uterine perforation occurred. After 72 successful hysteroscopic procedures, 58 patients had successful deliveries.

It is also worth noting that in a small, nonrandomized cohort study, 20 women underwent resection of septa, whereas 17 did not.[80] Seventy percent of the treated and 71% of the nontreated women subsequently delivered live infants. The numbers in this study were too small to allow one to state with certainty that a type 2 error was not made, but the success rates are remarkably similar to those reported by DeCherney et al.[79]

It is probable that we will continue to remove such lesions from women with a history of habitual abortion. All of these hysteroscopic procedures are clearly simpler and less invasive than the Tomkins or Jones metroplasty and have the obvious advantage of being performed on an outpatient basis.

Potential Therapeutic Applications of Hysteroscopy

Infertility, particularly unexplained infertility or that due to oligozoospermia or poor sperm–cervical mucus penetration, may now be managed with one form or another of gamete manipulation. Intrauterine insemination (IUI), in vitro fertilization (IVF), and gamete intrafallopian transfer (GIFT) are finding ever-wider roles in the treatment of infertility. Of these, GIFT may be of particular value in unexplained infertility and for women with hostile cervical mucus. Traditionally, GIFT does require the performance of laparoscopy. The essential component underlying all forms of gamete manipulation has been the juxtaposition of sperm and oocyte, initially in the laboratory for IVF and in the ampulla of the fallopian tube with GIFT.

We[81] demonstrated that it is simple to visualize and cannulate the fallopian tube with hysteroscopy in an office procedure that requires no anesthesia (see Fig 34–13). In 72 studied cycles, it was possible in all patients to deposit previously capacitated spermatozoa at the tubocornual junction. Our protocol called for synchronization of ovulation with a predetermined regimen of Provera–clomiphene citrate. No pregnancies resulted from this approach, and subsequent follow-up studies demonstrated that our stimulation regimen more often than not produced luteinized unruptured follicle syndrome. This approach, which we called SHIFT (synchronized hysteroscopic insemination of the fallopian tube), is technically feasible and, given effective ovarian stimulation, may open an avenue to the future that could, if successful, provide an alternative to GIFT.

CONCLUSIONS

Hysteroscopy is no longer a procedure looking for an indication. It has a small but definite role in the evaluation of the uterine cavity of patients with infertility or habitual abortion. As a result of improved optics in smaller-diameter instruments, hysteroscopy is also enjoying wider utilization as an office procedure, making it more accessible as a diagnostic modality. In addition, hysteroscopy offers an alternative approach to the management of intrauterine lesions (particularly fibroids, septa, and adhesions) and may find a place in alternative forms of gamete manipulation.

REFERENCES

1. Lindemann HJ: One hundred years of hysteroscopy. In: Siegler AM, Lindemann HJ (eds), *Hysteroscopy: Principles and Practice,* Philadelphia, Lippincott, 1984
2. Lyon SA: Intra-uterine visualization by means of hysteroscope. *Am J Obstet Gynecol* 90:443, 1964
3. Desormeaux AJ: De l'endoscopie et cec applications au diagnostic et au traitement des affections de l'urethre et de la venrie. Paris Balliere, 1855
4. Pantaleoni DC: On endoscopic examination of the cavity of the womb. *Med Press Circ* 8:26, 1869
5. Nitze M: Ueber eine neue Beleuchtungsmethods der Hohlen des menschilichen Korpers. *Med Pres Wien* 20:851, 1879
6. David C: *L'endoscopie uterine (hysteroscopie), applications au diagnostic et au traitement des affections intrauterine.* University of Paris, 1908. Thesis

7. Munde PF: *Minor Surgical Gynecology.* New York, Wood 1880

8. Reuter HJ: *One Hundred Years of Cystoscopy.* Tuttlingen, Richard Wolff, 1979

9. Van der Pas H: Historical aspects. In: Van der Pas H, Van Herendal B, Van Lith D, Keith L (eds), *Hysteroscopy.* Boston, MPP Press, 1983

10. Seibel MM: Simplified techniques of assisted reproduction. In: Seibel MM, Blackwell (eds), *Ovulation Induction.* New York, Raven, 1994

11. Steptoe PC: *Laparoscopy in Gynecology.* Edinburgh, Livingstone, 1967

12. ACOG Committee Opinion: Credentialling Guidelines for New Operative Procedures, No. 142, 1994

13. Society for Reproductive Surgeons: Guidelines for attaining privileges in gynecologic operative endoscopy. *Fertil Steril* 62:1118, 1994

14. Guidelines for training in operative endoscopy in the specialty of obstetrics and gynecology. Society of Obstetricians and Gynecologists of Canada Policy Statement. January 1993, No. 18. Ottawa, Canada K1S5NH

15. Valle RF, Sciarra JJ: Current status of hysteroscopy in gynecologic practice. *Fertil Steril* 32:619, 1979

16. Hamou J: Hysteroscopy and microhysteroscopy with a new instrument, the microhysteroscope. *Acta Eur Fertil* 12:1, 1981

17. Taylor PJ, Gordon AG: *Practical Hysteroscopy.* Oxford, England, Blackwell, 1993

18. Quinones CR, Albarado BA, Azmar RR: Tubal catheterization: Applications of a new technique. *Am J Obstet Gynecol* 114:674, 1972

19. Menken FS: Eine neues verfahren mit Vorrichtung zur Hysteroskopie. *Endoscopy* 3:200, 1971

20. Siegler AM, Valle RF, Lindemann HJ, Mencaglia L: *Therapeutic Hysteroscopy.* St. Louis, Mosby, 1990

21. Neuwirth RS, Amin HK: Excision of submucus fibroids with hysteroscopic control. *Am J Obstet Gynecol* 126:95, 1976

22. Leader A, Taylor PJ, Daudi FA: The value of routine rubella and syphylitic serology in the infertile couple. *Fertil Steril* 42:140, 1984

23. Hamou J, Taylor PJ: Panoramic, contract, and microcolpohysteroscopy in gynecologic practice. *Curr Probl Obstet Gynecol* 2:1, 1982

24. Taylor PJ: Diagnostic and operative hysteroscopy. In: Seibel MM (ed), *Infertility: A Comprehensive Text.* Norwalk, CT, Appleton & Lange, 1990: 363

25. Yuzpe AA, Gomel V, Taylor PJ, Rioux JE: Endoscopic documentation. In: Gomel V, Taylor PJ, Yuzpe AA, Rioux JE (eds), *Laparoscopy and Hysteroscopy in Gynecologic Practice.* Chicago, Year Book, 1986

26. Asherman JG: Amenorrhea traumaticum (atretica). *J Obstet Gynaecol Br Emp* 55:23, 1948

27. Knudston ML, Taylor PJ: Uberempfindlichkeitsreaktion auf Dextran 70 (Hyskon) wahrend einer Hysteroskopie. *Geburtshilfe Frauenheilkd* 36:263, 1976

28. Obstetrician convicted in sterilization death is placed on probation. *Ob/Gyn News* 9:4, 1974

29. Istre O, Bjoennes J, Naess R, Hornbask K, Formen A: Postoperative cerebral oedema after transcervical endometrial resection and uterine irrigation with 1.5% glycine. *Lancet* 344:1187, 1994

30. Taylor PJ, Leader A, Pattinson HA: Diagnostic hysteroscopy. In: Hunt RB (ed), *Atlas of Female Infertility Surgery.* Chicago, Year Book, 1986:182–197

31. Taylor PJ: *The Significance of Hysteroscopically Detected Intrauterine Adhesions in the Eumenorrheic Infertile Female.* Queen's University of Belfast, 1985. Thesis

32. Lindemann HJ: CO_2 hysteroscopy today. *Endoscopy* 11:94, 1979

33. Sullivan B, Kenney P, Seibel M: Hysteroscopic resection of fibroid with thermal injury to sigmoid. *Obstet Gynecol* 80:546, 1992

34. Salat-Baroux J, Hamou JE, Maillard G, Chouraqui A, Verges P: Microhysteroscopy complications. In: Siegler AM, Lindemann HJ (eds), *Hysteroscopy: Principles and Practice Philadelphia.* Philadelphia, Lippincott, 1984:112–118

35. Taylor PJ, Cumming DC, Hill PJ: Significance of intrauterine adhesions detected hysteroscopically in enumenorreic infertile women and the role of antecedent curettage in their formation. *Am J Obstet Gynecol* 139:239, 1981

36. Siegler AM, Kemmann E, Gentile GP: Hysteroscopic procedures in 257 patients. *Fertil Steril* 27:126, 1976

37. Taylor PJ, Cumming DC: Hysteroscopy in 100 patients. *Fertil Steril* 31:301, 1979

38. Taylor PJ, Gomel V: Endoscopy in the infertile patient. In: Gomel V, Taylor PJ, Yuzpe AA, Rioux JE (eds), *Laparoscopy and Hysteroscopy in Gynecologic Practice.* Chicago, Year Book, 1986:75

39. Malpas P: A study of abortion sequences. *J Obstet Gynaecol Br Emp* 45:932, 1938

40. Poland BJ, Miller JR, Jones DC, Trimble BK: Reproductive counselling in patients who have had a spontaneous abortion. *Am J Obstet Gynecol* 127:685, 1977

41. Gomel V, Taylor PJ: *Diagnostic and Operative Gynecologic Laparoscopy.* St. Louis, Mosby–Year Book, 1995

42. Taylor PJ, Cumming DC: Laparoscopy in the infertile female. *Curr Probl Obstet Gynecol* 2:3, 1979

43. Siegler AM: Hysterography and hysteroscopy in the infertile patient. *J Reprod Med* 18:143, 1977

44. Valle RF: Hysteroscopy in the evaluation of female infertility. *Am J Obstet Gynecol* 137:425, 1980

45. Labastida R, Dexeus S, Arias A: Infertility and hysteroscopy. In: Siegler AM, Lindemann HJ (eds), *Hysteroscopy: Principles and Practice.* Philadelphia, Lippincott, 1984:175

46. Snowden EU, Jarret JC, Dawood YM: Comparison of diagnostic accuracy of laparoscopy, hysteroscopy and hysterosalpingography in evaluation of female infertility. *Fertil Steril* 41:709, 1984

47. Zondek BM, Rozin S: Filling defects in the hysterogram simulating intra-uterine synechiae which disappear after denudation. *Am J Obstet Gynecol* 88:123, 1964

48. Loy RA, Weinstein FG, Seibel MM: Hysterosalpingography in perspective: The predictive value of oil soluble versus water soluble contrast media. *Fertil Steril* 51:170, 1989

49. Taylor PJ, Leader A, George RE, Fick G: Correlations between laparoscopic and hysteroscopic findings in 497 women with otherwise unexplained infertility. *J Reprod Med* 29:137, 1984

50. Balen FG, Allen CM, Siddle NC, Lees WR: Ultrasound contrast hysterosalpingography: Evaluation as an outpatient procedure. *Br J Radiol* 66:592, 1993

51. Hamou J, Salat-Baroux J: Advanced hysteroscopy and microhysteroscopy: Our experience with 1000 patients. In: Siegler AM, Lindemann HF (eds); *Hysteroscopy: Principles and Practice.* Philadelphia, Lippincott, 1984:63

52. Taylor PJ, Lewinthal D, Leader A, Pattinson HA: A comparison of dextran 70 with carbon dioxide as the distention medium for hysteroscopy in patients with infertility or requesting reversal of a prior tubal sterilization. *Fertil Steril* 47:861, 1987

53. Hamou J, Salat-Baroux J, Siegler AM: Diagnosis and treatment of intra-uterine adhesions by microhysteroscopy. *Fertil Steril* 39:321, 1983

54. Foix A, Bruno RO, Davision T, Lem AB: The pathology of postcurettage intra-uterine adhesions. *Am J Obstet Gynecol* 96:1027, 1966

55. Sugimoto O: Diagnostic and therapeutic hysteroscopy for traumatic intra-uterine adhesions. *Am J Obstet Gynecol* 96:1027, 1966

56. Schenker J, Margalioth EJ: Intra-uterine adhesions: An updated appraisal. *Fertil Steril* 37:593, 1982

57. Oelsner G, Ammon D, Insler V, Ferr DM: Outcome of pregnancy after treatment of intra-uterine adhesions. *Obstet Gynecol* 44:341, 1974

58. Buttram VC Jr, Reiter RC: Uterine leiomyomata: Etiology, symptomatology and management. *Fertil Steril* 36:433, 1981

59. Jones WAS: Obstetric significance of female genital anomalies. *Obstet Gynecol* 10:1039, 1957

60. Stirrat GM: Recurrent miscarriage. II. Clinical associations, causes and management. *Lancet* 363:728, 1990

61. Englund G, Ingleman-Sundberg A, Westin B: Hysteroscopy in diagnosis and treatment of uterine bleeding. *Gynaecologia* 143:217, 1957

62. Valle RF, Sciarra JJ: Intrauterine adhesions: Hysteroscopic diagnosis, classification, treatment, and reproductive outcome. *Am J Obstet Gynecol* 158:1459–1470, 1988

63. March CM, Israel R, March AD: Hysteroscopic management of intrauterine adhesions. *Am J Obstet Gynecol* 130:653, 1978

64. Fraser IS, Song JY, Jansen RPS, Ramsay P, Boogert T. Hysteroscopic lysis of intra-uterine adhesions under ultrasound guidance. *Gynaecol Endosc* 4:75, 1995

65. Georgakopoulos P: Placenta accreta following lysis of uterine synechia (Asherman's syndrome). *J Obstet Gynaecol Br Commonw* 81:730, 1974

66. Coddington CC, Collins RL, Shawker TH, et al: Long-acting gonadotropin hormone releasing hormone analogue used to treat uteri. *Fertil Steril* 45:624, 1986

67. Donnez J, Nicolle M: Hysteroscopic surgery. *Curr Opin Obstet Gynecol* 4:439, 1992

68. Brooks PG, Loffler FD, Serden SP: Resectoscopic removal of symptomatic intrauterine lesions. *J Reprod Med* 34:435, 1989

69. Corson SL, Brooks PG: Resectoscopic myomectomy. *Fertil Steril* 55:1041, 1991

70. Derman SG, Rehnstrom J, Neuwirth RS: The long-term effectiveness of hysteroscopic treatment of menorrhagia and leiomyomas. *Obstet Gynecol* 77:591, 1991

71. Donnez J, Gillerot S, Bourgonjon D, Clerckx F, Nisolle M: Neodymium:YAG laser hysteroscopy in large submucous fibroids. *Fertil Steril* 54:999, 1990

72. Indman P: Hysteroscopic treatment of menorrhagia associated with uterine leiomyomas. *Obstet Gynecol* 81:719, 1993

73. Istre O, Schiotz H, Sadik L, Vormdal J, Vangen O, Forman A: Transcervical resection of endometrium and fibroids. *Acta Obstet Gynecol Scand* 70:363, 1991

74. Itzkowic D. Submucous fibroids: Clinical profile and hysteroscopic management. *Aust N Z J Obstet Gynaecol* 33:63, 1993

75. Townsend DE, Fields G, McCausland A, Kauffman K: Diagnostic and operative hysteroscopy in the management of persistent postmenopausal bleeding. *Obstet Gynecol* 82:419, 1993

76. Robert M, Farrell SA: Hysteroscopic management of benign uterine tumors. *J SOGC* (in press).

77. Querleu D, Brasme TL, Parmentier D: Ultrasound-guided transcervical metroplasty. *Fertil Steril* 54:995, 1990

78. Valle JA, Lifchez A, Moise J: A simpler technique for reduction of uterine septum. *Fertil Steril* 56:1001, 1991

79. DeCherney AH, Russell JB, Giaebe RA, Pollen ML: Resectoscopic management of müllerian fusion defects. *Fertil Steril* 45:726, 1986

80. Coulam CB: Unexplained recurrent pregnancy loss. *Clin Obstet Gynecol* 29:999, 1986

81. Brooks JH, Mortimer D, Taylor PJ: Failure of hysteroscopic insemination of the fallopian tube in synchronized cycles. *J Fertil* (in press).

CHAPTER 35

Operative Laparoscopy

ROBERT B. HUNT

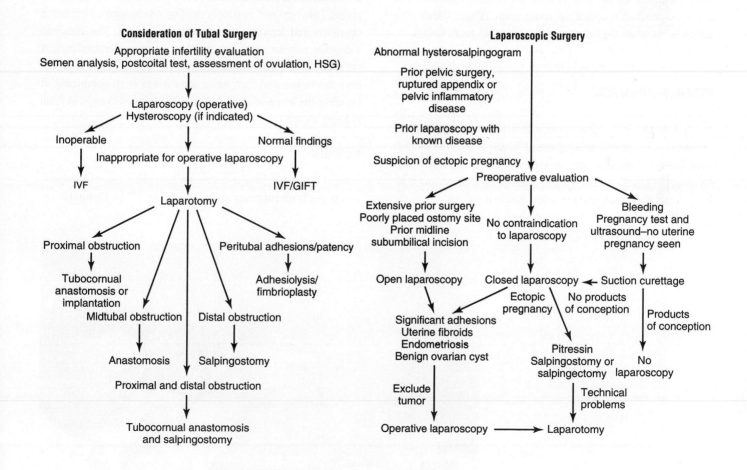

Consideration of Tubal Surgery

Appropriate infertility evaluation
Semen analysis, postcoital test, assessment of ovulation, HSG)

Laparoscopy (operative)
Hysteroscopy (if indicated)

Inoperable → IVF

Inappropriate for operative laparoscopy

Normal findings → IVF/GIFT

Laparotomy

Proximal obstruction → Tubocornual anastomosis or implantation

Peritubal adhesions/patency → Adhesiolysis/fimbrioplasty

Midtubal obstruction → Anastomosis

Distal obstruction → Salpingostomy

Proximal and distal obstruction → Tubocornual anastomosis and salpingostomy

Laparoscopic Surgery

Abnormal hysterosalpingogram

Prior pelvic surgery, ruptured appendix or pelvic inflammatory disease

Prior laparoscopy with known disease

Suspicion of ectopic pregnancy

Preoperative evaluation

Extensive prior surgery
Poorly placed ostomy site
Prior midline subumbilical incision → Open laparoscopy

No contraindication to laparoscopy → Closed laparoscopy

Bleeding
Pregnancy test and ultrasound–no uterine pregnancy seen → Suction curettage

Significant adhesions
Uterine fibroids
Endometriosis
Benign ovarian cyst → Exclude tumor

Ectopic pregnancy / No products of conception

Products of conception → No laparoscopy

Pitressin
Salpingostomy or salpingectomy → Technical problems

Operative laparoscopy ⟶ Laparotomy

Mistakes occur when a person is over-worked or over-confident.
William Feather

591

"The obituary of laparotomy for pelvic reconstructive surgery has been written; it is only its publication that remains."[1] These prophetic words are becoming a reality. Even some tubal anastomosis operations, the centerpiece of microsurgery, are being performed with laparoscopy.

OPERATING TEAM

To achieve excellence in laparoscopic surgery is a process. It requires attending workshops, observing surgeons accomplished in the techniques, practicing on models such as the Pelvi-Trainer (Fig 35–1), and being proctored until a satisfactory level of skill has been obtained. In addition to learning techniques, attention should be focused on the identification of retroperitoneal structures such as the rectum and ureters.

A great deal of effort must be expended to provide in-service training for the staff. A dynamic surgeon translates into a very enthusiastic operating room team. Video monitoring serves to maintain the interest of the operating room staff.

PATIENT PREPARATION

When feasible, it is advantageous to schedule a laparoscopic operation in the proliferative phase of the cycle but after menses have ceased. This principle lessens the chance of one's performing an operation on a woman who has conceived, and it allows the surgeon to operate in a less vascular pelvis.

Each patient receives an informed consent document at the time the operation is scheduled (Fig 35–2). She is asked to read it, initial each page, and return it to the surgeon's office before the operation. The consent then becomes a part of the permanent office record. The patient also receives instructions for either a 1- or 2-day intestinal preparation (Fig 35–3). The 2-day instructions are given if significant adhesions or severe endometriosis is suspected.

INSTRUMENTATION

Light Source and Photography

Superb light sources, video, and photographic capabilities are widely available (Fig 35–4). I take three sets of pictures, before and after. One set is given to the patient, one is sent to the referring physician, and one is kept in the patient's record. This policy makes sense from medical, public relations, and legal standpoints. I am opposed to simply making a videotape of the entire operation and handing the tape to the patient. The unedited videotape may be confusing and lead to misunderstandings. A satisfactory alternative is to tape the findings before the procedure has begun and then again after it has been completed. If possible, the surgeon's voice should be included to explain what is being shown.

Insufflator

A rapid flow insufflator is necessary to replace loss of intraperitoneal gas from cannulas and suction (Fig 35–5). Dramatic im-

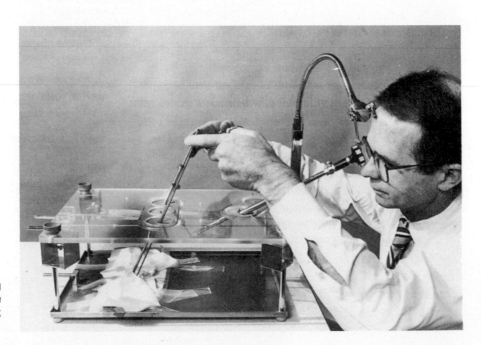

Figure 35–1. The Pelvi-Trainer is an excellent training model for suturing and other techniques that require fine eye-to-hand coordination (WISAP/USA, Tomball, TX 77375; 800-233-8448).

Purpose—Laparoscopy is an extremely valuable procedure in gynecology. It may be performed diagnostically or therapeutically, for example, to determine causes of pelvic pain or infertility, to divide adhesions, or to perform a tubal ligation. Pregnancy must be avoided during the menstrual cycle when the operation is to be performed.

Procedure—The operation is usually performed with the patient asleep (general anesthesia). Having attained satisfactory anesthesia, an instrument known as a cannula is inserted into the cervical canal and held in place with a tenaculum. These instruments enable the surgeon to position the uterus and thus aid in evaluation. An incision is made at the navel through which a telescope (laparoscope) is placed. One to three incisions are then made in the lower abdomen. These incisions aid the surgeon in moving structures in performing operative procedures. The incisions leave scars from one-quarter to one-half inch in length. To aid in visualization of pelvic and abdominal structures, the abdomen is inflated with gas to enlarge the space to be examined. Photographs are taken of the pelvic structures to augment the operative report. At the conclusion of the procedure, the gas is let out, all equipment is removed, and the abdominal wounds are closed with stitches. It is necessary sometimes to perform a dilatation and curettage (D&C) to assess the pelvic structures further. Laparoscopy may be performed as an outpatient procedure. In this case, the patient must arrange for someone to take her home.

Postoperative care—The patient will experience discomfort in her right shoulder due to referred pain from the right diaphragm created by the gas placed in the abdomen. The discomfort is usually gone within 2 days. There is invariably bruising and tenderness in the areas of the incisions. These usually disappear within 2 weeks.

Complications

1. Anesthesia: Anesthesiology has been refined so that it is a safe specialty. Anesthetic accidents do happen that may produce complications, however. The anesthesiologist will discuss these with you.
2. Phlebitis: The patient may experience tenderness at the site of the intravenous line. This responds to heat and is usually gone over several days. On occasion, a small lump will persist in that area.
3. Incisions: Occasionally, an incision will become infected or red-

dened. This should respond to warm showers or baths with gentle cleansing of the area with alcohol. If it does not respond within 2 days, the patient should notify Dr. Hunt.
4. Pelvic infections: The patient who has had previous pelvic infections or adhesions is predisposed to developing pelvic infections after any pelvic procedure. I usually administer an antibiotic to lessen the possibility of such an infection.
5. Allergic reactions: Several medications are used during hospitalization, including anesthetic agents, often antibiotics, and sometimes high-molecular-weight dextran, a solution made of sugar beets. Allergic reactions may develop to any of these agents.
6. Hemorrhage: When placing the various laparoscopic instruments through the abdominal wall or performing intraabdominal surgery, bleeding can occur. This is usually of a minor degree, but can be more serious and require major surgery to correct.
7. Gastrointestinal injuries: Injuries to the intestinal tract occur in approximately 1 per 500 procedures. They most often develop when placing the laparoscopic equipment through the navel because the surgeon cannot see what is within the abdominal cavity until the instrument has been placed. This is a major complication requiring immediate repair through a larger incision.
8. Failed procedure: Occasionally, I am unable to accomplish the procedure for any of a number of reasons.
9. Death: Each year, a few deaths are reported throughout the United States associated with laparoscopic procedures. They have been caused by such things as gas traveling to the lungs and infection. Fortunately, these are rare, but nevertheless, this procedure must be considered an operation with all its attendant complications.

Conclusion—I feel we have a very advanced operative team, including anesthesiologist, nurse anesthetists, and operating room nurses. Our equipment is modern. We are constantly aware of potential complications and are continually reviewing techniques to make all of our operative procedures safer.

(Modified from Hunt RB (ed): *Atlas of Female Infertility Surgery.* Chicago, Year Book, 1986, appendix A. Reprinted with permission.)

Figure 35–2. Consent form for laparoscopy.

provements have been made with insufflators. Some even warm the insufflated gas, and most provide high rates of flow. Care should be taken to avoid high intraperitoneal pressure. I find that 10 to 12 mm Hg pressure is ample in most operations, and I never exceed 15 mm Hg.

Laparoscope

Optics have improved dramatically. I use a 30° laparoscope, because I view the operative field directly through a lens equipped with a beam splitter to allow video monitoring. The distal lens of the laparoscope often fogs when it is first inserted into the abdomen. This is corrected by warming the lens or simply dipping the tip of the laparoscope in antiseptic cleanser (Phisohex) and wiping the lens clean with a dry sponge. Newer 2-mm office

laparoscopes offer too limited a view to be acceptable for operative laparoscopy.

Bipolar Coagulation

Bipolar forceps and generator are essential equipment and should be connected and tested before the operation begins (Figs 35–6 through 35–8). Bipolar forceps are extremely effective for coagulating small blood vessels. Using irrigation to flush away blood, the surgeon can identify the tip of the open vessel, lift it gently with the bipolar forceps, and apply current. Alternatively, the vessel to be divided is identified, coagulated, and then divided. It is important to remember that the tips of the bipolar forceps must be slightly separated to coagulate effectively. Narrow, well-insulated tips cause minimal thermal spread.

Bowel Preparation (1-Day)

1. Purchase one Fleet enema and one bottle of magnesium citrate from your pharmacy.
2. The day before surgery:

   Drink 1/2 bottle of magnesium citrate in the morning and 1/2 bottle in the afternoon.

   Breakfast—Light breakfast (for example, cold cereal or cream of wheat, juice, coffee).

   Lunch—Just liquids (such as custards, Jello, soups, cream of wheat, oatmeal).

   Dinner—Just clear liquids (examples include apple juice, bouillon, tea, ginger ale, coffee).

   Administer a Fleet enema to yourself 1 hour before bedtime.

   Nothing by mouth after midnight.

   Call if any questions!

Bowel Preparation (2-Day)

1. Purchase one Fleet enema, two bottles of magnesium citrate, and two 8-ounce cans of Ensure Plus from your pharmacy.
2. Two days before surgery:

   Drink 1/2 bottle of magnesium citrate in the morning.

   Breakfast—Light breakfast (for example, cold cereal or cream of wheat, juice, coffee).

   Lunch—Just liquids (such as custards, Jello, soups, cream of wheat, oatmeal).

   Dinner—Just clear liquids (examples include apple juice, bouillon, tea, ginger ale, coffee).
3. The day before surgery:

   Drink 1/2 bottle of magnesium citrate in the morning and 1/2 bottle in the afternoon.

   Clear liquids for each meal. Avoid milk products.

   Take one can of Ensure Plus with lunch and another with dinner.

   Administer a Fleet enema to youself 1 hour before bedtime.

   Nothing by mouth after midnight.

   Call if any questions!

Figure 35–3. Instruction for 1-day and 2-day intestinal preparations.

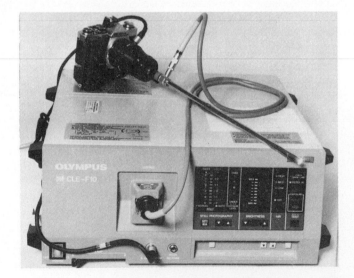

Figure 35–4. The Olympus halogen light source with built-in flash unit and associated laparoscope are excellent units. The xenon light source is model CLV-F10 (Olympus Corp., 4 Nevada Drive, Lake Success, NY 11042).

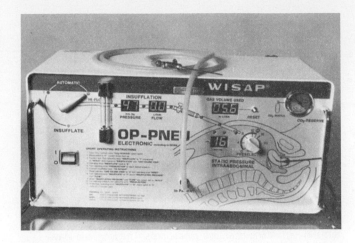

Figure 35–5. This rapid insufflator delivers between 1 and 6 L of gas per minute (WISAP/USA). The intraperitoneal pressure is set not to exceed 15 mm Hg. A less expensive and also superb unit is the Variflow (Laser, 1303 Keefer St, Tomball, TX 77375; 713-351-0424).

Endocoagulator

The endocoagulator is a helpful energy source (see Figs 35–7 and 35–8). The generator works by heating the tip of the endocoagulator probe to a predetermined temperature. An audio feature allows the operator to determine when the operating temperature, usually 100°C, is reached. I find the endocoagulator useful for contracting serosa of the distal tube to evert the tube at the time of salpingostomy.

Monopolar Electrosurgical Instrument

Sometimes monopolar electrosurgical technique is desirable during operative laparoscopy. For example, a monopolar needle electrode is effective for incising the uterine wall at the time of

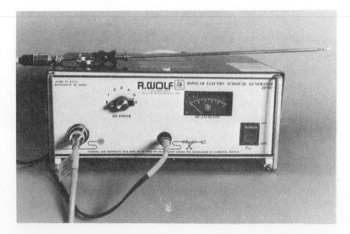

Figure 35–6. A Kleppinger bipolar forceps is connected to a Wolf bipolar generator (model 2075U, Richard Wolf Medical Instruments, 7046 Lyndon Avenue, Rosemont, IL 60018; 800-323-9653).

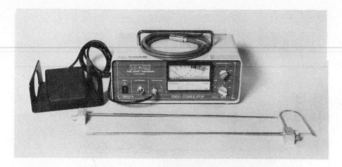

Figure 35–7. Endocoagulator generator, crocodile forceps, and point coagulator (WISAP/USA and Karl Storz, 10111 W Jefferson Blvd, Culver City, CA 90230; 800-421-0837, 213-558-1500, 800-252-2008 in California).

myomectomy for an intramural myoma or opening the fallopian tube at the site of an ectopic gestation. It is important to understand the physics of monopolar energy before using this modality and to select the correct waveform and power settings for a particular task.

Laser Energy

Many surgeons prefer to use lasers of various wavelengths for reconstructive procedures. These units are expensive but are very effective when the correct laser is used to perform an indi-

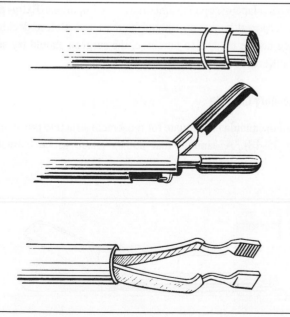

Figure 35–8. Top. Point coagulator (order no. 7515, WISAP/USA). **Middle.** Crocodile forceps (order no. 7510, WISAP/USA). **Bottom.** Kleppinger bipolar forceps (order no. 8383.24, Richard Wolf).

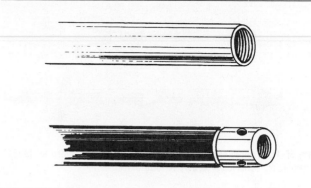

Figure 35–9. Top. Suction-irrigation cannula tip for the Aqua-Purator model (WISAP/USA). **Bottom.** Standard suction-irrigation cannula tip (order no. 8384.72, Richard Wolf; order no. 26178U, Karl Storz).

cated task. The operating room staff must have a thorough understanding of the physics of the particular type of laser being used, including safety issues. Ignoring these issues invites disaster.

Suction Irrigator

An efficient suction irrigator is essential (Figs 35–9 and 35–10). Adequate suction pressure and fluid flow must be available. Several manufacturers now offer excellent units.

Irrigation Fluids

I use 1.5% glycine or Ringer's lactate for irrigation. Glycine, a nonelectrolyte fluid, allows effective coagulation even when the target site is submerged. The circulating nurse attempts to maintain irrigating fluids at body temperature.

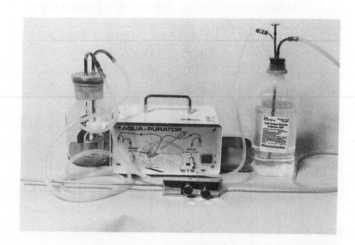

Figure 35–10. The Aqua-Purator in operational mode.

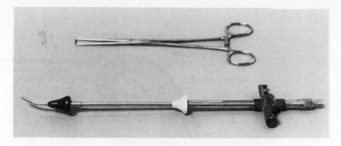

Figure 35–11. A Cohen cannula (order no. 8378, Richard Wolf; order no. 40-3510, Laser) and a tenaculum (order no. 8370.14, Richard Wolf).

Cervical Cannula

A standard laparoscopy cannula is used (Fig 35–11). Although adequate for most laparoscopic procedures, the newer uterine mobilizers, such as the Pelosi (Apple Medical Corp., Bolton, MA) are valuable for operations on the cul-de-sac, particularly when the uterus is retroverted.

Probes

These atraumatic rods are useful in moving intraabdominal viscera about at the time of exploration and for supporting organs when dissection is required (Fig 35–12).

Scissors

Great strides have been made by manufacturers in developing scissors that are sharp and user-friendly (Figs 35–13 and 35–14). New developments include a scissors with detachable tips or with shafts attached to a permanent handle. I prefer scissor tips that are rounded.

Graspers

The surgeon should have available a variety of graspers (Fig 35–15). Atraumatic graspers are very useful in fimbrial corrections, and Alyse and Kocher graspers are tremendously helpful for excision of endometrial implants.

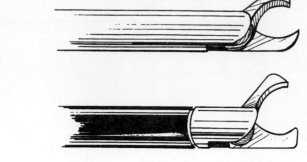

Figure 35–13. Top. Hooked scissors are excellent for opening a hydrosalpinx or opening the fallopian tube to remove an ampullary ectopic pregnancy (order no. 7652, WISAP/USA; order no. 26175 EH, Karl Storz; order no. 8384.02, Richard Wolf; order no. A5264, Olympus Corp; order no. 6614, Reznik Instruments, 7308 N Monticello, Skokie, IL 60076). **Bottom.** Standard dissecting scissors (order no. 8383.02, Richard Wolf).

Biopsy Instruments

Biopsy instruments are essential when some biopsies, such as those of the ovary, are performed (Fig 35–16). They are also quite useful for stripping adhesions from ovarian and peritoneal surfaces.

Needle Holders

A variety of needle holders are available (Fig 35–17). Suturing through a laparoscope is sometimes very important. Extra- and intracorporeal knot tying should be mastered. Before deciding which needle holders to purchase, the surgeon should try several different designs.

Secondary Cannula

A 5-mm cannula is adequate for most reconstructive procedures (Fig 35–18). A cannula that allows tissue to be extracted

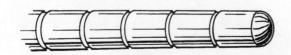

Figure 35–12. A palpation probe is calibrated in centimeters (order no. 7656-3, WISAP/USA; order no. 26175T, Karl Storz).

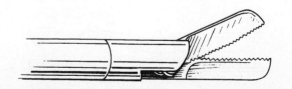

Figure 35–14. A serrated scissors is useful for cutting sutures (order no. 2617-PS, Karl Storz; order no. 7653, WISAP/USA).

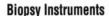

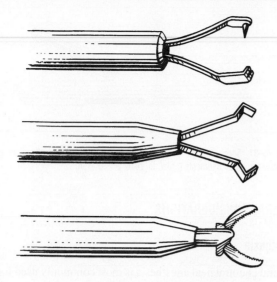

Figure 35–15. Top. Toothed grasping forceps are useful in stabilizing the fallopian tube during salpingostomy (order no. 26177G, Karl Storz). **Middle.** Ampullary dilator is helpful in dilating a phimotic fimbrial ostium (order no. 7651, WISAP/USA; order no. 8384.14, Richard Wolf). **Bottom.** An atraumatic grasping forceps is effective for lifting the fallopian tube by its serosa during delicate dissection (order no. 7655, WISAP/USA).

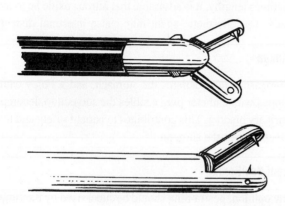

Figure 35–16. Top. A double-action biopsy forceps is excellent for removal of adhesions and for biopsies of ovaries and peritoneal surfaces (order no. 8383.10, Richard Wolf; order no. 6613, Reznik; order no. A5261, Olympus). **Bottom.** Single-action biopsy forceps has a spring-loaded handle that allows the surgeon to hold tissue without applying pressure to the handles. This feature is excellent for stabilizing the cut edge of an ovary while removing a cyst or fixing a cyst of Morgagni while the base is being coagulated and cut (order no. 7654, WISAP/USA).

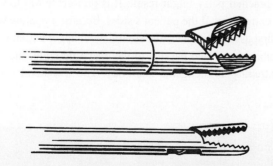

Figure 35–17. The 5-mm (top) and 3-mm (bottom) needle carriers are designed for placing intraabdominal sutures (order no. 7668-1 [5-mm] and 7688 [3-mm], WISAP/USA).

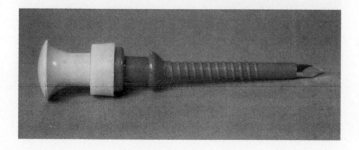

Figure 35–18. All-plastic 5-mm cannula (Apple Medical Corp., Bolton, MA 01740; 508-779-2926).

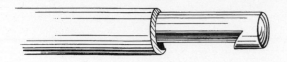

Figure 35–19. Tissue punch used for morcellation of large specimens such as a leiomyoma or an ovary (order no. 7674, WISAP/USA).

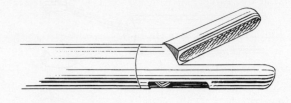

Figure 35–21. Spoon forceps used to remove tissue samples such as an ectopic pregnancy and tissue fragments (order no. 7675, WISAP/USA).

through it is important. If a 10-mm or larger cannula is used, the fascial and peritoneal defect should be closed if possible. This lessens the chance of an incisional hernia.

Morcellator

When large tissue specimens, such as a myoma, are resected, a morcellator may be used to remove the specimen from the abdomen (Figs 35–19 through 35–21). Morcellators come in a variety of sizes and have been greatly improved. Claw and spoon forceps are useful when removing these large specimens. Recently developed instruments facilitate this process immensely.

Tissue Retrieval Bags

Sometimes a large specimen, such as an endometrioma, is best removed by means of placement into a retrieval bag inserted through a secondary cannula, removal of the cannula, and bringing the mouth of the retrieval bag through the cannula site (Fig 35–22). A large instrument, such as a Kocher clamp, can then be passed through the mouth of the bag and the specimen removed. This method also avoids contamination of the abdominal wall.

GENERAL CONSIDERATIONS

Anesthesia

General endotracheal anesthesia is most commonly used for operative laparoscopic procedures. Because these operations are sometimes lengthy, it is advisable that nitrous oxide be avoided, because this anesthetic agent may cause intestinal distention.

Drainage

An orogastric tube deflates the stomach, and a Foley catheter equipped with catheter plug enables the surgeon to decompress the urinary bladder. This contributes to patient safety and to better visibility for the surgeon.

Patient Positioning

In my opinion, positioning should be supervised by the surgeon. Excessive abduction of upper extremities must be avoided, because brachial palsy might result. It is preferable to place the upper extremities at the patient's sides. Because I operate without a first assistant, I place the contralateral upper extremity on an armboard oriented parallel to the operating table, such that the extremity is alongside her body. The ipsilateral arm is

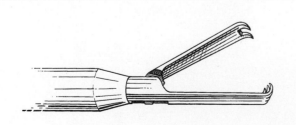

Figure 35–20. Claw forceps for removal of large tissue specimens such as leiomyoma, fallopian tube, or ovary (order no. 7672, WISAP/USA).

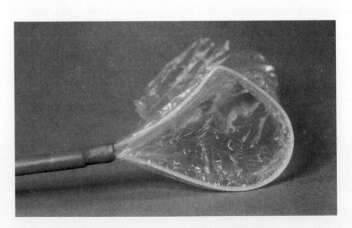

Figure 35–22. Tissue retrieval bag (Apple Medical Corp.).

tucked at her side. This position is safe, results in a much wider draped field, and prevents instruments from sliding onto the floor.

The lower extremities should be resting comfortably in Allen-type stirrups, such that the axis of the thigh is about 30° anterior to an imaginary line drawn along the patient's exposed trunk. The weight of the lower extremity is supported mostly by the heel.

Cannulas

The surgeon should use one, two, or as many secondary cannulas as necessary to allow safe dissection. In general, the lateral cannulas are placed lateral to the inferior epigastric vessels, cephalad enough to allow for easy accessibility to pelvic structures. I usually select 5-mm cannulas for secondary sites.[2] Two cannulas are inserted lateral to the respective inferior epigastric vessels and one cannula is inserted suprapubically (Fig 35–23).

Thermal Energy

Two important issues must be considered in the use of energy that is ultimately converted to heat. First, peritoneum is contracted by heat, with the effect that nearby structures attached to the peritoneum are drawn into the site of energy impact. Second, prolonged application of energy to a single site causes heat to be transmitted through adjacent tissue, which can damage a nearby structure. In the first instance, the surgeon incises the peritoneum between the planned site of impact and the nearby structure to be protected. This step prevents that structure from being drawn to the site of impact. In the second instance, the surgeon uses high-power density but releases it in short bursts; this lessens thermal spread.

Ovarian Cysts

Ovarian cysts often are emptied of fluid content before resection. It is important to drain the cysts in a controlled manner. One additional precaution against widespread intraperitoneal spill is to take the patient out of Trendelenburg position before draining the cyst. Any fluid leaked should then be contained in the pelvic cavity. After the cyst and fluid have been removed from the abdomen, the pelvis and abdomen are copiously irrigated.

OPERATIVE PROCEDURES

Salpingo-ovariolysis

Among the most common anatomic derangements encountered is adhesion formation. This condition may disturb the tubo-ovarian relation to such a point that ovum pick-up is impaired. These adhesions often can be removed efficiently by means of operative laparoscopy.

Typical pelvic findings are shown in Fig 35–24. Dissection begins in the posterior cul-de-sac. This is important because a cul-de-sac devoid of adhesions is necessary for effective suctioning. The key to safe and effective adhesiolysis is to place adhesions under tension.

The uterus is anteflexed with the uterine mobilizer enough to place the adhesions on stretch. Adhesions are coagulated, cut, and removed from the abdomen. Because adhesions are in layers, dissection begins superficially and continues until the floor of the pelvis has been reached (Figs 35–25 and 35–26).

Attention is next turned to the adnexa. For the sake of il-

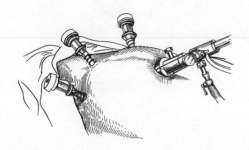

Figure 35–23. Placement of three secondary cannulas. *(From Hunt RB (ed): Atlas of Female Infertility Surgery. St. Louis, Mosby, 1992.)*

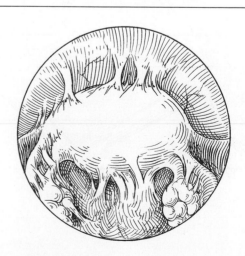

Figure 35–24. Characteristic appearance of pelvic adhesions.

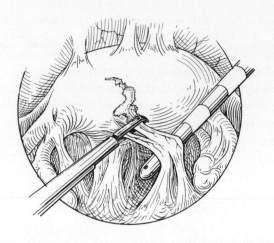

Figure 35–25. Broad adhesions are coagulated with crocodile forceps at 120°C.

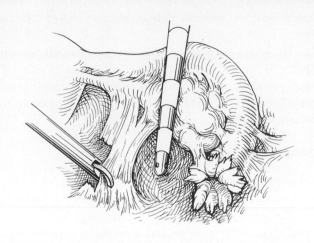

Figure 35–27. Coagulated adhesions are cut, which releases adnexal structures from the lateral pelvic sidewall.

lustration, attention is directed to the right adnexa. With the uterus flexed to the left and with the ureter in view, the ovary is lifted to place adhesions under tension. Adhesions are coagulated and released from the pelvic sidewall (Fig 35–27). It is important to cut the adhesions approximately 2 mm from their attachments to allow enough room to coagulate should bleeding occur. Dissection continues until the tube and ovary are totally freed from sidewall or intestinal adhesions. It is not usually necessary to enter the retroperitoneal space.

Attention is now directed toward the tube and ovary. With the tube lifted, the weight of the ovary places adhesions that bind the two structures together under tension, and these adhe-

sions are incised close to the fallopian tube (Figs 35–28 and 35–29).

To remove ovarian adhesions, one coagulates them and strips them away with a biopsy forceps (Figs 35–30 and 35–31). It is helpful to strip the adhesions parallel to the ovarian surface.

Irrigation is used to identify bleeding sites, and these are coagulated. It is important to minimize thermal damage to the ovarian cortex.

When adhesiolysis is complete on the right, attention is directed to the left adnexa. Often the surgeon must mobilize the rectosigmoid colon away from the left pelvic brim to allow adequate viewing of the left adnexa.

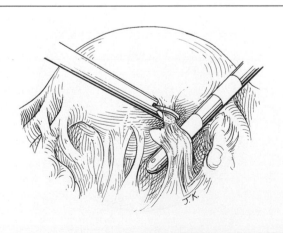

Figure 35–26. Adhesions are cut near the uterine serosa.

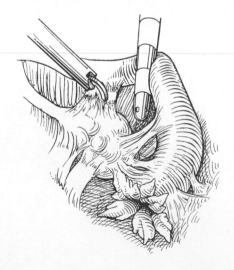

Figure 35–28. Adhesions are incised near the tubal serosa, releasing the fallopian tube from the ovary.

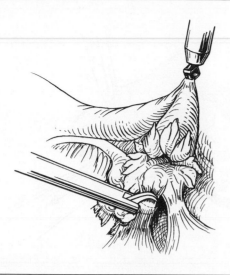

Figure 35–29. Tubal fimbriae are carefully released by means of sharp dissection.

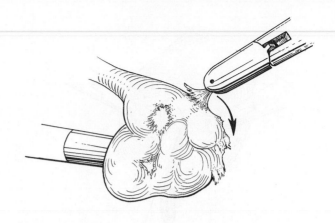

Figure 35–31. With a biopsy forceps, adhesions are stripped from the ovarian surface.

Salpingostomy

Figure 35–32 shows a hydrosalpinx after adhesiolysis has been completed. The distal fallopian tube is lifted anteriorly, and the surgeon dissects it free from the ovary to restore the original anatomic state. Sometimes the site of the tubo-ovarian ligament can be difficult to determine. The surgeon should stop the dissection when normal vascularity is reached.

My preferred method of opening the fallopian tube is to grasp it on either side, gently distend the tube by means of transcervical lavage, and incise it from the antimesenteric to the mesenteric side (Fig 35–33). It is essential to keep this incision short, usually no more than 1.5 cm in a hydrosalpinx that is 2.0

cm in diameter. An atraumatic instrument is inserted inside the tube approximately 2.0 cm and the mucosa is grasped (Fig 35–34). The lateral flaps are moved toward the proximal tube as the mucosa is gently retracted (Fig 35–35). Intussusception occurs, and the operation is completed with placement of a single suture of 4-0 material at the 12 o'clock position to prevent distal movement of the flaps. Lavage reveals patency. Alternatively, the flaps may be rotated externally with bipolar forceps disconnected from the power supply. Although the step is difficult to accomplish, the surgeon should attempt to suture each flap with a single suture (Fig 35–36). Tuboscopy may be performed to assess mucosal quality.

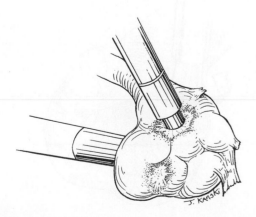

Figure 35–30. Adhesions attached to the ovary are coagulated with a point coagulator. Care is taken not to damage the ovarian cortex.

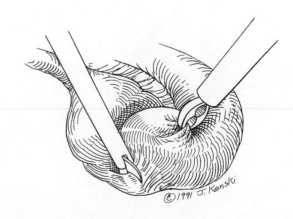

Figure 35–32. Salpingostomy. The distal tube is dissected sharply from the ovary. *(Copyright 1991 J. Kanski in Hunt RB (ed):* Atlas of Female Infertility Surgery. *St. Louis, Mosby, 1992.)*

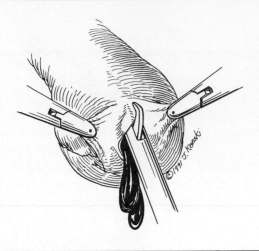

Figure 35–33. Salpingostomy. The salpingostomy is completed by means of eversion of the mucosa with a point coagulator at 100°C or by means of suturing with 4-0 polydioxanone (order no. Z-420, Ethicon, Rt 22 West, Somerville, NJ 08876; 201-524-0400). After the distal tube is mobilized the adhesiolysis is completed, a grasping forceps is placed on either side of the tube and gentle traction is applied to each forceps. A single incision is made with scissors from the mesenteric to the antimesenteric side of the tube. *(Copyright 1991 J. Kanski in Hunt RB (ed): Atlas of Female Infertility Surgery. St. Louis, Mosby, 1992.)*

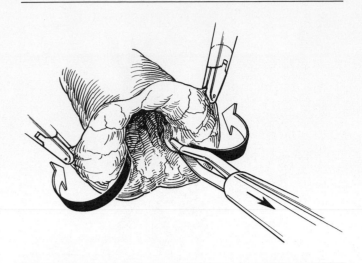

Figure 35–35. Salpingostomy. As gentle traction is applied, the mucosal flaps are slipped proximally, producing an intussusception. A single suture of 4-0 material is placed to fix the everted mucosa to the serosa.

Techniques for the Management of Endometriosis

Surgical management of endometriosis can be difficult. Endometriosis implants have an uncanny ability to invade pelvic tissues in the vicinity of important structures, such as the ureter or rectum. An example of advanced endometriosis is shown in Fig 35–37. The location of ureters and rectum is first deter-

mined. They may have to be dissected out. Next, adhesions are excised, beginning in the posterior cul-de-sac. Often vaginal or rectal probes are necessary to identify the vagina and rectum. Cul-de-sac dissection is greatly facilitated by marked anteversion of the uterus with a uterine mobilizer.

I am a strong proponent of excision of endometriotic im-

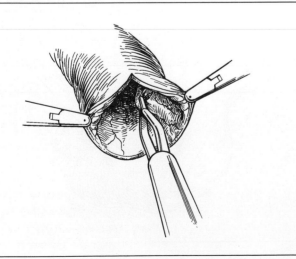

Figure 35–34. Salpingostomy. The mucosa is grasped with a deactivated bipolar forceps.

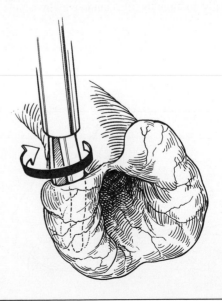

Figure 35–36. Salpingostomy. An alternative technique is to rotate the flaps outward and fix each everted flap with a 4-0 suture.

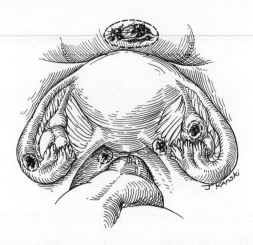

Figure 35–37. Endometriosis with peritoneal implants. *(From Hunt RB (ed): Atlas of Female Infertility Surgery. St. Louis, Mosby, 1992.)*

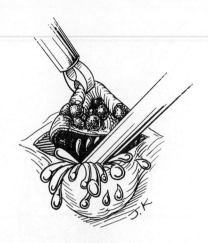

Figure 35–39. Endometriosis. The diseased peritoneum is lifted superiorly and dissected by means of aquadissection. *(From Hunt RB (ed): Atlas of Female Infertility Surgery. St. Louis, Mosby, 1992.)*

plants. I prefer bipolar coagulation only if the implant can be entrapped between the two paddles. Laser ablation may be used if the implant can be totally vaporized. Several modalities can be used to excise endometriotic implants, including bipolar coagulation and excision with a scissors, monopolar electrosurgery, endocoagulation and excision with a scissors, and laser excision. I prefer bipolar coagulation and scissors because of simplicity, economy, effectiveness, and safety.

The technique of excision with laser is shown in Figs 35–38 through 35–40. If I use a scissors, before making the incision I apply coagulation with slightly separated tips of bipolar forceps along the line of intended cutting. The lesion is circumscribed and underlying tissue is thinned out, coagulated, and in-

cised. Endometriotic tissue is next removed from the abdomen. Irrigation and bipolar coagulation as necessary complete that portion of the procedure.

A useful technique for ovarian biopsy is to grasp the lesion with a biopsy forceps and apply gentle traction on the biopsy forceps as the cannula is simultaneously advanced until the cannula is resting against the ovarian cortex surrounding the biopsy site. As more traction is applied with the forceps and additional pressure is applied to the ovarian cortex with the cannula, the lesion is pulled away, leaving a neat, round defect the size of the distal end of the cannula.

One removes endometriomas by grasping ovarian cortex overlying the endometrioma with a biopsy instrument. A second

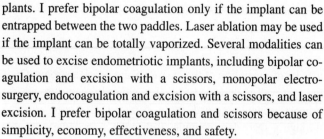

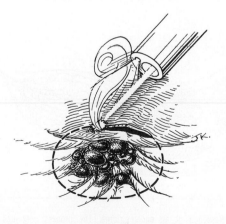

Figure 35–38. Endometriosis. An implant is circumscribed with a carbon dioxide laser. *(From Hunt RB (ed): Atlas of Female Infertility Surgery. St. Louis, Mosby, 1992.)*

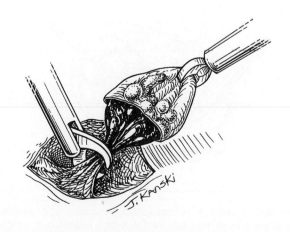

Figure 35–40. Endometriosis. The implant is excised and the peritoneum is left open. *(From Hunt RB (ed): Atlas of Female Infertility Surgery. St. Louis, Mosby, 1992.)*

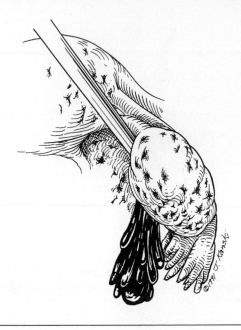

Figure 35–41. Resection of an endometrioma. The ovary is mobilized by aquadissection. *(Copyright 1991 J. Kanski in Hunt RB (ed): Atlas of Female Infertility Surgery. St. Louis, Mosby, 1992.)*

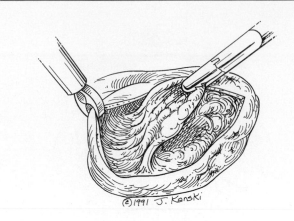

Figure 35–43. Resection of an endometrioma. The endometrioma is removed carefully by means of traction and countertraction. The surgeon must constantly observe tissue tension to avoid lacerating the ovary. *(Copyright 1991 J. Kanski in Hunt RB (ed): Atlas of Female Infertility Surgery. St. Louis, Mosby, 1992.)*

biopsy forceps grasps cortex overlying normal ovarian tissue. The scissors is brought through the midline cannula and an incision is made between the forceps. A plane is developed between the cyst and ovarian stroma, and the cyst is stripped away. It is extremely important to keep the forceps doing the stripping and the forceps supporting the ovary close together to prevent tearing the ovary. This means the surgeon must continually move the biopsy instrument tips such that they are close to the site of separation of the cyst wall and ovarian stroma. Once the cyst wall is dissected free, it is either brought through the primary cannula guided by a 5-mm laparoscope inserted through a secondary cannula or through a secondary cannula site, but with the lesion contained in a retrieval bag. A slightly modified technique is shown in Figs 35–41 through 35–45.

The ovarian defect is then carefully inspected. One accomplishes this step best by lifting the anterior ovarian flap with a

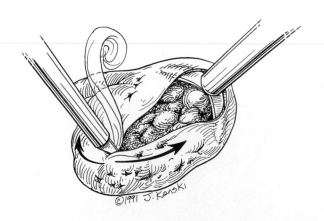

Figure 35–42. Resection of an endometrioma. The ovarian cortex overlying the endometrioma is incised with a knife electrode. A needle electrode, laser, or a scissors may be used. *(Copyright 1991 J. Kanski in Hunt RB (ed): Atlas of Female Infertility Surgery. St. Louis, Mosby, 1992.)*

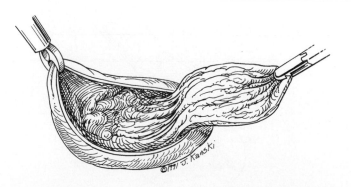

Figure 35–44. Resection of an endometrioma. The process continues until the endometrioma is completely removed from the ovary. *(Copyright 1991 J. Kanski in Hunt RB (ed): Atlas of Female Infertility Surgery. St. Louis, Mosby, 1992.)*

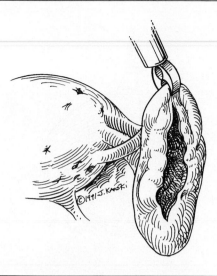

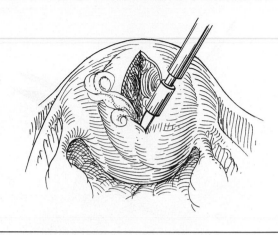

Figure 35–47. Myomectomy. The seromuscular incision is made with a needle or knife electrode. Laser or scissors may be used. *(From Hunt RB (ed):* Atlas of Female Infertility Surgery. *St. Louis, Mosby, 1992.)*

Figure 35–45. Resection of an endometrioma. The appearance of the ovary after the endometrioma has been excised. Suturing is usually not required. *(Copyright 1991 J. Kanski in Hunt RB (ed):* Atlas of Female Infertility Surgery. *St. Louis, Mosby, 1992.)*

biopsy forceps placed through the ipsilateral cannula, irrigating the ovarian stroma with an irrigator/aspirator placed through the midline cannula, and coagulating the vessels with a bipolar forceps inserted through the contralateral cannula. Suturing is infrequently required. If it is, sutures should be used sparingly and tied only tight enough to achieve coaptation.

Usually endometriomas rupture while the ovary is mobilized. If not, the endometrioma can be drained in a controlled manner. Any spilled endometriotic fluid must be removed to prevent adhesion formation and postoperative pain.

Myomectomy

Laparoscopic myomectomy continues to be controversial for women of reproductive age. In my view, removal of intramural fibroids that do not involve uterine vessels, fallopian tubes, rectum, or urinary bladder and not exceeding 5 cm in diameter can be removed by a skilled laparoscopist. Larger subserosal myomas can often be removed by means of laparoscopy.

Removal of an intramural myoma is shown in Figs 35–46 through 35–51. Up to 10 mL of dilute vasopressin (20 U in 100 mL saline solution) may be injected into the myometrium by

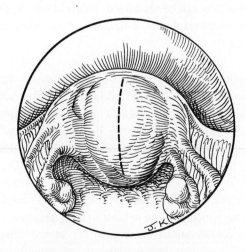

Figure 35–46. Myomectomy. An intramural myoma. *(From Hunt RB (ed):* Atlas of Female Infertility Surgery. *St. Louis, Mosby, 1992.)*

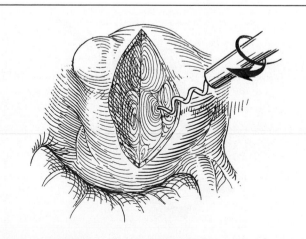

Figure 35–48. Myomectomy. A corkscrew is embedded in the myoma. *(From Hunt RB (ed):* Atlas of Female Infertility Surgery. *St. Louis, Mosby, 1992.)*

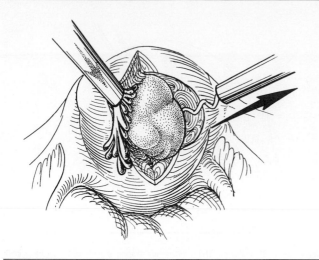

Figure 35–49. Myomectomy. The myoma is dissected from the pseudocapsule by means of traction and aquadissection. *(From Hunt RB (ed): Atlas of Female Infertility Surgery. St. Louis, Mosby, 1992.)*

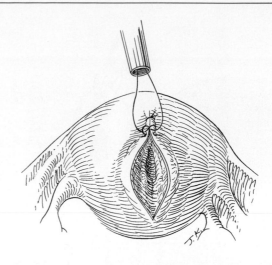

Figure 35–51. Myomectomy. The uterine defect is closed with sutures. *(From Hunt RB (ed): Atlas of Female Infertility Surgery. St. Louis, Mosby, 1992.)*

passing a 22-gauge spinal needle, connected to a 10-mL syringe by extension tubing, through the midline cannula. A linear incision is made over the myoma and deepened through the myoma and pseudocapsule. Uterine muscle and pseudocapsule are dissected off the myoma, and a corkscrew is fixed into the myoma. The myoma is leveraged anteriorly, and biopsy forceps positioned on either side of the midline are used to strip the uterine muscle and pseudocapsule off the myoma. When the final pedicle for the myoma is identified, it is coagulated and divided. The myoma can then be removed from the abdomen by means of morcellation.

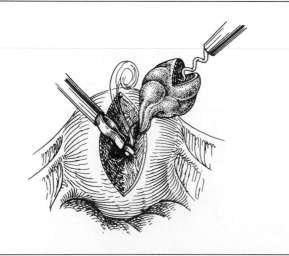

Figure 35–50. Myomectomy. The vascular pedicle of the myoma is desiccated and the myoma is removed. *(From Hunt RB (ed): Atlas of Female Infertility Surgery. St. Louis, Mosby, 1992.)*

Management of Ectopic Pregnancy

Ectopic pregnancy is a serious problem. With identification of women at increased risk for ectopic pregnancy, precise and timely determination of human chorionic gonadotropin (hCG) levels, and vaginal probe ultrasound, management of most ectopic pregnancies will become medical. Sometimes surgical intervention is warranted, and laparoscopic techniques are often applicable. Some ectopic pregnancies do not require treatment because they resolve on their own. Expectant management requires frequent determination of serum hCG levels and monitoring of signs and symptoms. One problem with surgical management of ectopic gestations is operating on them before they can be visualized. To avoid this, and to rule out spontaneous resolution, a period of observation may be warranted.

Early cornual pregnancies have been successfully removed by means of laparoscopy. A laparoscopist undertaking such a procedure should be skilled in suture techniques, have blood available if transfusion is anticipated, and be prepared for immediate laparotomy should this become necessary. In my opinion, an ectopic pregnancy in which a fetal heartbeat is detected by means of ultrasound should be managed surgically. Partial or complete salpingectomy also should be considered for inoperable lesions of the fallopian tube, recurrent ectopic pregnancy, or the patient's desire to have no more pregnancies. Two additional considerations are of great importance: monitoring hCG levels until they become normal and administration of immune globulin when indicated. To determine the most appropriate operation under these often tense circumstances, the surgeon must discuss these issues with the woman preoperatively.

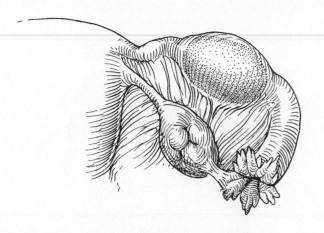

Figure 35–52. Ectopic pregnancy. An unruptured ampullary ectopic pregnancy. *(Copyright 1991 J. Kanski in Hunt RB (ed):* Atlas of Female Infertility Surgery. *St. Louis, Mosby, 1992.)*

To proceed otherwise invites calamity. Appropriate written informed consent should be obtained.

Management of an unruptured ampullary ectopic pregnancy is shown in Figs 35–52 through 35–57. A 22-gauge spinal needle is passed through a lower abdominal cannula, and 10 mL of dilute vasopressin (20 U per 100 mL of saline solution) is injected into the mesosalpinx. With the tube fixed, a monopolar electrode at 30 W pure cutting current is selected. A linear incision is made directly over the ectopic gestation and is deepened until the tubal lumen is entered. Sometimes a small gush of dark blood emits from the tube, but the bleeding usually stops abruptly. Vasopressin constricts the placental bed and usually controls bleeding from this site. Whereas co-

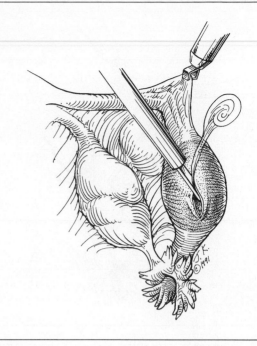

Figure 35–54. Salpingotomy for ectopic pregnancy. The tube is opened with a needle or knife electrode. A laser or scissors also may be used. *(Copyright 1991 J. Kanski in Hunt RB (ed):* Atlas of Female Infertility Surgery. *St. Louis, Mosby, 1992.)*

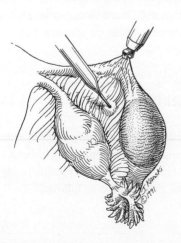

Figure 35–53. Salpingotomy for ectopic pregnancy. Two units of dilute vasopressin is injected into the mesosalpinx. *(Copyright 1991 J. Kanski in Hunt RB (ed):* Atlas of Female Infertility Surgery. *St. Louis, Mosby, 1992.)*

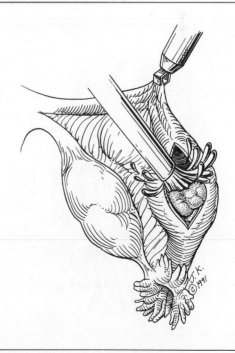

Figure 35–55. Salpingotomy for ectopic pregnancy. The ectopic gestation is dissected by means of a combination of aquatraction and aquadissection. *(Copyright 1991 J. Kanski in Hunt RB (ed):* Atlas of Female Infertility Surgery. *St. Louis, Mosby, 1992.)*

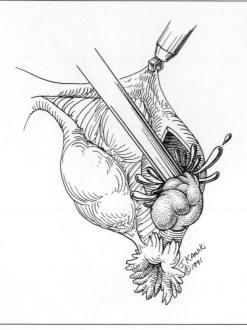

Figure 35–56. Salpingotomy for ectopic pregnancy. The ectopic pregnancy is removed. *(Copyright 1991 J. Kanski in Hunt RB (ed): Atlas of Female Infertility Surgery. St. Louis, Mosby, 1992.)*

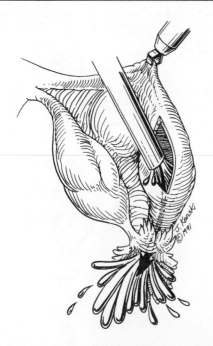

Figure 35–57. Salpingotomy for ectopic pregnancy. The tubal lumen is thoroughly lavaged. *(Copyright 1991 J. Kanski in Hunt RB (ed): Atlas of Female Infertility Surgery. St. Louis, Mosby, 1992.)*

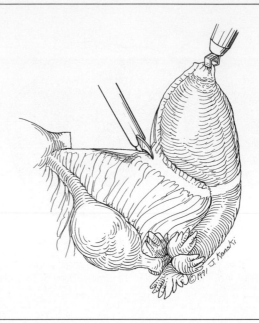

Figure 35–58. Partial salpingectomy. *(Copyright 1991 J. Kanski in Hunt RB (ed): Atlas of Female Infertility Surgery. St. Louis, Mosby, 1992.)*

agulation of the cut edge of the tube may require judicious application of bipolar energy, I refrain from coagulating tubal mucosa.

Once the tube is open, the surgeon should allow a few minutes for the products of conception to separate from tubal attachments. They are next removed by a combination of irrigation and gentle suction. Care is taken to ensure that all placental fragments are removed to prevent peritoneal implantation, which may lead to persistently elevated hCG titers. Generally, no suturing is required. Sometimes partial or complete salpingectomy is indicated. These are illustrated in Figs 35–58 and 35–59.

ADJUNCTIVE AGENTS

A substantial obstacle to satisfactory surgical outcome is postoperative adhesions. Many regimens have been tried through the years, and no ideal one has been identified. My current regimen for adhesion prevention is as follows.

Antiobiotics

Each woman receives prophylactic antibiotics, usually doxycycline. The patient is given 100 mg intravenously immediately preoperatively and 100 mg intravenously several hours later. To

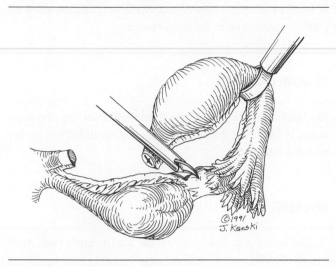

Figure 35–59. Complete salpingectomy. *(Copyright 1991 J. Kanski in Hunt RB (ed): Atlas of Female Infertility Surgery. St. Louis, Mosby, 1992.)*

lessen the problem of phlebitis, 10 mL of 4.2% sodium bicarbonate is mixed in the administration fluid bag that contains the dissolved doxycycline. Although no proof exists as to the efficacy of prophylactic antibiotics applied in this scenario, their use seems reasonable.[3,4]

Hydroflotation

At the completion of the operation, 2 L of warm Ringer's lactate is instilled intraperitoneally. Balanced salt solutions have been shown to be superior to normal saline solution when rabbit fallopian tubes are exposed to each.[5] This serves to float intraabdominal structures through eddy currents and differential densities of intraabdominal organs. For example, fatty epiploicae float, whereas the more dense ovary sinks. Early ambulation accentuates this process, causing organ separation during early healing. An additional advantage is that intraperitoneal gas is displaced from the abdomen at the time of wound closure, provided the Trendelenburg position is maintained to allow the gas to be exhausted from the secondary cannulas at the time the cannulas are removed. This technique essentially eliminates postoperative shoulder pain.

Steroids and Antihistamines

No consensus supports the effectiveness of steroids and antihistamines as adhesion preventives.[3,4] However, in view of their proved safety, and on the chance that they may help, I do add 20 mg of dexamethasone and 25 mg of promethazine to hydroflotation fluid.

Analgesics

I place 20 mg of bupivacaine in the hydroflotation fluid to lessen pain from peritoneal irritation. In addition, approximately 20 mg of bupivacaine is injected into abdominal wall incision sites.

SURGICAL RESULTS

Salpingo-ovariolysis

Gomel[6] reported results for 92 patients who underwent salpingo-ovariolysis by means of operative laparoscopy. Each patient had been infertile for at least 20 months and each was judged to have moderate to severe adhesions. Ovum pickup was either greatly hampered or impossible in every case. After operative laparoscopy each patient received follow-up care for at least 9 months. Fifty-four patients (59%) experienced at least one term pregnancy and 5 (5%) experienced an ectopic pregnancy. Among 123 patients undergoing salpingo-ovariolysis at laparotomy with an operating microscope, 28.4% delivered a term infant, and 3.3% experienced an ectopic pregnancy.[7]

Salpingostomy

The numbers of patients reported who have undergone salpingostomy by means of operative laparoscopy are small. Among nine patients so treated, four had intrauterine pregnancies.[8] Eight of these 9 patients had experienced tubal closure after salpingostomy by means of laparotomy.

Laparoscopic salpingostomy was performed on 38 patients.[9] Among these patients 10 (26%) became pregnant. The number of ectopic gestations and outcome of the pregnancies were not reported. Among 18 patients who underwent this procedure,[10] 6 (33%) had term pregnancies, 2 (11%) experienced ectopic pregnancies, and 1 (6%) had a spontaneous abortion.

Terminal salpingostomy by means of laparotomy with an operating microscope was performed on 143 patients.[7] Of these, 28 (19.6%) had term deliveries and 3 (2.1%) experienced ectopic pregnancies. Seventy-eight patients underwent the same procedure.[11] Fourteen (18%) did not participate in the follow-up study and were presumed not pregnant. Seventeen (22%) had viable pregnancies, and 4 (5%) had ectopic gestations.

Operations for Endometriosis

In the largest series of management of endometriosis by means of laparoscopy, a carbon dioxide laser was used. A combined series of 851 patients treated with this modality yielded the following pregnancy rates: 278 (7.6%) among 483 patients with mild endometriosis; 156 (51.3%) among 304 patients with moderate endometriosis; and 33 (52%) among 64 patients with severe disease.[12] Large series of destruction or resection of endometriosis by means of operative laparoscopic techniques other than the use of a carbon dioxide laser are yet to be published. Among 214 patients undergoing laparotomy for endometriosis, the conception rates were 70% for mild, 66% for moderate, and 61% for severe disease.[13] Among 107 patients treated similarly, conception rates were 75% for mild, 50% for moderate, and 33% for severe disease.[14] It should be noted, however, that in the former study, these percentages were based on life-table comparisons of cumulative pregnancy rates. In the latter study the investigators included only women who had not undergone previous surgical therapy for endometriosis. Therefore the reported results cannot be compared absolutely with the results for women who undergo operative laparoscopy.

Operations for Ectopic Pregnancy

That tubal pregnancies can be removed by means of operative laparoscopy has been clearly shown. Among 295 patients undergoing this procedure, only 14 (4.8%) required a second procedure to remove retained trophoblastic tissue. Seven of these underwent operative laparoscopy as the second procedure. Included in this series were 24 patients in whom the ectopic gestation occurred in a solitary tube. The fallopian tube was conserved, and each patient attempted a subsequent pregnancy. Of these 24, 11 (46%) had an intrauterine and 7 (29%) an ectopic pregnancy.[15]

CONCLUSIONS

Many laparoscopic techniques can be used to correct pelvic diseases that contribute to infertility. These procedures can be performed reproducibly with low complication rates by a skilled laparoscopist using properly designed and maintained equipment. The real question is whether these techniques applied to properly selected patients offer these patients a considerable advantage. The answer is an enthusiastic yes. Economically, the cost may be less than that of laparotomy.[16] Other important savings are the patient's ability to return home on the day of the operation in most instances, experience decidedly less discomfort, and resume full-time activities within 1 week. Pregnancy rates with laparoscopy appear to equal or better those obtained with laparotomy for salpingo-ovariolysis, salpingostomy, and management of endometriosis. A critic may argue correctly that our numbers are small and the follow-up period has been short. With this I agree, and I encourage those who perform operative laparoscopy to monitor carefully and report honestly the results

in terms of ectopic, aborted, and viable pregnancies, using all patients operated on as the denominator.

ACKNOWLEDGMENTS

My special thanks go to Jean Kanski-Bittl for the drawings, James F. Green for the photographs, and Sarah Jeffries for her editorial assistance.

REFERENCES

1. DeCherney AH: The leader of the band is tired. *Fertil Steril* 44:299, 1985
2. Hunt RB (ed): *Atlas of Female Infertility Surgery*. St. Louis, Mosby–Year Book, 1992
3. Holtz G: Prevention and management of peritoneal adhesions. *Fertil Steril* 41:497, 1984
4. Pfeffer WH: Adjuvants in tubal surgery. *Fertil Steril* 33:245, 1980
5. Blandau RJ: Comparative aspects of tubal anatomy and physiology as they relate to reconstructive procedures. *J Reprod Med* 21:7, 1978
6. Gomel V: Salpingo-ovariolysis by laparoscopy in infertility. *Fertil Steril* 40:607, 1983
7. Verhoeven HC, Hunt RB, Schlosser HW: Salpingostomy, fimbrioplasty, and adhesiolysis. In: Hunt RB (ed), *Atlas of Female Infertility Surgery.* Chicago, Year Book, 1986:302
8. Gomel V: *Recent Advances in Surgical Correction of Tubal Diseases Producing Infertility.* Chicago, Year Book, 1978
9. Mettler L, Giesel H, Semm K: Treatment of female infertility due to tubal obstruction by operative laparoscopy. *Fertil Steril* 32:384, 1979.
10. Leventhal JM: Laparoscopy in female infertility. In: Hunt RB (ed), *Atlas of Female Infertility Surgery*. Chicago, Year Book, 1986: 213.
11. Hunt RB, Cohen SM: Discussions of salpingostomy. *Current Problems in Obstetrics, Gynecology, and Fertility.* Vol. 9. Chicago, Year Book, 1986
12. Martin DC (ed): *Intra-abdominal Laser Surgery.* Memphis, Resurge, 1986
13. Rock JA: The conservative surgical treatment of endometriosis: Evaluation of pregnancy success with respect to the extent of the disease as categorized using contemporary classification systems. *Fertil Steril* 35:131, 1981
14. Buttram VC Jr: Conservative surgery for endometriosis in the infertile female: A study of 206 patients with implications for both medical and surgical therapy. *Fertil Steril* 31:117, 1979
15. Pouly JL, Mahnes H, Mage G, Canis M, Bruhat MA: Conservative laparoscopic treatment of 321 ectopic pregnancies. *Fertil Steril* 46:1093, 1986
16. Levine RL: Economic impact of pelviscopic surgery. *J Reprod Med* 30:655, 1985

CHAPTER 36

Technical Aspects of Tubal Surgery by Means of Laparotomy

ROBERT B. HUNT

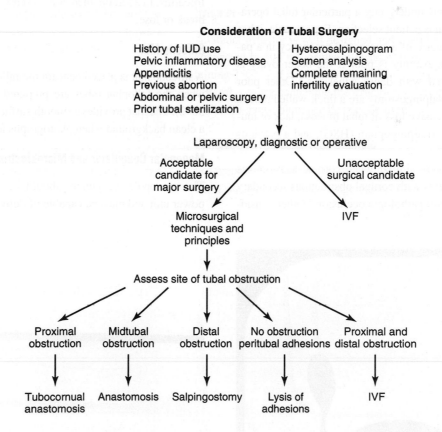

Consideration of Tubal Surgery

History of IUD use
Pelvic inflammatory disease
Appendicitis
Previous abortion
Abdominal or pelvic surgery
Prior tubal sterilization

Hysterosalpingogram
Semen analysis
Complete remaining
infertility evaluation

Laparoscopy, diagnostic or operative

Acceptable
candidate for
major surgery

Unacceptable
surgical candidate

Microsurgical
techniques and
principles

IVF

Assess site of tubal obstruction

Proximal
obstruction

Midtubal
obstruction

Distal
obstruction

No obstruction
peritubal adhesions

Proximal and
distal obstruction

Tubocornual
anastomosis

Anastomosis

Salpingostomy

Lysis of
adhesions

IVF

Nothing in life is to be feared. It is only to be understood.
Marie Curie

OPERATIVE PROCEDURES

Initiation of the Procedure

The patient enters the hospital on the day of the procedure. The appropriate evaluation for infertility has been completed. In addition, the patient has received and returned an informed consent sheet.[8] The previous afternoon she has taken one bottle of magnesium citrate to induce mechanical intestinal preparation, and she has refrained from taking anything by mouth after midnight. After the admission process is complete, blood and urine studies are performed, and the patient is taken to the surgical suite, where administration of intravenous fluid is started and final preparations are made.

Once either general endotrachael or regional anesthesia is induced, a pelvic examination is accomplished, a Foley catheter and intrauterine catheter are inserted, and a vaginal pack is positioned.

The abdomen is prepared. I prefer a Hunt-Acuna incision.[9] It gives excellent pelvic exposure, protects the ilioinguinal nerve from injury, and results in a less painful postoperative course than a Pfannensteil incision. If the patient has had a previous Pfannensteil incision, the Hunt-Acuna incision allows the surgeon to dissect in unscarred tissue. If the patient has a low midline scar, I use the midline incision.

Adhesiolysis

Once the peritoneal cavity is open, the surgeon performs a general abdominal exploratory procedure and identifies pelvic adhesions. The peritoneum in the lower abdomen and the anterior

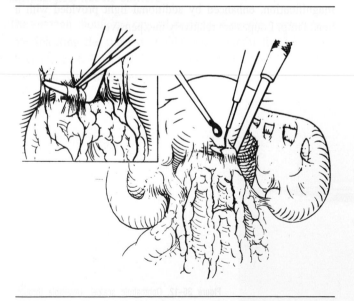

Figure 36–14. Posterior cul-de-sac dissection. Note bipolar coagulation (inset). *(From Hunt RB (ed): Atlas of Female Infertility Surgery. St. Louis, Mosby, 1992.)*

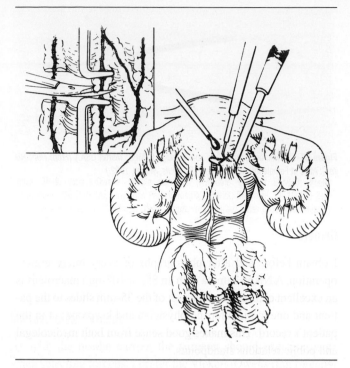

Figure 36–15. Omentopexy and partial omentectomy (inset). Intestine is protected from the unipolar electrode with a Teflon-coated dissecting rod. *(From Hunt RB (ed): Atlas of Female Infertility Surgery. St. Louis, Mosby, 1992.)*

and posterior cul-de-sac are cleared of intestinal and omental adhesions (Fig 36–14). Loupes may be used for this part of the operation. If the omentum appears unhealthy, it is resected, and each important omental vessel is ligated individually. If the omentum is healthy but adhesed, omentopexy is performed (Fig 36–15).

With dissecting rods and a needle electrode, the ovaries and fallopian tubes are dissected from the pelvic sidewall (Fig 36–16). It is unwise to use electrosurgery adjacent to the intestines. Sharp or, occasionally, blunt dissection is safer. Bleeding is controlled with bipolar coagulation.

Once adhesiolysis is competed, a Jackson-Pratt sump drain, connected to its own suction, is positioned in the posterior cul-de-sac and surgical gauze such as Kerlex is placed. The silicone mat may be laid over the gauze (Fig 36–17).

Pathologic Cornual Occlusion

In my experience, histologic studies of tissues removed because of cornual occlusion have revealed that the most common causes are salpingitis isthmica nodosa, endometriosis, and fibrosis. The concept of repair is to excise all abnormal tissue and restore patency by effecting a tension-free anastomosis or tubal implantation. I choose the latter procedure only if the entire intramural portion of the fallopian tube has been destroyed, an uncommon finding. Preferably the surgeon should personally re-

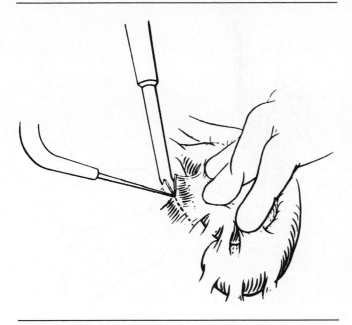

Figure 36–16. Mobilization of the right adnexa from the pelvic side wall. *(From Hunt RB (ed): Atlas of Female Infertility Surgery. St. Louis, Mosby, 1992.)*

view the HSGs, taking particular note of the intramural portion of the fallopian tubes.

Cornual Anastomosis

Approximately 3 mL of dilute vasopressin (20 U in 50 mL of Ringer's lactate) is injected into the cornu for hemostasis (Fig

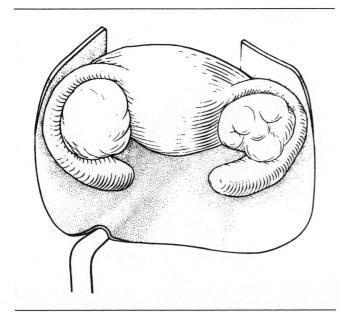

Figure 36–17. The pelvic structures are mobilized and exposed. *(From Hunt RB (ed): Atlas of Female Infertility Surgery. St. Louis, Mosby, 1992.)*

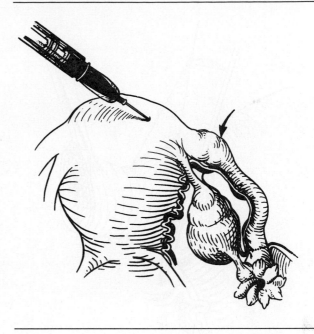

Figure 36–18. Dilute vasopressin is placed at the cornu. *(From Hunt RB (ed):* Atlas of Female Infertility Surgery. *St. Louis, Mosby, 1992.)*

36–18). With the aid of an operating microscope, the surgeon transects the fallopian tube in the midisthmus and dissects the proximal segment from the mesosalpinx until the uterotubal junction is reached. Care is taken to preserve the longitudinal vessels just beneath the tube. Bipolar coagulation is used for hemostasis. A peritoneal track is made over the fallopian tube, and the tube is divided with an iris scissors (Fig 36–19). Even though the tube may be patent at this level, it is seldom normal.

A 6-0 polypropylene suture is passed through the tube in a figure-of-eight pattern. The suture ends are held with a fine hemostat, and an incision is made around the circular muscle fibers surrounding the intramural tubal segment (Fig 36–20). When a 2-mm segment has been dissected, it is excised (Fig 36–21), and the intramural segment of fallopian tube again is checked to make certain it is free of fibrosis, has a healthy mucosa, and is patent (Fig 36–22). This dissection can be carried close to the uterine cavity if necessary, although this makes for a difficult anastomosis. Also, the surgeon may have to excise crescents of myometrium superiorly to improve visibility.

Working laterally, the surgeon separates the tube from its mesosalpinx until healthy tissue is encountered (Fig 36–23). Patency is documented by means of retrograde lavage with dilute indigo carmine (Fig 36–24).

Having prepared the tube for anastomosis, the surgeon places stay sutures of 6-0 nonabsorbable material to align the lumina. Great care must be taken to compensate for an asymmetrically located tubal ostium in the cornu as well as to keep

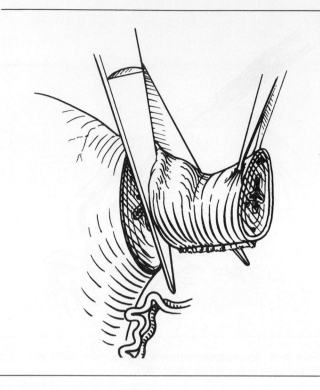

Figure 36–19. Proximal tube transected at its junction with the uterus. *(From Hunt RB (ed):* Atlas of Female Infertility Surgery. *St. Louis, Mosby, 1992.)*

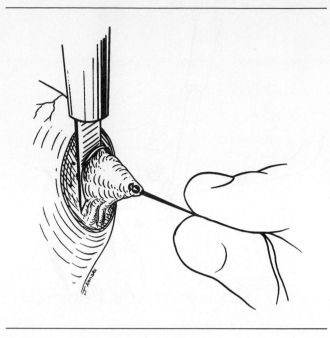

Figure 36–21. Intramural segment of the tube is excised. *(From Hunt RB (ed):* Atlas of Female Infertility Surgery. *St. Louis, Mosby, 1992.)*

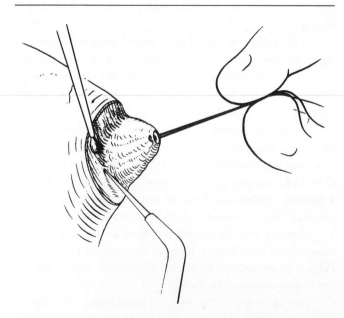

Figure 36–20. Intramural segment of the tube is dissected. *(From Hunt RB (ed):* Atlas of Female Infertility Surgery. *St. Louis, Mosby, 1992.)*

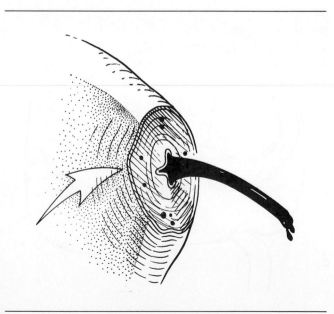

Figure 36–22. Tubal patency is established. *(From Hunt RB (ed):* Atlas of Female Infertility Surgery. *St. Louis, Mosby, 1992.)*

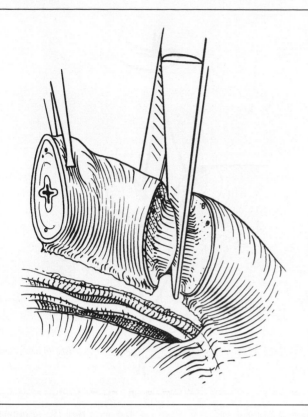

Figure 36–23. The tube is transected laterally. *(From Hunt RB (ed):* Atlas of Female Infertility Surgery. *St. Louis, Mosby, 1992.)*

the tubal lumina at the same level. When stay sutures are tightened, the lumina should align perfectly (Fig 36–25).

The anastomosis is then performed with sutures of 8-0 synthetic absorbable or nonabsorbable material. I prefer nylon on a 130-μm taper cut needle. Usually the tube is sutured in four places, avoiding the mucosa medially (Fig 36–26). A small amount of mucosa is incorporated if the ampullary segment is being sutured but the mucosa is avoided if the anastomosis involves only the isthmus.

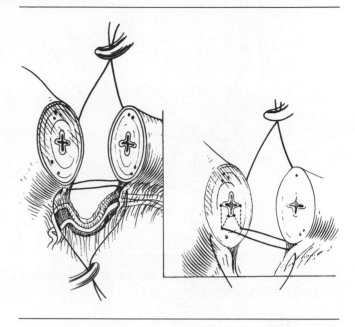

Figure 36–25. Stay sutures are placed. *(From Hunt RB (ed):* Atlas of Female Infertility Surgery. *St. Louis, Mosby, 1992.)*

After the inner layer and stay sutures are tied, the fallopian tube is tested for patency. A watertight anastomosis is not necessary, but patency must be confirmed. If the anastomosis is satisfactory, the uterine and tubal serosa are approximated with 8-0 material, and additional stay sutures are placed if desirable (Fig 36–27). A similar procedure is performed on the opposite side. After careful pelvic lavage, packing is removed, adjunctive agents are added, and the abdomen is closed.

Midtubal Anastomosis

The most frequent indication for isthmic-isthmic, isthmic-ampullary, or ampullary-ampullary anastomosis in my experience is reversal of a tubal ligation. The second most frequent indica-

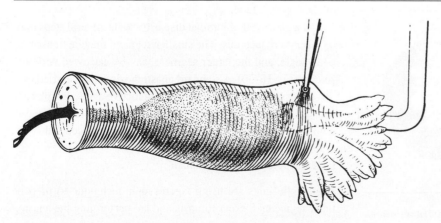

Figure 36–24. Patency is established. *(From Hunt RB (ed):* Atlas of Female Infertility Surgery. *St. Louis, Mosby, 1992.)*

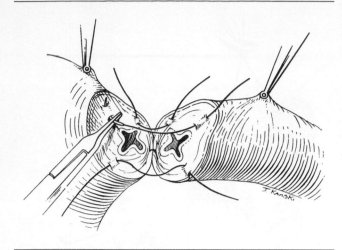

Figure 36–26. Inner layer of sutures is placed. *(From Hunt RB (ed):* Atlas of Female Infertility Surgery. *St. Louis, Mosby, 1992.)*

tion is tubal closure secondary to a previous ectopic pregnancy. The aim of the procedures is the same: to excise diseased tissue and perform a tension-free, precise anastomosis. Judgment is important. For example, the surgeon occasionally encounters an extensively diseased ampulla, requiring a compromise. Then it is necessary to adhere to the aforementioned concept, but leave enough ampulla for a successful pregnancy to occur. I believe the surgeon should leave at least 2 cm of ampulla with its fimbriae.

Studies have shown that the proximal fallopian tube adjacent to the ligation site is diseased in most patients.[10] I recommend removing 0.5 to 1 cm of tube when preparing the proximal segment for anastomosis. To prevent excessive luminal disparity, the surgeon should open the most medial portion of the lateral segment when the ligation involves the ampulla (Fig 36–28). It is seldom necessary to excise ampulla lateral to the site of ligation.

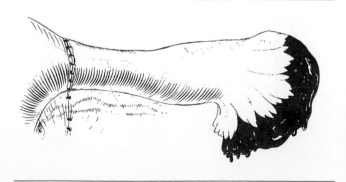

Figure 36–27. Anastomosis is completed. *(From Hunt RB (ed):* Atlas of Female Infertility Surgery. *St. Louis, Mosby, 1992.)*

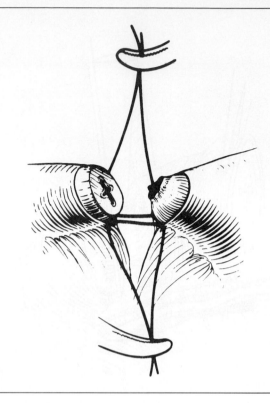

Figure 36–28. Tubal segments are prepared for anastomosis. *(From Hunt RB (ed):* Atlas of Female Infertility Surgery. *St. Louis, Mosby, 1992.)*

When the tubal segments have been prepared for anastomosis, stay sutures of 6-0 nonabsorbable material are placed, and the inner layer of 9-0 synthetic absorbable or nonabsorbable sutures is placed and tied (Fig 36–29). The surgeon should avoid the mucosa in the isthmic segment but may incorporate a small amount of mucosa in the ampullary segment. After stay sutures are tied, the tube is tested for patency and the serosa is approximated with 8-0 material. Additional stay sutures are placed if necessary. A similar procedure is carried out on the opposite tube.

If a great deal of luminal disparity exists, several steps may be taken to reduce this. The smaller segment may be transected at an angle, and the larger segment may be narrowed with 9-0 sutures (Fig 36–30). A standard anastomosis is then carried out.

The pelvic cavity is cleansed, adjunctive agents are placed, and the abdomen is closed. A follow-up HSG is obtained 4 months after the procedure if pregnancy has not occurred.

Laparoscopic Tubal Anastomosis

Some colleagues are using laparoscopic technique to prepare tubal segments for anastomosis and are performing the anastomosis through small incisions but with the aid of an operating

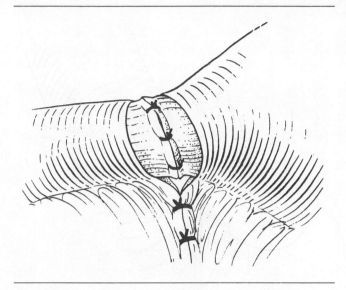

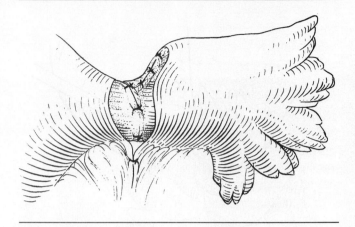

Figure 36–29. Inner layer of anastomosis is completed. *(From Hunt RB (ed): Atlas of Female Infertility Surgery. St. Louis, Mosby, 1992.)*

Figure 36–31. Inner layer of anastomosis is completed. *(From Hunt RB (ed): Atlas of Female Infertility Surgery. St. Louis, Mosby, 1992.)*

microscope.[11] Others are performing the entire procedure with laparoscopic technique. It is evident that new instruments need to be developed, and this is being accomplished. Whether the newer approaches will replace the conventional or minilaparotomy incisions remains to be determined.

Fimbrioplasty

Although a carbon dioxide laser may be used for fimbrioplasty, I prefer a microelectrode and microscissors. Aided by magnification, the surgeon carefully excises adhesions from the fallopian tube and ovary. Accessory fimbrial stalks, cysts of Mor-

gagni, and paratubal cysts are also removed when appropriate. If an accessory tubal ostium is present in the distal ampulla, the bridge of tissue separating it from the main ostium may be divided, converting the ostia into a single tubal ostium.

If fimbriae are covered by adhesions, the adhesions are gently excised; care is taken not to damage the fimbriae (Fig 36–32). Phimosis is corrected by means of an incision along the antimesenteric side of the tube (Fig 36–33).

When dissecting in the vicinity of the fimbriae, care must be taken not to grasp them but rather the serosa just proximal to them (Fig 36–34). The dissecting rod is a superb instrument for delineation and incision of mucosal bridges (Fig 36–35).

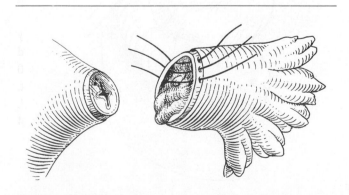

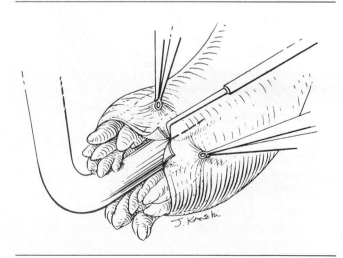

Figure 36–30. Correction of great luminal disparity. *(From Hunt RB (ed): Atlas of Female Infertility Surgery. St. Louis, Mosby, 1992.)*

Figure 36–32. Excision of scar tissue. *(From Hunt RB (ed): Atlas of Female Infertility Surgery. St. Louis, Mosby, 1992.)*

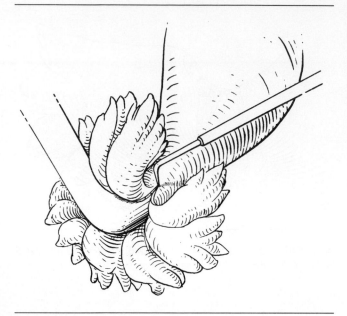

Figure 36–33. Correction of tubal phimosis. *(From Hunt RB (ed):* Atlas of Female Infertility Surgery. *St. Louis, Mosby, 1992.)*

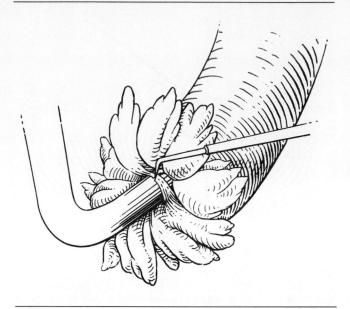

Figure 36–35. Division of mucosal bridge. *(From Hunt RB (ed):* Atlas of Female Infertility Surgery. *St. Louis, Mosby, 1992.)*

Salpingostomy

Once adhesiolysis has been accomplished (Figs 36–36 and 36–37), the fallopian tube is dissected from its respective ovary to restore proper tubo-ovarian anatomic relations (Fig 36–38). With the tube distended with dilute indigo carmine a single incision is made in the distal end of the tube. Fine hemostats are

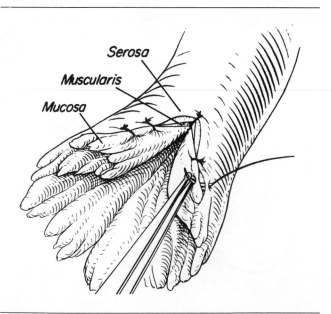

Figure 36–34. Fimbrioplasty nears completion. *(From Hunt RB (ed):* Atlas of Female Infertility Surgery. *St. Louis, Mosby, 1992.)*

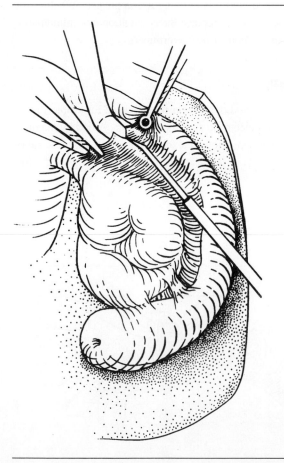

Figure 36–36. Division of adhesions between tube and ovary. *(From Hunt RB (ed):* Atlas of Female Infertility Surgery. *St. Louis, Mosby, 1992.)*

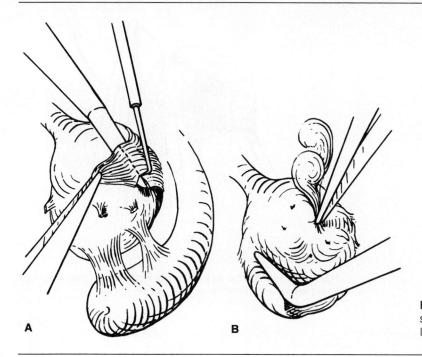

Figure 36–37. **A.** Excision of scar tissue. **B.** Shrinkage of small tufts of scar by means of bipolar coagulation. *(From Hunt RB (ed):* Atlas of Female Infertility Surgery. *St. Louis, Mosby, 1992.)*

used to evert the tubal flexus, and the mucosa is sutured with 6-0 absorbable or nonabsorbable material (Figs 36–39 through 36–43).

Bipolar Block

Many gynecologic surgeons believe concomitant cornual and distal fallopian tubal blockage is a contraindication to surgical correction. I disagree. My present policy is as follows. At the time of assessment laparoscopy, I perform adhesiolysis of all pelvic structures. I then open the distal ends of the fallopian tube and perform a tuboscopy. If the tubal mucosa appears to be in relatively satisfactory condition, I conclude the procedure with hysteroscopy to inspect the tubal ostia, and I attempt to open the proximal segment by means of tubal cannulation. If unsuccessful, I then schedule the patient for salpingostomy and cornual anastomosis 2 months later. In a small series of six patients, two delivered successfully. Among a series of eight patients who underwent correction of bilateral bipolar blocks there were two pregnancies.[12]

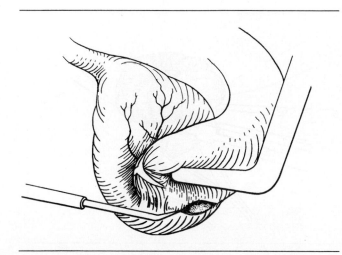

Figure 36–38. Mobilization of the distal end of a hydrosalpinx from the adjacent ovary. *(From Hunt RB (ed):* Atlas of Female Infertility Surgery. *St. Louis, Mosby, 1992.)*

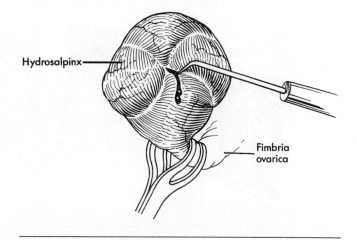

Figure 36–39. Stabilization of fimbria ovarica with a Babcock forceps, and opening of the distal tube with a microelectrode. A microscissors or laser may be used instead. *(From Hunt RB (ed):* Atlas of Female Infertility Surgery. *St. Louis, Mosby, 1992.)*

Hydrosalpinx

Fimbria ovarica

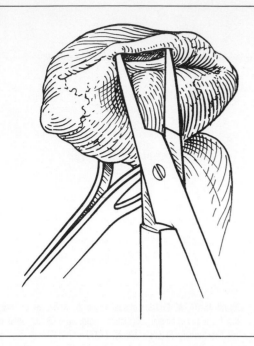

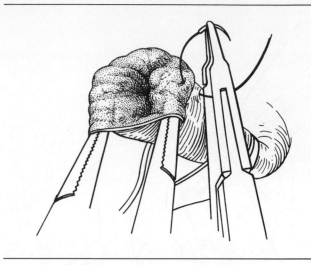

Figure 36–42. Fixation of mucosa to serosa with interrupted 6-0 sutures. *(From Hunt RB (ed):* Atlas of Female Infertility Surgery. *St. Louis, Mosby, 1992.)*

Figure 36–40. Enlargement of tubal opening with a fine hemostat. *(From Hunt RB (ed):* Atlas of Female Infertility Surgery. *St. Louis, Mosby, 1992.)*

RESULTS

Tubal Anastomosis

Cornual anastomosis has yielded excellent results. Among 43 women who underwent the procedure for reversal of sterilization, 26 (60%) achieved a pregnancy. There was one ectopic gestation.[13] Eighteen (64%) of 28 patients had term pregnancies after cornual anastomosis for mixed indications.[14] Among 48 patients who underwent the procedure for pathologic cornual occlusion, 27 (56%) had a term pregnancy. There were 3 (6%) ectopic pregnancies.[15] A series of 27 patients with pathologic cornual occlusion underwent microsurgical anastomosis. Of these 14 (53%) had viable pregnancies, and 3 (11%) had ectopic pregnancies.[16] I believe each patient with pathologic cornual occlusion should undergo an initial attempt, unless contraindicated, to establish patency by means of tubal cannulation guided with hysteroscopy or at the time of HSG.

Tubal anastomosis for reversal of a previous sterilization

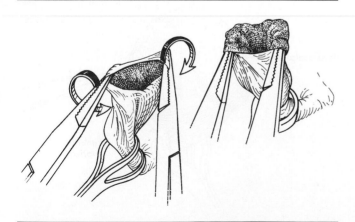

Figure 36–41. The mucosal flaps are grasped with fine hemostats and everted by means of rotation. *(From Hunt RB (ed):* Atlas of Female Infertility Surgery. *St. Louis, Mosby, 1992.)*

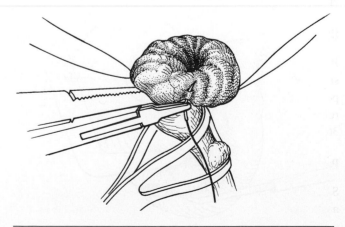

Figure 36–43. The process is continued until all mucosa is everted and fixed with sutures. *(From Hunt RB (ed):* Atlas of Female Infertility Surgery. *St. Louis, Mosby, 1992.)*

has superb overall results. Among 118 such patients, 93 (78.8%) patients achieved term pregnancies. Two (1.7%) experienced ectopic gestations.[15] Among 31 patients who underwent anastomosis to reverse previous sterilizations, 22 (71%) had intrauterine pregnancies; 19 (61%) delivered term infants.[17] Although none of these patients had ectopic pregnancies, the rate is generally thought to be approximately 5%.

Fimbrioplasty

Definitions of fimbrioplasty vary considerably. The word is sometimes used loosely to include correction of all distal tubal problems, including hydrosalpinges. Some series might include patients who undergo removal of adhesions from the fallopian tube that do not involve the fimbriae or patients with unilateral disease. Responsible reports should include only women with bilateral disease of the fimbriae or with an absent or inoperable opposite tube.

Among 130 patients who underwent fimbrioplasty and met the criteria just described, 39 (30.0%) achieved a term pregnancy. The rate of ectopic gestation was 3.2%.[18] Among 35 patients who underwent a procedure for disease that met the criteria, 21 (60%) achieved an intrauterine and 1 (3%) an ectopic pregnancy.[19,20]

ADHESION PREVENTION

Ischemia is a potent stimulus to intraabdominal adhesion formation.[21] All pelvic reconstructive procedures should be performed with this in mind. Another important fact is that peritoneal defects heal from the base and not from the edges.[22] Because of this valuable information, I discourage closure of peritoneal defects under tension, use of peritoneal grafts, and tying sutures tightly. In addition, several surgical procedures and therapeutic regimens have been devised to prevent postoperative adhesion formation.

Uterine Suspension

If the posterior cul-de-sac has been cleared of appreciable adhesions and the uterus is retroverted, the surgeon should consider performing a uterine suspension. I prefer triplication of the round ligaments, using No. 0 nonabsorbable material (Fig 36–44).

Peritoneal Platforms

Sometimes it is advisable to develop peritoneal platforms beneath each ovary after extensive adhesiolysis. I use 2-0 or 3-0 synthetic absorbable material (Fig 36–45). This procedure decreases the risk that the ovary will adhere to the pelvic side wall.

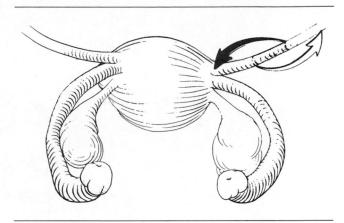

Figure 36–44. Triplication of round ligaments. *(From Hunt RB (ed):* Atlas of Female Infertility Surgery. *St. Louis, Mosby, 1992.)*

Omentopexy or Omentectomy

If the omentum is involved in extensive adhesions, the surgeon may remove the distal omentum or perform an omentopexy. The latter is reserved for patients with a relatively normal appearing omentum, and the former for those with a badly diseased one. If an omentectomy is performed, the surgeon must take care to ligate each omental artery individually to prevent postoperative hemorrhage (see Fig 36–15).

Irrigation

Saline solution produces edema of the fimbriae in the fallopian tubes of animals. Balanced salt solutions do not.[23] For this reason I use warm lactated Ringer's solution for irrigation; 5,000 U heparin is added to each liter of irrigant to prevent blood clots in the operative sites. Whereas blood clots alone do not produce adhesions, formation of clots in the presence of drying tissue does.[24] I leave 1 L of plain lactated Ringer's solution in the abdomen for hydroflotation at the conclusion of the procedure.

Steroids

In a controlled study, 2 g hydrocortisone was placed intraperitoneally after removal of ectopic pregnancies in one group of patients. Another second group received no steroids. A second-look laparoscopy 3 months later revealed fewer adhesions in the patients who received hydrocortisone.[25]

Although widely used at one time, steroids have not been shown in all animal studies to reduce the severity of adhesion.[26–28] The impetus for the use of steroids in North America came from a study in which dexamethasone and promethazine were used.[29] The study involved many different surgeons, institutions, and infertility operations and did not have a control group. The Horne regimen[29] consisted of 20 mg of dexametha-

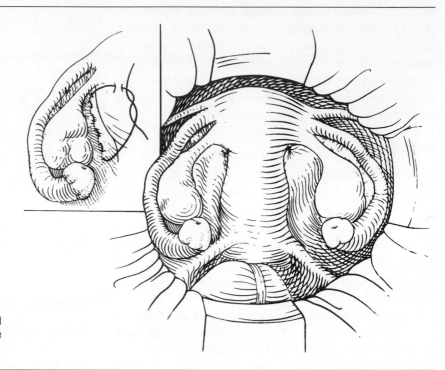

Figure 36–45. Placement of peritoneal platforms (inset) and appearance after placement. *(From Hunt RB (ed): Atlas of Female Infertility Surgery. St. Louis, Mosby, 1992.)*

sone and 25 mg of promethazine given intramuscularly preoperatively, intraperitoneally at completion of the operation, and every 4 hours intramuscularly for an additional 12 doses.

I use a modified Horne regimen that consists of 10 mg of dexamethasone and 12.5 mg of promethazine given intramuscularly preoperatively, intraperitoneally at the conclusion of the operation, and intramuscularly 4 hours postoperatively. Patients then receive seven additional doses orally every 4 hours.

High-Molecular-Weight Dextran

Intraperitoneal administration of high-molecular-weight dextran is used by some surgeons. Dextran has the ability to expand the volumes of intraperitoneal fluid by a factor of 5 to 1. If 100 mL of dextran is added to the intraperitoneal cavity at the completion of the operation, 500 mL results. This increase in volume produces hydroflotation, a desirable effect in prevention of adhesions. The regimen lessened adhesion formation in a multicenter study that included a control group.[30] Some surgeons believe dextran siliconizes peritoneal surfaces reducing risk for adhesions. High-molecular-weight dextran has not been approved for this use, however, and adverse reactions can occur. My colleagues and I have dropped dextran from use as a barrier to adhesions.

Antibiotics

Many surgeons use antibiotics in the perioperative period in reconstructive tubal operations. There has not been any proof that results are improved with this practice.[31] I administer 100 mg of doxycycline intravenously preoperatively and 100 mg postoperatively. The medication should be given in the antecubital vein if possible to prevent phlebitis. I usually continue doxycycline, 100 mg orally twice daily, until the patient is discharged.

Antiprostaglandins

Antiprostaglandins have been studied as possible adhesion preventives. The one that has received the most attention is ibuprofen. Results of animal studies have been inconsistent.[32] I do not use these agents.

Hydrotubation

One study showed a markedly improved pregnancy rate among patients who underwent multiple hydrotubations after salpingostomy.[33] This finding has not been reproduced by others, and most colleagues no longer use this practice.[31]

Barrier Methods

Several barrier methods to prevent adhesions have been developed. At this time, it is too early to determine effectiveness in prevention of adhesions in humans.[34]

Early Laparoscopy

Some surgeons have advocated that laparoscopy be performed as early as 8 days after adhesiolysis in the hope of separating postoperative adhesions before they have matured. One study showed a reduction in the rate of subsequent ectopic pregnancies but no increase in cumulative pregnancy rates when this practice was used.[35]

I previously performed laparoscopies 3 weeks after adhesiolysis for most patients. I no longer do this but recommend operative laparoscopy 12 to 18 months postoperatively, if indicated.

CONCLUSION

There have been enormous advances in the field of infertility. The most striking examples are IVF, gamete intrafallopian transfer (GIFT), ovulation induction methods, and medical therapy for endometriosis. Although not as sensational, evolutionary progress is being made in the surgical management of infertility. Examples are our better understanding of normal and abnormal peritoneal healing, judicious use of an operating microscope, and refinement of operative laparoscopic technique. We are proud of our contributions to reconstructive surgery for infertile women, but we are challenged by our failures. With continued assessment of these failures, our efforts, in concert with those of our colleagues in related fields, will result in a greater chance for infertile couples' ultimate goal—a healthy baby.

REFERENCES

1. Hulka JF: Adnexal adhesions: A prognostic staging and classification system based on a five-year survey of fertility surgery results at Chapel Hill, North Carolina. *Am J Obstet Gynecol* 144:141, 1982
2. Verhoeven HC, Berry H, Frantzen C, Schlosser HW: Surgical treatment for distal tubal occlusion. *J Reprod Med* 28:293, 1983
3. Henry-Suchet J, Testquiter L, Pez JP, Loffredo V: Prognostic value of tuboscopy vs hysterosalpingography before tuboplasty. *J Reprod Med* 29:609, 1984
4. Young PE, Egan JE, Barlow JJ, et al: Reconstructive surgery for infertility at the Boston Hospital for Women. *Am J Obstet Gynecol* 108:1092, 1970
5. Ozaras H: The value of plastic operations on the fallopian tubes in the treatment of female infertility. *Acta Obstet Gynecol Scand* 47:489, 1968
6. Musich JR, Behrman SJ: Surgical management of tubal obstruction at the uterotubal junction. *Fertil Steril* 40:423, 1983
7. Hunt RB (ed): *Atlas of Female Infertility Surgery.* Chicago, Year Book, 1986
8. Hunt RB: Informed consent for pelvic reconstructive surgery using the operating microscope and/or carbon dioxide laser. In: Hunt RB (ed), *Atlas of Female Infertility Surgery.* Chicago, Year Book, 1986:406–408
9. Hunt RB, Acuna HA: Pelvic preparation and choice of incision. In: Hunt RB (ed), *Atlas of Female Infertility Surgery.* Chicago, Year Book, 1986:125–142
10. Vasquez G, Winston RML, Boeckx W, Brosens I: Tubal lesions subsequent to sterilization and their relation to fertility after attempts at reversal: *Am J Obstet Gynecol* 138:86, 1980
11. Silva PD, Perkins HE: Improved combined laparoscopic and minilaparotomy technique to allow for reversal of extensive tubal sterilization. *J Am Assoc Gynecol Laparosc* 2:327, 1995
12. Hunt RB (ed): *Atlas of Female Infertility Surgery.* St. Louis, Mosby–Year Book, 1992
13. Winston RML: Reversal of tubal sterilization. *Clin Obstet Gynecol* 23:1261, 1980
14. Diamond E: A comparison of gross and microsurgical techniques for repair of cornual occlusion in infertility: A retrospective study, 1968–1978. *Fertil Steril* 32:370, 1979
15. Gomel V: An odyssey through the oviduct. *Fertil Steril* 39:144, 1983
16. Patton PE, Williams TJ, Coulam CB: Microsurgical reconstruction of the proximal oviduct. *Fertil Steril* 47:35, 1987
17. Hunt RB: Tubal anastomosis. In: Hunt RB (ed), *Atlas of Female Infertility Surgery.* Chicago, Year Book, 1986:265
18. Verhoeven HC, Hunt RB, Schlosser HW: Salpingostomy, fimbrioplasty, and adhesiolysis. In: Hunt RB, *Atlas of Female Infertility Surgery.* Chicago, Year Book, 1986:302
19. Patton GW Jr: Pregnancy outcome following microsurgical fimbrioplasty. *Fertil Steril* 37:150, 1982
20. Hunt RB, Cohen SM: Discussion of salpingostomy. In: Leventhal JM (ed), *Current Problems in Obstetrics, Gynecology and Fertility.* Vol 9. Chicago, Year Book, 1986:3
21. Ellis H: The cause and prevention of postoperative intraperitoneal adhesions. *Surg Gynecol Obstet* 133:497, 1971
22. Raftery AT: Regeneration of parietal and visceral peritoneum: An electron microscopical study. *J Anat* 115:375, 1973
23. Blandau RJ: Comparative aspects of tubal anatomy and physiology as they relate to reconstructive procedures. *J Reprod Med* 21:7, 1978
24. Ryan GB, Grobety J, Majno G: Postoperative peritoneal adhesions. *Am J Pathol* 65:117, 1971
25. Swolin K: Die Einwirkung von grossen, intraperitonealen Dosen Glukokortikoid auf die Bildung von postoperativen Adhäsionen. *Acta Obstet Gynecol Scand* 46:204, 1967
26. Liao S, Surhiro GT, McNamara JJ: Prevention of postoperative intestinal adhesions in primates. *Surg Gynecol Obstet* 137:816, 1973
27. Seitz HM Jr, Schenker JG, Epstein S, et al: Postoperative intraperitoneal adhesions: A double-blind assessment of their prevention in the monkey. *Fertil Steril* 24:935, 1973
28. diZerga GS, Hodgen GD: Prevention of postoperative tubal adhesions: Comparative study of commonly used agents. *Am J Obstet Gynecol* 136:173, 1980
29. Horne HW Jr, Clyman M, Debrovner C, et al: The prevention of postoperative pelvic adhesions following conservative operative treatment for human infertility. *Int J Fertil* 18:109, 1973
30. Adhesion Study Group: Reduction of postoperative pelvic adhesions with intraperitoneal 32% dextran 70: A prospective, randomized clinical trial. *Fertil Steril* 40:612, 1983

31. Hunt RB: Survey results. In: Hunt RB (ed), *Atlas of Female Infertility Surgery.* Chicago, Year Book, 1986:318–320

32. Holz G: Prevention and management of peritoneal adhesions. *Fertil Steril* 41:497, 1984

33. Grant A: Infertility surgery of the oviduct. *Fertil Steril* 22:496, 1971

34. Haney AF, Hesla J, Hurst BS, et al: Expanded polytetrafluoroethylene (Gore-Tex Surgical Membrane) is superior to oxidized cellulose (Interceed TC7) in preventing adhesions. *Fertil Steril* 63:1021, 1995

35. Trimbos-Kemper TCM, Trimbos JB, van Hall EV: Adhesion formation after tubal surgery: Results of the eight-day laparoscopy in 188 patients. *Fertil Steril* 43:395, 1985

CHAPTER 37

Laser Physics and Applications in Reproductive Medicine

YONA TADIR · MICHAEL W. BERNS

Physical Principles of Lasers
Laser-Tissue Interactions
Laser Safety
Lasers in Pelvic Reconstruction
Delivery Systems
Laser Laparoscopy
  Pelvic adhesiolysis
  Vaporization of endometriosis
  Terminal salpingostomy
  Uterosacral ligament ablation

Role of the Laser
  Tubal pregnancy
  Myomectomy
  Laser drilling
Hysteroscopic Laser Applications
Lasers in Micromanipulation
    of Gametes
  Sperm manipulations with optical trapping
  Oocyte manipulation: laser zona drilling (LZD)
    and laser-assisted hatching (LAH)
Photodynamic Therapy

The boundaries of laser applications in reproductive medicine expand rapidly. With the ongoing development of instruments and applications for minimally invasive therapy and assisted reproduction technology (ART), the range of laser treatments of women with infertility now spans a broad spectrum of applications.[1-3] This chapter describes the basic physics underlying lasers and laser-tissue interactions. Applications of lasers in pelvic reconstructive surgery and ART are reviewed, and progress in photodynamic therapy (PDT) as it relates to reproductive medicine is discussed.

PHYSICAL PRINCIPLES OF LASERS

Light is composed of packets of energy known as photons. Laser is an acronym for light amplification by the stimulated emission of radiation. Amplification by stimulated emission of radiation is the physical process that occurs within the laser tube. This physical process is discussed in more detail in the following section.

Light is an electromagnetic wave generated by atomic processes. The ground state for atoms represents their lowest state of energy, but atoms can be raised from this resting state to a higher energy level when they are excited with chemical, optical, or electrical energy. An excited atom quickly returns to its ground state and gives up its excess energy. This excess energy occurs in the form of the light particles called photons. The process is called *spontaneous emission of light.*

Laser light is coherent (parallel). Light from a light bulb radiates in all directions. As an observer walks away from it, the light becomes dimmer and dimmer; there is a direct mathematical relation between loss of light intensity and the distance of the observer from the source. In a laser, however, photons are emitted in parallel and in phase with each other—a property known as *coherence.*

Laser light is monochromatic (one wavelength, one color). Light emitted by a light bulb is white or yellowish white. It contains all colors and wavelengths in the visual portion of the electromagnetic spectrum and hence is polychromatic. In most cases, the number of photons in a laser beam is greater per unit area of emission than any other light source.

All light, regardless of its source, has four basic qualities: wavelength, frequency, velocity, and amplitude. *Wavelength,* the distance between two successive crests, determines the color of the light. By convention, a medical laser is referred to in terms of its wavelength in either nanometers (nm), micrometers (μm), or millimeters (mm). *Frequency,* expressed as cycles per second or hertz, is the number of waves passing a given point per second. Wavelength and frequency are inversely related. As wavelength increases or decreases, frequency decreases or increases. Higher frequencies (short wavelengths) such as cosmic, gamma, and x rays are high-energy waves. As such they are the most dangerous because, unlike laser light, they emit ionizing radiation, which disrupts molecular structure. *Velocity* is the speed of light, which is a constant. *Amplitude* is the height of the wave. The higher the wave, the greater is the power.

Although the details and purposes of lasers may vary greatly, their designs are similar. In discussions of different kinds of lasers, identification is made by the type of material inside the device that is going through the laser process (eg, ruby lasers, argon lasers, CO_2 lasers). The laser medium (gas, solid, or liquid) is contained in an optical cavity, or resonator, which is closed at both ends by mirrors. The optical axis of both mirrors coincides with the axis of the resonator. One end of the resonator has a pinhole through which the light produced exits as laser light. An exciting source (electrical, chemical, or mechanical) is applied to the atoms of the medium. The atoms are excited and spontaneously emit their photons in various directions. Many of these photons pass back and forth between the mirrors, hitting other excited atoms and stimulating them to release more photons—all with the same wavelength. Solid-state, diode-pumped lasers represent the latest developments in semiconductor technology. The diode laser is formed from a minute chip of gallium arsenide semiconductor material. It converts electricity to laser light with no mirrors.

Photons exit the pinhole as a beam of laser light, which can then be focused with a lens or a laser fiber to a finite spot. The spot size of the laser beam and its capability for adjustment are crucial to the application for which the laser is being used. Accordingly, when combined with other factors, laser energy produces different types of tissue interaction.

The three primary results of tissue interaction with lasers used for surgical applications are vaporization, excision, and coagulation. The power density of the laser beam determines the effects of the laser on tissue. Understanding the power density of a laser beam is the most important factor in effective use of any laser. The laser lens directs the energy of the laser beam

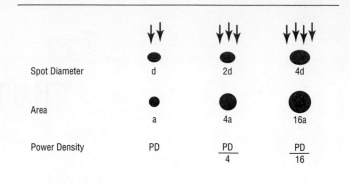

Figure 37–1. Power density as a function of spot size.

to a small spot (Fig 37–1). The concentration of energy per surface area of the spot is called its *power density* (or irradiance) expressed in W/cm^2. To determine approximate power density, clinicians use the following formula:

$$\text{Power density (PD)} = \frac{(\text{Power in watts}) \times 100}{(\text{Spot diameter in mm})^2} = W/cm^2$$

With an equal distribution of energy, the small spot size of the beam produces a greater concentration of energy per surface area and thus a greater power density than a large spot size. High power densities (small spot sizes) vaporize tissue layer by layer; however, if power density is too high, the depth of destruction is difficult to control. Low power densities (large spot sizes) are used to produce coagulation of tissue. The energy fluence of a laser beam consists of both power density and exposure time and is expressed as joules per unit surface area. One joule (J) equals 1 watt (W) times 1 second (s).

Lasers are generally operated in one of the following modes: continuous wave, pulsed, Q-switched, or mode-locked. In pelvic operations, a continuous-wave beam of constant power is usually used. In pulsed operation, pulsed pumping of the active medium results in relatively high-energy pulses at repetition rates from one to hundreds of pulses per second. The techniques of Q-switching and mode-locking often are used when pulses of extremely short duration are required.

LASER-TISSUE INTERACTIONS

The interaction of light with tissue can be described according to properties of absorption, reflection, scattering, and transmission.[4] For a laser to produce an effect on tissue, its beam must first be absorbed by the tissue. If it is transmitted through or reflected from tissue, the beam does not achieve its intended purpose. When light is scattered, it it absorbed over a broad area, diffusing its effects and possibly scattering light to places where it is not wanted (Fig 37–2). Other important considerations re-

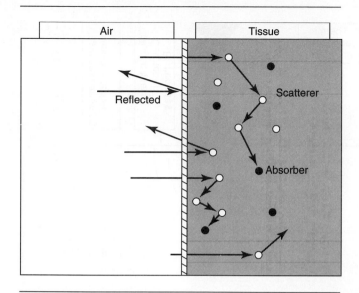

Figure 37–2. Light propagation through tissue. The photons are reflected, scattered, or absorbed.

garding laser tissue interactions include heat formation, photochemistry, photoablation, fluorescence, ionization, and plasma formation.

Absorption

The tissue molecules that absorb the light are usually referred to as *pigments*. Hemoglobin and water are two common body constituents that can function as pigments. Hemoglobin has a very high absorption in the violet and blue-green portions of the visible spectrum. Absorption declines in the red region of the spectrum, which is why hemoglobin is red (it does not absorb red light). This is the rationale for using an argon laser, which emits blue-green light for treating hemoglobin and hemosiderin containing lesions, such as endometriosis. Water, however, is absorbed maximally in the far infrared regions of the spectrum. Thus a carbon dioxide (CO_2) laser has a direct effect on any tissue in the body. A CO_2 laser removes cell layer by cell layer by votalizing the water. The selection of the correct laser for a particular clinical procedure requires an understanding of the absorptive as well as the reflective, scattering, and transmissive properties of the target tissue.

Heat

Laser light works primarily by causing molecular vibration, which produces heat. Controlling tissue heating is an important consideration for a laser surgeon. At 37°C to 60°C, tissue retracts, above 60°C there is protein denaturation and coagulation, from 90°C to 100°C carbonization and tissue burning occur. Above 100°C, the tissue is vaporized and ablated.[5] The physician should be able to stop the heating process at any one of

these thermal ranges to produce the desired clinical result. Moreover, for certain applications, such as ART, heat formation may be detrimental to gametes (in vivo or in vitro) and to sensitive organs such as the fallopian tubes (Fig 37–3).

Photochemistry

Certain molecules can function as photosensitizers. The presence of these photosensitizers in certain cells makes the cells vulnerable to light of an appropriate wavelength and intensity. The photosensitizers absorb the photons and are thereby elevated to an excited atomic state, subsequently reacting with a molecular substrate such as oxygen, producing singlet oxygen and causing irreversible oxidation of selected cellular components. This entire process occurs without the generation of heat. The most common clinical use of this process has been the management of cancer and precancerous tissue. Preliminary data suggest, however, that dysfunctional endometrial bleeding and endometriosis also may be treated. PDT is accomplished in a two-step procedure. The physician administers a photosensitizing agent either topically or intravenously. Once an optimal level in the target tissue is reached, the organ is illuminated with visible light tuned to 630 to 740 nm (depending on the photosensitizing agent). Photochemical changes induce cell necrosis within a few days through generation of highly reactive oxygen intermediates.

Fluorescence

Photon energy may be dissipated as the reemission of light. If this happens within 10^{-6} seconds after absorption, it is called *fluorescence*. Many of the photosensitizing dyes used to induce a photochemical reaction are fluorescent. This makes it possible for the physician to detect the cells containing the photosensitizer and, if needed, selectively damage these cells.

Photoablation

This tissue–laser light interaction can be described as breaking intermolecular bonds in polymeric chains. In this interaction, the tissue absorbs the high-energy ultraviolet photons that are produced by the excimer laser. The lasing material of the excimer laser is excited dimmers of unstable gases, usually a halogen and some rare elements. The ultraviolet photons generated by these lasers possess so much energy that they break apart molecular bonds before their energy can be dissipated as heat. The laser-treated tissue is reduced to its atomic constituents. Because ultraviolet radiation from 200 to 360 nm is well absorbed by most biologic tissue, the penetration depths are only a few microns with minimal thermal damage to adjacent tissue. Thus minimal thermal damage combines with the ability of excimer lasers to produce well-defined, nonthermal cuts. These effects can be used in assisted hatching.

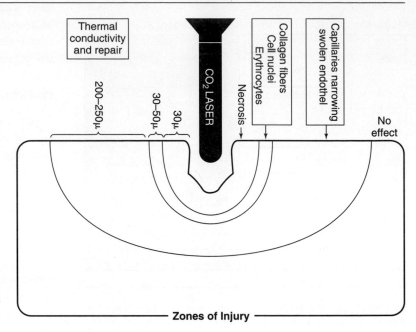

Figure 37-3. Zones of injury after exposure to CO₂ laser beam. (*Illustrated according to Ben-Bassat M, et al: A study of the ultrastructural features of the cut margin of skin and mucous membrane excised by carbon dioxide laser.* J Surg Res *21:77, 1976.*)

Ionization

Ionization is the ejection of an electron from an atom. It is generally believed that the individual photons generated from existing lasers do not have enough energy to cause the absorbing molecule to lose an electron. It is possible, however, to have absorption of more than one photon simultaneously in a multiphoton process.

Plasma Formation

Plasma formation is an effect that does not obey the basic laws of photobiology. With Q-switched (nanosecond) and short-pulsed (picosecond) lasers, it is possible to generate very high power densities (gigawatts/cm²) in focal spots of 25 to 50 microns. When these lasers are focused on a small spot of tissue, it is possible to generate a plasma that sometimes is referred to as the *fourth state of matter* because the properties of its gaseous cloud of free electrons are very different from those of solids, liquids, or gases. Because of the sudden production of an electrical field in 10^{-9} to 10^{-12} seconds, an intense acoustic shock wave is generated in the medium. At present, there are no clinical applications in reproductive medicine in which these effects are used.

LASER SAFETY

Unlike most standard surgical devices, a laser may harm surgeons and operating personnel as well as patients. Appropriate eye wear such as goggles with filters capable of protecting against the wavelength in use must be worn at all times. Oper-

ating room access must be controlled so that persons without appropriate eye wear do not enter. Surgical instruments in the field must be nonreflective, and operating room drapes must not be inflammable. Endotracheal tubes must either be metal or be wrapped with reflective tape to prevent ignition or melting.

Installation of a laser plume management system is a critical precaution. The system should be appropriate to the laser wavelength and clinical application, and it should always be used when the laser is in use. These systems are most typically called smoke evacuators and recirculation units. They are designed to remove effectively laser plume contaminants from the laser impact site to reduce risks of transmission of potentially hazardous particles to personnel in the room.[6]

LASERS IN PELVIC RECONSTRUCTION

Laser beams were introduced to gynecologic surgery in 1973.[7] Since then they have been used in minimally invasive therapy and used to study the physiologic aspects of reproduction. The incorporation of laser therapy is appealing because of its potential accuracy and high versatility. It was first introduced into pelvic reconstructive operations in the late 1970s and early 1980s, when the CO₂ laser (operating at 10,600 nm wavelength) was coupled to operative microscopes[8] and laparoscopes.[9,10] Later, specially designed rigid[11] and flexible[12] delivery systems for this laser, as well as other lasers (argon, operating at 540 nm[13]; neodymium: yttrium-aluminum-garnet [Nd:YAG], 1064 nm[14]; and frequency doubled [potassium titanyl phosphate, KTP, crystal] YAG at 532 nm[15] were developed and evaluated clinically. Further advancements in laser technology have introduced a large variety of other lasers in the ultraviolet, visible, or infrared range of the electromagnetic spectrum. These lasers are being assessed clinically and scientifically for various applications in reproductive medicine (Fig 37–4).

Numerous publications present conflicting data on the application of lasers in endoscopic surgery. Thus critical questions are being raised about the potential superiority of each of these lasers over conventional approaches.[16,17] Different criteria for patient selection, surgical skill, and personal bias could affect these data. There is no doubt that for certain applications, laser light may selectively interact with tissue (ie, pigmented endometriotic implants), cause minimal effect to surrounding tissue, and offer advantages over other techniques. However, most indications for operative laparoscopy can be managed without the use of a laser. An experienced endoscopist can take advantage of the special effects of the laser by alternating quickly between a small spot-size cutting beam and superficial vaporization by using a large spot or an electronically controlled laser beam scanner.[18] Some procedures can be performed by combining maneuvers of cutting and coagulation. This can be achieved with the use of contact fibers with different tip profiles or as the result of different tissue colors.[19] Controversies about the place of the laser in operative laparoscopy are anticipated, and one has to view the laser as an additional tool. In experienced hands a laser can offer advantages in properly selected indications.[20]

The incorporation of video equipment to endoscopic surgery contributed substantially to the increased interest in minimally invasive therapy.[21] The consequence in resolution dramatically enhanced the accuracy, and, therefore, the safety of this approach. The bright illuminating light used in endo-scopic surgery necessitated upgrading of the helium neon (He-Ne) aiming beam used with nonvisible lasers such as CO_2 and Nd:YAG. Concomitantly accuracy of CO_2 laser beam alignment, being delivered through long rigid tubes, enabled a reduction in the laser port of the laparoscope from the initial size of 8 mm to the currently available 5-mm channels.[22] Efficient use of an operative laser laparoscope requires direct coupling to the entire videoendoscopy unit in such a way that fast interchange from conventional accessories to the laser set-up does not require a waste of maneuvers and time.

DELIVERY SYSTEMS

A CO_2 laser, which is an ideal cutting and vaporization beam, is still the most commonly used laser in operative laparoscopy.[23] The beam is reflected by mirrors and is delivered mainly through a rigid set of tubes. Flexible hollow wave guides for CO_2 laser laparoscopy are available; however, for most indications, pelvic anatomy and surgical needs do not necessitate use of flexible instruments. Other lasers such as Nd:YAG, argon, and KTP are available for laparoscopic surgery. Various technical aspects that influence the development and the handling of these devices for laser endoscopy are described herein (Table 37–1).

CO_2 Laser

Laparoscopic application of the CO_2 laser through long and rigid channels requires lenses with 200 to 300 mm "back focal length" (BFL), which means a long focal depth. For example, if

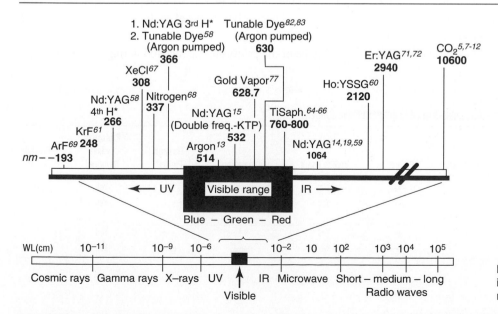

Figure 37–4. The electromagnetic spectrum. Lasers in clinical and experimental use in reproductive medicine. WL, wavelength; UV, ultraviolet; IR, infrared.

the minimum spot of the beam (at the focal point) after passing through the lens is about 1 mm in diameter, the beam remains relatively collimated 2 cm before and 2 cm behind the focal point with a diameter of approximately 1.1 mm. This means that power densities within the long range of the focal plane (which determine the effects of the laser beam on tissue) remain similar to those at the focal point.

To increase the effectiveness of a laser as a cutting and co-agulating tool, special lenses with different focal lengths are used. The distance between the lens and the focal point (the point where idealized light rays converge after passing through the lens) is termed the BFL.[24] The shorter the BFL of a given lens the smaller is the spot size (or waist) of a laser beam that passes through the lens and the smaller is the depth of focus. Depth of focus is defined as length along the beam direction of propagation where the laser beam possesses its smallest waist (for a given lens), and the beam is most collimated (ie, the beam of light in this region is neither diverging nor converging).

Indeed, one of the main advantages of the CO_2 laser is that varying the power density yields different effects on tissue. This is especially relevant in reproductive operations, in which minimizing heating and heat conductance prevents unwanted damage to adjacent tissues. The long focal length of the lenses used in rigid laser laparoscopes limits the achievable minimum spot size of the beam at the waist and results in lower power densities. In turn, using very low power densities can superficially ablate endometrial implants or cause serosal shrinkage needed for fimbrial eversion during salpingostomy.

Changes in power density can offer versatile tissue effects in this surgical modality. Minimal changes in power density can be obtained by means of sliding the lens in the endoscopic coupler (termed a *continuous variable defocus* [CVD] coupler). However, in view of the long BFL and the wide focal plane, these changes are minimal. A simple way to reduce power density is to reduce the power output of the laser source or move the joystick and reflect the beam on the inner cannula surface. The

emerging beam profile is crescent-shaped instead of round, but effects on tissue may be superficial as needed. Another innovative modality for superficial tissue ablation of relatively large areas (5 to 6 mm) with minimal thermal damage to the underlying layers is use of an electronic scanner.[18] When power output is reduced, superficial effects can safely be produced. This might be useful for procedures such as salpingostomy (Bruhat maneuver), ablation of endometriotic implants, and superficial ablation of the peritoneum over vital organs.

A CO_2 laser, unlike any other cutting tool, acts in noncontact mode. The lack of tactile feeling is unfamiliar to most surgeons and it takes some time to get used to. The collimated beam of light may cause damage to organs located behind the area treated with the laser. Several instruments and maneuvers protect against such damage. In general, these can be divided into mechanical and optical methods. Various types of rigid cannulas inserted at the suprapubic region usually contain a metal tongue at the distal end. This part is located behind the cutting area and prevents further delivery of the beam. Adding such a tongue to a single-puncture operative laparoscope is impossible because doing so may obstruct visibility. Several types of metal probes and hooks can be used as backstops when the beam is delivered through the operative laparoscope. Different tip profiles assist during tissue handling, and a channel for smoke evacuation is built into the device. It is important to note that in a single puncture operative laparoscope the laser port and the viewing lens are parallel to each other. When the target area is too close to the tip of the laser laparoscope the He-Ne aiming beam is invisible and activating the laser might cause damage to hidden organs.

Another way to protect deep pelvic organs from unwanted damage by a CO_2 laser beam is use of fluid that absorbs the light and acts as a backstop. This can be achieved as part of the on-going process of tissue irrigation or simply by application of the fluid at the lower pelvis, in the event that this is the area behind the dissected region.

One of the problems encountered during laser endoscopy

TABLE 37–1. EFFECTS AND TECHNICAL DETAILS OF VARIOUS LASERS USED IN REPRODUCTIVE SURGERY

Laser Type	Wattage (W)	Wavelength (μm)	Cutting*	Plume**	Visible Beam	Coagulation*	Through Fluids*	Protective Lenses Required	Flexible Fibers
CO_2	100	10.6	++++	++++	No	+	0	Yes	No[†]
Argon	20	0.458–0.515	++	++	Yes	++	+++	Yes	Yes
KTP	20	0.532	++	++	Yes	++	+++	Yes	Yes
Nd:YAG	20	1.064	+	+	No	++++	++++	Yes	Yes

*+, Possible; ++, good results; +++, very good; ++++, excellent.
**+–++++ (minimal–maximal).
[†]Flexible hollow wave guide.

is evacuation of the smoke produced during tissue vaporization without compromise of visibility and distention of the peritoneal cavity. Several methods can be used to allow smoke evacuation during laser laparoscopy: high-flow CO_2 gas insufflation; use of a synchronized laser-suction unit activated by the laser apparatus with preset suction delay; use of pressure valves designed to prevent the occurrence of excess pressure during high gas inflow; and use of a closed circuit of pumped, plastic tubing and filters that allows continuous filtration at high flow under constant gas pressure. Ports for smoke evacuation are a suction-irrigation probe that can be used as a backstop and smoke evacuator and a double channel in the second puncture probe.

Optical fibers made of silver halide crystals are capable of transmitting CO_2 laser energy.[25] Although transmission losses at low power levels are minimal, some limitations such as low flexibility, low cutting effects and high cost have prevented clinical use of flexible fiber optics in gynecologic endoscopy. When CO_2 gas is used for pneumoperitoneum, higher powers of CO_2 laser induce high gas temperatures that produce a larger spot size by means of an effect defined as *blooming*. This effect of the laser beam reduces power density at tissue and eliminates the pinpoint spot size needed for microdissection.[22,26] Clinically, this effect results in optimal cutting (vaporization) at low power settings and coagulation accompanying cutting at higher settings.

Flexible hollow wave guides for CO_2 laser laparoscopy are available.[27] However, pelvic anatomy and satisfactory organ visibility allow workable laser transmission through rigid wave guides.[28] Such probes allow the passage of the CO_2 laser beam via standard laparoscopes.

The principles of reconstructive microsurgical procedures on the pelvic organs (careful tissue handling and continuous irrigation) are relevant to laparoscopic surgical procedures. Suction irrigation probes were available before the era of laser laparoscopy. However, the increased need for fluid and smoke evacuation during laser operation necessitate instrument modifications such as surface abrasion (to prevent laser reflection), a variety of probe diameters, easy valve manipulation, and a dedicated port for fiber insertion (for visible and near infrared lasers). The correct handling of these multipurpose devices is important during laser laparoscopy, especially because they may also serve as backstops.

Nd:YAG, KTP, and Argon Lasers

Delivery of these laser beams (and others such as holmium:YAG, argon pumped dye, flash lamp pumped dye, and more) via optical fibers makes them potentially ideal energy sources for flexible endoscopy. Current technology in laser laparoscopy is based mainly on direct thermal effects on the target area. Some differences between such thermal systems exist. For example, Nd:YAG laser, which is in the near infrared range, is poorly absorbed by water and causes deep coagulating effects. However, when conical sculpted tips are used in a contact mode, cutting effects can become predominant. KTP laser (in which the Nd:YAG frequency is doubled by a potassium titanyl phosphate crystal, emitting at 532 nm) and argon laser (wavelengths 488 to 514 nm) fall in the visible range of the spectrum. Their absorption in water is poor, and tissue penetration is relatively high. However, because of its strong interaction with absorption centers embedded in the tissue (such as small pigmented endometrial implants), a continuous wave argon laser is useful in applications in which selective ablation is required. The KTP laser, operating at a similar wavelength but with higher power and in the pulsed mode, is a more efficient cutting tool.

For certain procedures, advantages of the Nd:YAG over the CO_2 laser include deeper penetration, improved hemostasis, and decreased plume formation. Effective transmission through fluids may be an advantage or a disadvantage depending on the type of procedure performed. The main disadvantages of Nd:YAG systems (compared with a CO_2 laser) are (1) the extent of tissue damage (similar to electrocautery), which may be critical in some areas (such as damage to the fallopian tube during a reconstructive procedure), and (2) the need for disposable fibers. Other lasers in the ultraviolet range such as xenon-chloride (XeCl) (308 nm) or nitrogen (337 nm), visible range such as the flash lamp dye (504/590 nm), infrared range such as Holmium: Yttrium Scandium Gallium Garnet (Ho:YSSG) (2120 nm) or erbium:YAG (2940 nm), and diode lasers in the visible and infrared range are available for clinical evaluation. Each of these lasers has different effects on tissue and may offer some advantages for specific applications. It is beyond the scope of this chapter to compare or evaluate all these new devices; however, it is expected that some of them will be used in the future when appropriate delivery systems are developed.

LASER LAPAROSCOPY: DELIVERY SYSTEMS, SURGICAL TECHNIQUES, AND CLINICAL APPLICATIONS

Almost all the pelvic reconstructive procedures that were performed with conventional or microsurgical techniques can be performed with a laparoscope. However, pregnancy rates may vary, and proper patient selection is still the most important factor in predicting outcome. If laser laparoscopy is performed, the instrument should be connected to a video system.[21] The final decision whether to use electrosurgical or laser techniques depends on the type and location of the diagnosed pathologic condition and the surgeon's expertise. Experienced surgeons are us-mass, adnexal pain, pregnancy-related symptoms, nausea, vomiting, breast tenderness, dizziness, shoulder pain, and passage of tissue. In addition, patients with ruptured ectopic pregnancies can experience syncope and hemorrhagic shock. Fortunately, as examination for and recognition of ectopic pregnancy have advanced over the last several decades, the ratio of ruptured to unruptured ectopic gestations at the time of diagnosis has decreased. However, it is important to realize that the patient population may alter the likely presenting symptom complex. In a 1994 report,[19] it was identified that among patients with nonemergency cases of ectopic pregnancy a patient who does not receive care at an infertility practice is more likely to have symptoms of pain and vaginal bleeding than a patient of an infertility practice, in spite of treatment by the same attending physicians. This may be the result of earlier testing initiated by women eager to identify whether they have been able to conceive.

Laboratory Studies

Tests used to diagnose ectopic pregnancies suggested at history and physical examination are shown in Table 38–4. The diagnoses that must be differentiated with these tests include a persistent corpus luteum (ruptured or unruptured), intrauterine pregnancy (viable gestation versus complete, incomplete, or threatened abortion), endometriosis, PID, degenerating fibroid,

appendicitis, adnexal torsion, and kidney stones. In addition, one of the most difficult diagnoses to make is a heterotopic pregnancy, in which one gestation may be a normal, viable intrauterine pregnancy and the other is an ectopic eccyesis. Although once extremely infrequent, this entity has increased in prevalence because of the increased use of fertility drugs.

Both urine and serum pregnancy tests are available. In the emergency department, urine tests are most frequently performed because the results can be available in minutes. Some tests are sensitive to human chorionic gonadotropin (hCG) levels as low as 50 IU/L, making the likelihood very small that a clinically significant ectopic pregnancy would not be identified. False-negative results can occur, however, because of dilution or the presence of an older ectopic pregnancy that is outgrowing its blood supply and thus making only small amounts of hCG. Both positive and negative results in clinically suspicious situations should be followed by acquisition of a serum sample to determine the level of the β subunit of hCG (β-hCG). In the future, it may be possible to assess a free β-subunit level (which is identifiable 3 to 4 weeks after conception[20]) or modifications of the β-hCG molecule to improve the discriminatory capability for ectopic pregnancy.

Probably the most common test used to identify the presence of an early pregnancy, its location, and its well-being is measurement of serum β-hCG levels. Titers of β-hCG are identifiable in serum beginning approximately 1 week after ovulation and continue to rise until approximately 10 menstrual weeks, at which time the mean level is 100,000 IU/L[21] (Fig 38–3). The false-negative rate (failure to identify an ectopic pregnancy) with this test was reported to be zero among 234 women with suspected ectopic gestations.[22] Among these women, 188 had negative pregnancy tests, and subsequent laparoscopy or laparotomy was avoided by 149 women. Women with positive pregnancy tests can be placed in a high-likelihood group and undergo further assessment to determine the location of the pregnancy.

In the past when the serum β-hCG level in our laboratory exceeded 6500 IU/L, abdominal pelvic ultrasound examination was used to identify the presence of an intrauterine pregnancy. In a series of 383 women with suspected ectopic pregnancies, lack of an intrauterine gestational sac with a β-hCG titer greater than 6500 IU/L was indicative of an ectopic pregnancy.[23] This test had 100% sensitivity and 86% positive predictive value. Although the precise level of β-hCG might vary from laboratory to laboratory, in our practice a patient with a possible ectopic pregnancy with a β-hCG level greater than 6500 IU/L and no intrauterine gestational sac was considered to have an ectopic pregnancy until proved otherwise. Such women should undergo laparoscopy for diagnosis.

For women with a suspected ectopic pregnancy but a β-hCG titer less than 6500 IU/L whose condition is clinically sta-

TABLE 38–4. DIAGNOSING ECTOPIC PREGNANCIES BY HISTORY AND PHYSICAL EXAMINATION

Sampling Period	No. of Patients	Doubling Time (days)
10–22 days after BBT nadir	57	1.4
11–21 days after administration of hCG	7[a]	1.7
11–32 days after insemination	27	1.9
0–20 days after detection of hCG	4	2.0
29–64 days after LMP	26	2.0
12–30 days after BBT shift	189	2.2
28–60 days after LMP	20	3.3
28–60 days after LMP	57	3.5[b]
13–20 days after BBT shift	18	1.5
13–25 days after BBT shift	26	1.9
13–30 days after BBT shift	30	2.2
13–39 days after BBT shift	35	2.7
28–35 days after LMP	17	1.4
28–42 days after LMP	35	2.2
28–49 days after LMP	40	2.5
28–56 days after LMP	42	2.9

BBT, basal body temperature; LMP, last menstrual period.
[a]One spontaneous abortion.
[b]Calculated from the author's data.
Modified from Pittaway DE, Reish RL, Wentz AC: Doubling times of human chorionic gonadotropin increase in early viable intrauterine pregnancies. Am J Obstet Gynecol 152:299, 1985.

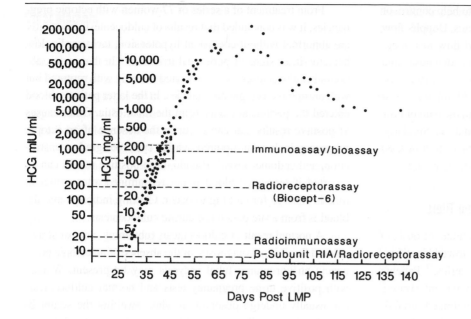

Figure 38–3. Limits of detection of blood and urine pregnancy tests. (*From Batzer FR: Hormonal evaluation of early pregnancy. Fertil Steril 34:1, 1980. Reprinted with permission of the publisher, The American Fertility Society.*)

ble, observation is appropriate. This includes serial determination of β-hCG level.[24-27] If with serial levels the titer exceeds 6500 IU/L, ultrasonography is performed to identify whether the pregnancy is intrauterine. The doubling time has been said to take 2 days, although ranges of 1.4 to 3.5 days have been identified (Table 38–5).[26] This variability may reflect the gestational age at which the observations are made or the viability of the developing embryo. In addition, it may reflect sampling bias, since peaks in serum β-hCG levels can be identified at 2- to 4-hour intervals.[28]

Ultrasonography

Ultrasound identification of an ectopic pregnancy has been most commonly performed with transvaginal ultrasonography.[29] Because transvaginal scanning allows close approximation of the ultrasound transducer to the posterior cul-de-sac, where the tubes are normally positioned, use of a higher frequency transducer is possible, thus providing greater resolution capability. As a result, it should now be possible to identify an ectopic gestation at transvaginal ultrasonography by the time the β-hCG titer reaches 3000 IU/L. (The clinician must remember that the absolute value of β-hCG for the discriminatory zone varies with the assay and the standard being used as well as with the quality and expertise of the ultrasound service.) With transvaginal scanning, sacs have been identified in the uterine cavity with β-hCG titers as low as 1000 IU/L and only 5 weeks from the date of the last menstrual period. However, in view of an expected doubling time of approximately 2 days when the β-hCG titers approximate the transabdominal and transvaginal discriminatory zones, a gain of only about 48 hours is achieved. Perhaps of equal or greater importance than the early detection of an intrauterine pregnancy is the greater likelihood of being able to identify an adnexal mass consistent with an ectopic pregnancy at transvaginal scanning.[30]

If the operator is experienced, Doppler flow studies of in-

TABLE 38–5. DOUBLING TIMES OF HUMAN CHORIONIC GONADOTROPIN IN EARLY PREGNANCY

Sampling Period (days)	No. of Patients	Doubling Time (days)
10–22 after BBT nadir	57	1.4
11–21 after administration of hCG	7[a]	1.7
11–32 after insemination	27	1.9
0–20 after detection of hCG	4	2.0
29–64 after LMP	26	2.0
12–30 after BBT shift	189	2.2
28–60 after LMP	20	3.3
28–60 after LMP	57	3.5[b]
13–20 after BBT shift	18	1.5
13–25 after BBT shift	26	1.9
13–30 after BBT shift	30	2.2
13–39 after BBT shift	35	2.7
28–35 after LMP	17	1.4
28–42 after LMP	35	2.2
28–49 after LMP	40	2.5
28–56 after LMP	42	2.9

BBT, basal body temperature; LMP, last mentrual period.
[a]One spontaneous abortion.
[b]Calculated from the authors' data.
From Pittaway DE, Reish RL, Wentz AC: Doubling times of human chorionic gonadotropin increase in early viable intrauterine pregnancies. Am J Obstet Gynecol 152:299, 1985.

into the myometrium perhaps predispose to subsequent cornual rupture. The likelihood of this occurrence depends in part on the amount of cornual tissue resected. It is our clinical practice to make only a very small cornual resection, 2 to 3 mm, if at all.

SUMMARY

Since the 1960s advances in the diagnosis of ectopic pregnancy have been achieved through the serial measurement of β-hCG levels and vaginal ultrasonography. Other techniques, including Doppler flow ultrasonography, are promising for continuing advances in the ability to identify ectopic pregnancies at an early gestational age before extensive tubal damage occurs. Great advances also have been made in the management of ectopic pregnancy. In contrast to radical procedures involving salpingectomy or salpingo-oophorectomy, many surgeons now perform conservative surgical procedures such as linear salpingostomy and segmental resection. Many of these procedures are performed at the time of laparoscopy rather than necessitating a laparotomy. Some surgeons now use chemotherapeutic agents such as methotrexate as initial therapy for an ectopic pregnancy, sometimes without performing laparoscopy to confirm the presumptive diagnosis of an ectopic pregnancy. Use of agents that impair ovarian steroidogenesis may be useful for nonsurgical management of ectopic pregnancies.

REFERENCES

1. Dorfman SF: Deaths from ectopic pregnancy, United States, 1979 to 1980. *Obstet Gynecol* 62:334, 1983
2. Dorfman SF, Grimes DA, Cates W, et al: Ectopic pregnancy mortality, United States, 1979 to 1980: Clinical aspects. *Obstet Gynecol* 64:386, 1984
3. Centers for Disease Control: Ectopic pregnancies, United States, 1970-1980. *MMWR Morb Mortal Wkly Rep* 33:2327, 1984
4. Mattingly RF: Ectopic pregnancy. In: TeLinde R (ed), *Operative Gynecology*, ed 5. Philadelphia, Lippincott, 1977:369
5. Westrom L: Effect of acute pelvic inflammatory disease on fertility. *Am J Obstet Gynecol* 121:707, 1975
6. Westrom L, Benatsson LH, Mardl PA: Incidence, trends, and risks of ectopic pregnancy in a population of women. *Br Med J* 282:15, 1981
7. Svensson L, Mardl P-A, Ahlgren M, Nordenskjold F: Ectopic pregnancy and antibodies to *Chlamydia trachomatis*. *Fertil Steril* 44:313, 1985
8. Brunham RC, Binns B, McDowell J, Paraskevas M: *Chlamydia trachomatis* infection in women with ectopic pregnancy. *Obstet Gynecol* 67:722, 1986
9. Ory HW, Women's Health Study: Ectopic pregnancy and intrauterine contraceptive devices: New perspective. *Obstet Gynecol* 57:137, 1981

10. Lavy G, Diamond MP, DeCherney AH: Ectopic pregnancy: Its relationship to tubal reconstructive surgery. *Fertil Steril* 47:543, 1987
11. Neumann HH, DeCherney A: Douching and pelvic inflammatory disease (letter). *N Engl J Med* 295:789, 1976
12. Chow W-H, Daling JR, Weiss NS, Moore DE, Soderstrom R: Vaginal douching as a potential risk factor for tubal ectopic pregnancy. *Am J Obstet Gynecol* 153:727, 1985
13. DeCherney AH, Cholst I, Naftolin F: Structure and function of the fallopian tubes following exposure to diethylstilbestrol (DES) during gestation. *Fertil Steril* 36:741, 1981
14. Majmudar B, Henderson PH, Semple E: Salpingitis isthmica nodosa: A high-risk factor for tubal pregnancy. *Obstet Gynecol* 62:73, 1983
15. Daling JR, Chow HW, Weiss NS, Metch BJ, Sodersom S: Ectopic pregnancy in relation to previous induced abortion. *JAMA* 253:1005, 1985
16. Russell JB: The etiology of ectopic pregnancy. *Clin Obstet Gynecol* 30:181, 1987
17. Shapiro BS, Diamond MP, DeCherney AH: Salpingoscopy: An adjunctive technique for evaluation of the fallopian tube. *Fertil Steril* 49:1076, 1988
18. Hershlag A, Diamond MP, DeCherney AH: Tubal physiology: An appraisal. *J Gynecol Surg* 5:3, 1989
19. Diamond MP, Wiser-Estin M, Jones EE, DeCherney AH: Failure of standard criteria to diagnose non-emergent ectopic pregnancies in a non-infertility patient population. *J Am Assoc Gynecol Laparosc* 1:131, 1994
20. Cole LA, Restrepo-Candelo H, Lavy G, DeCherney AH: HCG free β-subunit as marker of outcome of in vitro fertilization clinical pregnancies. *J Clin Endocrinol Metab* 64:1328, 1987
21. Batzer FR: Hormonal evaluation of early pregnancy. *Fertil Steril* 34:1, 1980
22. Schwartz RO, DiPietro DL: β-hCG as a diagnostic aid for suspected ectopic pregnancy. *Obstet Gynecol* 56:2, 1980
23. Romero R, Kadar N, Jeanty P, et al: Diagnosis of ectopic pregnancy: Value of the discriminatory human chorionic gonadotropin zone. *Obstet Gynecol* 66:357, 1985
24. Cartwright PS, DiPietro DL: Ectopic pregnancy: Changes in serum human chorionic gonadotropin concentration. *Obstet Gynecol* 63:76, 1984
25. Holman JF, Tyrey EL, Hammond CB: A contemporary approach to suspected ectopic pregnancy with use of quantitative and qualitative assays for the β-subunit of human chorionic gonadotropin and sonography. *Am J Obstet Gynecol* 150:151, 1984
26. Pittaway DE, Reish RL, Wentz AC: Doubling times of human chorionic gonadotropin increase in early viable intrauterine pregnancies. *Am J Obstet Gynecol* 152:299, 1985
27. Romero R, Kadar N, Copel JA, et al: The value of serial human chorionic gonadotropin testing as a diagnostic tool in ectopic pregnancy. *Am J Obstet Gynecol* 155:392, 1986
28. Owens OM, Ryan K, Tulchinsky D: Episodic secretion of human chorionic gonadotropin in early pregnancy. *J Clin Endocrinol Metab* 53:1307, 1971
29. Diamond MP, DeCherney AH: Distal segment tubal ectopic pregnancy after segmental resection for an isthmic ectopic. *J Reprod Med* 33:236, 1988

30. Shapiro BS: The nonsurgical management of ectopic pregnancy. *Clin Obstet Gynecol* 30:230, 1987

31. Estin MW, DeCherney AH, Diamond MP: Perils in the differentiation of a viable intrauterine pregnancy (IUP) from an ectopic eccyesis. *Gynecol Endosc* 2:223, 1994

32. Cartwright PS, Vaughn B, Tuttle D: Culdocentesis and ectopic pregnancy. *J Reprod Med* 29:89, 1984

33. Romero R, Copel JA, Kadar N, et al: Value of culdocentesis in the diagnosis of ectopic pregnancy. *Obstet Gynecol* 65:519, 1985

34. Matthews CP, Coulson PB, Wild RA: Serum progesterone levels as an aid in the diagnosis of ectopic pregnancy. *Obstet Gynecol* 68:390, 1986

35. Seppala M, Purhonen M: The use of HCG and other pregnancy proteins in the diagnosis of ectopic pregnancy. *Clin Obstet Gynecol* 30:148, 1987

36. Budowick M, Johnson TRB Jr, Gendry R, Parmley TH, Woodruff JD: The histopathology of the developing tubal ectopic pregnancy. *Fertil Steril* 34:169, 1980

37. Boyers SP, DeCherney AH: Isthmic ectopic pregnancy: Segmental resection as treatment of choice. *Fertil Steril* 44:307, 1985

38. Timonen S, Nieminen U: Tubal pregnancy, choice of operative method of treatment. *Acta Obstet Gynecol Scand* 46:327, 1967

39. Sherman D, Langer R, Herman A, Bukovsky I, Caspi E: Reproductive outcome after fimbrial evacuation of tubal pregnancy. *Fertil Steril* 47:420, 1987

40. DeCherney AH, Kase N: The conservative surgical management of unruptured ectopic pregnancy. *Obstet Gynecol* 54:451, 1979

41. DeCherney AH, Maheaux R, Naftolin F: Salpingostomy for ectopic pregnancy in the sole patent oviduct: Reproductive outcome. *Fertil Steril* 37:619, 1982

42. Oelsner G, Rabinovitch O, Morad J, Mashiach S, Serr DM: Reproductive outcome after microsurgical treatment of tubal pregnancy in women with a single fallopian tube. *J Reprod Med* 31:485, 1986

43. DeCherney AH, Diamond MP: Pregnancy following laparoscopic linear salpingostomy. *Obstet Gynecol* 70:948, 1987

44. Pouly JL, Mahnes H, Mage G, Canis M, Bruhat MA: Conservative laparoscopic treatment of 321 ectopic pregnancies. *Fertil Steril* 46:1093, 1986

45. Cartwright PS, Herbert CM III, Maxsom WS: Operative laparoscopy for the management of tubal pregnancy. *J Reprod Med* 31:589, 1986

46. DeCherney AH, Silidker JS, Mezer HC, Tarlatzis BC: Reproductive outcome following two ectopic pregnancies. *Fertil Steril* 43:82, 1985

47. Seifer DB, Silva PD, Grainger DA, Barber SR, Grant WD, Gutmann JM: Reproductive potential after treatment for persistent ectopic pregnancy. *Fertil Steril* 62:194, 1994

48. Seifer DB, Gutmann JN, Doyle MB, Jones EE, Diamond MP, DeCherney AH: Persistent ectopic pregnancy following laparoscopic linear salpingostomy obstetrics and gynecology. *Obstet Gynecol* 76:1121, 1990

49. Holtz G: Human chorionic gonadotropin regression following conservative surgical management of tubal pregnancy. *Am J Obstet Gynecol* 147:347, 1983

50. Kamrava MM, Taymor ML, Berger MJ, Thompson IE, Seibel MM: Disappearance of human chorionic gonadotropin following removal of ectopic pregnancy. *Obstet Gynecol* 62:486, 1983

51. Korhonen J, Stenman U-H, Ylöstälo P: Serum human chorionic gonadotropin dynamics during spontaneous resolution of ectopic pregnancy. *Fertil Steril* 61:632, 1994

52. Goldstein DP: Medical treatment of ectopic pregnancy. In: Seibel MM, Kiessling AA, Berstein J, Kevin SR (eds), *Technology and Infertility: Clinical, Psychosocial, Legal, and Ethical Aspects.* New York, Springer-Verlag, 1993:171

53. Tanaka T, Hayashi H, Kutsuzawa T, Fujimoto S, Ichinoe K: Treatment of interstitial ectopic pregnancy with methotrexate: Report of a successful case. *Fertil Steril* 37:851, 1982

54. Stovall TG, Ling FW: Some new approaches to ectopic pregnancy. *Contemp Ob/Gyn* 1992

55. Stovall TG, Ling FW, Gray LA, Carson SA, Buster JE: Methotrexate treatment of unruptured ectopic pregnancy: A report of 100 cases. *Obstet Gynecol* 77:749, 1991

56. Brown DL, Felker RE, Stovall TG, et al: Serial endovaginal sonography of ectopic pregnancies treated with methotrexate. *Obstet Gynecol* 77:406, 1991

57. Diamond MP, DeCherney AH: Surgical techniques in the management of ectopic pregnancy. *Clin Obstet Gynecol* 30:200, 1987

CHAPTER 39

Pelvic Adhesions and Infertility

CHARLA M. BLACKER · MICHAEL P. DIAMOND

Diagnosis
Pathophysiologic Process of
    Adhesion Formation
Prevention of Adhesions
Adjuvants for Adhesion Reduction
    Glucocorticoids, antihistamines, and
    nonsteroidal antiinflammatory
    agents

Nonsteroidal antiinflammatory agents
Anticoagulants
Fibrinolytic agents
Antibiotics
Calcium channel blockers
Mechanical barriers
Second-look laparoscopy
Conclusion

Adhesion reformation remains the most important unifying problem facing reproductive surgeons. Postoperative adhesions form after virtually every transperitoneal operation. The adhesions range from minimal scarring on the serosal surface to dense agglutination of nearly all structures. Adhesions are an important cause of failed surgical therapy. The economic consequences of the morbidity caused by adhesions has only recently been realized. In 1988, there were 281,982 hospitalizations in the United States during which lysis of adhesions was performed. According to one estimate, these hospitalizations were responsible for $1,179.9 million in medical costs.[1] However, even this number represents a gross underestimation. Such an estimate does not include outpatient and indirect costs such as time lost from work and loss of function as a result of chronic disability. It also does not include subsequent cost of treatment of adhesion-related infertility and pelvic pain.

Pelvic adhesive disease has been implicated in the causation of as many as 15% to 20% of cases of infertility. Presumably, fertility is impaired by adhesions that interfere with gamete transport or with ovum pick up secondary to altered spatial relation between the tube and ovary. The extent of in-

terference with fertility depends on the cause, extent, and thickness of the adhesions and the structures involved. Often there is associated pelvic disease such as endometriosis and tubal damage. Caspi et al[2] reported an inverse relation between grade of periadnexal adhesions and pregnancy rate in a study in which 101 patients undergoing reconstructive tubal operations for infertility participated. For a subgroup of 42 patients whose only identifiable lesion was periadnexal adhesions, salpingolysis was performed. Subsequent pregnancy rates were inversely related to adhesion grade before adhesiolysis. After adhesiolysis, patients with grade 1 adhesions had a pregnancy rate of 71.4% versus 20% in women with grade 4 adhesive disease.[2]

Because pelvic adhesive disease is an important issue for gynecologic surgeons, it is imperative that surgeons develop strategies to reduce postoperative development of adhesions, which includes both de novo adhesion formation and adhesion re-formation. This chapter presents our understanding of the pathogenesis of postoperative adhesion development and surgical techniques and adjuvant therapies currently used in attempts to eliminate development of adhesions.

DIAGNOSIS

There are currently no accurate noninvasive modalities for identification of pelvic adhesive disease. Hysterosalpingography (HSG) provides information about tubal patency and rugal patterns, but it allows only indirect assessment of adnexal adhesions. Retained contrast material on delayed images or loculation of contrast material may suggest peritubal adhesions; however, false-positive findings are not infrequent. Likewise, sonography, even when complemented by transuterine fluid instillation, may demonstrate echolucent pelvic loculations from adhesive disease, but does not depict abnormalities in most patients with pelvic adhesions. This means of identifying adhesions would be particularly inaccurate in the presence of cohesive adhesions (in which one structure is intimately attached to another without any intervening adhesive band), in which case there would be no space for loculation to occur. Thus, diagnosing intraperitoneal pelvic adhesions with certainty requires either laparoscopy or laparotomy.

Several scoring systems have been proposed for classification of pelvic adhesions. In 1982 Hulka[3] described a prognostic classification system based on a 5-year retrospective survey of the outcome of fertility operations at his institution. Two primary factors emerged: the extent of ovarian involvement and the nature (filmy or dense) of the adhesions before adhesiolysis. With this system the poorest prognoses for achievement of a spontaneous pregnancy occurred among patients with less than 50% of the ovarian surface visible at laparoscopy and those with adhesions classified as thick.[3]

The American Fertility Society (AFS) classification scheme is a modification of the scheme for adnexal adhesions provided in the Revised AFS Classification of Endometriosis (Fig 39–1). This scheme emphasizes the importance of the fimbriated ends of the fallopian tubes and bases the prognosis for conception on the score of the adnexa with the lease extensive abnormalities. The score is highly weighted to differentiate filmy from dense adhesions and does not incorporate cohesive adhesions.[4] In a 1994 report, the extent of interobserver variation in adhesion scores was assessed by review of 13 video tapes by 11 experienced gynecologic surgeons.[5] A statistically significant correlation did exist between the grading of video tapes by the surgeons; however, the degree of concordance was markedly improved with expansion of the number of sites specified within the pelvis (Fig 39–2).

Unfortunately, none of the scoring systems in use has been validated, so interpretation of research findings related to adhesion formation and prevention is difficult. Furthermore, even though a study may demonstrate a change in an adhesion score as assessed at the time of a second-look procedure, it may not reflect a true clinical difference in the extent of adhesive disease. In an attempt to address this important issue, a preliminary report was presented in which surgeons were asked their opinion on the contribution of adhesions to infertility and pelvic pain.[6,7] For each of these end points, even small reductions in numbers of adhesions was thought likely to have a statistically significant effect on improvement in fertility outcome or reduction of pelvic pain.

PATHOPHYSIOLOGIC PROCESS OF ADHESION FORMATION

Factors in the development of peritoneal adhesions can be classified into a limited number of causes—previous surgical trauma, infection, and inflammatory processes such as endometriosis or foreign-body reactions.

Adhesion formation represents an aberrant reaction to the normal healing process. To understand the pathogenesis of these aberrations, we must first understand the physiologic processes in the normal healing process. Unfortunately, our knowledge of these processes is very limited. After peritoneal injury, the microvasculature beneath the mesothelium becomes disrupted and releases vasoactive kinins and histamine. This produces increased capillary permeability with subsequent outpouring of serosanguineous fluid. Within 3 hours, this proteinaceous fluid coagulates, producing fibrinous bands, over and between abutting surfaces.[8] These fibrinous adhesions become infiltrated by monocytes, plasma cells, polymorphonuclear cells (PMNs), and histiocytes. In the absence of ischemia, fibrinolysis proceeds and the coagulum is lysed, probably within 72 hours.[9] Primitive mesothelial cells from the base of the wound form islands of regenerating mesothelium. Over the next 2 to 5 days, reepithelialization of the injured peritoneum occurs with a concomitant decrease in macrophage population.

Fibroblast proliferation and collagen synthesis are modulated by factors produced by macrophages and lymphocytes, including platelet-derived growth factor (PDGF), transforming growth factor-β (TGF-β), fibroblast growth factor (FGF), epidermal growth factor (EGF), interleukin-1 (IL-1), and tumor necrosis factor-α (TNFα). PDGF and TGFβ increase fibroblast collagen synthesis in other parts of the body,[10] whereas FGF and EGF have demonstrated in vitro activity in the mitogenesis of peritoneal tissue repair cells.[11] Because IL-1 and TNFα do not stimulate fibroblast proliferation or connective tissue in vitro, they are probably indirectly involved in adhesion formation, perhaps through secondary cytokines or arachidonic acid pathways.[12] These and other factors probably enhance adhesion formation by increasing collagen synthesis and cellular proliferation. Although the prostaglandins, especially prostaglandin E_2, are involved in normal and abnormal mesothelial repair, their mechanism of action does not involve fibroblast proliferation.[13]

During the normal healing process, fibrin deposition and fibrinolysis are in equilibrium. Factors that disrupt this equilib-

Patient's Name _____ Date _____ Chart # _____

Age _____ G _____ P _____ Sp Ab _____ VTP _____ Ectopic _____ Infertile Yes _____ No _____

Other Significant History (i.e. surgery, infection, etc.) _____

_____

HSG _____ Sonography _____ Photography _____ Laparoscopy _____ Laparotomy _____

	ADHESIONS	<1/3 Enclosure	1/3 - 2/3 Enclosure	>2/3 Enclosure
OVARY	R Filmy	1	2	4
	Dense	4	8	16
	L Filmy	1	2	4
	Dense	4	8	16
TUBE	R Filmy	1	2	4
	Dense	4*	8*	16
	L Filmy	1	2	4
	Dense	4*	8*	16

* If the fimbriated end of the fallopian tube is completely enclosed, change the point assignment to 16.

Prognostic Classification for Adnexal Adhesions

	LEFT		RIGHT
A. Minimal	_____	0-5	_____
B. Mild	_____	6-10	_____
C. Moderate	_____	11-20	_____
D. Severe	_____	21-32	_____

Treatment (Surgical Procedures): _____

_____

_____

_____

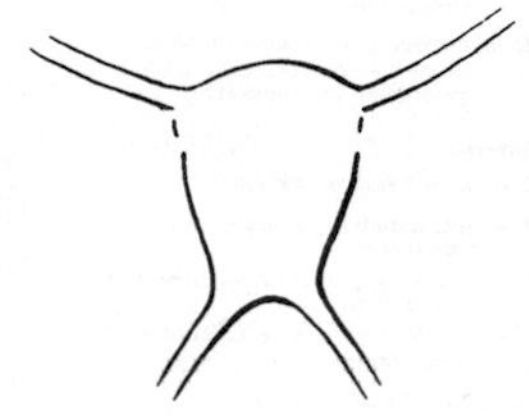

Prognosis for Conception & Subsequent Viable Infant**

_____ Excellent (> 75%)

_____ Good (50-75%)

_____ Fair (25%-50%)

_____ Poor (< 25%)

**Physician's judgment based upon adnexa with least amount of pathology.

Recommended Followup Treatment: _____

_____

Property of
The American Fertility Society

Additional Findings: _____

_____

_____

_____

_____

_____

DRAWING

L   R

For additional supply write to:
The American Fertility Society
2140 11th Avenue, South
Suite 200
Birmingham, Alabama 35205

Figure 39–1. American Fertility Society classification of adnexal adhesions. *(Courtesy of the American Fertility Society.)*

rium are those that suppress fibrinolytic activity or lead to excessive fibrin deposition. Predisposing factors for decreased fibrinolytic activity include tissue ischemia, devascularization, necrosis, and grafting or suturing of tissue to peritoneal defects. Ellis[14] concluded that ischemia and vascular injury are more important etiologic factors in postoperative adhesion formation than is serosal integrity. Ellis found consistent demonstration of fibrous adhesions in relation to areas of ischemia in rat intestine and peritoneum.[14] The fibrinolytic activity of peritoneum was characterized by Buckman et al.[15] Decreased fibrinolytic activity as measured with plasminogen activator activity (PAA) was associated with peritoneal grafts when compared with both normal peritoneum and deperitonealized but otherwise undamaged tissue surfaces. The low fibrinolytic activity was associated with fibrinous adhesions to the graft at 96 hours followed by fibrous adhesion formation at 2 weeks; these adhesions had not been present on either the normal peritoneum or deperitonealized but otherwise undamaged surfaces. Cecal abrasion and crushing were also associated with immediately depressed PAA and subsequent adhesion formation.[16]

The histologic and morphologic features of postsurgical adhesion formation in rats was described by Milligan and Raftery,[17] who used light and electron microscopic techniques. Adhesion formation began with a fibrin matrix that typically occurred during coagulation. This matrix was gradually replaced by vascular granulation tissue containing macrophages, fibroblasts, and giant cells. Early in this process there was no evidence of mesothelial cell attachment to the surface of the adhesion. The fibrin network was generally organized by day 5 and contained distinct bundles of collagen, fibroblasts, and mast

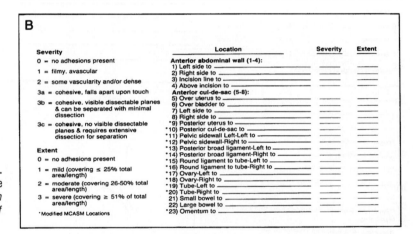

	ADHESIONS	< 1/3 Enclosure	1/3 - 2/3 Enclosure	> 2/3 Enclosure
OVARY	R Filmy	1	2	4
	Dense	4	8	16
	L Filmy	1	2	4
	Dense	4	8	16
TUBE	R Filmy	1	2	4
	Dense	4*	8*	16
	L Filmy	1	2	4
	Dense	4*	8*	16

* If the fimbriated end of the fallopian tube is completely enclosed. change the point assignment to 16.

B

Severity
0 = no adhesions present
1 = filmy. avascular
2 = some vascularity and/or dense
3a = cohesive, falls apart upon touch
3b = cohesive, visible dissectable planes & can be separated with minimal dissection
3c = cohesive, no visible dissectable planes & requires extensive dissection for separation

Extent
0 = no adhesions present
1 = mild (covering ≤ 25% total area/length)
2 = moderate (covering 26-50% total area/length)
3 = severe (covering ≥ 51% of total area/length)
* Modified MCASM Locations

Location	Severity	Extent
Anterior abdominal wall (1-4):		
1) Left side to		
2) Right side to		
3) Incision line to		
4) Above incision to		
Anterior cul-de-sac (5-8):		
5) Over uterus to		
6) Over bladder to		
7) Left side to		
8) Right side to		
*9) Posterior uterus to		
*10) Posterior cul-de-sac to		
*11) Pelvic sidewall Left-Left to		
*12) Pelvic sidewall-Right to		
*13) Posterior broad ligament-Left to		
*14) Posterior broad ligament-Right to		
*15) Round ligament to tube-Left to		
*16) Round ligament to tube-Right to		
*17) Ovary-Left to		
*18) Ovary-Right to		
*19) Tube-Left to		
*20) Tube-Right to		
21) Small bowel to		
22) Large bowel to		
*23) Omentum to		

Figure 39–2. A. American Fertility Society adhesion scoring method. **B.** More comprehensive adhesion scoring method. The asterisks in **B** indicate the sites most likely to be involved in tubal and ovarian adhesions. (*From Diamond MP et al: Improvement of interobserver reproducibility of adhesion sloping systems.* Fertil Steril *62:98, 1994.*)

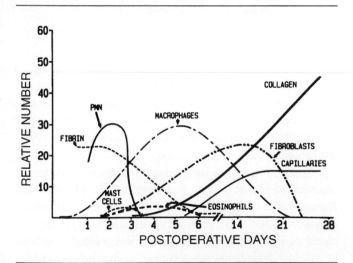

Figure 39–3. Changes in the relative number of cellular elements at the site of peritoneal injury during adhesion formation. (*From diZerega GS: Contemporary adhesion prevention.* Fertil Steril *61:219, 1994.*)

cells. Small vascular channels containing endothelial cells also were seen. During the next 5 days, fibroblasts within the developing adhesion became aligned and collagen deposition and organization advanced. By 2 weeks, relatively few cells were present, and these were predominately fibroblasts. At 1 to 2 months after injury, the collagen fibrils were organized into discrete bundles interposed by spindle-shaped fibroblasts and a few rare macrophages. Eventually the adhesion matured into a fibrous band, often covered by mesothelium and containing blood vessels and connective tissue fibers (Fig 39–3).[18]

Preexisting intraabdominal processes such as inflammation may influence intraperitoneal fibrinolysis. Vipond et al.[19] sampled the peritoneum of patients undergoing emergency operations for appendicitis or ruptured viscus and demonstrated reduced peritoneal PAA compared with that of patients undergoing elective operations. Similarly, a previous operation with a resultant reduction in tissue vascular supply may predispose a patient to adhesion development.

TABLE 39–1. RECOMMENDATIONS FOR ADHESION PREVENTION

I. Use the proper surgical technique
  Maintain as much vasculature as possible; do not leave devascularized tissue
  Keep tissues moist using wet sponges and irrigation
  Do not use gauze or dry sponges in the peritoneal cavity
  Eliminate foreign bodies
  Avoid excessive tissue handling
  Use finepoint electrocautery (or bipolar)-minimal cutting and coagulating current
  Do not use peritoneal grafts
  Minimize devitalization of tissues
  Avoid reactive sutures where possible
II. Achieve hemostasis
III. Use adjuvants for adhesion prevention where appropriate

PREVENTION OF ADHESIONS

The most effective method of reducing postoperative adhesions is to limit trauma at the time of the initial operative procedure. Careful surgical technique remains the cornerstone of adhesion prevention. A wide variety of suggestions can be made to try to optimize surgical outcome, but each must be applied in a clinically appropriate setting for the procedure (Table 39–1).

Powdered gloves must be thoroughly rinsed before use. Brief rinsing can cause clotting of the powder and lead to a severe postoperative peritoneal reaction with formation of extensive adhesions.[20] Tissue handling should be meticulous, irrigation should be copious, and residual clot and fibrin should be minimized. Attempts should be made to excise rather than incise adhesions, and hemostasis should be complete at the end of the procedure. Clamps and coagulation should be used as little as possible to minimize ischemic tissue effects.

Care should be taken to avoid drying or abrading serosal surfaces for fear of damaging peritoneal integrity. Irrigation rather than sponging should be used. Various irrigation solutions, from saline with heparin to Ringer's lactate, have been used. Tissue edema and petechial hemorrhages have been reported in tissues in contact with saline solution for prolonged periods. These changes have not been reported with Ringer's lactate and dextran.[21] For this reason, we prefer Ringer's lactate for intraoperative irrigation.

The choice of suture material may be relevant to reducing postoperative adhesion formation. Polyglycolic acid (Dexon) and polyglactin (Vicryl) reportedly produce only a mild foreign-body reaction as opposed to plain and chromic catgut, which are classically among the most reactive sutures.[22] Multifilament sutures may produce more tissue inflammation than monofilament sutures because foreign bodies adhere to multifilament suture. Polydioxanone (PDS), a newer synthetic monofilament absorbable suture material, has been reported to cause fewer ad-

hesions than multifilament sutures.[23,24] Neff et al, however, were unable to confirm the difference.[25]

Closure of peritoneal defects under tension or under other conditions that promote ischemia is more likely to result in adhesion formation in animal models than is leaving the defects open. DeCherney has advocated allowing linear salpingostomy incisions for ectopic to heal by secondary intention. However, adhesions are likely to develop in peritoneal defects of the lateral pelvic side wall that are left open. This occurred in one study after adhesiolysis in 72% of untreated, control sides.[26] Whether loose approximation of peritoneal or visceral edges with fine sutures of low tissue reactivity, under conditions unlikely to promote ischemia, predisposes to adhesion formation is unknown. Although conventional surgical techniques have emphasized closure of ovarian cortex defects with fine, nonreactive suture, operative laparoscopic procedures often have not involved reapproximation of peritoneal edges. Surprisingly the latter practice has been suggested to reduce postoperative adhesion formation. With rabbit models, Brumsted et al[27] and Meyer et al[28] documented fewer adhesions after ovarian operations when the cortex was left open compared with traditional microsurgical closure, a statistically significant difference. In spite of increased adhesion formation, ovarian function was not different among sutured or unsutured groups from that in nonsurgically treated controls. Given the increased use of endoscopic treatment of ovarian and other adnexal abnormalities and the inherent difficulty of laparoscopic suture placement, this finding, if confirmed in clinical trials, will have important implications.

The question of ovarian closure is of particular interest because laparoscopic treatment of endometriosis often involves excision of ovarian endometriomas. Canis et al[29] drained endometriomas in the dependent portion of the ovary, irrigated the cyst cavity, and left the cortex unsutured in 53 adnexae. Second-look laparoscopy revealed no evidence of deep endometriosis in 49 of the adnexae (92%) in which endometriomas > 3 cm were treated by laparoscopic stripping. However, de novo adhesion formation occurred in 4 of 19 (21%) of the treated adnexae and in 3 of 17 (17%) of the contralateral adnexae. Among the 34 adnexae in which endometriomas > 3 cm were accompanied by marked adhesions before the original operation, laparoscopic management of the endometriomas was associated with partial or complete recurrence of adhesions in 28 cases (82%). Although this rate does not compare unfavorably with the rate of adhesion formation after similar laparotomy procedures, it emphasizes the difficulty of eliminating adhesion reformation, especially in the presence of inflammatory conditions such as endometriosis.

Closure of the anterior peritoneum remains controversial. Tulandi et al[30] found no statistically significant difference in complication, wound healing, or adhesion rates with use of a

Pfannenstiel laparotomy incision with or without peritoneal suturing in infertility patients at the time of second-look laparoscopy. However, the study did not report the incidence of peritubal or periovarian adhesions, and the surgeons used chromic catgut suture for peritoneal closure.[30] Because of concern about ingress of blood and tissue products from the anterior abdominal wall into the pelvis during the immediately postoperative period, consideration should be given to closure of the peritoneum with fine, nonreactive suture material.

Electrocauterization has been widely used during microsurgical procedures because it allows meticulous hemostasis and precise tissue dissection. The use of minimal cutting and the delivery of coagulation currently through a fine point allow discrete coagulation of a bleeding point with little additional tissue destruction. A fine, bipolar forceps with minimal current also produces a small, discrete area of tissue destruction. Although the carbon dioxide laser has been used extensively for both laparoscopic and laparotomy procedures, neither animal nor human studies suggest that laser surgical technique has better results with respect to pregnancy rates after therapy for endometriosis or adhesiolysis than operations performed equally carefully with other modalities. Pittaway et al[31] compared the effect of use of a carbon dioxide laser with use of an electrocautery on postoperative intraperitoneal adhesion formation in rabbits. The investigators found no apparent difference, although they found that the ovaries seemed particularly prone to adhesions when either technique was used. Luciano et al[32] likewise found no difference in immediate tissue damage or chronic healing patterns in female rabbits when carbon dioxide laser or electromicrosurgical technique was used. On the other hand, Filmar et al[33] reported more particulate carbon in electromicrosurgical incisions and more pronounced and longer lasting foreign body reaction than in incisions made with a carbon dioxide laser.

In a comparison of continuous-wave with superpulsed carbon dioxide laser technique, it appears that the superpulsed carbon dioxide laser technique provoked less damage, but this modality has not been widely tested.[34] In a clinical comparison, Tulandi et al[35] reported no difference in intrauterine pregnancy rates when carbon dioxide laser or electromicrosurgical technique was used for reconstructive operations for hydrosalpinx (21.7% versus 22.7%). However, the interval between the operation and conception was shorter for the laser-treated group (3 months) than for the microelectrosurgically treated group (6.5 months).[35] In an animal study in which they compared electrosurgical, carbon dioxide laser, and Nd:YAG (neodymium: yttrium-aluminum-garnet) laser technique during operative laparoscopy, Luciano et al[36] found greater depth of thermal injury with the Nd:YAG laser. However, subsequent adhesion reformation was similar among all three treatment groups.[36] Although the use of lasers does not seem to decrease adhesion formation, some surgeons believe use of lasers facilitates performance of laparoscopic procedures.

With the advent of the carbon dioxide laser and other modern instruments, laparoscopic operations on the pelvic structures have become increasingly popular because of decreased hospitalization time and decreased postoperative pain. It also has been suggested that operative laparoscopy results in reduced postoperative adhesion development. Clinical studies examining adhesion formation and re-formation after laparoscopy have been limited and have not compared similar procedures performed at laparoscopy and laparotomy. Animal studies have been performed, but results may not apply to the human population. De novo adhesion formation after laparoscopy and laparotomy was compared by Filmar et al[37] in rats. Although the laparoscopy group had a greater mean area involved in adhesions, the difference was not statistically significant. The study was confounded by bleeding at the injury site in the laparoscopy group with no reference made about controlling hemostasis.[37]

Maier et al[38] compared use of a carbon dioxide laser at laparoscopy or laparotomy in a rabbit model. The investigators demonstrated lower adhesion scores at both the uterine horns and the side walls after adhesiolysis with both approaches, a statistically significant finding. The rabbits treated with laparoscopy, however, had fewer de novo adhesions than the laparotomy group, and the side-wall adhesions re-formed less often after laser laparoscopy than after laser laparotomy[38] (Fig 39–4).

The Operative Laparoscopy Study Group found that only 8 of 68 women (12%) developed de novo adhesions at sites not undergoing adhesiolysis during an initial operative laparoscopy[39] compared to 82 of 161 women (51%) treated by adhesiolysis during laparotomy.[40] During laparoscopic procedures, lysis of filmy, avascular adhesions was less likely to result in adhesion reformation (45.3%) than was lysis of dense or vascular adhesions (60.9%) or cohesive adhesions (79.3%). No such relation was identified after lysis of filmy, avascular as opposed to dense, vascular adhesions at laparotomy. Even with the advantages of a laparoscopic approach, however, adhesions remain troublesome; adhesions reformed at sites undergoing laparoscopic adhesiolysis in 66 of 68 women (91%) and 12% of women actually experienced worse adhesions after the operation.[39] Other groups have confirmed adhesion formation and re-formation after laparoscopic procedures.[41]

As the popularity of laparoscopic surgery increases, new instrumentation is being developed that may offer advantages over use of an electrocautery or laser for fertility surgery. The cavitron ultrasonic surgical aspirator (CUSA; Valleylab, Boulder, CO) combines tissue fragmentation, irrigation, and tissue

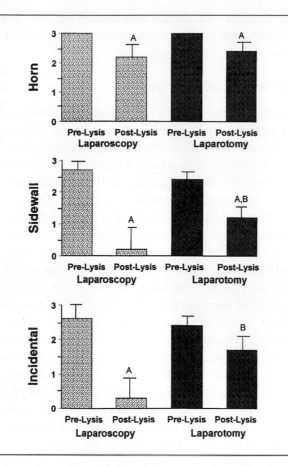

Figure 39–4. Extent of adhesion formation after adhesiolysis by laser laparoscopy and laparotomy. **A.** $P < .05$ compared with prelysis scores; **B.** $P < .05$ compared with postlysis scores after laparoscopy. (*After Maier DB et al: Laser laparoscopy versus laparotomy in lysis of pelvic adhesions.* J Reprod Med *37:965, 1992.*)

aspiration and allows dissection of water-dense tissue away from collagen-rich structures such as blood vessels, ureters, and nerves. It is possible that a CUSA may be applied in laparoscopic surgery for removal of undesired tissue (adhesions, myomas, endometriosis) with less risk of damage to vessels, intestine, and ureters compared with currently used modalities. Hurst et al[42] compared use of a CUSA with use of a Nd:YAG laser and bipolar cautery in an animal model. They found similar adhesion and inflammation scores in the CUSA and Nd:YAG group. Use of a bipolar cautery produced less inflammation on the uterine horn compared with use of a CUSA and subsequently less adhesions; however, dissection is not possible with a bipolar cautery. Because the CUSA may have important theoretic advantages for dissection and treatment of the pelvic side wall, additional studies assessing its use and safety in humans are necessary.

The ultrasonic scalpel is another instrument that has potential uses in surgery, producing good hemostasis and poten-

tially minimal tissue injury. In a comparative study of an ultrasonic scalpel electrocautery and a carbon dioxide laser, the ultrasonic scalpel produced less tissue injury on porcine skin than either of the other modalities.[43] Whether these observations are extendable to peritoneum remains to be established. Although no difference was found in adhesion formation in the rat uterine horn model, the ultrasonic scalpel caused increased coagulation necrosis for up to 14 days after the operation than did a conventional scalpel.[44] Because of better hemostasis, the ultrasonic scalpel may, nonetheless, offer advantages over a conventional scalpel in some reproductive operations, especially laparoscopy. Future studies will be necessary to document an advantage.

ADJUVANTS FOR ADHESION REDUCTION

Despite meticulous technique, adhesion reformation frequently occurs. In an attempt to reduce adhesion recurrence, several classes of adjuvants have been used. The possible mechanisms by which they may reduce adhesion formation include (1) reduction of the initial inflammatory response and subsequent proteinaceous exudate; (2) inhibition of coagulation; (3) promotion of fibrinolytic activity; (4) mechanical separation of peritoneal surfaces; and (5) inhibition of fibroblast proliferation (Table 39–2).

Glucocorticoids, Antihistamines, and Nonsteroidal Antiinflammatory Agents

Attempts to reduce the inflammatory response have involved use of corticosteroids, nonsteroidal antiinflammatory agents such as ibuprofen, and antihistamines. Corticosteroids have been used since the 1950's for prophylaxis against postoperative adhesions. Glucocorticoids suppress the inflammatory response to tissue injury by decreasing vascular permeability and stabilization of lysosome membranes. They inhibit the synthesis of histamine, which is released by mast cells, and antagonize the effect of histamine once it is released. The result is a decrease in the serofibrinous exudate. Glucocorticoids also have been reported to inhibit fibroblast migration and proliferation, although more recent studies have reported stimulation of fibroblast growth.[45] Administration of large doses of glucocorticoids effectively inhibits adhesion formation after peritoneal injury in small animals; however, their use has been associated with increased morbidity. Decreased immunologic capabilities increase risk for infection and impaired healing, resulting in increased risk for wound disruption.

Corticosteroids have been used frequently in combination with the antihistamine promethazine, which has a unique ability

TABLE 39–2. CLASSES OF ADJUVANTS USED IN AN ATTEMPT TO MINIMIZE THE OCCURRENCE OF POSTOPERATIVE ADHESIONS

Antibiotics
 Tetracyclines
 Cephalosporins
Anticoagulants
 Heparin
 Citrates
 Oxalates
Anti-inflammatory agents
 Corticosteroids
 Antihistamines
 Nonsteroidal antiInflammatory drugs
Calcium channel blockers
 Verapamil
 Nifedipine
 Diltiazem
Mechanical barriers
 Endogenous tissue
  Omental grafts
  Peritoneal grafts
  Fetal membranes
 Exogenous material
  Oxidized cellulose
  Dextran
  Crystalloid solutions
  Carboxymethylcellulose
  Chondroitin sulfate
  Poloxamer 407
  Oxidized regenerated cellulose (Interceed)
  Polytetrafluoroethylene (Gore-Tex surgical membrane)
  Hyaluronic acid
Fibrinolytic agents
 Plasminogen activator
 Fibrinolysin
 Streptokinase
 Urokinase
 Hyaluronidase

to inhibit increased vascular permeability induced by histamine, stabilize lysosomes, and inhibit fibroblast proliferation. Promethazine has not been examined for its ability to reduce adhesions when used alone. Replogle et al[46] found reduced incidence and severity of adhesion formation in patients treated with combination therapy of dexamethasone and promethazine given systemically pre- and postoperatively. Horne et al[47] reported similar favorable results using the same regimen after infertility operations; however, no control group participated in the study. A number of authors have questioned the efficacy of steroids in the prevention of postoperative adhesion formation. Gomel[48] reported no difference in quality or quantity of adhesions in rats subjected to pelvic trauma and treated with corticosteroids or saline irrigation. diZerega and Hodgen[49] found the combination of dexamethasone, promethazine, and ampicillin to be ineffective in controlled studies with rhesus monkeys subjected to

tubal operations. Other studies have not demonstrated a benefit of the use of this combination therapy in the prevention of adhesions.

Nonsteroidal Antiinflammatory Agents

Nonsteroidal antiinflammatory drugs (NSAIDs) inhibit synthesis of prostaglandins E and F, which are important mediators of the inflammatory response. Prostaglandins are produced by the PMNs and macrophages present at the site of inflammation or may result from platelet aggregation. They mediate many aspects of the postsurgical inflammatory response. Golan et al[13] found that addition of prostaglandins $F_{2\alpha}$ and E_2 into the peritoneal cavity of rats enhanced formation of adhesions to the injury site. Oxyphenbutazone administered perioperatively reduced adhesion formation in rats and monkeys,[9] but side effects from it and other first-generation antiprostaglandins allow only limited utility. Ibuprofen is better tolerated and has been shown to inhibit prostaglandin biosynthesis, platelet aggregation, and secretory activity, leukocyte migration, and phagocytosis and to suppress lysosome release.[50] Seigler et al[51] reported reduced severity of adhesions in rabbits treated with ibuprofen postoperatively. Results of animal investigations of adhesion prophylaxis are variable, perhaps because of varying dosage regimens. Nishimura et al[52a] noted significant reduction in adhesion formation after five doses of ibuprofen but not after two.

Although few studies have been performed with humans, Stangel et al[21] reported an improved postoperative course and higher pregnancy rates among patients treated with ibuprofen 400 mg three times a day for the first five postoperative days after laparotomy for infertility. Unfortunately, second-look appraisal of adhesion formation was not performed. These data suggest that inhibitors of prostaglandin synthesis or action may effectively reduce postoperative adhesion formation. However, devascularized sites are the most common sites for adhesion development secondary to decreased PAA, allowing persistence of fibrin and subsequent adhesiogenesis. Pharmacologic prevention of adhesion formation with NSAIDs or other adjuvants may depend on identification of an appropriate vehicle to deliver the drug to these relatively inaccessible sites.

Anticoagulants

Anticoagulants, specifically high-dose heparin given intraperitoneally or systemically, are associated with a decrease in adhesion formation. Side effects, including hemorrhage and wound disruption, have precluded its use. Although peritoneal irrigation with heparin solution has not been demonstrated to be effective in adhesion prevention, a synergistic effect was reported when small amounts of a heparin solution were used after application of oxidized, regenerated cellulose, Interceed (TC7)

(Johnson & Johnson, Arlington, TX) in an animal model.[52b] This observation was not confirmed in a human clinical trial.

Fibrinolytic Agents

Fibrinolytic agents reduce adhesion formation by means of both a direct effect on the fibrinous coagulum and by means of stimulation of PAA. At higher dosages, their use is associated with hemorrhagic complications. At lower dosages, fibrinolytic agents have been safely used in animal models. Recombinant tissue plasminogen activator has been shown to reduce the rate of formation of both primary and recurrent adhesions without reduction in wound strength in animal trials.[53,54] No bleeding complications were noted at the dosages used.

Antibiotics

Many women with pelvic adhesive disease do not have a clinical history of pelvic inflammatory disease; however, many of them have antibodies to *Chlamydia trachomatis*. Several studies have documented the association of chlamydial antibodies and tubal infertility.[21] Therefore, surgeons should be concerned about the persistence of such infections through the postoperative period as a source of postoperative adhesion formation. For this reason, systemic antibiotics, either tetracycline or broad-spectrum cephalosporins, are frequently administered prophylactically during the postoperative period. There is a very low incidence of postoperative infection during these procedures, however, and there is little evidence that the routine practice of administering systemic antibiotics decreases postoperative infection and subsequent adhesion formation rates. Increased peritoneal adhesions in a rat model have been associated with peritoneal irrigation with antibiotic-containing solutions,[21] and intraabdominal instillation of these solutions is not suggested.

Calcium Channel Blockers

Calcium channel blocking agents have been demonstrated to inhibit release of vasoactive substances, including histamine and prostaglandins E and F, and to prevent fibroblast penetration into fibrin matrices. Steinleitner et al[55] found reduced primary adhesion formation after postoperative administration of nifedipine, verapamil, or diltiazem to hamsters. Other investigators, however, have not been able to reproduce these results (M.P. Diamond et al, unpublished data, 1989).

Mechanical Barriers

Studies with animals have demonstrated that mechanical barriers can prevent adhesion formation by limiting tissue proximity during the initial phases of peritoneal repair.[56] Barriers for ad-

hesion prophylaxis are available in both liquid and solid preparations.

Liquid Preparations

Dextran can be manufactured in a variety of molecular weights; however, 32% dextran 70 (Hyskon) has been the most thoroughly researched. Its mechanism of adhesion reduction is thought to be (1) the siliconizing effect of dextran that coats raw surfaces and abrasions; (2) separation of tissues by means of a mechanical effect achieved by hydroflotation; and (3) indirect Hyskon-induced stimulation of PAA. Hyskon establishes an osmotic gradient, increasing the content of intraperitoneal fluid and decreasing tissue apposition.[57] Animal studies demonstrated reduced incidence or severity of adhesions in animals treated with intraperitoneal Hyskon.[58] However, some animal studies have not demonstrated the efficacy of Hyskon.

Two prospective, controlled, clinical studies of the use of Hyskon in infertility operations showed a statistically significant beneficial effect of Hyskon in the prevention of adhesion formation. Instillation of 250 mL of Hyskon or saline solution into the peritoneal cavity before closure was performed in women undergoing operations for distal tubal disease, endometriosis, or pelvic adhesions. At second-look laparoscopy performed 8 to 12 weeks later, fewer and less severe adhesions were found in the Hyskon-treated patients, particularly in the gravitationally dependent portions of the pelvis.[59] Likewise, Rosenberg and Board[60] reported lower adhesion scores for patients who received 200 mL of Hyskon intraperitoneally before closure in a randomized, prospective study of the use of Hyskon compared with Ringer's lactate. Other clinical studies, however, have not documented a beneficial effect of Hyskon on adhesion formation. A multicenter, prospective, randomized Swedish study[61] showed no improvement in adhesion formation rate after instillation of Hyskon compared with instillation of saline solution in evaluations at second-look laparoscopy 4 to 10 weeks later.[63] Jansen[62] likewise could document no improvement in adhesion scores in Hyskon-treated patients.

Serious side effects of Hyskon, including transient weight gain, vulvar edema, pleural effusion, and coagulopathy, have been reported. Anaphylactic shock or allergic symptoms occur in a small percentage of patients who receive Hyskon intraperitoneally. As newer modalities have been approved and because it is not approved for intraperitoneal use, Hyskon has been used with decreasing frequency.

Oelsner et al[63] compared other liquid barriers with Hyskon in an animal model. They found chondroitin sulfate superior to both carboxymethyl cellulose (CMC) or Hyskon in prevention of postsurgical adhesions. However, in a standardized rat model, Graebe et al[64] found CMC to be as effective as chondroitin sulfate and much better than Hyskon in prevention of adhesions. Because preventing adhesion re-formation may be more difficult than preventing de novo formation. Diamond et al[65] evaluated the ability of CMC to prevent adhesion re-formation in a rabbit horn model. They found that CMC reduced not only adhesion formation but also adhesion re-formation.

Viscous proteoglycans such as sodium hyaluronic acid (HA) polymers have been used with varying success to prevent adhesion formation. Several studies supported the efficacy of HA in the prevention of adhesion formation after tendon repair in animal models.[66,67] However, other studies showed no beneficial effect.[68] Grainger et al[69] studied four different formulations of HA in a rabbit model. None of the viscous solutions of HA resulted in a reduction of ovarian adhesions; however, a polymer slab of HA applied to the treated ovary resulted in reduced adhesion formation. Further trials are necessary to establish the efficacy of HA.

Poloxamer 407 is one of a family of polymers that demonstrates unusual physical characteristics. Aqueous solutions of poloxamer 407 exist as a viscous fluid at 4°C yet become a solid gel at body temperature. Preliminary studies by Leach et al[70] demonstrated a statistically significant reduction in de novo adhesion formation after pelvic trauma in rats treated with poloxamer 407. Other animal studies have shown equally promising results in prevention of adhesion reformation after adhesiolysis.[57] Preclinical and clinical trials of a solution of poloxamer 407 (Flowgel) are underway.

Solid Preparations

Solid barriers to adhesion formation include both endogenous and exogenous materials. The use of naturally occurring materials such as fetal membranes or peritoneal grafts has been abandoned because the use of devascularized tissues has been demonstrated to increase postsurgical adhesion formation. Oxidized regenerated cellulose was initially developed as a hemostatic material (Surgicel). Testing of this formulation in animals yielded mixed results, resulting in modification of the knit, weave, oxidation, and porosity of the fabric to form a new product, Interceed. This material adheres readily to serosal surfaces, gels to form a continuous surface within 8 hours, and is usually resorbed by the body within 3 to 4 days without evidence of foreign body reaction, as evidenced by the lack of giant cells. After promising results of animal studies in which reduced number and severity of adhesions were demonstrated after uterine or pelvic side-wall trauma,[71,72] human clinical trials confirmed reduced incidence, extent, and severity of postoperative adhesions at second-look laparoscopy in infertility patients undergoing lysis of bilateral pelvic side-wall adhesions.[26] In October 1989, Interceed received approval by the U.S. Food and Drug Administration (FDA) as the first adjuvant indicated for the reduction of postsurgical peritoneal adhesions. In addition to its usefulness during laparotomies, Interceed can be applied at laparoscopy.[72]

Clinical efficacy shown in the initial studies with Interceed was confirmed by a multicenter study performed in Japan. In a matched–side-wall comparison, use of Interceed was eight times more effective than an operation alone (control) in preventing adhesion re-formation or reducing severity.[73] Overall, the study in Japan suggested better outcome with Interceed than that found in the U.S. studies. Some differences in the application of the material may account for the improved results in Japan: (1) application of the Interceed beyond the perimeter of the surgical injury may provide a more effective barrier between perisurgical areas of inflammation and adjacent tissues; (2) staining of the Interceed to brown or black indicates a nonhemostatic area. Removal of the contaminated Interceed, establishment of hemostasis, and reapplication of fresh Interceed may have contributed to improved outcome.

Other animal and clinical trials have confirmed the necessity for completely hemostatic surgical fields with use of Interceed. In addition to increasing fibrin deposition per se, bleeding at a surgical site can compromise the ability of Interceed to reduce adhesion formation.[74] Application of Interceed after achievement of hemostasis reduced adhesion formation. This effect was enhanced when the material was moistened with heparin.[75] Use of a modified form of Interceed (nTC7) has been reported to decrease adhesion formation, even when hemostasis has not been achieved.

Gore-Tex surgical membrane (W.L. Gore, Flagstaff, AZ) is a permanent, inert microporous implant of expanded polytetrafluoroethylene. Measuring 0.1 mm in thickness, Gore-Tex was approved in 1983 for reconstruction of the peritoneum or pericardium. Minimal to no foreign body tissue response has been demonstrated after retrieval of the material as long as 8.75 years after implantation. Boyers et al[76] demonstrated the usefulness of Gore-Tex in reducing primary pelvic adhesion formation in a rabbit model. In an uncontrolled prospective clinical study by the Surgical Membrane Study Group,[77] Gore-Tex surgical membrane was placed at the time of adhesiolysis (8 patients) or at myomectomy (10 patients). Initial adhesion score was compared with that at second-look laparoscopy 2 to 6 weeks later, at the time of retrieval of the surgical membrane. A dramatic reduction in adhesion formation and re-formation was found[77] (Fig 39–5). A prospective, randomized trial of the use of Gore-Tex surgical membrane and Interceed to treat women with extensive bilateral adnexal adhesions demonstrated that both materials reduced adhesion re-formation in a statistically significant way as assessed at second-look laparoscopy; however, at that time, the Gore-Tex surgical site had significantly fewer adhesions.[78]

The extent to which efficacy would be maintained at the time of a third-look procedure remains to be determined. Supportive evidence was provided in a complicated, prospective,

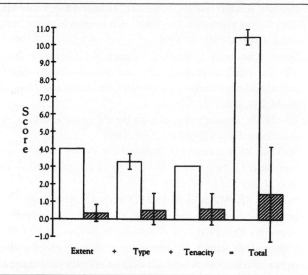

Figure 39–5. Adhesion scores after use of Gore-Tex surgical membrane after adhesiolysis or myomectomy. (*From the Surgical Membrane Study Group: pcophylaxis of pelvic sidewall adhesions with Gore-Tex surgical membrane: a multicenter clinical investigation.* Fertil Steril *57:921, 1992.*)

randomized, cross-over study with cynomolgus monkeys in which Grow et al[79] demonstrated that both Interceed and Gore-Tex surgical membrane reduced adhesion formation when compared with controls and that Gore-Tex led to fewer and less tenacious adhesions than Interceed. In this complex study, monkeys were either cycling regularly, receiving a gonadotropin-releasing hormone (GnRH) agonist (leuprolide acetate, Lupron depot; TAP Pharmaceuticals, Deerfield, IL), or receiving mifepristone (Roussel UCLAF, Paris, France) at the time of the second surgical procedure. Interestingly, animals that were hypoestrogenic at the time of the hysterotomy had significantly fewer adhesions at the time of the third-look operation.[80] If confirmed in other trials, hormonal manipulation before surgical procedures may be a useful tool for prevention of adhesion formation and re-formation.

Second-Look Laparoscopy

The concept of second-look laparoscopy (SLL) was introduced by Swolin[81a] in 1967 for the assessment of surgical technique and the effectiveness of adjuvant medications.[22] SLL has two other potential advantages: (1) provision of prognostic information regarding outcome and (2) therapeutic adhesiolysis of re-formed or de novo adhesions, vaporization of residual endometriosis, confirmation of tubal patency, or deagglutination of fimbria. Raj and Hulka[81b] reported no pregnancies in patients whose adhesions had worsened after adhesiolysis. Patients whose SLL reveals no improvement should

probably resort to alternatives such as in vitro fertilization or adoption instead of further surgical intervention, since prognosis may be poor.[81b]

The therapeutic value of SLL has been suggested to be limited to "early" SLL, when adhesions tend to be fine, filmy, avascular, and easily lysed as compared with years later. De-Cherney and Mezer[84] studied 61 randomly selected patients undergoing SLL. Of 20 patients undergoing early (4 to 16 weeks) SLL, 85% of patients had either no adhesions (25%) or filmy, avascular adhesions (60%). In the 41 late (16 to 19 months) SLL patients, only 36% of patients had either no (24%) or mild adhesions (12%), whereas 63% of women had dense, vascular adhesions. Some[81b,83,84] but not all[40] investigators have reported that adhesions at early SLL are more likely to be easily lysed with less bleeding than lysis of denser adhesions. The value of SLL in improving pregnancy rates, however, has yet to be established. Trimbos-Kemper et al[85] performed a third-look laparoscopy on patients who had undergone SLL with adhesiolysis. More than half of the adhesions that were separated at SLL did not recur, significantly less than in patients not undergoing SLL. Although this aggressive approach did not improve intrauterine conception rate, the incidence of ectopic pregnancy was lower among the SLL group.[85]

The optimal time for SLL has not been determined. Swolin recommended that the SLL be performed 6 weeks after the initial operation to allow management of the forming adhesions.[22] In a prospective study in which they evaluated the optimal time interval from the initial operation to SLL, Raj and Hulka[81b] reported increased bleeding at adhesiolysis when SLL was performed before 2 weeks or after 12 weeks. Before 2 weeks, granulation tissue from the laparotomy wound resulted in abdominal wall bleeding. After 12 weeks, newly formed adhesions were dense and bled easily at lysis. The authors determined the optimal time for SLL to be 4 to 8 weeks after the initial operation.[81b] Other investigators have not reported problems when SLL was performed at intervals less than 2 weeks.[40,84] In one report,[40] no difference in incidence or severity of adhesions was noted over the time interval from 7 to 70 days between the two operative procedures.

Potential disadvantages of SLL have been reported to be the morbidity, inconvenience, discomfort, and extra expense. Because it has yet to be proved that performance of SLL improves pregnancy outcome, surgeons should adopt an individualized approach to this issue.

CONCLUSION

When adhesions interfere markedly with organ function, such as tubal ovum pick-up, surgical management is the only proper treatment short of in vitro fertilization. Therefore, when performing operations for lysis of adhesions, all methods proved efficacious for adhesion prevention under those conditions should be considered. The degree of adhesion formation is related to the severity and type of tissue injury, ischemia being the strongest stimulus. Use of anticoagulants and fibrinolytic agents in high doses is dangerous, and use of steroids is unproved. Other antiinflammatory agents may have a role but have not yet been fully tested. Barrier methods appear promising, but research continues to find better adjuvants (or combinations of adjuvants) to prevent adhesion formation and reformation. The best treatment of adhesions is prevention. The best prevention is atraumatic tissue handling and meticulous surgical technique, regardless of the surgical approach. Newer modalities have only served to reemphasize the tenets of good surgical practice.

REFERENCES

1. Ray NF, Larsen JW, Stillman RJ, Jacobs RJ: Economic impact of hospitalizations for lower abdominal adhesiolysis in the United States in 1988. *Surg Gynecol Obstet* 176:271, 1993
2. Caspi E, Halperin Y, Bukovsky I: The importance of periadnexal adhesions in tubal reconstructive surgery for infertility. *Fertil Steril* 31:296, 1979
3. Hulka JF: Adnexal adhesions: A prognostic staging and classification system based on a five-year survey of fertility surgery results at Chapel Hill, North Carolina. *Am J Obstet Gynecol* 144:141, 1982
4. The American Fertility Society: The American Fertility Society classifications of adnexal adhesions, distal tubal occlusion, tubal ligation, tubal pregnancies, müllerian anomalies and intrauterine adhesions. *Fertil Steril* 49:944, 1988
5. Adhesion Scoring Group: Improvement of interobserver reproducibility of adhesion scoring systems. *Fertil Steril* 62:984, 1994
6. Diamond MP, Ackerman G, Bradshaw K, et al: The relationship of adhesions to pelvic pain. Presented at the International Congress of Gynecologic Endoscopy. October 18–23, 1994, New York, NY
7. Diamond MP, Ackerman G, Bradshaw AK, et al: When are the location, extent, and severity of adhesions significant enough to perform adhesiolysis in the infertile woman? Presented at the 4th Biennial Meeting of the International Society for Gynecologic Endoscopy. April 26–29, 1995, London, England
8. Jackson BB: Observations on intraperitoneal adhesions: An experimental study. *Surgery* 55:509, 1958
9. Holtz G: Prevention and management of peritoneal adhesions. *Fertil Steril* 41:497, 1984
10. Kovacs EJ: Fibrogenic cytokines: The role of immune mediators in the development of scar tissue. *Immunol Today* 12:17, 1991
11. Kovacs EJ, Brook B, Silber IA, Neuman JE: Production of fibrogenic cytokines by interleukin-2 treated peripheral blood leukocytes: Expression of transforming growth factor-β chain genes. *Obstet Gynecol* 82:29, 1993
12. Hershlag A, Otterness IG, Biven ML, Diamond MP, Polan ML: The effect of interleukin-1 on adhesion formation in the rat. *Am J Obstet Gynecol* 165:771, 1991
13. Golan A, Bernstein I, Wexler S, Neuman M, Bukovsky I, David MP: The effect of prostaglandins and aspirin—An inhibitor of prostaglandin synthesis—on adhesion formation in rats. *Hum Reprod* 6:251, 1991
14. Ellis H: The aetiology of post-operative abdominal adhesions: An experimental study. *Br J Surg* 50:10, 1963
15. Buckman RF, Buckman PD, Hufnagel HV, Gervin AS: A physiologic basis for the adhesion-free healing of deperitonealized surfaces. *J Surg Res* 21:67, 1976
16. Buckman RE, Woods M, Sargent L, Gervin AS: A unifying pathogenetic mechanism in the etiology of intraperitoneal adhesions. *J Surg Res* 20:1, 1976
17. Milligan DW, Raftery AT: Observations on the pathogenesis of peritoneal adhesions: A light and electron microscopical study. *Br J Surg* 61:274, 1974
18. diZerega GS: Contemporary adhesion prevention. *Fertil Steril* 61:219, 1994
19. Vipond MN, Whawell SA, Thompson JN, Dudley HAF: Peritoneal fibrinolytic activity and intra-abdominal adhesions. *Lancet* 335:1120, 1990
20. Utian WH: Adhesion prevention. *Fertil Steril* 41:785, 1985
21. Stangel JJ, Nisbet JD, Settles H: Formation and prevention of postoperative abdominal adhesions. *J Reprod Med* 29:145, 1984
22. Schwartz LB, Diamond MP: Formation, reduction, and treatment of adhesive disease. *Semin Reprod Med* 9:89, 1991
23. DeCherney A, Laufer N: The use of a new synthetic absorbable monofilament suture, polydioxanone (PDS), for surgery (abstract). *Fertil Steril* 39:401, 1983
24. Delbeke LO, Gomel V, McComb PF, Jetha N: Histologic reaction to four synthetic microsutures in the rabbit. *Fertil Steril* 40:248, 1983
25. Neff MR, Holtz GL, Betsill WL: Adhesion formation and histologic reaction with polydioxanone and polyglactin suture. *Am J Obstet Gynecol* 151:20, 1985
26. Interceed Adhesion Barrier Study Group: Prevention of postsurgical adhesions by Interceed (TC7) an absorbable adhesion barrier: A prospective, randomized multicenter clinical study. *Fertil Steril* 51:933, 1989
27. Brumsted JR, Deaton J, Lavigne E, Riddick DH: Postoperative adhesion formation after ovarian wedge resection with and without ovarian reconstruction in the rabbit. *Fertil Steril* 53:723, 1990
28. Meyer MR, Grainger DA, DeCherney AH, Lachs MS, Diamond MP: Ovarian surgery in the rabbit: Effect of cortex closure on adhesion formation and ovarian function. *J Reprod Med* 36:639, 1991
29. Canis M, Mage G, Wattiez A, Chapron C, Pouly JL, Bassil S: Second-look laparoscopy after laparoscopic cystectomy of large ovarian endometriomas. *Fertil Steril* 58:617, 1992
30. Tulandi T, Hum HS, Gelfand MM: Closure of laparotomy incisions with or without peritoneal suturing and second look laparoscopy. *Am J Obstet Gynecol* 158:536, 1988
31. Pittaway DE, Maxson WS, Daniell JF: A comparison of the CO_2 laser and electrocautery on postoperative intraperitoneal adhesion formation in rabbits. *Fertil Steril* 40:366, 1983

32. Luciano AA, Whitman G, Maier DB, Randolph J, Maenza R: A comparison of thermal injury, healing patterns, and postoperative adhesion formation following CO_2 electromicrosurgery. *Fertil Steril* 48:1025, 1987

33. Filmar S, Jetha N, McComb P, Gomel V: A comparative histologic study on the healing process after tissue transection. I. Carbon dioxide laser and electromicrosurgery. *Am J Obstet Gynecol* 160:1062, 1989

34. Barbot J: Impact of lasers on post-operative adhesions. *Prog Clin Biol Res* 381:65, 1993

35. Tulandi T, Farag R, McInnes RA, Gelfand MM, Wright CV, Vilos GA: Reconstructive surgery of hydrosalpinx with and without the carbon dioxide laser. *Fertil Steril* 42:839, 1984

36. Luciano AA, Frishman GN, Maier DB: A comparative analysis of adhesion reduction, tissue effects, and incising characteristics of electrosurgery, CO_2 laser, and Nd:YAG laser at operative laparoscopy: An animal study. *J Laparosc Endos Surg* 2:287, 1992

37. Filmar S, Gomel V, McComb PF: Operative laparoscopy versus open abdominal surgery: A comparative study on postoperative adhesion formation in the rat model. *Fertil Steril* 48:486, 1987

38. Maier DB, Nulsen JC, Klock A, Luciano AA: Laser laparoscopy versus laparotomy in lysis of pelvic adhesions. *J Reprod Med* 37:965, 1992

39. Operative Laparoscopy Study Group: Postoperative adhesion development after operative laparoscopy: Evaluation at early second-look procedures. *Fertil Steril* 55:700, 1991

40. Diamond MP, Daniell JF, Feste J, et al: Adhesion reformation and de novo adhesion formation following reproductive pelvic surgery. *Fertil Steril* 47:864, 1987

41. Redwine DB: Conservative laparoscopic excision of endometriosis by sharp dissection: Life table analysis of reoperation and persistent or recurrent disease. *Fertil Steril* 56:628, 1991

42. Hurst BS, Awoniyi CA, Stephens JK, Thompson LK, Riehl RM, Schlaff WD: Application of the cavitron ultrasonic surgical aspirator (CUSA) for gynecological laparoscopic surgery using the rabbit as an animal model. *Fertil Steril* 58:444, 1991

43. Hambley R, Hebda PA, Abell E, Cohen BA, Jegasothy BV: Wound healing of skin incisions produced by ultrasonically vibrating knife, scalpel, electrosurgery, and carbon dioxide laser. *J Dermatol Surg Oncol* 14:1213, 1988

44. Tulandi T, Chan KL, Arseneau J: Histopathological and adhesion formation after incision using ultrasonic vibrating scalpel and regular scalpel in the rat. *Fertil Steril* 61:548, 1994

45. Granat M, Schenken JG, Mor-Yosef S, Rosenkovitch E, Castellanos RC, Galili U: Effects of dexamethasone on proliferation of autologous fibroblasts and on the immune profile in women undergoing pelvic surgery for infertility. *Fertil Steril* 39:180, 1983

46. Replogle RL, Johnson R, Gross RE: Prevention of postoperative intestinal adhesions with combined promethazine and dexamethasone therapy: Experimental and clinical studies. *Ann Surg* 162:580, 1966

47. Horne HW, Clyman M, Debrovner C, Grigs G: The prevention of postoperative pelvic adhesions following conservative operative treatment for human infertility. *Int J Fertil* 18:109, 1973

48. Gomel V: Recent advances in surgical correlation of tubal disease producing infertility. *Curr Probl Obstet Gynecol* 1:10, 1978

49. diZerega GS, Hodgen GD: Prevention of postsurgical tubal adhesions: Comparative study of commonly used agents. *Am J Obstet Gynecol* 136:173, 1980

50. Gernaat CM, Stubbs DF: Clinical brochure for investigators studying ibuprofen and myocardial infarction. Kalamazoo, Michigan, The Upjohn Company, 1980

51. Seigler AM, Kontopoulos V, Wang CF: Prevention of postoperative adhesions in rabbits with ibuprofen, a non-steroidal antiinflammatory agent. *Fertil Steril* 34:46, 1980

52a. Nishimura K, Nakamura R, diZerega GS: Biochemical evaluation of postsurgical wound repair: Prevention of intraperitoneal adhesion formation with ibuprofen. *J Surg Res* 34:219, 1983

52b. Diamond MP, Linsky CB, Cunningham T, et al: Synergistic effects of Interceed (TC7) and heparin in reducing adhesion formation in the rabbit horn model. *Fertil Steril* 55:389, 1991

53. Menzies D, Ellis H: The role of plasminogen activator in adhesion prevention. *Surg Gynecol Obstet* 172:362, 1991

54. Doody KJ, Dunn RC, Buttram VC: Recombinant tissue plasminogen activator reduces adhesion formation in a rabbit uterine horn model. *Fertil Steril* 51:509, 1989

55. Steinleitner A, Lambert H, Henderson S: New modalities under development for adhesion prevention: Immunomodulatory agents and poloxamer barrier methods. *Prog Clin Biol Res* 381:235, 1993

56. Soules MR, Dennis L, Bosarge A, Moore DE: The prevention of postoperative pelvic adhesions: An animal study comparing barrier methods with dextran 70. *Am J Obstet Gynecol* 143:829, 1982

57. Greenberg M, Laverson NH: Postoperative adhesions: Etiology and prevention. In: Lauersen NL, Reyniak JV (eds), *Principles of Microsurgical Techniques in Infertility.* New York, Plenum, 1982:219

58. Dlugi AM, DeCherney AH: Prevention of postoperative adhesion formation. *Semin Reprod Endocrinol* 2:125, 1984

59. Adhesion Study Group: Reduction of postoperative pelvic adhesions with intraperitoneal 32% & dextran 70: A prospective, randomized clinical trial. *Fertil Steril* 40:612, 1983

60. Rosenberg SM, Board JA: High-molecular weight dextran in human infertility surgery. *Am J Obstet Gynecol* 148:380, 1984

61. Larsson B, Lalos O, Marsk L, et al: Effect of intraperitoneal instillation of 32% dextran 70 on postoperative adhesion formation after tubal surgery. *Acta Obstet Gynecol Scand* 64:437, 1985

62. Jansen RPS: Failure of intraperitoneal adjuncts to improve the outcome of pelvic operation in young women. *Am J Obstet Gynecol* 153:363, 1985

63. Oelsner G, Graebe RA, Pan S-B, et al: Chondroitin sulfate: A new intraperitoneal treatment for postoperative adhesion prevention in the rabbit. *J Reprod Med* 32:812, 1987

64. Graebe RA, Oelsner G, Cornelison TL, Pan S-B, DeCherney AH: An animal study of different treatment to prevent postoperative pelvic adhesions. *Microsurgery* 10:53, 1989

65. Diamond MP, DeCherney AH, Linsky CB, Cunningham T, Constantine B: Adhesion re-formation in the rabbit uterine horn model. I. Reduction with carboxymethylcellulose. *Int J Fertil* 33:372, 1988

66. Amiel D, Ishizue K, Billings E Jr, et al: Hyaluron in flexor tendon repair. *J Hand Surg* 14:837, 1989

67. Weiss C, Suros JM, Michalow A, Denlinger J, Moore M, Tejeiro W: The role of Na-hylan in reducing postsurgical tendon adhesions. II. *Bull Joint Dis Orthop Inst* 47:31, 1987

68. Meyers SA, Seaber AV, Glisson RR, Nunley JA: Effect of hyaluronic acid/chondroitin sulfate on healing of full thickness tendon lacerations in rabbits. *J Orthop Res* 7:683, 1989

69. Grainger DA, Meyer WR, DeCherney AH, Diamond MP: The use of hyaluronic acid polymers to reduce postoperative adhesions. *J Gynecol Surg* 7:97, 1991

70. Leach RE, Henry RL: Reduction of postoperative adhesions in the rat uterine horn model with poloxamer 407. *Am J Obstet Gynecol* 162:1317, 1990

71. Diamond MP, Linsky CB, Cunningham T, Constantine B, diZerega GS, DeCherney AH: A model for sidewall adhesions in the rabbit: Reduction by an absorbable barrier. *Microsurgery* 8:197, 1987

72. Diamond MP, Cunningham T, Linsky CP, DeCherney AH: Laparoscopic application of Interceed (TC7) in the pig. *J Gynecol Surg* 5:145, 1989

73. Sekiba K: Obstetrics and Gynecology Adhesion Prevention Committee: Use of Interceed (TC7) absorbable adhesion barrier to reduce postoperative adhesion formation in infertility and endometriosis surgery. *Obstet Gynecol* 79:518, 1992

74. Linsky CB, Diamond MP, DeCherney AH, diZerega GS, Cunningham T: Effect of blood on the efficacy of barrier adhesion reduction in the rabbit uterine horn model. *Infertility* 11:273, 1988

75. Wiseman DM, Kamp LF, Saferstein L, Linsky CB, Gottlick LE, Diamond MP: Improving the efficacy of interceed barrier in the presence of blood using thrombin, heparin or a blood insensitive barrier, modified Interceed (nTC7). *Prog Clin Biol Res* 381:205, 1993

76. Boyers SP, Diamond MP, DeCherney AH: Reduction of postoperative pelvic adhesions in the rabbit with Gore-Tex surgical membrane. *Fertil Steril* 49:1066, 1988

77. The Surgical Membrane Study Group: Prophylaxis of pelvic sidewall adhesions with Gore-Tex surgical membrane: A multicenter clinical investigation. *Fertil Steril* 57:921, 1992

78. March CM, Boyers SP, Franklin R, et al: Prevention of adhesion formation/reformation with the Gore-Tex surgical membrane. *Prog Clin Biol Res* 381:253, 1993

79. Grow DR, Seltman HJ, Coddington CC, Hodgen GD: The reduction of postoperative adhesions by two different barrier methods versus control in cynomolgus monkeys: A prospective, randomized crossover study. *Fertil Steril* 61:1141, 1994

80. Grow DR, Coddington CC, Seltman H, Hodgen GD: Role of hypoestrogenism or antiestrogens in adhesion formation after myometrial surgery in primates. Presented at the 50th Annual Meeting of the American Fertility Society. November 5–10, 1994, San Antonio, Texas

81a. Swolin K: Spontanneilung nach querresektion der tuba fallopii. *Acta Obstet Gynaecol Scand* 46:219, 1967

81b. Raj SG, Hulka JF: Second-look laparoscopy in infertility surgery; Therapeutic and prognostic value. *Fertil Steril* 38:325, 1982

82. DeCherney AH, Mezer HC: The nature of posttuboplasty pelvic adhesions as determined by early and late laparoscopy. *Fertil Steril* 41:643, 1984

83. Surrey MW, Friedman S: Second-look laparoscopy after reconstructive pelvic surgery for infertility. *J Reprod Med* 27:658, 1982

84. Daniell JF, Pittaway DE: Short-interval second-look laparoscopy after infertility surgery: A preliminary report. *J Reprod Med* 28:281, 1983

85. Timbos-Kemper TCM, Trimbos JB, van Hall EV: Adhesion formation after tubal surgery: Results of the eighth-day laparoscopy in 188 patients. *Fertil Steril* 43:395, 1985

PART IX

Reproductive Technology

CHAPTER 40

Embryo-Uterine Interactions During Implantation

JOHN THOMAS QUEENAN, JR · ASGERALLY T. FAZLEABAS

Embryo-Uterine Interactions During Implantation

Mechanisms of Implantation
Development of the Blastocyst
Stages of Implantation
  Hatching of the blastocyst
  Apposition
  Attachment
  Invasion
Structure of the Uterus and Decidualization

Pathologic Invasion
Clinical Assessment of Endometrial Receptivity
Lessons from In Vitro Fertilization and Oocyte Donation
  Endometrial effects of controlled ovarian hyperstimulation
  Hormone requirements for endometrial preparation
  Premature elevation of progesterone level
  Effect of embryo age
Conclusion

The nidation of the embryo within uterine endometrium is pivotal to the survival of all mammalian species. For implantation to occur, the necessity of having synchronization between the age of the embryo and the developmental stage of the endometrium has been shown in all species studied. The process is curiously fragile and given its importance poorly understood. Wilcox et al[1] reported that about 65% of conceptions end in unrecognized loss. Apposition of embryo and endometrium without invasion accounts for 45% of these losses, implantation failure occurs in 30%, and developmental failure after implantation is responsible for the remaining 25%. Since the inception of in vitro fertilization (IVF), programs have been reporting implantation rates that range between 5% and 15% per embryo transferred back to the uterus. Unfortunately this means that 85% to 95% of transferred embryos are not implanting. Satisfactory pregnancy rates are achieved only through the transfer of multiple embryos. Implantation is the least efficient process in reproduction and has been recognized as the rate-limiting step.

Considerable effort has been devoted to elucidating the mechanism of trophoblast-epithelium interaction and the ensuing invasion of the endometrium. Studies aimed at identifying the adhesion molecules responsible for the interaction between the embryo and the uterine surface epithelium may explain the first step in a chain of complex biochemical events that eventually result in maternal-fetal coupling. The complexity of the systems involved and the sanctity of the human embryo have made the study of implantation in humans a challenge. As a result, experimental models have arisen that display enormous creativity. There is a heavy reliance on animal models, and many observations have proved to be species specific. Innovative techniques have been used to isolate specific reproductive processes, such as pharmacologic induction of pseudopregnancy and asynchronous intraspecies embryo transfer. Advances are occurring rapidly with the application of modern techniques in molecular, cell, and developmental biology as well as tumor biology. Inventive laboratory methods like coculture and in vitro outgrowth culture have been applied to answer key questions without the presence of confounding maternal factors. Application of the rigorous work with animal models and advances in the field of animal husbandry have made the practice of IVF possible. The advent of assisted reproductive technology (ART) has brought considerable new information to light about implantation in humans.

MECHANISMS OF IMPLANTATION

Implantation is a series of interrelated events that lead to establishment of oxygen and nutrient exchange between the conceptus and the uterus. A logical beginning is the hatching of blastocyst from its surrounding zona pellucida. After hatching the process of implantation is ongoing, and an end point is difficult to discern. Invasive potential must be conserved throughout gestation that enables placental growth to match the increasing demands of the growing fetal unit. Unlike other cell-cell interactions that occur within organisms, implantation involves interaction between two immunologically distinct entities. The blastocyst may be destroyed by attack of maternal natural killer (NK) cells.[2] Understanding host tolerance to the semiallograft tissue of the conceptus is critical and yet remains elusive.

Much of our current knowledge of implantation is derived from animal experimentation owing to the obvious ethical problems with human studies. The uterine response to an implanting blastocyst is universal: increased permeability in the subepithelial capillaries surrounding the blastocyst,[3] glandular hypertrophy, stromal cell deciduation, and extracellular matrix (ECM) accumulation. After this initial response, implantation among mammals is extremely diverse,[4,5] to the point where it is almost species specific. It is paramount that the limitations of analogies between human implantation and that occurring in other mammals are thoroughly taken into account. Most experimental work has involved rodents, particularly rats and mice. Placentation in both rodents and humans is hemochorial,[6] in which invasion is most extreme. In both species, placentation concludes with the establishment of a chorioallantoic placenta with minimal separation between fetal and maternal blood supplies. These two systems share similar anatomic features of amniotic cavitation and formation of allantoic mesenchyme. Finally, there is similarity between the mice and humans in the organization of invading trophoblast cells.

Mouse trophoblasts form an invasive cone of proliferative cells. Invasion is carried out by multinuclear giant cells.[7] Cytotrophoblasts in human embryos fuse to form syncytiotro-

phoblasts, the invasive phenotype.[8] In both human and rodent models the syncytial cell mass is highly invasive,[7-9] capable of adhesion, cell migration, and phagocytosis. These syncytial cells release cytolytic agents that are central to the invasive process.[7,10,11] The human and rodent systems are characterized by a group of proliferating trophoblasts surrounded by terminally differentiated syncytial trophoblast cells. When the process concludes, fetal trophoblasts line the terminal placental vessels. It is cells of fetal origin that direct the functions of respiration, alimentation, and excretion for the fetus.

DEVELOPMENT OF THE BLASTOCYST

Several critical developmental events prepare an embryo for implantation. The stages of preimplantation embryogenesis are illustrated in Fig 40–1. After a 24-hour delay that precedes the

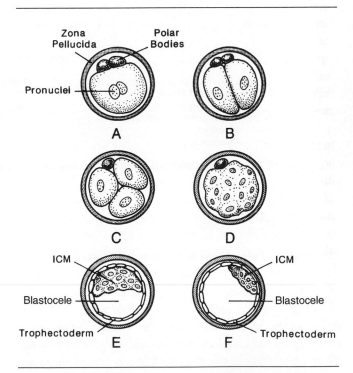

Figure 40–1. Stages of human preimplantation embryogenesis. **A.** The fertilized egg. The male and female pronuclei are present along with two polar bodies extruded during meiosis. A glycoprotein matrix, the zona pellucida, surrounds the egg. **B.** The two-cell embryo. After the first mitotic cleavage, two cells with diploid nuclei are present. **C.** The four-cell embryo. Three of the cells and one polar body are visible. **D.** Morula. After compaction, which occurs at the eight-cell stage, the delineation of individual blastomeres is no longer apparent. Tight junctions are forming at the outside of the embryo in preparation for blastulation. **E.** Early blastocyst. The blastocele forms within the intracellular space of the embryo. The outside cells of the embryo, the trophectoderm, seal the embryo so that solutes may be sequestered within, forming an osmotic gradient that promotes cavitation. The blastomeres have differentiated into trophectoderm and inner cell mass (ICM) cells. **F.** Expanding blastocyst. As more solutes are transported across the trophectoderm, the blastocele enlarges and the embryo expands.

first cell cleavage, cell number doubles every 12 hours.[12] The first 3 days of embryonic development are a period primarily concerned with increasing cell number. This is followed by differentiation into central blastomeres and peripherally aligned trophectoderm. During compaction, which occurs on the third day of gestation, blastomeres flatten against one another and form apical, tight junctions (Fig 40–1D). There is a change in cell morphology from spherical to cylindrical. A reorganization of organelles gives polarity to the cell, and this polarity determines the direction of proliferation and invasion. The blastomeres form a homogenous inner cell mass while the outer cells at the morula stage develop surface microvilli and glycoconjugates.[13] The trophectoderm eventually gives rise to the placenta and extraembryonic tissue, and the inner cell mass eventually forms the fetus. Active transport of solutes across the trophectoderm layer causes the blastocyst to expand during the fourth day of gestation because of fluid accumulation within the blastocele[14] (Fig 40–1F).

The inner cell mass undergoes differentiation into endoderm and ectoderm.[12] The outer trophectoderm cells undergo further specialization. Polar trophectoderm, that which covers the inner cell mass at the embryonic pole, forms an invasive ectoplacental cone. The mural trophectoderm, which lines the remainder of the blastocele, terminally differentiates into giant cells. In mice, these trophoblast giant cells invade the uterine endometrium.[8]

Early events in human embryogenesis are less well known. In the classic study by Hertig and Rock,[15] there is a peripheral layer of primitive syncytiotrophoblast, formed by the apparent fusion of trophectoderm cells, surrounded an inner layer of proliferating cytotrophoblast (Fig 40–3). Together these cells give rise to the structure of the primitive villi of the invading conceptus. Although the organization of rodent and human trophoblast differs (endoreplication of DNA versus cell fusion), both systems are characterized by proliferating mononuclear trophoblasts surrounded by terminally differentiated giant trophoblasts (syncytiotrophoblast). Trophoblasts are the first cell type to differentiate in mammalian embryos. They are endowed with a remarkable property: a transient ability to invade and migrate through other tissues.

STAGES OF IMPLANTATION

Human fertilization normally occurs in the ampullary portion of the fallopian tube. The embryo takes 3 days to traverse the tube and reach the uterus. The human blastocyst remains in the uterus for an additional 2 to 3 days before adhering to the uterine epithelium.[16] In humans, the blastocyst often takes several days to select an appropriate site for attachment. It most frequently becomes embedded in the posterior fundal portion of

the cavity. Whether this consistent placement reflects the effect of gravity while a person is in the supine position or some form chemoattraction is not known. At one point the early human blastocyst consists of 107 cells, of which 99 are trophoblasts and the remaining eight compose the inner cell mass.[17] This asymmetry suggests that the contribution of the inner embryonic cells is minimal with respect to implantation. Before implantation, the embryo has proceeded through six or seven cell divisions, compaction has occurred, and the blastocyst has undergone expansion, a process that aids hatching. A portion of the cytotrophoblast population differentiates into a syncytiotrophoblast which synthesizes large amounts of human chorionic gonadotropin (hCG). The precise time of hatching in humans is unclear.

Schlafke and Enders[8] described implantation as a process that takes place in three stages. After the blastocyst lodges in a crypt within the uterine folds, it hatches from the zona pellucida and then achieves (1) apposition to the uterine wall, (2) adhesion between the trophoblast and uterine epithelium, and (3) penetration of the epithelium, basement membrane, and the underlying stroma. During this process the nonadherent trophoblast cells acquire adherent and then invasive properties. In mice this happens within a few hours after the embryo hatches from the zona pellucida.[18,19]

Hatching of the Blastocyst

The blastocyst matures and leaves the zona during the process of hatching. This process occurs on day 5 after ovulation. The zona pellucida is composed of glycoproteins that surround the ovum throughout preimplantation embryogenesis. In addition to providing physical protection, these glycoproteins serve as species-specific sperm recognition molecules (eg, ZP-2, ZP-3) and induce the acrosome reaction after sperm binding.[20]

The emergence of the blastocyst from the zona is probably the result of at least three forces: a degradative enzyme on the blastocyst surface, enzymatic digestion by uterine secretions, and the physical expansion and contraction of the blastocele. A repeating pattern of blastocyst expansion and contraction is seen in mice and is potentially the means by which the blastocyst mechanically forces an opening in the zona pellucida. Mice have been shown to produce a trypsin-like enzyme known as strypsin, which is localized on the surface of blastomeres.[21] Its location correlates with the linear slit that forms during hatching in vitro. The uterus produces its own proteases, and there is evidence in mammals that these could participate in zonal lysis.[22] It appears that an absolute requirement for a uterine protease does not exist owing to the ability of blastocysts to hatch in culture.

Through a small slit-like opening in the zona, the trophectoderm cells squeeze out, producing a figure-eight shape during

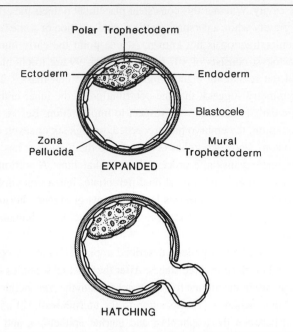

Figure 40–2. Hatching of the expanded blastocyst. A short time before implantation the zona pellucida is shed, allowing contact between the trophectoderm cells, now the trophoblast, and the uterine epithelia. Further cell differentiation of the trophectoderm into polar and mural trophectoderm forms a slit-like opening in the zona pellucida and progressively squeezes through it.

the intermediate stage of hatching (Fig 40–2). Once outside, these cells reexpand. The embryo on day 8 is at least twice the size of a day 5 blastocyst. Blastocyst expansion is one means by which the embryo and uterine epithelium are forced into closer contact. Embryos at this stage have yet to adhere and can be flushed from the uterus with a catheter for a period of 1 to 2 days.[23]

Apposition

Before attachment takes place a complex interchange of signals between the embryo and uterine lining takes place. Cytokines, growth factors, enzymes, peptide hormones, and cell surface lectins are certainly involved. The process starts 6 days after the luteinizing hormone (LH) surge and begins with the orientation of the blastyocyst within the lumen. In humans the embryonic site of apposition begins on day 5 or 6 with the trophectoderm immediately overlying the inner cell mass (Fig 40–3).

The progressive onset of adhesion begins when the embryo comes in contact with the receptive portion of the endometrium. During this period several conditions facilitate intimate contact between a trophoblast and uterine epithelium. Intrauterine fluid is absorbed by the uterus, bringing about collapse of the wall around the blastocyst. This stage coincides with the peak of uterine stromal edema, which may increase

contact between endometrium and the embryo within its cavity. Stromal edema may also loosen the interstitial matrices the trophoblast are to traverse.

The blastocyst contributes to this process by undergoing rapid proliferation and expansion. By increasing its size when lodged within a crypt or fold, the blastocyst achieves closer contact with the uterine lining. During this time the trophectoderm cells fuse to form a syncytium or aggregate to form cell columns that adhere to the uterus. In the underlying endometrium, blood vessels start to move toward the surface, eventually to facilitate nutrient and gas exchange.

Attachment

It stands to reason that the uterine surface epithelium is not adhesive for most of each menstrual cycle, nor should be the em-

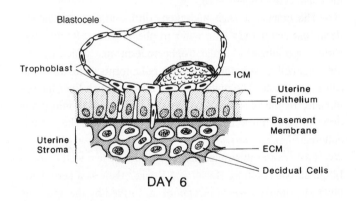

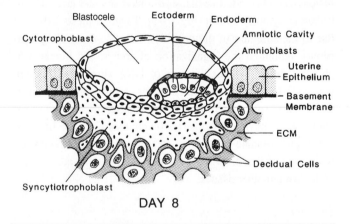

Figure 40–3. Implantation of the human blastocyst. On day 6 of pregnancy there is intrusive movement of the trophoblast cells past the uterine epithelial layer, through the basement membrane, and into the extracellular matrix (BCM) material that surrounds the decidual cells. By day 8 of pregnancy, some of the trophoblasts have fused to form a syncytium, which invades further through the basement membrane and into the stroma, and other trophoblasts near the inner cell mass (ICM) have become proliferative cytotrophoblast cells. Meanwhile, the ICM has undergone further development into an embryonic disk composed of endoderm, ectoderm, and amnioblasts with the beginnings of an amniotic cavity.

bryo throughout its journey from the follicle. Both undergo complex changes during the attachment phase that facilitate adhesion between two very distinct cell types. Completion of this phase can be demonstrated as the point in time after which flushing the uterus no longer yields embryos.

Cell interactions during preimplantation development are likely to require the expression of a variety of cell adhesion molecules at the cell surface. Campbell et al[24] pointed out that during the first 3 days of development the cells of an early embryo lack strong adhesion within themselves, a property that facilitates successful performance of blastomere biopsy. The first important change in cell adherence may come during compaction, when the cells are noticeably more closely apposed with one another.[25] The surfaces of human oocytes and the blastomeres have been shown to contain a mixture of cell adhesion molecules from all four main groups: integrins, selectins, immunoglobulins, and cadherins.[24]

The endometrial surface is covered with thick, negatively charged glycoproteins. A reduction in luminal surface negativity immediately precedes implantation.[26] There is considerable evidence in animal models that decreased thickness in the glycocalyx of the uterus confers receptivity to the endometrium.[27,28] In some species, these changes occur only at the site of embryo contact or only when an embryo is present. In addition, human trophoblasts cultured in vitro lose their proteolytic activity as the thickness of the extracellular matrix (ECM) increases.[29] This evidence suggests that thinning of the glycocalyx facilitates invasion and may unmask binding sites for trophoblasts. Muc-1, a highly glycosylated protein of the apical epithelial membrane, is downregulated at the time of initial attachment during implantation.[30] We recently obtained similar findings in a baboon model.[31] This supports the concept that Muc-1 may be a barrier to blastocyst adhesion that must be removed to allow embryonic-epithelial cell surface interaction.

The removal of barriers to implantation would result in a receptive endometrium. Studies have shown that opening of the putative window of implantation is associated with the development of projections known as pinopodes on the apical surface[32] and the expression of epithelial integrins.[33]

Pinopodes are progesterone-induced, ectoplasmic projections that perform endocytosis, pinocytosis, and reabsorption of fluid from the uterine lumen. Martel et al[32] observed the development of pinopodes starting on cycle day 18 and culminating by day 20. The appearance of pinopodes coincided with the window of implantation. By day 21 to day 22 the pinopodes had regressed. Psychoyos and Nikas[34] showed that these findings extend to clomiphene- and gonadotropin-stimulated cycles. These investigators found premature development of pinopodes, suggesting that these drugs could artificially advance the implantation window.

Lessey et al[33] described the distribution of different integrin subunits in the endometrium at various stages of the menstrual cycle. Integrins are heterodimeric transmembrane glycoproteins that interact with the ECM. Their differential expression in the endometrium is believed to be the only example of integrin modulation by steroid hormones. Studies have shown that the opening of the putative window for implantation is associated with the co-expression of two glandular epithelial integrins: $\alpha_4\beta_1$ and $\alpha_v\beta_3$.[35] Integrins are also found on the surface of human preimplantation embryos.[24] This interaction may be critical for stromal cell proliferation and differentiation and regulation of trophoblast invasion.[36,37] If integrins are present on both trophoblast and endometrial cell surfaces, adhesion may be mediated through bridging molecules like osteopontin, fibrinogen, or oncofetal fibronectin.[38] Clinical disorders in which fertility is impaired have been shown to have aberrant integrin expression. Abnormal endometrial integrin expression has been described in patients with endometriosis,[39,40] luteal-phase deficiency,[33] diethylstilbestrol (DES) exposure,[41] and idiopathic infertility.[42]

Invasion

Soon after attachment the trophoblast invades the epithelium. The breakdown of epithelial junctional complexes allows the trophoblast cells to migrate to the basement membrane and beyond.[43] This process occurs on day 8 and is illustrated in the lower half of Fig 40–3. Invasion requires penetration of the basement membrane. Further invasion into the decidualized stroma follows. The process culminates in penetration of the maternal spiral arteries within the uterus.

Human trophoblast invasion is a paradox. It proceeds rapidly and seemingly without control. Yet this type of invasion is by means of infiltration and insinuation. Cytotrophoblasts form cellular aggregates that invade the uterus initially in columns. Eventually these cells disperse and invasion proceeds individually.[44] Called intermediate trophoblasts, these cells possess the ability to pass through the inner third of the myometrial layer without causing hemorrhage, thrombosis, or necrosis. Once the trophoblasts are established, an inflammatory infiltrate is rarely seen in this process.

Trophoblast invasion has been compared with that of an aggressive metastatic carcinoma. Liotta et al[45] described the phenotypic change from carcinoma in situ to metastatic carcinoma that occurs when tumor cells acquire the ability to (1) attach to ECM proteins, (2) secrete proteases capable of degradation of these proteins, and (3) migrate through the degraded ECM and stroma.[45] Trophoblast activity in vitro demonstrates exteme degradative and proteolytic activity. Although rapidly invasive through epithelium, basement membrane, stroma, muscle and vasculature, trophoblast activity is regulated. Malignant transformation of these cells results in choriocarcinoma, yet the invasiveness of this disease is far less than that of a normal trophoblast during the first week of implantation.

Decidua is thought to have a modulating effect on trophoblast invasion. Implantation stage mouse blastocysts transplanted to ectopic sites invade without restraint.[46] This has been shown to occur regardless of the hormonal status of the female host, or even in males.[47] If the uterine epithelium is removed, blastocysts implant independent of any hormonal modulation.[48] In humans the sites of ectopic pregnancy, a life-threatening consequence of trophoblast invasiveness, are usually devoid of deciduate stroma. It is conspicuous that the only tissue in which trophoblast invasion does not occur indiscriminately is the natural implantation site, the uterine lining.

The decidua is rich with lymphoid cells, which may confer a barrier of immunoprotection for the blastocyst. Nidation is an immunologic paradox since antigenically foreign cells are being tolerated within an immunocompetent host environment.

The implanting blastocyst first encounters the uterine epithelium. Placentation requires that this protective layer be penetrated. The trophoblast encounters several other protective layers, each of different structure and composition. The epithelial basement membrane, stroma, myometrium, and uterine vasculature are all targets of the trophoblast. These cells therefore must carry an invasive strategy for each barrier it might encounter. Several studies have shown that trophoblast-secreted proteases play a crucial role in nidation. In mice, production of plasminogen activator by trophoblasts and blastocysts is synchronized with the time period of blastocyst invasion.[49] Implantation-defective mouse embryos have been found to secrete reduced amounts of plasminogen activator.[50] Cultured human trophoblasts secrete plasminogen activators with potent proteolytic activity.[51,52] Plasminogen activators catalyze the conversion of plasminogen to plasmin. Plasmin is an active protease of broad specificity; it is capable of direct degradation or activation of metalloproteinase zymogens. Therefore it is likely that secreted plasminogen activator catalyzes or initiates a cascade of extracellular proteolysis.

Within the endometrium, a basement membrane separates both liminal and glandular epithelial cells from the underlying stroma. This layer is normally a barrier to invasion yet contains type IV collagen and laminin, which are targets of the intrusive trophoblast. Studies in vitro suggest that a coordinate expression of matrix metalloproteinases (MMP), a family of enzymes that degrade components of the ECM, are important for trophoblast migration. Both the rodent and human trophoblasts secrete MMP-9 (gelatinase B) and MMP-2 (gelatinase A).[53] The invasive behavior of cytotrophoblasts in vitro was limited to those from early human gestations.

STRUCTURE OF THE UTERUS AND DECIDUALIZATION

Cycling endometrium is a complex environment of intracellular communication. The human endometrium exhibits a well-orchestrated repeating cycle of proliferation, differentiation, death, and renewal. The same cells programmed to slough in the absence of a blastocyst must also be able to nurture gestation for 40 weeks. The myriad of mediators involved in this recurring process includes cytokines, peptides, growth factors, and prostaglandins. The ability to establish a pregnancy with hormonal stimulation in the absence of functioning ovaries,[54] however, has demonstrated that estrogen and progesterone are the primary regulators of endometrial development.

After menses, the endometrium consists of simple tubular glands set within a vascular, cellular stroma. During the early proliferative phase of the menstrual cycle, the glands are small, straight, and round when seen in cross section. The endometrium is the primary target organ for ovarian steroids. Under the influence of estrogen, the glands multiply and their epithelium becomes taller and pseudostratified. By midsecretory phase, progesterone is abundant and intraglandular glycogen secretion reaches a peak. Stromal edema and spiral artery development reach a peak on day 22 or 23 in response to the presence of progesterone (Fig 40–4).

While the endometrium is acquiring its receptivity, the embryo is acquiring its invasiveness. The blastocyst normally implants during the midsecretory phase of the cycle. After implantation, glandular secretion continues and stromal edema persists. Fifteen days from ovulation, a fully formed decidua emerges, and almost the entire endometrial stroma is converted into pavement-like sheets of epithelial cells.[55] The decidua consists of three layers by the late luteal phase: compacta, spongiosa, and basalis. If implantation does not occur, the zona compacta and zona spongiosa are shed at menses. The basalis layer remains intact after menstruation, and a new endometrial lining is regenerated from this layer. Decidualization occurs only when the endometrium is sequentially exposed to estrogenic priming followed by progesterone stimulation. Fibroblastic stromal cells transform into large polygonal cells that contain glycogen and lipid. Clear cytoplasm becomes profoundly basophilic. The reaction takes several days and is first seen around stromal blood vessels.[56] Fibroblasts, mast cells, and stem cells are usually present within the stroma. During decidualization, macrophages and lymphocytes are transiently present.[57] The function of these cellular components ranges from protein synthesis to enzymatic degradation and phagocytosis.

The portion of the decidua directly beneath the site of implantation is called the decidua basalis. The basilis is invaded extensively by trophoblasts. A zone of fibrinoid degeneration occurs where the trophoblasts encounter the decidua. This re-

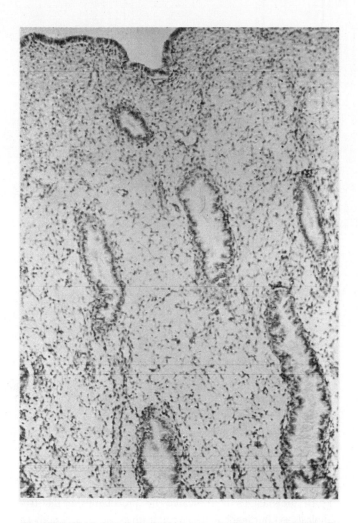

Figure 40–4. Histologic specimen of midsecretory endometrium, approximately day 22.

gion has been called Nitabuch's layer. When the integrity of the decidua is breached, as in placenta accreta, Nitabuch's layer is usually absent.[58] Ovarian steroids direct decidualization in humans, and a precise combination of estrogen and progesterone is critical for establishment of nidation.[59] The amount and degree of decidualization among species reflect the relative invasiveness of trophoblasts. More decidual tissue is made in species that have more intrusive trophoblasts.

Much of the knowledge concerning steroid hormone requirements for implantation comes from the study of delayed implantation in animals. In a number of species, embryos can lie dormant in the uterus for periods as long as 15 months before implantation is initiated. In other species, delayed implantation can be induced by means of postpartum suckling or ovariectomy on day 3 of pregnancy.[60] Delayed implantation is characterized by a marked decrease in DNA and protein synthesis by the blastocyst as it enters embryonic diapause. The embryo can be maintained at the blastocyst stage and the uterus in a neutral state by means of continuous progesterone injection into the

mother.[61] In mice, the endometrium is first primed with a basal level of estrogen and then maintained during a progesterone-dependent sensitization stage that is finally attenuated with an estrogen surge just before the blastocyst enters the uterus.[62] During the period of progesterone priming, the uterus shows suboptimal sensitivity for the decidual reaction. This allows the blastocyst to survive in dormancy. The subsequent action of a surge in estrogen level produces a state of uterine receptivity, followed in 36 hours by a state of uterine refractoriness.[63] During the latter period an environment develops that is hostile to the embryo and inhibitory to the decidual reaction.

It was once believed that after the window of implantation has closed, implantation is not possible. The antiprogesterone drug RU-486 given on day 1 of anticipated pregnancy in rats extends the receptive phase beyond normal timing and postpones establishment of uterine refractoriness.[64] An elegant demonstration of manipulation of the transfer window was recently reported by Beier et al.[65] In a rabbit model, 4-day postcoital blastocysts were transferred into recipients 4, 5, and 6 days after coitus. Normal synchrony achieved a 60% implantation rate, 1-day dysynchrony decreased the implantation rate to 35%, and 2-day dysynchrony prevented implantation. A second group of recipients received a 1-day regimen of progesterone antagonists. Transfer of 4-day postcoital blastocysts into a recipient 9 days after coitus yielded a 65% implantation rate. Transfer into recipients 12 days after coitus produced a 35% implantation rate. These findings have provided convincing evidence that the implantation window can be reopened pharmacologically. This represents a novel use of progesterone antagonists, which have achieved most of their notoriety as abortifacients, and has profound implications for eventual use in managing infertility in humans.

Our understanding of the implantation window comes from the cumulative experience with asynchronous transfers in animal models. Observations from the asynchronous transfer of embryos into the uteri of surrogate mothers suggest that the blastocyst can wait for the endometrium to become ready for implantation, for a limited period of time. On the other hand, a receptive endometrium cannot wait for the embryo to develop to the blastocyst stage.[66] This clearly indicates that the embryo must be at the blastocyst stage in the uterus and ready for implantation into the endometrium when the latter becomes receptive for the blastocyst. Once the receptive period is over, the endometrial environment becomes refractory, even toxic to the blastocyst.[67] The window of implantation refers to this short period of time of endometrial receptivity. The receptive phase in small mammals is usually less than 24 hours.[68] In primates the window of implantation is open for a longer duration. By transferring embryos into the fallopian tubes of surrogate mothers, Hodgen[69] showed that the receptive phase in primates is as long as 3 days. According to these and other findings, the steroid hormone requirements for implantation have been determined and are remarkably simple. However, the complex array of their actions in inducing autocrine and paracrine regulators within the human endometrium remains to be determined. In rodents, estrogen triggers several events that allow implantation to begin. It acts on the uterine epithelium, inducing it to secrete cytokines including epidermal growth factor (EGF), leukemia inhibitory factor (LIF), colony-stimulating factor 1 (CSF-1), heparin binding epidermal growth factor (HB-EGF), and interleukin-1B (IL-1B).[70] Transgene studies in which "gene knockouts" were used have suggested that of all these growth factors activated in response to the blastocyst signal, the absence of LIF alone prevents implantation.[71] Similar implantation blockades have been seen in CSF-deficient mice[72] and in mice treated with IL-1 receptor antagonist,[73] suggesting these factors may have critical importance in nidation.

On either side of the implantation window, the uterus is a hostile environment to an embryo. If placed into an environment without appropriate estrogen and progesterone preparation, the embryo does not implant. On the other hand, the trophoblast is remarkably invasive outside the uterus, either in culture or in ectopic implantation. Uterine function may be to limit invasion to maintain a balance between the needs of a rapidly growing pregnancy and the needs of the mother as host.

PATHOLOGIC INVASION

The uterus is cyclically permissive to an entrained program of trophoblast invasiveness. Placentation clearly is a tightly regulated phenomenon. Inadequate invasion results in failed implantation and early pregnancy loss, situations known to exist, yet which cannot be studied at the cellular level as they are occurring.

Examples of unrestricted trophoblast invasion include placenta accreta, ectopic pregnancy, and molar pregnancy. Postpartum hemorrhage and abruptio placentae are not currently attributed to a disorder in trophoblast invasiveness, but it stands to reason that there may be a contributing factor in some patients.

Ectopic pregnancies most frequently occur in the ampullary portion of the fallopian tube. An example of the inherently invasive nature of trophoblast cells is that embryonic implantations have occurred on the liver and spleen as well as in the retroperitoneum, cervix, and vagina.[74] Ectopic implantation is associated with copious hemorrhage. In normal gestation the endometrium gives rise to the decidual layer, which is thought to limit trophoblast invasion. Implantation in the fallopian tube lends support to this contention. Trophoblasts infiltrate the tubal

endosalpinx and then invade the lamina propria and muscularis. When trophoblasts encounter the peritoneal surface, invasion is redirected and proceeds in parallel to the long axis of the tube.[75] Rupture is the result of mechanical forces from the expanding mass and retroperitoneal hemorrhage. Pathologic trophoblast invasion has a predilection for attacking in sites of previous scarring, such as a fallopian tube with previous salpingitis or placenta accreta in the location of a previous uterine scar. These are areas where normal decidual formation is impaired.

It is now recognized that pregnancy-induced hypertension and preeclampsia have their pathogenesis in trophoblast invasion. Normal placentation ceases with complete trophoblast infiltration of the spiral arteries. Pregnancy requires an immediate threefold increase in uterine blood flow and an eventual tenfold increase in delivery of maternal blood to the placenta. The trophoblasts secrete their own matrix, and the walls of the spiral arteries are converted into tubes of fibrinoid material with embedded trophoblastic cells.[6] The structural integrity of the vessel is maintained, but the vessel wall is completely replaced by trophoblasts. In normal placentation, the diameter of the colonized vessel increases and the paucity of smooth muscle limits the ability of the vessel to constrict. The end result is development of dilated capacitance vessels. The changes in architecture allow for the greater requirements in blood flow. Brosens et al[76] suggested that this process changes the structure of the distal spiral arteries to the degree that they are set free from the vasomotor influences of the mother.

In pregnancies complicated by preeclampsia, the trophoblasts exhibit inadequate vascular invasion. In one study of the placental bed in patients with preeclampsia, no evidence of trophoblast-induced changes was seen in any myometrial segments of the spiral arteries.[77] The consequence of shallow invasion of uterine arterioles is poor perfusion of the placenta.[78] The hypoxia resulting from this poor perfusion can cause vascular endothelial cell damage and exacerbate the course of the disease.

CLINICAL ASSESSMENT OF ENDOMETRIAL RECEPTIVITY

The uterus is unique in that it is an internal organ with central tissues that are easily accessible for biopsy. Direct application of an ultrasound probe to this organ also is a noninvasive procedure. Unfortunately endometrial accessibility does not confer reliability in clinical testing. Assessment of endometrial receptivity has many shortcomings. Although the measures currently used are inaccurate for prediction of the receptive endometrium, they are more successful for identification of the nonreceptive state. If this negative condition can be predicted, corrective measures can be introduced before wasteful application of expensive technology.

Evaluation of the luteal phase is a critical part of the investigation for couples experiencing infertility or recurrent pregnancy loss. Luteal-phase deficiency was first described in 1949.[79] This disorder stems from inadequate ovarian progesterone production and results in failure of blastocyst implantation or inability to maintain an established pregnancy. The crucial role of ovarian progesterone has been demonstrated in animal models. In human gestation the need for progesterone is supported by a set of experimental observations that would be difficult to duplicate today. Women who were scheduled for pregnancy termination agreed to undergo luteectomy between 7 and 9 weeks' gestation.[80] All who underwent luteectomy at 7 weeks' gestation subsequently experienced abortions. None who underwent luteectomy at 9 weeks' gestation miscarried. This finding clearly demonstrated the timing of the luteal-placental shift in humans. In a follow-up study, supplemental progesterone was shown to salvage gestations after luteectomy was performed at 7 weeks' gestation.[81] The critical role of progesterone in implantation and maintenance of early gestation is not debated. A clinical syndrome of inadequate progesterone production by the corpus luteum explains many unfortunate clinical outcomes, especially among patients with symptoms and a luteal phase of 11 days or less. Unfortunately detection and treatment of luteal-phase defects have been a source of constant disagreement since this disorder was first described.

Clinical evaluation of luteal-phase deficiency is fraught with controversy. Serum progesterone levels would provide the most direct assessment of circulating hormone. However, luteal-phase progesterone secretion is pulsatile,[82] rendering serum determination inaccurate even with multiple blood draws. Although endometrial biopsy provides an indirect measurement of circulating levels, it does reflect an end-organ response to prolonged progesterone exposure. In a comprehensive review, biopsy was considered the preferred test to establish a diagnosis.[83] Many have called endometrial biopsy the "gold standard" against which all other dating modalities are to be measured.

Timing of the biopsy influences results, unfortunately there is no consensus about when this test should be performed. According to the original criteria established by Noyes et al,[84] a biopsy may be performed 2 to 3 days from the anticipated onset of the subsequent menstrual cycle or 11 to 13 days after ovulation. Results are interpreted by dating backward from subsequent menses or forward from ovulatory events. These two approaches may give different results for the same cycle. Pinpointing of ovulation is difficult, in part because of the many ways ovulation is determined (urine or serum LH measurements, basal body temperature (BBT) charts, ultrasound confirmation of follicular rupture). Some authors have advocated that biopsy on cycle day 20 would more accurately reflect endometrial status at the time of implantation.[85] Detection itself is complicated by inaccuracies inherent in the testing method used. Within one biopsy specimen on a single slide there can be regional differences in endometrial histologic features. Stromal elements and glandular components in the same field may not coincide, thereby introducing individual interpretation. At the time the criteria of Noyes et al were originally proposed, it was recognized that there was considerable interobserver variability. Several studies have shown that in addition to interobserver variability, testing accuracy is confounded by intercycle variation within the same patient.[86,87] Scott et al[88] showed an acceptable level of inter- and intraobserver variability among pathologists in a blinded study, but when the same pathologists later reexamined these specimens, a different endometrial date leading to a change in therapy was rendered in almost 40% of cases.

There is dispute in the literature whether a diagnosis of luteal-phase deficiency confers any risk to a patient. The prevalence of out-of-phase biopsies in an infertile population has been reported to be 3% to 20%.[89–91] A similar prevalence of out-of-phase biopsies has been reported among fertile women.[92,93] In settings in which this disorder has been correctly diagnosed, investigators have found no difference in fecundity among infertile patients with or without luteal-phase deficiency.[94,95] From the patient's standpoint, diagnosis is more uncomfortable and expensive than treatment. As a result treatment protocols have been empirical and uncontrolled. In a 1992 review, Karamardian and Grimes[96] concluded that uniform case definitions did not exist, diagnostic tests had not been validated by controlled trials, and no study to date had sufficient power to demonstrate benefit from treatment.

Transvaginal ultrasound examination provides rapid assessment of endometrial development, which could possibly be used to predict the outcome of embryo transfer. In one study of donor insemination in natural cycles, pregnancy did not occur when endometrial thickness was less than 6 mm.[97] Several studies of endometrial thickness in ART cycles have not shown a correlation between thickness and cycle outcome,[98–100] but many investigators have suggested that there is a minimum threshold of 5 to 8 mm below which no pregnancies have been observed.[101–103] Endometrial pattern can be assessed at the time of transvaginal ultrasound examination and may provide information of a higher predictive value. Several centers have reported higher pregnancy rates in cycles displaying a triple-line pattern versus a hyperechoic pattern.[104–106]

Uterine blood flow can be studied in a noninvasive manner with Doppler ultrasound. This modality is not in common use but can be added to most transvaginal ultrasound machines. In normal cycles, uterine blood flow rises in the luteal phase to coincide with the timing of implantation.[107] Two studies found Doppler patterns that were suggested to be predictive of pregnancy outcome. Steer et al[108] found a higher implantation rate and a higher incidence of multiple gestations among patients with higher uterine flow rates. Sterzik et al[109] found that no patients with absent diastolic flow after IVF sustained a successful conception. A 1995 prospective study of 196 IVF cycles demonstrated changes in uterine vascularity during different portions of a stimulation cycle, but no relation between uterine flow rates and pregnancy outcome was seen.[110] Larger studies with this modality are needed.

Establishment of a receptive endometrium is one of the main goals in the successful management of infertility. If lack of receptivity can be predicted, corrective measures could be applied before application of expensive procedures and technology. Currently all methods for determining uterine receptivity are blunt instruments at best. Their usefulness is limited by the fact that each test yields results thought to have positive and negative predictive value, which are within the confidence intervals of each other. Given the standard error of each detecting modality, intra- and interobserver variability, no method has emerged that has allowed reliable indentification of a receptive endometrium in a prospective manner.

LESSONS FROM IN VITRO FERTILIZATION AND OOCYTE DONATION

Developed initially as solution to tubal infertility, IVF has taught us that the 3 days an embryo spends in the fallopian tube are not critical to fertilization or implantation. Embryos can complete their development in vitro in a simple defined medium, a finding that suggests tubal factors act in only a permissive manner. The fallopian tube is invested with cilia, all of which beat in the direction of the uterus. Tubal function has traditionally been considered a means for achieving embryo transport. It may more accurately represent a safe holding zone that delays transport and allows the blastocyst time to divide and increase its cell number before presentation to the uterus.

Successful performance of IVF has brought about rapid advances in the practice of embryo culture. In spite of these advances implantation rates in IVF of individual embryos are disappointing and inferior to normal human fecundity. Satisfactory pregnancy rates have been achieved with the transfer of multiple embryos, at the expense of increased risk for multiple gestations. One problem is that embryos in tissue culture are not exposed to endometrially derived factors, which may enhance their ability to implant. Co-culture has been used at many centers in an attempt to provide a more physiologic environment for the embryo.

The final outcome measure of a successful IVF cycle is a thriving implantation. Considerable effort has been aimed at improving the efficiency of ART. Because implantation is a result of the synchronization of embryo quality with endometrial receptivity, conclusions that can be drawn from retrospective reviews of IVF cycles are limited. The development of donor egg programs has enabled many patients to overcome infertility. It has also provided a means by which complete separation of endometrial development and gametogenesis can be achieved. Controlling one of these variables allows closer examination of the effects on each of these two critical factors.

Endometrial Effects of Controlled Ovarian Hyperstimulation

Ovarian hyperstimulation with exogenous gonadotropins has become a routine part of infertility therapy. The large number of oocytes that can be obtained greatly increases the overall likelihood for pregnancy for infertile couples. A potential disadvantage of this therapy is that the supraphysiologic levels of preovulatory ovarian steroids appear to have detrimental effects on endometrial receptivity.[59,111,112] The fact that ovarian hyperstimulation has a detrimental effect on endometrial receptivity is supported by data that show pregnancy rates are lower and spontaneous abortion rates are much higher among patients who undergo hyperstimulation than among agonadal patients who receive donor eggs after exogenous hormonal priming[113] or among fertile women.[114] In spite of the high fertilization rates achieved in vitro, the "take home baby" rate after ovarian hyperstimulation remains low, especially when considered per embryo transferred.

Morphologic studies indicate that the luteal-stage endometrium is impaired by controlled ovarian hyperstimulation (COH).[115,116] This therapy induces considerable dysynchrony in the maturation of the glandular epithelium and stroma.[117] An abnormality in pinopode development also suggests that COH artificially advances the period of endometrial receptivity.[34]

The deleterious endometrial effect of COH has become evident with the success of donor egg programs. A persuasive demonstration was reported by Paulson et al,[113] who divided fertilized sibling oocytes between donors and recipients. These investigators controlled for age and egg quality. They showed consistently lower pregnancy rates among patients who were exposed to superovulation (donors) than among recipients who received exogenous hormones for endometrial preparation. Oocyte donation programs typically see implantation rates of 14% to 18%, which is considerable improvement over conventional IVF success on a per embryo basis.[118,119]

Hormone Requirements for Endometrial Preparation

One important lesson has been learned from the studies of endometrial preparation for recipients of donated eggs. The presence of a preimplantation embryo is not a prerequisite for endometrial priming as evidenced by the fact that cleaving embryos implant when transferred to a surrogate uterus prepared with exogenous estrogen and progesterone.

Ovum donation has allowed pregnancy in patients devoid of ovarian function. Exogenous steroids can be used to simulate the natural cycle in women with ovarian failure. Estrogen is required for endometrial proliferation and induction of progesterone receptors. An initial prerequisite was to determine the estrogen requirements for adequate endometrial proliferation. Navot et al[120] showed that the endometrium was amenable to a wide variation in duration of estrogen priming. The investigators saw no difference in implantation or pregnancy rates among recipients who received 5 days of estrogen versus those who had 35 days of treatment.

The wide range of estrogen exposure that produces a receptive endometrium should not be surprising. Studies of estrogen and progesterone levels during the normal menstrual cycle show wide variability from woman to woman.[121] It is also known that the follicular phase can be very flexible in length in fertile women. In contrast, excessive estrogen administered in the postovulatory period can prevent implantation.[122] In addition, high serum estradiol levels during ovarian hyperstimulation also have a detrimental effect on implantation.[111,112]

Patients who undergo cycles of hormone replacement as recipients of donated eggs typically have out-of-phase biopsy findings.[123] The most common finding is stromal-glandular dysynchrony with glands lagging behind appropriately dated stroma. Pregnancy rate is not compromised when the stromal date is in phase.

Premature Elevation of Progesterone Level

Premature surges in LH were a common problem in IVF before the widespread use of gonadotropin-releasing hormone (GnRH) agonists. The result was frequent cycle cancellation. GnRH agonists have virtually eliminated the possibility of an LH surge. However, progesterone level may still rise toward the end of an IVF cycle. The elevation is usually subtle, but there is concern that this may close the implantation window. The practical consequence of a subtle rise in progesterone level is controversial and has been reviewed.[124] Schoolcraft et al[125] reported a critical threshold of 0.9 ng/mL on the day of hCG administration. Patient levels higher than this had an 11% pregnancy rate, those with levels less than 0.5 ng/mL had a 54% pregnancy rate. Numerous other reports appeared citing elevated progesterone levels in association with lower pregnancy rates.[126,127] The donor egg model has been used to answer questions about egg quality versus endometrial disturbance as the cause of low pregnancy rates.

To examine the effects of elevated progesterone level on oocyte quality and endometrial maturation requires the separation of these two events. In an elegant demonstration by Hofmann et al,[128] 31% of oocyte donors who had elevated progesterone levels at the time of hCG administration participated in a study. Embryos from cycles with elevated progesterone levels had similar implantation and live delivery rates compared with cycles with normal progesterone levels. These results suggest that no harm is done to oocytes in a cycle with subtle progesterone elevation. This evidence indicates the endometrium sustains the adverse effects of an elevated progesterone level, yet the potential contribution by supraphysiologic estradiol levels must also be acknowledged.

Effect of Embryo Age

The rapid decline in fecundity after the age of 35 years has been widely observed. The absence of implantation or a single implantation that fails is tragic to patients who complete IVF. It is also a source of frustration to clinicians and embryologists that implantation rates are low even with the transfer of multiple embryos of apparently good quality. Morphologic integrity and rate of cleavage are valuable indices of embryonic potential but have proved to be of limited value in predicting successful outcomes.[129] A large portion of these failures can be attributed to factors not visible to the embryologist. A statistically significant increase in chromosomal abnormalities was seen among unfertilized oocytes from women older than 35 years.[130] Wramsby and Fredga[131] reported a high frequency of aneuploidy among mature oocytes obtained after IVF retrieval. In that report[131] almost 50% of oocytes examined were aneuploid, a finding that has been confirmed by others with different techniques.[132]

There is little doubt that advancing age has a detrimental effect on oocytes. Egg donation has extended the temporal boundaries of childbearing. The ability of the uterus to escape the consequences of aging is most convincing when one looks at the recent success of egg donation in menopausal patients.[133] However, many programs have also reported no differences in pregnancy rate or implantation rate among recipients 40 years and older versus those younger than 40 years.[134–136] The use of donated eggs has enabled women to conceive in their sixth decade. This has shown convincingly that menopause is an ovarian event, not a uterine one.

CONCLUSION

Embryonic implantation is the culmination of a highly complex sequence of tightly regulated events. Estradiol and progesterone have a central role in directing the changes that facilitate implantation. Early research sought to identify factors expressed at the time of implantation that were likely to be critical. It is now recognized that factors that are downregulated at the time of implantation may be just as important. Nidation is a difficult process to study in toto. Investigators need to isolate variables and control for many confounding factors. Once all the pieces of this puzzle are known, it will become clear that estrogen and progesterone initiate an intricate cascade of enzymes, secretory proteins, cytokines, and growth factors. The exact effects of each factor will be difficult to determine because of astounding complexity and perhaps immense redundancy, as has been clearly demonstrated in mouse studies in which transgene "knockout" technology was used.

Embryo quality and endometrial development are the two main determinants of successful nidation. All higher biologic systems function to enable these two determinants to function synchronously. No test allows accurate prediction of uterine receptivity, although there are several accurate indicators of uterine refractoriness. We must acknowledge that the lack of consistent success of IVF, GIFT, and insemination therapies may be related to problems at the level of implantation that we cannot yet diagnose. As our understanding of implantation broadens, we may be allowed to treat an implantation or preimplantation factor as a cause of infertility.

The initiation of placental morphogenesis is not fully understood, but advances are being made that are unraveling the mystery of this process. ART has provided powerful insights into the complex mechanisms that control reproduction and will certainly advance our knowledge of this fascinating phenomenon.

REFERENCES

1. Wilcox AJ, Weinberg CR, O'Connor JF, et al: Incidence of early loss of pregnancy. *N Engl J Med* 319:189, 1988
2. Lala PK, Kearns M, Parkar RS, Scodras J, Johnson S: Immunologic role of the cellular constituents of the decidua in maintenance of semiallogenic pregnancy. *Ann N Y Acad Sci* 476:183, 1986
3. Psychoyos A: The implantation window: Basic and clinical aspects. *Perspect Assist Reprod* 4:57, 1993
4. Wimsatt WA: Some comparative aspects of implantation. *Biol Reprod* 12:1, 1975
5. Finn CA: Species variation in implantation. *Biol Reprod* 7:253, 1980
6. Pijnenborg R, Robertson WB, Brosens I, Dixon G: Trophoblast invasion and the establishment of haemochorial placentation in man and laboratory animals (review article). *Placenta* 2:71, 1981
7. Ilgren EB: Control of trophoblastic growth (review article). *Placenta* 4:307, 1983
8. Schlafke S, Enders AC: Cellular basis of interaction between trophoblast and uterus at implantation. *Biol Reprod* 12:41, 1975
9. Enders A, Chavez DJ, Schlafke S: Comparison of implantation in

utero and in vitro. In: Glasser SR, Bullock DW (eds), *Cellular and Molecular Aspects of Implantation.* New York, Plenum, 1981: 365–382
10. Salomon DS, Sherman MI: Implantation and invasiveness of mouse blastocysts on uterine monolayers. *Exp Cell Res* 90:261, 1975
11. Glass RH, Aggeler J, Spindle A, Pedersen R, Werb Z: A model for implantation. *J Cell Biol* 96:1108, 1993
12. Gardner RL: Origin and differentiation of extraembryonic tissues in the mouse. *Int Rev Exp Pathol* 24:63, 1983
13. Ziomek CA, John MH: Cell surface interaction induces polarization of mouse 8-cell blastomeres at compaction. *Cell* 21:935, 1980
14. Benos DJ, Biggers JD, Balaban RS, Mills JW, Overstrom EW: Developmental aspects of sodium-dependent transport processes of preimplantation rabbit embryos. In: Graves JS (ed), *Regulation and Development of Membrane Transport Processes.* New York, Wiley, 1985:285–335
15. Hertig AT, Rock J: Two human ova of the pre-villous stage having a developmental age of about seven and nine days respectively. *Contrib Embryol* 31:65, 1945
16. Diaz S, Ortiz ME, Croxatto HB: Studies on the duration of ovum transport by the human oviduct. III. Time interval between the luteinizing hormone peak and recovery of ova by transcervical flushing of the uterus in normal women. *Am J Obstet Gynecol* 137:116, 1980
17. Hertig AT, Rock J, Adams EC: A description of 34 human ova within the first 17 days of development. *Am J Anat* 98:435, 1956
18. Sherman MI, Atienza-Samols S: In vitro studies of the surface adhesiveness of mouse blastocysts. In: Ludwig H, Tauber PF (eds), *Human Fertilization.* Littleton, MA, PSG, 1978:179–183
19. Jenkinson EJ, Wilson IB: In vitro studies of the control of trophoblast outgrowth in the mouse. *J Embryol Exp Morphol* 30:21, 1973
20. Bleil JD, Wasserman PM: Mammalian sperm-egg interaction: Identification of a glycoprotein in mouse egg zonae pellucidae possessing receptor activity for sperm. *Cell* 20:837, 1980
21. Perona RM, Wasserman PM: Mouse blastocysts hatch in vitro by using a trypsin-like proteinase associated with cells of mural trophectoderm. *Dev Biol* 114:42, 1986
22. Denker HW: Role of proteinases in implantation. *Prog Reprod Biol* 7:28, 1980
23. Buster JE, Bustillo M, Rodi IA, et al: Biologic and morphologic development of donated human ova recovered by nonsurgical uterine lavage. *Am J Obstet Gynecol* 153:211, 1985
24. Campbell S, Swann HR, Seif MW, Kimber SJ, Aplin JD: Cell adhesion molecules on the oocyte and preimplantation human embryo. *Hum Reprod* 10:1571, 1995
25. Fleming TP, Garrod DR, Elsmore A: Desmosome biogenesis in the mouse preimplantation embryo. *Development* 112:527, 1991
26. Morris JE, Potter SW: A comparison of developmental changes in surface charge in mouse blastocysts and uterine epithelium using DEAE beads and dextran sulfate in vitro. *Dev Biol* 103:190, 1984
27. Weitlauf HM: Biology of implantation. In: Knobil E, Neill J (eds), *Physiology of Reproduction.* New York, Raven, 1988:231–262

28. Enders AC, Schlafke S: Alterations in uterine luminal surface at the implantation site. *J Cell Biol* 75:70a, 1977

29. Kliman HJ, Feinberg RF: Human trophoblast extracellular matrix (ECM) interactions in vitro: ECM thickness modulates morphology and proteolytic activity. *Proc Natl Acad Sci USA* 87:3057, 1990

30. Hey NA, Graham RA, Seif MW, Aplin JD: The polymorphic epithelial mucin MUC-1 in human endometrium is regulated with maximal expression in the implantation phase. *J Clin Endocrinol Metab* 78:337, 1994

31. Hild-Petito S, Fazleabas AT, Julian JA, Carson DD: Mucin (Muc-1) expression is differentially regulated in uterine luminal and glandular epithelia of the baboon (*Papio anubis*). *Biol Reprod* 54:939, 1996

32. Martel D, Monier MN, Roche D, Psychoyos A: Hormonal dependence of pinopode formation at the uterine luminal surface. *Hum Reprod* 6:597, 1991

33. Lessey A, Damjanovich L, Coutifaris C, Castelbaum A, Abelda SM, Buck CA: Integrin adhesion molecules in the human endometrium. *J Clin Invest* 90:188, 1992

34. Psychoyos A, Nikas G: Uterine pinopodes as markers of uterine receptivity. *Assist Reprod Rev* 4:26, 1994

35. Lessey BA, Castelbaum AJ, Buck CA, Lei Y, Yowell CW, Sun J: Further characterization of endometrial integrins during the menstrual cycle and in pregnancy. *Fertil Steril* 62:497, 1994

36. Werb Z, Tremble PM, Behrendtsen O, Crowley E, Damsky CH: Signal transduction through the fibronectin receptor induces collagenase and stromelysin gene expression. *J Cell Biol* 109:877, 1989

37. Burrows TD, King A, Smith SK, Loke YW: Human trophoblast adhesion to matrix proteins: Inhibition and signal transduction. *Hum Reprod* 10:2489, 1995

38. Feinberg RF, Kliman HJ, Lockwood CJ: Oncofetal fibronectin: A trophoblast "glue" for human implantation? *Am J Pathol* 138:537, 1991

39. Bridges JE, Prentice A, Roche W, Englefield P, Thomas EJ: Expression of integrin adhesion molecules in endometrium and endometriosis. *Br J Obstet Gynaecol* 101:696, 1995

40. Lessey BA, Castelbaum AJ: Intergrins in the endometrium of women with endometriosis. *Br J Obstet Gynaecol* 102:347, 1995

41. Castelbaum AJ, Sawin SW, Bellardo LJ, Lessey BS: Endometrial integrin expression in women exposed to diethylstilbestrol in utero. *Fertil Steril* 63:1217, 1995

42. Lessey BA, Castelbaum AJ, Sawin SJ, Sun J: Integrins as markers of uterine receptivity in women with unexplained primary infertility. *Fertil Steril* 63:535, 1995

43. Nilson BD: Electron microscopic aspects of epithelial changes related to implantation. *Prog Reprod Biol* 7:70, 180

44. Aplin JD: Implantation, trophoblast differentiation and haemochorial placentation, mechanistic evidence in vivo and in vitro. *J Cell Sci* 99:681, 1991

45. Liotta LA, Rao CN, Wewer UM: Biochemical interactions of tumor cells with the basement membrane. *Annu Rev Biochem* 55:1037, 1986

46. Kirby DRS: The extra-uterine mouse egg as an experimental model. In: Raspe G (ed), *Schering Symposium on Mechanisms Involved in Conception*. Oxford, Pergamon, 1970:255–273

47. Porter DG: Observations on the development of mouse blastocysts transferred to the testis and kidney. *Am J Anat* 121:73, 1967

48. Cowell TP: Implantation and development of mouse eggs transferred to the uteri of non-progestational mice. *J Reprod Fertil* 19:239, 1969

49. Strickland S, Reich E, Sherman MI: Plasminogen activator in early embryogenesis: Enzyme production by trophoblast and parietal endoderm. *Cell* 9:231, 1976

50. Axelrod HR: Altered trophoblast functions in implantation-defective mouse embryos. *Dev Biol* 108:185, 1985

51. Martin O, Arias F: Plasminogen activator production by trophoblast cells in vitro: Effect of steroid hormones and protein synthesis inhibitors. *Am J Obstet Gynecol* 142:402, 1982

52. Queenan JT Jr, Kao LC, Arboleda CE, et al: Regulation of urokinase-type plasminogen activator production by cultured human cytotrophoblasts. *J Cell Biol* 262:10903, 1987

53. Librach CL, Werb Z, Fitzgerald ML, et al: 92-kD type IV collagenase mediates invasion of human cytotrophoblasts. *J Cell Biol* 113:437, 1991

54. Serhal PF, Craft IL: Ovum donation: A simplified approach. *Fertil Steril* 48:265, 1987

55. Wynn RM: Ultrastructural development of the human decidua. *Am J Obstet Gynecol* 118:652, 1974

56. Kennedy TG: Prostaglandins and uterine sensitization for the decidual cell reaction. *Ann N Y Acad Sci* 476:43, 1986

57. Padykula HA, Tansey TR: The occurrence of uterine stromal and intraepithelial monocytes and heterophils during normal late pregnancy in the rat. *Anat Rec* 193:329, 1979

58. Pritchard JA, MacDonald PC, Gant NF: *Williams Obstetrics*, ed 7. Norwalk, CT, Appleton-Century-Crofts, 1985:98–106

59. Gidley-Baird A, O'Neill C, Sinosich MJ, Porter RN, Pike RL: Failure of implantation in human in vitro fertilization and embryo transfer patients: The effect of altered progesterone/estrogen ratios in humans and mice. *Fertil Steril* 45:69, 1986

60. Van Blerkom J, Chavez DJ, Bell H: Molecular and cellular aspects of facultative delayed implantation in the mouse. In: Ciba Foundation Symposium: *Maternal Recognition of Pregnancy*. Amsterdam, Excerpta Medica, 1979:141

61. Evans CA, Kennedy TB: Blastocyst implantation in ovariectomized, adrenalectomized hamsters treated with inhibitors of steroidogenesis during the preimplantation period. *Steroids* 36:41, 1980

62. Shelesnyak MC: A history of research on nidation. *Ann N Y Acad Sci* 476:5, 1986

63. De Hertogh R, Ekka E, Vanderheyden I, Glorieux B: Estrogen and progesterone receptors in the implantation sites and interembryonic segments of rat uterus endometrium and myometrium. *Endocrinology* 119:680, 1986

64. Rider V, Heap RB, Wang MY, Feinstein A: Anti-progesterone monoclonal antibody affects early cleavage and implantation in the mouse by mechanisms that are influenced by genotype. *J Reprod Fertil* 79:33, 1987

65. Beier HM, Hegele-Hartung C, Mootz U, Beier-Hellwig K: Modifi-

cation of endometrial cell biology using progesterone antagonists to manipulate the implantation window. *Hum Reprod* 9:98 S, 1994

66. Doyle LL, Gates AH, Noyes RW: Asynchronous transfer of mouse ova. *Fertil Steril* 14:215, 1963

67. Yoshinaga K: Uterine receptivity for blastocyst implantation. *Ann N Y Acad Sci* 541:424, 1986

68. Adams CE: Factors affecting the success of egg transfer. In: Adams CE (ed), *Mammalian Egg Transfer* Boca Raton, CRC Press, 1982:175–183

69. Hodgen GD: Surrogate embryo transfer combined with estrogen-progesterone therapy in monkeys: Implantation, gestation, and delivery without ovaries. *JAMA* 250:2167, 1983

70. Cross JC, Werb Z, Fisher SJ: Implantation and the placenta: Key pieces of the development puzzle. *Science* 266:1508, 1994

71. Stewart CL, Karpur R, Brunet LJ, et al: Blastocyst implantation depends on maternal expression of leukaemia inhibitory factor. *Nature* 359:76, 1992

72. Pollard JW, Hunt JW, Wiktor-Jedrzejczak W, Stanley ER: A pregnancy defect in the osteopetrotic (*op/op*) mouse demonstrates the requirement for CSF-1 in female fertility. *Dev Biol* 148:278, 1991

73. Simon C, Frances A, Piquette GN, Zurawsky G, Deng W, Polan ML: The immune mediator interleukin-1 receptor antagonist (IL-1ra) prevents embryonic implantation. *Endocrinology* 134:521, 1994

74. Mishell DR: Ectopic pregnancy. In: Droegemueller W, Herbst AL, Mishell DR, Stenchever MA (eds), *Comprehensive Gynecology*. St. Louis, Mosby, 1987:406–439

75. Budowick M, Johnson TRB, Genadry R, Parmley TH, Woodruff JD: The histopathology of the developing tubal ectopic pregnancy. *Fertil Steril* 34:169, 1980

76. Brosens I, Robertson WB, Dixon HG: The physiological response of the vessels of the placental bed to normal pregnancy. *J Pathol Bacteriol* 93:569, 1967

77. Khong TY, DeWolf F, Robertson WB, Brosens I: Inadequate maternal vascular response to placentation in pregnancies complicated by pre-eclampsia and by small-for-gestational age infants. *Br J Obstet Gynecol* 93:1049, 1086

78. Zhou Y, Damsky CH, Chiu K, Roberts JM, Fisher SJ: Preeclampsia is associated with abnormal expression of adhesion molecules by invasive cytotrophoblast. *J Clin Invest* 91:950, 1993

79. Jones GES: Some newer aspects of management of infertility. *JAMA* 141:1123, 1949

80. Csapo AI, Pulkkinen MO, Ruttner B: The significance of the human corpus luteum in pregnancy maintenance. I. Preliminary studies. *Am J Obstet Gynecol* 112:1061, 1972

81. Csapo AI, Pulkkinen MO, Wiest WG: Effect of luteectomy and progesterone replacement therapy in early pregnant patients. *Am J Obstet Gynecol* 115:759, 1973

82. Fillicori M, Butler JP, Crowley WF Jr: Neuroendocrine regulation of the corpus luteum in the human: Evidence for pulsatile progesterone secretion. *J Clin Invest* 73:1638, 1984

83. McNeely M, Soules M: The diagnosis of luteal phase deficiency: A critical review. *Fertil Steril* 50:1, 1988

84. Noyes RW, Hertig AT, Rock J: Dating the endometrial biopsy. *Fertil Steril* 1:3, 1950

85. Castelbaum AJ, Wheeler J, Coutifaris CB, Mastroianni L Jr, Lessey BA: Timing of endometrial biopsy may be critical for accurate diagnosis of luteal phase deficiency. *Fertil Steril* 6:443, 1994

86. Balasch J, Vanrell JA, Creus M, et al: The endometrial biopsy for diagnosis of luteal phase deficiency. *Fertil Steril* 44:699, 1985

87. Li TC, Dockery P, Rogers AW, Cooke ID: How precise is histologic dating of endometrium using standard dating criteria? *Fertil Steril* 51:759, 1989

88. Scott RT, Snyder RR, Strickland DM, et al: The effect of interobserver variation in dating endometrial histology on the diagnosis of luteal phase defects. *Fertil Steril* 50:888, 1988

89. Jones GS: The luteal phase defect. *Fertil Steril* 27:351, 1976

90. Wentz AC: Diagnosing luteal phase inadequacy. *Fertil Steril* 37:334, 1985

91. Davidson BJ, Thrasher TV, Seraj IM: An analysis of endometrial biopsies performed for infertility. *Fertil Steril* 48:770, 1987

92. Balasch J, Creus M, Marquez M, Burzaco I, Varnell JA: The significance of luteal phase insufficiency on fertility: A diagnostic and therapeutic approach. *Hum Reprod* 1:145, 1986

93. Peters AJ, Riley RP, Coulam CB: Prevalence of out-of-phase endometrial biopsy specimens. *Am J Obstet Gynecol* 166:1738, 1992

94. Wentz AC, Kossoy LR, Parker RA: The impact of luteal phase inadequacy in an infertile population. *Am J Obstet Gynecol* 162:937, 1990

95. Driessen F, Holwerda PJ, Putte SCJ, Kremer J: The significance of dating an endometrial biopsy for the prognosis of an infertile couple. *Int J Fertil* 25:112, 1980

96. Karamardian LM, Grimes DA: Luteal phase deficiency: Effect of treatment on pregnancy rates. *Am J Obstet Gynecol* 167:1391, 1992

97. Gonen Y, Calderon M, Dirnfeld M, Abramovici H: The impact of sonographic assessment of the endometrium and meticulous hormonal monitoring during natural cycles in patients with failed donor artificial insemination. *Ultrasound Obstet Gynecol* 1:122, 1991

98. Fleischer A, Herber C, Sacks G, Wentz A, Entman S, James A: Sonography of the endometrium during conception and nonconception cycles of in vitro fertilization and embryo transfer. *Fertil Steril* 46:442, 1986

99. Ueno J, Oehninger S, Brzyski RG, Acosta AA, Philput CB, Muasher SJ: Ultrasonographic appearance of the endometrium in natural and stimulated in vitro fertilization cycles and its correlation with outcome. *Hum Reprod* 8:511, 1991

100. Coulam CB, Bustillo M, Soenkensen DM: Ultrasonic predictors of implantation after assisted reproduction. *Fertil Steril* 62:1004, 1994

101. Al-Shawaf T, Yang D, Al-Magid Y, Seaton A, Iketubosin F, Craft I: Ultrasonic monitoring during replacement of frozen/thawed embryos in natural and hormone replacement cycles. *Hum Reprod* 8:2068, 1993

102. Dickey R, Olar T, Curole D, Taylor D, Pye P: Relationship of endometrial thickness and pattern to fecundity in ovulation induction cycles: Effect of clomiphene citrate alone and in combination with human menopausal gonadotropins. *Fertil Steril* 58:756, 1993

103. Abdalla HI, Brooks AA, Johnson MR, Kirkland A, Thomas A, Studd JWW: Endometrial thickness: A predictor of implantation in ovum recipients? *Hum Reprod* 9:363, 1994

104. Khalifa E, Brzyski RG, Oehninger S, Acosta AA, Muasher SJ: Sonographic appearance of the endometrium: The predictive value for the outcome of in vitro fertilization in stimulated cycles: *Hum Reprod* 6:677, 1992

105. Gonen Y, Casper R: Prediction of implantation by the sonographic appearance of the endometrium during ovarian hyperstimulation for in vitro fertilization. *J In Vitro Fertil Embryo Transf* 8:115, 1991

106. Sher G, Herbert C, Maassarani G, Jacobs MH: Assessment of the late proliferative phase endometrium by ultrasonography in patients undergoing in vitro fertilization and embryo transfer. *Hum Reprod* 6:232, 1991

107. Kupesic S, Kurjak A: Uterine and ovarian perfusion during the periovulatory period assessed by transvaginal color Doppler. *Fertil Steril* 60:439, 1993

108. Steer CV, Campbell S, Tan SL, et al: The use of transvaginal color flow imaging after in vitro fertilization to identify optimum uterine conditions before embryo transfer. *Fertil Steril* 57:372, 1992

109. Sterzik K, Grab D, Sasse V, Hutter W, Rosenbusche B, Terinde R: Doppler sonographic findings and their correlation with implantation in an in vitro fertilization program. *Fertil Steril* 52:825, 1989

110. Bassil S, Magritte JP, Roth J, Nisolle M, Donnez J, Gordts S: Uterine vascularity during stimulation and its correlation with implantation in in vitro fertilization. *Hum Reprod* 10:1497, 1995

111. Forman R, Fries N, Testart J, Belaisch-Allart J, Hazout A, Frydman R: Evidence for an adverse effect of elevated serum estradiol concentrations on embryo implantation. *Fertil Steril* 49:118, 1988

112. Simon C, Cano F, Valbuena F, Remohi J, Pellicer A: Clinical evidence for a detrimental effect on uterine receptivity of high serum estradiol concentrations in high and normal responder patients. *Hum Reprod* 10:2432, 1995

113. Paulson RJ, Sauer MV, Lobo RA: Embryo implantation after human in vitro fertilization: Importance of endometrial receptivity. *Fertil Steril* 53:870, 1990

114. Liu HC, Jones HW, Rosenwaks A: The efficiency of human reproduction and in vitro fertilization and embryo transfer. *Fertil Steril* 49:649, 1988

115. Garcia JE, Acosta AA, Hsiu J-G, Jones HW Jr: Advanced endometrial maturation after ovulation induction with human menopausal gonadotropin/human chorionic gonadotropin for in vitro fertilization. *Fertil Steril* 41:31, 1984

116. Sterzik K, Dallenbach C, Schneider V, Sasse V, Dallenbach-Hellweg G: In vitro fertilization: The degree of endometrial insufficiency varies with the type of ovarian stimulation. *Fertil Steril* 50:457, 1988

117. Benadiva CA, Metzger DA: Superovulation with human menopausal gonadotropins is associated with endometrial-glandular desynchrony. *Fertil Steril* 617:700, 1994

118. Navot D, Bergh PA, Williams MA, et al: Poor oocyte quality rather than implantation failure as a cause of age related decline in female fecundity. *Lancet* 337:1375, 1991

119. Balmaceda JP, Alam V, Roszjtein D, et al: Embryo implantation rates in oocyte donation: A prospective comparison of tubal versus uterine transfers. *Fertil Steril* 57:362, 1992

120. Navot D, Anderson TL, Droesch K, Scott RT, Kreiner D, Rosenwaks Z: Hormonal manipulation of endometrial maturation. *J Clin Endocrinol Metab* 68:801, 1989

121. Landgren BM, Unden AL, Diczfalusy E: Hormonal profile of the cycle in 68 normally menstruating women. *Acta Endocrinol* 94:89, 1980

122. Morris JM, Wagenen G: Interception: The use of post-ovulatory oestrogens to prevent implantation. *Am J Obstet Gynecol* 115:101, 1973

123. Rosenwaks Z: Donor eggs: Their application in modern reproductive technologies. *Fertil Steril* 47:895, 1987

124. Queenan JT Jr, Muasher SJ: Is progesterone rise in the follicular phase detrimental to pregnancy outcome in ART? *Assist Reprod Rev* 4:16, 1994

125. Schoolcraft W, Sinton E, Schlenker T, Huynh D, Hamilton F, Meldrum D: Lower pregnancy rate with premature luteinization during pituitary suppression with leuprolide acetate and human menopausal gonadotropins. *Fertil Steril* 55:563, 1991

126. Silverberg KM, Burns WN, Olive DL, Riehl RM, Schenken RS: Serum progesterone levels predict success of in vitro fertilization/embryo transfer in patients stimulated with leuprolide acetate and human menopausal gonadotropins. *J Clin Endocrinol Metab* 73:797, 1991

127. Fanchin R, de Ziegler D, Taieb J, Hazout A, Frydman R: Premature elevation of plasma progesterone alters pregnancy rates of in vitro fertilization and embryo transfer. *Fertil Steril* 59:1090, 1993

128. Hofmann GE, Bentzien F, Bergh PA, et al: Premature luteinization in controlled hyperstimulation has no adverse effect on oocyte and embryo quality. *Fertil Steril* 60:675, 1993

129. Tarlatzis BC: Oocyte collection and quality. *Assist Reprod Rev* 2:16, 1992

130. Plachot M, Viega A, Montagut J, et al: Are clinical and biological IVF parameters correlated with chromosomal disorders in early life: A multicentric study. *Hum Reprod* 3:627, 1988

131. Wramsby H, Fredga K: Chromosome analysis of unfertilized human oocytes failing the cleavage after insemination in vitro. *Hum Reprod* 2:137, 1987

132. Munne S, Lee A, Rosenwaks Z, Grifo J, Cohen J: Diagnosis of major chromosome aneuploidies in human preimplantation embryos. *Hum Reprod* 8:2185, 1993

133. Antinori S, Versaci C, Gholami GH, Panci C, Caffa B: Oocyte donation in menopausal women. *Hum Reprod* 8:1487, 1993

134. Balmaceda JP, Bernadini L, Ciuffardi I, et al: Oocyte donation in humans: A model to study the effect of age on embryo implantation rate. *Hum Reprod* 9:2160, 1994

135. Check JH, Askari HA, Fisher C, Vanaman L: The use of a shared donor oocyte program to evaluate the effect of uterine senescence. *Fertil Steril* 61:252, 1994

136. Navot D, Drews MR, Bergh PA, et al: Age related decline in female fertility is not due to diminished capacity for the uterus to sustain embryo implantation. *Fertil Steril* 61:97, 1994

CHAPTER 41

Gamete Intrafallopian Transfer

ALEXANDER M. DLUGI · MICHAEL S. MERSOL-BARG · MACHELLE M. SEIBEL

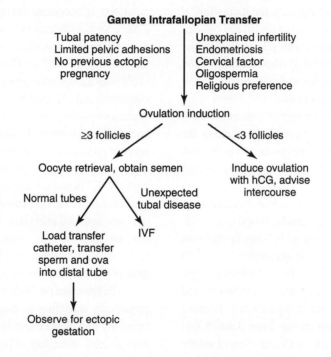

Gamete Intrafallopian Transfer

Tubal patency
Limited pelvic adhesions
No previous ectopic pregnancy

Unexplained infertility
Endometriosis
Cervical factor
Oligospermia
Religious preference

Ovulation induction

≥3 follicles

<3 follicles

Oocyte retrieval, obtain semen

Induce ovulation with hCG, advise intercourse

Normal tubes

Unexpected tubal disease

Load transfer catheter, transfer sperm and ova into distal tube

IVF

Observe for ectopic gestation

The first report in the United States literature of the successful transfer of human eggs into a patient's fallopian tube occurred in 1979.[1] Ovulation was enhanced with clomiphene citrate, 50 mg a day on cycle day 5 to 9. Artificial insemination was performed on cycle day 12, and a laparotomy was performed the following morning to reanastomose the ligated fallopian tubes. Six follicles were aspirated, at least one oocyte was identified, and the collected follicular fluid was equally divided and transferred into each reopened tube. A normal, single, term delivery followed.

The following year Kreitman and Hodgen reported on the reproductive potential of gamete tubal transfer in monkeys.[2] After tubal ligation, 55 monkeys mated before the day of anticipated ovulation. Laparoscopic oocyte retrieval was performed within 12 hours of ovulation, and the oocyte was injected into the ipsilateral fallopian tube proximal to the ligation. The monkeys mated again and 5 of the 31 (16%) conceived and delivered normal offspring. The study demonstrated the potential application of gamete transfer after surgical tubal occlusion and paved the way for more clinical applications. The first successful transfer of sperm and oocytes was performed in 1983.[3] Six patients with a history of pelvic inflammatory disease (PID) underwent ovarian stimulation and microsurgical repair at laparotomy immediately before anticipated ovulation. After sperm capacitation, the sperm were mixed with the oocytes in a small amount of culture medium and transferred into the repaired fallopian tubes. Among the four women treated, two conceived. One miscarried in the fifth postoperative week and the second continued to term without complication.

Also in 1983, the first United States center specializing in low ovum transfer was opened in a Catholic hospital in an attempt to overcome ethical objections to in vitro fertilization (IVF). Couples were instructed to have intercourse 24 and 30 hours after preovulatory injection of human chorionic gonadotropin (hCG). Laparoscopic oocyte retrieval followed, and the oocytes were transferred into the fallopian tubes. Because of poor results, moral theologians at the Pope John XXIII Medical-Moral Research and Education Center allowed semen also to be transferred, provided it was collected in a special perforated silicone polymer sheath so that neither contraception nor masturbation was used.[4] As with all the aforedescribed procedures, the gametes were transferred into blocked fallopian tubes.

Asch et al[5] were the first to report the use of gamete transfer in patients with unexplained infertility. The gametes, separated by an air space, were transferred by means of laparoscopic technique into the fimbriated end of a normal fallopian tube. These same investigators subsequently used minilaparotomy for the gamete transfer to assure optimum placement of the gametes. Since this original work, gamete intrafallopian transfer (GIFT) has evolved to become one of the most important assisted reproductive techniques (ART).

GIFT is a procedure in which preovulatory oocytes and washed sperm are transferred directly into the fallopian tubes. Because both gametes are placed at the most common site of human fertilization, GIFT is an attempt to assist fertilization and the natural physiologic process that leads to implantation of an embryo within the uterine cavity. Since the original description by Asch et al[5] in 1984, thousands of GIFT patient cycles have been reported in the literature.

PATIENT SELECTION

Before being considered for the GIFT procedure, every couple should undergo a thorough and complete infertility evaluation, including semen analysis, hysterosalpingography (HSG), timed endometrial biopsy, and possibly a postcoital test, although the latter test is becoming increasingly controversial. Diagnostic laparoscopy completes the evaluation, but some patients prefer to combine this procedure with a potentially therapeutic maneuver such as GIFT or IVF. One disadvantage of combining GIFT with a diagnostic procedure is that the pharmacologically stimulated and enlarged ovaries may interfere with thorough visualization of the pelvis and thus compromise the diagnostic aspect of the procedure. In addition, if an extensive endoscopic surgical procedure is indicated, it might have to be postponed to another time to not compromise the fragile ovaries or interfere with GIFT. Theoretic hazards such as laser plume and increased operative time with prolonged tissue exposure to carbon dioxide have not been analyzed. There are no statistically analyzed data on outcome after combined procedures. Therefore it remains unclear whether operative endoscopy performed at the time of GIFT influences pregnancy outcome.

The literature on GIFT does not document a breakdown of procedures according to diagnosis. Among 609 patients with infertility to which a cause had been ascribed, 205 (33.7%) had unexplained infertility (Table 41-1). Mild endometriosis (16.3%) and male-factor infertility (29.7%) (usually oligospermia) accounted for the two other largest diagnostic groups. Patients with disorders and patients with immunologic infertility in either partner that has not responded to less invasive measures and women with cervical-factor infertility or ovulatory dysfunction refractory to treatment might also benefit from GIFT. Some programs consider patients with unilateral tubal damage or with a sole ovary and tube on the contralateral side as candidates for this procedure. It has also been suggested that GIFT (clinical pregnancy rate of 34%) is appropriate treatment of couples with unexplained infertility after three failed cycles

TABLE 41–1. DISTRIBUTION OF DIAGNOSES AMONG PATIENTS WHO UNDERWENT GIFT

Diagnosis	No. of Patients
Unexplained infertility	205 (33.7)
Male-factor infertility	181 (29.7)
Polycystic ovary disease	1 (0.2)
Immune-factor infertility	7 (1.1)
Cervical-factor infertility	28 (4.6)
Anovulation	8 (1.3)
Endometriosis	104 (17.1)
Luteal-phase defect	2 (0.3)
Failed TID	10 (1.6)
Adnexal adhesions	49 (8.0)
Damage to one tube	8 (1.3)
Several factors	6 (1.0)

TID, therapeutic insemination with donor sperm.
Numbers in parentheses are percentages.

of controlled ovarian hyperstimulation (COH) and intrauterine insemination (IUI).[6]

Normalcy of at least one fallopian tube, if not both, has been emphasized by numerous authors as a prerequisite for GIFT.[7,8] One group specifically excluded any patient with a history of tubal disease or operation or with an apparent tubal abnormality at laparoscopy.[7] Other authors, however, have performed GIFT on patients with adnexal (including peritubal) adhesions.[9] Although the overall rate of ectopic pregnancy after GIFT is 1.5%, a primary concern is the risk for establishment of an ectopic pregnancy in an already compromised tube. Although the exact risk is unknown, the two ectopic pregnancies in one series of 276 cycles occurred in patients with tubal disease.[9] One patient had previously undergone bilateral neosalpingostomies with the remaining endosalpinx described as being grossly normal. The second patient had pelvic adhesions, a hydrosalpinx, and one "normal" tube. Clearly, caution should be exercised before transferring gametes into a possibly damaged fallopian tube.

Although GIFT is an alternative to IVF, unless pregnancy occurs it does not address the question whether the woman's oocytes are fertilizable by the man's spermatozoa. The answer may be of particular importance in cases of unexplained, immunologic, or male-factor infertility. The sperm penetration assay was recommended as a predictive test for successful IVF[10]; by extension, this could also apply to GIFT. Some investigators,[11] however, found this test to be of no predictive value in identifying couples who will or will not become pregnant through ART.

The results of simultaneous IVF and GIFT were reported for 16 couples.[12] Only one patient achieved a pregnancy with

GIFT. In addition, only four had any oocytes fertilized in vitro. The authors concluded that a substantial percentage of patients with infertility probably have spermatozoa or oocyte dysfunction. They suggested that GIFT be performed only for couples for whom there is conclusive proof that the woman's oocytes can be fertilized by the man's spermatozoa. Similarly, one pregnancy was reported among six couples with male-factor infertility and documented IVF.[13] Two of five women whose husbands' sperm did not fertilize the oocyte in vitro subsequently conceived when donor sperm were used. Three pregnancies occurred in nine cycles when IVF did not occur.[14] On the other hand, when supernumerary oocytes in a GIFT program were inseminated in vitro, there was no correlation between IVF and the likelihood of GIFT pregnancies; five women became pregnant even though the supernumerary oocytes did not become fertilized in vitro.[15] Combinations of zygote intrafallopian transfer (ZIFT) or GIFT with IVF (uterine) transfer were reported in 882 initiated cycles.[16] The clinical pregnancy rate was reported to be 34.7% per retrieval and 36.3% per embryo transfer with a 27.8% delivery per retrieval rate. Unfortunately, no information was reported regarding patient selection, indications for the procedure, or fertilization rate. In addition, there is no means by which to judge the efficacy of such combination procedures, because appropriate randomized, prospective studies have not been performed. The usefulness of an IVF cycle as a screening method before patient selection for GIFT is not clear. Nevertheless, until more information is available, an initial IVF cycle in cases of male-factor infertility or after several unsuccessful GIFT cycles appears warranted in evaluating sperm-egg interaction.

CONTROLLED OVARIAN HYPERSTIMULATION

The goal of any regimen of COH is to achieve growth of numerous follicles that yield numerous preovulatory oocytes suitable for transfer into the fallopian tube. Many protocols have been described, all virtually identical to those used for IVF cycles. Although use of human menopausal gonadotropin (hMG) alone is preferred by some authors, clomiphene citrate alone or in combination with hMG and follicle-stimulating hormone (FSH) with hMG also have been used (Table 41–2). FSH therapy after pituitary desensitization with a gonadotropin-releasing hormone (GnRH) agonist has proved to be efficacious.[17] This effect is most likely due to suppression of the LH surge with resultant fewer canceled cycles, allowing more patients to reach oocyte retrieval.

As with IVF cycles, no one protocol has proved to be more beneficial than another. One group reported the retrieval

TABLE 41–2. EXAMPLES OF FOLLICLE STIMULATION PROTOCOLS USED IN GIFT CYCLES

Stimulation	hCG (IU)	Criteria for hCG	Reference
hMG 150 IU beginning day 3	10,000	Two or more follicles ≥16 mm and estradiol level ≥300–500 pg/mL (1100–1840 pmol/L) for each main follicle	Asch et al[5]
Clomiphene 100 mg beginning on cycle day 3 or 4 for 5 days and hMG 150 IU starting on day 6 to 8 *or*	5000	?	Corson et al[4]
Clomiphene 100 mg beginning on day 3 or 4 for 5 days *or*	—	Spontaneous LH surge	"
hMG 150 IU beginning on day 3 or 4	5000	?	"
FSH 150 IU in AM, 150 IU in PM on cycle days 3 and 4 with hMG 150 IU daily from day 5 *or*	10,000	Two or more follicles ≥16 mm and estradiol ≥ 400 pg/mL (1470 pmol/L)	Molloy et al[8]
hMG 150 IU from day 3 or 5 *or* Clomiphene 100 mg daily from days 3 through 7 or days 5 through 9 *and*	10,000	"	"
hMG 150 IU from fourth day of clomiphene administration	5000	"	"
Clomiphene 100 mg daily from cycle days 2 through 6 and FSH 75 IU daily	5000	Two or more follicles ≥19 mm	Brooks et al[52]
Clomiphene 150 mg/day for 5 days starting on cycle day 3 *or* hMG 150–300 IU on day 3 *or*	5000	Two or more follicles ≥18–20 mm	Guastella et al[7]
Clomiphene 150 mg/day on days 3 through 7 and hMG from day 8 or 9	"		
Clomiphene 100 mg/day for 5 days starting 10 days before average cycle midpoint and hMG 150 IU starting on day 2 of clomiphene	5000	Given at optimal time *or* withheld if LH surge	Matson et al[14]
Clomiphene 100 mg/day for 5 days starting on cycle day 4 *and* hMG 75 on days 4 through 8 hMG 75–225 IU then continued	?	Sixth day of estradiol rise	Quigley et al[12]
Leuprolide acetate 1 mg/day for 14 days starting in midluteal phase, FSH 150–225 IU/day on cycle days 3 through 8 while continuing leuprolide 0.5 mg/day	10,000	Based on E₂ and ultrasound Leuprolide flare protocol	

of more oocytes when hMG was used alone or in conjunction with clomiphene as compared to clomiphene alone. In a later paper, the same authors[9] noted that 80% of cycles stimulated with clomiphene alone did not reach laparoscopy. They also noted that most of the GIFT pregnancies occurred when serum estradiol levels fell to 300 to 500 pg per preovulatory follicle, or when the mean serum estradiol level ws 1190 ± 18 pg/mL (4370 ± 60 pmol/L) (7 of 10 transfers). At higher (2683 ±

20 pg/mL [9850 ± 73 pmol/L]) levels of serum estradiol, more than half of early pregnancies were biochemical; that is, there was no clinical evidence. The two ectopic pregnancies in the series also fell into the group with high estradiol levels. Women of advanced reproductive age (>40 years) and women with polycystic ovary (PCO) disease present unique challenges that necessitate flexibility in management protocols.

THE PROCEDURE

Sperm Collection and Preparation

Sperm are typically collected by means of masturbation 2 to 2.5 hours before oocyte retrieval; some authors prefer a longer period of time before the actual transfer.[9] Patients who want to comply with the doctrines of the Roman Catholic church, can collect sperm during intercourse while using a perforated condom. In this way, neither contraception nor masturbation is used, and any ensuing pregnancy is an extension of the conjugal act.

The semen specimen is allowed to liquefy for 30 minutes. The sperm are then washed, centrifuged, and allowed to swim up to the final collectable pool. The media used for sperm washing vary according to the individual investigator. The following are examples:

1. Ham's F-10 with 10% fetal cord serum (1:3 vol/vol) containing streptomycin, 6000 U/10^4 mL and penicillin, 12,000 U/10^2 mL[5]
2. Ham's F-10 with 7.5% fetal cord serum[7]
3. Ham's F-10 with 7.5% patient serum containing penicillin G, 75 mg/L; streptomycin sulfate, 75 mg/L; calcium lactate, 252 mg/L; and sodium bicarbonate, 2.1 g/L at a pH of 7.35 and osmolarity of 280 to 285 mOsm[54]
4. Earle's medium[18]

No one method has proved to be superior to another, although it has been suggested that Percoll gradient centrifugation might yield sperm of better morphologic quality, as determined by means of transmission electron microscopic examination.[19] The final specimen is incubated at 95% air until ready for transfer catheter loading.

A semen analysis is performed during the preparation for GIFT. The Society for Assisted Reproductive Technologies (SART) database reports male-factor infertility based exclusively on the semen analysis on the day of the procedure. The SART criteria for male-factor infertility differ from those of the World Health Organization (WHO) (Table 41–3).

TABLE 41–3. CRITERIA FOR MALE-FACTOR INFERTILITY

Criterion	SART	WHO
Concentration	<20 million/mL	<20 million/mL
Motility	<40%	<50%
Normal morphology	Not included in criteria	<30%

Oocyte Retrieval

Thirty-four hours after administration of hCG, oocytes are retrieved. This is generally accomplished at laparoscopy with general anesthesia (Fig 41–1). More recently, however, ultrasound-guided transvaginal aspiration with conscious sedation has been used to retrieve the gametes from the ovary (Fig 41–2). Although no study has directly compared ultrasound-guided aspiration to the laparoscopic procedure, the benefits of the ultrasound technique appear to be those of decreased exposure to general anesthesia, decreased exposure of the gametes to pneumoperitoneum, and a higher number of oocytes retrieved. The increase in the number of oocytes retrieved is most likely due to better visualization of follicles; it is often not possible at laparoscopy to see follicles that are buried deep within the ovary. For a laparoscopic procedure, standard laparoscopic equipment and techniques are used. Several puncture sites may be necessary to attain access to all the ovarian follicles. These sites are usually placed lateral to the lower midline incision, either at the same level or higher. Both fallopian tubes may be cannulated later from a single right lower quadrant insertion of the aspirating cannula. We have found it easier, however, to use two separate insertions to facilitate cannulation of both tubes. Some programs replace all gametes into one fallopian tube rather than two with seemingly comparable results. The pelvis should be carefully assessed for appropriate placement of the aspirating cannula to minimize the number of puncture sites.

A historic alternative to laparoscopic retrieval is direct ovarian follicle aspiration through minilaparotomy. In this instance, a 2- to 3-cm transverse incision may be made at the level at which the uterine fundus reaches the anterior abdominal wall, as determined by bimanual pelvic examination. Once the peritoneal cavity is entered, the enlarged, fragile ovaries are often directly in view, and the individual follicles can be aspirated serially with the same needle used during a laparoscopic procedure. As the follicles shrink, the ovary often falls back into the pelvis. When this occurs, further aspirations may be technically difficult. Gently digital elevation of the suspensory ligament of the ovary or the ovary itself often restores the ovary to a more favorable position. Extreme care must be exercised to avoid bursting the follicle walls during this maneuver. Oocyte retrieval also may be performed by means of laparoscopy or ultrasound technique to avoid rupture of follicles; gamete transfer is performed at minilaparotomy.

Once the oocytes have been retrieved, they are placed in culture medium and graded for maturity. Culture media are as follows:

1. Ham's F-10 with 50% fetal cord serum under silicon oil
2. Ham's F-10 with 7.5% fetal cord serum[5]

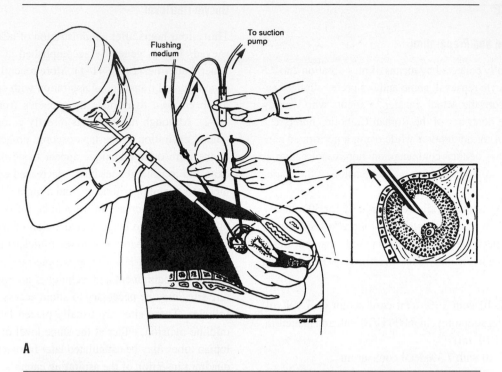

A

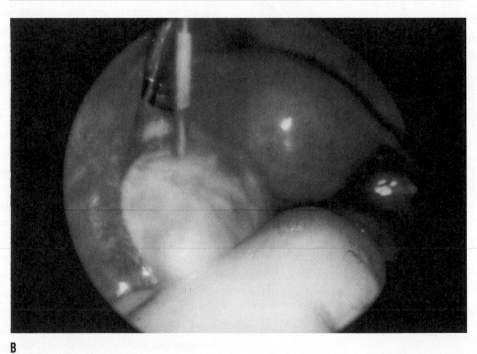

B

Figure 41–1. A. Laparoscopic oocyte retrieval. **B.** Needle entering a preovulatory follicle. *(A from Tan SL, Jacobs HS, Seibel MM: Infertility: Your Questions Answered. New York, Birch Lane Press, 1995.)*

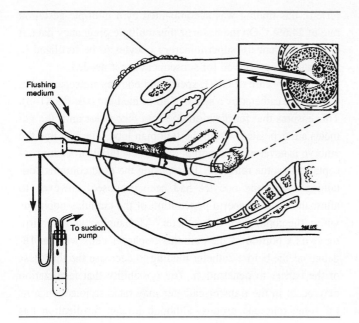

Figure 41–2. Ultrasound-guided transvaginal oocyte retrieval.

3. Menezo B$_2$ medium with 50% inactivated maternal serum[53]
4. Follicular fluid[54]
5. Ham's F-10[20]
6. Ham's F-10 with 50% maternal serum[8]
7. Earle's medium[18]
8. Human tubal fluid (HTF) medium[21]
9. B$_2$ medium (Fertility Technologies, Natick, MA)

Although most authors use prepared media, some place oocytes in a Petri dish containing clear follicular fluid, usually obtained from the first aspirated follicle. No advantage of this method or any other has been demonstrated thus far. A higher

pregnancy per retrieval rate (50% vs 21%), however, was reported by Fakih and Vijayakumar[22] in 131 GIFT cycles in which follicular fluid was used to capacitate sperm and as a transfer medium than when Ham's F-10 was used (29 cycles). Interestingly, the most important improvement in pregnancy rates occurred among couples with male-factor infertility. The pregnancy per retrieval rate was zero for the Ham's F-10 group and 44% for the follicular fluid group. A pregnancy was achieved with a motile sperm concentration as low as 1.5×10^6/mL. The authors suggested that when follicular fluid is used, GIFT can be performed even in the presence of severe oligozoospermia. When motile sperm concentrations fall to less than 1.5×10^6, however, the authors recommended documentation of fertilization in vitro with subsequent tubal embryo transfer. In this study either blood-free fresh or previously stored follicular fluid was used. The use of heterologous fluid, however, raises serious questions, particularly in terms of infection control.

Transfer

Some of the different types of transfer catheters available are as follows: Deseret Intracath (no 3132, Deseret Co, Sandy, UT); 16-gauge 24-inch Deseret Intracath; Semar Catheter (Wisap, Munich, West Germany); Teflon embryo transfer catheter (5F) with side-open tip cut off; Stirrable GIFT catheter (7F), and oocyte catheter (3F); 16-gauge end-hole Teflon catheter (HT Barnaby, Baltimore, MD); Cook Catheter (no. NRT 5.0-VT-50-P-NS-GIFT, Cook, Melbourne, Australia).

Methods of loading are described in Table 41–4 and Fig 41–3. Most authors use separate transfer catheters for each fallopian tube. The number of sperm transferred is generally 10,000 per fallopian tube, although one group reported 150,000 to 200,000. In cases of oligospermia, this number may be increased substantially with concentrations ranging from 200,000

TABLE 41–4. TRANSFER CATHETER LOADING

Reference	Space	Space (mm)	Sperm (μL)	Space (mm)	Oocytes (μL)	Space (mm)	End (μL)	Total Transferred Volume (μL)
Asch et al[55]	Air	None	5	5 air	25 medium	5 air	10 medium	50
Corson et al[7]	Medium	25 air	25	10 air	50 medium	10 air	25 medium	145
Guastella et al[53]	10 μL medium	20 air	25	20 air	30 medium	20 air	10 medium	135
Nemiro et al[54]	Follicular fluid	5 air	5–30	None	5–15 follicular fluid	5 air	5 follicular fluid	25–60
Confino et al[20]	4–5 μL of medium containing both oocytes and spermatozoa							4–5
Molloy et al[8]	Medium	5 air	50	None	25 medium	None	5 medium	85
Quigley et al[12]	Air	10 μL medium	?	Air	?	Air	5–10 medium	19–32
McGaughey and Nemiro[9]	Follicular fluid	5 air	4–15	None	1–2 follicular fluid	4–5	5 follicular fluid	100
Asch et al[5]	10 μL medium	5 air	25	5 air	40 medium	5 air	10 medium	100

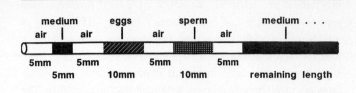

Figure 41–3. GIFT transfer catheter. Gametes are separated by air or medium.

to 800,000.[23] The number of oocytes transferred per tube is usually two to three, although as many as six have been used.[7] It is unclear whether only mature oocytes should be used or whether the transfer of immature oocytes has any detrimental effect. Furthermore, the ideal number has not been determined, although it has been suggested that the transfer of four oocytes results in a higher pregnancy rate than transfer of fewer oocytes. The pregnancy rate per cycle was 52.6% when three oocytes were transferred compared with 30.7% when only two were transferred. Penzias et al[24] conducted a retrospective review of 399 GIFT cycles. They found that women who received four or more oocytes were three times more likely to achieve a clinical pregnancy than those who received three or fewer. This is not surprising because women in whom four or more oocytes do not develop by definition have a poor response. The investigators found no statistically significant difference in pregnancy rate between the transfer of four versus the transfer of eight oocytes. Authors of another study also found that the number of oocytes transferred affected pregnancy rate. Successes were greatest (41.9%) with the transfer of five oocytes (7.1% for one, 10.0% for two, 32.9% for three, 33.6% for four oocytes trans-

ferred); this finding was accompanied by a multiple gestation rate of 24.6%.[25] On the basis of this multiple pregnancy data, it appears prudent for supernumerary oocytes to be fertilized in vitro and cryopreserved for subsequent use if needed.

In every case of GIFT, sperm and oocytes are separated in the transfer catheter by a space of air or medium (see Fig 41–3). This ensures that fertilization does not take place until the gametes are deposited within the fallopian tube. The fact that the embryo is never extracorporeal renders the GIFT procedure acceptable to some religions. Juxtaposing the fluid columns containing sperm and oocytes had been proposed, however, to allow the onset of sperm penetration of the cumulus oophorus within the confines of the catheter.[9] McGaughey and Nemiro[9] removed a portion of the cumulus oophorus cells with an 18-gauge needle before catheter loading to decrease the thickness of the barrier to penetration. The possibility that fertilization may occur in the transfer catheter may raise serious concerns for some religious groups, although human fertilization has been shown not to occur in vitro before 2 hours has elapsed.

The gametes are readily transferred into the fallopian tubes under laparoscopic visualization (Fig 41–4). The transfer catheter may be threaded down the aspirating cannula or through an appropriate-sized trocar cannula. With an atraumatic grasping forceps, the serosa is picked up and the fimbriated portion of the tube aligned with the advancing cannula. Straightening the tube often helps to identify its lumen, which typically is located near the antimesenteric border of the fallopian tube. It is important to approach the tube from an optimal angle to ensure proper placement of the cannula and the catheter within the tube. A flexible, maneuverable catheter had been described that may allow for easier entrance into the tubal ostium. The metal cannula is

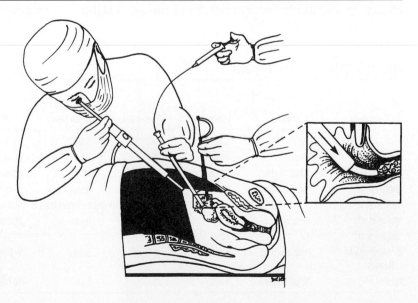

Figure 41–4. GIFT procedure. *(From Tan SL, Jacobs HS, Seibel MM: Infertility: Your Questions Answered. New York, Birch Lane Press, 1995.)*

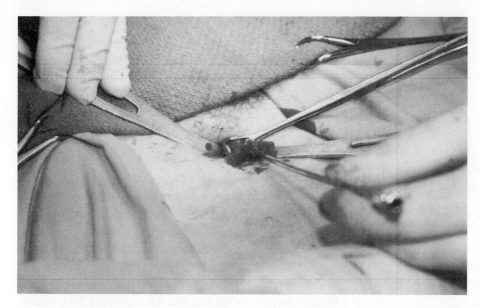

Figure 41–5. Gamete transfer by means of mini-laparotomy. (Courtesy Machelle M. Seibel, MD.)

placed in the tubal lumen to a distance of 1 to 2 cm. The catheter is then advanced another 1 to 2 cm beyond the end of the cannula, and the gametes are injected gently into the ampulla. The same process is then repeated for the other tube if desired.

Gamete transfer also is easily accomplished by means of minilaparotomy (Fig 41–5). A finger or an atraumatic tube holder can be used to elevate the tube and its fimbriated end into the opening of the incision. With direct visualization, the tubal lumen can be cannulated and the catheter threaded down to an appropriate position. This approach can always be used when laparoscopic cannulation is difficult. Scarring may make repeat procedures more difficult.

Though it has been common to transfer gametes into both fallopian tubes when available, Haines and O'Shea[26] in a poorly controlled, nonrandomized study compared pregnancy rates for 142 GIFT cycles in which bilateral transfer was used with 118 cycles in which unilateral transfer was used. There was no difference in pregnancy rates based on the approach to tubal cannulation. In theory, this would suggest an advantage to the unilateral approach because of a shorter operating and anesthesia time, decreased extracorporeal handling of the gametes, and the possible advantageous effects of decreased exposure of the gametes to the carbon dioxide environment required for cannulation of a second tube. Some authors have further suggested that transfer of gametes during GIFT be performed ipsilateral to the ovary with the most follicles.[27] In a retrospective analysis of 144 GIFT cycles, Ransom et al[28] recorded a cycle fecundity rate of 41.4% ($P = .042$, odds ratio = 2.39) among patients in whom gamete transfer was performed ipsilateral to the ovary that contained the greater number of follicles. The fecundity rate was 22.8% when transfer to the contralateral ovary was performed.[28] The authors speculated that the dominant ovary might contain higher concentrations of "embryotrophic factors" that would enhance conception. Although the concept may be appealing, further investigation with appropriately designed prospective, controlled, randomized clinical trials is needed to validate this theory. In contrast to the foregoing findings, other investigators noted that pregnancy occurred in 40.3% of cycles when both tubes were used compared with 21.6% when only one tube was used.[25]

One of the negative aspects of the GIFT procedure has been the requirement for the laparoscopic transfer of the gametes, necessitating abdominal incisions and general anesthesia. Consequently, some authors have suggested transferring the gametes with a hysteroscopic technique.[29,30] Possati et al[31] described their method of hysteroscopic GIFT with conscious sedation in the treatment of 27 patients. Gametes were retrieved by means of transvaginal ultrasound–guided puncture. The patients underwent sedation with diazepam 10 mg administered intramuscularly 15 minutes before the procedure. Atropine 0.5 mg intramuscularly was administered 30 minutes before oocyte retrieval and gamete transfer. With carbon dioxide insufflation, a 30° chorion hysteroscope with a 4-mm outer diameter sheath was used in conjunction with a flexible endoscopic catheter to deliver two to five oocytes and 100,000 to 200,000 sperm to one fallopian tube. The catheter was advanced 2 to 4 cm into the tubal lumen and the carbon dioxide distention was stopped 1 minute before gentle injection of the gametes. (Several studies have demonstrated a detrimental effect of carbon dioxide on mouse and human oocytes in terms of low cleavage and fertilization rates.[32–34]) No medium or air bubbles separated the gametes. The total volume placed into the tube was 60 to 100 μL. The authors reported a clinical pregnancy rate of 25.9% per cycle.

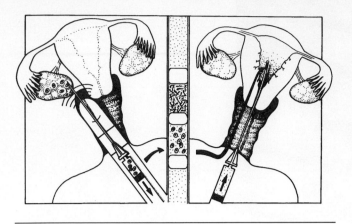

Figure 41–6. Gamete uterine transfer. (Courtesy Machelle M. Seibel, MD.)

Another study compared pregnancy rates after laparoscopic GIFT to rates after transvaginal ultrasound–guided GIFT.[35] Although the transvaginal GIFT clinical pregnancy rate of 20% was not statistically different from the laparoscopic GIFT pregnancy rate of 35%, it was not clear whether the small number of study patients might have masked a clinically significant detrimental effect. In a subsequent paper the authors[36] speculated that the decreased pregnancy rate might have been due to a smaller volume of fluid and decreased number of total sperm transferred into the tubes.

Several authors have reported placement of gametes into the uterine cavity (gamete uterine transfer) after transvaginal oocyte retrieval. This variation of GIFT is similar to IUI and therefore requires less technical experience than intrafallopian tube cannulation (Fig 41–6). Initial results are pregnancy rates of approximately 15%. Larger series are necessary to evaluate the ultimate role of this technique, but its simplicity is enticing.

RESULTS

A comparison of annual U.S. and Canadian GIFT outcomes submitted to SART from 1990 through 1993 is shown in Table 41–5. The number of medical centers offering GIFT and reporting outcomes to SART rose rapidly in the 1980s, but the number has leveled since 1991. One hundred eighty programs voluntarily reported their data to SART in 1993. Thus far in the 1990s, 20,690 cycles have been initiated; 16,913 of these initiated cycles (81.7%) led to the transfer of gametes; 5700 clinical pregnancies resulted from women having gametes transferred (33.7%); and 4485 women who had gametes transferred had a delivery (26.5%) with one of every three deliveries resulting in multiple births. The trend in outcomes reported was consistent over all years. Although the number of programs reporting results remained stable from 1992 to 1993, the number of cycles initiated dropped for the first time this decade (13.5%). Data for 1994, yet to be published, will clarify this downward trend should one exist. The ectopic pregnancy rate was 1.5% per transfer. Table 41–6 shows the effect of women's age and male-factor infertility on the outcome of GIFT in 1993. As with other forms of assisted reproduction, the cycle cancellation rate was higher for women older than 40 years in the absence of male-factor infertility (27.5% vs 13.0%), and the delivery rate per retrieval was lower (11.8% vs 32.32%) than for women younger than 40 years. The same was true in the presence of male-factor infertility (delivery rate per retrieval, 8.9% vs 29.1%). These reports had a similar trend for 1990–1992. During the same reporting period, the ZIFT pregnancy per retrieval rate was 24.4% (1993), 213.8% (1992), 24.4% (1991), and 21.3% (1990).[15,37–39]

The cause of infertility has some bearing on the success of GIFT (Table 41–7) as reported in the early literature on GIFT. Patients with mild endometriosis or unexplained infertility appear to fare well. Pregnancy rates per cycle of 26% (27 cycles)

TABLE 41–5. COMPARISON OF ANNUAL U.S. AND CANADIAN GIFT PROCEDURE OUTCOMES REPORTED TO SART

	1993	1992	1991	1990
No. of programs reporting	180	176	166	135
No. of cycles initiated	4992	5767	5492	4439
Cancellation rate (%)	15.8	16.2	19.2	15.5
No. of retrievals	4202	4837	4474	3750
No. of transfers	4138	4712	4371	3692
No. of clinical pregnancies (%/transfer)	1472 (35.6)	1621 (34.4)	1515 (34.7)	1093 (29.6)
No. of deliveries (%/transfer)	1182 (28.6)	1273 (26.7)	1188 (26.6)	842 (22.8)
Pregnancy loss rate (%)	20.6	16.9	21.6	19.0
No. of ectopic pregnancies (%/transfer)	61 (1.5)	61 (1.3)	44 (1.0)	54 (1.5)
Singleton birthrate (%)	64.5	67.3	66.0	66.0

TABLE 41–6. EFFECT OF WOMEN'S AGE AND MALE-FACTOR INFERTILITY ON OUTCOME FOR 1993 GIFT CYCLES REPORTED TO SART

Patient Category	No. of Retrievals	Cancellation Rate (%)	Percentage of Transfers per Retrieval	No. of Pregnancies	No. of Deliveries[a]	Percentage of Deliveries per Retrieval
Woman <40 y, no male factor	2805	13.0	98.7	1106	903	32.2
Woman ≥40 y, no male factor	635	27.5	97.6	136	54	8.5
Woman <40 y, male factor	605	13.0	99.0	210	176	29.1
Woman ≥40 y, male factor	157	20.3	95.5	20	14	8.9

[a]Deliveries with at least one liveborn infant.

for unexplained infertility, 66.6% for mild endometriosis (three cycles), and 66.6% (nine cycles) for adhesions were reported for patients who did not conceive after conventional donor insemination. No pregnancies were achieved among patients with hostile cervical mucus or male-factor infertility. Of two pregnancies in three patients with adnexal adhesions, one ended in a miscarriage and the second resulted in an ectopic pregnancy. A favorable clinical pregnancy rate per retrieval was reported for patients with unexplained infertility (27%). In the latter study,[8] poorer rates were noted in the presence of oligospermia (15%), endometriosis (0%), and cervical factor problems (0%). One of two patients with immune-factor infertility conceived, as did two of three with ovulatory dysfunction. Eight of 20 patients with adnexal adhesions or tubal disease also were successful in achieving intrauterine pregnancy. In a follow-up study, the authors reported continued success among patients with unexplained infertility (37.5% rate of pregnancy per transfer), pelvic adhesions (50%), and tubal disease (33.3%).[9] Lower rates were found among patients with endometriosis (28.5%), oligospermia (16.6%), and cervical factor infertility (14.2%). No pregnancies occurred among patients who were anovulatory or had an immune factor. No pregnancy was achieved with GIFT

TABLE 41–7. PREGNANCY RATES (%) BASED ON CAUSE OF INFERTILITY

Reference	Unexplained	Endometriosis	Cervical Factor	Male Factor	Adhesions
Quastella et al[53]	66.6	26.0	0	0	66.6
Nemiro et al[54]	27.0	0.0	0	15.0	40.0
McGaughey and Nemiro[9]	37.5	28.5	14.2	16.6	50.0
Blackledge et al[23]	—	—	—	0	—
Imodemhe et al[18]	40.0	26.0	—	21.0	—
Medical Research International[38]	47.0	30.0	—	36.0	—

among 9 patients whose partners had oligospermia (<12 × 10⁶/mL), and 4 of 9 couples in which the man had a normal sperm count conceived.[40] These data must be interpreted with caution, because the total number of patients in each diagnostic category is low. In addition, diagnostic criteria are not strictly defined, as evidenced by conflicting data about outcome among patients with endometriosis.

Prognostic factors relating to successful outcome of GIFT have been the subject of several studies. Nelson et al[41] in a retrospective review of 54 consecutive GIFT cycles found that sperm motility, the number of oocytes transferred, and the age of the woman had bearing on outcome. When the woman's age was bracketed into groups younger than 34, 34 to 40, and older than 40 years, there was a negative linear trend in pregnancy rate: 37.0%, 32.1%, and 20%. With regard to semen values, only motility in the initial screening specimen and the specimen used for GIFT before processing showed a statistically significant association with initiation of pregnancy. When stratified at the 50% level, pregnancy rates comparing greater than 50% motility with 50% motility or less in the first specimen were 35.0% and 21.7%. For the second specimen the pregnancy rates were 34.5% and 24.0%. Although increasing numbers of other semen defects (concentration, morphology) had an inverse correlation with pregnancy, no other factor was related to outcome, including the results of a zona-free hamster egg penetration test. This is in contrast to the findings of Rodriguez-Regau et al,[42] who found a statistically significant correlation between pregnancy rate and both sperm concentration and sperm motility. A diagnosis of endometriosis regardless of stage did not appear to impede pregnancy outcome. In contrast, in a matched control follow-up study with 114 patients with endometriosis and 214 controls who underwent GIFT, Guzick et al[25] found a lower pregnancy rate per retrieval (47.2% vs 32.5%) and delivery rate per retrieval (35.5% vs 23.75%) among patients with endometriosis, regardless of the stage of the disease (relative risk = 0.69). The number of oocytes transferred affected pregnancy rate; the highest rate of 41.9% occurred with transfer of five oocytes (7.1% for 1, 10.0% for 2, 32.9% for 3, 33.6% for 4 oocytes transferred). This was accompanied by a multiple gestation rate of 24.6%. Finally, pregnancy occurred in 40.3% of cycles when both tubes were used compared with 21.6% when only one tube was used. Other authors have found contradictory results.

In a study of 710 cycles of laparoscopic GIFT, Jansen et al[43] found that the most important variables associated with the chance of conception were age of the woman, number of oocytes transferred, and number of previous cycles of assisted conception attempted without success. In contrast, with the exception of lower pregnancy rates with oligospermia, the diagnosis was unimportant as was the duration of prior infertility. More recently, Bopp et al[44] reviewed a series of 1826 GIFT cycles to determine the effect of age on outcome. Although the number of oocytes transferred did not differ among the age groups studied, the cancellation rate was higher among women 40 to 43 years of age (24.8%) and 44 to 45 (31.4%) compared with women 25 to 39 years of age (15.1%). More important, the delivery rate per retrieval among women 40 to 43 years of age was significantly lower (12.2%) than that for women 25 to 39 years of age (21.5%). Among women 44 to 45 years of age, the rate was 4.2%. To compensate for the effect of age, one group suggested transfer of a higher order of oocytes.[45] In 73 GIFT cycles initiated in 48 women 40 years of age or older, the overall viable pregnancy rate per transfer was 14.9%; no woman older than 43 years conceived. The clinical pregnancy rate per transfer was higher among patients who received more than five oocytes (37%) than among those who received five or fewer oocytes (10%), a statistically significant difference.

A 1994 study[46] showed the impact of tubal abnormalities on GIFT outcome. In this prospective, observational study of 201 GIFT cycles performed for 146 women with endometriosis, the presence of more than two tubal abnormalities (fimbrial agglutination or phimosis, tubal convolutions, diverticula, sacculations, or peritubal adhesions) lowered the pregnancy rate across all stages of endometriosis in a statistically significant way. These results, however, must be viewed with caution. The overall pregnancy rate range reported in this study was 62% for severe endometriosis to 75% for mild endometriosis. Pregnancy was not defined by the authors (chemical or clinical pregnancy), so comparison to SART data is not possible. There were no ectopic pregnancies reported in the 201 cycles, which is lower than the figure reported by SART. Perhaps the tubal abnormalities observed do not directly reflect diminished tubal function or structure. The overall very high pregnancy rates lend support to this interpretation. Although the pregnancy rates were lower in the presence of more than two tubal abnormalities, the effect of any single abnormality on outcome was not described. This type of information is useful in aiding the surgeon to improve patient selection for GIFT.

The question has been raised about the efficacy of GIFT relative to less invasive treatment such as ovarian stimulation with human menotropins with or without IUI. To that end, Wessels et al[47] in a randomized, prospective study followed 200 patients who received either GIFT or treatment with hMG followed by IUI or intercourse. A thorough infertility evaluation was performed, and all patients with male-factor infertility were excluded from the study, as were those with tubal disease. The ongoing pregnancy rate among the GIFT group (26.7%) was higher than that among the conventional treatment group (9.7%), a statistically significant difference. These results must be viewed with caution, however, because the ovarian stimulation in the conventional treatment group was not as aggressive as in the GIFT group, and the distribution of infertility factors between the two groups was not defined, leading to the potential for study bias. In addition, no differentiation was made between the intercourse and IUI subgroups. Nevertheless, GIFT appeared to be more efficacious among women with endometriosis and anovulation. Similar results were reported for patients with idiopathic infertility, immunologic factors, unfavorable cervical mucus, and multiple infertility factors.

Another similar study[48] followed patients undergoing 257 cycles of superovulation-IUI with 54 concurrent cycles of GIFT or pronuclear stage transfer (PROST, used primarily for male-factor infertility). The superovulation-IUI group acted as the control and was matched to the treatment groups according to age and diagnosis. Patients for whom the conventional therapy was not successful were eligible to switch to either GIFT or PROST. Each infertility factor was equally represented among the study groups. The pregnancy rate for couples with male-factor infertility was higher for patients who underwent GIFT/PROST only (78.6%) than that for couples who underwent superovulation-IUI only (30.8%), a statistically significant difference. The patients with endometriosis or unexplained infertility tended toward higher pregnancy rates with GIFT/PROST (69.2% and 83.3%, respectively) than with conventional treatment (41.2% and 40.0%). Of more interest, however, was the finding that patients who underwent superovulation-IUI had a statistically significantly lower initial cycle and cumulative fecundity rate than patients who underwent GIFT/PROST. The superovulation-IUI initial cycle fecundity rate was 0.21 compared with 0.59 for patients for whom previous conventional treatment had failed who then underwent GIFT/PROST and 0.47 for the GIFT/PROST only group. The cumulative probability of achieving pregnancy after four or more cycles of superovulation-IUI was 0.41 compared with 0.74 for the GIFT/PROST only group and 0.80 for the

GIFT/PROST after superovulation-IUI group after three or more complete treatment cycles.

Molloy et al[49] conducted a retrospective examination of pregnancy outcome for patients who returned for subsequent GIFT procedures. In 2941 initial cycles, the clinical pregnancy rate per retrieval was 31.0%. For patients seeking a second GIFT pregnancy, the rate was 34.7%, and for those seeking a third pregnancy, the rate was 42.7%, both statistically significantly higher than the initial cycle rate. The likelihood of achieving pregnancy after the first oocyte retrieval increased from 34.3% in the initial pregnancy to 39.7% in the second pregnancy to 53.6% in the third pregnancy. These data suggest that a successful GIFT pregnancy is advantageous in terms of achieving subsequent GIFT conceptions. Interestingly, for patients whose initial pregnancy did not result in a livebirth, the livebirth rate for second and later pregnancies was lower (62.1%) than that for patients who had a livebirth with the initial pregnancy (74.2%), a statistically significant finding. The authors suggested that this might be the result of poor embryo quality or deficient uterine performance, because there was no difference in demographic characteristics or in the number of oocytes retrieved or transferred.

MODIFICATIONS OF GAMETE INTRAFALLOPIAN TRANSFER

How can infertile couples counseled to undergo ART be assured that the cause of infertility does not lie in the process of fertilization? A disadvantage of GIFT is that fertilization is verified only if pregnancy occurs. This means that two of every three couples who complete GIFT cannot exclude the possibility that their cycle failed because of an error in fertilization. To identify such couples, innovations in the GIFT procedure have been proposed and implemented. These modifications, in order of progressive embryonic development, include PROST, ZIFT, and tubal embryo transfer (TET). A combination of GIFT with IVF during the same cycle also has been used. In couples with oligospermia, for whom the answer to this question is particularly relevant, it was proposed that fertilization be allowed to take place in vitro.[23] If fertilization were under way, as judged by the presence of two pronuclei 18 hours after insemination of an oocyte, the pronuclear oocytes would be transferred into the fallopian tubes by means of GIFT. Among five patients who underwent this modified procedure, only one demonstrated IVF of one of four oocytes. Three of another woman's oocytes were fertilized by donor sperm. No pregnancies were reported. On the other hand, one twin pregnancy was achieved in a patient whose serum contained sperm antibodies. Three oocytes were fertilized in vitro and the zygotes later transferred into one fallopian tube.[50] Although fertilization is confirmed and the early embryo is allowed to be nurtured in its natural physiologic environment with this technique, it remains to be determined whether the method improves pregnancy rates compared with conventional GIFT or IVF protocols. Again, because of extracorporeal fertilization, objections may be raised for religious reasons by couples seeking GIFT.

The SART registry for 1990 through 1993 reports that 96% of women who underwent oocyte retrieval for GIFT had gametes transferred into at least one fallopian tube. Two percent did not have gametes transferred because of bilateral tubal disease or inability to retrieve at least one mature oocyte. Over the same reporting period, 84% of women who underwent oocyte retrieval for any of the modified procedures (PROST, ZIFT, or TET) had at least one fertilized oocyte transferred. If one assumes that a similar proportion of women did not have a transfer of fertilized oocytes for the same reasons as did those with GIFT (2%), it may be suggested that the remaining 14% of women did not have a transfer because of abnormal fertilization or lack of fertilization. This further suggests to clinicians that for one in seven couples GIFT may fail because of a problem with fertilization.

During the years 1990 through 1993, the overall clinical pregnancy rate per transfer for modified procedures was 29.9% compared with 33.7% for GIFT. Similarly, the overall rates of delivery per transfer were 23.4% and 25.5% respectively. Single births accounted for two thirds of all deliveries for both treatments. This comparison of outcomes suggests GIFT may offer little if any benefit over PROST, ZIFT, or TET. Failure to identify fertilization problems through GIFT puts couples with these problems at risk for delaying or never undergoing more appropriate treatment such as intracytoplasmic single-sperm injection (ICSI).

Although the foregoing hypothesis is plausible, it must be viewed with caution. Epidemiologic factors such as duration of infertility, single or combinations of infertility factors present, number of cycles attempted per patient, and age of patient are not accounted for in SART reporting. The lack of confident epidemiologic and statistical analysis introduces a large, but unquantifiable degree of bias in the interpretation of the success of these treatments. Comparison of treatment necessitates prospective, randomized, controlled trials which have yet to be conducted. The crude observational data reported by SART and within the body of scientific literature leads clinicians to flounder in developing guidelines intended to optimize patient selection for appropriate procedures.

Intratubal insemination has been proposed as an extension to intracervical and intrauterine insemination.[51] In this procedure, only sperm are placed within the fallopian tube under laparoscopic or ultrasound guidance. Five pregnancies were achieved among 20 women undergoing 28 such treatment cycles. In a similar vein, hysteroscopic insemination of the fallopian tube has been described.[16] No pregnancies were achieved in 52 cycles. More extensive experience with these methods is required before judgment can be passed concerning their efficacy.

SUMMARY

The rationale for performing GIFT is that it allows gametes to be placed directly into the natural physiologic environment appropriate for fertilization. The placement of several ova retrieved from pharmacologically stimulated ovaries may increase the likelihood that one will be fertilized. Potentially defective ovum pick-up mechanisms in the fallopian tube are bypassed. Similarly, introduction of motile spermatozoa within the ampulla of the tube may overcome compromised sperm transport and hostile cervical mucus.

Many centers that provide ART have observed outcomes with IVF similar to those with GIFT or its modifications. Some centers have discontinued offering GIFT in favor of IVF because the latter procedure is less invasive, requires less anesthesia, offers shorter duration of recovery, and verifies fertilization. It may be argued that the current indications for GIFT and its modifications introduce bias toward more favorable results compared with IVF. For example, patients undergoing diagnostic laparoscopy as part of the infertility evaluation are frequently offered GIFT at the time of their procedure. IVF is not usually offered to couples at the time of laparoscopy. Couples who eventually elect to undergo IVF usually have experienced a period of follow-up care after laparoscopy. In the follow-up period, some couples conceive without further intervention and never undergo IVF. In contrast, couples who undergo GIFT at the time of laparoscopy have no follow-up period. ART was conducted at the time of laparoscopy. How many couples would have conceived after laparoscopy had GIFT not been performed? There is currently no clear answer to this question. It is safe to assume that at least some couples would have conceived in the follow-up period. Although GIFT may have assisted these couples to conceive in a shorter time relative to laparoscopy, they would have conceived on their own regardless of GIFT. In this scenario, how would outcome of GIFT compare with outcome of IVF if all couples had the same interim follow-up time before undergoing either form of ART? This answer also is not known. This favorable bias contributes to overestimation of success observed with GIFT, ZIFT, TET, and PROST treatments.

Advocates of GIFT and its modifications may reply to the criticisms as follows:

1. Observational data at their medical centers suggest success is greater with GIFT than with IVF.

2. Less laboratory equipment, space, and technical expertise are needed with GIFT, making it an easier service to provide at reduced patient cost relative to IVF.

3. Innovations in office microlaparoscopy with local anesthesia and intravenous sedation provide additional reduced cost in terms of eliminating use of an operating room and the expense of general anesthesia.

Although the pregnancy rate after GIFT is certainly respectable, it remains to be defined whether it is statistically better than that achieved with standard IVF cycles. Some combination of sequential GIFT and IVF cycles may ultimately prove to be the best approach to investigate the intricacies of sperm-egg interaction while maintaining a high therapeutic value.

REFERENCES

1. Shettles LB: Ova harvest with in vivo fertilization. *Am J Obstet Gynecol* 133:845, 1979
2. Kreitman O, Hodgen GD: Low tubal ovum transfer: An alternative to in vitro fertilization. *Fertil Steril* 34:374, 1980
3. Tesarik J, Pilka L, Dvorak M, et al: Oocyte recovery, in vitro insemination and transfer into the oviduct after its microsurgical repair at a single laparotomy. *Fertil Steril* 39:472, 1983
4. McLaughlin DS, Troike DE, Tegenkamp TR, et al: Tubal ovum transfer: A Catholic approved alternative to in vitro fertilization. *Lancet* 1:214, 1987
5. Asch RN, Ellsworth LR, Balmaceda JP, Wong PC: Pregnancy after translaparoscopic gamete intrafallopian transfer. *Lancet* 2:0134, 1984
6. Ranieri M, Beckett VA, Marchant S, Kinis A, Serhal P: Gamete intra-fallopian transfer or in-vitro fertilization after failed ovarian stimulation and intrauterine insemination in unexplained infertility? *Hum Reprod* 10:2023, 1995
7. Corson SL, Batzer F, Eisenberg E, et al: Early experience with the GIFT procedure. *J Reprod Med* 31:219, 1986
8. Molloy D, Speirs A, du Plessis Y, McBain J, Johnston I: A laparoscopic approach to a program of gamete intrafallopian transfer. *Fertil Steril* 47:289, 1987
9. McGaughey RW, Nemiro JS: Correlation of estrogen levels with oocytes aspirated and with pregnancy in a program of clinical tubal transfer. *Fertil Steril* 48:98, 1987
10. Rogers BJ: The sperm penetration assay: Its usefulness reevaluated. *Fertil Steril* 43:821, 1985
11. Wolf DP, Sokoloski JE, Quigley MM: Correlation of human in vitro fertilization with the hamster egg bioassay. *Fertil Steril* 40:53, 1983
12. Quigley MM, Sokoloski JE, Withers DM, Richards SI, Reis JM: Simultaneous in vitro fertilization and gamete intrafallopian transfer. *Fertil Steril* 47:797, 1987

13. Grunert GM, Gibbons W, Rodriguez-Riqau LJ, Steinberger E: Combined gamete intrafallopian transfer (GIFT) and in vitro fertilization in male factor infertility. Presented at the 5th World Congress on In Vitro Fertilization and Embryo Transfer, April 1987, Norfolk, VA

14. Chang SP, Ng HT, Chen SC, Tzeng CR: Early experience with a combined procedure of GIFT and IVF. Presented at the 5th World Congress on In Vitro Fertilization and Embryo Transfer, April 1987, Norfolk, VA

15. Matson PL, Yovich JM, Bootsma BD, Spittle JW, Yovich JL: The vitro and fertilization ability of human sperm capacitated by swim up and Percoll gradient centrifugation. Presented at the 43rd Annual Meeting of the American Fertility Society, 1987, Reno, NV

16. Society for Assisted Reproductive Technology, The American Society for Reproductive Medicine: Assisted reproductive technology in the United States and Canada: 1993 results generated from the American Society for Reproductive Medicine/Society for Assisted Reproductive Technology registry. *Fertil Steril* 64:13, 1995

17. Hull MGR, Armatage RJ, McDermott A: Use of follicle-stimulating hormone alone (urofollitropin) to stimulate the ovaries for assisted conception after pituitary desensitization. *Fertil Steril* 62:997, 1994

18. Imodemhe DAG, Wafik AA, Chan RCW: Gamete intrafallopian transfer (GIFT): The Solimon Fakeeh Hospital preliminary experience. Presented at the 5th World Congress on In Vitro Fertilization and Embryo Transfer, April 1987, Norfolk, VA

19. Tanphaichitr N, Agulnick A, Seibel MM, Taymor ML: Comparison of the in vitro fertilization rate by human sperm capacitation by multiple-tube swim-up and Percoll gradient centrifugation. *J In Vitro Fertil Embryo Transf* 5:119, 1988

20. Confino E, Friberg J, Gleicher N: A new stirrable catheter for gamete intrafallopian tube transfer (GIFT). *Fertil Steril* 46:1147, 1986

21. Quinn P, Kerin JF, Warnes GM: Improved pregnancy rate in human in vitro fertilization with the use of a medium based on the composition of human tubal fluid. *Fertil Steril* 44:493, 1985

22. Fakih H, Vijayakumar R: Improved pregnancy rates and outcome with gamete intrafallopian transfer when follicular fluid is used as a sperm capacitation and gamete transfer medium. *Fertil Steril* 53:515, 1990

23. Blackledge DG, Matson PC, Willcox DC, et al: Pro-nuclear stage transfer and modified gamete intrafallopian transfer techniques for oligospermic cases. *Med J Aust* 145:173, 1986

24. Penzias AS, Alper MM, Oskowitz SP, Berger MJ, Thompson IE: Gamete intrafallopian transfer: Assessment of the optimal number of oocytes to transfer. *Fertil Steril* 55:311, 1991

25. Guzick DS, Yao YAS, Berga SL, et al: Endometriosis impairs the efficacy of gamete intrafallopian transfer: Results of a case-control study. *Fertil Steril* 62:1186, 1994

26. Haines CJ, O'Shea RT: The effect of unilateral versus bilateral tubal cannulation and the number of oocytes transferred on the outcome of gamete intrafallopian transfer. *Fertil Steril* 55:423, 1991

27. Penzias AS, Alper MM, Oskowitz SP, Berger MJ, Thompson IE: Comparison of unilateral and bilateral tubal transfer in gamete intrafallopian transfer (GIFT). *J In Vitro Fertil Embryo Transf* 8:276, 1991

28. Ransom MX, Corsan GH, Garcia AJ, Doherty KA, Kemmann E: Tubal selection for gamete intrafallopian transfer. *Fertil Steril* 61:386, 1994

29. Wurfel W, Krusmann G, Rothenaicher M, Hirsch P, Krusmann W: Pregnancy following intratubal gamete transfer by hysteroscopy. *Geburtshilfe Frauenheilkd* 48:401, 1988

30. Risquez F, Boyer P, Rolet F, et al: Retrograde tubal transfer of human embryos. *Hum Reprod* 5:185, 1990

31. Possati G, Seracchiolo R, Melega C, Pareschi A, Maccolini, Flamigni C: Gamete intrafallopian transfer by hysteroscopy as an alternative treatment for infertility. *Fertil Steril* 56:496, 1991

32. Pabon JE Jr, Findley WE, Gibbons WE: The toxic effect of short exposures to the atmospheric oxygen concentration on early mouse embryonic development. *Fertil Steril* 51:896, 1989

33. Hayes MF, Sacco AG, Savoy-Moore RT, Magyar DM, Endler GC, Moghissi KS: Effect of general anesthesia on fertilization and cleavage of human oocytes in vitro. *Fertil Steril* 48:975, 1987

34. Boyers SP, Lavy G, Russell JB, DeCherney AH: A paired analysis of in vitro fertilization and cleavage rates of first- versus last-recovered preovulatory human oocytes exposed to varying intervals of 100% CO_2 pneumoperitoneum and general anesthesia. *Fertil Steril* 48:969, 1987

35. Jansen RPS, Anderson JC: Transvaginal versus laparoscopic gamete intrafallopian transfer: A case-controlled retrospective comparison. *Fertil Steril* 59:836, 1993

36. Jansen RPS, Anderson JC: Nonsurgical gamete intrafallopian transfer. *Semin Reprod Endocrinol* 13:72, 1995

37. The American Fertility Society, Society for Assisted Reproductive Technology: Assisted reproductive technology in the United States and Canada: 1992 results generated from the American Fertility Society/Society for Assisted Reproductive Technology registry. *Fertil Steril* 62:1121, 1994

38. Medical Research International, Society for Assisted Reproductive Technology (SART), The American Fertility Society: In vitro fertilization-embryo transfer (IVF-ET) in the United States: 1990 results from the IVF-ET registry. *Fertil Steril* 57:15, 1992

39. The American Fertility Society, Society for Assisted Reproductive Technology: Assisted reproductive technology in the United States and Canada: 1991 results from the Society for Assisted Reproductive Technology generated from the American Fertility Society registry. *Fertil Steril* 59:956, 1993

40. Yovich JC, Matson PL, Turner SR, Richardson P, Yovich JM: Limitation of gamete intrafallopian transfer in the treatment of male infertility. *Med J Aust* 144:444, 1986

41. Nelson JR, Corson SL, Batzer FR, et al: Predicting success of gamete intrafallopian transfer. *Fertil Steril* 60:116, 1993

42. Rodriguez-Rigau LJ, Ayala C, Grunert GM, et al: Relationship between the results of sperm analysis and GIFT. *J Androl* 10:139, 1989

43. Jansen RPS, Anderson JC, Birrell WRS, et al: Outpatient gamete intrafallopian transfer: 710 cases. *Med J Aust* 153:182, 1990

44. Bopp BL, Alper MM, Thompson IE, Mortola J: Success rates with gamete intrafallopian transfer and in vitro fertilization in women of advanced maternal age. *Fertil Steril* 63:1278, 1995

45. Qasim SM, Karacan M, Corson GH, Shelden R, Kemman E: High-order oocyte transfer in gamete intrafallopian transfer patients 40 or more years of age. *Fertil Steril* 64:107, 1995

46. Fakih H, Marshall J: Subtle tubal abnormalities adversely affect gamete intrafallopian transfer outcome in women with endometriosis. *Fertil Steril* 62:799, 1994

47. Wessels PH, Cronje HS, Oosthuizen AP, Trumpelmann MD, Grobler S, Hamlett DK: Cost-effectiveness of gamete intrafallopian transfer in comparison with induction of ovulation with gonadotropins in the treatment of female infertility: A clinical trial. *Fertil Steril* 57:163, 1992

48. Robinson D, Syrop CH, Hammitt DG: After superovulation-intrauterine insemination fails: The prognosis for treatment by gamete intrafallopian transfer/pronuclear stage transfer. *Fertil Steril* 57:606, 1992

49. Molloy D, Doody ML, Breen T: Second time around: A study of patients seeking second assisted reproduction pregnancies. *Fertil Steril* 64:546, 1995

50. Devroey P, Braechmans P, Smitz J, et al: Pregnancy after trans-laparoscopic zygote intrafallopian transfer in a patient with sperm antibodies. *Lancet* 1:1329, 1986

51. Berger GS: Intratubal insemination. *Fertil Steril* 48:328, 1987

52. Brooks JH, Taylor PJ, Mortimer D: Synchronized hysteroscopic insemination of the fallopian tube (SHIFT). Presented at the 5th World Congress on In Vitro Fertilization and Embryo Transfer, April 1987, Norfolk, VA

53. Guastella G, Comaretto G, Palermo R, et al: Gamete intrafallopian transfer in the treatment of infertility: The first series at the University of Palermo. *Fertil Steril* 46:417, 1986

54. Nemiro JS, McGaughey RW: An alternative to in vitro fertilization embryo transfer: The successful transfer of human oocytes and spermatozoa to the distal oviduct. *Fertil Steril* 46:644, 1986

55. Asch H, Balmaceda JP, Ellsworth L, Wong PC: Preliminary experiences with gamete intrafallopian transfer (GIFT). *Fertil Steril* 45:366, 1986

CHAPTER 42

In Vitro Fertilization

NERI LAUFER · ALEX SIMON · ARYE HURWITZ · ISAAC Z. GLATSTEIN

In Vitro Fertilization

Infertile couple considered for in vitro fertilization

Patient Selection
    Tubal disease
    Endometriosis
    Male factor
    Unexplained infertility
    Immunologic causes

Patient Evaluation
    Laparoscopy and hysterosalpingography
    Semen analysis and culture
    Vaginal culture, rubella screen, HIV
    Psychologic evaluation and support
    Counsel couple on alternatives, low
      success rates, costs risks, and
      emotional impact

Baseline ultrasound

Monitor follicle development   Sperm collection

Natural cycle E2, LH, Prog   Husband versus Fresh versus
Stimulated cycle | Ultrasound   donor | frozen

Oocyte retrieval   Sperm preparation

Ultrasound   Layering Percoll
Laparoscopy   Swim up

Oocyte maturation ⟶ Fertilization ⟵ Sperm capacitation

Oocyte freezing In vivo: Microinjection
or donation   GIFT   Zona drilling
           Intravaginal
           culture

In vitro

No cleavage   Embryo

Discuss how many Adoption Egg donation Embryo freezing ⟶ Embryo transfer
IVF cycles to attempt

The first successful human pregnancies and births after in vitro fertilization (IVF) were reported by Steptoe and Edwards in 1978[1] and by Lopata et al in 1980.[2] This achievement was a culmination of scientific efforts that stretched over nearly a century. Walter Heape in 1891 was the first to demonstrate the possibility of recovering a preimplantation-stage embryo from flushing a rabbit oviduct and transferring the embryo to a foster mother, in which normal development continued.[3] As a result of Heape's pioneering work and successful embryo transfers in other species, scientific interest focused on culturing embryos in the laboratory. Hammond[4] in 1949 developed a complex medium that supported the growth of eight-cell mouse embryos to blastocysts, and Whitten[5] in 1956 demonstrated that a simple, chemically defined medium could be equally effective. The discovery of sperm capacitation by Austin[6] and Chang[7] in 1951, coupled with simple culture techniques, resulted in the first successful fertilization of rabbit eggs in vitro, reported by Chang in 1959.[8]

The birth of Louise Brown, the first IVF–embryo transfer (ET) baby, in 1978, triggered a succession of medical, biologic, and technical developments that have simplified the procedure, increased its efficiency, and expanded its indications. In the late 1970s and early 1980s, IVF-ET was transformed from an experimental procedure to one that is integral to the reproductive endocrinologist's practice. It has become a medical discipline in which clinicians and reproductive biologists team closely to treat patients and gain better insights into problems associated with human reproduction, and it has dramatically affected almost all the traditional infertility treatment modalities.

PATIENT SELECTION

Originally, IVF was developed for patients with absent or irreparably damaged fallopian tubes.[2] As IVF evolved and became more widely available, its indications broadened. Currently, in addition to tuboperitoneal-factor infertility, IVF is performed for women with infertility due to such disorders as endometriosis, unexplained infertility, immunologic infertility, and male-factor infertility. IVF also is used whenever oocyte donation is indicated and in some patients with polycystic ovarian (PCO) disease in whom routine induction of ovulation is associated with a high risk for the development of ovarian hyperstimulation syndrome (OHSS). In addition, IVF-ET is used to treat fertile couples who participate in a program of preimplantation diagnosis of affected embryos.

The minimal requirements for IVF are that the patient has a normal uterine cavity, a source of oocytes, and enough sperm to achieve fertilization, either by means of routine insemination or by assisted fertilization techniques. Although IVF may be an alternative in therapy for most infertility disorders, it may not always be the best treatment. Therefore it is imperative that the infertility evaluation be thorough, that alternative therapies be considered, and that success rates for all forms of treatment be discussed candidly with the couple.

Tubal Disease

Advances in microsurgical techniques have resulted in excellent outcomes for many types of tubal dysfunction. As a result, for obstructed fallopian tubes, surgical treatment still has to be considered. However, the success of surgical repair depends on the extent of tubal destruction.[9] When the fimbriae are preserved and the tube is not dilated, lysis of adhesions may be followed by pregnancy in more than 50% of patients.[10] In contrast, when the fimbriae are closed, a neosalpingostomy must be performed, resulting in a favorable outcome in only 15% to 20% of patients.[9] For comparison, a single cycle of IVF results in pregnancy in approximately 20% of women. However, fewer than 10% of patients with dense adnexal adhesions, fixation of the ovary and tube, absence of fimbriae, bipolar disease, and presence of a hydrosalpinx greater than 30 mm diameter become pregnant after surgical repair.[11]

Sterilization procedures that retain more than 6 cm of fallopian tube and preserve the fimbriae are best reversed with microsurgical anastomosis. A midsegment tubal anastomosis offers a pregnancy rate of more than 60%, whereas a tubocornual anastomosis results in pregnancy in 45% to 50% of patients.[9,10] Even several cycles of IVF cannot match these success rates. Patients initially treated with a microsurgical procedure who do not conceive are best treated with IVF, because the success rate for repeat tuboplasty after microsurgical procedure is less than 10%.[12] Eighty-five percent of intrauterine pregnancies occur within 2 years of repair of distal tubal obstruction. Therefore, after a surgical procedure, it is important to wait an appropriate length of time for pregnancy to occur before initiating IVF.

Endometriosis

Endometriosis is present in 20% to 40% of women with infertility.[13] The mechanism of infertility in severe disease is mechanical obstruction of the fallopian tubes and encasement of the ovaries. In mild disease, the cause of the infertility is less clear.[14] However, pregnancy rates of 50% occur with no treatment in the 6 months after diagnostic laparoscopy.[15–18]

Infertility due to moderate and severe endometriosis treated with surgical correction combined with either danazol or a gonadotropin-releasing hormone (GnRH) agonist results in pregnancy rates of more than 50% among women with moderate endometriosis and 30% to 40% for those with severe disease.[13] When conception does not occur within an adequate follow-up interval, IVF should be considered.

Unexplained Infertility

According to generally accepted criteria of unexplained infertility, the incidence rate approximates 10% to 15% of all couples seeking treatment of infertility. The diagnosis should be made only after it has been shown that the woman ovulats regularly, has patent fallopian tubes, and shows no evidence of tuboperitoneal factor. In addition, it is imperative that the woman has a partner with normal sperm production and function as tested by means of sperm analysis, postcoital test, and sperm penetration assay, or hemizona assay.[19]

Follow-up studies have shown that spontaneous pregnancies do occur among couples with unexplained infertility. Twenty percent of the women become pregnant each year for 3 years, with a cumulative pregnancy rate of 58% after 4 years.[16,19] Several treatment modalities have been suggested to increase the fecundity rate of patients with the diagnosis of unexplained infertility, but most of them are empirical. Only menotropin treatment combined with intrauterine insemination (IUI) has been found to be valuable, with a cumulative pregnancy rate of 23% after three menotropin cycles and 45% after seven cycles.[18,20] These pregnancy rates are comparable to the success rate among patients with unexplained infertility who undergo IVF. Therefore, it has been advocated that patients with unexplained infertility be treated for three to six cycles with menotropins and IUI before attempting IVF.[20] When treatment with human menopausal gonadotropin (hMG) fails, IVF should be attempted. In that case, the IVF cycle serves not only as a treatment cycle but also as a diagnostic tool. Because the definite proof of normal oocyte and sperm function is the achievement of fertilization, it has been suggested that the diagnosis of unexplained infertility be made only after a successful IVF. When no fertilization occurs in repeat cycles, either an oocyte abnormality or a sperm defect exists. This calls for the use of cross-over gamete donation[21] or gamete micromanipulation[22] to overcome the problem.

Male-Factor Infertility

For patients with oligoteratoasthenozoospermia, IVF offers the possibility of introducing a sufficient number of spermatozoa into the vicinity of the oocyte to result in fertilization. Although a lower fertilization rate can be anticipated among these patients, once fertilization occurs, implantation rates may be normal.[23] However, because fertilization rates are lower among oligospermic couples, the pregnancy rate per cycle is markedly reduced.

The hamster-egg penetration test described by Yanagi-machi et al[24] in 1976 is considered useful in screening sperm before IVF. Although in most cases a positive result correlates well with human oocyte fertilization, among patients with oligozoospermia the test is less predictive. Among normospermic couples, 90% of those with a normal hamster-egg penetration test achieve IVF. Sperm penetration assays are useful before IVF as a screen for unexplained infertility, but oligozoospermic couples should not be rejected from attempts at IVF solely on the basis of a poor result of this test. The results of the hemizona assay, which is used to evaluate the ability of the sperm to attach to the zona pellucida of unfertilized human oocytes, were found to be in good correlation with a sperm's fertilizing potential in vitro.[26–28] These tests can serve as a predictive tool for IVF and allow the appropriate mode of treatment to be chosen in couples referred for IVF. It has become clear that although IVF is a successful solution in certain conditions, most couples with male-factor infertility do not benefit from its conventional application. Gamete micromanipulation, developed toward the end of the 1980s, offers an excellent solution to most couples with male-factor infertility in whom conventional IVF is anticipated to fail or is not applicable at all.

Immunologic Causes

The presence of antisperm antibodies in the female reproductive tract or on the sperm surface adversely affects fertility.[29] Antibodies directed against the sperm tail and midpiece can alter sperm motility, and antibodies directed against the sperm head can affect sperm-oocyte interaction.[30]

Women with antisperm antibodies fertilize fewer oocytes than do those whose sera do not contain antibodies to sperm.[31,32] Some of these patients have abnormal binding to the zona pellucida.[33] As a result, their fertilization rate is decreased. If IVF is performed in a woman with antisperm antibodies, it is important that her serum not be used in preparation of the medium. If the oocytes do fertilize, the expected implantation rate of these embryros is identical to that among patients with tubal disease.[29] If the fertilization rate is poor or if fertilization does not occur, gamete micromanipulation by means of intracytoplasmic sperm injection (ICSI) can alleviate the problem.

INDUCTION OF FOLLICULAR GROWTH

The first pregnancies achieved by IVF in humans were produced with oocytes from unstimulated natural cycles.[1,2] The disadvantages of this approach were the need for frequent measuring of blood or urine luteinizing hormone (LH) level, the need for a 24-hour commitment of staff and facilities, a low (0 to 60%) chance of aspirating at least one oocyte, and a low mean number of oocytes aspirated per patient.[34] This approach was abandoned in 1981, when it was shown that ovulation induction with clomiphene citrate coupled with either a naturally occurring LH surge or administration of human chorionic gonadotropin (hCG) resulted in an 8% rate of viable pregnancies and the first twin gestation.[34,35]

Since the early 1980s, the number of ovulation induction protocols in IVF has grown to include those with protection from an LH surge and an increased number of agents used for induction of follicle development. These agents include clomiphene citrate, hMG, "pure" urinary-derived follicular stimulating hormone (u-FSH), recombinant FSH (r-FSH), GnRH and its agonist or antagonist derivatives, and growth hormone (GH) as cotreatment of ovulation induction. Although advances in hormone monitoring and embryo culture combined with ultrasound-guided retrieval have made the natural cycle an option,[36] particularly for women younger than 35 years, GnRH agonists have become a fundamental drug in most protocols. The availability of natural-cycle IVF and the many treatment protocols that follow allow individualization of treatment for patients who do not respond to one method.

Treatment Protocols in Which GnRH Agonists Are Not Used

Clomiphene Citrate-hMG

Use of clomiphene citrate alone, 50 to 150 mg/day on cycle days 5 to 9, was abandoned after a very short time and replaced by clomiphene citrate-hMG (CC-hMG) regimens that capitalize on the synergistic effect of the two agents. Clomiphene, 50 to 100 mg/day, is given from cycle days 2 to 6 or 5 to 9; hMG, 2 to 4 ampules (75 u-FSH; 75 u-LH), is added from day 2, 5, or 7 for 3 to 4 days. When at least one follicle reaches a diameter greater than 18 to 20 mm, hMG is discontinued and hCG is administered.[37-39]

In a summary of almost 1000 IVF pregnancies from Australia and New Zealand between 1979 and 1984 and published by the Australian National Perinatal Statistics Unit in 1985, CC-hMG was used in more than 75% of cycles.[40] The overall pregnancy rate reported for use of these agents was in the range of 15% to 17% per aspiration, or 20% per transfer[38,41] with a 25% multiple pregnancy rate.[37] The pregnancy rate nearly doubled to more than 30% if the oocyte aspiration followed an endogenous LH surge rather than the administratiaon of hCG.[37] In another report, no difference was found between spontaneous LH surge and exogenous hCG administration, but the best results were obtained when the addition of hMG to clomiphene citrate was tailored to individual responses.[38] When hMG cycles were compared with cycles with CC-hMG regimens, the latter demonstrated the following: (1) a faster growth rate, so that at time of aspiration, follicles are larger and easier to aspirate; (2) a higher estradiol response; (3) a large preovulatory progesterone rise;

(4) a high percentage of LH initiation; and (5) a higher frequency of poor or abnormal endocrine response.[42] Manipulation of the initiation of CC-hMG to day 2 or day 4 of the cycle did not change any of these disadvantages; a spontaneous LH surge occurred in nearly 50% of patients on day 2 and in 36.5% of patients on day 4. Conception rates did not differ between the groups.[43]

One must bear in mind that a considerable body of data exists to suggest that clomiphene citrate may have undesirable effects on the reproductive tract. This estrogen antagonist seems to have a dose-dependent antiestrogenic effect on the endometrium[44] and is associated with decreased levels of endometrial cytosol estrogen receptors.[45] It was demonstrated that clomiphene citrate administered in the follicular phase induces premature secretory changes in the rabbit oviduct and uterine mucosa[46] and the human endometrium.[47] Asynchronous endometrial development may interfere with uterine receptivity and early stage of implantation. In view of the possible detrimental effect of clomiphene citrate on the endometrium, oocyte,[48] and steroidogenesis by the corpus luteum,[49,50] several authorities preferred the use of menotropins alone for IVF. These potentially adverse effects of clomiphene citrate do not occur when the medication is given to oocyte donors and the oocytes are transferred to the recipient's endometrium.[51] Nevertheless, analysis of abundant data on the success rate of the regimens in which menotropin is used alone or in combination with clomiphene citrate do not substantiate a clear advantage of one treatment over the other.[52-55]

hMG-FSH

Mild ovarian stimulation with hMG for oocyte retrieval in IVF was pioneered by Steptoe[39] but later abandoned. The first viable pregnancies resulting from the use of ovulation induction with hMG were assisted by Jones et al[56] This group used a relatively small dosage of hMG (approximately 10 ampules per cycle) with the objective of maturing about three large follicles. hCG is administered either 28, 36, or 52 to 60 hours after discontinuation of hMG, depending on the individual response. Use of this regimen in more than 400 cycles resulted in an average of 2.3 mature cleaving oocytes, a pregnancy rate of about 25%, an abortion rate of 26.5%, and a cancellation rate of 15% due to either low response or premature LH surge.[57] We have chosen to intervene more aggressively in the normal cycle with a higher dose of hMG, starting with 3 ampules/day from day 3 of the cycle for 5 days followed by the same dose or higher according to the patient response.[58,59] This high-dose hMG treatment was initiated at the time of follicular recruitment to obtain four to five large follicles. The minimal criteria for hCG administration 24 hours after the last hMG injection are at least two follicles with diameter greater than 1.5 cm and estradiol levels exceeding 500 pg/mL (1840 pmol/L). With this regimen, it was possible to obtain an average of six mature oocytes with 18% clinical pregnancies per transfer and a 15% abortion rate. Other groups using a similar protocol reported an 11% to 31% clinical pregnancy rate with an abortion rate of about 18%.[60-62]

Pure u-FSH was introduced in the late 1980s.[63] It is used either in combination regimens with hMG[64] or alone[65] followed by hCG. In a preliminary report of the comparison of various combinations of hMG-FSH, a higher pregnancy rate was reported among patients undergoing their first IVF attempt with a combination of hMG-FSH (30%) than among those receiving u-FSH alone (21%).[60] In an extended study of more than 1300 cycles, the highest pregnancy rate (25%) was achieved in combination 1 (2 ampules hMG + 2 ampules u-FSH on day 3 or 4 and 2 ampules hMG thereafer), in which u-FSH was used to augment the recruitment phase.[66] The success rate was lower for the fixed protocol of 2 ampules of hMG/day (21.5%) and lowest (17%) for 2 ampules of u-FSH. Similarly, the viable pregnancy rate was low (12.2%) for 2 ampules of u-FSH and high (18%) for combination 1, although not statistically significant. It was suggested that the addition of FSH to hMG at the beginning of the treatment cycle mimics the normal menstrual cycle by improving the FSH/LH ratio and by providing a healthier intrafollicular environment for oocyte development because of a decrease in the androgen-to-estrogen ratio and a lower testosterone level.[67] However, prospective, randomized studies[68] comparing the u-FSH and hMG protocols found a significantly lower rate of cancellation cycles for the u-FSH treatment protocol, but no significant difference regarding pregnancy rate. Similarly, data from the IVF registry in the United States[54,55] demonstrated no difference in cancellation and clinical pregnancy rates between the hMG and u-FSH/hMG protocols.

It is concluded that hMG and u-FSH regimens seem to offer the same clinical conception rate per transfer (20%) as CC-hMG cycles but are associated with a lower clinical abortion rate (18% versus 25%) and consequently a slightly higher number of livebirths. The occurrence of a spontaneous LH surge is twice as likely in CC-hMG cycles (30%) as in hMG cycles (15%), necessitating close LH monitoring, and is probably associated with a higher rate of canceled cycles.

Use of GnRH Agonists in Ovulation Induction

One of the difficulties encountered when menotropins are used to stimulate the growth of several follicles is asynchronous development. Follicles mature at different rates because not all are at the same developmental stage when menotropin treatment is started. Follicular development is a random event that begins at least 60 days before the onset of the FSH rise that indicates the beginning of a menstrual cycle.[69] This development is not gonadotropin dependent and occurs even in women with gonadotropin deficiencies. When menotropins are administered, some follicles are more advanced than others and therefore are of different sizes producing varying quantities of estrogen.[70] Because occytes must be aspirated simultaneously, not all are ready for fertilization.

An additional problem with endogenous pituitary secretion is premature LH release. Under ordinary circumstances the pituitary gland responds to sustained elevations of estrogen levels with a positive feedback of LH secretion. Although this physiologic response is necessary for a single ovulation to occur, an LH surge before administration of hCG in stimulated cycles can result in ovulation before egg retrieval or premature luteinization of the follicular cells and secretion of progesterone, which can adversely affect endometrial receptivity. In addition, even if ovulation does not occur prematurely, exposure to high levels of LH before ovulation can have detrimental effects on the developing oocyte.[71]

GnRH agonists, which produce a hypogonadotrophic hypogonadal state through their desensitization effect on the pituitary gland, offer an excellent solution to the disadvantages of menotropin treatment alone. The use of GnRH agonists concomitantly with menotropins for ovulation induction was found to be more efficient than use of menotropins alone. It was observed that a combination of menotropins and GnRH agonists was associated with an enhanced follicular recruitment, better follicular synchrony, and an almost total elimination of the endogenous LH surge.[72-76] In IVF cycles, administration of GnRH agonists resulted in an increased number of fertilizable oocytes and a higher conception rate per cycle of treatment.[76,77] It was speculated that better interfollicular synchronization could be achieved when treatment with GnRH agonists was begun in the mid-late luteal phase and that this effect was brought about by the abolishment of the premenstrual FSH secretion responsible for the process of follicular recruitment.[78] Evidence of interfollicular synchronization is demonstrated by a better cohort of oocytes with higher fertilization and cleavage rates.[78] These advantages of GnRH agonist treatment are hampered by the need for a higher dose of menotropins for ovulation induction and by the deleterious effect of the drug on progesterone production by the corpus luteum.[79] In rats a GnRH agonist was found to exert a direct antiovarian effect, reducing ovarian LH and FSH receptor levels.[80] Thus the ovarian resistance to administration of exogenous menotropins as well as the luteolytic effect of GnRH agonists may be the result of either the abolishment of pulsatile endogenous gonadotropins or a direct inhibitory effect of the analog on the ovary.

Suppression of endogenous gonadotropin secretion has both the advantage of preventing premature LH secretion and the benefit of extending the follicular phase, resulting in higher estradiol levels and the retrieval of increased numbers of oocytes. However, such treatment exposes the patient to an increased risk for the development of OHSS. Although the incidence of OHSS in hMG-alone protocols was 0.7%,[81] the incidence was significantly higher (6.6%) in IVF cycles in which a GnRH agonist protocol was used. Other complications reported in association with GnRH agonist treatment are cyst formation originating from a growing follicle that does not ovulate because of pituitary blockade and abolition of the feedback mechanism.[82,83] These cysts develop in about 15% of treatment cycles and demonstrate no tendency to recur in repeated cycles.[83,84] They can manage by means of cycle cancellation, aspiration or waiting for regression under GnRH agonist treatment. We prefer to aspirate cysts transvaginally because adverse effects such as cyst enlargement, disturbed normal follicular development, and an increased hMG requirement are anticipated to occur if cysts are left in situ.[85,86] Once a cyst is aspirated, exogenous gonadotropin treatment can be initiated without affecting cycle outcome.

It has been suggested that patients with PCO disease may benefit from treatment with GnRH agonists. Owen et al[87] observed a higher fertilization rate when a GnRH agonist was used in PCO disease. This was a statistically significant finding that indicated the achievement of better-quality oocytes when the tonic LH secretion was abolished by the agonist. Other investigators observed no difference in cycle outcome irrespective of the type of stimulation used to treat these patients.[88] In addition, it has been suggested that patients with high tonic LH levels suffer from lower pregnancy rates and increased abortion rates.[89] This finding was attributed to the possible adverse effect of the high LH levels on the developing oocytes during the follicular phase. These patients demonstrated a significant reduction in abortion rate when a GnRH agonist was used concomitantly during controlled ovarian stimulation.[90]

GnRH Agonist Protocols

GnRH agonists can be administered as daily subcutaneous injections, via nasal spray, or can be given intramuscularly as a depot preparation (Table 42–1). Different regimens for induction of ovulation have been designed to combine GnRH agonists as concomitant treatment. These include long, short, and ultrashort protocols (Fig 42–1).

GnRH agonists, especially the depot preparation, have a detrimental effect on the corpus luteum that results in a luteal-phase defect. This adverse effect is brought about by either abolition of LH secretion or a direct inhibitory impact of the agonist on ovarian cells. Therefore, it is advocated that cycles in which GnRH agonists are used should be supported with either progesterone or hCG during the luteal phase.

Long Protocol. In the long protocol, menotropin treatment is started only after downregulation of the pituitary gland is achieved. Desensitization of the pituitary gland is accomplished with administration of a GnRH agonist either from the midluteal phase of the preceding cycle or from the early follicular phase of the actual treatment cycle. Desensitization, determined by an estradiol level less than 30 pg/mL (110 pmol/L) is usually achieved after 10 to 14 days of agonist treatment. The agonist can be given either as depot preparation, daily injections, or as nasal spray and should be continued concomitantly with ovulation induction until hCG administration.

When the long protocol started in the early follicular phase was compared with initiation in the midluteal phase, it was found that profound ovarian suppression was achieved within a shorter period of time with the midluteal protocol.[79] However, this advantage of the midluteal protocol was hampered by the higher dose of hMG needed for an adequate response and a lower number of mature oocytes, leading to considerably fewer embryos available for transfer. However, the pregnancy rate was similar between the groups, and the outcome of the pregnancies did not differ.

Although the long protocol can be used to treat most patients, some patients, known as "poor responders," may have unfavorable outcomes with such treatment. This may be attributed to the longer suppression and exposure to the agonist, which may exert a direct antigonadal effect. These patients may be better treated with different GnRH agonist protocols.

TABLE 42–1. GnRH AGONISTS USED FOR IN VITRO FERTILIZATION

Compound	Trade Name	Half-life	Potency	Administration
Leuprolide acetate [D-Leu^6-Pro^{9}NEt]GnRH	Lupron	90 min	20–30	Subcutaneous microcapsules
Triptorelin [D-Trp^6]GnRH	Decapeptyl	30 min	144	Subcutaneous microcapsules
Buserelin [D-Ser(But)^6-Pro^{9}NEt]GnRH	Suprefact	80 min	20–40	Subcutaneous nasal spray
Goserelin [D-Ser(But)^6-AzaGlyc^{10}]GnRH	Zoladex	4.5 h	50–100	Implant
Nafarelin [D-Nal(2)^6]GnRH	Synarel	3–4 h	200	Nasal spray

1. Long protocol

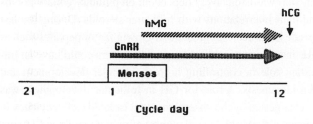

2. Short protocol

3. Ultrashort protocol

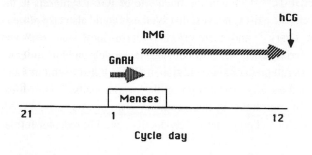

Figure 42–1. Schematic representation of three alternative GnRH agonist treatment protocols.

Short Protocol, or "Flare-Up," Protocol. With this protocol, the agonist is administered from the first or second day of the treatment cycle and menotropins are added on the third day of the cycle. It is called a flare-up protocol because the menotropin treatment takes advantage of the initial endogenous release of gonadotropins that characterizes the stimulatory phase of the GnRH agonist. As with the long protocol, the agonist is discontinued when hCG is administered.

Some prospective studies[91,92] have shown that there was no difference in pregnancy rate when either a long or a short protocol was used. However, several retrospective studies and large prospective studies demonstrated that the long protocol is associated with retrieval of more fertilizable oocytes and a markedly higher pregnancy rate, irrespective of the type of agonist, used when compared with the short protocol.[79] Although a better ovarian response and a higher pregnancy rate were reported with the long protocol, this treatment was associated with a higher dose of hMG needed for adequate response. This protocol is usually reserved for low responders, in whom the flare-up effect seems to enhance the action of gonadotropin.

Ultrashort Protocol. The ultrashort protocol was originally developed for use by poor responders.[93] With this protocol, GnRH agonist is administered for only 3 days in the early follicular phase, days 2, 3, and 4. As with the short protocol, it takes advantage of the initial surge of gonadotropin secretion induced by the agonist. Use of this protocol was associated with lower LH and estradiol levels on the day of hCG administration than use of the CC-hMG protocol.[94] Suppression of LH in the late follicular phase leads to optimal maturity of collected ocytes, improved embryo quality, and greater likelihood of implantation. Because high levels of estradiol in the late follicular phase have been associated with failure of implantation and pregnancy loss, lower estradiol levels at this stage may be of advantage in respect to uterine receptivity. The ultrashort protocol has proved to be of advantage compared with the long protocol in respect to the length of the treatment cycle and the amount of menotropin needed. However, premature ovulation and cycle cancellation are still troublesome with the ultrashort protocol compared with short and long protocols. We use the ultrashort protocol as a last resort for low responders who do not produce adequate follicular growth with other modes of stimulation.

GnRH Antagonist

One of the disadvantages of use of GnRH agonists for downregulation is the length of time required for the effect to occur and the need for an increased hMG dose for achievement of an adequate response. By altering the amino acid substitutions in the native GnRH molecule, antagonists can be synthesized that have high-affinity binding to the GnRH receptor without any agonistic properties. The first antagonist preparations had the tendency to cause histamine release concomitantly with the blocking effect and therefore had limited clinical application. New substances, namely Nal-Glu and Cetrorelix, which lacked this undesired effect were developed and successfully used by women during controlled ovarian stimulation. Experience with the GnRH antagonist Nal-Glu in monkeys and humans shows that the LH surge can be suppressed and that follicular maturation is not affected.[95] Furthermore, it has been shown that administration of the antagonist during the late follicular phase postpones the LH surge[96,97] and abolishes the positive feedback of estradiol during the periovulatory period.[98] These findings led to the use of GnRH antagonists in cycles of ovulation induction. Several studies have indicated that the antagonist prevents a premature LH surge and subsequent luteinization.[95,99] The main advantages of the antagonist are the achievement of an immediate suppression of gonadotropin release and that the unwanted stimulatory phase associated with GnRH agonist administration is avoided. For ovulation induction cycles, the antagonist can be used only for several days in the late follicular phase until hCG administration.[100] Compared with cycles in which the agonist is used, treatment cycles in which an antagonist is used are shorter and require a lower amount of hMG. In addition, expenses are lower and treatment proves to be much more comfortable for patients.[100] Because treatment with the new generation of GnRH antagonists in ovarian stimulation is promising, it seems that in the near future these drugs will be widely used and substituted for GnRH agonists in protocols of ovulation induction.

Recombinant Human FSH

Recombinant DNA technology enables the transfection of both α and β subunit genes of FSH into Chinese hamster ovary cells. After transfection, these cells express the hormone and synthesize intact recombinant human FSH (r-FSH).[101] Studies showed that r-FSH lacks intrinsic LH activity and exhibits high specific FSH bioactivity compared with a highly purified u-FSH preparation.[101,102] Administration of r-FSH is safe with no antibody formation and has led to normal pregnancies and healthy babies.[103,104] Normal folliculogenesis and estradiol production from androgen precursors is an LH-dependent process. Because r-FSH preparation contains no LH activity, concomitant use of r-FSH with GnRH agonist, producing a hypogonadotropic hypogonadal state was questioned.[103] However, successful ovarian stimulation in IVF cycles indicate that when GnRH agonist is used, a minimal amount of circulating LH still exists and is sufficient for an adequate ovarian response. When r-FSH was used in gonadotropin-deficient women, multiple follicular growth to the preovulatory stage was achieved, whereas estrogen and androgen concentrations in serum and follicular fluid remained low.[105,106] Although the importance of estrogen-deficient milieu in the development potential of fertilized preovulatory oocytes needs further investigation, the results of these studies substantiate the existence of the two-cell theory in the ovary.

The present source of commercial FSH preparations, the urine of postmenopausal women, carries the risk of protein, bacterial, and viral contamination. Recombinant FSH avoids such contamination risks and offers a highly purified preparation with a remarkable batch-to-batch consistency. In addition, because r-FSH is highly purified and devoid of protein contamination, it is well tolerated when given subcutaneously. Thus self-administration will simplify the treatment cycle for both the patient and the staff. In the future, r-FSH will replace other commercial preparations of urinary-origin gonadotropins.

Although hCG can effectively replace LH when indicated, the longer half-life of hCG may have undesirable effects and lead to OHSS when used to induce ovulation in overstimulated ovaries. In the future, the introduction of recombinant LH with a half-life shorter than that of hCG may overcome this disadvantage of the latter drug.

Growth Hormone

Until recently it was believed that the regulation of ovarian function was exclusively dependent on pituitary gonadotropins and their interrelations with follicular steroids. During the last decade it has been suggested that growth factor peptides such as GH, insulin, and insulin-like growth factors could have an important role in controlling normal follicular development and steroidogenesis. A role for GH in follicular development was first suggested by the observation that isolated GH deficiency in teenage girls could delay the onset of puberty and that GH substitution could reverse this condition.[107] It is currently thought that this effect of GH is mediated by insulin-like growth factor I (IGF-I).[108] Although the main site of IGF-I synthesis is the liver, data exist to suggest that synthesis could also take place in the ovary[109] and therefore may have local autocrine and paracrine functions.[108] In both animal models and human granulosa cell preparations, addition of GH or IGF-I to cultures amplified gonadotropin action on the ovarian cells.[110] This effect was demonstrated by augmentation of aromatase activity, 17-β estradiol and progesterone production, and LH receptor formation.

Triggered by these observations has been a growing interest in the potential use of exogenous GH as an adjuvant agent in ovulation induction with menotropins. Using this combination to treat hypogonadotrophic women who had been previously resistant to hMG, several investigators[111,112] found a significant augmentation of ovarian response and reduction of gonadotropin requirement. It was suggested that because these patients had tonically low IGF-I levels, the addition of GH resulted in an increased level of IGF-I in both the plasma and follicular fluid, improving ovarian response. However, in randomized, placebo-controlled studies, when GH was supplemented in patients with normal ovulation undergoing IVF, no beneficial effect was noted in GH-treated patients compared with a placebo group.[113,114] GH co-treatment with menotropins was suggested to be beneficial in patients with PCO disease as it reduced the hMG dose needed for an adequate response, decreased the duration of the follicular phase, and increased the number of retrieved oocytes.[115] This positive effect is considered to evolve from an increased level of IGF-I and a decreased level of androstenedione in the follicular fluid induced by GH.[116] However, these studies included only a small number of patients and must be extended before any firm conclusions can be drawn. Current evidence on the use of GH as an adjuvant treatment in poor responders appears inconclusive. Although some studies demonstrated a beneficial effect in respect to ovarian response and clinical outcome (Fig 42–2), others did not find treatment with GH valuable for poor responders.[117]

The dosage of GH varies in different protocols. It is usually 6 to 12 IU given subcutaneously every other day starting on the first and ending at the seventh day of hMG administration (a total of four injections). Some authors use GH in daily dose of 0.1 IU/kg concomitant with hMG administration until follicular maturation is achieved.

Taken together it may be concluded that GH supplementation is beneficial mostly for patients with hypogonadotrophic hypogonadism (HH) who are hypoestrogenic and who demonstrate low IGF-I levels. Patients with normal ovulation may not benefit from treatment even if they undergo suppression by GnRH agonists, whereas some poor responders may take advantage of GH supplementation.

CLINICAL MONITORING OF OVULATION INDUCTION

Monitoring in Clomiphene and HMG-only Cycles

An optimal system of ovulation induction is probably the most important factor affecting the success of IVF, because it determines the quality of oocytes, the completeness of endometrial responsiveness, and corpus luteum function. The two most widely used peripheral markers for monitoring ovarian activity in IVF and ovulation induction are estradiol-17β to assess follicular development (mostly in combination with ovarian ultrasonography) and progesterone as a marker of luteinization and corpus luteum function. Some centers also measure LH in the urine or serum as a means of intercepting a premature surge.

The programmed succession of steps involved in follicular growth and maturation, as well as in endometrial development, are maintained through a delicate balance of steroidal and nonsteroidal signals. Because of this apparent complexity it is necessary to weigh the relative importance of these steroid markers and to determine whether estradiol and progesterone are sufficient by themselves to act on their main target organ, the endometrium, to induce morphologic and functional changes compatible with successful embryo implantation. Women with primary ovarian failure who conceive after the transfer of donated embryos to the uterus serve as a unique model to address this issue. We[118,119] and others[120,121] who work with oocyte donation have demonstrated conclusively that artificially induced endometrial maturation is coupled with functional receptivity. Pregnancies that result from the transfer of donated embryos to fallopian tubes demonstrate that it is possible artificially to mimic functional changes within the tubes that support normal growth and propagation of an embryo to the implantation site solely by means of administration of estradiol progesterone.[122] These clinical trials clearly suggest that serum levels of the two markers might be sufficient to assess follicular growth and endometrial responsiveness if they are properly interpreted. The monitoring and consequent titration of medication in the original embryo-donation protocols were geared to mimic an unstimulated cycle. During the normal ovulatory cycle, follicular growth is linear and is paralleled by an increase in circulating estradiol. In these cycles, ultrasound measurement of follicles correlated well with serum estradiol levels, and both these variables were shown to be equally effective predicators of follicular growth.[123,124] In natural cycles, 95% of circulating estradiol was shown to emanate from the growing follicle[125]; ovulation occurs at the fairly narrow range of 22 to 27 mm in diameter.[126]

In induced cycles, the normal monofollicular quota is disturbed, producing radical changes in the intraovarian milieu.[127] When serum estradiol levels and follicle size, determined with ultrasound, were correlated in normally ovulating women treated with clomiphene for IVF, both increased linearly, but the correlation between separate pooled values was lower than that reported for the normal cycle.[128] Similarly, in hMG cycles for IVF, no correlation was found between serum estradiol level and the size of the largest follicle.[129] We found that estradiol level alone on the day of hCG administration could not be used to differentiate between women developing one large (greater than 15 mm) follicle (635±47 pg/mL [2330±172 pmol/L]) and those developing several large follicles (687±86 pg/mL [2520±315 pmol/L]).[126] The mean follicular volume did not differ in these

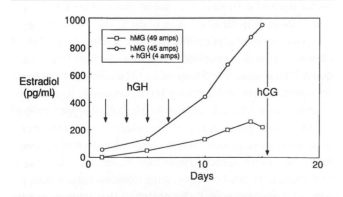

Figure 42–2. Ovarian estradiol response to growth hormone and hMG stimulation in a low-responding patient (12 IU/day of hGH is administered).

cycles. We concluded that the individual follicle contributes more to peripheral estradiol levels in monofollicular cycles than in multifollicular cycles. This observation, coupled with our demonstration that mature oocytes are not necessarily aspirated from large follicles, strongly suggests asynchrony between follicular growth and functional maturation.

The crucial decision in every IVF cycle is the timing of hCG administration, which triggers the cascade of luteal-phase events. Premature administration disrupts preovulatory follicular development and results in failure to ovulate.[130] Delay in hCG administration is associated with a reduced fertilization rate and an increased percentage of degenerated oocytes because of prolonged oocyte retention in follicles undergoing atresia.[131] Because of close monitoring in IVF cycles, further insight has been gained into ovulation induction, and better criteria have been established for timing of hCG administration and cancellation of cycles.

The absolute level of estradiol at the time of hCG administration seems to play an important part in IVF success. Low responders have been shown to do poorly, and arbitrarily high cutoff levels have been retrospectively correlated with better success rates. In the Norfolk program, high responders (>600 pg/mL [2200 pmol/L]) had a higher conception rate than low responders (<300 pg/mL [1100 pmol/L]) (23% and 15%, respectively).[132] With the same protocol of ovulation induction, cycles that did not reach an estradiol level greater than 700 pg/mL (2570 pmol/L) were aborted.[133] A higher conception rate was shown with CC-hMG cycles when estradiol levels were more than 1000 pg/mL (3670 pmol/L) on the day of hCG administration (20% versus 4%, respectively) and 17% and 13% in high-dose hMG IVF cycles.[62] Similar findings were reported for estradiol levels exceeding 1000 pg/mL (3670 pmol/L) in "programmed" cycles (50% and 5.6%, respectively).[134] In a retrospective analysis of 242 IVF cycles of high-dose hMG and ultrasound-guided aspiration, a higher cutoff point (1500 pg/mL [5510 pmol/L]) was associated with a doubling of conception rate (20.5% and 10.4%, respectively; $P < .05$).[135] It is concluded that absolute estradiol levels greater than 1000 pg/mL (3670 pmol/L) in CC-hMG cycles, greater than 800 pg/mL (2940 pmol/L) for high-dose hMG, and greater than 500 to 700 pg/mL (1840 to 2570 pmol/L) in low-dose hMG cycles, are associated with a better clinical conception rate.

Monitoring in Cycles Managed with GnRH Agonists and hMG

The addition of GnRH agonists to ovulation induction regimens in IVF has gained widespread acceptance. The introduction of this treatment has led to higher pregnancy rates, larger numbers of oocytes retrieved, and a decrease in cancellations due to premature LH surge. Specifically, comparing the ovarian response to GnRH agonist–hMG with the traditional hMG treatment re-

TABLE 42–2. COMPARISON OF OVARIAN RESPONSE DURING OVULATION INDUCTION WITH AND WITHOUT GnRH AGONIST

Factor Measured	GnRH Agonist+hMG	hMG	Probability
Age (y)	33.6±4	32.4±3.8	NS
hMG dose (ampule)	32.7±12.4	26.2±11.7	.01
Peak estradiol level (pg/mL)[a]	2281±1067 (8370±3920)	1828±817 (6710±3000)	.02
No. of oocytes retrieved	14.5±6.2	10.9±4.3	.001
No. of embryos produced	9.7±4.0	8.2±2.8	.014
Oocytes fertilized (%)	70.6	77.4	.036

Values are mean ± standard deviation.
NS, not significant.
[a]Numbers in parentheses are Systems International conversion (pmol/L).
Adapted from Benshushan A, et al: The effect of gonadotropin-releasing hormone agonist on embryo quality and pregnancy rate following cryopreservation. Fertil Steril 59:1065, 1993. Reprinted with permission of the publisher, The American Fertility Society.

vealed an increase in gonadotropin consumption, higher estradiol levels on the day of hCG administration, and increased numbers of oocytes and embryos (Table 42–2).[136] Furthermore, a meticulous meta-analysis demonstrated that with the use of the GnRH agonist there was a significant increase in the number of ampules of hMG used, the number of oocytes retrieved, and the number of clinical pregnancies achieved with no change in the rate of spontaneous abortions or pregnancies after cryopreservations.[76,137,138] There are conflicting results concerning the optimal mode of GnRH agonist suppression before hMG administration: the long protocol (2 weeks in either the luteal or follicular phase) or the flare-up protocol (starting in the follicular phase 3 to 5 days before the addition of hMG). Nevertheless, most IVF units have adopted long suppression (usually midluteal) as the first line of treatment because the results were superior to the results obtained with the flare-up protocol.[139] Attempts have been made to predict the best suppression protocol on the basis of individual estradiol response to the GnRH agonist given daily in the first 4 days of the cycle.[140]

Once ovarian suppression has been reached with a GnRH agonist, the patient receives hMG in a step-up[136] or a step-down[140] technique. The timing of hCG administration depends on follicular size and estradiol levels; however, there are no strict criteria for these determinants. The follicular size required for hCG administration may differ widely. Some workers require at least one to three follicles larger than 16 mm in diameter or three to five follicles larger than 15 mm.[140–142] Other centers require at least two or three follicles larger than 18 mm.[143–146] Forman et al[141] demonstrated that pregnancy rates were independent of the number of follicles larger than 14 mm on day of hCG administration. This finding explains the similar results among the various IVF centers despite different criteria.

The situation concerning the desired estradiol level on the day of hCG administration is less clear. Most centers have determined a minimal threshold of estradiol below which the chances of achieving a pregnancy are grim. Thus either hCG is withheld or the patient continues to receive additional hMG treatment. Specifically, some authors require at least 650 pg/mL (2390 pmol/L)[147] or 1000 pg/mL (3670 pmol/L).[145,148] Others require 200 pg/mL (734 pmol/L) per follicle larger than 14 mm.[142,149] Moreover, all programs have set a maximal level of estradiol above which the risk for OHSS increases markedly, and either the dose of hCG is decreased or hCG is withheld. According to Forman et al,[141] if estradiol level is more than 2000 pg/mL (7340 pmol/L) and there are more than 15 follicles larger than 12 mm in diameter, hCG is withheld. Our unit has adopted the following requirements for hCG administration in IVF: at least two to three follicles larger than 18 mm, a minimal estradiol level of 500 pg/mL (1840 pmol/L), and a maximum estradiol level of 5000 pg/mL (18,360 pmol/L). To avoid OHSS we use a modification of the algorithm described by Navot et al[149] Briefly, up to 2500 pg/mL (9180 pmol/L), 10,000 U of hCG is given; between 2500 and 5000 pg/mL (9180 and 18,360 pmol/L), the dose of hCG is reduced to 5000 or 2500 U; and above 5000 pg/mL (18,360 pmol/L), hCG is withheld or ovulation is induced with 2500 U, after which aspiration of the follicles and cryopreservation of embryos is performed.

Considerable attention has been focused on the effect of increased progesterone levels before hCG administration on oocyte quality, embryo quality, and pregnancy rate. Several investigators suggested that elevated progesterone levels were associated with decreased pregnancy rates in IVF cycles.[149,150] When the cutoff point for elevated progesterone level was set at 0.9 ng/mL (2.9 nmol/L), Fanchin et al[151] demonstrated that although both groups had similar numbers of oocytes retrieved with identical cleavage rates, the group with high progesterone levels had lower ongoing pregnancies per ET compared with the low progesterone level group (14% versus 28%). Similarly, when the cutoff levels of progesterone were set at 1 ng/mL (3.2 nmol/L), Check et al[152] found a decrease in pregnancy rate among the high progesterone group compared with the control (7.2% versus 14.4%). Nevertheless, the authors showed that in their oocyte donation program there was no difference in pregnancy rate whether or not the oocytes were exposed to high progesterone levels (13.7% versus 14.4%). Moreover, Silverberg et al[153] also demonstrated that the pregnancy rates in subsequent frozen-thawed cycles were similar whether or not the oocytes were obtained with an elevated progesterone level (>0.9 ng/mL [2.9 nmol/L]). The authors concluded that an elevated progesterone level does not adversely affect the quality of oocytes.

When the progesterone level was set at more than 1.1 ng/mL (3.5 nmol/L) on the day of hCG administration, Hof-

mann et al[154] found identical numbers of mature oocytes, fertilization rate, polyspermia rate, and embryo grade from women with and without an elevated progesterone level. Since oocyte recipients from both groups achieved similar pregnancy rates, the authors concluded that the decrease in clinical pregnancy rate among women with elevated progesterone levels is due to a yet undetermined factor that results in impairment of the endometrium as a result of premature luteinization with no substantial deleterious effects on the oocytes. Yovel et al[155] found that when the progesterone cutoff levels were set at 1.9 ng/mL (6.0 nmol/L), there was an adverse effect on oocyte and embryo quality. According to those authors, it may be assumed that high progesterone levels (> 1.9 ng/mL [6.0 nmol/L]) are deleterious to the oocytes, yet modest progesterone elevations (> 1 ng/mL) (3.2 nmol/L) are sufficient to cause unfavorable changes in the endometrium and not the oocytes.

That assumption notwithstanding, there is no consensus concerning the effect of elevated progesterone level on pregnancy rate. In a 1994 report Givens et al[142] showed that when cutoff progesterone level was set at 0.9 ng/mL (2.9 nmol/L) on the day of hCG administration, more oocytes were retrieved with a higher percentage of mature oocytes in the high progesterone group and a slight decrease in fertilization rate. Nevertheless, in terms of embryo cleavage and implantation rate there was no difference between the groups.

It is yet to be determined whether elevated progesterone levels truly represent premature luteinization or indicate appropriate preovulatory hormonal secretion from the theca of multiple stimulated follicles. Because of conflicting data, in our program, as long as the estradiol level is rising appropriately we do not cancel the cycle or cryopreserve embryos in the face of elevated progesterone levels.

Over the past several years with the improvement in transvaginal ultrasonography, increasing interest has been focused on means of determining the probability of implantation based on the ultrasound appearance of the endometrium on the day of hCG administration. It was suspected that the appropriate ultrasound appearance would indirectly reflect endometrial receptivity. If criteria could be set, decisions could be made about when to perform ET or cryopreserve the embryos for later transfer under artificially induced cycles. Several investigators found that the pregnancy rates were positively correlated with an endometrial thickness greater than 9 mm on the day of hCG administration or 1 day later.[145,156] Other authors demonstrated negligent pregnancy rates when the endometrial thickness was less than 10 mm.[157] Moreover, the same authors[158] found that in oocyte donation cycles, an endometrium thicker than 10 mm correlates well with improved conception rates (38.7% versus 9%). In contrast, others found no correlation between pregnancy rate and endometrial thickness,[146] yet judging from the literature there seems to be more solid evidence supporting the use of en-

Becton-Dickinson, Lincoln Park, NJ) in Earle's medium supplemented with a synthetic serum substitute (Irvine Scientific, Santa Ana, CA) and are placed in the center well for preincubation.

The mammalian oocyte undergoes a complex series of structural and metabolic changes before ovulation. These include the resumption of meiosis, the breakdown of the germinal vesicle, and the extrusion of the first polar body concurrent with cytoplasmic and membrane maturation.[232] In grading oocytes, an immature oocyte has a sparse cumulus, a tightly packed corona, an absent polar body, and possibly a germinal vesicle. Mature oocytes have an expanded, puffy cumulus, an expanded corona, and a polar body. Postmature oocytes have an expanded but scant cumulus, an expanded but often partially lost corona, and a polar body[233] (Fig 42–7). It is unclear if it is necessary or even desirable to assess the maturity of the oocyte with an inverted microscope because of the potential detrimental effects of pH and osmolarity shifts during observation. We have found that in some cases, there is poor correlation between the morphology of the corona and cumulus and the actual maturity of the oocyte.[234] In the absence of a precise determination of the meiotic state of the oocyte, it has been empirically determined that an in vitro culture period of 5 to 8 hours between oocyte aspiration and insemination optimizes fertilization and cleavage rates.[235] Fully immature oocytes can be preincubated for as long as 36 hours to await the extrusion of the polar body; however, these oocytes have relatively low rates of fertilization.

Sperm Preparation and Insemination

The semen specimen is obtained by means of masturbation into a sterile container that is free of embryo-toxic substances. If the man is known to have seminal plasma antisperm antibodies, it has been suggested that ejaculation into a vessel containing medium enriched with 50% serum combined with rapid processing will increase the fertilization rate, presumably by avoiding binding of antibody to the sperm surface.[236] After collection, the specimen is allowed to liquefy, and an assessment of sperm number and motility is made. We prefer to use a Makler sperm-counting chamber (Sefi Instruments, Israel) because of its ease of use and good reproducibility.

Various techniques have been described to process semen for IVF, but a common goal is the production of a specimen of high count and motility that is free of seminal proteins and microbial contamination. In the swim-up technique, the specimen is diluted with insemination media and centrifuged twice. The resultant pellet containing the spermatozoa is overlaid with media. During a 1-hour incubation, the motile fraction swim into the media and are isolated.

The use of a Percoll gradient has been recommended for specimens of low count or motility. This technique uses a modified colloidal silica medium to separate cells present in the ejaculate by their specific density and generally improves the semen characteristics, yielding a better specimen for insemination. In this method, discontinuous gradients are produced by

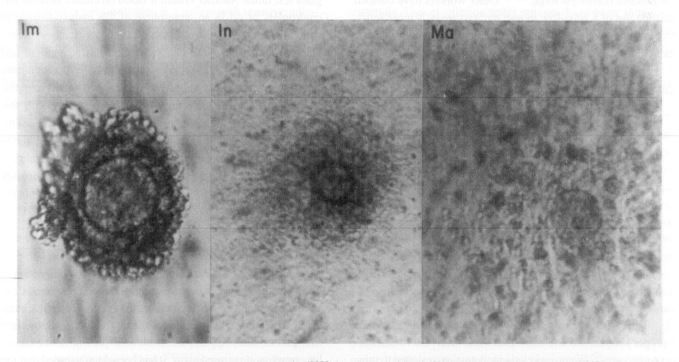

Figure 42–7. The morphology of oocyte-corona-cumulus complex (OCCC) in a woman treated with hMG-GnRH agonist. Three main types of OCCC are identified: (*Im,* Immature OCCC—tight corona and cumulus of a few layers only; (*In,* intermediate OCCC—partly dispersed cumulus and corona; Ma, mature OCCC—advanced cumulus and corona dispersal allowing visualization of the zona pellucida (original magnification × 200).

means of pipetting 1-mL aliquots of 95%, 50%, and 75% Percoll in a centrifuge tube. Semen is placed on top of the gradient, and the specimen is centrifuged at 300 g for 20 to 30 minutes. The sediment and the lower portion are collected and washed twice to remove any residual Percoll.[237] Although isotonic gradients may be used, it has been claimed that hyperosmotic gradients improve the resolution of separation.[238] A further modification of this method, the mini-Percoll, was developed for cases of severe oligoasthenozoospermia (total motile count less than 5×10^6 and uses reduced volumes of Percoll.[239] Studies comparing use of the Percoll gradient with the swim-up approach have demonstrated that although Percoll gradients increase motile fraction, fertilization rates were identical with both preparations.[240]

The actual minimal sperm density requirement to achieve fertilization is unknown. Normally, insemination is performed at a concentration of 50,000 to 250,000 sperm/mL when no male factor for the infertility exists. In poor semen samples, 500,000 or even 1 million sperm/mL have been used. Some reports, however, have indicated a paradoxic decrease in fertilization rates with increasing sperm numbers, perhaps from a buildup of toxic metabolites.[241] According to a strict criterion proposed by Kruger et al[242] to enhance the predictive value of sperm morphology, preparations containing less than 4% normal forms had a fertilization rate of 7.6%, preparations with 4% to 14% normal forms fertilized 63.9% of oocytes, and preparations with more than 14% normal forms fertilized approximately 90% of oocytes.[242] However, it must be emphasized that fertilization and conception can occur even when the morphology approaches zero normal forms.[243]

A variety of methods have been described to enhance the IVF capability of poor semen specimens. These include preincubation of semen with maternal follicular fluid, use of glass wool column filtration, and treatment of spermatozoa with TEST yolk medium.[244–246] The exact role of these methods, however, in enhancing IVF success rates must be clarified. In specimens with very low numbers of sperm, short of gamete micromanipulation, it has been suggested that haremization of multiple eggs in a single insemination dish, use of microdrop inseminations with very high sperm concentrations, and fertilization of oocytes in capillary tubes with as few as 500 sperm per oocyte may enhance the fertilization potential of these samples.[247] An additional, inexpensive option is to pool sequential ejaculates collected from oligozoospermic men to increase the number of motile sperm available for insemination.[248]

Fertilization

The fusion of spermatozoa and egg represents the culmination of a series of events that results in a union of gametes. Initially, a sperm traversing the male reproductive tract undergoes a mat-

uration process in which it acquires motility. At ejaculation, the sperm undergoes capacitation whereby its plasma membrane is altered in such a manner as to cause hyperactivation. This poorly understood activity results in a vigorous, motile sperm, which may now penetrate the cumulus oophorus and bind to the zona pellucida by means of a series of binding proteins. After this binding step, the sperm undergoes the acrosome reaction whereby fusion of the outer acrosomal membrane and the sperm plasma membrane occurs, resulting in release of hydrolytic enzymes from the sperm head overlying the nucleus. This release of acrosin and hyaluronidase from vesicles in the anterior region of the sperm head allows the sperm to penetrate the zona pellucida and gain entry into the perivitelline space. At this point, the sperm encounters and fuses with the vitelline membrane through action of microvilli on the egg surface. These steps of fertilization invoke the cortical reaction, whereby cytoplasmic, membrane-bound granules are released from the egg into the perivitelline space, resulting in a hardening of the zona pellucida. The subsequent alterations in the zona pellucida architecture constitute a block to prevent additional sperm entry. This impediment to polyspermy may also be mediated by a change in membrane depolarization, constituting an additional sperm barrier.[249]

In most clinical IVF programs, including ours, oocytes are harvested in the morning, inseminated in the early afternoon after a period of preincubation, and examined the following morning for evidence of fertilization. Cumulus or corona cells are dislodged with gentle pipetting to enable optimal visualization of fertilization. The ova are examined carefully for the appearance of the second polar body and the presence of two pronuclei. After confirmation of fertilization, the oocytes are transferred to growth media. The visualization of a third pronucleus is a contraindication to subsequent ET, even though these embryos may undergo rapid cleavage and assume a completely normal appearance.[250] Cellular vacuoles may be mistaken for pronuclei, and normal embryos may be inadvertently discarded. It has therefore been suggested that the presence of nucleoli be used as a criterion for a pronucleus.[251] Occasionally, inseminated oocytes contain only a single pronucleus. Various authors have reported the incidence of this finding to encompass 1.6% to 5.9% of oocytes after insemination.[252,253] In one study, chromosomal analysis of four- to eight-cell embryos resulting from single pronucleated nuclei revealed a diploid complement 80.5% of the time.[254] In a study of 312 postinsemination single pronucleated oocytes serially examined, a second pronucleus was observed in 25% of oocytes 4 to 6 hours after the initial viewing, with a similar cleavage pattern to control di-pronucleated oocytes. In addition, pregnancies and livebirths were reported from patients who had single embryos transferred that originated from oocytes with a single pronucleus 16 to 18 hours after insemination. It has therefore been recommended that single pronucleated oocytes be reinspected for a second pronu-cleus; if the second pronucleus is present, the oocyte is treated as viable.[254]

The topic of re-insemination of unfertilized oocytes is an unresolved one. Some authorities advocating an additional attempt at fertilization 18 to 24 hours after insemination, and others do not.[255–258] It has also been proposed that secondary insemination be performed only on oocytes that were immature at the initial retrieval. It has been suggested that oocytes that have failed conventional IVF are candidates for ICSI. The efficacy, safety, and clinical utility of this approach, however, remain to be validated.

Assessment of Embryo Quality

After oocyte collection, a culture period of 48 hours brings most fertilized eggs to the four-cell stage or beyond. The challenge at this point is to determine which embryos are best suited for transfer and which, if any, should be cryopreserved. Currently, this evaluation of embryo viability is performed on the basis of morphologic appearance of the embryo at light microscopy. Several grading systems have been postulated to evaluate embryo quality. These descriptive methods evaluate several basic criteria: cleavage rate, number of blastomeres per embryo, blastomere size, and degree of fragmentation and granularity.[259,260] Although these criteria have been found useful in the theoretic assessment of embryo quality, in practice, there has been no strong, consistent correlation between embryo quality as evaluated on the basis of gross morphology and the likelihood of implantation.[261] It has been demonstrated that slowly dividing embryos and those with poor morphologic appearance may undergo normal development.[262] A further morphologic aspect of embryo assessment is the presence of multinucleated blastomeres.[263,264] It has been postulated that this finding has an adverse effect on implantation rate, although this area needs further exploration.

Besides its limitations in predicting embryo quality, morphologic evaluation requires experience and is essentially a subjective analysis. In an effort to evaluate embryos objectively, a number of methods have been described that measure the functional capacity of an embryo. For example, it is known that embryos preferentially consume pyruvate during early cleavage and that consumption of glucose and excretion of lactate are greater in embryos that develop normally compared with those that are growth retarded.[265] Ultramicrofluorometric assays that measure these metabolic factors are potentially valuable tools in determining embryo quality.[266] Another approach to embryo assessment is measurement of various secreted factors that have been found to correlate with its likelihood of implantation. Platelet-activating factor, a soluble substance released by embryos, has been found to be secreted in higher quantities in association with pregnancy, but this correlation is not absolute.[267] The utility of measuring interleukin-1 and other immunomodulatory factors in embryo culture media as a means of assessing viability has been described.[268] These results, however, have not been substantiated by others.[269]

Several novel approaches to testing embryo viability have been suggested. These include use of fluorescent markers that pass through the cell membrane, are hydrolyzed by esterases, and emit fluorescein and the use of fluorimetry with the reduced form of nicotinamide-adenine dinucleotide (NADH) to assess embryo metabolism after pyruvate pulses are given to starved two-cell mouse embryos.[270] Because of safety concerns, it is likely that these invasive methods will remain experimental techniques for use in animal models.

Embryo Co-culture

Several centers have described the use of co-culture systems to aid in embryonic maturation and development. A co-culture is defined as the addition of nonembryonic cells to a defined milieu. The impetus for the development of co-culture techniques has been frustration due to the relatively stable but low take-home baby rate at most centers even after many years of IVF experience. It has been postulated that it may be of benefit in human IVF to replicate the physiologic environment of the fallopian tube by exposing embryos to layers of cells during growth and cleavage.[271] Investigators found that growing oocytes and embryos in co-culture enhanced embryo morphology, increased the number of cells per embryo, and allowed more embryos to reach the blastocyst stage compared with control embryos grown under standard conditions.[272,273]

Multiple types of co-culture systems have been described. Autologous co-culture involves use of maternally derived cells such as endometrial, granulosa, or even cumulus-mass cells to nurture embryonic growth.[272,274,275] Heterologous co-cultures of human oviductal cells obtained from women undergoing hysterectomy and even interspecies systems such as fetal bovine uterine fibroblasts, bovine oviductal cells, and green monkey kidney epithelium have been employed.[276,277] An interesting sequential system designed to mimic in vivo conditions has been described in which early pronuclear-stage embryos are initially grown on human tubal cells until the eight-cell stage and are then transferred to an endometrial feeder layer.[278]

The mechanism of action of these support cells is a matter of debate. Some authorities postulate that the feeder cells work by means of a negative conditioning mode by means of elimination of toxic substances deleterious to the embryo, such as hypoxanthanine and excess proteins. The positive conditioning argument is that co-culture is of benefit to embryos by means of secretion as of yet undefined embryotrophic substances.

Critics of the co-culture method argue that the addition of

a foreign biologic variable to the delicate balance of the embryo is potentially harmful. Heterologous and nonhuman cells may transmit pathogens. The system is relatively labor-intensive, expensive, and the cells have a definite life span. In addition, the issues of batch-to-batch reproducibility and quality control have not been adequately addressed.

Clinical results with human embryos grown in co-culture have emphasized the improvement in embryo quality, but the effects on pregnancy and take-home baby rate remain unclear. A recent randomized trial demonstrated that the culture of human embryos on Vero cells did not result in increased pregnancy rates among patients undergoing initial IVF treatments.[279] However, authors of another study that enrolled 90 patients with multiple previous failures of fertilization grew the embryos on homologous endometrial cells. The investigators found higher implantation and pregnancy rates than in previous cycles.[274] These authors postulated that co-culture may increase implantation rates by allowing embryos to remain viable in culture for longer periods and therefore help select the best quality embryo for transfer.

In summary, the use of co-cultures to support embryonic growth appears to be an exciting development in the field of embryo culture. Many urgent questions need to be answered, such as which subset of patients will likely benefit, how to simplify and standardize culture conditions, and how to ensure the safety of this technique. The exact mechanism of how co-cultures enhance embryonic development needs to be addressed. The coming years will surely see intense research into these questions.

Genetic Aspects of In Vitro Fertilization

A plausible explanation for poor efficiency of IVF may be the relatively large number of chromosomal abnormalities found in human gametes. Several reviews summarizing the data on the karyotyping of thousands of oocytes concluded that the overall frequency of oocytes with abnormal chromosomal complements is between 24% and 35%.[280,281] Errors most commonly are aneuploidy, diploidy, and structural abnormalities. Most of these studies were performed on oocytes that failed fertilization and subsequently underwent cytogenetic analysis. The few studies that investigated uninseminated oocytes demonstrated that the incidence of abnormalities in this fresh cohort is probably no greater than in inseminated, unfertilized oocytes.[282, 283] In contrast, studies on human spermatozoa have yielded aneuploidy rates of approximately 9%.[284]

It has been argued that clinical factors of IVF, such as the cause of infertility, use of gonadotropins for ovarian stimulationa, and addition of a GnRH agonist to the stimulation protocol may affect the incidence of chromosomal anomalies. However, studies have not shown any correlation between these clinical variables and the incidence of chromosomally abnormal oocytes.[283,285,286] Most, but not all, studies do demonstrate an increased incidence of aneuploidy with age older than 35 years.[281,287,288]

Data on the chromosomal complement of human embryos have been forthcoming in recent years (Table 42–3). The most common abnormalities are aneuploidy, mosaicism, and structural alterations. A common feature to all these studies has been

TABLE 42–3. SUMMARY OF 11 PUBLISHED CHROMOSOMAL ANALYSIS STUDIES ON HUMAN PREIMPLANTATION EMBRYOS

Author	Year	No. of Embryos Analyzed	Type of Embryo	Technique	Percentage Abnormal
Angell et al[289]	1986	15	Research[a]	Karyotype	26
Plachot et al[290]	1987	68	Spare[b]	Karyotype	23
Wimmers and Van der Merne[291]	1988	55	Reject[b,c] Spare	Karyotype	74
Papadopoulos et al[292]	1989	35	Research[c] Spare	Karyotype	40
Bongso et al[293]	1991	91	Reject	Karyotype	32
Zenzes et al[294]	1992	76	Spare	Karyotype	87
Edirisinghe et al[295]	1992	22	Reject[c] Spare	Karyotype	41
Benkhalifa et al[296]	1993	54	Reject	FISH	30
Munne et al[297]	1993	30	Reject[c] Spare	FISH	70
Jamieson et al[298]	1994	195	Reject[c] Spare	Karyotype	30
Munne et al[299]	1994	131	Reject	FISH	56.5

FISH, fluorescent in situ hybridization.
[a]Embryos donated by fertile volunteers undergoing sterilization.
[b]Poor-quality embryos deemed not suitable for transfer.
[c]Embryos not transferred due to lack of cryopreservation facilities.

the finding that there is virtually no correlation between the karyotype of the embryo and either its morphologic appearance or its rate of cleavage. It has been postulated that once an oocyte is activated into division, it has the inherent capacity to divide irrespective of its chromosomal composition until activation of the embryonic genome at the eight-cell stage.[281] Most studies that investigated the chromosomal complement of human embryos used karyotype analysis to evaluate the metaphase spread. The recent application of fluorescent in situ hybridization (FISH) has enabled investigators to use labeled probes to target specific chromosomes. Although no information is available concerning chromosomal structure, and only probes to the chromosomes of interest are visualized, this is the technique of choice for determining interphase chromosome status. With the high rates of mosaicism found in FISH studies, an important unanswered question is the extent of mosaicism in normally developing embryos and if this is a routine event in the developmental process.[297] This question can only be satisfactorily answered by studies on large numbers of normal human embryos, rather than on rejected or arrested embryos.

Cryopreservation

In large part because of the success of IVF and ICSI in producing large numbers of high-quality embryos, a parallel technology has evolved to allow long-term storage of embryos. Subsequent to the initial report of a human pregnancy after cryopreservation, thawing and transfer of an eight-cell embryo, thousands of livebirths have been achieved.[300] Frozen embryos ranging from the zygote to the blastocyst stage have yielded successful pregnancies. As a direct result of this freezing technology, the ability to store supernumerary embryos has resulted in fewer numbers of fresh embryos transferred, limiting multiple pregnancy rates. Freezing allows multiple transfers as a result of a single oocyte retrieval, yielding a higher overall pregnancy rate with less expense and risk to the patient.[301] Embryo transfer in a subsequent cycle also protects the embryo from the potentially deleterious hyperestrogenic environment encountered in the stimulated cycle of retrieval. Cryopreservation of biopsied embryos will enhance the flexibility of preimplantation diagnosis studies. Some authors have demonstrated that for patients at risk for OHSS, the elective freezing of all embryos resulted in a significant decrease in the incidence and severity of OHSS.[302,303]

One of the basic tenets in cryobiology is the prevention of lethal intracellular ice formation during the cooling process.[304] It has been found that the use of a cryoprotectant that penetrates the cells causes intracellular dehydration and prevents ice crystal formation within the embryo proper. A variety of cryoportectants have been described and used with success for human embryos. Glycerol, dimethylsulfoxide

(DMSO), and 1,2 propanediol are examples of cryoprotectants that permeate cells. Sucrose, a nonpermeable cryoprotectant, remains in the extracellular space. Frequently, both a permeable and a nonpermeable agent are used in conjunction in embryo freezing. In general, the choice of cryoprotectant is largely dictated by the developmental stage of the embryo. 1,2 Propanediol appears to be the most effective agent for early stage embryos, DMSO for four- to eight-cell embryos, and glycerol for blastocysts.

Several methods have evolved to freeze human embryos. The most commonly used technique in human IVF involves slow cooling with either DMSO or 1,2 propanediol as a cryoprotectant. The basic principles are similar for both substances in that the embryo is exposed to the cryoprotectant and equilibrated at room temperature. The embryos are then transferred to ampules or straws and placed in a programmable biologic freezing apparatus, where they are cooled at a rate of $-2°C/min$ to $-6°C$. Seeding, a process whereby a precooled forceps is placed on the ampule to initiate freezing and avoid excess supercooling, is then performed. After further freezing, the embryos are placed into liquid nitrogen. A prospective, randomized study comparing DMSO and 1,2 propanediol found that cryopreservation with DMSO yielded the highest likelihood of embryo survival and the highest implantation rates.[305] A caution, however, is that each cryopreservation program should adhere to the technique that works best in their experience.

The vitrification method involves ice-free cryopreservation of embryos by suspending them in high-solute concentrations followed by plunging into liquid nitrogen in which the solutions become viscous and solidify in a glass-like state. This essentially eliminates ice crystal formation, obviates use of a programmed freezing apparatus, and greatly simplifies the entire process.[306] Ultrarapid freezing, a modification of standard vitrification, uses high concentrates of cryopreservant together with sucrose. In this simplified approach, embryos are dehydrated in DMSO and sucrose and immersed directly into liquid nitogen. Human pregnancies have been reported with this method, but the rate of embryo survival after thawing is low. So far, a distinct advantage over the slow freezing method has not been demonstrated.[307]

Cryopreserved, thawed embryos may be transferred either in a natural cycle in which LH surge and ultrasound examination are used to predict ovulation or in an artificial cycle with a GnRH agonist to downregulate pituitary function and sequential estrogen and progesterone replacement. In our cryopreservation program we rely on the latter protocol. Timing of transfer should be planned to maximize synchronization between the embryonic stage of development and endometrial maturity.

It is generally accepted that thawed embryos should have an intact zona pellucida and at least half the original number of intact blastomeres before transfer.[308] Studies examining the factors related to a successful freeze-thaw cycle concluded that embryo quality and patient age are the primary factors involved in determining pregnancy rate.[309–311] The day of LH surge, peak estradiol level, number of embryos transferred, and length of cryopreservation had no effect on pregnancy rate. It was also found that frozen sibling embryos derived from a prior success-ful IVF cycle were more likely to initiate a pregnancy than em-bryos derived from a nonpregnant cycle, probably reflecting better embryo quality in the cohort that leads to pregnancy.[310]

Data from the American Fertility Society/Society for Assisted Reproductive Technology Registry from 1992 demon-strated that 83.5% of programs offered cryopreservation proce-dures.[312] Clinical pregnancy rate was 15.3% of procedures, and total delivery rate was 11.6% of procedures. One group reported that cryopreservation resulted in an increase in the cumulative pregnancy rate from 23.5% to 37.1% comparing with preg-nancy from a retrieval cycle alone with pregnancy for which cryopreservation also was used.[313]

In contrast to the relative success of embryo cryopreserva-tion, freezing of human oocytes has been disappointing. Al-though there are scattered reports of pregnancies resulting from frozen human oocytes, many obstacles need to be overcome be-fore this technique is perfected.[314] Concerns have been raised about the potential rise in aneuploidy rates with oocyte freezing secondary to the sensitivity of the delicate microtubule appara-tus to temperature changes.[304] In cryopreserved inseminated mouse oocytes, the frequency of polyploidy was higher than in a control group.[315] Other unresolved concerns involving oocyte freezing are parthenogenetic activation of oocytes by cryo-preservants, premature induction of zona activation resulting in reduced fertilization rates, and overall low oocyte survival rate.[316] Because of the tremendous potential involved in oocyte cryopreservation, this field will surely gather much attention in the coming years.

In Vitro Maturation

One of the most important disadvantages in IVF is the need for controlled ovarian hyperstimulation and its attendant risks to obtain a pool of fertilizable oocytes. An ideal situation would be to obtain ovarian tissue from women not exposed to go-nadotropin stimulation, isolate primordial oocytes, and grow them to maturity in vitro until fertilization. In this manner, any woman with functioning ovarian tissue could use her vast pool of primordial oocytes to provide material for fertilization. An-other disadvantage is the need for a fresh, healthy source of meiotically competent oocytes. This limiting factor prohibits women whose ovaries no longer function properly because of age, disease, or premature failure from providing mature ga-metes for insemination. If in vitro maturation becomes a reality however, ovary cryopreservation would allow these women to

store a pool of follicles for future use.[317] Tremendous progress in the mouse model in recent years has enabled us to think of these goals as a possibility rather than a fantasy. Several groups have reported successful maturation of murine oocytes in vitro.[318–320] Various systems have been suggested, including use of collagen-coated membranes to support the growth of granulosa-oocyte complexes and the technique of whole follic-ular culture. Spears et al[321] reported on the successful growth of primary mouse follicles in vitro to the graafian stage. The folli-cles were then ovulated with exposure to LH and fertilized and had normal embryo development and viable offspring in host animals.[321] It also was reported that primordial follicles ob-tained from juvenile mouse ovaries were cryopreserved, thawed, and transplanted into host mice. After mating, the host animals produced offspring derived from the frozen-thawed pri-mordial follicles as proved by genetic markers.[322]

Despite tremendous enthusiasm and interest generated by these advances in animal models, we must recognize that the human system certainly operates under a different set of rules, not the least of which is the larger size of human oocytes, and its unique oxygen and nutrient requirements. In addition, the fac-tors that control the resumption of meiosis from its state of ar-rest in humans are poorly understood. However, the potential medical and social benefits to be obtained if this technology were available would be immense. This enthusiasm, however, must be tempered with moral responsibilities that will surely arise as a result of implementation of these techniques should and if they become reality.

Embryo Transfer

The rate-limiting step in an IVF program is successful implanta-tion of transferred embryos in the uterine cavity. Based on data from the 1992 SART survey,[312] 87.5% of all patients who under-went an oocyte retrieval had embryos available for transfer, but only 21.1% of patients conceived as a result of the ET. Although tremendous advances have been made in nearly all aspects of as-sisted reproduction, the basic method of human ET remains es-sentially unchanged since its initial descriptions.[323–325]

The function of the procedure is to safely place cultured embryos within the uterine cavity, where they undergo the process of implantation. To achieve this end, the clinician should be aware of several considerations. First, timing of ET is critical in regard to the stage of embryo development. Although the transfer of human zygotes as soon as 1 day after oocyte re-trieval and as late as day 5 with blastocysts have resulted in pregnancies and livebirths, most programs choose to perform ET at the four- to eight-cell stage on day 2 or 3 after retrieval.[326] Dawson et al[327] demonstrated that delaying ET to day 3 postin-semination led to a higher implantation rate than after day 2 transfer (23% versus 19%, $P < .05$), although pregnancy rates were similar for both groups. Additional studies, including a prospective, controlled trial by Huisman et al,[328] confirmed that there was no significant difference in pregnancy rates when ET was performed on day 2, 3, or 4 after retrieval. Our center routinely performs ET 48 hours after oocyte retrieval, at approximately the four-cell stage. Some authors suggest that under suboptimal laboratory conditions, the embryos could be transferred as early as 1 day after insemination with no detrimental effect on pregnancy rate.[329]

The state of endometrial development is thought to be important in the timing of ET. The optimal synchronicity between embryonic development and uterine receptivity has been termed the window of embryo transfer. Using data derived from the model of ovum donation, we and others have shown this window to be optimal from day 17 to day 19 of an idealized cycle.[118,330] Subsequently, several centers have demonstrated that ultrasound evaluation of the endometrium to assess conditions of uterine receptivity is useful for the prediction of implantation outcome.[146,163,164] These investigators concluded that measurements of echogenic pattern, as well as assessment of uterine blood flow, is useful in determining endometrial receptivity. Future applications using both transvaginal color Doppler flow and with bio- and histochemical markers of uterine receptivity hold great promise in the objective assessment of endometrial receptivity.[165]

The issue of the optimal number of embryos to transfer in a single fresh cycle has undergone an evolutionary thought process. In the early years of IVF, it was not uncommon to transfer many embryos in a single fresh cycle to maximize the likelihood of conception. However, studies have shown a clear relation between number of high-quality embryos transferred and occurrence of multiple gestations. Staessen et al[331] demonstrated that embryos transferred at the four-cell stage had higher implantation rates than morphologically comparable two-cell embryos and that heavily fragmented embryos had poor implantation rates. Overall, the authors concluded that the multiple pregnancy rate increased in a significant way with the number of good-quality embryos transferred.[331] These iatrogenic high-order gestations have been found to present risk for increased obstetrical and neonatal complications.[332]

Appreciation of the risks involved in multiple transfer, combined with advances in laboratory culture techniques that enable the growth of better-quality embryos, has encouraged the trend in recent years to limit the number of embryos transferred. Several centers have documented that elective transfer (that is, when there are more than two good-quality embryos to choose from) of two embryos in a select population of patients younger than 35 years versus transfer of three or four embryos resulted in similar pregnancy rates.[333,334] Twinning rates among the two-embryo group ranged from 11% to 26%, and higher-order gestations were eliminated. Triplet rates among the group

receiving three or four embryos ranged from 14% to 18%. The incidence of quadruplets among the group receiving four embryos was 4%. In addition to entirely eliminating the possibility of high-order pregnancies, the policy of limiting ET in selected patients to two embryos has the additional benefit of increasing the numbers of good-quality embryos available for cryopreservation, thawing, and transfer in a future cycle.[335] Usually, we do not transfer more than three fresh embryos for women younger than 35 years. However, among older patients, the likelihood of achieving a pregnancy decreases, and one should tailor the number of transferred embryos to the individual patient.

Some authorities have advocated the utility of a mock ET trial in a cycle preceding the actual IVF-ET procedure.[62] In a prospective, controlled, randomized study, patients who underwent mock transfer had a higher pregnancy rate than those who did not undergo this procedure (22.8% versus 13.1% $P = .02$).[336] Advocates of this mock ET claim that it affords several advantages over a blind transfer. First, it decreases the subsequent number of difficult ETs, a factor that has consistently been shown to decrease pregnancy rate.[337] It allows an exact measurement of the length of the uterine cavity and may reveal a stenosed cervical canal, which is potentially amenable to dilation before an actual treatment cycle. A distorted canal can also be identified and a "road map" delineated in anticipation of the actual ET. In addition, mock ET allows selection of the most appropriate ET catheter for the patient's anatomy. Finally, mock ET acclimatizes the patient to the upcoming procedure and may therefore help to reduce stress.

A wide variety of ET catheters have been developed but all have either a side port or an end opening. Soft polytetrafluoroethylene (PTFE; Teflon) or silicone catheters such as the Wallace or the Jones need a rigid outer sleeve for introduction into the cervical canal. In contrast, Tomcat or Frydman catheter is semirigid, usually made for polyethylene, and does not require use of an introducer.[338] A modification of the Frydman, the TDT catheter, consists of a set containing catheter with a plastic-coated metal mandrel that can be adjusted to the cervical canal. The embryos are loaded into an ultrathin tube, which is passed into the catheter after removal of the metal mandrel. One advantage of this method is easy ultrasound visualization of the metal portion during difficult transfers.

Several studies have explored the issue of pregnancy rate in regard to choice of ET catheter. Although some authors have demonstrated that catheter type may influence pregnancy rate, others have not duplicated these results.[339–341] We recommend that each IVF program be proficient with the use of several catheter types should the need arise in treatment of a patient to resort to an alternative catheter. For technically difficult transfers, it has been suggested that a full bladder, use of a tenaculum to straighten the cervix, assistance of a cervical introducer, or performance of the procedure with ultrasound guidance may alleviate transfer difficulty.[338,342] If none of these maneuvers is successful in introducing the embryos into the uterus, the cycle can still be salvaged by means of tubal ET with laparoscopic guidance.

The embryos are suspended in medium supplemented with a high serum content to enhance viscosity and to facilitate transfer. Our program transfers embryos with 90% maternal serum in Earle's media. Although increased viscosity may increase the ease of transfer, it has not been found to increase pregnancy rate.[343] The use of human serum albumin for transfer media has also been described.[344] Typically, the embryos are loaded in a small volume of medium (10 to 20 μL) with 1-cm columns of air and medium on either side. Studies have shown that the volume of transfer medium is critical to the pregnancy rate, higher volumes being detrimental.[336] This bracketing of the embryonic column with small air bubbles can help track their movement with ultrasound and has been demonstrated not to have an adverse effect on pregnancy rate.[345]

A study investigating the retention of dye after mock ET concluded that dye was extruded from the external ostium in 57% of patients for whom cervical mucus was not aspirated before the ET compared with 23% of patients for whom cervical mucus was completely aspirated ($P = .01$).[346] This suggests that gentle, atraumatic aspiration of cervical mucus reduces dye expulsion and may therefore aid in the retention of embryos after ET. Efficacy in terms of increased pregnancy rate with this technique remain to be established.

The patient's position during ET has been postulated to be important.[347] However, the consensus is that the patient's position is not a factor in determining pregnancy rate.[342] Therefore, we routinely use the dorsal lithotomy position, which is the most comfortable for the patient. Before transfer, the cervix should be visualized with a bivalve speculum, which is moistened with medium. Extreme care should be taken not to use gels, lubricants, talcum powder, or other potentially embryotoxic substances during ET.

The precise location at which to inject the embryos within the uterine cavity has been a matter of debate. Some studies suggest that low uterine transfer may yield a higher pregnancy rate than high fundal transfer.[348] In addition, other authors have suggested that high fundal transfer may predispose patients to an increased rate of ectopic pregnancy.[349] It is recommended that the embryos be gently injected at least 1 cm proximal to the uterine fundus. After injection, the catheter should be carefully removed and passed to the embryologist for inspection of retained embryos. Although most authorities advocate immediate transfer of retained embryos, some recommend delaying the procedure until the following day.[350]

The overwhelming majority of ETs are performed via the transcervical route. However, in patients with distorted cervical anatomy in which the usual maneuvers are unsuccessful, alter-

native methods have been described. The Towako technique is a transvaginal, transmyometrial approach to ET. This procedure, performed with ultrasound guidance, had a reported clinical pregnancy rate of 31% during stimulated cycles among 104 patients who previously had not conceived with at least two cycles of IVF after difficult transfers.[351] Other authors have described a perurethral approach to ET.[352]

The duration of bed rest after ET does not affect conception rate. Complications of ET itself are rare, although there has been a case report of an agonadal patient experiencing severe PID and a tubo-ovarian abscess after ET without prior oocyte aspiration.[353]

A novel area of research has focused on the use of fibrin as biologic glue in an attempt to cause retention of embryos within the uterine cavity after ET.[354] Although one study showed that the addition of aprotinin-fibrin sealant resulted in a lower ectopic pregnancy rate than for a control group, there was no improvement in intrauterine pregnancy rate.[355]

THE LUTEAL PHASE

The assessment of luteal function in IVF programs has gone through two different periods. The first was from the beginning of the 1980s until 1987 in which clomiphene citrate, hMG only, and the combination of both was used for ovarian stimulation. During the period morphologic and hormonal characterization of the luteal phase was performed, and late luteal-phase deficiency was documented in a large proportion of patients. However, supplementation with either hCG or progesterone did not improve the results. The second period is from 1987 to the present, in which a GnRH agonist is introduced to ovulation induction combined with menotropins. In these regimens, luteal-phase deficiency is universal and supplementation mandatory.

The Luteal Phase in Clomiphene Citrate and hMG-only Cycles

We compared the pattern of luteal-phase progesterone and estradiol in patients who underwent hMG stimulation without follicular aspiration with that of women who underwent IVF with a similar ovulation induction regimen and progesterone supplementation. The length of the luteal phase did not differ between these two groups; it was 14.4 and 15.8 days, respectively. Similarly, the pattern of progesterone and estradiol did not differ between nonconceptual cycles of aspirated and nonaspirated cycles. In cycles resulting in a continuing IVF pregnancy, however, a sharp decline in both estradiol and progesterone serum levels occurred from day 8 to day 12 of the luteal phase, with a subsequent increase in these hormones with the establishment of pregnancy. This pattern was highlighted when successful IVF cycles were compared with findings for a failed IVF group in which the women were implanted with the same number of morphologically normal, cleaved embryos. The pattern of declining estradiol and progesterone levels in the latter half of IVF conceptual cycles is in sharp contrast to the hormonal pattern of conception cycles in similarly treated women not undergoing IVF. Among these women a continuous rise in both estradiol and progesterone levels was shown to take place from the midluteal phase onward.[356] Similar observations on a nadir of progesterone production in the late luteal phase also were demonstrated in CC-hMG cycles.[357,358]

The hormonal pattern demonstrating a luteal-phase deficiency is coupled with morphologic evidence of endometrial luteal-phase defects in 28% to 87% of IVF cycles (Table 42–4). Endometrial biopsies performed in the early luteal phase demonstrate luteal-phase deficiency in 28% to 76% of patients.[359-363] However, biopsies performed early, approximately at the time of ET, are infrequently inaccurate in revealing maximal endometrial maturation. We therefore evaluated the luteal phase by means of endometrial biopsy 11 to 13 days after hCG administration or initiation of an LH surge in 25 stimulated patients who did not undergo ET.[365] Nineteen patients (76%) had luteal-phase deficiency ranging from 3 to 7 days (see Table 42–4). It has been suggested that the inadequate endometrial maturation observed in stimulated IVF cycles is a consequence of the supraphysiologic levels of sex steroids, which cause modifications in endometrial receptor dynamics. However, analysis of the relation of estradiol level to endometrial histologic findings in our work demonstrated that 66% of patients with estradiol levels greater than 1000 pg/mL (3670 pmol/L) had an in-phase biopsy result, whereas 26% with out-of-phase biopsy results had an estradiol level greater than that on day 0. These findings were corroborated in a similar study of GnRH agonist cycles[366] and support the assertion that to achieve optimal results in ovulation induction cycles one should intentionally aim for high estradiol levels. Luteal-phase deficiency could also be caused by inadequate hCG production by the embryo. Serum estradiol, progesterone and β-hCG levels were measured

in viable pregnancies, clinical abortions, biochemical pregnancies, and nonconception cycles.[367] hCG level started to increase in a significant way earlier in viable pregnancies than in clinical abortions. This finding suggested that delayed hCG production may be a sign of embryopathy. We found that estradiol levels on day 11 to 12 after hCG administration, at the nadir of β-hCG levels, are predictive of IVF outcome. It was found that estradiol levels on these days were higher in conception cycles (294±20-pg/mL [1080±70 pmol/L]) than in failed ones (72±11 pg/mL, [260±40 pmol/L]) a statistically significant difference. An estradiol level greater than 100 pg/mL (370 pmol/L) on day 11 that increases on day 14 is an early sign of corpus luteum rescue by means of conception. These observations on the luteal phase and early conception strongly suggest that inappropriate follicular stimulation may result in an increased rate of embryos defective in their biosynthetic ability, impaired corpus luteum function, and abnormal endometrial development.

The Luteal Phase After Use of GnRH Agonists

Luteal-phase defects after GnRH agonist–hMG stimulation were first described by Smitz et al[368] in 1987. They demonstrated that 8 days after administration of hCG a dramatic drop in serum progesterone and estradiol occurred, leading to corpus luteum insufficiency. They later demonstrated that this drop could be attributed to a prolonged blockade of pituitary LH secretion after discontinuation of the GnRH agonist throughout the luteal phase. Multiple corpora lutea produced from massive ovarian stimulation by hMG are devoid of LH stimulation and undergo premature luteolysis.[369] In addition to this indirect effect of GnRH agonists, they also probably have a direct inhibitory action on the ovaries. Pellicer and Miro[370] demonstrated in vitro reduction in progesterone production by granulosa cells obtained from buserelin-hMG cycles compared with cells obtained from CC-hMG cycles. Direct action of agonists on the ovary is possible because GnRH binding sites on human granulosa cells have been demonstrated[371] and GnRH agonist was shown to inhibit progesterone secretion in cultured human granulosa cells.[372] The luteal-phase defect associated with the use of GnRH agonists is demonstrated not only by low luteal serum hormone levels but also by endometrial biopsy findings that show a delay in development in almost half of samples.[373]

Unlike CC-hMG or hMG-only cycles, in which supplementation of the luteal phase has not been proved to be necessary or to affect conception rate, in GnRH agonist–hMG cycles, supplementation is mandatory, as was demonstrated in several prospective, randomized studies.[374,375] Supplementation with either hCG, progesterone, or combined progesterone and estradiol has been suggested as a possible treatment. hCG is used as a surrogate for the deficient LH. hCG 2500 IU every 3 days

TABLE 42–4. LUTEAL-PHASE ENDOMETRIAL BIOPSY FINDINGS IN STIMULATED IVF CYCLES

Author	Day of Endometrial Biopsy	No. of Patients	Abnormal Dating (%)
Frydman et al[359]	17	25	28
Garcia et al[360]	14–16	22	73
Cohen et al[361]	16–18	19	63
Sterzik et al[362]	16	16	79
Forman et al[363]	16	12	75
Salat-Baroux et al[364]	21	32	35
Graf et al[365]	23–25	25	76

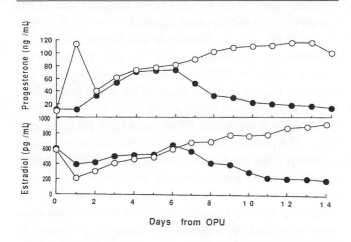

Figure 42–8. Comparison between progesterone and estradiol levels in hCG-supplemented (∘) and unsupplemented (•) GnRH-agonist–induced cycles. OPU, ovum pick-up. *(Adapted from Bellaisch-Allart J, et al: The effect of hCG supplementation after combined GnRH-a/hMG treatment in an IVF program. Hum Reprod 5:163,1990.)*

reestablished an in-phase endometrium for more than 90% of patients undergoing late luteal-phase biopsies[374] (Fig 42–8). In a large randomized study Belaisch-Allart et al[374] evaluated the effect of hCG supplementation and demonstrated that 1500 IU every 4 days, following the ovulatory dose of hCG, resulted in a doubling of conception rate from 9.3% to 18.7%. hCG treatment is associated with a greater risk for severe OHSS (4% to 15%) than the usual 1% observed with GnRH agonist cycles) and should therefore be withheld from patients with a high pre-ovulatory estradiol level (>2500 pg/mL [9180 pmol/L]) or when a large crop of oocytes is aspirated (more than 15 to 20 oocytes).[375] No clear benefit of hCG over progesterone supplementation was demonstrated. Progesterone may be administered orally, intramuscularly, or intravaginally and together with estrogen.

A French multicenter, double-blind, randomized study with 525 patients compared the effect of an oral preparation of dydrogesterone with that of placebo. The study did not show an increase in pregnancy rate with this supplementation in GnRH agonist–hMG cycles. When use of oral tablets of micronized progesterone was compared with use of hCG, a higher pregnancy rate was observed with the latter.[374] However, comparisons between hCG and natural progesterone injection demonstrated similar results and no statistically significant improvement with hCG.[376] It seems therefore that the administration of progesterone by the oral route is ineffective and that either intramuscular injection or intravaginal application is the most effective with the least side effects. Use of the vaginal route increases patient comfort compared with injection and is not associated with local intolerance such as pruritus or greasy

discharge. We use either 50-mg intramuscular injections of progesterone in oil daily or 600 mg (200 mg three times a day) of micronized progesterone tablets vaginally. With intramuscular injections, serum progesterone levels are expected to be about 25 ng/mL (80 nmol/L) and with vaginal application 15 ng/mL (48 nmol/L).

The exact role of estradiol in the luteal phase of mammals is undetermined. It is not clear if in addition to progesterone, estradiol also should be supplemented. Because of the observation of low estradiol levels in the late luteal phase of GnRH agonist–hMG cycles supplemented by progesterone only, Smitz et al[368] studied the potential benefit of adding estradiol valerate 6 mg a day starting on the 6th day after hCG administration. They found this protocol to have a luteolytic effect because estradiol and progesterone levels were lower between days 14 and 21 of the luteal phase in the estradiol valerate and progesterone supplement group compared with the progesterone-alone group with no improvement in pregnancy rate. Even when this dose of estradiol valerae was reduced to 2 mg a day, no change in IVF results was shown.[377] In a prospective, randomized study Devroey et al[378] compared use of vaginal micronized progesterone with use of vaginal progesterone plus estradiol and demonstrated that a similar ongoing pregnancy rate was achieved by the two groups. On the basis of these observations, it seems that the addition of an estrogen preparation in the luteal phase has no proved beneficial effect. Therefore we do not use estrogen in GnRH agonist protocols.

RESULTS AND OUTCOME

Since the first birth of an IVF child in 1987, assisted reproductive technology has undergone considerable development, particularly in the scope of ovulation induction and oocyte retrieval. According to the World Collaborative Reports,[379,380] there is a growing tendency to use GnRH agonists in stimulation regimens (52% in 1989; 71.5% in 1990). Most oocyte retrievals are performed with transvaginal ultrasound with increasing tendency (59% in 1986; 97.5% of all recoveries in 1990).[381] Nevertheless, although newer regimens have simplified the treatment cycle, a breakthrough in clinical outcome since the introduction of GnRH agonist treatment protocols has not been observed. Table 42–5 demonstrates the increasing numbers of retrievals, clinical pregnancies, and deliveries in the United States in the years 1985 through 1990.[52–55,382] Although the pregnancy rates obtained with the GIFT procedure (25% to 30% per retrieval) is higher than that resulting from IVF-ET (12% to 19%), there has been no substantial improvement within the last several years in each of the treatment modalities.

Confusion exists concerning success rates because of a lack of standard definitions. Some centers report pregnancies as

TABLE 42–5. IVF AND GIFT OUTCOME IN THE UNITED STATES (1985–1990)

Year	No. of Retrievals	No. of Clinical Pregnancies (%)[a]	No. of Livebirths (%)
IVF-ET			
1985	2892	337 (11.7)	257 (8.9)
1986	3365	485 (14.4)	311 (9.2)
1987	8725	1367 (15.7)	991 (11.4)
1988	13,647	2243 (16.4)	1657 (12.1)
1989	15,392	2811 (18.3)	2104 (13.7)
1990	16,405	3057 (18.6)	2345 (14.3)
GIFT			
1987	1968	492 (25.0)	362 (18.4)
1988	3080	846 (27.5)	654 (21.2)
1989	3652	1112 (29.6)	848 (23.2)
1990	3750	1093 (29.2)	842 (22.4)

[a]Percentages are per retrieval.

any positive pregnancy test. Others report only pregnancies that have an ultrasound diagnosis of viable fetus. Approximately 20% of pregnancies are chemical pregnancies, and this artificially inflates success rate.[40] For any statistical calculation, clinical pregnancy should be considered as one with appropriately rising β-hCG levels and the presence of a gestational sac in the uterine cavity documented with ultrasound. As indicated in Table 42–5, and further substantiated by the data presented in Table 42–6, the livebirth rate for IVF is considerably less than the clinical pregnancy rate; it is approximately 75% of all clinical pregnancies. The spontaneous abortion rate is 19% to 22%,[55,379,383] and although somewhat higher than for the fertile population, it is comparable to the rate among infertile women.[384] The woman's age seems to have a statistically significant effect on outcome of the cycle (Table 42–7). IVF attempts in women older than 40 years comprise 10% to 15% of treatment cycles[52,53,379]; the clinical pregnancy rate for this group is only 8% for IVF and 19% for GIFT cycles. The livebirth rate, however, is 4% and 9% for the same treatment modalities. This 50% decline in the rate of clinical pregnancies to deliveries stems from the increased abortion rate associated with advancing age (Table 42–7).

The French National IVF registry in an evaluation of data from 1986 to 1990 demonstrated that when the infertility diagnosis was considered, the highest pregnancy rate per recovery was observed for attempts involving donor semen (22.6%). The lowest rate was observed in cases of male-factor infertility (13.4%). Other diagnoses, including endometriosis, pure tubal-factor infertility, and unexplained infertility were associated with approximately the same rates (18.9%, 18.9%, and 18.5%, respectively).[381] However, when fertilization took place, the

pregnancy rate per ET for male-factor infertility was 23.7%, comparable with that for other diagnoses.

Each IVF cycle is independent, and the probability of implantation does not change from cycle to cycle. The French statistics from 1986 to 1990 demonstrated that the pregnancy rate per ovum pick-up increased from 18.3% in the first cycle to 67.7% for the sixth one (Table 42–8).

Ectopic gestation after ET occurs in 4% to 5% of pregnancies.[379,380] It probably occurs because of the inadvertent transfer of embryos into the fallopian tube at time of uterine embryo transfer, or it may result when an embryo "floats" into a damaged tube and implants. To prevent this complication, it is recommended that the cornual ends of the tubes be cauterized when laparoscopic evaluation detects damage too severe to attempt further repair. Heterotopic pregnancies are reported to occur at a rate of 1% of clinical IVF pregnancies, which is much higher than the 1:30,000 among the general population. Factors that may contribute to the complication are the transfer of multiple embryos, deep insertion of the transfer catheter, and the use of viscous medium for transfer.

Pregnancy rates increase when larger numbers of embryos are replaced (Table 42–9). However, this rate plateaus if more than three embryos are transferred, increasing the risk of a multiple-gestation pregnancy. Therefore, many IVF units are now transferring no more than three oocytes in GIFT, three zygotes in zygote intrafallopian transfer (ZIFT), and three embryos in IVF-ET. Nevertheless, the number of embryos to be transferred can be modified according to the grade of their morphologic quality and the patient's age.

Pregnancies that progress to viability are complicated only by the risk of multiple gestation. The multiple gestation rate seems to be comparable in the various reports (19% to 21% per ET for twins, 3% to 4.5% for triplets, and 0.2% to 0.4% for quadruplets) and stable during the last several years. The French National IVF registry reported that twin pregnancies were found in 23% to 24% of the delivered gestations during the years 1988 through 1990; multiple pregnancies (triplets and more) complicated 4.3% to 5.8% of deliveries for the same period of time.[381] In the World Collaborative Report from 1991, the rates of twin, triplet, and quadruplet gestations were 20.9%, 4.2%, and 0.4%.[379] These rates were comparable to those reported in the World Collaborative Report from 1989.[380] The multiple gestation rate for GIFT cycles was 26% to 27% and was comparable in its distribution to the rate for IVF-ET cycles.[55,380]

When multiple births are excluded, the risk for premature delivery (26 to 28 weeks) is 12.8%[379] and is not higher than that for the general population. The risk for prematurity among multiple pregnancies conceived in vitro is 49% for twins and 92% for triplets.[378] The cesarean section rate among IVF pregnancies

TABLE 42–6. CLINICAL PREGNANCY AND DELIVERY RATES OF SEVERAL REGISTRIES

Registry	1988			1989			1990			1991		
	No. of Ova Picked-up	No. of Pregnancies[a] (%)	No. of Deliveries[a] (%)	No. of Ova Picked-up	No. of Pregnancies (%)	No. of Deliveries[a] (%)	No. of Ova Picked-up	No. of Pregnancies (%)	No. of Deliveries (%)	No. of Ova Picked-up	No. of Pregnancies (%)	No. of Deliveries[a] (%)
FIVNAT (France)	13,336	2214 (16.6)	1587 (11.9)	17,591	3149 (17.9)	2270 (12.6)	17,818	3213 (18.7)	2337 (13.6)	26,951	4922 (18.3)	3634 (13.5)
Australia	7930	1063 (13.4)	745 (9.4)	7228	1003 (13.9)	652 (9.0)				6558	727 (11.0)	517 (7.8)
USA	13,647	2115 (15.5)	1638 (12.0)	15,392	2811 (18.3)	2104 (13.7)	16,405	3057 (18.6)	2345 (14.3)	21,083	4017 (19.1)	3215 (15.2)
UK	8514	1354 (15.9)	775 (9.1)							10,774	2186 (20.3)	1604 (14.9)
Total	43,427	6746 (15.5)	4745 (10.9)	40,211	6963 (17.3)	5026 (12.5)	33,586	6270 (18.7)	4682 (13.9)	65,396	11,852 (18.1)	8970 (13.7)
World Collaborative Report	81,691				13,362 (16.4)	8784 (10.8)				82,299	14,908 (18.1)	11,094 (13.5)

[a] Absolute number of pregnancies or deliveries; percentage is expressed per ovum pick-up.

TABLE 42–7. OUTCOME OF IVF AND GIFT BY AGE (US REGISTRY 1989–1990)

Age (y)	No. of ET Cycles	No. of Clinical Pregnancies (%)[a]	Abortion Rate (%)[b]	No. of Deliveries (%)[a]
IVF-ET				
30–34	2718	610 (22.4)	19	485 (17.8)
35–39	2693	474 (17.6)	24	352 (13.1)
≥40	947	72 (7.6)	35	39 (4.1)
GIFT				
30–34	1315	458 (4.8)	15	297 (22.7)
35–39	1043	293 (28.1)	20	223 (21.4)
≥40	348	67 (19.2)	42	32 (9.2)

[a]Percentage is expressed per ET.
[b]Rate of abortions is expressed as percentage of clinical pregnancies.

was 45% to 55%, but bias on the part of obstetricians in performing early cesarean delivery probably accounts for this figure.[384,385] The perinatal mortality rate (stillbirths and deaths in the first 7 days of life was 45 per 1000 births in Australia, 27 per 1000 in Great Britain, and 22 per 1000 in Israel. The perinatal mortality rate in the general population is 10 to 15 per 1000 births. Multiple pregnancy rate and the higher mean maternal age for patients undergoing IVF-ET cycles appear to be important factors contributing to this high rate of perinatal mortality.

Serious congenital malformations were found among 2.1% of the total births in both the U.S. registry and the World Collaborative Report from 1991. In the Israel National Registry (1982 through 1989) the malformation rate was 2.5%, comparable to the 2.2% reported in the Australian collaborative series (1979 through 1989).[383] In all instances the malformation rate does not differ substantially from the general population of newborns. Similarly, although several cases of chromosomal anomalies have been reported, patients undergoing IVF do not seem to be at increased risk.[380]

TABLE 42–8. PREGNANCY RATES ACCORDING TO CYCLE RANK

Rank	No. of Cycles	Clinical Pregnancies		
		No.	Percentage per Recovery	Cummulative Percentage
1	25,666	4689	18.3	18.3
2	15,021	2563	17.1	32.3
3	8576	1523	17.8	44.3
4	4846	816	16.8	53.6
5	2774	458	16.5	61.2
6	1514	252	16.6	67.7
7	847	126	14.9	72.5
8	456	75	16.4	77.6
≥9	618	95	15.4	80.6

(Compiled from the French National IVF Registry.)[381]

The pregnancy rate after replacement of frozen-thawed embryos was reported to be 10% to 12%.[54,55,386] Among 382 clinical pregnancies from 3290 replacements of frozen-thawed embryos, 8% were ectopic and 23% ended in spontaneous abortion to give a livebirth rate of 9%.[54] As for IVF babies, there is no increased risk for serious malformations among newborns resulting from frozen-thawed embryos compared with the risk among general population of newborns.

MICROMANIPULATION OF GAMETES

It has become clear that although IVF is capable of providing successful solutions for certain conditions, at the same time limitations in solving other infertility problems remain. Male-factor infertility in particular has been one of the fields in which only a small fraction of men with oligozoospermia have benefited from IVF while most are not helped with the technique.[387]

The three main forms of sperm characteristics associated with male-factor infertility are oligozoospermia, teratozoospermia, and asthenozoospermia. A combination of all three disorders is usually present. Union of the gametes either in vivo or in vitro requires successful penetration of the layers surrounding the oocyte. In oligozoospermia, the statistical likelihood that a sufficient number of sperm cells capable of traversing the cumulus oophorus and zona pellucida is reduced. Even though some normal sperm are released, the man is functionally infertile. For these patients, IVF offers the possibility of introducing a sufficient number of sperm cells into the vicinity of the oocyte. In spite of these improved conditions, low fertilization rates and low pregnancy rates have been reported for male-factor infertility. This failure has been shown to be directly related to abnormalities of sperm cell morphology and motility.[387]

In recent years the technology of micromanipulation of gametes has improved. It is now possible to circumvent the oocyte barriers to sperm penetration and greatly reduce the number of sperm cells needed to achieve fertilization.

Three micromanipulative strategies have been suggested to improve the fertilization ability of spermatozoa: zona-opening procedures, subzonal insertion of sperm cells, and sperm microinjection into the ooplasm (Fig 42–9). Of these three techniques, the last is the most successful and is, therefore, currently the recommended approach to male-factor infertility.

Zona-Opening Procedures

The first attempts at zona opening were based on animal data that indicated that the zona pellucida poses a substantial barrier to sperm penetration. Zona-intact mouse eggs require exposure to many thousands of sperm to assure fertilization, but eggs denuded of their zonae can be fertilized by as few as three sperm. The frequency with which zona-free eggs implant, however, is

TABLE 42–9. PREGNANCY RATES ACCORDING TO THE NUMBER OF EMBRYOS TRANSFERRED*

No. of Embryos	1987 (10,470)		1988 (11,339)		1989 (13,332)	
	(%) ET	(%) Pregnancy Rate	(%) ET	(%) Pregnancy Rate	(%) ET	(%) Pregnancy Rate
1	22.5	9.6	19.6	9.8	18.0	9.1
2	22.1	18.1	18.4	16.5	17.9	18.1
3	28.2	26.4	23.5	26.7	26.2	27.5
4	20.8	31.8	30.8	29.8	28.7	29.5
≥5	6.4	39.6	7.7	32.1	9.2	32.9

(Compiled from the French National IVF Registry.)[381]

drastically reduced.[388] This finding demonstrates that zona removal is not an acceptable approach to enhancing egg penetration. While investigating these issues in a mouse model, Gordon and Talansky[389] developed a new procedure they called *zona pellucida drilling*. This technique involves placement of cumulus-free eggs in a micromanipulation device and the use of a fine stream of acid Tyrode's solution (pH 2.3) to dissolve a small hole in the zona. The result is controlled formation of a gap in the zona with minimal oocyte damage. When zona-drilled mouse oocytes were subjected to IVF with normal sperm concentrations, the fertilization rate increased threefold over the rate for zona-intact controls, and the rate of polyspermy was only 2.1% (1% in normal IVF). Reduction of sperm concentration to 10^2 to 10^3 cells/mL demonstrated that zona drilling increased the efficacy of fertilization by a factor of about 100.[389]

The studies with mice justified efforts to use zona drilling in the clinical setting. The first such clinical trial involved 10 couples who had previously suffered total failure of fertilization in at least one previous IVF cycle. Drilling of 47 oocytes resulted in damage to 16 (34%), and 10 (32%) of the surviving 31 oocytes were fertilized. The rate of polyspermy for the drilled eggs was high (50%). Three embryo transfers of cleaved oocytes were performed, but no pregnancies were achieved.[390] This trial demonstrated the sensitivity of human oocytes to acid Tyrode's solution and suggested that unlike in mice, the human block to polyspermy is at the level of the zona pellucida rather than the oolemma. Malter and Cohen[391] overcame some of the problems of the zona drilling procedure by using a modified mechanical dissection technique called *partial zonal dissection* (PZD). This technique entails making a slit in the zona pellucida with a microneedle to expose the membrane of the oocyte plasma to direct contact with spermatozoa. Using this procedure for male-factor infertility, Malter and Cohen[391] reported an increased fertilization rate of 79% as compared to 53% among nontreated controls. This process led to the establishment of the first three pregnancies following PZD. These investigators noted that although polyspermy occurred relatively frequently after PZD (12% to 26% of treated oocytes), it was not as pronounced as had been reported after other methods of drilling. The same group later reported on a larger study,[392] which supported the use of methylprednisolone during the first 4 days after retrieval. Similar results were reported by others,[393] although the success rate of fertilization and normal cleavage depend on sperm morphology and on the total motile sperm cell number in the ejaculate.[394,395] Unfavorable results were obtained when the sperm used for insemination contained less than 6% spermatozoa with normal morphology or if total motile sperm cell concentration was less than 5 million/mL.

The most important limitation of mechanical PZD is inability to produce standardized and uniform holes. The average slit after PZD is rectangular, 10 to 20 mm long and 2 to 5 mm wide (Fig 42–10). An optimal opening must be large enough to allow interaction between sperm cells and oolemma and small enough not to increase the likelihood of polyspermic fertiliza-

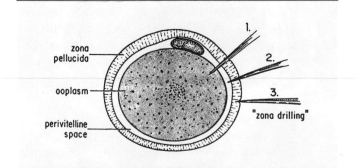

Figure 42–9. Schematic representation of the three main methods used in micromanipulative enhancement of fertilization, sperm injection into the ooplasm; 2, subzonal insertion of sperm cells; 3, zona-opening procedures.

The first decade of IVF has primarily involved standardization of the routine procedure. The second decade should be considered the one in which a breakthrough in the treatment of male-factor infertility has evolved. The development of gamete micromanipulation techniques and especially ICSI not only offers new hope to many couples with male-factor infertility but also opens an exciting new field to enable a better understanding of the fertilization process.

Assisted Hatching

One of the prerequisite processes that occurs before implantation is hatching of the blastocyst from its shell, the zona pellucida. The hatching process involves both mechanical and chemical reactions, which eventually lead to zona pellucida thinning followed by rupture and blastocyst hatching.[425] It was suggested that failure of embryos to hatch and implant contributes to the inefficiency of clinical IVF, resulting in a limited pregnancy rate. Both laboratory and clinical findings support this hypothesis. It has been observed that embryos with a good prognosis for implantation have a reduced zonal thickness, presumably in preparation for hatching. In addition, microsurgically fertilized embryos with artificial gaps in the zona appear to have higher implantation rates.[426] These promising results observed in embryos generated from oocytes that underwent microsurgically assisted fertilization encourage the use of the assisted hatching technique. This procedure entails the introduction of holes in the zona pellucida of intact embryos before their transfer to the uterine cavity to assist hatching and eventually to increase implantation rate. These gaps in the zona pellucida can be made either mechanically,[427] chemically by dissolving the zona pellucida with acid Tyrode's solution,[426] or by laser drilling.[400] In a prospective, randomized trial, Cohen et al[426] demonstrated that assisted hatching with chemical zonal drilling is most effective in embryos with thick zonae (≥15 μm). The rate of embryonic implantation among a group that underwent selective zonal drilling was 25%, significantly higher than the rate among the nontreated control group (18%). In addition, it has been shown that selective assisted hatching appeared most effective for women older than 38 years (implantation rate of 15% compared with 5% among controls) and for those with elevated basal FSH levels (>15 IU/mL) (implantation rate of 26% as compared to 10% in controls). These results suggest that there may be an association between age, FSH level, and the physical or chemical properties of the zona pellucida that interferes with the physiologic hatching process. Therefore, although assisted hatching may be used successfully, its clinical applications should be considered on a patient-to-patient basis taking into account the patient's age, basal FSH level, and the thickness of the zona pellucida of the embryo.

PREIMPLANTATION GENETIC DIAGNOSIS

Preimplantation genetic diagnosis may be used by couples at high risk for transmitting a genetic defect who would like to assure the birth of a healthy child. It involves removal and analysis of single cells, obtained at biopsy of in vitro fertilized embryos. Such an early-stage diagnosis allows selective transfer of unaffected embryos to the uterus, avoiding the need for therapeutic abortion.

Embryo Biopsy

The biopsy may be performed at various stages of development before implantation, including first polar bodies,[428] blastomeres,[429] or trophectoderm cells[430] (Fig 42–12). By means of analysis of the first polar body it is possible to determine the genotype of the oocyte and avoid the fertilization of genetically abnormal germ cells. The polar body can be removed with minimal adverse effect on fertilization and embryo development. However, it does not allow analysis of paternal alleles and is uninformative when crossing over occurs (most frequent in telomeric genes).

Blastomere biopsy at the early cleavage stage is the method used at most centers that perform preimplantation genetic diagnosis. It involves zona pellucida opening followed by cell sampling. Various protocols for isolation of individual blastomeres in mouse and human embryos have been evaluated. It has been concluded that the eight-cell stage (day 3 after insemination) is the most suitable stage for diagnosis and that up to two blastomeres may be removed without affecting further development.[431,432] The zona pellucida may be opened with either mechanical force, or it may be dissolved with acid Tyrode's solution. Once the zona is opened, the embryonic cells are either aspirated by means of gentle suction, displaced by gentle flow of medium, or removed by means of squeezing the zona at some distance from the hole.[433]

Sampling of trophectoderm cells at the blastocyst stage provides additional cells for diagnosis (10 to 30 cells) and may be ethically more acceptable, because the material is extraembryonic. However, currently the technique cannot be used because only a small proportion of embryos reach the blastocyst stage in vitro and only a small number of these successfully implant in the uterus.

Genetic Analysis

The limited material for analysis and the narrow window for diagnosis places stringent demands on the sensitivity, reliability, and speed of the genetic assay to be used for preimplantation genetic diagnosis. Polymerase chain reaction (PCR) and FISH are highly sophisticated molecular techniques for this purpose.

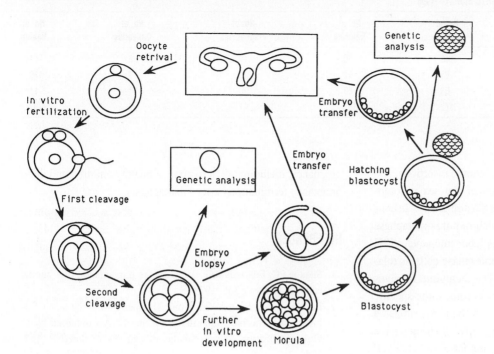

Figure 42–12. Schematic representation of the various options for preimplantation genetic diagnosis.

Polymerase Chain Reaction

The PCR is an in vitro method for the enzymatic synthesis of specific DNA sequences. Two oligonucleotide primers are used that hybridize to opposite strands and flank the region of interest in the target DNA. A repetitive series of cycles involving template denaturation, primer annealing, and extension of the annealed primer by Taq DNA polymerase results in the accumulation of a specific fragment the termini of which are defined by the 5′ ends of the primers. Because the primer extension products synthesized in one cycle can serve as a template in the next, the number of target DNA copies doubles at every cycle, accumulating exponentially.

The PCR is a highly specific and relatively rapid method. It is almost an ideal tool for detection of mutations in single blastomeres obtained at biopsy by use of allele specific fragments, restriction fragment analysis, heteroduplex formation, and other molecular techniques. There have been a number of reports demonstrating amplification of DNA fragments from unfertilized oocytes and single blastomeres, enabling preimplantation diagnosis of a variety of genetic disorders, such as Duchenne muscular dystrophy, sickle cell anemia, hemophilia A, Lesch-Nyhan syndrome, cystic fibrosis, and ornithine transcarbamylase.[434-439]

We have developed a PCR-based method that allows determination of the RhD blood type of early-cleavage-stage embryos.[440] This genetic assay may be used when alloimmunization is a risk factor and the father is an RhD-positive het-

erozygote. In such cases, preimplantation RhD typing allows the selective transfer of only RhD-negative embryos, avoiding complications due to mother-fetus RhD-incompatibility (Fig 42–13).

Fluorescence in Situ Hybridization

The FISH technique can be used for the detection of chromosomal abnormalities, such as change in number and structure, in-

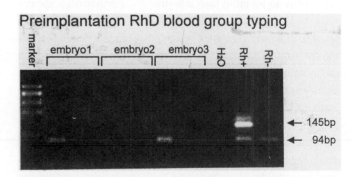

Figure 42–13. RhD typing of early cleavage stage embryos by means of single blastomere analysis. Amplified products obtained from blastomeres obtained at biopsy and their media blanks. According to the band pattern obtained, the single cells were typed as RhD-positive if they had two bands of 94bp (internal control) and 145bp (RhD-specific sequence) or as RhD-negative, if they had only one band of 94bp (embryos 1 and 3). Absence of any band was considered a failure in amplification (embryo 2). Genomic DNA of RhD-positive and RhD-negative subjects as well as ddH$_2$O were used as positive and negative controls, respectively.

TABLE 42–10. PREIMPLANTATION DIAGNOSIS BY EMBRYO BIOPSY—1995

Diagnosis	No. of Patients	No. of Cycles	No. of Transfers	No. of Pregnancies	No. of Deliveries	No. of Babies
X-linked (PCR)	35	46	40	10	8	11
X-linked (FISH)	44	63	52	11	7	10
Single gene defects	58	63	60	20	11	11
Total	137	172	152	41	26	32

cluding aneuploidy, polyploidy, large deletions, insertions, and translocations, and for the identification of the sex chromosomes for gender determination in single blastomeres.[441] In contrast to standard karyotype analysis, which requires metaphase chromosomes, is time consuming, and is labor intensive, FISH may be applied on either metaphase or interphase cells, is relatively rapid, and is simple to perform. The technique involves hybridization of fluorescent labeled chromosome-specific probes to the nuclear DNA. When such a probe is hybridized a bright colored dot is generated by each copy of chromosome present in the nucleus. By counting the number of dots per cell one can detect changes in chromosome number or stucture. The FISH technique allows one to focus on specific chromosomes but is unsuitable for karyotype analysis. The FISH procedure includes four basic steps: (1) probe labeling, (2) preparation of the single cell sample (fixation and permeabilization), (3) hybridization of the probe to the sample, (4) detection of the tagged chromosome by means of fluorescence microscopy. Each of these steps must be optimized for successful analysis. Failure to do so results in a decreased signal-to-noise ratio, leading to loss of sensitivity and misdiagnosis.

The introduction of directly labeled probes and improved methods for nuclear spreading have increased hybridization efficiencies in single cells and have reduced the time of the genetic assay to no more than 6 hours.[442,443] Furthermore, the development of additional fluorochromes, use of combinatorial fluorescence, and computer imaging has made it possible to visualize simultaneously different chromosomes. Labeling each probe with a different fluorochrome makes it possible, for example, to detect chromosomes X, Y, 21, 18, and 13, which account for most chromosomal abnormalities in prenatal clinics, in a single hybridization experiment.[444,445]

Multicolor FISH not only may be used for selective screening of affected embryos among high-risk couples but also may be considered a diagnostic tool for patients undergoing infertility treatment, especially when abnormal embryo development occurs.[446,447] By the beginning of 1995, 172 preimplantation genetic diagnostic procedures had been performed by means of embryo biopsy in 13 centers around the world (Table 42–10); 152 resulted in ET. Of these 41 resulted in clinical pregnancy, including 32 deliveries of healthy children and three pregnancy terminations after misdiagnosis.

REFERENCES

1. Steptoe PC, Edwards RG: Birth after re-implantation of a human embryo. *Lancet* 2:366, 1978
2. Lopata A, Johnston JWH, Hoult IJ, Speirs AI: Pregnancy following intrauterine implantation of an embryo obtained by in vitro fertilization of a preovulatory egg. *Fertil Steril* 33:117, 1980
3. Heape W: Preliminary note on the transplantation and growth of mammalian ova within a uterine foster-mother. *Proc R Soc* 48:457, 1891
4. Hammond J: Culture of mouse embryos using an egg-saline medium. *Nature* 163:28, 1949
5. Whitten WK: Culture of tubal mouse ova. *Nature* 177:96, 1956
6. Austin CR: Observations of the penetration of the sperm into the mammalian egg. *Aust J Sci Res* 134:581, 1951
7. Chang MC: Fertilization capacity of spermatozoa deposited in the fallopian tubes. *Nature* 168:697, 1951
8. Chang MC: Fertilization of rabbit ova in vitro. *Nature* 184:406, 1959
9. Soules MR: Infertility surgery. In: DeCherney AH (ed), *Reproductive Failure*. New York, Churchill Livingstone, 1986:58
10. Bateman BG, Nunley WC, Kitchen JK: Surgical management of distal tubal obstruction: Are we making progress? *Fertil Steril* 48:523, 1987
11. Trimbos-Kemper TCM, Trimbos JB, Van Hall EV: Conscientious evaluation of tubal surgery results. In: DeCherney AH (ed), *Reproductive Surgery*. Chicago, Year Book, 1987:112
12. Thie JL, Williams TJ, Coulam CB: Repeat tuboplasty compared with primary microsurgery for postinflammatory tubal disease. *Fertil Steril* 45:784, 1986
13. Webster BW, Wentz AC, Maxson WS: Endometriosis. In: DeCherney AH (ed), *Reproductive Surgery*. Chicago, Year Book, 1987:89
14. Seibel MM, Berger MJ, Weinstein FG, et al: The effectiveness of danazol on subsequent fertility in minimal endometriosis. *Fertil Steril* 38:534, 1982
15. Olive DL, Haney AE: Endometriosis. In: DeCherney AH (ed), *Reproductive Failure*. New York, Churchill Livingstone, 1986:141

16. Rousseau S, Lord J, Lepage Y, Campenhout JV: The expectancy of pregnancy for "normal" infertile couples. *Fertil Steril* 40:768, 1983

17. Haney AF, Hughes CL, Whitesides DB, Dodson WC: Treatment independent, treatment associated pregnancies after additional therapy in a program of in vitro fertilization and embryo transfer. *Fertil Steril* 47:634, 1987

18. Dodson WC, Whitesides DB, Hughes CL, Easley HA, Haney AF: Superovulation with intrauterine insemination in the treatment of infertility: A possible alternative to gamete intrafallopian transfer and in vitro fertilization. *Fertil Steril* 48:441, 1987

19. Simon A, Laufer N: Unexplained infertility: A reappraisal. *Assist Reprod Rev* 3:26, 1993

20. Simon A, Avidan B, Mordel N, et al: The value of menotrophins treatment for unexplained infertility prior to an in-vitro fertilization attempt. *Hum Reprod* 6:222, 1991

21. Ezra Y, Simon A, Laufer N: Defective oocytes: A new subgroup of unexplained infertility. *Fertil Steril* 58:24, 1992

22. Benshushan A, Ezra Y, Simon A, Gordon JW, Laufer N: Subzonal insertion, a possible treatment for "defective oocytes." *J Assist Reprod Genet* 10:98, 1993

23. Mahadevan MM, Trounson AO: The influence of seminal characteristics on the success rate of human in vitro fertilization. *Fertil Steril* 42:400, 1984

24. Yanagimachi R, Yanagimachi H, Rogers BJ: The use of zona-free animal ova as a test system for the assessment of the fertilizing capacity of human spermatozoa. *Biol Reprod* 15:471, 1976

25. Rogers BJ: The usefulness of the sperm penetration assay in predicting IVF success. *J In Vitro Fert Embryo Transf* 3:209, 1986

26. Burkman LJ, Coddington CC, Franken DR, et al: The hemizona assay (HZA): Development of a diagnostic test for the binding of human spermatozoa to the human hemizona pellucida to predict fertilization potential. *Fertil Steril* 49:688, 1988

27. Liu DY, Lopata A, Johnston WIH, et al: A human sperm–zona pellucida binding test using oocytes that failed to fertilize in vitro. *Fertil Steril* 50:782, 1988

28. Oehninger S, Coddington CC, Scott R, et al: Hemizona assay: Assessment of sperm dysfunction and prediction of in vitro fertilization outcome. *Fertil Steril* 51:665, 1989

29. Aybaliotis B, Bronson R, Rosenfeld D, Cooper G: Conception rates in couples where autoimmunity to sperm is detected. *Fertil Steril* 43:739, 1985

30. Bronson R, Cooper G, Rosenfeld D: Sperm antibodies: Their role in infertility. *Fertil Steril* 42:171, 1984

31. Clarke GN, Lopata A, Johnston WIH: Effect of sperm antibodies in females on human in vitro fertilization. *Fertil Steril* 46:435, 1986

32. Mandelbaum SL, Diamond MP, DeCherney AH: Relationship of antisperm antibodies to oocyte fertilization in in vitro fertilization–embryo transfer. *Fertil Steril* 47:644, 1987

33. Bronson RA, Cooper GW, Rosenfeld DL: Sperm-specific isoantibodies and autoantibodies inhibit the binding of human sperm to the human zona pellucida. *Fertil Steril* 38:724, 1982

34. Trounson AO, Leeton JF, Wood C, Webb J, Wood J: Pregnancies in humans by fertilization in vitro and embryo transfer in the controlled ovulatory cycle. *Science* 212:681, 1981

35. Wood C, Trounson AO, Leeton JF, et al: Clinical features of eight pregnancies resulting from in vitro fertilization and embryo transfer. *Fertil Steril* 38:22, 1982

36. Seibel MM, Kearnan M, Kiessling A: Parameters that predict success for natural cycle in vitro fertilization. *Fertil Steril* 63:1251, 1995

37. Kerin JF, Warner GM, Quinn PJ, et al: Incidence of multiple pregnancy after in vitro fertilization and embryo transfer. *Lancet* 2:537, 1983

38. Lopata A: Concepts in human in vitro fertilization and embryo transfer. *Fertil Steril* 40:289, 1983

39. Edwards RG: In vitro fertilization and embryo replacement: Opening lecture. *Ann N Y Acad Sci* 442:1, 1985

40. In vitro fertilization pregnancies, Australia and New Zealand 1979–1984. Sydney, National Perinatal Statistics Unit, 1985

41. Marrs RP, Vargyas JM, Saito H, et al: Clinical applications of techniques used in human in vitro fertilization research. *Am J Obstet Gynecol* 146:477, 1983

42. Kerin J, Quinn P, Herriot D, Wilson L, Stone B: Effects of follicle induction on ovary and endometrium. In: DeCherney AH (ed), *The Control of Follicle Development, Ovulation and Luteal Function: Lessons from In Vitro Fertilization.* New York, Raven, 1987:112

43. Mahadevan MM, Fleetman J, Taylor PJ, Leader A, Pattinson AH: The effect of the day of initiation of ovarian stimulation on the day of luteinizing hormone surge and the outcome of in vitro fertilization. *Fertil Steril* 47:976, 1987

44. Lamb EJ, Colliflower WW, Williams JW: Endometrial histology and conception rate after clomiphene citrate. *Obstet Gynecol* 39:389, 1972

45. Kokko E, Janne O, Kauppil A, Vihko R: Cyclic clomiphene citrate treatment lowers cytosol estrogen and progestin receptor concentrations in the endometrium of postmenopausal women on estrogen replacement therapy. *J Clin Endocrinol Metab* 52:345, 1981

46. Birkenfeld A, Weber-Benndorf M, Mootz V, Beier HM: Effects of clomiphene on the functional morphology of oviductal and uterine mucosa. *Ann N Y Acad Sci* 442:153, 1985

47. Birkenfeld A, Navot D, Levij IS, et al: Advanced secretory changes in the proliferative human endometrial epithelium following clomiphene citrate treatment. *Fertil Steril* 45:462, 1986

48. Laufer N, Pratt B, DeCherney AH, Naftolin F, Merino M, Markert CL: The in vivo and in vitro effects of clomiphene citrate on ovulation, fertilization, and development of cultured mouse oocytes. *Am J Obstet Gynecol* 147:633, 1983

49. Laufer N, Barr I, Lewin A, et al: Clomiphene inhibits progesterone secretion of human granulosa luteal cells in long term culture. Proceedings of the 4th World Congress on IVF, Oct, 1985, Melbourne, Australia

50. Olsson JH, Nilsson L, Hillensjo T: Effect of clomiphene isomers on progestin synthesis in cultured human granulosa cells. *Hum Reprod* 2:463, 1987

51. Seibel MM: The effect of clomiphene citrate on human preovula-

tient in vitro fertilization using transvaginal oocyte retrieval and local anesthesia. *N Engl J Med* 312:1639, 1985

172. Booker M, Parsons J: The perurethral technique for ultrasound directed follicle aspiration in an in vitro fertilization and embryo transfer programme: A report of 636 patient cycles. *Br J Obstet Gynecol* 97:499, 1990

173. Parsons J, Pampiglione JS, Sadler AP, Booker MW, Campbell S: Ultrasound directed follicle aspiration for oocyte collection using the perurethral technique. *Fertil Steril* 53:97, 1990

174. Lewin A, Laufer N, Rabinowitz R, Margalioth EJ, Bar I, Schenker JG: Ultrasonically guided oocyte collection under a local anesthesia: The first choice method for in vitro fertilization—A comparative study with laparoscopy. *Fertil Steril* 46:257, 1986

175. Dellenbach P, Nisand I, Moreau L, et al: Transvaginal sonographically controlled ovarian follicle puncture for egg retrieval. *Lancet* 1:1467, 1984

176. Hammarberg K, Enk L, Nilsson L, Wikland M: Oocyte retrieval under the guidance of a vaginal transducer: Evaluation of patient acceptance. *Hum Reprod* 2:487, 1987

177. Gohar J, Lunenfeld E, Potashnik G, Glezerman M: The use of sedation only during oocyte retrieval for in vitro fertilization: Patients' pain self-assessments versus doctor's evaluations. *J Assist Reprod Genet* 10:476, 1993

178. Lavy G, Restrepo-Candelo H, Diamond M, Shapiro B, Grunfeld L, DeCherney AH: Laparoscopic and transvaginal ova recovery: The effect on ova quality. *Fertil Steril* 49:1002, 1988

179. Jamieson ME, Fleming RF, Kader S, Ross KS, Yates RW, Coutts JR: In vivo and in vitro maturation of human oocytes: Effects on embryo development and polyspermic fertilization. *Fertil Steril* 56:93, 1991

180. Corson SL, Batzer FR, Gocial B, et al: Is paracervical block anesthesia for oocyte retrieval effective? *Fertil Steril* 62:133, 1994

181. Godoy H, Erard P, DeMunck L, et al: Comparison of two local anesthetics in transvaginal ultrasound-guided oocyte retrieval. *Hum Reprod* 8:1093, 1993

182. Coetsier T, Dhont M, De Sutter P, Merchiers E, Versichelen L, Rosseel MT: Propofol anaesthesia for ultrasound guided oocyte retrieval: Accumulation of the anaesthetic agent in follicular fluid. *Hum Reprod* 7:1422, 1992

183. Boyers SP, Lavy G, Russell JB, DeCherney AH: A paired analysis of in vitro fertilization and cleavage rates of first- versus last-recovered preovulatory human oocytes exposed to varying intervals of 100% CO_2 pneumoperitoneum and general anesthesia. *Fertil Steril* 48:969, 1987

184. Schoeffler PF, Levron JC, Jany L, Brenas FJ, Pouly JL: Follicular concentration of fentanyl during laparoscopy for oocyte retrieval: Correlation with in vitro fertilisation results. *Anesthesiology* 69:A663, 1988

185. Bailey-Pridham DD, Reshef E, Drury K, Cook CL, Hurst HE, Yussman MA: Follicular fluid lidocaine levels during transvaginal oocyte retrieval. *Fertil Steril* 53:171, 1990

186. Chetkowski RJ, Nass TE: Isofluorane inhibits early mouse embryo development in vitro. *Fertil Steril* 49:171, 1988

187. Kingsland CR, Taylor CT, Aziz N, Bickerton N: Is follicular flushing necessary for oocyte retrieval? A randomized trial. *Hum Reprod* 6:382, 1991

188. Ben-Shlomo I, Schiff E, Levran D, Ben-Raphael Z, Mashiach S, Dor J: Failure of oocyte retrieval during in vitro fertilization: A sporadic event rather than a syndrome. *Fertil Steril* 55:324, 1991

189. Howe RS, Wheeler C, Mastroianni L, Blasco L, Tureck R: Pelvic infection after transvaginal ultrasound-guided ovum retrieval. *Fertil Steril* 49:726, 1988

190. Curtis P, Amson M, Keith E, Bernard A, Shaw RW: Evaluation of the risk of pelvic infection following transvaginal oocyte recovery. *Hum Reprod* 6:1294, 1991

191. Evers JL, Larsen JF, Gnany GG, Siec UV: Complications and problems in transvaginal sector scan-guided follicle aspiration. *Fertil Steril* 49:278, 1988

192. Dicker D, Ashkenazi J, Feldberg D, Levy T, Dekel A, Ben-Raphael Z: Severe abdominal complications after transvaginal ultrasonographically guided retrieval of oocytes for in vitro fertilization and embryo transfer. *Fertil Steril* 59:1313, 1993

193. Bergh C, Lundkvist O: Clinical complications during in vitro fertilization treatment. *Hum Reprod* 7:625, 1992

194. Schenker JG, Ezra Y: Complications of assisted reproductive technologies. *Fert Steril* 61:411, 1994

195. Meldrum DR: Antibiotics for vaginal oocyte aspiration. *J In Vitro Fert Embryo Transf* 6:1, 1989

196. Tureck RW, Garcia CR, Blasco L, Mastroianni L: Perioperative complications arising after transvaginal oocyte retrieval. *Obstet Gynecol* 81:590, 1993

197. Scoccia B, Marcovici I: Uterine abscess after ultrasound-guided ovum retrieval in an in vitro fertilization-embryo transfer program: Case report and review of the literature. *J Assist Reprod Genet* 9:285, 1992

198. Van Hoorde GJ, Verhoeff A, Zeilmaker GH: Perforated appendicitis following transvaginal oocyte retrieval for in-vitro fertilization and embryo transfer. *Hum Reprod* 7:850, 1992

199. Neuwinger J, Todorow S, Wildt L: Ureteral obstruction: a complication of oocyte retrieval. *Fertil Steril* 61:787, 1994

200. Steptoe PC, Edwards RG, Purdy JM: Clinical aspects of pregnancies established with cleaving embryos grown in vitro. *Br J Obstet Gynaecol* 87:757, 1980

201. Borland RM, Biggers JD, Lechene CP, Taymor ML: Elemental composition of fluid in the human fallopian tube. *J Reprod Fertil* 58:479, 1980

202. Menezo YJ, Khatchadourian CJ: The laboratory culture media. *Assist Reprod Rev* 1:136, 1991

203. Loutradis D, John D, Kiessling AA: Hypoxanthine causes a 2-cell block in random-bred mouse embryos. *Biol Reprod* 37:311, 1987

204. Warikoo PK, Bavister BD: Hypoxanthine and cyclic adenosine 5′ monophosphate maintain meiotic arrest of rhesus monkey oocytes in vitro. *Fertil Steril* 51:886, 1989

205. Quinn P, Kerin JF, Warnes GM: Improved pregnancy rate in human in vitro fertilization with the use of a medium based on the composition of human tubal fluid. *Fertil Steril* 44:493, 1985

206. Muggleton-Harris AL, Findlay I, Whittingham DG: Improvement of the culture conditions for the development of human preimplantation embryos. *Hum Reprod* 5:217, 1990

207. Brinster RL: Studies on the mouse embryo development in vitro I, II, III. *J Exp Zool* 49:158, 1965

208. Whitten WK: Culture of tubal ova. *Nature* 179:1081, 1957

209. Flynn TH, Hillman N: Lipid synthesis from U-14 C glucose in preimplantation mouse embryos in culture. *Biol Reprod* 10:315, 1978

210. Pratt HPM: Phospholipid synthesis in the preimplantation mouse embryo. *J Reprod Fertil* 58:247, 1980

211. Yovich JL, Edirisinghe WR, Yovich JM, Stanger JD, Matson PL: Methods of water purification for the preparation of culture media in an IVF-ET programme. *Hum Reprod* 3:245, 1988

212. Menezo Y, Testart J, Perrone D: Serum is not necessary in human in vitro fertilization, early embryo culture, and transfer. *Fertil Steril* 42:750, 1984

213. Caro CM, Trounson A: Successful fertilization, embryo development and pregnancy using a chemically defined culture medium containing no protein. *J In Vitro Fert Embryo Transf* 3:215, 1986

214. Shirley B, Wortham JW, Witmyer J, Condon-Mahony M, Fort G: Effects of human serum and plasma on development of mouse embryos in culture media. *Fertil Steril* 43:129, 1985

215. Ball GD, Coulam CB, Field CS, Harms RW, Thie JT, Byers AP: Effect of serum source on human fertilization and embryonic growth parameters in vitro. *Fertil Steril* 44:75, 1985

216. Ashwood-Smith MJ, Hollands P, Edwards RG: The use of albuminar 5 (TM) as a medium supplement in clinical IVF. *Hum Reprod* 4:702, 1989

217. Pool TB, Martin JE: High continuing pregnancy rates after in vitro fertilization–embryo transfer using a medium supplemented with a plasma protein fraction containing alpha and beta globulins. *Fertil Steril* 61:714, 1994

218. O'Neill C, Collier M, Ammit AJ, Ryan JP, Saunders DM, Pike IL: Supplementation of in-vitro fertilisation culture medium with platelet activating factor. *Lancet* 1:769, 1989

219. Gardner HG, Kaye PL: Insulin stimulates mitosis and morphological development in mouse preimplantation embryos in vitro. *Reprod Fertil Dev* 3:79, 1991

220. Harvey MB, Kay PL: Mouse blastocysts respond metabolically to short term stimulation by insulin of IGF-1 through the insulin receptor. *Mol Reprod Dev* 29:253, 1991

221. Caro CM, Trounson A, Kirby C: Effect of growth factors in culture medium on the rate of mouse embryo development and viability in vitro. *J In Vitro Fert Embryo Transf* 4:265, 1987

222. Fishel S, Jackson P, Webster J, Faratia B: Endotoxins in culture medium for human in vitro fertilization. *Fertil Steril* 49:108, 1988

223. Davidson A, Vermesh M, Lobo RA, Paulson RJ: Mouse embryo culture as quality control for human in vitro fertilization: One versus the two-cell model. *Fertil Steril* 49:516, 1988

224. Davidson A, Vermesh M, Lobo RA, Paulson RJ: The temporal effects of changes in in vitro fertilization culture media on the one-cell mouse embryo system. *J In Vitro Fert Embryo Transf* 5:149, 1988

225. Montoro L, Subias E, Young P, Baccaro M, Swanson J, Sueldo C: Detection of endotoxin in human in vitro fertilization by the zona free mouse embryo assay. *Fertil Steril* 54:109, 1990

226. Fleming TP, Pratt HP, Braude PR: The use of mouse preimplantation embryos for quality control of culture reagents in human in vitro fertilization programs: A cautionary note. *Fertil Steril* 47:858, 1987

227. Pickering SJ, Braude PR, Johnson MH, Cant A, Currie J: Transient cooling to room temperature can cause irreversible disruption of the meiotic spindle in the human oocyte. *Fertil Steril* 54:102, 1990

228. Abramczuk JW, Lopata A: Incubator performance in the clinical in vitro fertilization program: Importance of temperature conditions for the fertilization and cleavage of human oocytes. *Fertil Steril* 46:132, 1986

229. Cohen J, Talansky B, Alikani M: Laboratory techniques for handling gametes and embryos. *Br Med Bull* 46:643, 1990

230. Chetkowski RJ, Nass TE, Matt DW, et al: Optimization of hydrogen ion concentration during aspiration of oocytes and culture and transfer of embryos. *J In Vitro Fert Embryo Transf* 2:207, 1985

231. Daya S, Kohut J, Gunby J, Younglai E: Influence of blood clots in the cumulus complex on oocyte fertilization and cleavage. *Hum Reprod* 5:744, 1990

232. Plachot M, Mandelbaum J: Oocyte maturation, fertilization and embryonic growth in vitro. *Br Med Bull* 46:675, 1990

233. Veeck LL, Wortham JW, Witmyer J, et al: Maturation and fertilization of morphologically immature human oocytes in a program of in vitro fertilization. *Fertil Steril* 39:594, 1983

234. Laufer N, Tarlatzis BC, DeCherney AH, et al: Asynchrony between human cumulus-corona cell complex and oocyte maturation after human menopausal gonadotrophin treatment for in vitro fertilization. *Fertil Steril* 42:366, 1984

235. Trounson AO, Mohr LR, Wood C, Leeton JF: Effect of delayed insemination on in vitro fertilization, culture and transfer of human embryos. *J Reprod Fertil* 64:285, 1982

236. Elder KT, Wick KL, Edwards RG: Seminal plasma anti-sperm antibodies and IVF: The effect of semen sample collection into 50% serum. *Hum Reprod* 5:179, 1990

237. Ng FL, Liu DY, Baker HW: Comparison of Percoll, mini-Percoll, and swim-up methods for sperm preparation from abnormal semen samples. *Hum Reprod* 7:261, 1992

238. La Calle JF: Human spermatozoa selection in improved discontinuous Percoll gradients. *Fertil Steril* 56:737, 1991

239. Ord T, Patrizio P, Marell E, Balmeceda JP, Asch R: Mimi-Percoll: A new method of semen preparation for IVF in severe male factor infertility. *Hum Reprod* 5:987, 1990

240. Englert Y, Bergh M, Rodesch C, Bertrand E, Biramane J, Legreve A: Comparative auto-controlled study between swim-up and Percoll preparation of fresh semen samples for in-vitro fertilization. *Hum Reprod* 7:399, 1992

241. Wolf DP, Byrd W, Dandekar P, Quigley MM: Sperm concentration and the fertilization of human eggs in vitro. *Biol Reprod* 31:387, 1984

242. Kruger TF, Acost AA, Simmons KF, Swanson RJ, Matta JF,

Oehninger SO: Predictive value of abnormal sperm morphology in in vitro fertilization. *Fertil Steril* 49:112, 1988

243. Seibel MM, Zilberstein M: The shape of semen morphology. *Hum Reprod* 10:247, 1995

244. Veeck L: TES and Tris (TEST)-yolk buffer systems, sperm function testing, and in vitro fertilization. *Fertil Steril* 58:484, 1992

245. Ghetler Y, Ben-Nun I, Kaneti H, Jaffe R, Gruber A, Fejgin M: Effect of sperm preincubation with follicular fluid on the fertilization rate in human in vitro fertilization. *Fertil Steril* 54:944, 1990

246. Katayama KP, Stehlik E, Roesler M, Jeyendran RS, Holmgren WJ, Zaneveld LJ: Treatment of human spermatozoa with an egg yolk medium can enhance the outcome of in vitro fertilization. *Fertil Steril* 52:1077, 1989

247. van der Ven HH, Hoebbel K, Al-Hasani S, Diedrich K, Krebs D: Fertilization of human oocytes in capillary tubes with very small numbers of spermatozoa. *Hum Reprod* 4:72, 1989

248. Tur-Kaspa I, Dudkiewicz A, Con E, Gleicher N: Pooled sequential ejaculates: A way to increase the total number of motile sperm from oligozoospermic men. *Fertil Steril* 54:906, 1990

249. Wassarman PM: The biology and chemistry of fertilization. *Science* 235:553, 1987

250. Plachot M: Choosing the right embryo: Challenge of the nineties. *J In Vitro Fert Embryo Transf* 6:193, 1989

251. Van Blerklom J, Bell H, Henry G: The occurrence, recognition, and developmental fate of pseudo-multipronuclear eggs after in vitro fertilization of human oocytes. *Hum Reprod* 2:217, 1987

252. Plachot M, Mandelbaum J, Junca AM, de Grouchy J, Salat-Baroux J, Cohen J: Cytogenetic analysis and developmental capacity of normal and abnormal embryos after IVF. *Hum Reprod* 4:99, 1989

253. Muechler EK, Graham MC, Huang K, Partridge AB, Jones K: Parthenogenesis of human oocytes as a function of vacuum pressure. *J In Vitro Fert Embryo Transf* 6:335, 1989

254. Staessen C, Janssenswillen C, Devroey P, Van Steirteghem A: Cytogenetic and morphological observations of single pronucleated human oocytes after in vitro fertilization. *Hum Reprod* 8:221, 1993

255. Boldt J, Howe AM, Butler WJ, McDonough PG, Padilla SL: The value of oocyte insemination in human in vitro fertilization. *Fertil Steril* 48:617, 1987

256. Trounson A, Webb J: Fertilization of human oocytes following reinsemination in vitro. *Fertil Steril* 41:816, 1984

257. Ben-Raphael Z, Kopf GS, Blasco L, Tureck RW, Mastroianni L: Fertilization and cleavage after insemination of human oocytes in vitro. *Fertil Steril* 45:58, 1986

258. Ashkenazi J, Feldberg D, Dicker D, Shelef M, Goldman GA, Goldman JA: Reinsemination in human IVF with fresh versus initial semen: A comparative study. *Eur J Obstet Gynecol Reprod Biol* 34:97, 1990

259. Steer CV, Mills CL, Tan SL, Campbell S, Edwards RG: The cumulative embryo score: A predictive technique to select the optimal number of embryos to transfer in an in vitro fertilization and embryo transfer programme. *Hum Reprod* 7:117, 1992

260. Visser DS, Fourie F: The applicability of the cumulative embryo score system for embryo selection and quality control in an in vitro fertilization/embryo transfer programme. *Hum Reprod* 8:1719, 1993

261. Grillo JM, Gamerre M, Lacroix O, Noizet A, Vitry G: Influence of the morphological aspect of embryos obtained by in vitro fertilization on their implantation rate. *J In Vitro Fertil Embryo Transf* 8:317, 1991

262. Bolton VN, Hawes SM, Taylor CT, Parsons JH: Development of spare human preimplantation embryos in vitro: An analysis of the correlations among gross morphology, cleavage rates, and development to the blastocyst. *J In Vitro Fertil Embryo Transf* 6:30, 1989

263. Hardy K, Winston RML, Handyside AH: Binucleate blastomeres in preimplantation human embryos in vitro: Failure of cytokinesis during early cleavage. *J Reprod Fertil* 98:549, 1993

264. Jackson KV, Clarke RN, Nureddin A, Hornstein MD, Rein MS, Friedman AJ: Transfer of embryos with multinucleated blastomeres is associated with lower implantation rates in IVF patients. *Fertil Steril* (Suppl):171, 1992

265. Gott AL, Hardy K, Winston RML, Leese HJ: Non-invasive measurement of pyruvate and glucose uptake and lactate production by single human preimplantation embryos. *Hum Reprod* 5:104, 1990

266. Conaghan J, Hardy K, Handyside A, Winston RML, Leese HJ: Selection criteria for human embryo transfer: A comparison of pyruvate uptake and morphology. *J Assist Reprod Genet* 10:21, 1993

267. Collier M, O'Neill C, Ammit AJ, Saunders DM: Measurement of human embryo-derived platelet-activating factor (PAF) using a quantitative bioassay of platelet aggregation. *Hum Reprod* 5:323, 1990

268. Sheth KV, Roca GL, Al-Sedairy ST, Parhar RS, Hamilton CJ, Jabbar F: Prediction of successful embryo implantation by measuring interleukin-1-alpha and immunosuppressive factors in preimplantation embryo culture fluid. *Fertil Steril* 55:952, 1991

269. Hardy RI, Anderson DJ, Hill JA: Lack of correlation between interleukin-1-alpha in preimplantation culture media and pregnancy outcome. *Fertil Steril* (Suppl):139, 1993

270. Hardy RI, Biggers JD, Golan DE: Use of NADH laser fluorimetry for the metabolic assessment of oocyte and embryo quality. *Proc Soc Gynecol Invest* 3:133, 1994

271. Bongso A, Ng SC, Fong CY, Ratnam S: Cocultures: A new lead in embryo quality improvement for assisted reproduction. *Fertil Steril* 56:179, 1991

272. Saito H, Hirayama T, Koike K, Saito T, Nohara M, Hiroi M: Cumulus mass maintains embryo quality. *Fertil Steril* 62:555, 1994

273. Wiemer KE, Hoffman DI, Maxson WS, et al: Embryonic morphology and rate of implantation of human embryos following co-culture on bovine oviductal epithelial cells. *Hum Reprod* 8:97, 1993

274. Jayot S, Parneix I, Verdaguer S, Discamps G, Audebert A, Emperaire C: Coculture of embryos on homologous endometrial cells in patients with repeated failures of implantation. *Fertil Steril* 63:109, 1995

275. Freeman MR, Whitworth CM, Hill GA: Granulosa cell co-

culture enhances human embryo development and pregnancy rate following in-vitro fertilization. *Hum Reprod* 10:408, 1995

276. Wiemer KE, Cohen JSRW, Malter HE, Wright G, Godke RA: Coculture of human zygotes on fetal bovine uterine fibroblasts: Embryonic morphology and implantation. *Fertil Steril* 52:503, 1989

277. Bongso A, Soon-Chye N, Sathananthan H, Lian NP, Rauff M, SR: Improved quality of human embryos when co-cultured with human ampullary cells. *Hum Reprod* 4:706, 1989

278. Bongso A, Fong CY, Ng SC, Ratnam S: The search for improved culture systems should not be ignored: Embryo co-culture may be one of them. *Hum Reprod* 8:1155, 1993

279. Sakkas D, Jaquenoud N, Leppens G, Campana A: Comparison of results after in vitro fertilized human embryos are cultured in routine medium and in coculture on Vero cells: A randomized study. *Fertil Steril* 61:521, 1994

280. Pellestor F: Frequency and distribution of aneuploidy in human female gametes. *Hum Genet* 86:283, 1991

281. Zenzes MT, Casper RF: Cytogenetics of human oocytes, zygotes, and embryos after in vitro fertilization. *Hum Genet* 88:367, 1992

282. Tarin JJ, Gomez E, Pellicer A: Chromosome anomalies in human oocytes in vitro. *Fertil Steril* 55:964, 1991

283. Gras L, McBain J, Trounson A, Kola I: The incidence of chromosomal aneuploidy in stimulated and unstimulated (natural) uninseminated human oocytes. *Hum Reprod* 7:1396, 1992

284. Martin RH, Balkan W, Burns K, Rademaker AW, Lin CC, Rudd NL: The chromosome constitution of 1000 human spermatozoa. *Hum Genet* 63:305, 1983

285. Plachot M, Veiga A, Montagut J, et al: Are clinical and biological IVF parameters correlated with chromosomal disorders in early life: A multicentric study. *Hum Reprod* 3:627, 1988

286. Delhanty JD, Penketh RJ: Cytogenetic analysis of unfertilized oocytes retrieved after treatment with the LHRH analogue, buserelin. *Hum Reprod* 5:699, 1990

287. Pellestor F, Sel B: Assessment of aneuploidy in the human female by using cytogenetics of IVF failures. *Am J Hum Genet* 42:274, 1988

288. Angell RR: Aneuploidy in older women. *Hum Reprod* 9:1199, 1994

289. Angell RR, Templeton AA, Aitken RJ: Chromosome studies in human in vitro fertilization. *Hum Genet* 72:333, 1986

290. Plachot M, Junca A-M, Mandelbaum J, Grouchy J, Salat-Baroux J, Cohen J: Chromosome investigations in early life. II. Human preimplantation embryos. *Hum Reprod* 2:29, 1987

291. Wimmers MS, Van der Merwe JV: Chromosome studies on early human embryos fertilized in vitro. *Hum Reprod* 3:894, 1988

292. Papadopoulos G, Templeton AA, Fisk N, Randall J: The frequency of chromosome anomalies in human preimplantation embryos after in vitro fertilization. *Hum Reprod* 4:91, 1989

293. Bongso A, Ng SC, Lim J, Fong CY, Ratnam S: Preimplantation genetics: Chromosomes of fragmented human embryos. *Fertil Steril* 56:66, 1991

294. Zenzes MT, Wang P, Casper RF: Chromosome status of untransferred (spare) embryos and probability of pregnancy after in vitro fertilization. *Lancet* 340:391, 1992

295. Edirisinghe WR, Murch AR, Yovich J: Cytogenetic analysis of

human oocytes and embryos in an in vitro fertilization programme. *Hum Reprod* 7:230, 1992

296. Benkhalifa M, Janny L, Vye P, Malet P, Boucher D, Menezo Y: Assessment of polyploidy in human morulae and blastocysts using co-culture and fluorescent in-situ hybridization. *Hum Reprod* 8:895, 1993

297. Munne, Lee A, Rosenwaks Z, Grifo J, Cohen J: Diagnosis of major chromosome aneuploidies in human preimplantation embryos. *Hum Reprod* 8:2185, 1993

298. Jamieson ME, Coutts JR, Connor JM: The chromosome constitution of human preimplantation embryos fertilized in vitro. *Hum Reprod* 9:709, 1994

299. Munne S, Grifo J, Cohen J, Weier H: Chromosome abnormalities in human arrested preimplantation embryos: A multiple-probe FISH study. *Am J Hum Genet* 55:150, 1994

300. Trounson A, Mohr L: Human pregnancy following cryopreservation, thawing, and transfer of an eight cell embryo. *Nature* 305:707, 1983

301. Kahn JA, von During V, Sunde A, Sordal T, Molne K: The efficacy and efficiency of an in vitro fertilization programme including embryo cryopreservation: A cohort study. *Hum Reprod* 8:247, 1993

302. Wada I, Matson PL, Troup SA, Morroll DR, Hunt L, Lieberman BA: Does elective cryopreservation of all embryos from women at risk of ovarian hyperstimulation syndrome reduce the incidence of the condition? *Br J Obstet Gynaecol* 100:265, 1993

303. Pattinson HA, Hignett M, Dunphy C, Fleetham JA: Outcome of thaw embryo transfer after cryopreservation of all embryos in patients at risk of ovarian hyperstimulation syndrome. *Fertil Steril* 62:1192, 1994

304. Friedler S, Giudice LC, Lamb EJ: Cryopreservation of embryos and ova. *Fertil Steril* 49:743, 1988

305. Van der Elst J, Camus M, Van den Abbeel E, Maes R, Devroey P, Van Steirteghem AC: Prospective randomized study on the cryopreservation of human embryos with dimethylsulfoxide or 1, 2-propanediol protocols. *Fertil Steril* 63:92, 1995

306. Rall WF, Fahy GM: Ice-free cryopreservation of mouse embryos at −196 C by vitrification. *Nature* 313:573, 1985

307. Gordts S, Roziers P, Campo R, Noto V: Survival and pregnancy outcome after ultrarapid freezing of human embryos. *Fertil Steril* 53:469, 1990

308. Trounson A: Preservation of human eggs and embryos. *Fertil Steril* 46:1, 1986

309. Lieberman BA, Troup SA, Matson PL: Cryopreservation of embryos and pregnancy rates after IVF. *Lancet* 340:116, 1992

310. Lin YP, Cassidenti DL, Chacon RR, Soubra SS, Rosen GF, Yee B: Successful implantation of frozen sibling embryos is influenced by the outcome of the cycle from which they were derived. *Fertil Steril* 63:262, 1995

311. Schalkoff ME, Oskowitz SP, Powers RD: A multifactorial analysis of the pregnancy outcome in a successful embryo cryopreservation program. *Fertil Steril* 59:1070, 1993

312. Assisted reproductive technology in the United States and Canada: 1992 results generated from the American Fertility Soci-

ety/Society for Assisted Reproductive Technology Registry. *Fertil Steril* 62:1121, 1994

313. Fugger EF, Bustillo M, Dorfmann AD, Schulman JD: Human preimplantation embryo cryopreservation: Selected aspects. *Hum Reprod* 6:131, 1991

314. Chen C: Pregnancy after human oocyte cryopreservation. *Lancet* 1:884, 1986

315. Bouquet M, Selva J, Auroux M: The incidence of chromosomal abnormalities in frozen-thawed mouse oocytes after in-vitro fertilization. *Hum Reprod* 7:76, 1992

316. Trounson AO: Cryopreservation. *Br Med Bull* 46:695, 1990

317. Spears N: In vitro growth of oocytes. *Hum Reprod* 9:969, 1994

318. Eppig JJ, Schroeder AC: Capacity of mouse oocytes from pre-antral follicles to undergo embryogenesis and development to live young after growth, maturation, and fertilization in vitro. *Biol Reprod* 41:268, 1989

319. Eppig JJ: Growth and development of mammalian oocytes in vitro. *Arch Pathol Lab Med* 116:379, 1992

320. Nayudu PL, Osborn SM: Factors influencing the rate of preantral and antral growth of mouse ovarian follicles in vitro. *J Reprod Fertil* 95:349, 1992

321. Spears N, Boland NI, Murray AA, Gosden RG: Mouse oocytes derived from in vitro grown primary ovarian follicles are fertile. *Hum Reprod* 9:527, 1994

322. Carroll J, Gosden RG: Transplantation of frozen-thawed mouse primordial follicles. *Hum Reprod* 8:1163, 1993

323. Kerin JF, Jeffery R, Warnes GM, Cox LW, Broom TJ: A simple technique for human embryo transfer into the uterus. *Lancet* 2:726, 1981

324. Leeton J, Trounson A, Jessup D, Wood C: The technique for human embryo transfer. *Fertil Steril* 38:156, 1982

325. Jones HW, Acosta AA, Garcia JE, Sandow BA, Veeck L: On the transfer of conceptuses from oocytes fertilized in vitro. *Fertil Steril* 39:241, 1983

326. Bolton VN, Wren ME, Parsons JH: Pregnancies after in vitro fertilization and transfer of human blastocysts. *Fertil Steril* 55:830, 1991

327. Dawson KJ, Conaghan J, Ostera GR, Winston RML, Hardy K: Delaying transfer to the third day post-insemination, to select non-arrested embryos, increases development to the fetal stage. *Hum Reprod* 10:177, 1995

328. Huisman GJ, Alberda AT, Leerentveld RA, Verhoeff A, Zeilmaker GH: A comparison of in vitro fertilization results after embryo transfer after 2, 3, and 4 days of embryo culture. *Fertil Steril* 61:970, 1994

329. Quinn P, Stone BA, Marrs RP: Suboptimal laboratory conditions can affect pregnancy outcome after embryo transfer on day 1 or 2 after insemination. *Fertil Steril* 53:168, 1990

330. Navot D, Scott RT, Droesch K, Veeck LL, Liu HC, Rosenwaks Z: The window of embryo transfer and the efficiency of human conception in vitro. *Fertil Steril* 55:114, 1991

331. Staessen C, Camus M, Bollen N, Devroey P, Van Steirteghem AC: The relationship between embryo quality and the occurrence of multiple pregnancies. *Fertil Steril* 57:626, 1992

332. Seoud M, Toner JP, Kruithoff C, Muasher SJ: Outcome of twin, triplet, and quadruplet in vitro fertilization pregnancies: The Norfolk experience. *Fertil Steril* 57:825, 1992

333. Vauthier-Brouzes D, Lefebvre G, Lesourd S, Gonzales J, Darbois Y: How many embryos should be transferred in in vitro fertilization? A prospective randomized study. *Fertil Steril* 62:339, 1994

334. Staessen C, Janssenswillen C, Van den Abbeel E, Devroey P, Van Steirteghem AC: Avoidance of triplet pregnancies by elective transfer of two good quality embryos. *Hum Reprod* 8:1650, 1993

335. Nijs M, Geerts L, van Roosendaal ESBG, Vanderzwalmen P, Schoysman R: Prevention of multiple pregnancies in an in vitro fertilization program. *Fertil Steril* 59:1245, 1993

336. Mansour R, Aboulghar M, Serour G: Dummy embryo transfer: A technique that minimizes the problems of embryo transfer and improves the pregnancy rate in human in vitro fertilization. *Fertil Steril* 54:678, 1990

337. Shaker AG, Fleming R, Jamieson ME, Yates RW, Coutts JR: Assessments of embryo transfer after in vitro fertilization: Effects of glyceryl trinitrate. *Hum Reprod* 8:1426, 1993

338. Friedler S, Lewin A, Schenker JG: Methodology of human embryo transfer following assisted reproduction. *J Assist Reprod Genet* 10:393, 1993

339. Wisanto A, Janssens R, Deschacht J, Camus M, Devroey P, Van Steirteghem AC: Performance of different embryo catheters in a human in vitro fertilization program. *Fertil Steril* 52:79, 1989

340. Gonen Y, Dirnfeld M, Goldman S, Koifman M, Abramovici H: Does the choice of catheter for embryo transfer influence the success rate of in-vitro fertilization? *Hum Reprod* 6:1092, 1991

341. Diedrich K, van der Ven H, Al-Hasani S, Krebs D: Establishment of pregnancy related to embryo transfer techniques after in vitro fertilization. *Hum Reprod* 4(suppl):111, 1989

342. Hurley VA, Osborn JC, Leoni MA, Leeton J: Ultrasound guided embryo transfer: A controlled trial. *Fertil Steril* 55:559, 1991

343. Menezo Y, Arnal F, Humeau C, Ducret L, Nicollet B: Increased viscosity in transfer medium does not improve pregnancy rates after embryo replacement. *Fertil Steril* 52:680, 1989

344. Khan I, Staessen C, Devroey P, Van Steirteghem AC: Human serum albumin versus serum: A comparative study on embryo transfer medium. *Fertil Steril* 56:98, 1991

345. Krampl E, Zegermacher G, Eichler C, Obruca A, Strohmer H, Feichtinger W: Air in the uterine cavity after embryo transfer. *Fertil Steril* 63:366, 1995

346. Mansour RT, Aboulghar MA, Serour GI, Amin YM: Dummy embryo transfer using methylene dye. *Hum Reprod* 9:1257, 1994

347. Knutzen V, Stratton CJ, Sher G, McNamee PI, Huang T T, Soto-Albors C: Mock embryo transfer in the early luteal phase, the cycle before in vitro fertilization and embryo transfer: A descriptive study. *Fertil Steril* 57:156, 1992

348. Waterstone J, Curson R, Parsons J: Embryo transfer to the low uterine cavity. *Lancet* 337:1413, 1991

349. Nazari A, Askari HA, Check JH, O'Shaughnessy A: Embryo transfer technique as a cause of ectopic pregnancy in in vitro fertilization. *Fertil Steril* 60:919, 1993

350. Visser DS, Fourie F, Kruger HF: Multiple attempts at embryo

transfer: Effect on pregnancy outcome in an in vitro fertilization and embryo transfer program. *J Assist Reprod Genet* 10:37, 1993

351. Kato O, Takatsuka R, Asch RH: Transvaginal-transmyometrial embryo transfer: The Towako method—Experiences of 104 cases. *Fertil Steril* 59:51, 1993

352. Parsons JH, Bolton VN, Wilson L, Campbell S: Pregnancies following in vitro fertilization and ultrasound directed surgical embryo transfer by perurethral and transvaginal techniques. *Fertil Steril* 48:691, 1987

353. Sauer MV, Paulson RJ: Pelvic abscess complicating transcervical embryo transfer. *Am J Obstet Gynecol* 166:148, 1992

354. Feichtinger W, Barad D, Feinman M, Barg P: The use of two-component fibrin sealant for embryo transfer. *Fertil Steril* 54:733, 1990

355. Feichtinger W, Strohmer H, Radner KM, Goldin M: The use of fibrin sealant for embryo transfer: Development and clinical studies. *Hum Reprod* 7:890, 1992

356. Dlugi A, Laufer N, DeCherney AH, et al: The periovulatory and luteal phase of conception cycles following IVF. *Fertil Steril* 41:530, 1984

357. Lejeune B, Camus M, Deschacht J, Leroy F: Differences in the luteal phase after failed or successful IVF-ET. *J In Vitro Fert Embryo Transf* 3:358, 1986

358. Mahadevan MM, Leader A, Taylor PJ: Effects of low dose hCG on corpus luteum function after embryo transfer. *J In Vitro Fert Embryo Transf* 2:190, 1985

359. Frydman R, Testart J, Giacomini P, et al: Hormonal and histological study of the luteal phase in women following aspiration of the preovulatory follicle. *Fertil Steril* 38:312, 1982

360. Garcia J, Jones GS, Acosta A, Wright G: Corpus luteum function after follicle aspiration for oocyte retrieval. *Fertil Steril* 36:565, 1981

361. Cohen JJ, Debache C, Pigeau F, et al: Sequential use of clomiphene citrate, hMG and hCG in human IVF. II. Study of luteal phase adequacy following aspiration of preovulatory follicles. *Fertil Steril* 42:360, 1984

362. Sterzik K, Dallenbach C, Schneider V, et al: IVF: The degree of endometrial insufficiency varies with the type of ovarian stimulation. *Fertil Steril* 50:457, 1988

363. Forman RG, Eychenne B, Nessmann C, et al: Assessing the early luteal phase in IVF cycles: Relationships between plasma steroids, endometrial receptors and endometrial histology. *Fertil Steril* 51:310, 1989

364. Salat-Baroux J, Giacomini P, Cornet D: Study of the luteal phase after IVF (abstract). *Fertil Steril* 41:16S, 1984

365. Graf M, Reyniak VPB, Laufer N: Histologic evaluation of the luteal phase in women following follicle aspiration for oocyte retrieval. *Fertil Steril* 49:616, 1988

366. Balasch J, Inmaclada J, Marquez M, Vanrell J: Hormonal and histological evaluation of the luteal phase after combined GnRH-a/gonadotropin treatment for superovulation and luteal phase support in IVF. *Hum Reprod* 6:914, 1991

367. Tarlatzis BC, Laufer N, DeCherney A, et al: The value of b-hCG estradiol and progesterone levels in predicting pregnancy outcome in IVF cycles. *J In Vitro Fert Embryo Transf* 1:143, 1984

368. Smitz J, Devroey P, Braeckmans P, et al: Management of failed

cycles in an IVF/GIFT program with the combination of GnRH analog and hMG. *Hum Reprod* 2:309, 1987

369. Smitz J, Devroey P, Camus MJD, et al: The luteal phase and early pregnancy after combined GnRH-a/hMG treatment for superovulation in IVF or GIFT. *Hum Reprod* 3:585, 1988

370. Pellicer A, Miro F: Steroidogenesis in vitro of human granulosa luteal cells pretreated in vivo with GnRH-a. *Fertil Steril* 54:590, 1990

371. Latouche J, Crumeyrolle-Arias M, Jordan D, et al: GnRH receptor in human granulosa cells: Anatomical localization and characterization by auto radiographic study. *Endocrinology* 125:1739, 1989

372. Tureck RW, Mastroianni L, Blasco L, Strauss JF: Inhibition of human granulosa cells progesterone secretion by a gonadotropin releasing hormone agonist. *J Clin Endocrinol Metab* 54:1078, 1982

373. Smith EM, Anthony FW, Gadd SC, Masson GM: Trial of support treatment with human chorionic gonadotropin in the luteal phase after treatment with buserelin and human menopausal gonadotropins in women taking part in an in vitro fertilization program. *Br Med J* 298:1483, 1989

374. Bellaisch-Allart J, De-Muozon J, Lapouterle C, Mayer M: The effect of hCG supplementation after combined GnRH-a/hMG treatment in an IVF program. *Hum Reprod* 5:163, 1990

375. Herman A, Ron-El R, Golan A, Nachum H, Soffer Y, Caspi E: Pregnancy rate and ovarian overstimulation after luteal hCG in IVF stimulated with GnRH-a. *Fertil Steril* 53:92, 1990

376. Van Steirteghem AC, Smitz J, Camus M, Wisanto A, Bourgain C, Devroey P: The luteal phase after in vitro fertilization and related procedures. *Hum Reprod* 3:161, 1988

377. Lewin A, Benshushan A, Mezker E, Yanai N, Schenker JG: The role of estrogen support during the luteal phase of IVF-ET cycles: A comparative study between progesterone alone and estrogen and progesterone support. *Fertil Steril* 62:121, 1994

378. Devroey P, Smitz J, Bourgain C, Van Steirteghem AC: Only micronized progesterone is needed to substitute the luteal phase in stimulated cycles. *Contracept Fertil Sex* 20:1, 1992

379. Cohen J, de Mounzon J, Lancaster P: World Collaborative Report: VIIIth World Congress on In Vitro Fertilization and Alternate Assisted Reproduction. Oct, 1993, Kyoto, Japan

380. Testart J, Plachot M, Mandelbaum J, Salat-Baroux J, Frydman RCJ: World collaborative report on IVF-ET and GIFT: 1989. *Hum Reprod* 7:362, 1992

381. FIVNAT (French In Vitro National): French national registry: Analysis of 1986 to 1990 data. *Fertil Steril* 59:587, 1993

382. Medical Research International, The American Fertility Society Special Interest Group: In vitro fertilization/embryo transfer in the United States: 1985 and 1986 results from the National IVF-ET Registry. *Fertil Steril* 49:212, 1988

383. AIH National Perinatal Statistics Unit, Fertility Society of Australia: Assisted conception Australia and New Zealand 1989. Sydney, Australian Fertility Society, 1991

384. Sepalla M: The world collaborative report on in vitro fertilization and embryo replacement: Current state of the art in January 1984. *Ann N Y Acad Sci* 442:558, 1984

385. Frydman R, Belaisch-Allart J, Fries N, et al: An obstetric assessment of the first 100 births from the in vitro fertilization program at Clamart, France. *Am J Obstet Gynecol* 154:550, 1986

386. Van Steirteghem AC, Van Den Abbeel E: World results of human embryo cryopreservation. In: Mashiah S, Ber-Raphael Z, Laufer N, Schenker JG (eds), *Advances in Assisted Reproductive Technologies.* New York, Plenum, 1990:601

387. Acosta AA, Oehninger S, Morshedi M, Swanson RJ, Scott R, Irianni F: Assisted reproduction in the diagnosis and treatment of the male factor. *Obstet Gynecol Surv* 44:1, 1988

388. Thadani VM: Mice produced from eggs fertilized in vitro at a very low sperm:egg ratio. *J Exp Zool* 219:277, 1982

389. Gordon JW, Talansky BE: Assisted fertilization by zona drilling: A mouse model for correction of oligospermia. *J Exp Zool* 239:347, 1986

390. Gordon JW, Grunfeld L, Garrisi GJ, Talansky BE, Richards C, Laufer N: Fertilization of human oocytes by sperm of infertile males after zona-pellucida drilling. *Fertil Steril* 50:68, 1988

391. Malter HE, Cohen J: Partial zona dissection of human oocytes: A nontraumatic method using micromanipulation to assist zona pellucida penetration. *Fertil Steril* 51:139, 1989

392. Cohen J, Malter H, Wright G, Kort HJM, Mitchell D: Partial zona dissection of human oocytes when failure of zona pellucida penetration is anticipated. *Hum Reprod* 4:435, 1989

393. Laufer N, Simon A: Treatment of male infertility by gamete micromanipulation. *Hum Reprod* 7(Suppl 1):73, 1992

394. Simon A, Younis J, Lewin A, Bartoov B, Schenker JG, Laufer N: The correlation between sperm cell morphology and fertilization after zona pellucida slitting in subfertile males. *Fertil Steril* 56:325, 1991

395. Cohen J, Talansky BE, Malter H, et al: Microsurgical fertilization and teratozoospermia. *Hum Reprod* 6:118, 1991

396. Palanker D, Ohad S, Lewis A, et al: Technique for cellular microsurgery using the 193-nm excimer laser. *Lasers Med Surg* 11:580, 1991

397. Laufer N, Palanker D, Shufaro Y, Safran A, Simon A, Lewis A: The efficacy and safety of zona pellucida drilling by a 193 nm excimer laser. *Fertil Steril* 59:889, 1993

398. Feichtinger W, Strohmer H, Fuhrberg P, et al: Photoablation of oocyte zona pellucida by erbium-yag laser for in-vitro fertilisation in severe male infertility. *Lancet* 339:811, 1992

399. Antinori S, Versaci C, Fuhrberg P, Panci C, Caffa B, Gholami GH: Seventeen live birth after the use of an erbium-yytrium aluminium garnet laser in the treatment of male factor infertility. *Hum Reprod* 9:1891, 1994

400. Stohmer H, Feichtinger W: Successful clinical application of laser for micromanipulation in an in-vitro fertilization program. *Fertil Steril* 58:212, 1992

401. Obruca A, Strohmer H, Sakkas D, et al: Use of lasers in assisted fertilization and hatching. *Hum Reprod* 9:1723, 1994

402. Gordon JW, Laufer N: Application of micromanipulation to human in vitro fertilization. *J In Vitro Fert Embryo Transf* 5:57, 1988

403. Mann JR: Full term development of mouse eggs fertilized by a spermatozoon microinjected under the zona pellucida. *Biol Reprod* 38:1077, 1988

404. Ng SC, Bongso A, Ratnam SS, et al: Pregnancy after transfer of multiple sperm under the zona. *Lancet* 2:790, 1988

405. Fishel S, Antinori S, Jackson P, Johnson J, Rinaldi L: Presentation of six pregnancies established by sub-zonal insemination. *Hum Reprod* 6:124, 1991

406. Cohen J, Alikani M, Malter HE, Adler A, Talansky BE, Rosenwaks Z: Partial zona dissection or subzonal sperm insertion: Microsurgical fertilization alternatives based on evaluation of sperm and embryo morphology. *Fertil Steril* 56:696, 1991

407. Imoedemhe DAG, Sigue AB: Subzonal multiple sperm injection in the treatment of previous failed human in vitro fertilization. *Fertil Steril* 59:172, 1993

408. Bongso TA, Sathananthan H, Wong PC, et al: Human fertilization by microinjection of immotile spermatozoa. *Hum Reprod* 4:175, 1989

409. Soong YK, Lai YM, Chang SY, Wang ML, Chang MY, Lee CL: A successful pregnancy after subzonal insertion with epididymal sperm and coculture on Vero cell monolayer. *Fertil Steril* 59:1308, 1993

410. Silber SJ, Nagy ZP, Liu J, Godoy H, Devroey P, Van Steirteghem AC: Conventional in-vitro fertilization versus intracytoplasmic sperm injection for patients requiring microsurgical sperm aspiration. *Hum Reprod* 9:1705, 1994

411. Markert CL: Fertilization of mammalian eggs by sperm injection. *J Exp Zool* 228:195, 1983

412. Lanzendorf SE, Maloney MK, Veeck LL, Slusser J, Hodgen GD, Rosenwaks Z: A preclinical evaluation of pronuclear formation by microinjection of human spermatozoa into human oocytes. *Fertil Steril* 49:835, 1988

413. Goto K, Kinoshita A, Takuma Y, Ogawa K: Birth of calves after the transfers of oocytes fertilized by sperm injection. *Theriogenology* 35:205, 1991

414. Iritani A, Hosoi Y: Microfertilization by various methods in mammalian species. In: Yoshinaga K (ed), *Development of Preimplantation Embryos and Their Environment.* New York, Alan R. Liss, 1989:220

415. Palermo G, Joris H, Devroey P, Van Steirteghem A: Pregnancies after intracytoplasmic injection of single spermatozoon into an oocyte. *Lancet* 2:17, 1992

416. Van Steirteghem AC, Liu J, Joris H: Higher success rate by intracytoplasmic sperm injection than by subzonal insemination: Report of a second series of 300 consecutive treatment cycles. *Hum Reprod* 8:1055, 1993

417. Van Steirteghem AC, Nagy Z, Joris H, et al: High fertilization and implantation rates after intracytoplasmic sperm injection. *Hum Reprod* 8:1061, 1993

418. Payne D, Flaherty SP, Jeffrey R, Warnes GM, Matthews C: Successful treatment of severe male factor infertility in 100 consecutive cycles using intracytoplasmic sperm injection. *Hum Reprod* 9:2051, 1994

419. Tsirigotis M, Yang D, Redgment CJ, Nicholson N, Pelekanos M, Craft IL: Assisted fertilization with intracytoplasmic sperm injection. *Fertil Steril* 62:781, 1994

420. Palermo G, Joris H, Camus M, Devroey P, Van Steirteghem A: Sperm characteristics and outcome of human assisted fertiliza-

tion by subzonal insemination and intracytoplasmic sperm injection. *Fertil Steril* 59:826, 1993

421. Devroey P, Liu J, Nagy Z, Tournaye H, Silber SJ, Van Steirteghem AC: Normal fertilization of human oocytes after testicular sperm extraction and intracytoplasmic sperm injection. *Fertil Steril* 62:639, 1994

422. Shrivastav P, Nadkarni P, Wensvoort S, Craft I: Percutaneous epididymal sperm aspiration for obstructive azoospermia. *Hum Reprod* 9:2058, 1994

423. Nagy Z, Liu J, Cecile J, Silber S, Devroey P, Van Steirteghem A: Comparison of fertilization, embryo development and pregnancy rates after intracytoplasmic sperm injection using ejaculated, fresh and frozen-thawed epididymal and testicular spermatozoa. *Fertil Steril* 63:808, 1995

424. Van Steirteghem A, Liu J, Nagy P, et al: Therapies in male-factor infertility. *Hum Reprod* 9 (Suppl 3):6, 1994

425. Cohen J: Assisted hatching of human embryos. *J In Vitro Fert Embryo Transf* 8:179, 1991

426. Cohen J, Alikani M, Trowbridge J, Rosenwaks Z: Implantation enhancement by selective assisted hatching using zona drilling of human embryos with poor prognosis. *Hum Reprod* 7:685, 1992

427. Cohen J, Elsner C, Cort H, et al: Impairment of the hatching process following IVF in the human and improvement of implantation by assisted hatching using micromanipulation. *Hum Reprod* 5:7, 1990

428. Verlinsky Y, Ginsberg N, Lifchez A, Valle J, Moise J, Strom CM: Analysis of the first polar body: Preconception genetic diagnosis. *Hum Reprod* 5:826, 1990

429. Hardy K, Handyside AH: Biopsy of cleavage stage human embryos and diagnosis of single gene defects by DNA amplification. *Arch Pathol Lab Med* 116:388, 1992

430. Dorkas A, Sargent IL, Ross CRLG, Barlow DH: Trophectoderm biopsy in human blastocysts. *Hum Reprod* 5:821, 1990

431. Hardy K, Martin LK, Leese HJ, Winston RM, Handyside AH: Human preimplantation development in-vitro is not adversely affected by biopsy at the 8-cell stage. *Hum Reprod* 5:708, 1990

432. Handyside AH, Lesko JG, Tarin JJ, Winston RML, MRH: Birth of a normal girl after in-vitro fertilization and preimplantation diagnosis testing for cystic fibrosis. *Lancet* 327: 905, 1992

433. Tarin JJ, Handyside AL: Embryo biopsy strategies for preimplantation diagnosis. *Fertil Steril* 59:943, 1993

434. Monk M, Kenealy MR, Mohadjerani S: Detection of both the normal and mutant alleles in single cells of individuals heterozygous for the sickle cell mutation—prelude to preimplantation diagnosis. *Prenat Diag* 13:45, 1993

435. Coutelle C, Williams C, Handyside AH, Hardy K, Winston RML, Williamson R: Genetic analysis of DNA from single human oocytes: A model for preimplantation diagnosis of cystic fibrosis. *BMJ* 229:22, 1989

436. Pickering SJ, McConnell JM, Johnson MH, Braude PR: Reliability of detection by polymerase chain reaction of sickle cell-containing region of the beta-globin gene in single human blastomeres. *Hum Reprod* 7:630, 1992

437. Liu J, Lissens W, Devroey P, Van Steirteghem A, Liebaers I: Efficiency and accuracy of polymerase-chain-reaction assay for cystic fibrosis allele DF508 in single cell. *Lancet* 339:1190, 1992

438. Morsy M, Takeuchi K, Kaufman R, Veeck L, Hodgen GD, Beebe SJ: Preclinical models for human pre-embryo biopsy and genetic diagnosis. II. Polymerase chain reaction amplification of deoxyribonucleic acid from single lymphoblasts and blastomeres with mutation detection. *Fertil Steril* 57:431, 1992

439. Avner R, Laufer N, Safran A, Kerem B, Friedmann A, Mitrani-Rosenbaum S: Preimplantation diagnosis of cystic fibrosis by simultaneous detection of the W1282X and DF508 mutations. *Hum Reprod* 9:1676, 1994

440. Avner R, Reubinoff BE, Simon A, et al: Management of RhD isoimmunization by preimplantation genetic diagnosis. *Mol Hum Rep* 2:60, 1996

441. Coonen E, Dumoulin JCM, Ramaekers FCS, Hopman AHN: Optimal preparation of preimplantation embryo interphase nuclei for analysis by fluoresence in-situ hybridization. *Hum Reprod* 9:533, 1994

442. Pierce KE, Kiessling AA, Brenner CA, Seibel M, Zilberstein M: Diagnosis of chromosome balance in embryos from a patient with a balanced translocation. Presented at the 51st Annual Meeting American Society for Reproductive Medicine, April, 1995, Seattle, WA

443. Munne S, Weier HU, Stein J, Grifo J, Cohen J: A fast and efficient method for simultaneous X and Y in situ hybridization of human blastomeres. *J Assist Rep Genet* 10:82, 1993.

444. Ried T, Landes G, Dackowski W, Klinger K, Ward D: Multicolor fluoresence in situ hybridization for the simultaneous detection of probe sets for chromosomes 13,18,21,X and Y in uncultured amniotic fluid cells. *Hum Mol Genet* 1:307, 1992

445. Delhanty JDA, Griffin DK, Handyside AH, Atkinson GHG, Pieters HEC, Winston RM: Detection of aneuploidy and chromosomal mosaicism in human embryos during preimplantation sex determination by fluorescent in situ hybridization (FISH). *Hum Mol Genet* 2:1183, 1993

446. Harper J, Robinson F, Duffy S, et al: Detection of fertilization in embryos with accelerated cleavage by fluorescent in-situ hybridization (FISH). *Hum Reprod* 9:1733, 1994

447. Coonen E, Harper J, Ramaerkers FCS, et al: Presence of chromosomal mosaicism in abnormal preimplantation embryos detected by fluorescence in situ hybridisation. *Hum Genet* 94:609, 1992

CHAPTER 43

Assisted Fertilization Techniques

ANDRÉ C. VAN STEIRTEGHEM · INGEBORG LIEBAERS · PAUL DEVROEY

Assisted Fertilization Procedures
Clinical Evaluation of ICSI
   Patient selection and counseling
   Ovarian stimulation and oocyte handling
   Semen evaluation and preparation
   Intracytoplasmic sperm injection procedure

Oocyte damage and pronuclear status
   after ICSI
Embryo development, transfer, and freezing
Obstetric outcome, prenatal diagnosis,
   and follow-up study with the children
Summary

In vitro fertilization and embryo transfer (IVF-ET) has been extremely successful for the alleviation of long-standing infertility due to female factors such as tubal infertility and severe endometriosis and for couples with unexplained infertility. IVF has been less successful for the treatment of male-factor infertility.[1,2] Other innovative approaches to the management of male-factor infertility, such as tubal replacement of oocytes and spermatozoa (gamete intrafallopian transfer [GIFT]) or the tubal replacement of normally fertilized oocytes (zygote intrafallopian transfer [ZIFT]) failed to render the treatment more successful.[3,4] To overcome these limitations, several corrective measures have been proposed. These measures include in vitro insemination with a higher number of progressively motile spermatozoa,[5,6] modification of the insemination procedures,[6–8] glass-wool column filtration of semen,[9] discontinuous Percoll gradient centrifugation,[10,11] in vitro metabolic stimulation of recovered spermatozoa,[12,13] and the use of micromanipulation.[14]

At our center IVF results for couples with male-factor infertility were markedly lower than for couples with tubal infertility.[15] Fertilization did not occur in approximately one third of cycles.[15] Methods of improving fertilizing potential by stimulating sperm function in vitro failed to improve results.[16–18] All centers of reproductive medicine see some couples with andrologic infertility, which cannot be helped with conventional IVF treatment. Furthermore, a large number of couples are unacceptable candidates for IVF, because they have an insufficient number of progressively motile spermatozoa with normal morphology (about 500,000) available to achieve successful insemination. This includes patients with obstructive and nonobstructive spermatozoa.

ASSISTED FERTILIZATION PROCEDURES

The clinical introduction of assisted fertilization was based on experimental work performed over the last few decades. Pronuclei were formed when immotile spermatozoa were microinjected directly into the ooplasm of hamsters' and other rodents' oocytes.[19,20] Markert[21] reported the formation of zygotes after injection of sonicated mouse spermatozoa into the ooplasm of mouse oocytes. Barg et al[22] injected immobilized mouse spermatozoa treated with calcium ionophore A23817 into the perivitelline space of a large number of mouse oocytes and did not observe fertilization. A few years later Mann[23] reported fertilization and term development after subzonal insertion of a single motile mouse spermatozoon incubated for up to 2 hours in glucose-containing medium. Lacham et al[24] reported a higher fertilization rate after injection of a single motile spermatozoon treated with dibutyryl cyclic guanosine monophosphate (dbcGMP) and imidazole into the perivitelline space of mouse oocytes. The enhancement of acrosome reaction and the results of subzonal insemination of a single spermatozoon in mouse eggs revealed that the acrosome reaction can be induced by both biochemical and physical stimuli. The highest percentage of acrosome-free spermatozoa were obtained by combining the incubation in medium containing dbcGMP and imidazole with electroporation. After microinjection of eggs, high fertilization (70%), in vitro development to the blastocyst stage, and implantation and development to term after transfer into pseudopregnant mice were recorded.[25]

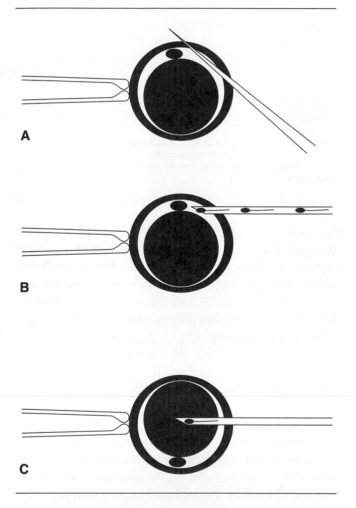

Figure 43–1. Techniques of assisted fertilization. **A.** Partial zonal dissection (PZD). An opening is made in the zona pellucida with a glass micropipette. The oocyte is inseminated with spermatozoa as in conventional IVF. **B.** Subzonal insemination (SUZI) of a metaphase II oocyte. The holding pipette (left) immobilizes the oocyte, and a variable number of spermatozoa are injected into the perivitelline space by means of an injection pipette (right). **C.** Intracytoplasmic single-sperm injection (ICSI) into a metaphase II oocyte. The oocyte is immobilized with the polar body at the 6 o'clock position by means of a holding pipette. A single immobilized spermatozoon is aspirated into the injection pipette and injected deep into the cytoplasm of the oocyte after penetration of the zona pellucida and the oolemma.

In parallel with assisted fertilization in animals, several studies reported the injection of human spermatozoa into the perivitelline space of hamster oocytes.[26–28] Human spermatozoa also have been injected successfully into the cytoplasm of human oocytes.[29] Other reports described injection of several spermatozoa into the perivitelline space to allow relatively natural sperm selection to occur.[14,30]

Assisted fertilization procedures have been used to treat couples with severe male-factor infertility who cannot be helped with conventional IVF. The strategy has been to reduce or remove the barrier to fertilization in vitro by disrupting the zona pellucida, allowing sperm direct access to the perivitelline space of the oocyte. The first such technique was partial zonal dissection (PZD) (Fig 43–1A), in which a small slit is made in the zona pellucida to allow sperm passage through to the oolemma. The results of PZD were generally found to be unsatisfactory and associated with erratic but generally low fertilization rates.[31,32] The next technique to gain temporary enthusiasm was subzonal insemination (SUZI) (Fig 43–1B). In that procedure several (between 3 and 20) motile spermatozoa are injected through the zona pellucida into the perivitelline space. The monospermic fertilization rate with SUZI was low, about 20% of all metaphase II oocytes into which spermatozoa were injected.[31,33–37] The overall success with PZD and SUZI was limited. Normal fertilization occurred in only two thirds of patients receiving these treatments. Even then, one or two eggs were all that were fertilized. As such, pregnancy and live-birth rates were unacceptably low.[37–43]

In 1992, our group reported the first pregnancies and births to result from replacement of embryos generated by a novel assisted fertilization procedure known as intracytoplasmic single-sperm injection (ICSI).[44] The ICSI technique involves injection of a single spermatozoon through the zona pellucida directly into the oocyte (Fig 43–1C). Before our clinical success, ICSI had been used successfully only to obtain live offspring from rabbits and cattle.[45] Two other IVF centers had attempted ICSI on a series of 143 human oocytes. They reported the transfer of four zygotes into two women and of 11 cleaved embryos into seven others, none of whom became pregnant.[42,46] Our experience with ICSI has been that the fertilization rate is considerably better than after SUZI, and also leads to the production of more embryos capable of achieving implantation.[36,37,47,48] Thus ICSI has been adopted as the technique of choice when assisted fertilization is necessary.

CLINICAL EVALUATION OF ICSI

Between 1991 and 1995, we had the opportunity to perform and evaluate more than 4500 ICSI cycles involving more than

30,000 oocytes. Our large experience has allowed us to analyze our data critically. The following summary reviews patient selection and counseling, ovarian stimulation and oocyte handling, semen evaluation and preparation, the ICSI procedure itself, oocyte damage and pronuclear status after ICSI, embryo development, transfer, and freezing, and results of obstetric outcome, prenatal testing, and a report of a prospective follow-up study of children born after ICSI.

Patient Selection and Counseling

A total of 4688 couples with long-standing infertility were selected for treatment with ICSI. The study consisted of several categories of couples. The ICSI procedure could not be performed in 119 cycles (2.5%) either owing to an absence of cumulus-oocyte complexes or metaphase II oocytes (48 cycles) or because no spermatozoa were available for the microinjection procedure (71 cycles). The ICSI procedure was performed in 4569 cycles.

The ICSI procedure was performed with spermatozoa from the ejaculate in 88% of the cycles in which couples had undergone one or more cycles of conventional IVF with no or poor fertilization after juxtaposition of the cumulus-oocyte complexes with at least 200,000 progressively motile spermatozoa per milliliter. Other ICSI cycles were performed on couples with semen values too impaired to be accepted for conventional IVF; that is, fewer than 500,000 progressively motile spermatozoa in the total ejaculate after semen preparation.

Couples with azoospermia due to obstruction also are candidates for ICSI. Sperm can either be aspirated from the epididymis (5% of our cycles) or obtained from testicular biopsies (7% of the cycles). Epididymal spermatozoa are typically used when patients have congenital bilateral absence of the vas deferens or failed vasoepididymostomy or vasovasostomy.[49–52] Both fresh and frozen thawed sperm appear to be relatively comparable. Testicular spermatozoa also can be used for ICSI. Indications include obstructive azoospermia and failure to retrieve motile spermatozoa from the epididymis, nonobstructive azoospermia due to germ-cell aplasia (Sertoli-cell-only syndrome), or maturational arrest.[52–57] Frozen thawed testicular spermatozoa yield substantially lower success rates than fresh testicular samples or those obtained when epididymal spermatozoa are used.

Initially, the ICSI procedure was clinically unproved, and ethics committee review and approval were required. Couples were fully informed about the novelty of the ICSI procedure, the uncertainty of its outcome, and the many unknown aspects surrounding the procedure. After extensive counseling, those who agreed to the procedure signed a consent form to have prenatal diagnosis and to participate in a prospective follow-up

study involving children born after ICSI.[58–64] The details of the epidemiologic data are described at the end of this chapter.

Ovarian Stimulation and Oocyte Handling

Ovarian stimulation was performed with gonadotropin-releasing hormone (GnRH) agonists, human menopausal gonadotropin (hMG), and human chorionic gonadotropin (hCG). Administration of the agonist was started on day 1 or 21 of the menstrual cycle. When serum estradiol concentration was 40 pg/mL (147 pmol/L) or less and serum progesterone concentration was 0.3 ng/mL (1 nmol/L) or less and when ovarian structures at ultrasound examination were less than 8 mm in diameter, ovarian stimulation was initiated with 150 hMG IU/day for 4 days in most instances. The hMG dose was subsequently individualized according to the rate of serum estradiol increment and ultrasound measurements of follicular diameter.[65–71] Blood samples were assayed for estradiol, progesterone, luteinizing hormone (LH), and follicle-stimulating hormone (FSH) beginning on the fifth day of gonadotropin treatment. When serum estradiol level exceeded 1000 pg/mL (3670 pmol/L) and when at least three follicles 18 mm or more in diameter were found at ultrasound examination, ovulation was induced with 10,000 IU of hCG. Oocyte retrieval was performed 36 hours after hCG administration by means of ultrasound-guided transvaginal aspiration. The luteal phase was supported with either natural micronized progesterone, 600 mg per day intravaginally in three divided does, starting on the day after the hCG injection or injection of 1500 IU of hCG on days 4, 8, and 12 after the hMG injection.[65–71] Because success rates are higher when more oocytes are retrieved, women 36 years and younger have the highest success rates. Women 40 years and older have fewer deliveries, although the fertilization rate is similar at all ages.

Our experience is drawn from a total of 61,048 cumulus-oocyte complexes retrieved during 4718 cycles (a mean of 12.9 complexes per cycle). In most cases, the cumulus and the corona cells were well dispersed.

Cumulus and corona cells are removed by means of a combination of enzymatic and mechanical procedures. The steps include a 1-minute incubation in HEPES-buffered Earle's medium containing 60 IU/mL hyaluronidase followed by aspiration of the cumulus-oocyte complexes in and out of hand-drawn glass pipettes with two different diameters (250 to 300 μm initially followed by a 200-μm opening. Oocytes are then rinsed several times in droplets of HEPES-buffered Earle's and B₂ medium and carefully observed under an inverted microscope at 200× magnification. Observations include assessment of the zona pellucida, the oocyte, and the presence or absence of a germinal vesicle or a first polar body.[72] Of the 61,048 cumulus-oocyte complexes, 95% contained an oocyte with an intact zona pellucida of which 81% contained metaphase II oocytes that had extruded the first polar body, 10% contained germinal-vesicle-stage oocytes, and 4% contained metaphase I oocytes that had undergone breakdown of the germinal vesicle but had not yet extruded the first polar body. The metaphase II oocytes are then incubated in 25-μL microdrops of B$_2$ medium covered by mineral oil at 37°C in an atmosphere of 5% oxygen, 5% carbon dioxide, and 90% nitrogen. The ICSI procedure is then performed.[72]

Semen Evaluation and Preparation

Semen analysis and preparation constitute an extremely important aspect of ICSI. Sperm used in a particular cycle may have originated from any level of the male reproductive tract and may have been previously frozen. In addition, the absolute numbers of sperm involved are often much lower than levels in conventional IVF.

During the evaluation before treatment, semen analysis and a semen selection procedure should be performed if possible to verify whether enough preferentially motile spermatozoa are present to perform ICSI. Semen assessment in our laboratory is performed according to the recommendations of the World Health Organization,[73] except for sperm morphology, which is assessed with the strict criteria.[74] Semen values are considered normal if the volume of the ejaculate is at least 2 mL, sperm concentration is at least 20×10^6/mL, progressive sperm motility is at least 40%, and normal sperm morphology is at least 14%. The distribution of characteristics of the freshly ejaculated semen used in 4035 ICSI cycles revealed that all three semen values were abnormal in 46% of the cycles, two semen values were abnormal in 29% of the cycles, one semen value was abnormal in 17% of the cycles, and all three semen values were normal in 9% of the cycles. Most of the couples with normal semen values had had previous conventional IVF treatments that failed.

The preparation of the ejaculated sperm for ICSI involves the following steps: removal of the seminal fluid by means of washing with culture medium, centrifugation at 1800g for 5 minutes, and removal of the supernatant; passage through two or three layers of a discontinuous Percoll gradient; and a final concentration step immediately before the injection procedure.[72,75–77]

Epididymal sperm is usually recovered from the most proximal part of the caput of the epididymis in a microsurgical procedure. During microsurgical epididymal sperm aspiration, several sperm fractions are collected into separate tubes. Sperm fractions with similar concentration and motility are pooled and then treated in the same way as ejaculated semen. Whenever possible, a part of the freshly recovered sperm should be frozen for later use to avoid a surgical procedure in subsequent cycles.[72,76]

Testicular spermatozoa are isolated from a testicular biopsy specimen, which is usually obtained by means of surgical excisional biopsy performed with general anesthesia. The testicular biopsy specimen is transferred to a Petri dish with HEPES-buffered Earle's medium and shredded into small pieces with sterile microscope slides on the heated stage of a stereomicroscope. The presence of spermatozoa is assessed on the inverted microscope. The pieces of the biopsy tissue are removed, and the medium is centrifuged at 300g for 5 minutes. The pellet is then resuspended for the ICSI procedure.[72,76,78]

Intracytoplasmic Sperm Injection Procedure

Microtool preparation and the actual microinjection procedure are the central components of ICSI. They have been described in detail in several publications.[47,48,72] Holding and injection pipettes are made from washed borosilicate glass capillary tubes that are first pulled on a horizontal microelectrode puller and then sharpened at the end of the injection pipette with a microgrinder and microforge. The injection pipette has a 5 to 6 μm inner and a 7 to 8 μm outer diameter. The holding pipette has a 10 to 20 μm inner and a 60 to 80 μm outer diameter. Both needles are bent to an angle of about 40° to allow them to be used parallel to the injection dish.

Eight droplets of 5 μL HEPES-buffered Earle's medium are placed on the bottom of the injection dish surrounding a central droplet of medium with 10% polyvinylpyrrolidone and 1 μL of the resuspended sperm droplet. The ICSI procedure is performed on the heated stage of an inverted microscope at 400× magnification using the Hoffman modulation contrast system. The holding and injection pipettes are fixed into a tool holder and connected to a micrometer-type microinjector. The movement of the pipettes is coordinated with two coarse positioning manipulators and two three-dimensional hydraulic remote-control micromanipulators.

A single, living, immobilized spermatozoan is aspirated, tail first, into the injection pipette. The oocyte is fixed with the holding pipette; care is taken that the polar body is situated at the 6 o'clock position. The injection pipette is pushed through the zona pellucida and into the cytoplasm at the 3 o'clock position, and the sperm is delivered with the smallest possible amount of medium.[79] Orienting the oocyte in this way minimizes the risk that the injection pipette will damage the metaphase plate. It is useful to aspirate the cytoplasm gently into the injection pipette before the sperm injection to be certain the tip of the pipette has penetrated the oolemma rather than simply indenting it.

After injection the oocytes are washed and stored in 25-μL microdrops of B$_2$ medium in a Petri dish and stored at 37°C in an incubator containing 5% carbon dioxide, 5% oxygen, and 90% nitrogen.

Oocyte Damage and Pronuclear Status after ICSI

Sixteen to eighteen hours after ICSI, oocytes are inspected for intactness and fertilization.[80] The number and aspect of polar bodies and pronuclei are recorded. Oocytes are considered to be normally fertilized when two individualized or fragmented polar bodies are present together with two clearly visible pronuclei that contain nucleoli. In 4569 cycles ICSI was performed on 48,393 metaphase II oocytes (a mean of 10.6 oocytes per cycle). The number of intact oocytes was 43,332 (89.5% of the oocytes that received injections). One can anticipate that the oocyte will be damaged or the zona pellucida will break in approximately 10% of instances. The mean number of successfully injected oocytes was 9.5 per treatment. Normally fertilized oocytes result in nearly 71% of oocytes that receive successful injections, 63.5% of metaphase II oocytes, and 50.3% of retrieved cumulus-oocyte complexes. Abnormal fertilization occurs in 3.3% (1419) of intact pronuclear oocytes, and 4.6% (2010) of intact oocytes demonstrate three pronuclei. Unlike in conventional IVF, one-pronucleus oocytes resulting from ICSI generally do not demonstrate change when reassessed for pronuclear status a few hours after the initial observation.[81] If these abnormally fertilized oocytes cleave, they are not transferred, because they are likely to be parthenogenetically activated as a result of mechanical or chemical factors. The occasional finding of three-pronucleus oocytes after injection of a single spermatozoon into the ooplasm is probably caused by nonextrusion of the second polar body at the time of fertilization.

Damage and pronuclear status after ICSI were analyzed for the four types of sperm (ejaculated, fresh and frozen-thawed epididymal, and testicular) used to perform ICSI (Table 43–1). The percentage of oocytes that remain intact after ICSI varies between 89.1% and 91.8% and is similar for the four different types of spermatozoa. The percentage of oocytes fertilized normally (two pronuclei) varies between 53.4% and 64.8%. The

normal fertilization rate for ICSI is higher when ejaculated sperm is used than when other types of sperm are used, a statistically significant difference. The percentage of oocytes with one pronucleus after ICSI varies between 2.8% and 4.2%. The percentage of oocytes with three pronuclei after ICSI varies between 4.0% and 5.6%. There is no statistically significant difference in the abnormal fertilization rates for the four different types of spermatozoa used.

The exceptional circumstance in which no oocytes that receive injections normally fertilize occurs when only one metaphase II oocyte is available for ICSI, only totally immotile spermatozoa are available for the injection, gross abnormalities are present in the oocytes, round-headed spermatozoa are injected, and all oocytes are damaged in the injection procedure. Most of these patients achieve fertilization in a subsequent cycle.[82]

Embryo Development, Transfer, and Freezing

After successful fertilization, pregnancy potential depends on embryo cleavage of the two-pronucleus oocytes after a further 24 hours of in vitro culture. The cleaving embryos should be scored according to equality of size of the blastomeres and number of anucleate fragments and further classified into three categories according to the percentage of anucleate fragments: excellent, type A embryos (without anucleate fragments); good-quality, type B embryos (between 1% and 20% of the volume filled with anucleate fragments); and fair-quality, type C embryos (between 21% and 50% anucleate fragments). Cleaved embryos with less than half of their volume filled with anucleate fragments are eligible for transfer. Supernumerary embryos with less than 20% anucleate fragments are cryopreserved on day 2 or day 3 after oocyte retrieval by means of a slow-freezing protocol with dimethylsulfoxide.[83–85]

In our experience, the total number of embryos of sufficient quality to be transferred, that is, those with less than 50% anucleate fragments, was 24,507 (79.8% of the two-pronucleus oocytes, 56.6% of the oocytes that received successful injections, 50.6% of the metaphase II oocytes, and 40.1% of the retrieved cumulus-oocyte complexes.

The percentages of two-pronucleus oocytes that developed to excellent, good-quality, and fair-quality embryos for the different types of spermatozoa used for ICSI are summarized in Table 43–2. One-way analysis of variance showed a significantly different distribution in percentages of good-quality embryos for the four types of spermatozoa. The percentages of embryos actually transferred or frozen as supernumerary embryos was similar for the four types of spermatozoa and varied between 62.6% and 65.1% of the two-pronucleus oocytes.

Embryo replacement was possible in 4227 of the 4569 treatment cycles with ICSI (92.5%). This can be considered a

TABLE 43–1. SPERM ORIGIN AND DAMAGE AND PRONUCLEAR STATUS OF OOCYTES AFTER ICSI (1991–1995)

| | Ejaculated | Epididymal | | Testicular |
		Fresh	Frozen-thawed	
No. of oocytes receiving ICSI	41,912	1747	929	3805
Percentage of oocytes intact	89.5	89.7	91.8	89.1
Percentage of injected oocytes with				
One pronucleus	2.8	4.2	3.3	4.1
Two pronuclei	64.8 [a]	58.5 [b]	54.7 [a]	53.4 [a,b]
Three pronuclei	4.1	5.0	5.6	4.0

[a,b] $P<0.001$ by one-way analysis of variance.

TABLE 43-2. SPERM ORIGIN AND EMBRYO DEVELOPMENT AFTER ICSI (1991–1995)

| | | Epididymal | | |
	Ejaculated	Fresh	Frozen-thawed	Testicular
No. of two-pronucleus oocytes	27,161	1022	508	2030
Percentage excellent embryos	6.9	7.1	3.7	6.0
Percentage good-quality embryos	59.0 [a]	49.0 [a]	48.0 [a]	47.0 [a]
Percentage fair-quality embryos	15.0	14.5	17.7	18.7
Percentage transferred or frozen embryos	65.1	63.9	62.6	62.6

[a] $P<0.01$

high transfer rate because it represents couples with previous fertilization failure in conventional IVF, ejaculated sperm too poor to be included in IVF, or men with obstructive or nonobstructive azoospermia. As indicated in Table 43–3, the percentage of transfers was not different among the four groups of sperm used for ICSI; the transfer rate varied from 88.3% to 93.0%. The overall pregnancy rate per transfer and the pregnancy rate per number of embryos transferred were similar for the four types of sperm. Especially high pregnancy rates were noticed when elective transfer of two or three embryos was performed.[85,86]

Obstetric Outcome, Prenatal Diagnosis, and Follow-Up Study with the Children

Because of the novelty and the many unknown aspects of ICSI, couples in our program were counseled extensively and asked to adhere to genetic counseling, prenatal testing, and participation in a prospective clinical follow-up study involving the children.[58–64]

As of February 1996, 705 prenatal diagnoses had been obtained about pregnancies resulting from ICSI. Among these 705 samples obtained through either chorionic villus sampling

(CVS) or amniocentesis, 11 (1.6%) de novo chromosomal anomalies were found. Six were sex-chromosomal aberrations (three 47,XXY; one 47,XXX; one 47,XYY; and one mosaic 46,XX/47,XXX). The remaining chromosomal anomalies were two trisomy 21 and three unbalanced translocations. These data suggest there might be a slightly increased risk of sex-chromosomal anomalies among children conceived after ICSI as compared with the prevalence among the general population or at prenatal diagnosis performed because of maternal age. Two abnormal postnatal karyotypes were also observed: one trisomy 21 and one 47,XXY.

As of February 1996, among 1123 children born after ICSI, 28 (2.5%) serious malformations leading to functional impairment or necessitating surgical treatment had been observed. This malformation rate is similar to the numbers found in population surveys or among children born after assisted procreative procedures other than ICSI.[63]

Although there is no indication of an increase in serious congenital malformations after replacement of embryos obtained after ICSI, it is important to continue this careful prospective follow-up study with the children in different centers practicing ICSI. This is one of the goals of the Task Force on ICSI established by the European Society of Human Reproduction and Embryology.[60]

SUMMARY

The limited potential to achieve successful pregnancy outcomes in the presence of severe male-factor infertility has been one of the limitations of assisted reproduction. As a result of ICSI, this limitation has been greatly overcome. Nevertheless, despite this breakthrough in the management of male-factor infertility, children resulting from the ICSI procedure must be followed postpartum so that future patients may receive thorough counseling.

TABLE 43-3. SPERM ORIGIN AND OUTCOME OF EMBRYO TRANSFERS AFTER ICSI (1991–1995)

| | | Epididymal | | |
	Ejaculated	Fresh	Frozen-thawed	Testicular
No. of cycles	4035	145	77	314
Transfer rate (%)	93.0	91.7	88.3	91.1
Pregnancy rate per transfer (%)	35.9 (3751)	45.1 (133)	32.4 (68)	33.9 (286)
One embryo	12.5 (312)	25.0 (4)	12.5 (8)	9.7 (31)
Two embryos	22.5 (494)	29.4 (17)	9.1 (11)	24.3 (37)
Two embryos (elective)	41.9 (733)	31.6 (19)	40.0 (5)	26.9 (26)
Three embryos	38.2 (1068)	51.2 (41)	33.3 (15)	38.0 (71)
Three embryos (elective)	45.3 (838)	53.3 (30)	52.9 (17)	39.6 (48)
More than three embryos	32.7 (306)	50.0 (22)	33.3 (12)	43.8 (73)
Pregnancy rate per cycle (%)	33.3	41.4	28.6	30.1

Values in parentheses are numbers of cycles.

ACKNOWLEDGMENTS

The authors are indebted to their many clinical, scientific, nursing and technical colleagues of the Centre for Reproductive Medicine and the Centre for Medical Genetics. Viviane De Wolf typeset the manuscript. This work is supported by several grants from the Belgian Fund for Medical Research. The children follow-up program was supported by an unconditional grant from Organon International.

REFERENCES

1. Mahadevan MM, Trounson AO: The influence of seminal characteristics on the success rate of human in vitro fertilization. *Fertil Steril* 42:400, 1984

2. Yovich JL, Stanger JD: The limitations of in vitro fertilization from males with severe oligospermia and abnormal sperm morphology. *J In Vitro Fertil Embryo Transf* 1:172, 1984

3. Tournaye H, Camus M, Khan I, Staessen C, Van Steirteghem AC, Devroey P: In-vitro fertilization, gamete- or zygote intra-fallopian transfer for the treatment of male infertility. *Hum Reprod* 6:263, 1991

4. Tournaye H, Devroey P, Camus M, Valkenburg M, Bollen N, Van Steirteghem AC: Zygote intrafallopian transfer or in vitro fertilization and embryo transfer for the treatment of male-factor infertility: A prospective randomized trial. *Fertil Steril* 58:344, 1992

5. Oehninger S, Acosta AA, Morshedi M, et al: Corrective measures and pregnancy outcome in in vitro fertilization in patients with severe sperm morphology abnormalities. *Fertil Steril* 50:283, 1988

6. Ord T, Patrizio P, Balmaceda JP, Asch RH: Can severe male factor infertility be treated without micromanipulation? *Fertil Steril* 60:110, 1993

7. Van der Ven H, Hoebbel K, Al-Hasani S, Diedrich K, Krebs D: Fertilization of human oocytes in capillary tubes using very low number of spermatozoa: A new treatment of severe oligozoospermia? *Ann Urol* 23:317, 1989

8. Hammit DG, Walker DL, Syrop CH, Miller TM, Bennet MR: Treatment of severe male-factor infertility with high concentrations of motile sperm by microinsemination in embryo cryopreservation straws. *J In Vitro Fertil Embryo Transf* 8:101, 1991

9. Van der Ven HH, Jeyendran RS, Al-Hasani S, et al: Glass wool column filtration of human semen: Relation of swim-up procedure and outcome of IVF. *Hum Reprod* 3:85, 1988

10. Ord T, Patrizio P, Marello E, Balmaceda JP, Asch RH: Mini-Percoll: A new method of semen preparation for IVF in severe male factor infertility. *Hum Reprod* 5:987, 1990

11. Sapienza F, Verheyen G, Tournaye H, et al: An auto-controlled study in in-vitro fertilization reveals the benefit of Percoll centrifugation to swim-up in the preparation of poor-quality semen. *Hum Reprod* 8:1856, 1993

12. Yovich JM, Edirisinghe WR, Cummins JM, Yovich JL: Preliminary results using pentoxifylline in a pronuclear stage tubal transfer (PROST) program for severe male factor infertility. *Fertil Steril* 50:179, 1988

13. Yovich JM, Edirisinghe WR, Cummins JM, Yovich JL: Influence of pentoxifylline in severe male factor infertility. *Fertil Steril* 53:715, 1990

14. Laws-King A, Trounson A, Sathananthan H, Kola I: Fertilization of human oocytes by microinjection of a single spermatozoon under the zona pellucida. *Fertil Steril* 48:637, 1987

15. Tournaye H, Devroey P, Camus M, et al: Comparison of in-vitro fertilization in male and tubal infertility: A 3 year survey. *Hum Reprod* 7:218, 1992

16. Tournaye H, Janssens R, Camus M, Staessen C, Devroey P, Van Steirteghem A: Pentoxifylline is not useful in enhancing sperm function in cases with previous in vitro fertilization failure. *Fertil Steril* 59:210, 1993

17. Tournaye H, Janssens R, Verheyen G, Camus M, Devroey P, Van Steirteghem A: An indiscriminate use of pentoxifylline does not improve in-vitro fertilization in poor fertilizers. *Hum Reprod* 9:1289, 1994

18. Tournaye H, Janssens R, Verheyen G, Devroey P, Van Steirteghem A: In vitro fertilization in couples with previous fertilization failure using sperm incubated with pentoxifylline and 2-deoxyadenosine. *Fertil Steril* 62:574, 1994

19. Uehara T, Yanagimachi R: Microsurgical injection of spermatozoa into hamster eggs with subsequent transformation of sperm nuclei into male pronuclei. *Biol Reprod* 15:467, 1976

20. Thadani VM: A study of hetero-specific sperm-egg interactions in the rat, mouse and deer mouse using in vitro fertilization and sperm injection. *J Exp Zool* 212:435, 1980

21. Markert CL: Fertilization of mammalian eggs by sperm injection. *J Exp Zool* 228:195, 1983

22. Barg PE, Wahrman MZ, Talansky BE, Gordon JW: Capacitated, acrosome-reacted but immotile sperm, when microinjected under the mouse zona pellucida, will not fertilize the oocyte. *J Exp Zool* 237:365, 1986

23. Mann JR: Full-term development of mouse eggs fertilized by a spermatozoon microinjected under the zona pellucida. *Biol Reprod* 38:1077, 1988

24. Lacham O, Trounson A, Holden C, Mann J, Sathananthan H: Fertilization and development of mouse eggs injected under the zona pellucida with single spermatozoa treated to induce the acrosome reaction. *Gamete Res* 23:233, 1989

25. Palermo G, Van Steirteghem A: Enhancement of acrosome reaction and subzonal insemination of a single spermatozoon in mouse eggs. *Mol Reprod Dev* 30:339, 1991

26. Lasalle B, Courtot AM, Testart J: In vitro fertilization of hamster and human oocytes by microinjection of human sperm. *Gamete Res* 16:69, 1987

27. Martin RH, Ko E, Rademaker A: Human sperm chromosome complements after microinjection of hamster eggs. *J Reprod Fertil* 84:179, 1988

28. Lanzendorf S, Maloney M, Ackerman S, Acosta A, Hodgen G: Fertilizing potential of acrosome-defective sperm following microsurgical injection into eggs. *Gamete Res* 19:329, 1988

29. Lanzendorf SE, Maloney MK, Veeck LL, Slusser J, Hodgen GD,

Rosenwaks Z: A preclinical evaluation of pronuclear formation by microinjection of human spermatozoa into human oocytes. *Fertil Steril* 49:835, 1988

30. Lasalle B, Testart J: Human sperm injection into the perivitelline space (SI-PVS) of hamster oocytes: Effect of sperm pretreatment by calcium-ionophore A23187 and freezing-thawing on the penetration rate and polyspermy. *Gamete Res* 20:301, 1988

31. Cohen J, Adler A, Alikano M, et al: Assisted fertilization and abnormal sperm function. *Semin Reprod Endocrinol* 11:83, 1993

32. Fishel S, Dowell K, Timson J, Green S, Hall J, Klentzeris L: Micro-assisted fertilization with human gametes. *Hum Reprod* 8:1780, 1993

33. Imoedemhe DAG, Sigue AB: Subzonal multiple sperm injection in the treatment of previous failed human in vitro fertilization. *Fertil Steril* 59:172, 1993

34. Lippi J, Mortimer D, Jansen RPS: Subzonal insemination for extreme male factor infertility. *Hum Reprod* 8:939, 1993

35. Palermo G, Joris H, Devroey P, Van Steirteghem AC: Induction of acrosome reaction in human spermatozoa used for subzonal insemination. *Hum Reprod* 7:248, 1992

36. Palermo G, Joris H, Derde M-P, Camus M, Devroey P, Van Steirteghem AC: Sperm characteristics and outcome of human assisted fertilization by subzonal insemination and intracytoplasmic sperm injection. *Fertil Steril* 59:826, 1993

37. Van Steirteghem A, Liu J, Nagy Z, et al: Use of assisted fertilization. *Hum Reprod* 8:1784, 1993

38. Cohen J, Malter H, Wright H, Kort H, Massey J, Mitchell D: Partial zona dissection of human oocytes when failure of zona pellucida penetration is anticipated. *Hum Reprod* 4:435, 1989

39. Cohen J, Talansky BE, Malter H, et al: Microsurgical fertilization and teratozoospermia. *Hum Reprod* 6:118, 1991

40. Cohen J, Alikani M, Adler A, et al: Microsurgical fertilization procedures: The absence of stringent criteria for patient selection. *J Assist Reprod Genet* 9:197, 1992

41. Fishel S, Timson J, Lisi F, Rinaldi L: Evaluation of 225 patients undergoing subzonal insemination for the procurement of fertilization in vitro. *Fertil Steril* 57:840, 1992

42. Ng S-C, Bongso A, Ratnam SS: Microinjection of human oocytes: A technique for severe oligoasthenoteratozoospermia. *Fertil Steril* 56:1117, 1991

43. Van Steirteghem A, Nagy Z, Liu J, et al: Intracytoplasmic sperm injection. *Baillieres Clin Obstet Gynaecol* 8:85, 1994

44. Palermo G, Joris H, Devroey P, Van Steirteghem AC: Pregnancies after intracytoplasmic injection of single spermatozoon into an oocyte. *Lancet* 340:17, 1992

45. Iritani A: Micromanipulation of gametes for in vitro assisted fertilization. *Mol Reprod Dev* 28:199, 1991

46. Veeck LL, Oehninger S, Acosta AA, Muasher SJ: Sperm microinjection in a clinical in vitro fertilization program. Proceedings of the 45th Annual Meeting of the American Fertility Society, 1989, San Francisco

47. Van Steirteghem AC, Liu J, Joris H, et al: Higher success rate by intracytoplasmic sperm injection than by subzonal insemination: Report of a second series of 300 consecutive treatment cycles. *Hum Reprod* 8:1055, 1993

48. Van Steirteghem AC, Nagy Z, Joris H, et al: High fertilization and implantation rates after intracytoplasmic sperm injection. *Hum Reprod* 8:1061, 1993

49. Silber SJ, Nagy ZP, Liu J, Godoy H, Devroey P, Van Steirteghem AC: Conventional in-vitro fertilization versus intracytoplasmic sperm injection for patients requiring microsurgical sperm aspiration. *Hum Reprod* 9:1705, 1994

50. Tournaye H, Devroey P, Liu J, Nagy Z, Lissens W, Van Steirteghem A: Microsurgical epididymal sperm aspiration and intracytoplasmic sperm injection: A new effective approach to infertility as a result of congenital bilateral absence of the vas deferens. *Fertil Steril* 61:1045, 1994

51. Devroey P, Silber S, Nagy Z, et al: Ongoing pregnancies and birth after intracytoplasmic sperm injection with frozen-thawed epididymal spermatozoa. *Hum Reprod* 10:903, 1995

52. Silber SJ, Nagy Z, Liu J, et al: The use of epididymal and testicular spermatozoa for intracytoplasmic sperm injection: The genetic implications for male infertility. *Hum Reprod* 10:2031, 1995

53. Devroey P, Liu J, Nagy Z, Tournaye H, Silber SJ, Van Steirteghem AC: Normal fertilization of human oocytes after testicular sperm extraction and intracytoplasmic sperm injection. *Fertil Steril* 62:639, 1994

54. Silber SJ, Van Steirteghem AC, Liu J, Nagy Z, Tournaye H, Devroey P: High fertilization and pregnancy rate after intracytoplasmic sperm injection with spermatozoa obtained from testicle biopsy. *Hum Reprod* 10:148, 1995

55. Devroey P, Liu J, Nagy Z, et al: Pregnancies after testicular sperm extraction and intracytoplasmic sperm injection in non-obstructive azoospermia. *Hum Reprod* 10:1457, 1995

56. Tournaye H, Camus M, Goossens A, et al: Recent concepts in the management of infertility because of non-obstructive azoospermia. *Hum Reprod* 10(Suppl 1):115, 1995

57. Tournaye H, Liu J, Nagy P, et al: Correlation between testicular histology and outcome after intracytoplasmic sperm injection using testicular spermatozoa. *Hum Reprod* 1:127, 1996

58. Bonduelle M, Desmyttere S, Buysse A, et al: Prospective follow-up study of 55 children born after subzonal insemination and intracytoplasmic sperm injection. *Hum Reprod* 9:1765, 1994

59. Bonduelle M, Legein J, Derde M-P, et al: Comparative follow-up study of 130 children born after intracytoplasmic sperm injection and 130 children born after in-vitro fertilization. *Hum Reprod* 10:3327, 1995

60. Bonduelle M, Hamberger L, Joris H, Tarlatzis BC, Van Steirteghem AC: Assisted reproduction by intracytoplasmic sperm injection: An ESHRE survey of clinical experiences until 31 December 1993. *Hum Reprod Update* (CD-ROM) 1: no. 3, 1995

61. Bonduelle M, Legein J, Buysse A, et al: Prospective follow-up study of 423 children born after intracytoplasmic sperm injection. *Hum Reprod* 11:1558, 1996

62. Liebaers I, Bonduelle M, Legein J, et al: Follow-up of children born after intracytoplasmic sperm injection. In: Hedon B, Bringer J, Mares P (eds), *Fertility and Sterility: A Current Overview.* Proceedings of the 15th World Congress on Fertility and Sterility, September 17–22, 1995, Montpellier, France. London, England, Parthenon, 1995:409–412

63. Liebaers I, Bonduelle M, Van Assche E, Devroey P, Van Steirteghem A: Sex chromosome abnormalities after intracytoplasmic sperm injection. *Lancet* 346:1095, 1995

64. Wisanto A, Magnus M, Bonduelle M, et al: Obstetric outcome of 424 pregnancies after intracytoplasmic sperm injection. *Hum Reprod* 10:2713, 1995

65. Smitz J, Devroey P, Camus M, et al: The luteal phase and early pregnancy after combined GnRH-agonist/HMG treatment for superovulation in IVF or GIFT. *Hum Reprod* 3:585, 1988

66. Smitz J, Devroey P, Camus M, Wisanto A, Khan I, Van Steirteghem AC: Gonadotropin treatment in patients with previously failed stimulations for in vitro fertilization. *Infertility* 12:73, 1989

67. Smitz J, Bourgain C, Devroey P, Camus M, Wisanto A, Van Steirteghem AC: Endocrinologia y morfologia del endometrio en la fase luteinica tras superovulacion mediante analogos de la GnRH. In: Calaf J (ed), *GnRH y Analogos en Medicina Reproductiva*. Barcelona, Espaxs, 1990:163–188

68. Smitz J, Van Dessel A, Camus M, et al: Comparison of different dosage regimens of LHRH analogues in GIFT, ZIFT or IVF. In: Brosens I, Jacobs HS, Runnebaum B (eds), *LHRH Analogues in Gynaecology*. Carnforth, England, Parthenon, 1990:35–41

69. Smitz J, Devroey P, Faguer B, Bourgain C, Camus M, Van Steirteghem AC: A prospective randomized comparison of intramuscular or intravaginal progesterone as a luteal phase and early pregnancy supplement. *Hum Reprod* 7:168, 1992

70. Smitz J, Van den Abbeel E, Bollen N, et al: The effect of gonadotropin-releasing hormone (GnRH) agonist in the follicular phase on in-vitro fertilization outcome in normo-ovulatory women. *Hum Reprod* 7:1098, 1992

71. Smitz J, Bourgain C, Van Waesberghe L, Camus M, Devroey P, Van Steirteghem AC: A prospective randomized study on oestradiol valerate supplementation in addition to intravaginal micronized progesterone in buserelin and HMG induced superovulation. *Hum Reprod* 8:40, 1993

72. Van Steirteghem AC, Joris H, Liu J, et al: Protocol for intracytoplasmic sperm injection. *Hum Reprod Update* (CD-ROM) 1: no. 3, 1995

73. World Health Organization: WHO Laboratory Manual for the Examination of Human Semen and Sperm Cervical Mucus Interaction. Cambridge, Cambridge University Press, 1992

74. Kruger TF, Menkveld R, Stander FSH, et al: Sperm morphologic features as a prognostic factor in in vitro fertilization. *Fertil Steril* 46:1118, 1986

75. Liu J, Nagy Z, Joris H, Tournaye H, Devroey P, Van Steirteghem AC: Intracytoplasmic sperm injection does not require special treatment of the spermatozoa. *Hum Reprod* 9:1127, 1994

76. Nagy Z, Liu J, Janssenswillen C, Silber S, Devroey P, Van Steirteghem A: Using ejaculated, fresh, and frozen-thawed epididymal and testicular spermatozoa gives rise to comparable results after intracytoplasmic sperm injection. *Fertil Steril* 63:808, 1995

77. Nagy ZP, Liu J, Joris H, et al: The result of intracytoplasmic sperm injection is not related to any of the three basic sperm parameters. *Hum Reprod* 10:1123, 1995

78. Verheyen G, De Croo I, Tournaye H, Pletincx I, Devroey P, Van Steirteghem AC: Comparison of four mechanical methods to retrieve spermatozoa from testicular tissue. *Hum Reprod* 10:2956, 1995

79. Nagy ZP, Liu J, Joris H, et al: The influence of the site of sperm deposition and mode of oolemma breakage at intracytoplasmic sperm injection on fertilization and embryo development rates. *Hum Reprod* 10:3171, 1995

80. Nagy ZP, Liu J, Joris H, Devroey P, Van Steirteghem A: Timecourse of oocyte activation, pronucleus formation and cleavage in human oocytes fertilized by intracytoplasmic sperm injection. *Hum Reprod* 9:1743, 1994

81. Staessen C, Janssenswillen C, Devroey P, Van Steirteghem AC: Cytogenetic and morphological observations of single pronucleated human oocytes after in-vitro fertilization. *Hum Reprod* 8:221, 1993

82. Liu J, Nagy Z, Joris H, et al: Analysis of 76 total fertilization failure cycles out of 2732 intracytoplasmic sperm injection cycles. *Hum Reprod* 10:2630, 1995

83. Van Steirteghem AC, Van der Elst J, Van den Abbeel E, Joris H, Camus M, Devroey P: Cryopreservation of supernumerary multicellular human embryos obtained after intracytoplasmic sperm injection. *Fertil Steril* 62:775, 1994

84. Van der Elst J, Camus M, Van den Abbeel E, Maes R, Devroey P, Van Steirteghem AC: Prospective randomized study on the cryopreservation of human embryos with dimethylsulfoxide or 1,2-propanediol protocols. *Fertil Steril* 63:92, 1995

85. Staessen C, Nagy ZP, Liu J, et al: One year's experience with elective transfer of two good quality embryos in the human in-vitro fertilization and intracytoplasmic sperm injection programmes. *Hum Reprod* 10:3305, 1995

86. Staessen C, Janssenswillen C, Van den Abbeel E, Devroey P, Van Steirteghem AC: Avoidance of triplet pregnancies by elective transfer of two good quality embryos. *Hum Reprod* 8:1650, 1993

CHAPTER 44

Preimplantation Genetics and Preimplantation Diagnosis

MOSHE ZILBERSTEIN · MACHELLE M. SEIBEL

What Can Be Done?
Polar-body biopsy
Preembryo biopsy
Polymerase chain reaction
Fluorescent in situ hybridization
What Should Be Done?

The ambition of medicine traditionally has been to prevent and eliminate disease. The recent unprecedented advances in understanding the genetic basis of human diseases have raised our hopes and expectations even higher. Techniques emanating from various disciplines (bacteriology, virology, cell biology, and molecular biology) allow rapid identification of human genes and mutations. Because of the potential impact of expanded genetic knowledge, the Human Genome Project has been developed. It is a testimony to the formidable scientific and financial commitment of the United States to mapping, cloning, and sequencing the 3.3 billion DNA base pairs that constitute the human genome. Similarly large-scale efforts have been established in Europe. The proclaimed aspiration of these outstanding endeavors is to benefit humankind by providing an understanding of many human diseases that originate in faulty genes.[1] The prediction is that first this will lead to more accurate ways of screening and diagnosing genetic diseases. It is hoped that the information may be applied to specific genetic cures for many diseases.[2]

Assisted reproductive technology (ART) concurrently has become streamlined and simplified because of advances such as transvaginal egg retrieval, intracytoplasmic single-sperm injection (ICSI) (see Chapters 42 and 43), and other micromanipulation techniques.[3,4] Embryo freezing and improved implantation rates improve overall success. The convergence of ART and genetics led to the newly emerging field of *preimplantation genetics*. This frontier of medicine—the genetic make-up of the human embryo—is shrouded with clinical, ethical, legal, and political issues that make it highly controversial.[5] The objective of this chapter is to describe preimplantation diagnosis. Although only a few centers around the world offer this technology, preimplantation diagnosis is rapidly evolving and will probably become more widespread in coming years.

The two principal components of preimplantation genetics are preimplantation diagnosis and germ-line gene therapy.[5] The first is a modality of the present and near future; the latter is predicted by some to emerge in the distant future.[6] A high level of anxiety has been expressed specifically about germ-line gene therapy to the point of condemnation and the crafting of anticipatory policies by some political and professional authorities.[6,7]

The imminent implementation of preimplantation diagnosis into ART practice is a source of excitement for some and a source of anxiety for others.[5,8] At the core of this mixed reaction lies the illusion created by the media and practitioners alike that "everything is possible" and therefore "anything that can be done will be done."[8] It seems appropriate for this chapter to address the pertinent social and ethical issues that are integral to preimplantation genetic diagnosis (PGD) before describing its technical aspects. It is surprising that these two issues—the technical and the ethical—are usually presented separately by different authors from different disciplines (ART practitioners present the technical aspects, ethicists or attorneys present the ethical and legal). PGD is presented by prominent practitioners of ART as the ultimate prenatal medicine and potentially also the ultimate in disease prevention.[9] Because of the need to both establish clear indications and consider ethical implications, preimplantation diagnosis is introduced as an extension of amniocentesis and chorionic villus sampling (CVS), merely drawing prenatal screening and diagnosis to an earlier stage of embryo development.[10] Although this new technique soothed some concerns about the consequences of prenatal diagnosis (that is, pregnancy termination after implantation), it also raised many old and new public concerns regarding embryo research.

On the one hand, some authors believe that practitioners have demonstrated appropriate sensitivity; for example, the editorial opinion in the journal *Nature* was, *"Given the proper delicacy with which physicians working in these fields approach these issues (and the supervision of ethical committees), fear that whole societies will suddenly be overwhelmed by novel methods of reproduction are needless self-induced nightmares."*[8] Many others believe, however, that *"for all the worried talk about genetic engineering over the last two decades, it is surprising how quietly plans for the genetic diagnosis of human embryos have developed."*[11] In this way, the introduction of preimplantation diagnosis into mainstream prenatal diagnosis renewed the longstanding debate over the morality of prenatal diagnosis per se.[12–15] It is beyond the scope of this chapter to detail the different sides in this debate, nor is it our intention to promote a certain position regarding preimplantation diagnosis in this context. When we initiated the preimplantation diagnosis program at the Faulkner Centre for Reproductive Medicine, we were very much aware of the controversy. We also recognized the unique opportunity to develop a paradigm for the introduction of novel technology in reproduction. Our aim was to develop governing principles that would establish the groundwork for later oversight when and if it occurred.

PGD is currently an experimental procedure. Therefore it must comply with and be subjected to the same restrictions applicable to similar research propositions.[16] When our center established similar programs in the past, namely the gamete donation program, a voluntary ethics advisory board was formed to serve as a testing ground and a sounding board for ideas and technology. Team members were able to observe the reflection

of their ideas among this pluralistic body of experts and scholars. We have found the forum of an ethics advisory board an outstanding instrument for ongoing development of ethical concepts applicable to the local milieu in which the clinic practices. Issues such as informed consent, indications for PGD, patient selection, and specific patient requests such as sex selection were presented to the group. After most of the ethical ground was explored with the ethics advisory board, the team presented an investigational protocol to the institutional review board and obtained the appropriate approval.

Before offering PGD, our team presented the procedure to our immediate public. Using a small grant from New England Regional Genetic Group (NERGG) and our personal funding, we invited a wide range of experts, disability groups, students, general public, reproductive endocrinologists, geneticists, ethicists, legal experts, health policy experts, and patients to an open forum. To avoid flagrant conflicts of interest or bias we allowed the NERGG social and ethics committee to choose the faculty to attract participants with opposing views. The course was aimed at discussion of PGD: What can be done? What should be done? After presenting a short introduction of what can be done, the dialogues throughout most of the day continued in informal presentations and workshops[17] that discussed what should be done. Such interaction with the community before the introduction of new technology allowed us to understand its need and place among our immediate potential patients. It also allowed us to build some level of mutual trust and ongoing dialogue.

One should be cognizant that for the initiation of a successful PGD program one needs to have in place a successful ART program with personnel capable of using micromanipulation techniques to inject sperm into eggs and to obtain polar bodies and single blastomeres for diagnosis. ICSI is becoming common in many programs. The more difficult requirements to implement in PGD programs are the establishment of sophisticated and accurate molecular diagnostic capability for single cells and the ability to counsel patients appropriately for such testing.[10]

WHAT CAN BE DONE?

PGD was originally devised to allow couples with known inherited disease the opportunity to test eggs before fertilization or test embryos before transfer and implantation. The state of the art to date requires use of in vitro fertilization (IVF) systems. Embryo flushing[18,19] from the uterus after in vivo fertilization but before implantation is not yet developed into a valid option because of the risk that some fertilized eggs may not be flushed out.[9,18,19] To understand the premise on which PGD is performed one must be familiar with the biologic processes from which a human preembryo emerges.[20] During fertilization, the egg and the sperm unite to form a preembryo. Until this occurs, each gamete contains half the number of chromosomes and hence one half the genetic material needed to constitute the newly formed preembryo. Fertilization is a complex biochemical and molecular process that occurs after natural penetration or mechanical insertion of a sperm into an egg. In the past the limited availability of gametes and embryos for research hindered our understanding of egg maturation, fertilization, and implantation. However, novel developments in ART and advances in micromanipulation provided new insights into these processes. With understanding of the putative mechanisms involved in human gamete interaction and embryo development, implementation of PGD became feasible.[3,20]

Meiosis is the type of cell division that occurs only in germ cells. Progenitor diploid (46 chromosomes) germ cells produce haploid (23 chromosomes) gametes. Halving the chromosome number is achieved by means of a single chromosomal duplication followed by two successive meiotic nuclear divisions. The first meiotic division (meiosis) is called a *reduction division* because it reduces the chromosomal complement from diploid to haploid. At the first stage of meiosis (prophase) each chromosome has replicated and comprises two sister chromatids attached at the centromere. During prophase, homologous chromosomes pair along their entire length and into proximity by a process called *synapsis*. The chromosomes condense and become visible under the light microscope. New combinations of linked genes occur as a result of exchanging reciprocal segments of their homologous pairs of chromosomes by crossing over (recombination). During meiosis the sister chromatids remain attached at the centromere, which does not divide the individual chromosomes randomly. Chromosomes that originally came from the mother or the father move independently to either pole to form cells with haploid sets of chromosomes and double the amount of DNA. Meiosis II proceeds after a brief interphase similar to that of mitosis except that DNA synthesis and replication (*s* phase) does not occur.

The genetic consequences of meiosis are (1) reduction of the diploid set of chromosomes to haploid, (2) segregation of the genes so that each like gene of the original pair ends in a different gamete, (3) independent segregation of homologous chromosomes so that each gamete inherits some chromosomes from the mother and the father (that is, the individual from whom the gametes originate), (4) crossover between homologous chromosomes so that each chromosome possesses some genes from the mother and some from the father. Much of the development of the oocyte occurs during fetal life. Proliferation of diploid germ cells is limited in the human female embryo to the first few months after conception. Approximately 7 million oocytes are produced during fetal life (Fig 44–1). They are arrested as prophase-I primary oocytes and remain so until they

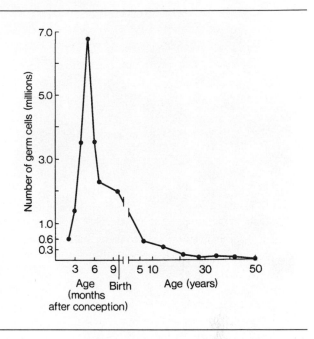

Figure 44–1. Number of germ cells at various ages after conception. (*From Baker TG, Wai Sum O: Development of the ovary and oogenesis. Clin Obstet Gynecol 3:3, 1976.*)

are recruited just before ovulation after the woman reaches reproductive maturity.

By the time a female newborn is delivered, the number of primary oocytes within her ovaries declines to approximately 4 million. Therefore, during most of their life-span, human eggs are immature and arrested in prophase of the first meiotic division. Just before ovulation a cohort of 10 to 20 eggs undergo oocyte maturation, a sequence of events that result in germinal vesicle breakdown and resumption of meiosis I. The products of meiosis result in unequal cytoplasmic division. Most of the cytoplasm and its organelles go to the secondary oocyte. A much smaller amount surrounds the nucleus of the first polar body, which contains half the chromosomes. The presence of a polar body defines a mature metaphase-II oocyte (Fig 44–2).

Meiosis II is complete only with fertilization and the formation of the second polar body, which allows the oocyte to possess the correct amount of chromatin. The chromosomes of the oocyte and those delivered by the sperm each become pronuclei surrounded by a nuclear membrane. The pronuclei fuse in the fertilized oocyte to produce a diploid zygote that divides by mitosis to form two diploid daughter cells (blastomeres). This is the first of a series of cleavage divisions that initiate embryo development. The first cleavage of human zygotes occurs 16 hours after fertilization, and the second cleavage requires approximately 12 more hours. These first two cleavages are believed to be the result of maternal mRNA expression. The preembryonic genome is believed to be expressed only after the four-cell stage.

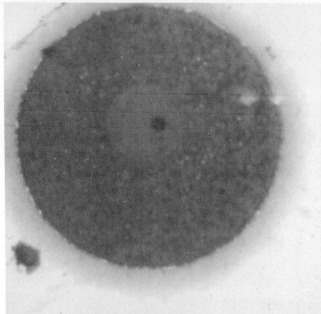

A

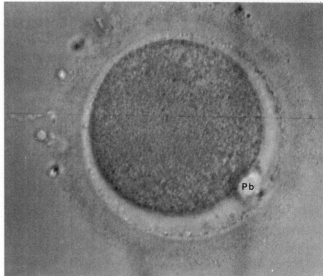

B

C

Figure 44–2. Stages of oocyte maturation. **A.** General vesicle stage oocyte. **B.** Metaphase-I oocyte with chromatin plate (arrow). Note the absence of both the nuclear membrane and a polar body. **C.** Metaphase-II oocyte with a polar body (Pb) in the perivitelline space.

The term *preembryo* includes the developmental stages that start with the first cell and end approximately 14 days after fertilization (Fig 44–3). Approximately 3 days after fertilization the preembryo contains up to eight blastomeres, a number that doubles over the next day or two. During early zygote and preembryo cell divisions the blastomeres are loosely attached to each other. As the preembryo develops further into the morula stage, the blastomeres adhere tightly to each other. Until the morula stage, each blastomere is multipotential and theoretically can give rise to a complete embryo.[21] Beyond the morula stage, the preembryo blastomeres begin to acquire designations to become specific entities. A distinct inner cell mass gives rise to the embryo. Trophoectoderm cells (outer cell mass) produce the fetal component of the placenta. During most of the developmental period (up to the blastocyst stage), the preembryo travels unattached between the fallopian tube and the uterine cavity.

Implantation is the process of preembryo attachment to the endometrium and its subsequent embedding into the uterine lining. This process is usually completed 8 to 9 days after fertilization. By approximately 14 days after fertilization, all the cells of the preembryo assume a designation to become either part of the placenta or part of the embryo proper. The preembryo stage ends approximately 2 weeks after fertilization when the preembryo becomes an embryo.

The availability of human oocytes and embryos provided by ART produced the opportunity for PGD to become an option for prenatal diagnosis. The access gained unfortunately is inherently expensive because it entails examination of material from IVF protocols, after superovulation and transvaginal ultrasound-guided needle aspiration. Most of the physical risks associated with PGD stem from the medication and the procedure[17,22,23]; they are risks that remain acceptably low.

There are three basic approaches to obtain a specimen for PGD: (1) polar-body biopsy of the unfertilized oocyte; (2)

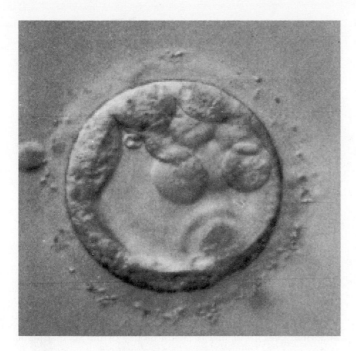

Figure 44–3. Human blastocyst.

results in a 6% rate of spontaneous nonscreened pregnancies. These detriments contraindicate the use of uterine lavage until they can be overcome. Because only some eggs or preembryos are affected (the proportion affected depends on the nature of the disorder), several must be examined to ensure that at least one unaffected egg or preembryo is identified for transfer.

Interestingly, although patients undergoing PGD are not infertile, even experienced centers such as Hamersmith Hospital and University College, London, have found that in one third of all cycles, only one embryo is considered suitable for transfer.[25,26] In this context it seems clear that for most patients the objective should be to obtain the highest possible number of eggs and preembryos. This is why most PGD medication protocols incorporate superovulation protocols that include typical luteal-phase gonadotropin-releasing hormone (GnRH) agonists and gonadotropins (Fig 44–4).

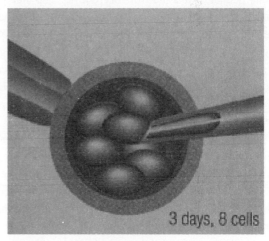

3 days, 8 cells

A

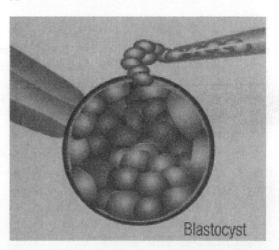

Blastocyst

B

Figure 44–4. PGD. **A.** Blastomere biopsy. **B.** Trophoectoderm biopsy (*From Carson SA, Buster JE: Diagnosis and treatment before implantation: The ultimate prenatal medicine. Contemp OB/GYN 40(12):71,1995.*)

biopsy of the preembryo after fertilization,[9,24] when blastomeres are nondifferentiated and multipotent; (3) biopsy of the later stage preembryo at a developmental stage when cells are further differentiated (Figs 44–4 and 44–5). The last biopsy approach involves removal of trophoectoderm cells that are destined to become the part of the placenta derived from the fetus (the trophoectoderm) and allows avoidance of embryonic cells (inner cell mass). Polar-body biopsy and embryo biopsy require use of ovarian stimulation, transvaginal oocyte retrieval, and IVF followed by micromanipulation of the egg or preembryo, respectively.[3,19] Trophoectoderm biopsy is aimed at retrieval preimplantation preembryos from the uterine cavity after natural spontaneous fertilization in vivo or after ovarian stimulation and spontaneous in vivo fertilization.[18,19] It is comparatively inexpensive and less demanding and requires less involvement on the part of patients than the other two procedures. Biopsy of the trophoectoderm allows removal of 10 to 30 cells.

Attempts to achieve accurate molecular diagnosis with multiple cells is more likely to be correct than attempts to make a diagnosis with one or two cells because the former approach allows duplication of all results. The combined experience with uterine lavage, albeit scanty, confers promise. Among 15 recovered and transferred blastocysts, nine produced clinical pregnancies, and seven resulted in livebirths. Another shortcoming of uterine lavage for PGD is the unexplained fact that gonadotropin superovulation treatment does not increase the yield of recovered blastocysts.[19,24] Failure to recover all the embryos

Polar-Body Biopsy

Polar-body biopsy is used to determine the genetic status of the first polar body. In the absence of crossing over between sister chromatids, the genetic material in the polar body is theoretically complementary to that in the pronucleus of the egg. If one attempts to identify mutant alleles of an autosomal recessive disorder such as cystic fibrosis (*CF*) carried by the mother, identification of the mutant allele in the first polar body would suggest a normal *CF* allele in the egg. Eggs that contain the normal allele can be selected and fertilized in vitro. First-polar-body biopsy confers, therefore, the advantage of diagnosis before fertilization. This timing of micromanipulation, diagnosis, and selection has the potential to alleviate the ethical and social distress that surrounds prenatal diagnosis and pregnancy termination.[16,17]

The polar-biopsy specimen can be obtained by means of either aspiration or extrusion of the first polar body from inside the zona pellucida of a preovulatory oocyte. The unfertilized oocyte is secured onto a holding pipette so that the polar body is located on the upper pole of the oocyte. The polar body is then gently sucked into a beveled micropipette inserted through the zona pellucida (Fig 44–5). Alternatively, the polar body can be forced out through an adjacent slit in the zona pellucida. Extrusion of the polar body is achieved by means of pressure applied to the intact part of the zona with the micropipette. The polar body is then transferred into the appropriate microtube or slide for processing or fixation. This maneuver does not appear to directly affect the ability of the oocyte to become fertilized.[27,28] After the genetic material in the polar body is examined, the oocytes deemed unaffected are presented to sperm, and the fertilized eggs are transferred into the uterus.[28] Molecular analysis of the polar body can be performed with DNA methods[27] or fluorescent in situ hybridization (FISH).[29] The stage at which analysis of the polar body is being performed shows both the advantages and the shortcomings of the technique.

Because the diagnosis is achieved before fertilization occurs, polar-body biopsy may be more acceptable to many who would otherwise object to manipulation of fertilized eggs. If proved efficient, first-polar-body biopsy not only will allow direct prefertilization diagnosis but also will contribute to the success rate of IVF by producing the opportunity to avoid fertilization of oocytes that harbor genetic errors.[29] Use of first-polar-body biopsy is limited because it is technically difficult and only allows examination of the maternal genetic contribution to the preembryo. Furthermore, although the first polar body contains only one allele of each pair, at that stage of meiosis each allele is replicated and is represented on each sister chromatid. If crossing over occurs, then chromatids exchange segments and the secondary oocyte may carry an allele that is also represented in the first polar body (and may be the abnormal gene). For that reason a biopsy of the second polar body or blastomere biopsy may be needed for confirmation. This second biopsy obviates the main advantage of first-polar-body analysis.[30]

Polar-body diagnosis has been used for sex determination, diagnosis of the F508 mutation of *CF* and to identify ZZ 1 antitrypsin deficiency.[27,28,31] Analysis of the polar body was performed by means of DNA amplification with polymerase chain reaction (PCR). PCR failure occurred in 14 of 83 instances. Recently the same group of investigators[32] described the possible application of polar-body biopsy in the diagnosis of aneuploidy in oocytes. Because most aneuploidy emanates from nondysjunction events during maternal meiosis, this approach may decrease the age-related risk for chromosomal abnormalities and potentially increase success rates. To date, polar-body diagnosis of aneuploidy is still inefficient and not routinely performed for screening.[32]

Preembryo Biopsy

Attempts have been made to perform biopsy on preembryos at a later stage of development.[33–35] At the morula stage (16 to 32 cells) the blastomeres of the preembryo are compact. To release blastomeres from the preembryo special decompaction buffers devoid of Ca^{2+} and Mg^{2+} ions must be used. Despite the technical feasibility of morula decompaction and either aspiration or slicing of five or six blastomeres, the survival of the morulas on which biopsies were performed was severely compromised.[36] These animal experiments led to disenchantment with the technique, and morula biopsies have not been performed on humans.

Five days after IVF, blastocysts can be obtained for biopsy. At this stage the preembryo comprises 100 to 300 cells and is

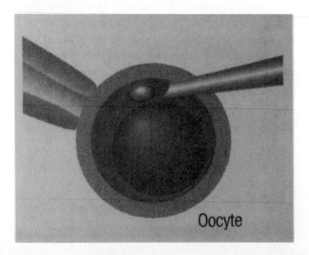

Oocyte

Figure 44–5. Polar-body biopsy (*From Carson SA, Buster JE: Diagnosis and treatment before implantation: The ultimate prenatal medicine. Contemp OB/GYN 40(12):71,1995.*)

further differentiated. One can differentiate the inner cell mass that will develop into the embryo proper and the trophoectoderm that will produce the fetal counterpart of the placenta. Therefore, trophoectoderm cells that have been subjected to biopsy can be analyzed in a manner similar to CVS. The most appropriate method to obtain trophoectoderm cells is herniation (spontaneous or induced) of the blastocyst at the pole opposite the inner cell mass.[37] In animal experiments 10 to 30 cells have been obtained from the murine blastomere with minimal damage to the preembryo as assessed with vital stains.[38] A similar method was used to obtain trophoectoderm cells from human preembryos.[34] It appears that up to 10 cells can be removed from the trophoectoderm with no apparent deleterious effect on either the ability of the preembryo to produce human chorionic gonadotropin (hCG) or to develop further. The availability of this number of cells for analysis improves the accuracy and the quality of genetic diagnosis.[10]

Trophoectoderm biopsy allows analysis of relatively abundant extraembryonic cells that are not themselves progenitors of fetal tissue but represent the genetic composition of the embryo. In the future, when and if the shortcomings of trophoectoderm biopsy are resolved, this may become the preferred method for the development of biochemical and metabolic analysis of some disorders in vitro, because the trophoectoderm expresses much of the embryonic genome. The paramount disadvantage of trophoectoderm/blastocyst biopsy is the dismal associated pregnancy rate.[38,39] It takes a zygote about 5 days to develop into a blastocyst. Afterward, 12 to 24 additional hours are needed for trophoectoderm hatching.[30] To eliminate the time needed for blastocyst herniation, direct one-step methods were developed whereby the trophoectoderm is directly aspirated from within the zona.[30] By the time diagnosis is achieved 1 to 3 days later, the endometrium may be less receptive to implantation of the transferred blastocyst. Developing uterine lavage as a viable option will allow access to the blastocyst without the need for culture and could overcome the deleterious effects of delayed transfer.

Blastomere biopsy is by far the most prevalent method of obtaining preembryo stem cells for PGD.[25] Blastomere biopsy is performed on cleavage-stage preembryos 3 days after IVF and culture. The first pregnancies were achieved in England after such biopsies and sex determination by means of DNA techniques.[40,41] Studies have demonstrated that 25% of the cell mass of the preembryo can be removed safely.[42] This percentage provides practical clinical information with reference to the stage of preembryo development at the time of biopsy. Only one cell can be obtained from a four-cell preembryo. An eight-cell preembryo tolerates biopsy of two blastomeres, which allows repetition of tests for intraassay control.[42,43] Another approach to obtain two blastomeres has been reported in which two subsequent biopsies, one at the eight-cell stage and a second in the blastocyst stage were compatible with normal blastocyst development.[35] Several different biopsy methods were reviewed to obtain blastomeres from four- and eight-cell embryos.[24,30]

All these techniques are variations of either aspiration methods or extrusion/displacement methods. Aspiration can be achieved by means of direct penetration through an intact or acid-treated zona. Displacement of blastomeres is accomplished by means of slitting the zona and extruding the blastomeres through the slit either by pushing on the zona at a remote location or by making a second hole in the zona and injecting fluid into the subzonal space. Survival rates among mouse embryos subjected to biopsy with different techniques are similar, but the survival rate of cells subjected to biopsy appears better after the displacement technique.[43] Our center has primarily used displacement extrusion methods. The survival of four-cell preembryos after biopsy is controversial[26,44,45]; however, the removal of one or two cells from eight-cell preembryos does not interfere with embryo development or metabolism.[42]

A summary of PGD results through the spring of 1995 revealed that pregnancy rates are comparable with IVF results: 197 cycles resulted in 171 preembryo transfers (86%) and 50 pregnancies (25% per cycle, 29% per transfer, 34% per patient). All together 34 babies have been born in 28 deliveries.[34] Among the 149 patients and 197 cycles, 90 patients (132 cycles) underwent the procedure for sex determination (22 babies born), and 59 patients (65 cycles) underwent the procedure to avoid single-gene defects (12 babies born). The procedure was performed for a wide variety of disorders, including cystic fibrosis, Lesch-Nyhan syndrome, fragile X syndrome, Ducheune muscular dystrophy, Tay-Sachs disease, hemophilia, and RhD blood typing. Our group was the first to report an attempt to use PGD for detection of an unbalanced translocation (chromosome 5:8). Two embryos were transferred, but unfortunately pregnancy did not occur.[46]

The field of molecular diagnosis is evolving quickly. Emerging diagnostic methods requiring ever smaller sample sizes are becoming part of the routine diagnostic repertoire. Given the small amount of DNA (6 pg) in a single cell, and the limitation that a single cell contains only one set of mostly noncondensed chromosomes, PGD poses a technical challenge.[10] The two most common diagnostic techniques are PCR and FISH.

Polymerase Chain Reaction

PCR is used to amplify specific DNA sequence mass 10^5 to 10^6 times, even if they exist in only minute amounts among a mixture of DNA.[47] Two oligonucleotide primers must be synthesized. The primers are short single strands of DNA with complementary base sequences to each end of the targeted piece of DNA to be amplified. Primers are added in excess to the DNA extract in which the targeted sequence is present (that is, the sequence that is part of a mutated gene). Heat is used to denature the DNA; cooling then allows the primers to hybridize to their complementary sequences. The synthetic oligonucleotides flank the targeted strand and in the presence of DNA polymerase and an abundance of nucleotides, they prime and bring about the polymerization and synthesis of the piece of DNA between them. These series of three steps; denaturation, hybridization (primers to DNA), and polymerization are repeated many times, exponentially amplifying the DNA sequence between the two primers. For n cycles the DNA amount is increased 2^n. This method was first used to amplify a short segment of the β globin gene in the diagnosis of sickle cell anemia; less than 1 mg of genomic DNA was used as the original sample.[48]

The application of PCR technology to PGD was initially sex determination. Two main concerns were identified that are pertinent to single-cell diagnosis in biopsied blastomeres: (1) the risk of error due to contamination by cells and DNA and (2) the sensitivity and retaining specificity of PCR amplification of the minute (6 pg) amount of DNA derived from a single blastomere. These issues were addressed by means of mathematical modeling to suggest that PGD by means of PCR analysis necessitates confirmation later in pregnancy with more conventional prenatal diagnostic methods, that is, amniocentesis or CVS.[49] Since the initial attempt to identify sex by means of PCR amplification of Y chromosome sequences,[40,41] various techniques have been used to safeguard against misdiagnosis when PCR amplification of four chromosome sequences is used to identify sex.[40,41] Duplex PCR coamplification has been used to amplify concurrently both X and Y chromosome-specific DNA sequences[50] so that failure to amplify will affect both X and Y sequences, making technical error more easily detectable. With this approach, selective failure of one copy or one sequence has been observed.[50]

Nested primer PCR has been used to identify sex, δ F 508 *CF* mutations, and Tay-Sachs disease. This technique involves a second round of PCR amplification after the first set of primers, increasing the amount of the target DNA sequence. The second PCR reaction locates a new set of primers internal to the first pair of primers. This technique increases the sensitivity of DNA amplification and allows identification of as little as 1 pg of DNA in the sample.

To confirm further diagnoses through PCR analysis, heteroduplex formation analysis can be performed. When single strands of DNA are mixed with either normal strands or abnormal strands and allowed to form complexes, two different complexes can be formed. Homoduplexes are made from exact complementary strands and can be either normal or abnormal. Heteroduplexes are formed by means of reannealing of mismatched strands. Heteroduplexes migrate more slowly on an electrophoresis gel and are easily detected. The heteroduplex technique is based on detection of different-sized DNA complexes formed when the final PCR product is mixed with equal amounts of either homozygous normal or homozygous abnormal DNA. For example, if the sample is analyzed for diagnosis of cystic fibrosis,[51] each normal homozygous sample has two strands with normal alleles. Heterozygous carriers possess one normal and one mutant strand, and each of the two strands from homozygous abnormal carriers contains two abnormal alleles.

Until the spring of 1995, 22 babies were born after blastomere biopsy and DNA diagnosis. Eleven were born after sex identification and 12 after specific diagnosis of single-gene disorders.[25] Identification of δ F508 *CF* is the most prevalent diagnosis attempted. Specific diagnosis is being developed for Ducheune muscular dystrophy,[52] Tay-Sachs disease,[53] fragile X syndrome,[25] RhD blood typing,[54] and hemophilia A.[25] Ninety-five percent of the cycles in which specific diagnosis of a single-gene disorder was attempted, yielded embryos deemed suitable for transfer. The pregnancy rate was 34%. PCR technology currently seems the only valid approach to the diagnosis of single-gene disorders. The thrust of technical development is aimed at improving sensitivity, reliability, accuracy, and prevention of contamination. Efforts are made to overcome PCR amplification failures and allele drop-out or preferential amplification due to amplification of one allele and not the other.[55,56] Concerns linger regarding the possibility of misdiagnosis, especially of autosomal dominant disorders. One of the approaches to reduction of contamination by DNA of sperm attached to the zygote is the use of ICSI rather than conventional insemination.[57]

The clinical consequences of PCR failure and DNA contamination have been reviewed.[10] Failure to detect a mutant allele would result in transfer of an embryo that is phenotypically normal but actually carries the mutant gene as a heterozygote (carrier). Failure of the normal allele in a heterozygote results in avoiding the transfer altogether (the preembryo is assumed abnormal). An opportunity for a normal pregnancy is missed, but no long-term consequences occur. Contamination with DNA not related to the zygote results in the transfer of an abnormal preembryo that is assumed to be normal.

Other promising developments in this area are concentrated on the effort to increase the number of diagnoses that can be obtained from a single cell. This endeavor is in anticipation of further use of PGD as a screening tool. Efforts are made to achieve multiplex PCR diagnoses by means of augmentation of the amount of DNA generated for analysis. A large fraction of the genomic DNA of a single cell can be amplified randomly in excess of 30 copies by the use of primer extension preamplification.[58] This DNA can be used for diagnostic techniques that require several reactions or to probe for several different disorders. A different avenue is the possibility of cell recycling.[59] In this approach, FISH and PCR analysis are performed consecutively. Fluorescent PCR combines fluorescent primers and modification of PCR analysis. It has been shown to be a highly sensitive method of simultaneous identification of sex and the *CF* gene in somatic cells. This method allows simultaneous DNA fingerprinting of single cells that may allow accurate detection of DNA contamination.[55] To date, these new methods have not yet found their way into clinical use in PGD.

Fluorescent In Situ Hybridization

More laboratories are using an alternative molecular method primarily to identify sex and chromosomal abnormalities.[46,59-62] FISH at present cannot be used for single-gene detection. Many cycles are performed with FISH to detect age-related chromosomal aneuploidy. According to one report[63] FISH analysis of chromosomes X, Y, 13, 18, and 21 was accomplished in 200 PGD cycles resulting in 33 pregnancies and seven healthy babies.

Traditional cytogenetic methods are not appropriate for single blastomere analysis. Obtaining a karyotype requires examination of cells arrested at metaphase by means of first a mitogenic factor (mitosis-stimulating agent like phytohemagglutinin) and then a dilute solution of colchicine to prevent completion of nuclear and cytoplasmic division. Although it is possible to obtain single cells at metaphase karyotyping of single blastomeres, it is not feasible for technical reasons.[64,65] Karyotyping has the advantage of conferring the ability to examine all the chromosomes concurrently and detect subtle chromosomal rearrangements. In the future, it might be possible to cryopreserve cleavage-stage preembryos that have been subjected to biopsy and culture the blastomere to increase the number of cells available for genetic analysis.[66] If these circumstances materialize, then karyotyping may become a valid option. FISH analysis allows detection of targeted DNA sequences in the interphase nucleus with labeled chromosome specific probes. After the blastomere is obtained it is fixed to a glass slide, and its DNA is denatured. The labeled probe is allowed to hybridize to the interphase or metaphase chromosome. The label is then developed to fluoresce and demarcate a specific chromosome or segment of a chromosome.[67] FISH can be performed simultaneously with several probes in which multiple fluorochromes are used. Metaphase staining has been developed to allow detection of all chromosomes.[68] This is a promising technique that cannot yet be used in PGD. Detection of severe chromosomal aneuploidy in preimplantation embryos is almost routinely used at some centers.[62]

Because a large proportion of abnormal embryos can be detected with FISH, the number of embryos suitable for transfer is reduced. Some authors have suggested a skewed gender ratio (60:40, male:female) among blastomeres subjected to biopsy.[25] For genetic reasons FISH is used mostly for sex selection, specifically to avoid the transfer of male preembryos affected with X-linked disorders.[25] Several groups of investigators have tried to increase the number of selected-sex embryos to undergo biopsy (primarily efforts to increase the number of female embryos). This theoretically can be achieved by means of preselection of X-carrying sperm cells before fertilization.[25]

Most methods available for gender selection on the level of the sperm are not efficient. The more efficient methods involve use of dyes that intercalate into the DNA, a fact that raises concerns regarding potential mutagenicity. Using novel cosmid probes, our group was able to detect several unbalanced reciprocal translocations in somatic cells and in blastomeres subjected to biopsy.[46] A combination of primer extension preamplification to increase the amount of available genomic DNA from single cells and comparative genomic hybridization may be used in the future for the detection of unbalanced translocation.[69]

FISH analysis of blastomeres allows direct detection of X and Y chromosomes but also has been shown to be efficient in detecting autosomal chromosomes 18, 13, 21, and 16. This increased power of detection prompted some centers to offer preembryo biopsy to women at advanced age undergoing IVF and multiplex FISH screening of embryos for X, Y, 21, 18, 13, and 16. The rationale behind the screening was obvious albeit controversial. The advantage is reduction of the chance that parents will encounter age-related chromosomal abnormalities at the time of amniocentesis. In addition, because chromosomal abnormalities underlie 50% to 80% of early pregnancy loss, it is conceivable that avoiding the transfer of chromosomally abnormal preembryos will increase the success rate of IVF at advanced maternal age. The controversy, however, stems from the perception that using PGD for screening at this stage of fertility treatment imposes a technologic imperative rather than a response to a genuine need. For PGD to be used as a primary screening modality, it must have an accuracy rate close to 100% to obviate amniocentesis. Even at an experienced center, only a small number of embryos (only one embryo in one third of cycles) was deemed suitable for transfer.[25] A higher rate of chromosomal mosaicism[62] was observed among human preembryos. Some reports suggest technical shortcomings of FISH analysis of single blastomeres that preclude conclusive diagnosis in approximately 10% of blastomeres analyzed.[31] Taken together these issues behoove the practitioner to exercise caution when presenting PGD as a screening test in the context of traditional IVF for the treatment of patients at advanced maternal age. Special counseling is mandatory in face of the currently less than perfect sensitivity of FISH analysis.

WHAT SHOULD BE DONE?

Rapid developments in molecular genetics hold formidable promise for streamlining PGD. It is predicted that PGD will find its deserved legitimate niche within the choices of prenatal diagnostic modalities. The primary objective of PGD is to avoid conception of abnormal embryos in couples at high genetic risk. About 200 X-linked conditions can be avoided with use of the currently available techniques of sex selection and transfer of unaffected females. This approach, however, results in many instances of avoidance of transfer of healthy males. In many such disorders females may express abnormal phenotype. Many of the X-linked disorders have been discovered, and direct testing methods are being developed that could be used in the future to manage specific X-linked disorders. Hectic efforts are invested diligently to locate and identify the genes and mutations that bring about single-gene disorders, allowing more diagnoses to be made on single cells.

To date it seems that PGD is not a valid screening modality to manage conditions such as advanced maternal age because it adds a great deal of risk and it is not yet accurate enough to justify the expense. PGD may be more appropriate as a screening tool for women at advanced maternal age already undergoing IVF with appropriate counseling. In the near future without adding substantial risk to the embryos, several common chromosomal abnormalities can be identified. This approach will confer another theoretic advantage of improving IVF results by avoiding chromosomally abnormal preembryos. This is because most early pregnancy losses after IVF are probably the results of such disorders.

FISH diagnosis has proved promising in the management of infertility due to pregnancy losses by patients who carry chromosomal translocations. The fertility of these patients is compromised because of reduced fecundity that stems from the low ratio of normal zygotes that they conceive. Appropriate counseling about the accuracy of diagnosis should be provided. The patient should understand that when pregnancy ensues other methods of confirming prenatal diagnosis will be pursued (CVS or amniocentesis). In these circumstances, PGD can be used to increase the likelihood that pregnancy will proceed to term and to reduce the risk for finding unbalanced fetuses at CVS or amniocentesis.

It was suggested that PGD may reduce the trauma and emotional consequences of pregnancy termination and therefore would be more acceptable for many couples who otherwise have to avoid procreation with their own gametes. Although this premise is logical, our experience shows that with the current state of the art in PGD and with current efficiency and accuracy, this approach is difficult to implement. The counseling is difficult and emotionally charged, because it has to be clear to the patients that after an expensive and risky procedure (most of the couples are not infertile) there is not 100% confidence that the embryo they carry is free of abnormality. It should also be explained that it is possible that the embryo will carry the very specific disorder for which PGD was used in the first place. This risk albeit much smaller than before PGD became possible is not totally eliminated. All PGD protocols require follow-up tests by other means of prenatal diagnosis. In the minds of many practitioners, PGD is the extension of other traditional prenatal diagnostic methods. It has been shown that a substantial number of women find embryonic diagnosis more acceptable than CVS when pregnancy is at risk for a genetic disorder.[70]

As PGD is streamlined in the near future and its accuracy and efficiency improve, it will become the ultimate practical tool to realize many of the goals of new developments in human genetics to benefit humankind.

REFERENCES

1. Watson JD: Foreword. *National Center for Human Genome Research Annual Report I-FY.* Department of Health and Human Services, Public Health Service. Bethesda, MD, National Institutes of Health, 1990
2. Garver KL, Garver B: The Human Genome Project and eugenic concerns. *Am J Hum Genet* 54:148, 1994
3. Winston RML, Handyside AH: New challenges in human in vitro fertilization. *Science* 260:932, 1993
4. Tan SL: Simplifying in-vitro fertilization therapy. *Curr Opin Obstet Gynecol* 6:111, 1994
5. Pergament E, Bonnicksen A: Preimplantation genetics: A case for prospective action. *Am J Med Genet* 52:151, 1994
6. Bonnicksen AL: National and international approaches to human germ-line gene therapy. *Politics Life Sci* Feb:1, 1994
7. Grabowski GA, Whitsett JA: Gene therapy. In: Nelson WE (ed), *Nelson Textbook of Pediatrics.* Philadelphia, Saunders, 1996: 321–326
8. Opinion: More fuss about genetics and embryos (editorial). *Nature* 367:99, 1994
9. Carson SA, Buster JE: Diagnosis and treatment before implantation: The ultimate prenatal medicine. *Contemp OB/GYN* 40(12): 71, 1995
10. Simpson JL, Carson SA, Buster JE, Elias S: Single-cell genetic diagnosis: Molecular methods and pitfalls. *Semin Reprod Endocrinol* 12:196, 1994
11. Bonnicksen A: Genetic diagnosis of human embryos. *Hastings Center Report* July–August (Suppl):S5–S11, 1992
12. Mori M, Brambati B, Tului L: Prenatal diagnosis today: The current ethical controversy over reproductive medicine—Prenatal diagnosis. *Hum Reprod* 10:765, 1995
13. Gordon JW: Debate: Prenatal diagnosis today: The morality of prenatal diagnosis. *Hum Reprod* 10:767, 1995
14. Schafer D, Arnemann J, Brude E, Baumann R: Prenatal diagnosis today: Society must decide about prenatal diagnosis. *Hum Reprod* 10:767, 1995

15. Wertz DC, Fletcher JC: A critique of some feminist challenges to prenatal diagnosis. *J Women Health* 2:173, 1993

16. Robertson JA: Ethical and legal issues in preimplantation genetic screening. *Fertil Steril* 57:1, 1992

17. Wertz DC: Ethical and social issues in preimplantation genetic diagnosis. *Genet Res* 8:17, 1996

18. Formigli L, Roccio C, Belloti G, et al: Non-surgical flushing of the uterus for pre-embryo recovery: Possible clinical application. *Hum Reprod* 5:329, 1990

19. Carson SA, Smith AL, Scoggan JL, et al: Superovulation fails to increase human blastocyst yield after uterine lavage. *Prenatal Diagn* 11:513, 1991

20. Zilberstein M, Seibel MM: Fertilization and implantation. *Curr Opin Obstet Gynecol* 6:184, 1994

21. Mottla GL, Adelman MR, Hall JL, Gindoff PR, Stillman RJ, Johnson KE: Lineage tracing demonstrates that blastomeres of early cleavage-stage human preembryos contribute to both trophoectoderm and inner cell mass. *Hum Reprod* 10:384, 1995

22. Bennett SJ, Waterstone JJ, Cheng WC, Rearsons J: Complications of transvaginal ultrasound directed follicle aspiration: A review. *J Assist Reprod Genet* 10:72, 1993

23. Feichtiger W: Results and complications of IVF therapy. *Curr Opin Obstet Gynecol* 6:190, 1994

24. Carson SA, Buster JE: Biopsy of gametes and preimplantation embryos in genetic diagnosis. *Semin Reprod Endocrinol* 12:184, 1994

25. Harper JC: Preimplantation diagnosis of inherited disease by embryo biopsy: An update of the world figures. *J Assist Reprod Genet* 13:90, 1996

26. Krzyminska VB, Lutjen J, O'Neill C: Assessment of the viability and pregnancy potential of mouse embryos biopsied at different preimplantation stages of development. *Hum Reprod* 5:203, 1990

27. Verlinsky Y, Reditsky S, Evsikov S, et al: Preconception and preimplantation diagnosis of cystic fibrosis. *Prenat Diagn* 12:103, 1992

28. Verlinsky Y, Ginsberg N, Lifchez A: Analysis of the first polar body: Preconception genetic diagnosis. *Hum Reprod* 5:826, 1990

29. Dyban A, Freidine M, Severova E, Cieslak J, Ivakhnenko V, Verlinsky Y: Detection of aneuploidy in human oocytes and corresponding first polar bodies by fluorescent in situ hybridization. *J Assist Reprod Genet* 13:73, 1996

30. Tarin JJ, Handyside AH: Embryo biopsy strategies for preimplantation diagnosis. *Fertil Steril* 59:943, 1993

31. Grifo J: Preconception and preimplantation genetic diagnosis: Polar body, blastomere, and trophoectoderm biopsy. In: Cohen J, Malter HE, Tolanski BE, Grifo J (eds), *Micromanipulation of Human Gametes and Embryos.* New York, Raven, 1992:223–249

32. Verlinsky Y, Cieslak J, Freidine M, et al: Polar body diagnosis of common aneuploidies by FISH. *J Assist Reprod Genet* 13:157, 1996

33. Bolton VN, Wren ME, Parson JH: Pregnancies after in vitro fertilization and transfer of human blastocysts. *Fertil Steril* 55:830, 1991

34. Dorkas A, Sargent IL, Gardner RL: Human trophoectoderm biopsy and secretion of chorionic gonadotropin. *Hum Reprod* 6:1453, 1991

35. Muggleton-Harris AL, Glazier AM, Pickering S, Wall M: Genetic diagnosis using polymerase chain reaction and fluorescent in-situ hybridization analysis of biopsied cells from both the cleavage and blastocyst stages of individual cultured human preimplantation embryos. *Hum Reprod* 10:183, 1995

36. Van Blerk M, Nijs M, Van Steirteghem AC: Decompaction and biopsy of late mouse morulae: Assessment of in vitro and in vivo developmental potential. *Hum Reprod* 6:1298, 1991

37. Carson SA, Gentry WL, Smith AL, et al: Trophoectoderm microbiopsy in murine blastocysts: Comparison of four methods. *J Assist Reprod Genet* 10:427, 1993

38. Menezo Y, Nicollet B, Herbaut N, et al: Freezing co-cultured human blastocysts. *Fertil Steril* 58:977, 1992

39. Dawson KJ, Rutherford AJ, Winston NJ, et al: Human blastocyst transfer: Is it a feasible proposition? *Hum Reprod* 145(Suppl):44, 1988

40. Handyside AH, Pattinson JK, Penketh RJ, Delhanty JD, Winston RM, Tuddenham EG: Biopsy of human preimplantation embryos and sexing by DNA amplification. *Lancet* 1:347, 1989

41. Handyside AH, Kontogianni EH, Hardy K, Winston RM: Pregnancies from biopsied human preimplantation embryos sexed by Y-specific DNA amplification. *Nature* 344:768, 1990

42. Hardy K, Martin KL, Leese HJ, Winston RML, Handyside AH: Human preimplantation development in vitro is not adversely affected by biopsy at the 8-cell stage. *Hum Reprod* 5:708, 1990

43. Roudebush WE, Kim JG, Minhas BS, Dodson MG: Survival and cell acquisition rates after preimplantation embryo biopsy: Use of two mechanical techniques and two mouse strains. *Am J Obstet Gynecol* 162:1084, 1990

44. Wilton LJ, Show JM, Trounson AO: Successful single cell biopsy and cryopreservation of preimplantation mouse embryos. *Fertil Steril* 51:513, 1989

45. Wilton LJ, Trounson AO: Biopsy of preimplantation mouse embryos: development of micromanipulated embryos and proliferation of single blastomeres in vitro. *Biol Reprod* 40:145, 1989

46. Pierce KE, Kiessling AA, Brenner CA, Seibel MM, Zilberstein M: Preimplantation genetic diagnosis of chromosome balance in embryos from a patient with balanced translocation. Presented at the Annual Meeting of the American Society for Reproductive Medicine, October 1995, Seattle

47. Mullis KB: The unusual origin of the polymerase chain reaction. *Sci Am* 262:64, 1990

48. Saiki RK, Scharf S, Faloona F, et al: Enzymatic amplification of β-globin genomic sequences and restriction site analysis for diagnosis of sickle cell anemia. *Science* 230:1350, 1985

49. Navidi W, Arnheim N: Using PCR in preimplantation genetic disease diagnosis. *Hum Reprod* 6:836, 1991

50. Grifo JA, Tang Y, Cohen J, et al: Pregnancy after embryo biopsy and amplification of DNA from X and Y chromosomes. *JAMA* 268:727, 1992

51. Handyside AH, Lesko JG, Tarin JJ, et al: Birth of a normal girl after in vitro fertilization and preimplantation diagnostic testing for cystic fibrosis. *N Engl J Med* 327:905, 1992

52. Liu J, Lissens W, Van Broeckhoven C, et al: Normal pregnancy after preimplantation DNA diagnosis of dystrophin gene deletion. *Prenatal Diagn* 15:351, 1995

53. Gibbons WE, Gitlin SA, Lazendorf SE, Kaufmann RA, Slotnick RN, Hodgen GD: Preimplantation genetic diagnosis for Tay Sachs disease: Successful pregnancy after pre-embryo biopsy and gene amplification by polymerase chain reaction. *Fertil Steril* 63:723, 1995

54. Avner R, Reubinoff BE, Simon A, et al: Management of RhD isoimmunization by preimplantation genetic diagnosis. *Hum Reprod* 1996

55. Findley I, Quirke P, Hall J, Rutherford A: Fluorescent PCR: A new technique for PGD of sex and single-gene defects. *J Assist Reprod Genet* 13:96, 1996

56. Gitlin SA, Lanzendorf SE, Gibbons WE: Polymerase chain reaction amplification specificity: Incidence of allele dropout using different DNA preparation methods for heterozygous single cells. *J Assist Reprod Genet* 13:107, 1996

57. Liu J, Lissens W, Devroey P, Liebaers I, Van Steirteghem A: Birth after preimplantation diagnosis of the cystic fibrosis delta F 508 mutation by polymerase chain reaction in human embryos resulting from intracytoplasmic sperm injection with epididymal sperm. *JAMA* 272:1858, 1994

58. Zhang L, Cui X, Schmitt K, Hubert R, Navidi W, Arnheim H: Whole genome amplification from single cells: Implications for genetic analysis. *Proc Natl Acad Sci USA* 89:5847, 1992

59. Rechitsky S, Freidine M, Verlinsky Y, Storm CM: Allele dropout in sequential PCR and fish analysis of single cells (cell recycling). *J Assist Reprod Genet* 13:115, 1996

60. Delhanty JDA, Griffin DK, Handyside AH, et al: Detection of aneuploidy and chromosomal mosaicism in human embryos during preimplantation sex determination by fluorescent in situ hybridization (FISH). *Hum Mol Genet* 2:1183, 1993

61. Verlinsky Y: Preimplantation genetic diagnosis (editorial). *J Assist Reprod Genet* 13:87, 1996

62. Munne S, Lee A, Rosenwaks Z, Grifo J, Cohen J: Diagnosis of major chromosome aneuploidies in human preimplantation embryos. *Hum Reprod* 8:2185, 1993

63. Harper JC, Coonen E, Handyside AH, Winston RML, Hopman AHN, Delhanty JDA: Mosaicism of autosomes and sex chromosomes in morphologically normal monospermic preimplantation human embryos. *Prenatal Diagn* 15:41, 1994

64. Geber S, Winston RML, Handyside AH: Proliferation of blastomeres from biopsied cleavage stage human embryos in vitro: An alternative to blastocyst biopsy for preimplantation diagnosis. *Hum Reprod* 10:1492, 1995

65. Plachot M, Mandelbaum J, Junca AM, et al: Cytogenetic analysis and developmental capacity of normal and abnormal embryos after IVF. *Hum Reprod* 4:99, 1989

66. Kallionemi A, Kallionemi O-P, Suder D, et al: Comparative genomic hybridization for molecule cytogenetic analysis of solid tumors. *Science* 258:818, 1992

67. Kola I, Wilton L: Preimplantation embryo biopsy: Detection of trisomy in a single cell biopsied from a four-cell mouse embryo. *Mol Reprod Dev* 29:16, 1991

68. Korf B: Molecular diagnosis. *N Engl J Med* 332:1218, 1995

69. Coonen E, Dumolin J, Dressen J, Bras M, Geraedts J, Evers J: Clinical application of FISH for sex determination of embryos in preimplantation diagnosis of X-linked diseases. *J Assist Reprod Genet* 13:133, 1996

70. Miedzybrodzka Z, Templeton A, Dean J, Haites N, Mollison J, Smith N: Preimplantation diagnosis or chorionic villus biopsy? Women's attitudes and preferences. *Hum Reprod* 8:2192, 1993

CHAPTER 45

Ovum Donation

MARK A. DAMARIO · ZEV ROSENWAKS

Evaluation for Ovum Donation

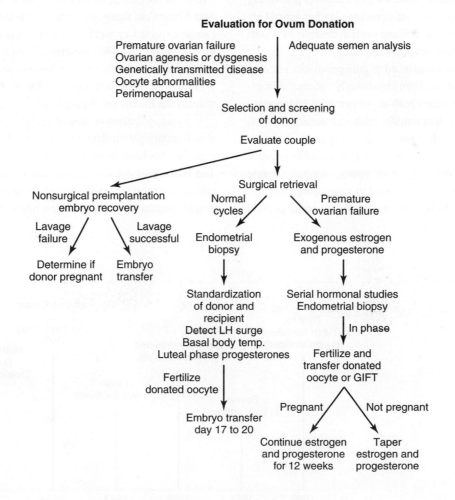

In vitro fertilization (IVF) and assisted reproductive technology (ART) represent important breakthroughs in the field of reproductive medicine. These techniques not only have alleviated infertility for people who previously had no hope of conceiving but also have provided an opportunity to study the microenvironment of the human oocyte and the subtleties of gamete interaction and early embryonic development. Oocyte donation is a successful outgrowth of this technology and also provides an elegant in vivo model for the study of human reproduction. Oocyte donation involves the transfer of oocytes or embryos from a fertile donor to a phenotypically matched recipient with the goal of achieving fertilization (either in vitro or in vivo) that results in a subsequent gestation.

For women previously thought to have irreversible sterility, oocyte donation provides an option for achieving pregnancy, including women with either absent or hypoplastic gonads and those with premature ovarian failure or ovarian failure after medical treatment. Those at risk for transmitting a genetic disorder may choose oocyte donation as a means of preventing disease in their offspring. Oocyte donation also has proved effective for women with diminished ovarian reserve in whom prior attempts at IVF have been unsuccessful.

Oocyte donation has continued to gain popularity since its introduction in 1983. It has been consistently successful in establishing viable pregnancies both in women with endogenous ovarian function and in functionally agonadal women. In fact, many clinics report a higher per transfer pregnancy rate with oocyte donation than with conventional IVF, possibly because the donated ova are obtained from young, normally fertile women and the embryos are transferred to a physiologically optimal endometrial bed. In light of this success, more than 2000 oocyte donation cycles are initiated annually in IVF programs in the United States and Canada.[1]

HISTORICAL PERSPECTIVE

Although the use of donor oocytes and embryos to alleviate human infertility is relatively recent, work with animals has been under investigation for at least a century (Fig 45–1). Although Heape[2] described the first successful transfer of a fertilized ovum in a rabbit in 1890, soon thereafter experimentation was expanded to a number of other species. In 1951, Wilett et al[3] described the first successful bovine embryo transfer. Refinements of this technology led to the successful routine use of donor embryo transfer in the cattle industry.[4]

In animals, the success of embryo transfer depends on accurate synchronization of the estrus cycles of donor and recipient within the temporal window of maximal endometrial receptivity. For success in mice, this window of transfer is no more than 6 hours[5]; in sheep, accurate synchronization of up to 2 days can be expected to yield a relatively high pregnancy rate (approximately 75%).[6] Nevertheless, if asynchrony exceeds three or more days, only 8% of ewes become pregnant. The situation is similar for cattle; asynchrony of more than 2 days markedly reduces the likelihood of pregnancy.[7]

Synchronization of animal cycles is achieved through hormonal manipulation designed to align the estrus cycles of the pair. This has been facilitated with cryopreservation technology. The techniques not only allow transfer of thawed embryos in subsequent recipient cycles but also eliminate the need for geographic proximity of the donor-recipient pair.

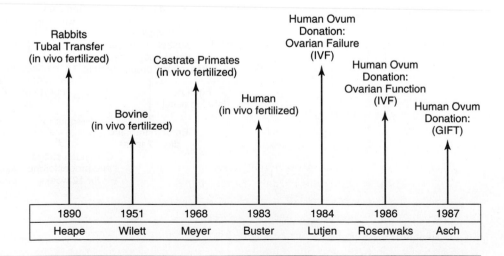

Figure 45–1. Milestones of ovum donation.

Meyer et al[8] described the first successful embryo donation procedure in castrated primates in 1968. This was soon followed by other reports of viable pregnancies in castrated monkeys who received steroidal hormone replacement. Hodgen[9] described the transfer of monkey embryos fertilized in vivo obtained by means of uterine lavage to long-castrated female recipients who underwent a regimen of sequential estrogen and progesterone replacement. Four viable pregnancies were obtained in 11 attempts, confirming that exogenous steroids may allow development of a receptive endometrial environment for maximal implantation efficiency. This study also suggested that with hormonal priming and donated ova, it would be possible for women without ovarian function to conceive.

The first human pregnancy resulting from oocyte donation was reported by Buster et al[10] This technique entailed intracervical insemination of a healthy female volunteer with sperm obtained from the husband in an infertile couple on or about the day of the donor's luteinizing hormone (LH) peak. After in vivo fertilization in the reproductive tract of the donor, the early conceptus was retrieved by means of transcervical uterine lavage performed on days 5 to 7 after the donor's LH peak during the perinidatory period. If obtained, the pre-embryo was then transcervically transferred to the primed recipient. The objective of this procedure was to synchronize the LH peaks of donor and recipient to within plus or minus 2 days. Buster et al[11] reported two pregnancies in the first five embryo transfers in which this technique was used; however, the efficiency of obtaining fertilized ova from the inseminated volunteers ranged from 0 to 75%.

Formigli et al[12] reported their experience with nonsurgical recovery of donor fertilized ova transferred to synchronized recipients. In their series of 56 uterine lavages, 23 ova were obtained and 17 fertilized ova were transferred, resulting in 8 viable pregnancies. Pregnancy rates were reported to be 12.5% per uterine lavage and 41% per transfer with a single conceptus, demonstrating the relatively high efficiency of this technique, since the embryo implantation rate seemed to exceed that of IVF. However, the potential risk of transmission of infectious diseases, technical difficulties, and the possibility of a retained pregnancy in the donor have limited the application of this technique.[13]

The transfer of donor oocytes fertilized in vitro to appropriately synchronized recipients is a technique more practical for clinical application. Trounson et al[14] reported the first pregnancy after IVF of a donated oocyte with intrauterine embryo transfer to a synchronized recipient; unfortunately the pregnancy ended in spontaneous abortion at 16 weeks. Rosenwaks et al[15] reported the first successful term delivery after natural cycle oocyte donation. Meticulous care was taken to synchronize the recipient's LH surge with the administration of human

chorionic gonadotropin (hCG) and oocyte retrieval from the donor (Fig 45–2).

Lutjen et al[16] described the first successful pregnancy in a patient with ovarian failure after IVF of a donated oocyte with intrauterine embryo transfer and steroid replacement therapy. Hormonal replacement therapy in this recipient consisted of oral estradiol valerate along with intravaginal progesterone suppositories to mimic the endogenous steroidal milieu of a normal ovulatory cycle. Estrogen and progesterone therapy were then withdrawn at 12 weeks and 19 weeks of gestation, respectively. Donated oocytes also have been successfully used by recipients undergoing tubal transfer procedures. Asch et al[17] described the successful application of gamete intrafallopian transfer (GIFT) with donated ova in six of eight patients with premature ovarian failure who underwent a steroid replacement protocol. Likewise, patients treated by Yovich et al[18] achieved pregnancies by means of zygote intrafallopian transfer (ZIFT) for ovum donation.

PATIENT SELECTION AND INDICATIONS

Oocyte donation can be used successfully for a number of clinical indications (Table 45–1). Essentially, oocyte donation may be used for women with primary or secondary ovarian failure; for women who do not respond well to ovarian stimulation, which often results in a limited harvest or poor quality oocytes; and for women with known or suspected abnormalities of the oocyte. Women with ovarian failure compose one of the largest groups of patients who seek oocyte donation, although for most patients the underlying cause of the ovarian failure is unknown. Identifiable causes of ovarian failure include chemotherapy or pelvic irradiation for the treatment of malignant disease, surgical extirpation, autoimmune disorders, and gonadal dysgenesis (Table 45–2).

Conditions that may necessitate oocyte donation in the presence of ovarian function include (1) repeatedly unsuccessful IVF or GIFT cycles secondary to persistently poor oocyte or embryo quality or repeated fertilization failure of apparently normal oocytes and spermatozoa; (2) anatomically inaccessible ovaries that make oocyte retrieval either difficult or impossible; and (3) genetic abnormalities in which the woman fears transmitting an autosomal dominant, X-linked trait or chromosomal rearrangement to her offspring.

With the development of sophisticated ultrasound-guided oocyte aspiration techniques, few patients fall into the category of having ovarian inaccessibility. Patients whose ovaries are located high in the pelvis and have substantial associated adhesions rarely might be considered candidates for ovum donation. Multiple failures of conventional IVF may be attributed to

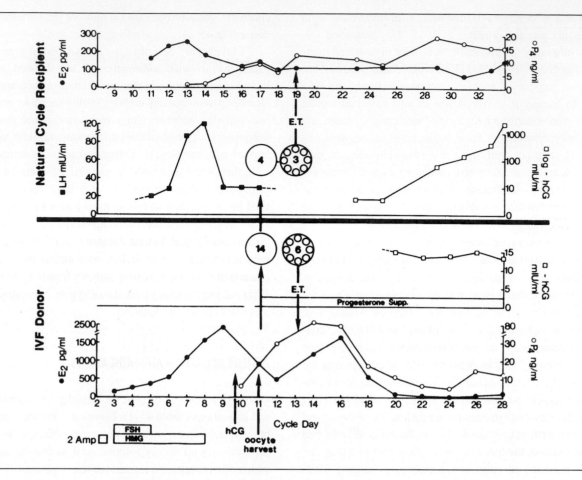

Figure 45–2. Oocyte donation of excess oocytes (from a patient undergoing IVF) to a natural-cycle recipient. The day of LH surge is defined as day 14. Four oocytes were inseminated with the spermatozoa of the recipient's husband. Three embryos were transferred on day 19 of the recipient's cycle. An eight-cell conceptus was the most advanced embryo transferred.

oocyte abnormalities, poor folliculogenesis in response to stimulation, or repeated absence of fertilization with seemingly normal gametes (after coexisting male-factor infertility is ruled out). Whereas it is clear that oocyte donation should be implemented early in the course of treatment of a patient who has demonstrated repeatedly poor follicular development or repeated fertilization failure, the question remains when one should resort to oocyte donation if IVF is consistently unsuccessful after repeated attempts with apparently normal harvest of ova.

It has been well established that advancing maternal age (older than 40 years) has a negative effect on fertility potential in general and the prognosis for success after IVF. Our recent experience demonstrates a well-defined linear diminution in embryo implantation in older women. We believe this phenomenon is primarily due to oocyte senescence; that is, diminished ovarian reserve, rather than uterine aging. Measurable declines

in ovarian reserve and fertility rates are initially seen about 15 years before the climacteric period and drop precipitously after the age of 40 years. These women are rapidly becoming the largest group seeking oocyte donation.

Diminished ovarian reserve is a normal physiologic phenomenon observed in women during their perimenopausal years. Incipient ovarian failure is usually seen in the latter part of the fifth decade of life. At times, however, it also can occur in younger women. Ovarian reserve can be assessed with determinations of basal follicle-stimulating hormone (FSH) and estradiol levels early in the follicular phase (day 3). Elevated FSH (≥20 mIU/mL) or estradiol concentrations (≥75 pg/mL [280 pmol/L]) may be indicative of incipient ovarian failure and predict a markedly diminished likelihood of success after IVF and related therapies among women who are older than 36 years.[19,20]

Diminished ovarian reserve is manifested by an elevation of day 3 FSH levels, which may be a result of reduced secretion

TABLE 45–1. INDICATIONS FOR OOCYTE DONATION

Ovarian agenesis or dysgenesis
    Pure gonadal dysgenesis (46,XX)
    Turner's syndrome (45,X)
    Turner-like mosaic (variable karyotype)
    Swyer's syndrome (46,XY)
Premature ovarian failure
    Idiopathic
    Autoimmune
    Iatrogenic (surgical ablation, radiation therapy, chemotherapy)
    Environmental (infection, drugs)
    Resistant ovary syndrome
Genetically transmitted disease
    Maternal autosomal dominant
    Autosomal recessive, both partners
    X-linked recessive
    Balanced chromosomal translocations
Surgically inaccessible ovaries
Oocyte abnormalities
Diminished ovarian reserve

of inhibin by the germ cell–depleted ovaries. Increased serum estradiol level on day 3 also appears to predict a poor outcome after use of ART. It is theorized that elevated levels of early follicular phase estradiol may be caused by accelerated follicular recruitment resulting from an elevation in pituitary FSH in the late luteal phase of the preceding cycle.

We analyzed 1249 gonadotropin-stimulated cycles of 782 women (mean age, 36 years). The patients were treated at our center without gonadotropin releasing-hormone (GnRH) agonist downregulation. Basal day 3 FSH and estradiol concentrations were determined concomitantly in the cycle of stimulation. Elevations of either FSH or estradiol level both independently influenced IVF outcome.[21] The ongoing pregnancy rate per retrieval in this series dropped from 21.1% among women with day 3 FSH concentrations less than 10 mIU/mL to 10.0% among women whose day 3 FSH levels were greater than 20 mIU/mL. Likewise, the ongoing pregnancy rate per retrieval fell from 23% when day 3 estradiol level was less than 30 pg/mL (110 pmol/L) to 10.2% when estradiol level was more than 75 pg/mL (280 pmol/L). Further analysis of these data revealed that the mean basal FSH level did not differ from that of women with day 3 estradiol levels less than 30 pg/mL (110 pmol/L), between 30 and 75 pg/mL (110 and 280 pmol/L), and more than 75 pg/mL (280 pmol/L). Women with a high basal estradiol level rarely exhibited a concomitant elevation in FSH level because of apparent feedback inhibition. In short, meaningful interpretation of basal hormonal values in the context of ovarian reserve requires concurrent determination of both FSH and estradiol levels on day 3 of an unstimulated cycle. Both tests allow accurate prognostication of IVF outcome,

providing important markers for patient counseling and expectations. It should be emphasized that a mildly elevated estradiol level (>75 pg/mL [280 pmol/L] and <100 pg/mL [370 pmol/L]) may be normal for younger women (<35 years).

A number of other tests have been devised for indirect assessment of ovarian reserve. Navot et al[22] described a clomiphene challenge test for prospective assessment of fecundity potential; FSH, LH, and estradiol are measured at baseline (days 2 to 3) and again (days 9 to 11) after administration of 100 mg of clomiphene citrate daily for 5 days. Among 51 women 35 years and older with unexplained infertility and normal baseline FSH determinations, 18 had an exaggerated FSH response of 26 mIU/mL or more (>2 standard deviation [SD] greater than the control values) on days 9 through 11. Patients with this exaggerated FSH response were considered to have diminished ovarian reserve, and subsequently only 1 of 18 (6%) conceived. This was compared with the findings among patients with a normal response and anticipated normal ovarian reserve ($n = 33$), 14 (24%) of whom conceived. The authors proposed that there may be a disparity between the estradiol and inhibin secretory capacity of granulosa cells, which can explain the inappropriately high FSH levels in response to a clomiphene challenge. Padilla et al[23] reported that the early estradiol response to leuprolide acetate administered in a flare protocol during controlled ovarian hyperstimulation (COH) for IVF also was an appropriate prognosticator for diminished ovarian reserve. Patients who exhibited elevated estradiol levels by cycle day 3 or 4 followed by a fall in estradiol levels by cycle day 4 or 5 demonstrated higher embryo implantation rates and ongoing pregnancy rates than patients who either lacked a marked early estradiol response or exhibited a persistent estradiol elevation through cycle day 5.

TABLE 45–2. CAUSES OF PREMATURE OVARIAN FAILURE

Chromosomal abnormalities
    Forms of gonadal dysgenesis
Autoimmune disorders
    Type I polyglandular autoimmunity—hypoparathyroidism, chronic mucocutaneous candidiasis, Addison's disease, alopecia, malabsorption syndromes, pernicious anemia
    Type II polyglandular autoimmunity—Addison's disease, autoimmune thyroid disease, diabetes mellitus
Physical causes
    Irradiation
    Chemotherapeutic agents
    Viral agents
    Surgical extirpation
Congenital thymic aplasia
Galactosemia
17-Hydroxylase deficiency
Resistant ovary syndrome
    Defects in gonadotropin action (receptor or postreceptor defects)
Idiopathic causes

Patients with diminished ovarian reserve generally develop fewer oocytes and achieve lower peak estradiol levels even with exogenous gonadotropin stimulation.[24] Although fertilization does not seem to be impaired, implantation efficiency per embryo transfer is diminished. This impaired implantation appears to be related to oocyte (and consequently embryo) quality and not to endometrial environment, that is, uterine aging.

Evaluation of ovarian function is key to counseling a patient about her prognosis and expectations. Determination of FSH and estradiol levels on day 3 of the menstrual period is a simple and established method of assessment of fecundity potential. It should be emphasized, however, that no baseline marker or functional test is absolute; the final arbiter of potential outcome is the actual response to ovarian stimulation. Patients with elevated day 3 gonadotropin or estradiol levels do not, in general, have good results after conventional treatment and should be appropriately counseled and directed toward ovum donation.

EVALUATION OF POTENTIAL OVUM RECIPIENTS

As a rule, programs that practice ovum donation are referral centers. When appropriate, patients should already have undergone a complete infertility evaluation. However, the need may arise to complete this evaluation, which should include a comprehensive medical examination and documentation of age of menarche and onset of secondary sexual development.

The onset of amenorrhea should be documented and the patient questioned regarding possible exposure to environmental toxins, chemotherapy and radiation therapy. A careful review of systems should be conducted with particular regard to possible symptoms of endocrinologic or autoimmune disease. A complete physical examination should include a careful assessment of pelvic structures and a search for evidence of other endocrinopathies or autoimmune disease. Patients with typical features of Turner's syndrome (short stature, webbed neck, cubitus valgus, high-arched palate) should be identified. Serial elevations in FSH and LH level should be confirmed. A karyotype is indicated to rule out sex chromosome abnormalities, such as XO mosaicism or the presence of a Y-bearing cell line. General endocrinologic studies should include thyroid function tests, morning fasting blood glucose measurement, serum calcium and phosphorus determination, and an adrenocorticotropic hormone (ACTH) stimulation test or 8 AM serum cortisol level. Testing for autoimmune disease may include a complete blood cell count (CBC) to screen for pernicious anemia, rheumatoid factor, and an antinuclear antibody. Antiovarian, antithyroid, and antiadrenal antibodies may also be determined.

All donor oocyte recipients undergoing hormonal replacement cycles should undergo a thorough physical examination, including a breast examination and assessment of blood pressure before the start of estrogen therapy. A Papanicolaou (Pap) smear should be obtained. Cervical cultures for *Neisseria gonorrhoeae, Chlamydia trachomatis,* and *Mycoplasma hominis* should be obtained. Blood type, antibody screen, CBC, and rubella titers should be documented. In addition, potential donor recipients and their partners should undergo screening for human immunodeficiency virus (HIV), hepatitis B and C, and syphilis. The male partner should undergo semen analysis to rule out coexisting male-factor infertility.

Hysterosalpingography (HSG) is recommended to assess the normality of the uterine cavity and to perform a trial transfer to determine the uterine depth and ease of future embryo transfers. Transvaginal ultrasonography can be used to identify uterine and ovarian abnormalities and to monitor endometrial thickness during therapy.

Psychologic screening and counseling of the recipient couple is important to determine their emotional preparedness. It is particularly important to identify any ambivalence toward the process. It may also be important to discuss other issues, including feelings about disclosure and any anxiety surrounding the treatment.

In most programs, recipients without endogenous ovarian function usually undergo a preparatory cycle before the actual cycle of embryo transfer to assess the adequacy of the replacement regimen. Serial serum estradiol and progesterone determinations are obtained and a midluteal endometrial biopsy is performed and dated according to the criteria of Noyes et al[25] Glandular-stromal disparity is frequently seen, but this does not appear to impair successful implantation and pregnancy. We have found that biopsies on cycle days 20 to 22 frequently display the glandular architecture of day 17 or 18 and a characteristic stroma consistent with days 21 to 23. The histologic specimen of a typical early biopsy performed on day 21 is shown in Fig 45–3. The subnuclear vacuolization and linear arrangement of nuclei characteristic of day 18 architecture are juxtaposed with edematous stroma suggestive of day 21 to 22 endometrium. This asynchrony occurs despite seemingly adequate progesterone absorption. In contrast, late luteal biopsies in subsequent cycles in these same patients undergoing the same replacement protocol have characteristically revealed the glandular maturation and pseudodecidual stromal change of day 25 to 26 endometrium. Therefore, early development of the endometrial glands seems to frequently lag behind development of the stroma, although the endometrium appears to catch up in the late luteal phase in exogenous hormonal replacement protocols. For this reason, we perform one endometrial biopsy (day 20 to 22) in a preparatory cycle and defer other testing unless there is dysynchronous development of the stroma. Patients with en-

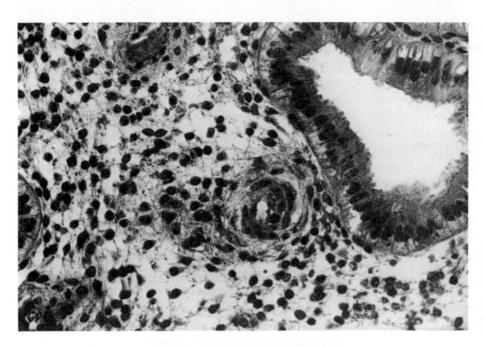

Figure 45–3. Histologic specimen from an endometrial biopsy performed on cycle day 21 after estrogen and progesterone replacement in a patient with ovarian failure. Subnuclear vacuolization and linear arrangement of nuclei characteristic of day 18 glands are juxtaposed with edematous stroma and periarteriolar cuffing characteristic of day 22 to day 23.

dogenous ovarian function usually undergo a similar preparatory cycle and midluteal endometrial biopsy after downregulation with GnRH agonists. In rare instances in which frozen-thawed embryos are to be replaced in a natural cycle, a late luteal-phase biopsy is performed to confirm the adequacy of corpus luteum function.

EVALUATION AND SCREENING OF OOCYTE DONORS

The main limiting factor in establishment and operation of a donor oocyte program is the availability of donors. Donors can be anonymous or not; donors who are not anonymous may include sisters and designated people who are not relatives.

Anonymous gamete donation has been the traditional practice in sperm donation. Many couples who undergo egg donation prefer this approach to maximize confidentiality. Anonymous donors may include volunteers willing to undergo ovarian stimulation and oocyte retrieval for the sole purpose of ovum donation, IVF patients who are willing to donate a portion of their oocytes, and patients scheduled for tubal sterilization who agree to undergo preoperative ovarian stimulation and oocyte harvest at the time of their anticipated surgical procedure. The availability of embryo cryopreservation techniques, however, has reduced the number of IVF patients willing to donate some of their oocytes; most elect to have their excess embryos cryopreserved for possible future replacement. Nevertheless, the op-

portunity to defray a portion of the cycle costs by contributions from the recipient may be attractive for some patients.

A review of our experience at The Center for Reproductive Medicine and Infertility at The New York Hospital–Cornell Medical Center between 1900 and 1995 revealed that 72% of donors were paid anonymous volunteers. It is interesting to note, however, that 14% were IVF patients and 14% were sisters (Fig 45–4). Moreover, it appears that older recipients are more likely to use eggs from anonymous donors, presumably because fewer of these recipients have available younger sisters.

All prospective oocyte donors must undergo a thorough screening process that includes a detailed history and physical examination, psychologic evaluation, and genetic screening. It is desirable to include a psychologist, a genetic counselor, and a physician in the screening process. Published guidelines are available from the American Society for Reproductive Medicine (formerly the American Fertility Society) that describe the recommended evaluation of potential oocyte donors.[26] Updated modifications are available in textbooks on the subject.[27]

Donors who are younger than 34 years are usually preferable not only to maximize success rates but also more importantly to minimize the risk for fetal chromosomal abnormalities and spontaneous miscarriages. Furthermore, using eggs from younger donors obviates routine amniocentesis or chorionic villus sampling. In selected instances, however, older donors may be acceptable if appropriate genetic counseling regarding the

dosage to four patches (0.4 mg) every other day. On the day before the planned oocyte retrieval, the recipient discontinues the leuprolide acetate injections and begins daily intramuscular injections of progesterone-in-oil at a dose of 25 mg (cycle day 15), increasing to 50 mg per day the next day. At this point, transdermal estradiol patches are decreased to 0.2 mg every other day, and daily oral doses of methylprednisolone (16 mg) and tetracycline (250 mg four times a day) are administered to the recipient for 4 days beginning on cycle day 15. Embryo transfer (of 3-day-old embryos) is performed on day 19 of the recipient's cycle.

DONOR STIMULATION AND OOCYTE RETRIEVAL

Gonadotropin stimulation begins on day 3 of the donor's menstrual cycle in a manner identical to that used by patients attempting to conceive through routine IVF. Decisions regarding the specific stimulation protocol should be based on contemporary criteria used within the particular IVF program. Monitoring and decisions regarding the timing of hCG administration and oocyte retrieval should be identical to the standard IVF criteria. During office visits, donors are kept separate from routine IVF patients (the potential recipient) to preserve anonymity.

Our primary ovarian stimulation protocol involves a combination of human menopausal gonadotropins (hMG) and purified FSH. Most patients initially undergo pituitary downregulation with a GnRH agonist begun in the midluteal phase. In our standard protocol, leuprolide acetate is started at a dosage of 1.0 mg subcutaneously daily with a decrease to 0.5 mg daily when gonadotropin therapy is begun. Gonadotropins are administered beginning on day 3 of the menstrual period (2 to 3 ampules [150–225 IU] daily) for most younger donors. We use a stepdown approach to stimulation, that is, decreasing the gonadotropin dosage once follicular recruitment is achieved. Careful monitoring is undertaken with serial serum estradiol determinations and transvaginal ultrasound examinations. Particular care should be taken to minimize development of OHSS in donors. Some younger donors are extremely sensitive to gonadotropin and require lower doses to avoid hypersensitivity. Once appropriate follicular and hormonal criteria have been met, hCG is administered (5000 to 10,000 IU). Oocyte retrieval is scheduled for about 35 hours after hCG administration.

Oocyte retrieval is routine and may be performed either laparoscopically or by means of an ultrasound-guided transvaginal technique. For patients not undergoing tubal sterilization, the latter procedure should be used exclusively because it does not require general anesthesia. Throughout the cycle, the donor should be advised to use barrier contraception to minimize the risk of pregnancy.

After a preincubation period of 2 to 8 hours, the donated ova are inseminated with the recipient's partner's sperm in vitro. Micromanipulation may be used when appropriate, as dictated by the husband's semen profile. Standard embryology laboratory procedures are undertaken, and the resultant embryos are either cryopreserved or incubated until transfer to the synchronized recipient, 48 to 72 hours after retrieval (Fig 45–7). Assisted hatching is performed on the donor embryos according to criteria established in our embryology laboratory.[40]

DONOR AND RECIPIENT SYNCHRONIZATION

Because ovarian and endometrial events are dissociated in donor IVF cycles, effective synchronization of embryonic development in the donor and endometrial development in the recipient is essential. Clinical experience has indicated that a maximally efficient window of transfer exists and implantation efficiency is compromised when embryo transfer is performed outside this window. We evaluated the implantation efficiency of embryo transfers performed on different luteal days in 52 ovum donation cycles.[41] Two- to 12-cell embryos were transferred between days 16 and 24 of hormonally and histologically defined recipient cycles. Of 37 transfers performed on days 17 to 19, 15 (40%) resulted in an ensuing pregnancy, 12 of which (32%) reached viability. None of the 11 patients who underwent transfer on days 20 to 24 conceived. Four patients who underwent transfer on day 16 also were unsuccessful. Analysis of transfers with two or more embryos, at least one of which was considered to be of good quality (grades 1 to 2), in the suggested window of endometrial receptivity (days 17 to 19) revealed that 63% of such cycles were indeed successful. These results suggest a high efficiency for the in vitro fecundity of donor ova provided that optimal conditions are attained.

When cryopreserved embryos are used, synchronization between donor and recipient is straightforward. The recipient is prepared with exogenous estrogen and progesterone as outlined earlier; the first day of progesterone administration is designated day 15. The frozen pronuclear embryos are thawed on day 16, incubated overnight, and transferred on day 17 at the two- to four-cell stage. (Recipients with intact ovarian function either may be treated with exogenous hormone replacement or may undergo embryo transfer in the natural cycle, provided that luteal-phase adequacy has been documented. Embryo thawing and subsequent transfer are timed according to the recipient's LH surge.) Salat-Boroux et al[42] described 4 of 12 successful cycles (33%) in which cryopreserved donated embryos were transferred to recipients with ovarian failure undergoing hormonal replacement. The investigators transferred one- to four-

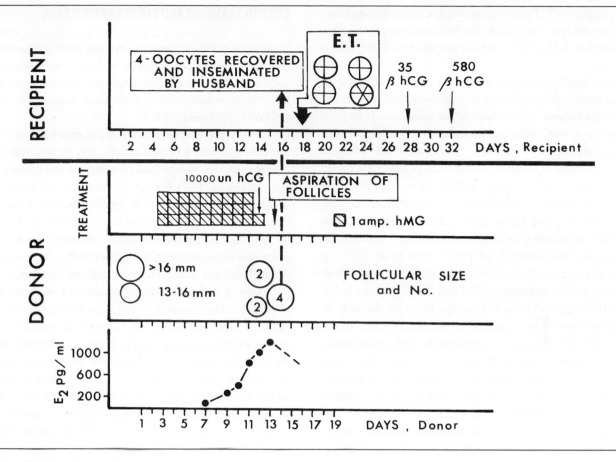

Figure 45–7. Synchronization between a recipient with ovarian failure and a matched donor. A singleton pregnancy was established after the transfer of four embryos in the four- to six-cell stage on cycle day 19. Cycle day 1 of the donor corresponds to cycle day 3 of the recipient. ET, embryo transfer; hCG, human chorionic gonadotropin; hMG, human menopausal gonadotropin; E_2, estradiol.

cell stage frozen and thawed embryos in each instance on the second day of the recipient's progesterone therapy.

The generally poorer success rates with cryopreserved embryos in assisted reproduction has led most practitioners to prefer using fresh embryo or oocyte transfers. Various approaches have been developed to aid in synchronization of the donor and recipient. Several investigators have looked at the feasibility of artificially prolonging the follicular phase of the recipient. We examined three experimental protocols to induce endometrial maturation in women with ovarian failure.[43] A short follicular phase protocol consisted of only 6 days of oral estrogen before the addition of progesterone. A long follicular phase protocol consisted of oral estrogen administration for 3 to 5 weeks before introduction of progesterone. In selected patients undergoing the accelerated protocol, supraphysiologic progesterone (150 mg/day) was given. We found that even very short or long estradiol exposure yielded normal endometrial maturation after the addition of progesterone. The supraphysiologic doses of progesterone also appeared to enhance endometrial maturity in the accelerated cycles.

Younis et al[44] also studied the effect of a prolonged artificial follicular phase on endometrial development in preparation for ovum donation. Patients received oral estradiol and estriol (2:1 ratio in a dose of 4 mg/day) for 21, 28, or 35 days. Late follicular and midluteal endometrial biopsies (day 21) were performed. All late follicular biopsies showed normal proliferative endometrium; the midluteal biopsies revealed adequate secretory endometrium consistent with 18.6, 21.8, and 18.6 days in the respective groups. Substantial glandular-stromal dysynchrony was not observed. Artificially prolonging the follicular phase did not seem to have an adverse effect on endometrial histologic composition. The same investigators[45] studied the effect of a prolonged artificial follicular phase on clinical outcome. After varying estrogen stimulations of 4 to 11 days, 12 to 19 days, and 20 to 29 days before initiation of progesterone therapy, the clinical pregnancy rates were 7.7%, 52%, and

7.7%, respectively. These findings suggest that unlike endometrial morphologic composition, the functional receptivity of the endometrium is less permissive to manipulations of the follicular phase.

Synchronization of donor-recipient cycles in which the recipient has a normal cycle may be even more troublesome. Initial efforts focused on coordinating the midcycle LH surge of the recipient with follicular maturation, hCG administration, and oocyte retrieval for the donor.[15] Serhal and Craft[46] offered a simplified approach in which women with normal cycles started taking estradiol valerate (2 mg orally) three or four times a day starting early in the cycle. No specific synchronization efforts were undertaken, and the recipients continued to take estrogen for 2 to 4 weeks before the donor oocytes became available. Intramuscular administration of progesterone-in-oil (100 mg daily) was initiated the day before the donor's egg collection. Five of 7 patients undergoing GIFT and 2 of 10 patients undergoing IVF conceived using this strategy. However, the study involved a relatively small number of patients. It is also known that ovulation is not always suppressed by oral administration of micronized estradiol and intramuscular injection of progesterone at these dosages. Sauer et al[47] reported five instances of spontaneous ovulation during 200 cycles (2.5%) of hormonal replacement ovum donation cycles in women who were previously believed to be functionally agonadal. Three of these cycles were canceled because of inappropriate timing of spontaneous ovulation.

Our approach is to render cycling women functionally agonadal with a GnRH agonist.[38] It is important to note that because the donor's follicular phase may be shortened by gonadotropin therapy, estrogen replacement in the recipient should ideally begin a few days before the donor's expected menses. The length of the recipient's follicular phase does not appear to be critical and can be adjusted to accommodate the duration of the donor's stimulation. Progesterone is initiated the day before donor egg retrieval, allowing embryo transfer on cycle day 18 (for 2-day-old embryos) or day 19 (for 3-day-old embryos) into a receptive endometrial milieu. It must be emphasized that although transfer is performed on day 18 or 19, the early embryo must continue to develop in vivo to the blastocyst stage when it hatches from the zona pellucida and implants 2 to 4 days after transfer. Thus transfer of blastocyst stage embryos would theoretically be performed on day 20 or 21 to ensure synchronization. This correlates with the classic findings of Croxatto et al[48] who showed that in spontaneous cycles, embryo implantation most likely takes place 5 to 7 days after ovulation. In the case of donor oocyte GIFT cycles, the laparoscopic transfer of gametes is generally performed on cycle day 15, coincident with the initiation of progesterone administration. This practice allows transport of any resulting embryos to the recipient's endometrial cavity by cycle day 18 or 19.

EMBRYO TRANSFER AND POSTTRANSFER CARE

In donor oocyte IVF, appropriately timed embryo transfer in the recipient is usually performed by means of routine transcervical catheterization. Other approaches are possible; pregnancies have been reported after pronuclear stage tubal transfer (PROST), GIFT, and ZIFT.[49]

After embryo transfer, the recipient rests for about 30 to 60 minutes, after which normal activity may be resumed. The recipient continues estrogen and progesterone replacement during the luteal phase. The adequacy of hormonal administration and absorption is documented with serial measurements of the patient's hormone levels. A serum β-hCG level may be obtained 10 to 12 days after embryo transfer. If the test is positive the replacement regimen is continued. In a failed cycle, medication is discontinued and is followed by withdrawal bleeding.

After a successful donor oocyte IVF–embryo transfer (IVF-ET) cycle, the onset of placental steroidogenesis is heralded by a marked increase in the pregnant recipient's serum estradiol and progesterone levels; at this point the dosage of the replacement hormones may be halved. Steroid concentrations are reassessed in the following week. If a continued rise is detected, replacement therapy is unnecessary after the 12th week of gestation. Estradiol and progesterone levels are monitored for at least 1 week after medication is discontinued to ensure adequacy of placental steroidogenesis.

Once the luteoplacental shift has occurred, the patient is referred to an obstetrician for continued prenatal care. An early sonographic evaluation is advised to confirm normal intrauterine implantation, fetal viability, and to evaluate possible multifetal gestations. Donor oocyte recipients older than 40 years should be considered at high risk because there may be an increase in obstetric complications in older women.[50]

OUTCOME OF OOCYTE DONATION

Oocyte donation has continued to be an effective form of treatment for both women with and women without ovarian failure who have been unsuccessful with conventional IVF. Because oocytes generally are obtained from young, fertile donors and the resulting embryos are transferred to an optimized, physiologically primed endometrial bed, the success rates in many programs actually exceed those of conventional IVF. An analysis of the 1993 IVF Registry of the Society for Assisted Reproductive Technology (SART) supported this trend.[1] Programs in the United States and Canada reported a total of 2766 cycles of oocyte donation initiated during that year, of which 2368 went to retrieval (14.4% cancellation rate). A total of 2446 embryo transfers were performed, and in some instances a single donor's oocytes were used for more than one recipient. These findings revealed a 36.6% clinical pregnancy rate and 29.3% delivery rate per transfer. These statistics are clearly favorable when viewed in the context of overall IVF clinical pregnancy and delivery rates of 25.9% and 20.9% per transfer.

Several interesting points regarding factors that affect the success of ovum donation are apparent. First, it appears that success does not diminish appreciably with the advancing age of the recipient. Sauer et al[51] reported on 65 patients 40 years or older who underwent oocyte donation and found that the pregnancy rate for this group approximated that of women younger than 40 years. Abdalla et al[52] did report a steady drop in pregnancy rate with advancing age of the oocyte recipient in an initial report; however, when this group expanded their database after 259 cycles, they did not find a difference in the pregnancy rates between age groups.[53] We evaluated our results after 250 ovum donation transfers (Table 45–4) and did not find any appreciable decrease in clinical pregnancy rate, ongoing pregnancy rate, or embryo implantation rate with advancing age. The ongoing pregnancy rate per transfer among patients 40 years and older was 48% compared with 50% among patients 34 years and younger. However, there was a small, but not statistically significant, drop in implantation rate per embryo with advancing age of the recipient.

Ovum donation has been used successfully for women who have been unsuccessful with prior IVF cycles. Burton et al[54] reported on treatment of 32 women who previously had only a 2.5% clinical pregnancy rate and no livebirths after 119 standard IVF cycles. With oocyte donation, these women were able to achieve a 24% clinical pregnancy rate in 45 cycles. Remohi et al[55] also reported that oocyte donation can be successful in women who typically exhibit a low response to ovarian stimulation.

Ovum donation has been used successfully in the setting of tubal transfers. Borrero et al[56] reported on a series of 19 patients with premature ovarian failure who underwent GIFT with donated oocytes. The authors reported a 58% clinical pregnancy rate among this group. Balmaceda et al[57] described a prospective, randomized comparison between uterine and tubal transfer in their oocyte donation program. All embryos were transferred at the two- to four-cell stage 44 to 48 hours after insemination whether or not transfer was planned to be intrauterine or intratubal. Transfers were performed on the third day of progesterone replacement in the recipient. Pregnancy rates were equivalent after uterine transfers (54%) and tubal transfers (58%) in this series.

There may be a higher incidence of obstetric complications in pregnancies resulting from ovum donation. Pados et al[58] reported a 35% incidence of uterine bleeding in the first trimester, a 33% incidence of maternal hypertension, and a 12% incidence of intrauterine growth retardation in a series of 52 pregnancies resulting from oocyte donation, which included eight sets of twins. The cesarean section rate was 63%, with a high percentage of elective procedures (54%). The advanced maternal age of some of these patients and the increased incidence of multiple gestations may be contributing factors in these increased risks.

OOCYTE DONATION AS AN IN VIVO MODEL FOR EARLY REPRODUCTIVE PROCESSES

Because there is an inherent dissociation of perinidatory embryonic and endometrial events in donor oocyte IVF, these two variables can be independently studied and manipulated. This has afforded a detailed scientific model for analyzing various processes in human reproductive physiology, particularly uterine versus oocyte senescence and the definition of the optimal window of embryo transfer.

We examined the efficiency of transfer of early donor embryos replaced on different luteal days of a primed recipient in an attempt to demarcate the temporal interval of maximal endometrial receptivity.[41] Optimum implantation efficiency was observed when transfers were performed on days 17 to 19 of the recipient's replacement cycle. No pregnancies resulted when embryos were transferred on cycle day 16 or after cycle day 20. In a later study, Navot et al[59] did document pregnancies after embryo transfers on luteal day 1 (recipient's day 15) to luteal day 6 (recipient's day 20), suggesting that the interval of endometrial receptivity may actually be longer than previously thought, although the precise width of this window has not yet been fully defined.

Oocyte donation has also served as an excellent model for examining the luteoplacental shift and attainment of placental steroidogenic competence in early pregnancy. In the early 1970s, Csapo et al[30,31] estimated that placental takeover of steroidogenesis generally occurs during the eighth week of gestation, according to studies with pregnant women who underwent luteectomy. We further examined this issue with a group of nine patients with ovarian failure who achieved pregnancies through ovum donation.[60] These patients received a constant

TABLE 45–4. PREGNANCY OUTCOME BY AGE OF RECIPIENT

	Recipient Age (y)		
	≤34	35–39	≥40
Mean age of donor (y)	28.8	28.5	28.6
No. of transfers	32	56	162
No. of clinical pregnancies per transfer	18 (56)	37 (66)	93 (57.4)
No. of ongoing pregnancies per transfer	16 (50)	35 (62)	78 (48.1)
Embryo implantation rate (%)	34.4	31.6	28.1

Numbers in parentheses are percentages.
Data from The Center for Reproductive Medicine and Infertility at The New York Hospital-Cornell Medical Center (1989–1994).

dosage of exogenous estradiol and progesterone during the luteal phase and throughout early gestation. Serum estradiol and progesterone levels were measured at 2- and 5-day intervals throughout the first trimester. Despite constant hormone replacement, statistically significant increases in serum estradiol and progesterone levels were recorded about 25 and 34 days after transfer, respectively. Regression analyses of estradiol and progesterone levels with gestational age suggested an intersection with basal hormonal levels approximately 3 weeks after transfer. These findings suggested that the onset of placental steroidogenesis occurred during the fifth gestational week, as calculated by the last menstrual period, rather than in the eighth gestational week as previously reported.

Salat-Baroux et al[61] examined levels of hCG, estradiol, and progesterone in patients with ovarian failure undergoing oocyte donation with fresh versus frozen embryos. This team found that hCG and estradiol levels were higher after fresh embryo transfers up to the fifth gestational week, a statistically significant difference. They speculated that this difference may be attributed to either a reduction in the blastomere number of frozen and thawed embryos or possibly a decrease in the metabolic activity of these particular embryos.

Ovum donation has proved to be a useful model in addressing controversy about the age-related decline in female fecundity and the relative importance of uterine as opposed to ovarian factors. Sauer et al[62] suggested that the successful implantation of oocyte donation for women older than 40 years demonstrates that the endometrium of an older woman retains its receptivity to implantation with proper steroid replacement therapy. This group also reported that there was no diminution in the embryo implantation rate among women older than 40 years who underwent ovum donation cycles compared to younger recipients.[51] Navot et al[63] also examined the relative roles of diminished oocyte quality and endometrial inadequacy in the age-related decline in fecundity. In a group of ovum donation patients 40 years and older, only 8 patients (5.3%) became pregnant in 150 previous cycles of ovulation induction and only 2 (3%) pregnancies were achieved in 60 previous cycles of conventional IVF. In contrast, after 50 ovum donation cycles, a 56% clinical pregnancy rate and a 30% delivery rate were recorded. Pregnancy outcomes among younger IVF patients were compared with those among their respective older recipients, who shared oocytes from the same cohort. There were no statistically significant differences in clinical pregnancy and delivery rates between the younger donors and their older recipients. These observations suggest that poor oocyte quality rather than endometrial factors is responsible for the poor reproductive outcome associated with advancing age. Using a similar model, we demonstrated that uterine factors may actually affect age-related fecundity.[64] Twenty-four younger IVF

TABLE 45–5. COMPARISON OF PREGNANCY OUTCOME AND IMPLANTATION EFFICIENCY AMONG YOUNGER IVF DONORS AND THEIR RESPECTIVE OLDER RECIPIENTS

Number	IVF Donors	Recipients	Significance
Number	24	24	—
Oocytes retrieved[a]	8.8 ± 4.0	7.2 ± 1.8	NS
Oocytes fertilized	109/173 (63)	127/211 (60)	NS
Embryos transferred[a]	3.0 ± 1.0	3.6 ± 0.7	$P < .05$
Embryos implanted	31/73 (42)	22/86 (26)	$P < .05$
Ongoing pregnancies	15/24 (62)	14/24 (58)	NS

NS, not significant.
Numbers in parentheses are percentages.
[a]Mean ± standard deviation.

patients who donated half of their oocytes were studied along with their respective older donor oocyte recipients (Table 45–5). The mean age of the donors and recipients was 32.3 and 40.0 years, respectively. Despite the similarity in the ongoing pregnancy rate for donors (62%) and recipients (58%), a statistically significant decrease occurred in embryo implantation rate in the recipients (26%) compared with the donors (42%). This suggests that there may be a subtle decrease in implantation efficiency among older donor oocyte recipients, although the transfer of multiple embryos may compensate for these elusive uterine factors.

GESTATIONAL SURROGACY

The use of a gestational surrogate (gestational carrier) to carry a genetically unrelated embryo was first described by Utian et al[65] in 1985. This group then reported on a series of 39 cycles in which a gestational carrier aided women undergoing IVF who had no functional uterus.[66] The primary indication for infertile couples seeking third-party involvement by a gestational carrier was either a surgically or congenitally absent uterus or a uterus that was nonfunctional because of surgical damage or developmental abnormalities. Other indications have included a history of placenta accreta, cervical incompetence, and various severe medical problems that would be life-threatening if the woman were to carry a pregnancy.

Gestational surrogacy should be differentiated from conventional (or traditional) surrogacy. In conventional surrogacy the pregnancy is the product of the gestational mother's oocyte and the sperm of the husband in the infertile couple. The surrogate is expected to relinquish her genetic child. In gestational surrogacy, the embryo is the genetic product of the egg and sperm of the infertile couple and it is transferred to the uterus of the gestational carrier, who has no genetic relation to the offspring.

Because the distinction between a gestational surrogate carrier and a conventional surrogate carrier is based on the source of the oocyte, the legal and ethical responsibilities of the gestational surrogate are less complicated. This is primarily because the gestational surrogate has no genetic relation to the offspring and serves only as a host for the duration of pregnancy and delivery. However, the legal relationships of the gestational surrogate are still not universally established and vary from state to state. Several states and countries have made any type of surrogacy illegal, and in some cases it is considered a criminal offense.

Marrs et al[67] reported on their experience with a large gestational carrier program. All women seeking treatment had either a surgically absent uterus or a uterus deemed incapable of sustaining a pregnancy. The infertile couples underwent assessment of ovarian function, tests for sexually transmitted diseases (including HIV infection), and semen evaluation. Surrogates were required to be younger than 35 years, have a normal medical and obstetric history, and have delivered at least one naturally borne child. Normality of the uterus was confirmed by means of ultrasonography or HSG. Surrogates were evaluated for ovulatory and luteal function by means of hormonal monitoring and endometrial biopsy. Screening for sexually transmitted diseases was undertaken. In addition, a full psychologic evaluation was performed. After a detailed discussion of the risk of participation with each party, a legal contractual agreement was obtained.

The type of stimulation used for the infertile woman (ovum donor) was determined by the natural synchrony of the two participants. If spontaneous synchrony was close, a leuprolide acetate flare protocol was used. If adjustments were necessary, a leuprolide acetate downregulation protocol was used. Ovulatory synchrony was satisfied when hCG was administered to the stimulated donor within 24 hours of the spontaneous LH surge of the surrogate in her natural cycle. If an LH surge did not occur within 24 hours of hCG administration, hCG also was administered to the surrogate if follicle maturation was determined by means of ultrasonography and hormonal evaluation. If the LH surge and hCG timing were more than 48 hours out of synchrony, all ova were collected, fertilized, and cryopreserved, and subsequent frozen-thawed embryo replacement cycles were performed according to the natural ovulation of the surrogate.

Among 45 infertile couples who underwent 81 cycles of treatment with the aid of a gestational carrier, there were 29 cycles of intrauterine transfer of fresh embryos, 18 ZIFTs of fresh embryos, and 34 cycles of embryo transfer with frozen and thawed embryos. Nineteen clinical pregnancies (23%) occurred, of which 15 (18%) resulted in ongoing pregnancies. There were no statistically significant differences in clinical outcomes between the various assisted reproduction procedures or in the clinical pregnancy rate between the donors who were younger than 39 years (23%) and those 39 years and older (24%).

We have begun a gestational surrogate program at The New York Hospital-Cornell Medical Center. We have found that rendering the host functionally agonadal with GnRH agonist therapy followed by programmed hormone replacement facilitates synchronization of both participants. The use of a hormone replacement cycle rather than the natural cycle in the host also greatly diminishes the risk of untimely spontaneous conception in a surrogate who has not practiced adequate contraception during her treatment cycle.

ETHICAL ISSUES

Oocyte donation raises a number of ethical and legal issues that are discussed in detail in Chapters 47 and 48. Clarification of the intent of all involved parties is essential, particularly concerning rearing rights and responsibilities for the offspring. Only three states (Oklahoma, Texas, and Florida) have enacted legislation that addresses issues related to children from oocyte donation.[68] To avoid misunderstanding, both donors and recipients should be fully counseled regarding the legal implications of participation, and informed consent should be obtained. The agreement should clearly state that the donors relinquishes all rearing rights and duties for the offspring, which are to be assigned to the recipient couple.

It is reasonable for oocyte donors to be compensated for the direct and indirect expenses of participation. However, compensation should not be so large as to constitute an inducement and deter the donor from the altruistic nature of donation. It also remains unclear who should bear the costs if a complication occurs in a donor who has undergone ovarian stimulation and oocyte retrieval solely for the purpose of oocyte donation. These responsibilities remain legally untested. However, several insurance companies do offer riders to medical insurance policies specifically designed to cover oocyte donors. It is incumbent on programs to emphasize to recipients that they are responsible for the medical costs of the donor.

Concerns about unintended consanguinity and the undesirable genetic consequence of multiple donation from a single donor has led The American Society for Reproductive Medicine to recommend that if donors are to be used repeatedly, care should be taken to assure that no more than ten offspring are born from any one donor. It seems unlikely that this situation would arise in oocyte donation.

Although the principal indication for oocyte donation has been the treatment of infertile women with premature ovarian failure, perhaps greater potential exists to extend the reproductive potential of women who have undergone natural menopause. Several studies have demonstrated the applicability and effectiveness of oocyte donation extended to women in their 40s.[51,62] Successful pregnancies and deliveries have occurred among women older than 50 years.[69,70] Although no serious complications were described in these reports, not enough data have been accumulated to assure safety for both mother and offspring. Sauer et al[69] recommended extensive medical screening for oocyte donation candidates older than 50 years. However, because pregnancy experience is limited in this age group, it is not known if this type of testing would preclude increased maternal or fetal complications. Little is known about the psychologic effects of childbearing in advanced years or whether patients are physically and emotionally equipped for caring for a newborn infant and ensuing other parenting challenges.

The limiting factor in most oocyte donation programs continues to be the relative shortage of oocytes, that is, donors. As technology develops, particularly the capability to culture and maintain immature oocytes, novel sources of oocytes may become available. Use of cadaveric tissue[71] or oocytes obtained from aborted fetuses[72] has been proposed. Continued careful ethical consideration of these evolving techniques and emerging ideas is warranted.[27]

REFERENCES

1. Society for Assisted Reproductive Technology, American Society for Reproductive Medicine: Assisted reproductive technology in the United States and Canada: 1993 results generated from the American Society for Reproductive Medicine/Society for Assisted Reproductive Technology Registry. *Fertil Steril* 64:13, 1995
2. Heape W: Preliminary note on the transplantation and growth of mammalian ova within a uterine foster mother. *Proc R Soc Lond* 48:457, 1890
3. Wilett EL, Black WG, Casida LE, et al: Successful transplantation of a fertilized bovine ovum. *Science* 113:247, 1951
4. Seidel GE, Jr: Superovulation and embryo transfer in cattle. *Science* 211:351, 1981
5. Beatty RA: Transplantation of mouse eggs. *Nature* 168:995, 1951
6. Rowson LEA, Moor RM: Embryo transfer in the sheep: The significance of synchronizing estrus in the donor and recipient animal. *J Reprod Fertil* 11:201, 1966
7. Rowson LEA, Lawson RAS, Moor RM, Baker AA: Egg transfer in the cow: Synchronization requirements. *J Reprod Fertil* 28:427, 1972
8. Meyer RK, Wolf RC, Arslan M: Implantation and maintenance of pregnancy in progesterone-treated ovariectomized monkeys (*Macaca mulatta*). In: Hofer H (ed), *Proceedings of the Second International Congress of Primatology*. Vol 2. 1968, Atlanta, GA, Karger, Basel/New York, pp. 30–35
9. Hodgen GD: Surrogate embryo transfer combined with estrogen-progesterone therapy in monkeys. *JAMA* 250:2167, 1983
10. Buster JE, Bustillo M, Thorneycroft IH, et al: Non-surgical transfer of an in-vivo fertilized donated ovum to an infertility patient. *Lancet* 1:816, 1983
11. Buster JE, Bustillo M, Thorneycroft IH, et al: Nonsurgical transfer of in vivo fertilized donated ova to five infertile women: Report of two pregnancies. *Lancet* 2:223, 1983
12. Formigli L, Formigli G, Roccio C: Donation of fertilized uterine ova to infertile women. *Fertil Steril* 47:162, 1987
13. Sauer MV: Retained pregnancy complicating donor ovum transfer. *Int J Gynecol Obstet* 29:83, 1989
14. Trounson A, Leeton J, Besanko M, et al: Pregnancy established in an infertile patient after transfer of a donated embryo fertilized in vitro. *Br Med J* 286:835, 1983
15. Rosenwaks Z, Veeck LL, Liu H-C: Pregnancy following transfer of in vitro fertilized donated oocytes. *Fertil Steril* 45:417, 1986
16. Lutjen P, Trounson A, Leeton J, et al: The establishment and maintenance of pregnancy using in vitro fertilization and embryo donation in a patient with primary ovarian failure. *Nature* 307:174, 1984
17. Asch RH, Balmaceda JP, Ord T, et al: Oocyte donation and gamete intrafallopian transfer in premature ovarian failure. *Fertil Steril* 49:263, 1988
18. Yovich JL, Blackledge DG, Richardson PA, et al: PROST for ovum donation. *Lancet* 1:1209, 1987
19. Scott RT, Toner JP, Muasher SJ, et al: Follicle-stimulating hormone levels on cycle day 3 are predictive of in vitro fertilization outcome. *Fertil Steril* 51:651, 1989
20. Licciardi FL, Liu H-C, Rosenwaks Z: Day 3 estradiol serum concentrations as prognosticators of stimulation response and pregnancy outcome in patients undergoing in vitro fertilization. *Fertil Steril* 64:991, 1995
21. Rosenwaks Z, Davis OK: Implantation efficiency and egg donation in women with elevated FSH concentration and advanced chronological age. In: Schats R, Schoemaker J (eds), *Ovarian Endocrinopathies: The Proceedings of the 8th Reinier de Graaf Symposium*. New York, Parthenon, 1993:49–55
22. Navot D, Rosenwaks Z, Margalioth EJ: Prognostic assessment of female fecundity. *Lancet* 19:645, 1987
23. Padilla SL, Smith RD, Garcia JE: The Lupron screening test: Tailoring the use of leuprolide acetate in ovarian stimulation for in vitro fertilization. *Fertil Steril* 56:79, 1991
24. Jones HW Jr, Jones GS, Andrews MC, et al: The program for in vitro fertilization at Norfolk. *Fertil Steril* 38:14, 1982
25. Noyes RW, Hertig AT, Rock J: Dating the endometrial biopsy. *Fertil Steril* 1:3, 1950
26. The American Fertility Society: Guidelines for gamete donation: 1994. *Fertil Steril* 62:105S, 1994
27. Seibel MM, Crockin SL (eds): *Family Building Through Egg and Sperm Donation: Medical, Legal and Ethical Issues.* Sudbury, MA: Jones & Bartlett, 1996
28. Whittemore AS, Harris T, Intyre J, and the Collaborative Ovarian Cancer Group: Characteristics related to ovarian cancer risk: Col-

laborative analysis of 12 US case-control studies. II. Invasive epithelial ovarian cancers in white women. *Am J Epidemiol* 136: 1184, 1992

29. Seibel MM, Kiessling A: Compensating egg donors: Equal pay for equal time? *N Engl J Med* 328:737, 1993

30. Csapo AI, Pulkkinen MO, Wiest WG: Effects of luteectomy and progesterone replacement therapy in early pregnant patients. *Am J Obstet Gynecol* 115:759, 1973

31. Csapo AI, Pulkkinen MO, Kaihola HL: The effect of estradiol replacement therapy on early pregnant luteectomized patients. *Am J Obstet Gynecol* 117:987, 1973

32. Rosenwaks Z: Donor eggs: Their application in modern reproductive technologies. *Fertil Steril* 47:895, 1987

33. Stumpf PG, Maruca J, Santen RJ, Demers LM: Development of a vaginal ring for achieving physiologic levels of 17β-estradiol in hypoestrogenic women. *J Clin Endocrinol Metab* 54:208, 1982

34. Droesch K, Navot D, Scott R, et al: Transdermal estrogen replacement in ovarian failure for ovum donation. *Fertil Steril* 50:931, 1988

35. Davis OK, Rosenwaks Z: The impact of in vitro fertilization on the treatment of castrate women. *Semin Reprod Endocrinol* 8:313, 1990

36. Lutjen PJ, Findlay JK, Trounson AO, et al: Effect on plasma gonadotropins of cyclic steroid replacement in women with premature ovarian failure. *J Clin Endocrinol Metab* 62:419, 1986

37. Navot D, Laufer N, Kopolovic J, et al: Artificially induced endometrial cycles and establishment of pregnancies in the absence of ovaries. *N Engl J Med* 314:806, 1986

38. Meldrum DR, Wisot A, Hamilton F, et al: Artificial agonadism and hormone replacement for oocyte donation. *Fertil Steril* 52:509, 1989

39. Seibel MM: Toward reducing risks and costs of egg donation: A preliminary report. *Fertil Steril* 64:199, 1995

40. Cohen J, Alikani M, Trowbridge J, Rosenwaks Z: Implantation enhancement by selective assisted hatching using zona drilling of human embryos with poor prognosis. *Hum Reprod* 7:685, 1992

41. Navot D, Scott RT, Droesch K, et al: The window of embryo transfer and the efficiency of human conception in vitro. *Fertil Steril* 55:114, 1991

42. Salat-Baroux J, Cornet D, Alvarez S, et al: Pregnancies after replacement of frozen-thawed embryos in a donation program. *Fertil Steril* 49:817, 1988

43. Navot D, Anderson TL, Droesch K, et al: Hormonal manipulation of endometrial maturation. *J Clin Endocrinol Metab* 68:801, 1989

44. Younis JS, Mordel N, Ligovetsky G, et al: The effect of a prolonged artificial follicular phase on endometrial development in an oocyte donation program. *J In Vitro Fertil Embryo Transf* 8:84, 1991

45. Younis JS, Mordel N, Lewin A, et al: Artificial endometrial preparation for oocyte donation: The effect of estrogen stimulation on clinical outcome. *J Assist Reprod Genet* 9:222, 1992

46. Serhal PF, Craft IL: Ovum donation: A simplified approach. *Fertil Steril* 48:265, 1987

47. Sauer MV: Spontaneous ovulation in functionally agonadal women prior to oocyte donation: Incidence and remedies for avoiding cancellation. *J Assist Reprod Genet* 10:381, 1993

48. Croxatto HB, Diaz S, Fuentealba B, et al: Studies on the duration of egg transport in the human oviduct. I. The time interval between ovulation and egg recovery from the uterus of normal women. *Fertil Steril* 23:447, 1972

49. Abdalla HJ, Leonart T: Cryopreserved zygote intrafallopian transfer for anonymous oocyte donation. *Lancet* 1:835, 1988

50. Naeye RL: Maternal age, obstetric complications and the outcome of pregnancy. *Obstet Gynecol* 61:210, 1983

51. Sauer MV, Paulson RJ, Lobo RA: Reversing the natural decline in human fertility: An extended clinical trial of oocyte donation to women of advanced reproductive age. *JAMA* 268: 1275, 1992

52. Abdalla HI, Baber R, Kirkland A, et al: A report on 100 cycles of oocyte donation: Factors affecting the outcome. *Hum Reprod* 5:1018, 1990

53. Abdalla H, Burton G, Kirkland A, et al: Factors affecting outcome in 259 cycles of ovum donation. *Hum Reprod* 6(Suppl): 114, 1991

54. Burton G, Abdalla HI, Kirkland A, Studd JWW: The role of oocyte donation in women who are unsuccessful with in-vitro fertilization treatment. *Hum Reprod* 7:1103, 1992

55. Remohi J, Vidal A, Pellicer A: Oocyte donation in low responders to conventional ovarian stimulation for in vitro fertilization. *Fertil Steril* 59:1208, 1993

56. Borrero C, Remohi J, Ord T, et al: A program of oocyte donation and gamete intra-fallopian transfer. *Hum Reprod* 4:275, 1989

57. Balmaceda JP, Alam V, Roszjtein D, et al: Embryo implantation rates in oocyte donation: A prospective comparison of tubal versus uterine transfers. *Fertil Steril* 57:362, 1992

58. Pados G, Camus M, Van Steirteghem A, et al: The evolution and outcome of pregnancies from oocyte donation. *Hum Reprod* 9:538, 1994

59. Navot D, Bergh PA, Williams M, et al: An insight into early reproductive processes through the in vivo model of ovum donation. *J Clin Endocrinol Metab* 72:408, 1991

60. Scott R, Navot D, Liu H-C, Rosenwaks Z: A human in vivo model for the luteoplacental shift. *Fertil Steril* 56:481, 1991

61. Salat-Baroux J, Cornet D, Alvarez S, et al: Hormonal secretions in singleton pregnancies arising from the implantation of fresh or frozen embryos after oocyte donation in women with ovarian failure. *Fertil Steril* 57:150, 1992

62. Sauer MV, Paulson RJ, Lobo RA: Preliminary report on oocyte donation extending reproductive potential to women over 40. *N Engl J Med* 323:1157, 1990

63. Navot D, Bergh PA, Williams MA, et al: Poor oocyte quality rather than implantation failure as a cause of age-related decline in female fertility. *Lancet* 337:1375, 1991

64. Sultan KM, Neal GS, Cholst I, et al: Uterine factors influence implantation in an oocyte donation program. Presented at the 50th Annual Meeting of the American Fertility Society, November 5–10, 1994, San Antonio, Texas

65. Utian WH, Sheean L, Goldfarb JM, Kiwi R: Successful pregnancy after in vitro fertilization and embryo transfer from an infertile woman to a surrogate. *N Engl J Med* 313:1351, 1985

66. Utian WH, Goldfarb JM, Kiwi R, et al: Preliminary experience with in vitro fertilization-surrogate gestational pregnancy. *Fertil Steril* 52:633, 1989

67. Marrs RP, Ringler GE, Stein A, et al: The use of surrogate gestational carriers for assisted reproductive technologies (ART). *Am J Obstet Gynecol* 168:1858, 1993

68. The American Fertility Society: American law and assisted reproductive technologies. *Fertil Steril* 62(Suppl):8, 1994

69. Sauer MV, Paulson RJ, Lobo RA: Pregnancy after age 50: Application of oocyte donation to women after natural menopause. *Lancet* 341:321, 1993

70. Antinori S, Versaci C, Gholami GH, et al: Oocyte donation in menopausal women. *Hum Reprod* 8:1487, 1993

71. Seibel MM: Cadaveric ovary donation. *N Engl J Med* 330:796, 1994

72. Shusan A, Schenker JG: The use of oocytes obtained from aborted fetuses in egg donation programs. *Fertil Steril* 62:449, 1994

CHAPTER 46

Cryopreservation and Infertility

PATRICK QUINN · PIERRE JOUANNET · RENE FRYDMAN · ANDRÉ C. VAN STEIRTEGHEM ·
J. P. WOLF · F. CZYGLIK · E. VAN DEN ABBEEL

Historical Overview of Cryopreservation
  Sperm freezing
  Embryo freezing
  Oocyte freezing
Concepts
Cryopreservation in Animal Reproduction
Cryopreservation of Human Spermatozoa
  Technical procedures
  Influence of cryopreservation on sperm function
  Clinical use of cryopreserved semen

Cryopreservation of Human Embryos
  Embryo survival after thawing
  Survey of cryopreservation of
    human embryos
  Clinical importance of these techniques
  The fate of supernumerary cryopreserved
    embryos
Oocyte Freezing
Ethical Considerations

HISTORICAL OVERVIEW OF CRYOPRESERVATION

Sperm Freezing

The first studies of the effect of very low temperatures on human spermatozoa were performed by Spallanzani in 1776,[1] and the concept of sperm banking was discussed about a century later by Mantegazza.[2] It was known in the early 1940s that some spermatozoa could survive after freezing, and cryopreservation of spermatozoa became possible when Rostand[3] discovered the cryoprotective role of glycerol for biologic structures in 1946 and when Polge et al[4] successfully used this procedure in 1949. The technique was rapidly and extensively used to breed farm animals, but application to humans was not undertaken for some time. Bunge and Sherman[5] first observed in 1953 that human sperm, frozen in dry ice and later thawed, were able to fertilize and induce normal embryonic development. In the following years only a few births were reported after insemination with stored sperm. The first births after freezing of human spermatozoa with glycerol in liquid nitrogen were reported in 1964.[6] The same year it was shown that dimethylsulfoxide (DMSO) was toxic to spermatozoa.

In the 1970s there was a gradual emergence of national and commercial cryobanks for semen. In the United States, the hope of obtaining "fertility insurance" before vasectomy led to the development of commercial banks, and some banks also were established in university hospitals. In France, the first Centre d'Etude et de Conservation du Sperme (CECOS) was set up in 1973. The American Association of Tissue Banks was founded in 1976, and the first international meeting on human semen cryopreservation was held in Paris in 1978.

The concept of using frozen donor sperm for artificial insemination was not clearly understood in many countries until recently. It is only since the risk of disease transmission was demonstrated, especially transmission of acquired immunodeficiency syndrome (AIDS),[7] that it has been recommended that only frozen semen be used for therapeutic insemination with donor sperm (TID), because this procedure provides the necessary controls to contain this risk.

Embryo Freezing

Embryo cryopreservation was first performed successfully in mice.[8] The methods were later adapted to preserve embryos of other animal species at low temperature, and they became established means of commercially banking cattle and sheep embryos. In mice, this procedure allowed genetic conservation of different strains. For mice and other animal species embryo cryopreservation is reliable and safe with respect to genetic stability and occurrence of malformations at birth.

The techniques used to freeze human embryos were based on those used for animals. The first human pregnancy was reported after transfer of an eight-cell embryo frozen in DMSO. The pregnancy aborted at 24 weeks because of an obstetric complication.[9] The first pregnancies and livebirths with the DMSO protocol were reported in the mid 1980s.[10,11] Around the same time, the first birth after successful conservation at low temperature of a blastocyst frozen in glycerol was reported.[12] In addition to those with the DMSO and glycerol protocols, pregnancies were reported with the use of propanediol as cryoprotective agent.[13]

Oocyte Freezing

In contrast to embryo freezing, fewer experimental data are available concerning oocyte freezing. Only three groups have reported pregnancies and the birth of four children after transfer of a previously frozen fertilized oocyte.[14–16] The survival rate after thawing was reduced in three protocols, and polyploidy was substantially increased.[15] More recent studies have centered on problems of fertilization and embryonic development associated with oocytes subjected to cryopreservation and ways to alleviate these problems.[17–19]

CONCEPTS

Long-term storage of biologic structures requires the arrest of cellular and molecular activity while the integrity of the structures necessary to restore normal cell function is maintained. This can be done by means of removal of water from the cell with either lyophilization or by freezing; however, the former may be mutagenic. Lowering the temperature induces an important decrease or a complete stop of cell metabolism. Freezing and thawing can be toxic either directly through physical or chemical modifications of the cell or indirectly because of damage to the cell structures by ice crystals. The phenomena accompanying freezing and thawing are summarized in Fig 46–1. Basic aspects and consequences of low-temperature preservation have been extensively reviewed elsewhere.[20] The main consequence of freezing is the phase modification of water. The first event is the nucleation or formation of the first ice crystal at a temperature below the equilibrium freezing point. In biologic systems, nucleation begins in the extracellular environment usually between $-5°C$ and $-15°C$. The difference between equilibrium and nucleation temperature is *supercooling*. The degree of supercooling may be decreased by inducing physical seeding, which is the initiation of nucleation at a controlled temperature near the equilibrium point.

During freezing, the proliferation of ice crystals induces the development of a solid phase, whereas the solute concentration increases in the portion that remains liquid. Because of membrane permeability and the freezing rate, this leads to cell dehydration and shrinkage and increased concentration of intracellular solute. Cell dehydration may be avoided by rapid freezing, but this does result in nucleation of large amounts of intracellular ice, which may damage the cell structure. Partial dehydration of the cells before freezing may reduce intracellular crystallization, for example, by means of incubation of the cells in a sucrose solution. During thawing, an osmotic shock may occur when water returns to the cell. Other damage may be the consequence of crystallization of the amorphous intracellular ice.

The addition of cryoprotective agents (CPAs) has been shown to diminish considerably the deleterious effect of freezing and thawing. These organic solvents modify the physical properties of a solution by lowering its freezing point. When they replace intracellular water, CPAs reduce the adverse consequences of phase change during crystallization and fusion. Their action depends on their ability to penetrate the membranes and on their degree of toxicity to the cell. To prevent this toxicity, CPAs are often added to the solution at a very low temperature. Another way to avoid cell damage is to produce vitrification instead of water crystallization. Vitrification is the formation of amorphous ice, which can be achieved with very rapid freezing or use of a very high concentration of CPA.

The success of the freezing storage thawing procedure depends on many factors. Some are linked to the cell, such as cell size, surface-to-volume ratio, membrane permeability, and resistance to osmotic or cold shock. Other factors are technical, such as the nature and concentration of the CPA, and the rate of freezing and thawing. The various factors cannot be efficiently combined with a mathematical formula, and the pragmatic approach of gamete and embryo cryopreservation has shown that optimum conditions have not yet been well defined and may be very different from one cell to another.

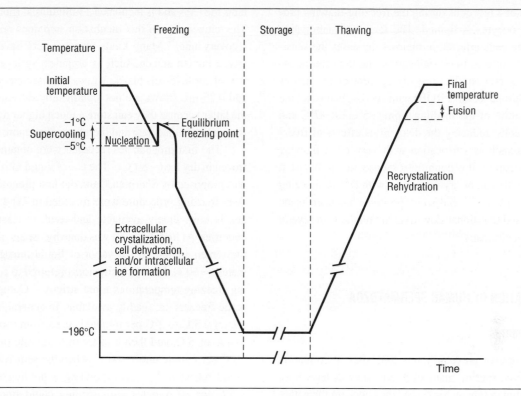

Figure 46–1. Schematic depiction of events occurring at the cell level during freezing and thawing. In this example the sample is not seeded, so supercooling is important before nucleation.

CRYOPRESERVATION IN ANIMAL REPRODUCTION

Cryopreservation of spermatozoa has been widely developed in domestic animal species.[21] The protocol used is derived mainly from the method initially proposed by Polge et al[4] Because cryopreservation allows almost indefinite conservation of semen, numerous sperm banks have been established, allowing dramatic improvement in techniques of reproduction of domestic animals by means of genetic selection, preservation of various disappearing species, and development of some new ones, such as cows that produce abundant milk and that resist bad climatic conditions. Furthermore, progress in gene transfer has emphasized the interest in cryopreservation of breeds of genetic significance.

Semen of more than 50 different species has been frozen successfully. Artificial insemination with frozen semen in cattle is widely practiced; more than 90% of dairy animals are reproduced by this technique in developed countries. There is a great variability among species and among males with respect to freezability of semen, however.[22] In pigs, for instance, birth rates after artificial insemination with frozen sperm are about 10% less than those obtained with fresh semen,[23] whereas in mares this level drops to 50% of the controls.[21,22]

Techniques for the cryopreservation of embryos have been used successfully in at least nine species of domestic animals, including cows, rabbits, and mice. These are described in detail elsewhere.[24–27] Only minor changes have been introduced in the procedures. One modification is the use of sucrose before cooling the embryos and during the thawing process as an osmotic aid during dilution of the CPA.[13,27]

Hormonal stimulation of ovaries and the ability to increase by several times the mean number of viable embryos produced per cycle have led to advances in embryo cryopreservation. Under optimal conditions, the resulting pregnancy rate among cattle is only 10% lower than with fresh embryo transfer. The economic aspects are important because this technique allows the development of embryos of defined genetic origins in "surrogate cows." This may eventually help find a solution to the problem of disease transmission by embryos (such as bovine diarrhea virus), because evidence exists that several types of viruses are unable to cross the zona pellucida of frozen-thawed embryos.[28]

Cryopreservation of oocytes also has been proposed. In 1977, Whittingham[29] reported the first study of fertilization of unfertilized mouse oocytes previously stored at −196°C. Although survival of embryos is good because they can accommodate the loss of a few cells during the freezing-thawing procedure, that of oocytes is limited. The fact that mammalian oocytes are large cells arrested in meiosis increases the sensitivity of the cell skeleton to crystallization and the osmotic effects of cryopreservation. The use of cryoprotectant such as DMSO and 1,2-propanediol (PROH) with sucrose decreases the seeding temperature of the medium from $-5°C$ to $-7°C$ and dehydrates the cells, reducing the deleterious effects of freezing. Techniques such as vitrification with very rapid freezing are under investigation. It is doubtful if mouse, rabbit, hamster, and primate oocytes can be cryopreserved with DMSO freezing and thawing protocols,[29–33] but some progress has been made with ultrarapid and traditional slow-freezing methods in several species, including humans.[18,34–37]

CRYOPRESERVATION OF HUMAN SPERMATOZOA

Technical Procedures

Since the first human pregnancy reported after insemination with cryopreserved sperm,[5] many different methods have been used to freeze human semen. Variations may concern the nature of the cryoprotective agent, the dilution medium, the temperature of CPA added to the semen, the semen container, the cooling, freezing, and thawing rates, and the storage temperature.[38]

Technical procedures have been progressively improved in a pragmatic way. In most instances, they were not evaluated with study of the fertilization rate of cryopreserved sample but by means of establishment of the recovery or cryosurvival rate, which is the ratio of the percentage of motile sperm observed after thawing to the percentage of motile sperm in fresh semen multiplied by 100. The choice of technique may be a function of the cryopreservation activity of a given center. A sperm bank that freezes many samples every day can use sophisticated methods, whereas a small center uses simple and inexpensive procedures.

Glycerol is the CPA most commonly used. It has a better cryoprotective effect than DMSO or ethylene glycol.[39,40] A final concentration of 6% to 8% glycerol gives the best postthaw motility and velocity of spermatozoa.[41] Although glycerol may be used alone, diluting it in a semen extender that contains proteins and sugars seems to allow better recovery of postthaw motility[42,43] and should be recommended. Many different media have been described, most of them containing egg yolk, sucrose or glucose, citrate, glycine, and antibiotics.[39,44] A comparative study found that the best recovery rate of sperm motility was obtained with the following buffer: 48% TEST (a mixture of TES and TRIS buffers), 30% citrate, 20% egg yolk, and 2% fructose.[42]

Usually, the semen is diluted 1:1 in an extender that contains the CPA and is incubated 15 minutes at room temperature. The temperature of this incubation step does not influence the recovery rate.[39] Many kinds of containers have been used to freeze human semen, such as ampules, syringes, pellets, and 0.5-mL or 0.25-mL plastic straws. The recovery rates for 0.5- and 0.25-mL straws are not significantly different.[45] We prefer the latter because they can store a much higher number of doses from a single ejaculate and therefore allow more inseminations.

The first pregnancies recorded were obtained with semen frozen in dry ice ($-80°C$).[5] The use of liquid nitrogen ($-196°C$) was proposed by Sherman,[46] and the first pregnancies after this deep-freezing procedure were recorded in 1964.[6] Liquid nitrogen is now widely available and used, at least in developed countries. At first, freezing was done by means of suspension of the semen sample in the vapor of liquid nitrogen at approximately $-60°C$. Later investigators preferred to control the cooling freezing temperatures more strictly.[40] Computerized automatic freezers are readily available. In general, a slow cooling rate of 0.5°C to 2°C per minute is used from room temperature to 4°C or 5°C, and then a faster freezing rate of 3°C to 5°C or 10°C per minute until $-80°C$, when the semen is plunged into liquid nitrogen.[40,47,48] Incorporating a holding temperature of $-5°C$ for 10 minutes with seeding could improve postthaw sperm motility and the ability to penetrate zona-free hamster oocytes.[49] Thawing is done by means of bringing the semen to room temperature or to 37°C for 10 to 15 minutes before insemination.

Influence of Cryopreservation on Sperm Function

Whatever the CPA and the technique, the most important and spectacular effect of freezing on sperm is loss of motility.[39,41,42,49] It is mainly due to the cold shock, but dilution in cryoprotective medium before freezing is also partly responsible.[50] The mean motility recovery rate is between 60% and 70% according to most studies but can be very different from one sample to another depending on initial sperm concentration, motility, and morphology.[44] In a study of 15,364 insemination cycles with frozen semen, the most predictive variable of conception rate was postthaw motility[51] (Fig 46–2).

The main cellular alterations responsible for the loss of motility do not seem to be at the axonemal level; it is possible to restore normal movement of demembranated bull spermatozoa after freezing and thawing.[52] Loss of motility is more probably related to plasma membrane damage, which has been described in electron microscopic studies.[53–57] Important modifications of the acrosomal structure are also frequently observed, but the ability of frozen sperm to penetrate zona-free hamster oocytes is not altered over that of fresh spermatozoa.[49,57] The mechanisms of sperm membrane cryoinjury are not well understood. It has been suggested that hyperproduction of superoxide radicals may

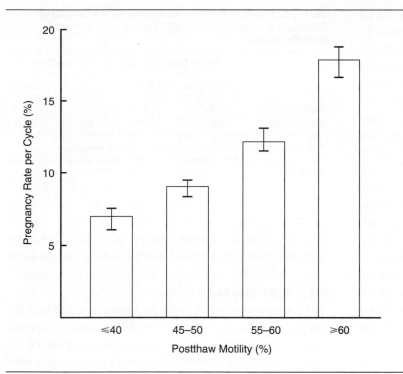

Figure 46–2. The influence of spermatozoa postthaw motility on pregnancy rate. These results were obtained from a program of artificial insemination with 1,438 donor ejaculates. (*From Mayaux et al,[51] reproduced with permission.*)

be responsible.[58,59] The demonstration of a beneficial effect of adding dithiothreitol to the cryoprotective medium on sperm motility and viability recovery rate after freezing supports this hypothesis.[60] There is no evidence of genetic alteration of spermatozoa with freezing, and the risks of abortion or malformation are not higher with frozen than with fresh sperm.[61–63]

Clinical Use of Cryopreserved Semen

In cattle breeding, the use of frozen semen allows genetic control of reproduction. Such possibilities were advocated by some of the pioneers who used frozen semen in humans. In 1964, one of them was predicting a "genetic improvement through germinal choice to achieve human betterment of mind and body."[63] Fortunately, such strange, controversial, and unrealistic views were not widely adopted, and the clinical developments of human semen banking have been limited mainly to preserving fertility of men undergoing voluntary sterilization or treatment of malignant disease and to TID to manage infertility.

Semen Autopreservation

Semen autopreservation may be considered when a man is to be sterilized either intentionally, as in the case of vasectomy, or as a consequence of treatment, mainly chemotherapy and radiation therapy. Accompanying the development of vasectomy in the United States, commercial banks were established in the 1960s. After that, controversy arose about the efficiency of this proce-

dure to restore fertility compared with vasovasostomy. Unfortunately, no clear data are available in the literature on these subjects. In France, about 500 men every year store their semen before vasectomy in the various CECOS banks. The sperm is stored only if the freezing test on each ejaculate is positive; that is, if more than 2×10^6 spermatozoa per 0.25-mL straw have progressive motility after thawing. The test is positive for only 70% of men, although most of them are fertile when they request a vasectomy.[64] As a rule, 50 straws are stored for each man, and usually two or three ejaculates are sufficient to supply this stock.[64]

In France a little more than 1% of vasectomized men use their frozen semen. This low figure may be explained by the fact that most vasectomies are performed for stable couples with children. If the number of men who use their semen after vasectomy is so small, and "if the storage of first semen does not guarantee future fertility,"[65] one can wonder if it is necessary to store semen before a vasectomy. The CECOS experience shows that even if frozen semen should not be considered fertility insurance, the delay together with various contacts with the medical team caused by the need to collect several ejaculates before the operation may help give men time to think about and discuss their options and thus strengthen their decision whether to undergo vasectomy. Having a "fertility potential" may also have some psychologic benefit even if men never use their stored semen.[66]

In the year after chemotherapy, the frequency of azoospermia varies from 14% for men with testicular tumors to 79% for those with Hodgkin's disease.[67] Semen freezing may offer the ability to preserve the fertility potential of young men with malignant disease. Unfortunately, semen quality is often altered in such men, and the minimum number of motile spermatozoa in a thawed straw estimated necessary to result in pregnancy is obtained in only a few.[68,69] No pregnancy was achieved with autopreserved semen when sperm concentration was less than 40%[68,70] or 55%[67] of the initial ejaculate. In the CECOS of Paris-Bicetre, the freezing test found more than 2×10^6 motile spermatozoa per thawed straw among 40% of men with Hodgkin's disease ($n = 580$) and 16% of men with testicular tumors ($n = 560$).[67] The very low number of pregnancies achieved with frozen sperm of such patients (Table 46–1) may be explained by this poor quality. This was well demonstrated by Czyglik,[67] who did not observe a pregnancy when less than 0.5×10^6 spermatozoa per straw were motile after thawing. On the other hand, pregnancy rates were identical to those observed in TID when the straw contained more than 2×10^6 motile spermatozoa after thawing (Table 46–2).

There is a clear need to improve semen autopreservation. At the CECOS Paris-Bicetre, 13% of the men whose semen was successfully frozen used it afterward, and 40% declared that they would have used it if necessary. New techniques must be developed to allow better cryopreservation of the fertilizing abilty of sperms. In addition, in vitro fertilization (IVF) might facilitate fertilization and normal fetal development with thawed semen of poor quality. The recent widespread and rapidly expanding use of intracytoplasmic sperm injection (ICSI) to treat many forms of male infertility[75] is certain to alleviate many of the problems of storage of semen with low-quality fertility potential when traditional forms of artificial conception (TID, IVF) are used.

A final question regarding autopreservation is the influence of long-term storage on the fertilizing ability of sperm.[71,72,74] In 1973, a substantial decline was reported in the motility of sperm thawed after 3 years in storage.[73] This result was not confirmed by others, who found that motility of sperm cryopreserved for more than 10 years remained remarkably sta-

TABLE 46–1. OVERVIEW OF THE USE OF SEMEN AUTOPRESERVED BY MEANS OF FREEZING (VASECTOMY EXCLUDED)

Reference	Period Under Study	Total Number of Men	Number of Men Using Their Semen	Number of Pregnancies
71	1969–1979	183	16	0
72	1973–1978	113	15	4
73	1975–1984	24	4	1
74	1976–1984	ND	22	8

ND, no data.

TABLE 46–2. PREGNANCY RATES PER INSEMINATION CYCLE ACCORDING TO THE QUALITY OF THAWED SEMEN PRESERVED BEFORE CHEMOTHERAPY OR RADIATION THERAPY

	Number of Motile Spermatozoa per Thawed Straw (10^6)			
	<0.5	0.5–2	>2	Control[a]
Pregnancy rate (%)	0	3	11	10.4
Number of cycles	106	159	267	5022

[a] Control values are the result of a therapeutic insemination with donor sperm program.
From Sanger WG, et al: Feasibility of semen cryopreservation in patients with malignant disease. JAMA 244:789, 1980.

ble.[76] Several men with cancer became fathers after their wives were inseminated with semen stored for more than 10 years.

Use of Frozen Donor Semen in TID

TID is widely used to help infertile couples have children. Because several studies have shown higher pregnancy rates with fresh semen, however, the use of cryopreserved semen has been increasing rather slowly. In a survey conducted in 1979, only 12.7% of physicians who were practicing TID in the United States used frozen semen.[77] A survey conducted in 1987 by the Office of Technology Assessment (OTA) of the U.S. Congress revealed that frozen semen was used by 78% of physicians.[78] The threat of transmission of human immunodeficiency virus (HIV) through semen[7] has made the use of quarantined and tested frozen semen from male partners or donors mandatory.

In France, since the early 1980s the nationwide CECOS network located in university hospitals receives about 3000 requests for TID every year, representing about 90% of these procedures.[79] The experience in France clearly demonstrates the advantages of using frozen semen: better organization of semen collection and screening of donors; disassociation of semen collection and TID to preserve donors' anonymity; the possibility of storing and transporting semen, allowing several inseminations to be performed per cycle or allowing a couple to conceive several children from the same donor; greater choice of phenotype characteristics; and better medical control of donor screening in specialized centers and better knowledge of results.

On the last point, the results of the last OTA survey are informative. In 1986 The American Fertility Society recommended genetic screening of potential donors,[80] but in 1987 less than half of U.S. physicians did this, and did it inefficiently in many cases.[78] Genetic screening is not always easy, however. Of 676 potential fertile donors interviewed by a geneticist and karyotyped between 1973 and 1983 in the CECOS Paris-Bicetre, 2.6% were excluded for cytogenetic reasons and 3.4% for genetic reasons.[81] It appears that much of the difficulty lies in the subjectivity of the decision to reject donors.[81] The authors concluded that donors should be classified into the following three categories:

1. Those rejected because of genetic risk regarded as being too high
2. Those accepted without any particular conditions, whose semen can be used for every recipient
3. Those accepted under certain conditions because of a moderate genetic risk factor, whose semen can be used only for recipients without the same risk factor.

Of course such a policy can be set up in all cases, but it is easier to apply when the geneticist and a center using frozen semen collaborate closely.[81]

One main advantage of cryopreservation is that it offers the maximum guarantee of avoiding the transmission of sexual diseases. Of course, semen donors may be screened for medical history of sexually transmitted disease (STD) and bacteriologic tests may be performed on the sample used, but a complete evaluation cannot be performed on the day of donation.[82] Furthermore, it is well known that seropositivity for the HIV antibody may be delayed.[83] Therefore it is necessary to establish a quarantine between the collection and use of donated semen. According to the recommendations of the U.S. Food and Drug Administration (FDA) and the Centers for Disease Control and Prevention (CDC), this quarantine should last 6 months.[84] The American Fertility Society modified its guidelines accordingly,[85] and the CECOS network is following the same practice. Donors must be screened for risk factors for HIV infection. Blood samples are to be taken at the time of semen collection and 6 months after. The semen can be used only if both samples are negative for HIV antibodies.[86]

If the primary purpose of a fertility clinic is to establish safe pregnancy,[84] only frozen semen should be used as long as simple and rapid tests are not available to detect STD in fresh samples. To establish pregnancy as quickly as possible, it is important to recruit large numbers of donors to use the semen with the best potential fertilizing ability, to improve cryotechnology to reduce alterations in spermatozoa induced by freezing, or both. When both male and female factors are taken into account

and when similar numbers of viable spermatozoa are used for TID, the pregnancy rates with fresh and frozen semen are similar.[38] Apart from semen quality and its vulnerability to cryopreservation, other factors such as timing of insemination and ovulation, the number of oocytes ovulated, and the age of the female recipient have been reported to influence pregnancy rates when frozen semen is used.[38]

CRYOPRESERVATION OF HUMAN EMBRYOS

Embryo Survival after Thawing

The stage at which human embryos should be frozen to obtain optimal results is controversial[87–89]; recommendations have included blastocyst,[90] eight-cell stage,[91] and pronucleate egg[13] using glycerol, DMSO, and PROH, respectively. In the experience of one group, no differences were found between DMSO and PROH (Table 46–3). Embryo survival was correlated with morphologic features.[92] Optimum success was obtained by selecting one-cell embryos or two- and four-cell embryos with a favorable appearance.[93] Differences in ability to implant were not found between intact and nonintact embryos. Pregnancy was reported even if less than half the cells were intact after thawing.[94] The follicular response of the embryo recipient also influences success. Cleaving embryos had a higher chance of survival and implantation in women with four to seven follicles.[95] Although several reports suggested that pregnancy rates tend to be higher for cryopreserved embryos in women who did not receive agonist therapy than in those who did,[95] others have reported no differences.[96,97] The pregnancy rate per frozen embryo has been reported not to decrease with increased length of storage[98] (Table 46–4).

Survey of Cryopreservation of Human Embryos

A survey was conducted on human embryo and oocyte cryopreservation up to December 1986. The results, presented at the fifth world congress on IVF, summarized the experience of 24 centers.[99] As indicated in Table 46–5, about half of the 3577

TABLE 46–3. PREGNANCIES AFTER REPLACEMENT OF FROZEN-THAWED EMBRYOS

			Pregnancies			
			No./Embryo			
Freezing Medium	No./Transfer	%	Replaced	%	Thawed	%
PROH	16/132	12.1	16/153	9.9	16/461	3.5
DMSO	25/204	12.3	25/281	8.9	25/759	3.3
Totals	41/336	12.2	41/434	9.3	41/1220	3.4

Outcome of 41 pregnancies: 19 healthy children born, including seven children from the donation program; 15 continuing pregnancies; 7 (early) abortions.
From Frydman R, et al: An obstetric assessment of the first 100 births from in vitro fertilization. Am J Obstet Gynecol 154:550, 1986.

TABLE 46–4. INFLUENCE OF LENGTH OF STORAGE OF CRYOPRESERVED EMBRYOS ON PREGNANCY RATE

Length of Cryostorage (months)	No. of Thawed Embryos	Transferred Embryos (% of thawed embryos)	Thawing Cycles	Pregnancies (% thawing cycles)
<3	341	239 (70.1)	245	31 (12.6)
4–6	185	137 (74.1)	109	13 (11.9)
7–12	72	48 (66.7)	41	4 (9.8)
13–24	19	16 (84.2)	12	2 (16.7)
Total	617	440 (71.3)	387	50 (12.9)

From Frydman R, et al: An obstetric analysis of 50 consecutive pregnancies after transfer of human cryopreserved embryos. Am J Obstet Gynecol 160:209, 1989.

frozen and thawed embryos were judged suitable for transfer. They had a 4.6% chance to implant. A pregnancy rate of 13.4% per replacement was achieved. The abortion rate (26.4%) was similar to that in IVF and gamete intrafallopian transfer (GIFT).

The most recent data from the Assisted Reproductive Technology Registry of the American Society for Reproductive Medicine[100] indicate very similar results from IVF programs surveyed in the United States and Canada in 1993. Thus from 6869 frozen embryo transfer procedures reported, 13.3% deliveries per procedure ensued. Of the 267 programs reporting results, 234 (87.6%) reported transfer of cryopreserved embryos. A transfer resulted from 93% of the thawing procedures. When donor cryopreserved embryos were used, the pregnancy and delivery rates were 22% and 17% per thaw, respectively. These higher rates with donated embryos may reflect their origin from donor women who had already conceived babies from the fresh, sibling embryos and did not wish to retain their cryopreserved embryos for their own use.

Clinical Importance of These Techniques

There is a positive correlation between the pregnancy rate per transfer and the number of embryos transferred. The pregnancy rate varies from 18% when only one embryo is transferred to approximately 30% for three embryos.[101] Multiple pregnancies occur with a frequency of 2% in natural cycles but reach 20% after replacement of two or more embryos in IVF cycles.[102]

The perinatal mortality for multiple pregnancies is about 10 times greater than for singleton gestations. Therefore, it is

TABLE 46–5. SURVEY OF RESULTS OF HUMAN EMBRYO CRYOPRESERVATION

Result	Number
Embryos frozen and thawed	3577
Embryos replaced	1794
Transfers	1219
Pregnancies	163
Abortions	43
Births or continuing pregnancies	123

From Van Steirteghem A, Van Den Abbeel: Survey on cryopreservation. Ann N Y Acad Sci 541:571, 1988.

recommended that the number of fresh embryos replaced in the course of the IVF cycles (three or four) be reduced to avoid the disadvantage of multiple pregnancies. The remaining (supernumerary) embryos are cryopreserved for later use. Even so, in GIFT the number of oocytes replaced should be limited to three or four. The remaining oocytes can be inseminated, and if they fertilize and cleave normally, they can be cryopreserved.

Freezing may be justified as a means to meet a couple's short-term procreative goal. It may be acceptable to the extent that it allows either the transplantation of embryos during the woman's subsequent cycle or successive transplantations in the case of failure without the necessity for further surgical intervention and without destroying the embryos not immediately transplanted. It has also been proposed that all the embryos obtained should be frozen and in this way possibly avoid their replacement in hyperstimulated cycles, which could adversely affect implantation. For a given number of embryos, however, there was no significant difference in pregnancy rates when they were all immediately transferred or when they were frozen and replaced successively.[103] Only the multiple pregnancy rate varies in these different circumstances.

Transfers can be carried out either in spontaneous cycles or in highly stimulated cycles in anovulatory patients (Fig 46–3). Substitutive hormonal therapy after desensitization by a gonadotropin-releasing hormone (GnRH) agonist also is used.[104] Exact embryo-endometrium synchrony seems to give the best results in terms of pregnancy per transfer. Transfer of embryos cryopreserved at later stages of development (eight-cell or blastocyst) should preferably be done in cycles where the temporal stage of the reproductive tract is less advanced than that of the embryos to compensate for the slower rates of embryonic development in vitro.[105] Transfer takes place between 0 and 3 hours after thawing. Usually, pronucleate embryos are cultured for 1 day after thawing before transfer. However, it has been shown that higher pregnancy rates result if the thawed zygotes are transferred after short-term culture for a few hours or are cocultured overnight on bovine oviductal epithelial cells.[106] There would seem to be little physiologic benefit in prolonging the culture of thawed zygotes before transfer.[105]

The perinatal outcome of 50 pregnancies resulting from

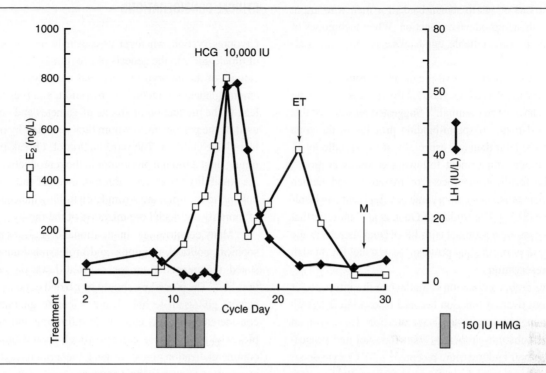

Figure 46–3. Concentrations of estradiol-17β and luteinizing hormone (LH) during the transfer cycle of a cryopreserved blastocyst. The patient received human menopausal gonadotropin (HMG), 150 IU daily, from day 8 to day 12 of the cycle. On day 14 ovulation was induced by the administration of 10,000 IU human chorionic gonadotropin (HCG). The frozen and thawed blastocyst was replaced on day 22. No pregnancy occurred.

the transfer of human embryos that had been cryopreserved for up to 2 years was reported.[98] Early pregnancy losses after the use of these embryos did not appear different from those in IVF pregnancies transferring fresh embryos. One serious fetal abnormality was recorded. Thirty-one healthy babies were born from 28 pregnancies, and a further seven pregnancies were in progress. The cesarean section rate for these deliveries was only slightly higher than that in the general population.

The Fate of Supernumerary Cryopreserved Embryos

The de facto existence of extra embryos raises ethical problems of their possible conservation by means of freezing, their donation to another patient, and their destruction without invasive examination.[107]

The donation of embryos from one couple to another is possible, but although the technical aspects of these manipulations are relatively straightforward, the ethical dimensions are complicated. The donation of frozen embryos, however, should not be regarded any differently from the donation of fresh embryos, as is performed with uterine lavage procedures. Frozen embryos would most probably be donated when several embryos are obtained in an IVF cycle, and pregnancy, especially multiple gestations, results from the transfer of the fresh embryos. Such a couple might then donate their frozen embryos to a less fortunate couple. The somewhat higher pregnancy rates

from donated cryopreserved embryos[100] that may reflect their origination from IVF cycles that resulted in a pregnancy from the transfer of the fresh embryos has been mentioned previously.

Recent concern has centered on the lapsing of storage time limits for cryopreserved embryos in many IVF centers and the inability to contact the original biologic providers of the embryos, resulting in "orphaned" embryos.[108] These problems appear to have originated because of nonenforceable consent agreements and lapses in rigorous contact with the patients concerning the disposition of their embryos. Strict time limits and well-defined criteria for cryopreservation and thawing, as well as storage time, such as those that apply in Denmark[109] (1-year storage time and destruction or donation of the embryos to research after the storage time elapses) is one way to lessen these problems.

OOCYTE FREEZING

Oocyte freezing is clearly useful from a practical standpoint, similar to that outlined for embryo freezing. Furthermore, in some countries it might be more acceptable on ethical grounds than freezing and thawing embryos. It also would be beneficial to young women at risk for losing ovarian function because of chemotherapy, a surgical procedure, or certain pelvic diseases.

This would be analogous to semen banks for men who are at risk for losing their reproductive function. When techniques of oocyte freezing become reliable, egg banks can offer similar alternatives.

Despite early reports of five pregnancies from three IVF centers using cryopreserved oocytes,[14–16] the success rates using this procedure have been minimal.[110] Suggested reasons for this have included damage to sperm-binding proteins in the zona pellucida, cytoskeletal damage, especially at the spindle level, and other cytologic impairment following cryopreservation.[17] Defects in the fertilization process of frozen-thawed human oocytes and their subsequent embryonic development can be alleviated with ICSI.[18,19] The studies of Gook et al[109] indicate that a slow freeze–fast thaw protocol with PROH and sucrose as the CPAs might be a promising protocol to pursue for human oocyte cryopreservation.

Oocyte or embryo donation can alleviate the infertility of patients without ovarian function because of ovarian dysgenesis, premature menopause, or surgical castration. These women require steroid substitution therapy with estradiol and progesterone to make their endometrium receptive.[112–115] Oocyte donation also can be indicated for patients with functional ovaries who have repeated ovarian stimulation failures, failed fertilizations in the course of several IVF cycles, the presence of genetic risk factor, or a medical contraindication to undergoing oocyte retrieval.

Oocytes and embryos can be donated by volunteers, patients undergoing laparoscopic sterilization, and women who are willing to donate their excess oocytes and embryos after IVF. A difficulty in a donation program consists in the synchrony between the ovarian cycles of donor and recipient. If this synchrony is not present at the time donated material is available, the embryo can be cryopreserved to be replaced at an appropriate time in the course of a subsequent cycle,[116,117] or steroid replacement therapy after ovarian downregulation with a GnRH analog can be used. The availability of an adequate embryo cryopreservation program increases the likelihood of establishing a donor program (Table 46–6).

ETHICAL CONSIDERATIONS

Cryopreservation, whatever its uses may be, results in a period of timelessness in the genesis of life. It may bring out the "reification" of the embryo in vitro and the risks of disassociation among gamete production, fertilization, and pregnancy. It may lead to the production of stocks of gametes and embryos to be used by the persons from whom they issued or by others to help them have children. The introduction of a break in the normal timing or of a foreign procreator in the reproductive process and the possibility for society (through medical and scientific technology) to control it are strongly disturbing the classic concepts of morality and social organization of the family.

Many countries and international organizations and philosophical, political, religious, and professional authorities have stated recommendations or enacted laws on cryopreservation.[118–120] The procedure should be carried out only in approved centers giving all technical and scientific guarantees and are considered to be fully capable of informing and assisting couples who apply. These centers, which should operate without commercialization, must respect the principles that regulate procreation in vitro in their country.

The ethical questions that concern cryopreservation of spermatozoa and oocytes are similar. When either is frozen to preserve the fertility potential of a given person, the only questions are who is allowed to use the gamete and when? The simple and logical answer is that the person who produced the cell is the only one able to decide its use, and that should be, of course, to procreate. This would deny the use of cryopreserved gametes after the death of the donor—for example, if the remaining partner wanted to have the child of the deceased individual. To permit this would change the purpose of cryopreservation, which is to preserve the fertility potential of the donor. As a rule, respect for the dignity of this person would allow him or her the right to decide on the use of the gametes, and, of course, this can be done only if the person is alive unless proper informed consent is obtained before the donor's death. Thus the question arises whether gametes should be cryopre-

TABLE 46–6. PREGNANCIES AFTER OOCYTE AND EMBRYO DONATION

Replacement	No. of Pregnancies/No. of Transfers		
	Primary Ovarian Failure[a]	Functional Ovaries[a]	Ovarian Function Unknown[b]
Fresh oocytes or embryos			
Intrauterine	7/30	6/25	—
GIFT	1/20	—	—
ZIFT	3/8	0/1	—
Cryopreserved embryos	4/23	5/17	9/29

GIFT, gamete intrafallopian transfer; ZIFT, zygote intrafallopian transfer.
[a] Summarized at the Center for Reproductive Medicine at the Vrje Universiteit, Brussels.
[b] From reference 38.

served only for people facing possible sterility or be preserved for anyone who would like to procreate at any time.

When gametes are cryopreserved for donation, fewer specific issues arise. It can be emphasized that because freezing offers the best condition for detailed screening of donors and for precise matching of donors and recipients, all programs of gamete donation should use only frozen specimens.

Embryo cryopreservation raises different questions because it concerns a unique entity able to develop into a human being. Human embryos should not be frozen independently of the desire for parenthood. The technique should be considered only as an extension of IVF for infertile couples. It is freezing not for convenience but as part of infertility treatment.

According to the French National Ethical Committee and most other national ethics bodies, embryos may be cryopreserved only for a limited period of time and related to the immediate project of having a child, not as part of an indeterminate parenthood program. This time limit has been limited to no more than 1 year except for medical reasons in some centers and countries. In other facilities and countries, a limit of 10 years or the reproductive life span of the couple has been stipulated as the storage time.[96,108] In the experience of the Clamart and Brussels groups, most patients ask for transfer of the remaining frozen embryos in the 6 months after unsuccessful transfer of a fresh one. This assures that freezing is only a prolongation of IVF. If pregnancy results from the transfer of fresh embryos, the remaining cryopreserved embryos are usually used by the couple within several years in an attempt to complete their family without the requirement for another stimulation cycle to produce embryos.

During the limited period of preservation, frozen embryos belong to the genitor couple. The couple may request to have the embryos transferred in a later cycle, to destroy them with or without allowing them to be subjected to scientific research, or to donate them to another infertile couple. Problems arise when the time limit is exceeded and the embryos have not been reclaimed or contact with the patients is lost and the cryopreserved embryos become abandoned.[108]

After the birth of a child and if a couple still has stored embryos, the question arises whether it is acceptable to transfer the embryos to attempt a second pregnancy. Although we did suggest in the first edition of this book that the idea of a stock of embryos subjected to the hazards of parental desire must be rejected, perhaps a more tolerant approach to the desires of infertile couples could be accommodated. Nevertheless, strict adherence to informed consent, time limits of storage and the disposition of the cryopreserved embryos, whether the patients can be contacted or not, is desirable. Our clinical experience indicates that after the first pregnancy, most patients desire a second baby. In Clamart, however, nine problems arose among 150 couples. These occurred when the couple abandoned the proj-

ect, or when a second pregnancy was unfeasible, for example, because of separation, illness, or death of one or both partners. In such cases should the embryos be destroyed when both genitors cannot agree on donation?

We believe that gamete and embryo freezing are intended to help sterile people have children. Several principles should guide our thinking. One of the most important is that human gametes and embryos are the products of the human body and cannot be commercialized. Cryopreservation will lead to the birth of many children and, as is the case for atomic energy, this gametic energy must be regulated to avoid catastrophes. Unfortunately, some catastrophes have occurred. Society must define the rules; however, the medical community is not merely a technician but is concerned with the conception and progress of humanity. As such, medical scientists and clinicians must offer society guidelines based on their experience and on their projections, however inchoate, of future capabilities.

Note added in proof. In a report (Tucker M, Wright G, Morton P, Shanguo L, Massey J, Kort H: Preliminary experience with human oocyte cryopreservation using 1,2-propanediol and sucrose. *Hum Reprod* 11:1513, 1996) of the clinical outcome of human oocyte cryopreservation using the methodology outlined by Gook et al,[111] good fertilization rates (65%) by ICSI and embryo development in vitro were obtained. However, the cryosurvival of freshly collected oocytes was low (25%) and although three pregnancies were initiated after five embryo transfers, none were ongoing. The authors comment that oocyte cryosurvival must be improved to make this procedure worthwhile for clinical use.

REFERENCES

1. Spallanzani L: Opuscoli di fisca spermamtici, animale e vegatabile, opuscule. II. Osservaziioni, a sperienze intorno ai vermicelli dell'uomo et degli animali. Modena, Italy, 1776
2. Mantegazza J. Fisiologia sullo sperma umano. *Rendic Reale Instit Lomb* 3:183, 1866
3. Rostand J: *Cole R Acad Sci Paris* 222:1534, 1946
4. Polge C, Smith AU, Parkes AS: Revival of spermatozoa after vitrification and dehydration at low temperature. *Nature* 164:664, 1949
5. Bunge RG, Sherman JK: Fertilizing capacity of frozen human spermatozoa. *Nature* 172:767, 1953
6. Perloff WH, Steinberger E, Sherman JK: Conception with human spermatozoa frozen by nitrogen vapor technique. *Fertil Steril* 15:501, 1964
7. Stewart GJ, Tyler JPP, Cunningham AL, et al: Transmission of human T-cell lymphotropic virus type III (HTLV-III) by artificial insemination by donor. *Lancet* 2:581, 1985
8. Whittingham DG: Survival of mouse embryos frozen to $-196°C$ and $-269°C$. *Nature* 178:411, 1972

9. Trounson A, Mohr L: Human pregnancy following cryopreservation, thawing and transfer of an eight-cell embryo. *Nature* 305:707, 1983

10. Zeilmaker GH, Alberda AT, Van Gent I, Rijkmans CMPM, Drogendijk AC: Two pregnancies following transfer of intact frozen-thawed embryos. *Fertil Steril* 42:293, 1984

11. Downing BG, Mohr LR, Trounson AO, Freeman LE, Wood C: Birth after transfer of cryopreserved embryos. *Med J Aust* 142:409, 1985

12. Cohen J, Simon RF, Fehily CB, et al: Birth after replacement of hatching blastocyst cryopreserved at expanded blastocyst stage. *Lancet* 1:647, 1985

13. Lassalle B, Testart J, Renard JP: Human embryo features that influence the success of cryopreservation with the use of 1,2-propanediol. *Fertil Steril* 44:645, 1985

14. Chen C: Pregnancy after human oocyte cryopreservation. *Lancet* 1:884, 1986

15. Al-Hasani A, Diedrich K, Van Der Ven H, et al: Cryopreservation of human oocytes. *Hum Reprod* 2:695, 1987

16. Van Uem JFHM, Siebzehnrubl ER, Schuh B, et al: Birth after cryopreservation of unfertilized oocytes. *Lancet* 1:752, 1987

17. Gook DA, Osborn SM, Bourne H, Johnston WIH: Fertilization of human oocytes following cryopreservation: Normal karyotypes and absence of stray chromosomes. *Hum Reprod* 9:684, 1994

18. Gook DA, Schiewe MC, Osborn SM, Asch RH, Jansen RPS, Johnston WIH: Intracytoplasmic sperm injection of human oocytes cryopreserved using 1,2-propanediol. *Hum Reprod* 10:2637, 1995

19. Kazem R, Thompson LA, Srikantharajah, et al: Cryopreservation of human oocytes and fertilization by two techniques: In-vitro fertilization and intracytoplasmic sperm injection. *Hum Reprod* 10:2650, 1995

20. McGrath JJ: Preservation of biological material by freezing and thawing. In: Shitzer H, Eberhart C (eds), *Heat Transfer in Medicine and Biology.* New York, Plenum, 1985:185–238

21. Renard JP, De Rochambeau H, Lauverq JJ: Utilization of gamete and embryo banking for the preservation and study of genetic resources in farm animals. *Proc Vth World Congress of Animal Production* 1:66, 1983

22. Nishikawa Y: Studies on the preservation of raw and frozen horse semen. *J Reprod Fertil* 23:99, 1975

23. Paquignon M, Bussiere J, Bariteau F, Courot M: Effectiveness of boar semen under practical conditions of artificial insemination. *Theriogenology* 14:217, 1980

24. Ciba Foundation Symposium 52. The freezing of mammalian embryos. Elliott K, Whelan J (eds) Amsterdam, Excerpta Medica, 1979

25. Whittingham DG: Principles of embryo preservation. In: Ashwood-Smith MJ, Farrant J (eds), *Low Temperature Preservation in Medicine and Biology.* Baltimore, University Park Press, 1980: 65–83

26. Whittingham DG, Leibo SP, Mazur P: Survival of mouse embryos frozen to −196°C and −269°C. *Science* 178:411, 1972

27. Renard JP, n'Guyen B-X, Garnier V: Two-step freezing of two-cell rabbit embryos after partial dehydration at room temperature. *J Reprod Fertil* 71:573, 1984

28. Eaglesome MD, Mitchell D, Betteridge KJ, et al: Transfer of embryos from bovine leukaemia virus-infected cattle to uninfected recipients: preliminary results. *Vet Rec* 3:122, 1982

29. Whittingham DG: Fertilization in vitro and development to term of unfertilized mouse oocytes previously stored at −196°C. *J Reprod Fertil* 49:89, 1977

30. De Mayo FJ, Rawlins RG, Dukelow WR: Xenogenous and in vitro fertilization of frozen/thawed primate oocytes and blastomere separation of embryos. *Fertil Steril* 43:295, 1985

31. Critser JK, Arneson BW, Aaker DV, Ball GD: Cryopreservation of hamster oocytes: Effects of vitrification or freezing on human sperm penetration of zona-free hamster oocytes. *Fertil Steril* 46:277, 1986

32. Al-Hasani S, Tolksdorf A, Diedrich K, Van Der Ven H, Drebs D: Successful in vitro fertilization of frozen-thawed rabbit oocytes. *Hum Reprod* 1:309, 1986

33. Glenister PH, Wood MJ, Kirby C, Whittingham DG: Incidence of chromosome anomalies in first cleavage mouse embryos obtained from frozen-thawed oocytes fertilized in vitro. *Gamete Res* 16:205, 1987

34. Nakagata N: High survival rate of unfertilized mouse oocytes after vitrification. *J Reprod Fertil* 87:479, 1989

35. Tateno H, Kamiguchi Y, Mikamo K: A freezing and thawing method of hamster oocytes designed for both the penetration test and chromosome assay of human spermatozoa. *Mol Reprod Dev* 33:202, 1992

36. Wood MJ, Barros C, Candy C, Carrol J, Melendez J, Whittingham DG: High rates of survival and fertilisation of mouse and hamster oocytes after vitrification in dimethyl sulphoxide. *Biol Reprod* 49:489, 1993

37. Rayos AA, Takahashi Y, Hishinuma M, Kanagawa H: Quick freezing of unfertilized mouse oocytes using ethylene glycol with sucrose or trehalose. *J Reprod Fertil* 100:123, 1994

38. Quinn P: Cryopreservation. In: Marrs RP (ed), *Assisted Reproductive Technologies.* Boston, Blackwell, 1993:89–107

39. Mahadevan M, Trounson AO: Effect of cryopreservation media and dilution methods on the preservation of human spermatozoa. *Andrologia* 15:355, 1983

40. Serafini P, Marrs RP: Computerized staged-freezing technique improves sperm survival and preserves penetration of zona-free hamster ova. *Fertil Steril* 45:854, 1986

41. Pilikian S, Czyba JC, Guerin JF: Effect of various concentrations of glycerol on post-thaw motility and velocity of human spermatozoa. *Cryobiology* 19:147, 1982

42. Weidel L, Prins GS: Cryosurvival of human spermatozoa frozen in eight different buffer systems. *J Androl* 8:42, 1987

43. Harrison RF, Shepard BL: A comparative study in methods of cryoprotection for human semen. *Cryobiology* 17:25, 1980

44. David G, Czyglik F: Tolérance à la congélation du sperme humain en fonction de la qualité initiale du sperme. *J Gynecol Obstet Biol Reprod* 6:601, 1977

45. Emperaire JC, Czyglik F: Semen freezing in 0.15 and 0.25-mL straws. In: David G, Price WS (eds), *Human Artificial Insemination and Semen Preservation.* New York, Plenum, 1980: 161–166

46. Sherman JK: Improved methods of preservation of human sper-

matozoa by freezing and freezing-drying. *Fertil Steril* 14:49, 1963

47. Mahadevan M, Trounson AO: Effect of cooling, freezing and thawing rates and storage condition on preservation of human spermatozoa. *Andrologia* 16:52, 1984

48. Thachil JV, Jewett MAS: Preservation techniques for human semen. *Fertil Steril* 35:546, 1981

49. Critser JK, Husebenda AR, Aaker DW, Arneson BW, Ball GD: Cryopreservation of human spermatozoa. I. Effect of holding procedure and seeding motility, fertilizing ability and acrosome reaction. *Fertil Steril* 47:656, 1987

50. Serres C, Jouannet P, Czyglik F, David G: Effects of freezing on spermatozoa motility. In: David G, Price WS (eds), *Human Artificial Insemination and Semen Preparation*. New York, Plenum, 1980:147–160

51. Mayaux MJ, Schwartz D, Czyglik F, David G: Conception rate according to semen characteristic in a series of 15,364 insemination cycles: Results of a multivariate analysis. *Andrologia* 17:9, 1985

52. Lindemann CB, Fisher M, Lipton M: A comparative study of the effects of freezing and frozen storage on intact and demembranated bull spermatozoa. *Cryobiology* 19:20, 1982

53. Pedersen H, Lebech PE: Ultrastructural changes in human spermatozoa after freezing for artificial insemination. *Fertil Steril* 22:125, 1971

54. Escalier D, Bisson JP: Quantitative ultrastructural modification in human spermatozoa after freezing. In: David G, Price WS (eds), *Human Artificial Insemination and Semen Preservation*. New York, Plenum, 1980:107–122

55. Mahadevan MM, Trounson AO: Relationship of fine structure of sperm head to fertility of frozen human semen. *Fertil Steril* 41:287, 1984

56. Heath E, Jeyendran RS, Perez-Pelaez M, Sobrero AJ: Ultrastructural categorization of human sperm cryopreserved in glycerol and in TESTCY. *Int J Androl* 8:101, 1985

57. Serafini PC, Hauser D, Moyer D, Marrs RP: Cryopreservation of human spermatozoa: Correlation of ultrastructural sperm head configuration with sperm motility and ability to penetrate zona-free hamster ova. *Fertil Steril* 46:691, 1986

58. Jones R, Mann T: Damage to ram spermatozoa by peroxidation of endogenous phospholipids. *J Reprod Fertil* 50:261, 1977

59. Aitken RJ, Clarkson JS: Cellular basis of defective sperm function and its association with the genesis of reactive oxygen species by human spermatozoa. *J Reprod Fertil* 81:459, 1987

60. Rao B, David D: Improved recovery of post thaw motility and vitality of human spermatozoa cryopreserved in the presence of dithiothreitol. *Cryobiology* 21:536, 1984

61. Schwartz D, Mayaux MJ, Guichard-Moscato ML, Czyglik F, David G: Abortion rate in AID and semen characteristics: A study of 1345 pregnancies. *Andrologia* 18:292, 1986

62. Federation CECOS, Matte JF, Le Marec B: Genetic aspects of artificial insemination by donor (AID): Indication, surveillance and results. *Clin Genet* 23:132, 1983

63. Sherman JK: Research on frozen human semen: Past, present and future. *Fertil Steril* 15:486, 1964

64. Jouannet P, Jardin A, Czyglik F, David G, Fourcade R: Conserva-

tion du sperme et vasectomie. *Seminaire d'Uronephrologie*. no. 5. Paris, Masson, 1979:113–120

65. Behrman SJ: The preservation of semen. *Fertil Steril* 24:396, 1973

66. Delaisi de Parseval G, Jouannet P: Semen storage, delayed fatherhood and vasectomy. In: *Psychosomatic Obstetrics and Gynaecology*. Leiden, Boerhaave Committee for Postgraduate Medical Education, 1985:45–50

67. Czyglik F: Prévention des sterilites introgenes par la congélation du sperme. In: *33rd Assises Francaises de Gynecologie*. Paris, Masson, 1987:265–276

68. Sanger WG, Armitage JO, Schmidt MA: Feasibility of semen cryopreservation in patients with malignant disease. *JAMA* 244:789, 1980

69. Bergman S, Howards S, Sanger W: Practical aspects of banking patients' semen for future artificial insemination. *Urology* 13:408, 1979

70. Scammel GE, Stedronska J, Edmonds DK, et al: Cryopreservation of semen in men with testicular tumors of Hodgkin's disease: Results of artificial insemination of their partners. *Lancet* 2:31, 1985

71. Czyglik F, Auger J, Albert M, David G: L'autoconservation du sperme avant thérapeutique sterilisante. *Nouv Presse Med* 11:2749, 1982

72. Rhodes EA, Hoffman DJ, Kaempfer SH: Ten years' experience with semen cryopreservation by cancer patients: Follow-up and clinical considerations. *Fertil Steril* 44:512, 1985

73. Smith K, Steinberger E: Survival of spermatozoa in a human sperm bank, *JAMA* 223:774, 1973

74. Friedman S, Broder S: Homologous artificial insemination after long-term semen cryopreservation. *Fertil Steril* 35:321, 1981

75. Flaherty SP, Matthews CD (eds): Intracytoplasmic sperm injection: The revolution in male infertility. *Reprod Fertil Dev* 7:1, 1995

76. David G, Czyglik F: Apparent improvement in human semen after long-term storage. In: Andre J (ed), *The Sperm Cell*. The Hague, Martinus Nijhoff, 1983, pp 29–32

77. Currie Cohen M, Luttrell L, Shapiro S: Current practice of artificial insemination by donor in the United States. *N Engl J Med* 300:585, 1979

78. *Artificial Insemination Practice in the U.S.: Summary of a 1987 Survey*. Washington, DC, Office of Technology Assessment, 1988

79. David G: Artificial insemination by donor (AID). In: Steinberger E, Frajese G, Steinberger A (eds), *Reproductive Medicine*. New York, Raven, 1984:319–326

80. American Fertility Society: New guidelines for the use of semen donor insemination: 1986. *Fertil Steril* 46(Suppl 2):95S, 1986

81. Selva J, Leonard C, Albert M, Auger J, David C: Genetic screening for artificial insemination by donor (AID). *Clin Genet* 29:389, 1986

82. Maslola L, Guinan ME: Screening to reduce transmission of sexually transmitted diseases in semen used for artificial insemination. *N Engl J Med* 314:1354, 1986

83. Ranki, Krohn K: Long latency precedes over seroconversion in sexually transmitted human immunodeficiency virus infection. *Lancet* 2:589, 1987

84. Centers for Disease Control: Semen banking, organ and tissue

transplantation, and HIV antibody testing. *MMWR Morb Mortal Wkly Rep* 37:57, 1988

85. American Fertility Society: New guidelines for the use of semen donor insemination: 1990. *Fertil Steril* 53(Suppl 1):13S, 1990

86. Ball GD: Acquired immune deficiency syndrome and the fertility clinic. *Fertil Steril* 45:172, 1988

87. Trounson A, Jones G: Freezing of embryos: Early vs late stages. *J Assist Reprod Genet* 10:179, 1993

88. Veeck LL: Freezing of embryos: Early vs late stages. *J Assist Reprod Genet* 10:181, 1993

89. Van Steirteghem AC, Van den Abbeel E: Freezing of embryos: Early vs late stages. *J Assist Reprod Genet* 10:185, 1993

90. Cohen J, Simons FR, Edwards RG, Fehilly CB, Fishel SB: Pregnancies following the frozen storage of expanding human blastocysts. *J In Vitro Fertil Embryo Transf* 2:59, 1985

91. Freeman L, Trounson A, Kirby C: Cryopreservation of human embryos: Progress on the clinical use of the technique in human in vitro fertilization. *J In Vitro Fertil Embryo Transf* 3:53, 1986

92. Mandelbaum J, Junca AM, Plachot P, et al: Human embryo cryopreservation, extrinsic and intrinsic parameters of success. *Hum Reprod* 2:709, 1987

93. Testart J, Lassalle B, Forman RG, et al: Factors influencing the success rate of human embryo freezing in an in vitro fertilization and embryo transfer program. *Fertil Steril* 48:107, 1987

94. Veiga A, Calderon G, Barri PN, Corleu B: Pregnancy after the replacement of a frozen thawed embryo with <50% intact blastomeres. *Hum Reprod* 2:321, 1987

95. Testart J: Development and clinical application of embryo cryopreservation. *Hum Reprod* 3:Suppl, 70, 1988

96. Quinn P: Success of oocyte and embryo freezing and its effect on outcome with in vitro fertilization. *Semin Reprod Endocrinol* 8:272, 1990

97. Oehninger S, Toner JP, Veeck LL, et al: Performance of cryopreserved pre-embryos obtained in in vitro fertilization cycles with or without gonadotropin-releasing hormone agonist. *Fertil Steril* 57:620, 1992

98. Frydman R, Forman RG, Belaisch-Allart J, et al: An obstetric analysis of 50 consecutive pregnancies after transfer of human cryopreserved embryos. *Am J Obstet Gynecol* 160:209, 1989

99. Van Steirteghem A, Van Den Abbeel E: Survey on cryopreservation. *Ann N Y Acad Sci* 541:571, 1988

100. Society for Assisted Reproductive Technology, American Society for Reproductive Medicine: Assisted reproductive technology in the United States and Canada: 1993 results generated from the American Society for Reproductive Medicine/Society for Assisted Reproductive Technology registry. *Fertil Steril* 64:13, 1995

101. Edwards RG, Steptoe PC: Current status of in vitro fertilization and implantation of human embryos. *Lancet* 2:1265, 1973

102. Frydman R, Belaisch-Allart J, Fries N, et al: An obstetric assessment of the first 100 births from in vitro fertilization. *Am J Obstet Gynecol* 154:550, 1986

103. Frydman R, Forman RG, Belaisch-Allart J, Hazout A, Testart J: An assessment of alternative policies for embryo transfer in an IVF-ET program. *Fertil Steril* 50:466, 1988

104. Frydman R, Bouchard P, Parneix I: Les agonistes de la LHRH ont-ils un role dans le cycle de transfert des embryons congelés. *Contrib Fertil Sex* 16:29, 1988

105. Quinn P: Cryopreservation of embryos and oocytes. In: Keye WR, Chang RJ, Rebar RW, Soules MR (eds), *Infertility. Evaluation and Treatment.* Philadelphia, Saunders, 1995:821–840

106. Wiker S, Tucker M, Wiemer K, et al: Co-culture of thawed human embryos. In: Rodriguez AO, Baumgartner W, Burgos-Briceno L (eds), Fertility and sterility, progress in research and practice. *Proceedings of the XIV World Congress on Fertility and Sterility.* Nov. 1992, Carnforth, Parthenon Publishing, Caracas, Venezuela 1994:407–414

107. Jouannet P: Reflexion à propos des problèmes ethiques soulevés par la congélation d'embryons humains. *Med Sci* 2: 345, 1986

108. Saunders DM, Bowman MC, Grierson A, Garner F: Frozen embryos: Too cold to touch? The dilemma ten years on. *Hum Reprod* 10:3081, 1995

109. Andersen CY, Westergaard LG, Grinsted J, et al: Frozen embryos: Too cold to touch? Frozen pre-embryos in Denmark. *Hum Reprod* 11:703, 1996

110. Mandelbaum J, Jones AM, Plachot M, et al: Cryopreservation of human embryos and oocytes. *Hum Reprod* 3:117, 1988

111. Gook DA, Osborn SM, Johnston WIH: Cryopreservation of mouse and human oocytes using 1,2-propanediol and the configuration of the meiotic spindle. *Hum Reprod* 8:1101, 1993

112. Lutjen P, Trounson A, Leeton J, et al: The establishment and maintenance of pregnancy using in vitro fertilization and embryo donation in a patient with primary ovarian failure. *Nature* 307: 174, 1984

113. Navot D, Laufer N, Kopolovic J, et al: Artificially induced endometrial cycles and establishment of pregnancies in the absence of ovaries. *N Engl J Med* 314:806, 1986

114. Rosenwaks Z: Donor eggs: Their application in modern reproductive technologies. *Fertil Steril* 47:895, 1987

115. Devroey P, Braeckmans P, Camus M, et al: Pregnancies after replacement of fresh and frozen-thawed embryos in a donation program. In: Feichtinger W, Kemeter P (eds), *Future Aspects of Human in Vitro Fertilization.* Berlin, Springer-Verlag, 1987:133

116. Van Steirteghem AC, Van Den Abbeel E, Braeckmans P, et al: Pregnancy with a frozen-thawed embryo in women with primary ovarian failure. *N Engl J Med* 317:113, 1987

117. Van Steirteghem AC, Van Den Abbeel E, Camus M, et al: Cryopreservation of human embryos obtained after gamete intrafallopian transfer and/or in vitro fertilization. *Hum Reprod* 2:309, 1987

118. Warnock M: *Report of the Committee of Inquiry into Human Fertilization and Embryology.* London, Her Majesty's Stationary Office, 1984

119. Avis du Comite National d'Ethique: La Fabrique du corps humain: Avis de recherche sur l'embryon. *Acte Sud-INSERM,* 1987

120. American Fertility Society Ethics Committee: Ethical considerations of the new reproductive technologies. *Fertil Steril* 53(Suppl 2):109S, 1990

CHAPTER 47

Legal Aspects of Infertility

LORI B. ANDREWS · AMI S. JAEGER

Constitutional Dimensions of Procreation
Embryo Research and Development of Infertility Therapies
   Fetal research
   Embryo transfer
   Excess embryos
Informed Consent
   Considerations for IVF
   Considerations for cryopreservation
   Considerations for embryo donation
Single Parenthood

Physician Involvement
Quality Assurance
   Personnel qualifications
   Screening
Record-Keeping and Confidentiality
   Record-keeping
   Confidentiality
Legal and Biologic Parentage
Payment to Third Parties
The Law, Responsibility, and New Reproductive Therapies

Medical practice involving the diagnosis and treatment of infertility is influenced by a variety of factors, ranging from community attitudes to the personal moral judgments of the patients and the health care professionals involved. Not the least of the factors affecting medical efforts to overcome infertility is the law. Statutes, regulations, judicial decisions, and constitutional protection of the right to privacy to make procreative decisions can profoundly influence which infertility services are offered and in what manner. The law in some cases shapes the standards by which health care professionals must practice; in other instances, it influences the rights and responsibilities of the infertile couple and of society with respect to the resulting child.

CONSTITUTIONAL DIMENSIONS OF PROCREATION

There is a strong moral and legal basis in our society for protection of autonomy in reproductive decisions. Decisions about whether or when to have children are thought to be a matter of personal private concern, not a subject of governmental mandate. Such decisions are protected by the U.S. Constitution under the right to privacy.

The constitutional protection of reproductive decisions was addressed by the U.S. Supreme Court as early as 1942 in *Skinner v Oklahoma,*[1] which struck down an Oklahoma statute authorizing the sterilization of habitual criminals convicted of crimes involving moral turpitude. The court stated, "[W]e are dealing with legislation which involves one of the basic civil rights of man. Marriage and procreation are fundamental to the very existence and survival of the race."[2]

In a later series of cases involving contraception and abortion, the Supreme Court delineated how an individual's decision whether or not to bear or beget a child was constitutionally protected from governmental interferences.[3] The court deemed childbearing and childrearing rights as "far more precious than property rights."[4] The court wrote, "[I]f the right of privacy means anything it is the right of the individual, married or single, to be free of unwarranted governmental intrusion into matters so fundamentally affecting a person as the decision whether to bear or beget a child."[5] For a governmental regulation that infringes on reproductive decisions to be upheld as constitutional, it must be necessary to further a compelling state interest, and it must regulate in the least restrictive manner possible.[6]

In reality, it is hard to imagine a state interest strong enough to justify a law prohibiting a person from choosing to become a parent. "The decision ranks in importance with any other a person may make in a lifetime; an attempt to imagine state interests that would justify governmental intrusions amounting to a practical prohibition on procreation and childbearing takes us out of our experience and into an imaginary world of Malthusian nightmare."[7] Various commentators and legislators have set forth particular state interests that they argue would justify regulating alternative reproduction. These include the fetus's interest in being free from pain; the potential child's interest in being physically and mentally healthy; the adult participant's interest in being free from undue physical and psychologic risk; the individual's interest in making decisions about his or her own body; the individual's and couple's interest in reproductive and parental autonomy; the donor's and surrogate's interest in being free from manipulation by other people; doctors' and researchers' interests in meeting their professional obligations to help patients and to further scientific knowledge; and society's interests in retaining values and maintaining institutions such as the family.[8]

The constitutional right to privacy protects the decision to reproduce coitally because of the biologic and social importance of being a parent.[9] The rationales for reproductive autonomy similarly extend to decisions to reproduce noncoitally.[10] The New Jersey Supreme Court in the landmark *Baby M* case, which dealt with a child conceived by means of artificial insemination of a surrogate mother, noted that alternative reproduction methods fall within the constitutional right of privacy.[11]

This right serves as the backdrop against which government actions (such as the adoption of state or federal laws) must be measured. It is a basis on which health care professionals and patients can challenge legislation that prohibits or otherwise restricts research or clinical practice in the area of medically assisted reproduction. It also provides the framework that guides the actions and decisions of individuals who use new technologies and of practitioners who provide them. For example, proposed state laws banning surrogate parenting are not the least restrictive means of regulating surrogate parenting and so may be declared unconstitutional.[12] Similarly, total prohibition of embryo transfer under existing embryo research bans would probably be invalid as an unconstitutional interference with the fundamental right to procreate.[13]

EMBRYO RESEARCH AND DEVELOPMENT OF INFERTILITY THERAPIES

In vitro fertilization (IVF) is the keystone of new reproductive technologies. It is one of the principal therapies for infertility and it makes other reproductive innovations (such as surrogate gestational motherhood) possible. The development of IVF became a reality through research with embryos. Improved IVF pregnancy rates and the development of other infertility treatments will occur as such research continues. Yet the permissibility of undertaking such investigations is guided by state and federal laws (known as "fetal research laws") that govern research with conceptuses.

Fetal Research

Used in the broadest sense, *fetal research* includes any untested or unproved procedure involving embryos or fetuses. According to the medical definition, a human embryo becomes a fetus at about the end of the eighth week of fertilization.[14] In contrast, statutory language generally defines a fetus as any product of conception, which means the fertilized egg, zygote, morula, blastocyst, embryo, and fetus. Thus many statutes that regulate fetal research would apply equally to what a physician would categorize as embryo research.

Just as the statutes cover a broad developmental range of fetuses, they cover a broad range of activities that affect not only basic research but also the introduction of reproductive technologies into the clinical setting. With their advent, these technologies opened a vast range of therapies for infertility. They also opened up a window of opportunity for research on the embryo.[15] Extracorporeal embryos provide an opportunity for observation and discovery of disease or developmental processes that have no clinical application in the treatment of infertility. For example, embryo research could be important "for developing or testing contraceptives, studying early forms of malignant cancer, providing an in vitro screening system for teratogens, studying the mechanisms by which chromosomal abnormalities are produced, understanding normal and abnormal cell growth and differentiation. . . ."[16] Embryo research could also lead to better understanding of genetic disease, genetic screening, and gene therapy.[17] What should be the source of embryos to be used in research? Should only spare embryos produced in attempts to treat infertility be used, or should some be produced specifically for research purposes? Society must balance the potential scientific and social gains from such investigations with the ethical and moral value in protecting the embryo as the symbolic potential of human life. Statutory enactments have attempted to formulate a regulatory framework for these ethical issues.[18]

As of early 1994, 25 states have laws specifically aimed at regulating fetal research.[19] Of these 25 laws, 24 impose some restriction on experimentation with live fetuses ex utero,[20] 6 prohibit or impose sanctions aimed at prohibiting any type of research on a live fetus,[21] and 12 prohibit nontherapeutic research on live fetuses.[22] The Louisiana statute prohibits an IVF embryo from being "farmed or cultured solely for research purposes or any other purposes."[23]

Some of these statutes were originally enacted as sections of an abortion statute. For example, of the 25 fetal research statutes, 13 apply to research performed on fetuses or embryos that are the product of an abortion.[24] This distinction becomes important as reproductive and genetic diagnostic technologies are introduced into the clinical setting. For example, if embryo lavage is considered to be an abortion, these statutes could regulate in vivo fertilization followed by embryo transfer.

By performing new techniques, physicians begin to bridge the gap between research and accepted clinical procedures. Some commentators argue that IVF, despite a decade of clinical application, is experimental because its long-term medical, psychologic, and social effects have not been determined.[25] A more common viewpoint is that IVF is now an accepted clinical practice rather than an experimental technology. Some of the more recently applied adjuncts to IVF, such as embryo cryopreservation, preimplantation embryo genetic diagnosis, donation of embryos and oocytes, and in vivo fertilization followed by embryo transfer, are sufficiently novel and untested to be considered research, however.

Clinicians' involvement with embryos can be differentiated from that of researchers who do not intend to transfer the embryo to a uterus and whose inquiries go beyond the treatment of infertility. The former usually perform transfers to initiate pregnancy, and so safety to the potential offspring should be a concern to them.[26]

Merely because physicians use a research procedure to treat infertility, however, does not exempt them from federal and state regulations on fetal research. Federal regulations cover the conceptus starting with implantation[27]; thus they would not address techniques such as IVF or in vivo fertilization followed by embryo transfer. An additional set of regulations, however, bans funding of research involving IVF unless reviewed by the Ethics Advisory Board of the federal department of Health and Human Services. The term of the Ethics Advisory Board has expired and has not been reconstituted. There has been a de facto ban on federally funded IVF research. Upon taking office in January 1993, President Clinton signed an executive order lifting the ban on use of fetal tissue for research.[28]

A 19-member panel appointed by the National Institutes of Health in 1994 issued recommendations concerning what types of research involving experimentation on human embryos should and should not be federally funded.[29] The panel found techniques such as cloning and the creation of chimeras to be unacceptable.[30] Studies of preimplantation diagnosis and the fertilization process, though, were deemed acceptable.[31] Soon after the panel made its recommendations, President Clinton issued a directive banning federal funding for research that created embryos solely for research purposes.[32] This directive does not bar the use of spare embryos in research, that is, embryos that may be left over from IVF procedures.

State laws extend beyond governmentally funded research and could affect privately funded investigation and the private clinical practice of a number of infertility techniques involving embryos. Of the 25 states with such laws, at least 7 prohibit research involving preimplantation embryos.[33] These statutes probably do not apply to IVF, which is now generally considered to be standard medical practice, and arguably is not experimental. The laws, however, could restrict extensions of IVF such as cryopreservation, preimplantation diagnosis, or embryo donation. A few states specifically address IVF in their fetal research statutes. For example, New Mexico defines clinical research to include research involving human IVF.[34] Illinois, on the other hand, specifically exempts IVF from the prohibition on fetal research.[35]

Embryo Transfer

In vivo fertilization followed by embryo transfer is not as well developed as is IVF, and thus statutory restrictions on embryo research affect in vivo fertilization differently. In this procedure, a second woman is artificially inseminated with the sperm of the husband of an infertile woman. Five days later the embryo is flushed out of the second woman by means of lavage and is implanted into the wife.[36] Because embryo lavage may be considered an abortion (since it involves removing the embryo from the uterus), the procedure could run afoul of laws banning research on preimplantation embryos and laws that ban research on a fetus in connection with an abortion.[37] These statutes could prohibit in vivo fertilization followed by embryo transfer or cryopreservation.

Excess Embryos

In the course of IVF or in vivo fertilization a woman may produce more eggs and embryos than she can safely use for reproductive purposes. Questions arise whether these materials can be cryopreserved, discarded, donated to another woman, or used for research. The answer depends on statutory regulation and the wishes of the couple. The laws regulating fetal research before or after a planned abortion would not affect cryopreservation after IVF because neither procedure involves an aborted fetus.[38] Because cryopreservation is still an experimental procedure, however, laws in nine states that prohibit fetal research even in instances in which there is no abortion could prohibit its use.[39] Although regulation might be justified on the grounds that the goal of such legislation is to protect the resulting child, harm to the embryo itself would not justify a state ban on this technique.[40]

A second option the couple or individual may have is to discard any excess embryos. There are several reasons why a couple would make that choice; for example, the woman might not want to risk multiple pregnancies, or the embryo may show cellular damage. After genetic testing is conducted on embryos, the embryo could be allowed to expire to avoid the birth of a child with a disability. No law explicitly requires all fertilized eggs and preimplantation embryos to be transferred to a uterus[41]; however, several statutes imply that physicians could be prosecuted for discarding embryos. The Louisiana law that defines an embryo as "an in vitro fertilized human ovum"[42] states, "The use of a human ovum fertilized in vitro is solely for the support and contribution of the complete development of human in utero implantation."[43] A further provision states, "A viable in vitro fertilized human ovum . . . shall not be intentionally destroyed by any natural or other juridical person or through the actions of any other such person."[44] Thus under this statute, it seems that discarding embryos produced through IVF is prohibited.

A separate provision within the Louisiana statute creates responsibilities for the physician. It provides that "[a]ny physician or medical facility who causes in vitro fertilization of a human ovum in vitro will be directly responsible for the in vitro safekeeping of the fertilized ovum."[45] This statute forces physicians and health care institutions to be cautious in introducing new therapies because of the increased statutory responsibilities. The creation of extra liabilities and responsibilities impedes the availability of IVF and its adjuncts.

A Kentucky statute allows public medical facilities to conduct IVF "as long as such procedures do not result in the intentional destruction of a human embryo."[46] Thus the law seems to require medical institutions to donate excess IVF embryos for implantation.

An earlier Illinois law created a similar responsibility for physicians performing IVF.[47] It raised so many questions about their duties and liabilities that a physician and couple he was treating brought suit against the Illinois Attorney General and the prosecuting attorney to prevent its enforcement.[48] In response, the defendants indicated they would not prosecute physicians for all potential risks to the embryo. A physician would be in violation of the law only if he or she willfully harmed the embryo through abuse, mutilation, extermination, or destructive laboratory experimentation. Even these limitations put a chill on IVF programs. Subsequently the law was amended to provide an exception for IVF.[49] Unless cryopreservation is considered to be part of IVF, however, the law may make embryo freezing a criminal offense.

Physicians and clinics also face liability for discarding an embryo without the permission of the couple. That right belongs to the couple. In a 1973 case, physicians at Columbia Presbyterian Hospital in New York City attempted IVF of a woman's egg with her husband's sperm. Without consulting with the physician or the couple, the department chairman removed the culture and destroyed it. The couple sued the department chairman and the hospital's trustees, charging conversion of personal property and intentional infliction of emotional distress.[50] The jury rejected the property claim but awarded plaintiffs damages for emotional distress.

A third option a couple has with respect to excess embryos is to sell or donate them to another woman. Sixteen states prohibit a woman from selling an embryo for experimentation[51]; 9 prohibit the donation of embryos or a fetus for research purposes.[52] As embryo transfer after IVF or in vivo fertilization becomes standard clinical practice, these regulations would no longer restrict donation.

The restriction on the sale or donation of embryos for research must be differentiated from the bans in three states that restrict such sale or donation for any purpose.[53] The primary distinction is that, even if in vivo fertilization followed by embryo transfer were to become standard clinical procedure, the latter laws would still restrict the sale or donation of embryos.

In Illinois, a physician and IVF patients challenged the constitutionality of an Illinois statute banning embryo and fetal research.[54] The statute allowed IVF but did not allow embryo donation, embryo freezing, or experimental prenatal diagnostic procedures. The federal district court for the northern district of Illinois held that banning research on conceptuses violated the U.S. Constitution because it impermissibly infringed on a woman's fundamental right to privacy and was impermissibly vague because it did not define the terms *experimentation* and *therapeutic*.[55]

A fifth circuit opinion questioned the continued validity of the statutory bans on embryo and fetal research.[56] The court declared unconstitutional an earlier Louisiana law that forbade experimentation on living or dead aborted fetuses unless the experimentation was therapeutic.[57] The court concluded that the word *experimentation* was impermissibly vague,[58] because physicians do not and cannot differentiate clearly between medical experiments and medical tests.[59] The court noted that "even medical treatment can be reasonably described as both a test and an experiment."[60] In light of the opinion, the Louisiana legislature drafted a new statute; whether it reconciles these distinctions remains to be seen through litigation.

Although the Louisiana statute prohibits the sale of eggs and embryos produced through IVF,[61] it allows embryo donation.[62] It states, "If the in vitro fertilization patients renounce, by notarial act, their parental rights for in utero implantation, then the in vitro fertilized human ovum shall be available for adoptive implantation in accordance with written procedures of the facility where it is housed or stored."[63] No payment will be made to either party. A further provision prohibits the culture of human ovum fertilized in vitro for research "or any other purposes."[64] The statute still seems to ban embryo research. Thus it seems that excess embryos may be donated but only for implantation in another woman. Furthermore, the statute does not seem to resolve the ambiguity between research and treatment called into question by the fifth circuit case.

INFORMED CONSENT

The ultimate decision regarding the use of infertility therapies lies with the individual or couple. There is a legal basis for allowing a patient to decide which treatment plan to undergo. Founded both in statutory and case law, the doctrine of informed consent protects the patient's decision making and right to control her or his body.[65] It is the legal and ethical duty of the physician to communicate with the patient so that the patient fully understands the treatment options.

The informed consent doctrine requires health care professionals to provide sufficient information so that patients can make a knowledgeable decision about whether to proceed with a proposed procedure.[66] Studies show that patients benefit both physically and psychologically from having such information. These benefits include furthering self-determination, checking against unnecessary or inappropriate procedures, aiding physician decision making, improving the physician-patient relationship, and speeding recovery.[67] The goal of the communication is to ensure that patients receive relevant information so that they can evaluate the proposed procedure objectively and then apply personal values to reject or accept the recommendation.[68]

Early court decisions on informed consent held physicians liable for operating on patients without their consent. By the late 1950s and early 1960s the courts' notion of informed consent included the requirement that patients must be told about the risk of a proposed procedure to make an informed decision.[69] Current doctrine requires a physician to discuss the patient's condition; the availability, risks, and alternatives of diagnostic procedures; and the availability, risks, and alternatives of treatment procedures.

Health care professionals providing infertility therapies should provide extensive information to the couple on the nature and risks as well as the potential success of the proposed procedure. Alternative means of treatment also should be discussed. The couple should be counseled together and individually to assure that one partner is not being pressured to undergo

certain therapies. The institution should provide its success rates, because these differ widely for various programs, some programs not yet reporting a pregnancy.[70] Information should be given to patients concerning embryo discard, storage, donation, research, and cost to themselves.[71] The couple should be counseled to prepare a directive for embryo disposition in the event of divorce or death. The information should include which techniques are available; data on the risk of infection, spontaneous abortion, stillbirth, and so forth; an explanation of the psychologic risks of participating in the procedures; and the type and purpose of research if it is being conducted. Federal law requires each assisted reproductive technology program to report pregnancy success rates to the U.S. Centers for Disease Control and Prevention (CDC), which shall make the information publicly available. The same law requires the CDC to develop a model program to be carried out by the states for the certification of embryo laboratories.[72] Finally, the discussion should be concluded with solicitation of what the couple wants.

Considerations for IVF

In addition to the general types of information regarding risks, alternatives, and so forth that must be disclosed about all proposed procedures, each reproductive technique raises special informed consent considerations. For example, the IVF protocol involves stimulation of a woman's ovaries. This has resulted in some women's providing as many as 17 or more eggs per laparoscopic procedure.[73] If all eggs were fertilized and reimplanted into the woman's uterus, the risks of multiple pregnancies to her and to the potential offspring would be great. Usually only three or four embryos are implanted; hence the couple must decide what they want done with the excess embryos. The couple may decide to implant all the embryos (at which point the risks of multiple gestation should be explained, as should the possibility and risks of multi-fetal reduction), freeze the embryos for subsequent implantation, terminate them, donate them to another woman,[74] or donate them for research. Whereas clinics previously limited the couple's choice to implantation or termination, donation is now common.[75]

Considerations for Cryopreservation

If the couple is considering cryopreservation, the physician should explain to them the institution's policies on how long preservation is allowed, the survival rate of embryos after thawing, and any physical or psychologic risks to the resulting child that freezing might entail. The couple should also be asked for a written directive regarding the fate of the embryos if they divorce, decide against implantation, or if one or both die. If both die or if they file for divorce without directives about what will be done with the embryos, it is unclear who should make the decision regarding the embryos' future. The issue of what should be done with the embryos of a couple going through a divorce was addressed by the Supreme Court of Tennessee.[76] That court held that when the preferences of the couple are unclear or are in dispute and when no prior agreement exists concerning disposition, the interests of the individuals in using the frozen embryos must be weighed.[77] In addition, the court held that the party seeking to avoid procreation should prevail.[78] In contrast to the approach suggested by Tennessee case law, Louisiana, by appointing the physician as temporary guardian, might make him or her responsible for embryo disposition decisions.[79]

In contrast, a New York Supreme Court held that the woman had the right to control the future outcome of embryos she produced with her husband. Maureen and Steven Kass underwent six cycles of IVF but did not achieve a pregnancy. When Maureen petitioned for divorce, five embryos had been frozen. The couple had signed two consent agreements. One provided that in the event of a divorce, any stored embryos would be included in a property settlement as directed by a divorce court. The other agreement provided that if the parties could not decide the disposition of the embryos, the embryos would be donated for research. The only contested issue in the divorce was possession of the embryos. Maureen intended to implant the embryos (she wanted to gestate the embryos herself); Steven intended to donate the embryos for research.

The court stated that embryos are not persons and that they are not property. However, the judge recognized that the people who provided the gametes have a property interest in the embryos. The judge refused to consider dividing the embryos. He wrote that it was simplistic—"a sidestepping of the real issue—a determination of which party has the right to decide the embryos' fate." He gave possession of the embryos to the divorcing wife, entrusting her with the right to control their destiny.

In rejecting the rights of the divorcing husband, the court noted that a man (whether or not married) cannot control the conception or continuance of a pregnancy. The woman has the sole right to use contraceptives or to terminate a pregnancy. "The fact is that an in vivo husband's rights and control over the procreative process ends with ejaculation."[80] The court wrote that there is no legal, ethical, or logical difference between in vivo and in vitro fertilization. "It matters little whether the ovum/sperm union takes place in the private darkness of a fallopian tube or the public glare of a petri dish."[81]

The court differentiated the case from *Davis v Davis*.[82] In *Davis,* the court recognized the man's constitutional right to avoid procreation and balanced his right against his ex-wife's right to procreate. In contrast, the court in *Kass*[83] did not recognize the man's right not to procreate, hence it did not balance the man's right (to not procreate) against the woman's right to procreate.

The court did not consider the man's support obligations or other legal claims he may have had against his ex-wife. The issues should be decided by a court if and when a pregnancy (and livebirth) occurs. However, the court wrote that the potential for parenthood must not remain open-ended. Maureen must implant the embryos in a medically reasonable time.

If cryopreservation becomes more common, it might be considered negligent for a physician to discard embryos. For example, if 5 embryos are produced, 3 are implanted, and the other 2 destroyed but the 3 implanted embryos do not develop into a pregnancy, the woman might claim that her physician negligently interfered with her chances of producing a child by discarding the additional embryos rather than freezing them.[84] This could be especially critical if the eggs are obtained as the result of a "last chance" operation (for example, before a woman undergoes radiation therapy or hysterectomy).

Considerations for Embryo Donation

The physician should discuss the risks involved with embryo donation with the donors. There are two types of donors: those who have completed their families and are donating embryos so another woman may have a family and women undergoing infertility treatments who, through therapy procedures, have produced excess embryos. Women who have fulfilled their own childbearing needs should be counseled about the physical risks associated with embryo donation, such as infection, permanent scarring, and other side effects. In addition to these physical risks, women who undergo infertility therapy must be counseled on the psychologic risks of donation. First the physician should make sure there is no coercion of the woman or the couple to donate an embryo; participation in an IVF program should not be limited to women or couples who agree to donate excess embryos. Second, the physician must counsel the woman to consider the emotional risk of donation in case she herself does not achieve a pregnancy. Donors also should consider the risk of the resulting child's potential emotional reaction on learning of the existence of a biologic parent with whom he or she will have no contact.

These considerations for IVF, cryopreservation, and embryo donation arise in addition to the required informed consent disclosures. They point to the increased complexity of decision making in the area of medically assisted reproduction compared with that with other medical advances, because they involve caretaking decisions for potential or newly created life, in addition to the preservation of an existing life.

SINGLE PARENTHOOD

Originally intended to assist married couples, the new reproductive technologies can be used to facilitate single parenthood.

Single men may hire a surrogate; single women may be artificially inseminated. Most artificial insemination statutes assume that a married couple will be using the procedure, but none makes it illegal for an unmarried woman to do so.[85] The Ohio and Oregon statutes specifically acknowledge that a single woman might use donor sperm.[86]

No laws prohibit the insemination of unmarried women. Even if a state passed such a law it would be unlikely to be upheld as constitutional. The constitutional protection of reproductive decisions extends to individuals as well as married couples.[87] A single woman denied artificial insemination at a clinic affiliated with a state or federal institution that will only inseminate a married couple can claim that her privacy right to make procreative decisions and her equal protection right are violated by the clinic's policies. This has already happened in one case. The clinic associated with a state university settled the suit by agreeing to drop the marriage requirement and consider the woman as a candidate for insemination.[88]

The insemination of single women brings into question traditional notions of family.[89] It raises issues such as whether it is in the child's best interests to have two parents and whether a single parent can meet the physical and emotional needs of a child, especially if the parent will have to work to support the child. However, studies of children in single-parent, woman-headed families have found that these children have comparable cognitive abilities to those raised in two-parent homes.[90] In addition, children in single-parent homes have a level of self-esteem that is at least equal to that of children in two-parent families.[91] Children raised in lesbian-headed households do not differ from other children in gender-role behavior or sexual orientation.[92]

Societal interests, even those that concern the definition of family or suggest community intolerance, are not compelling enough to prohibit the insemination of single women. One court stated in a case involving an unmarried woman undergoing artificial insemination, "We wish to stress that our opinion in this case is not intended to express any judicial preference toward traditional notions of family structure or toward providing a father where a single woman has chosen to bear a child."[93]

The focal point of case law concerning artificial insemination of single women has been paternity. An Ohio law tries to clarify this issue by providing that if an unmarried woman is artificially inseminated, "the donor shall not be treated in law or regarded as the natural father."[94] In contrast, a New Jersey case involving the home insemination of a single woman held that the man who provided the semen was the legal father of the child.[95] This decision was based on a unique set of facts (the donor, who was the woman's boyfriend, sued for visitation rights), so it does not provide much guidance for other cases. The court held that the boyfriend who provided the sperm was the legal father and granted him visitation rights. In reaching its

decision, the court differentiated this case from previous artificial insemination cases because "there is no married couple [and because] there is no anonymous donor."[96] The court found that, "If an unmarried woman conceives a child through artificial insemination from semen from a known man, that man cannot be considered to be less a father because he is not married to the woman."[97] The court also stated that the decision was consistent with judicial policy "favoring the requirement that a child be provided with a father as well as a mother."[98] This decision has been read narrowly; there have been no cases in which an anonymous sperm donor has been held liable for child support against his wishes.

Similar issues are raised in the context of egg donation. In contrast to their laws on artificial insemination, few states have given legal recognition to the intentions of the parties with regard to rearing the children born of such arrangements. Only five states have statutes defining the rearing rights of oocyte donors and recipients.[99] Each of these statutes irrebuttably presumes that a child resulting from egg donation is the child of the couple who consented to receive the donated egg.[100]

PHYSICIAN INVOLVEMENT

Physician involvement in artificial insemination by donor (AID) is not medically necessary; nonetheless, some statutory enactments require physician supervision. (Although the medical term has evolved to be therapeutic insemination by donor [TID], in legal language it is still AID, and that term is used in this chapter.) Arguably, this could clarify the parental status of the parties involved. At least 16 of the related statutes assume that AID will be performed by or under the supervision of a "licensed physician," "certified medical doctor," or person "duly authorized to practice medicine."[101] Because AID is a relatively simple procedure[102] and involves minimal risk, the statutes that require medical assistance raise questions about whether its performance by someone other than a physician (such as a husband, lover, donor, or friend) has different legal consequences that prevent the consenting husband from taking on, and the consenting donor from relinquishing, parental rights and responsibilities. For example, the California artificial insemination statute states, "[I]f, under the supervision of a licensed physician and with the consent of her husband, a wife is inseminated artificially with the semen donated by a man who is not her husband, the husband is treated in law as if he were the natural father of a child thereby conceived."[103] This type of statutory language raises questions about whether the consenting husband is the legal father when a physician is not involved in the procedure.[104] In that case, however, more general statutory provisions regarding paternity would usually give paternity rights to the husband.

The statutory requirement for physician supervision, however, can cause problems when AID performed by a nonphysician involves an unmarried woman. Some unmarried women have trouble finding physicians who will agree to perform the procedure for them.[105] Their alternative is to find a donor through a network of friends and acquaintances. In one case, an unmarried woman privately selected a sperm donor and performed the insemination in her home by herself.[106] The sperm donor was listed as the father on the child's birth certificate. He filed an action to establish paternity and visitation rights. The appellate court scrutinized the statute, which said, "The donor of semen provided to a licensed physician for use in artificial insemination of a woman other than the donor's wife is treated in law as if he were not the natural father of a child thereby conceived."[107] The court held that because the semen was not provided to a physician, the donor was the legal father, and granted him visitation rights.

The court noted that "nothing inherent in artificial insemination requires the involvement of a physician."[108] Physician involvement "might offend a woman's sense of privacy and reproductive autonomy, might result in burdensome costs to some women, and might interfere with a woman's desire to conduct the procedure in a comfortable environment such as her own home or to choose the donor herself."[109] A fourth reason for not using the services of a physician, not mentioned by the court, is that some people believe that the medical screening of donors by infertility clinics is inadequate, and thus they wish to choose their own donors.[110] The court also gave two reasons why physician involvement might be appropriate, however. The physician could obtain a medical history of the donor and screen him. Also, the physician "can serve to create a formal, documented structure for the donor-recipient relationship to avoid misunderstandings between the parties."[111] These reasons are particularly applicable to situations in which AID is used as part of a surrogate parenting arrangement.

QUALITY ASSURANCE

Personnel Qualifications

Traditionally patients have relied on the tort system to ensure a minimal level of quality by bringing a medical malpractice claim. The guidelines of professional organizations such as The American Fertility Society (AFS) and the American Association of Tissue Banks (AATB) regarding the performance of reproductive techniques are evidence of the standard of care that must be met. A Louisiana law codifies such standards by specifically addressing the qualifications of professionals and standards for facilities performing IVF[112]: the facilities must meet "the standards of the American Fertility Society and the Ameri-

can College of Obstetrics and Gynecologists"; the director of the facility must be a "medical doctor licensed to practice medicine in this state and possessing specialized training and skill in in vitro fertilization"; and the physicians performing the technique are required to act "in conformity with the standards established by the American Fertility Society or the American College of Obstetricians and Gynecologists." In contrast, no state laws specifically set forth qualifications for personnel who are involved with artificial insemination or surrogate motherhood.

Screening

The statutes that address reproductive technology have generally paid no attention to medical, genetic, and psychologic screening of the participants. The development of surrogate motherhood has caused lawmakers to consider the issue and to rethink previous law about donor insemination to address screening in that context as well.[113] Medical and genetic screening of donors is necessary to protect the health of recipients and the resulting children. A psychologic assessment may be necessary to determine whether the participants are informed and are voluntarily and competently entering into alternative reproduction.

At least 10 statutes address sperm donor screening. Laws in Idaho and Oregon provide that a person who knows he has a genetic defect or venereal disease may not be a sperm donor,[114] but they provide no requirement that the donors be screened. The Idaho law does require that sperm donors be screened for human immunodeficiency virus (HIV).[115] Under an Ohio law,[116] the donor of fresh semen must undergo a physical examination, give a medical and genetic history, and be tested for blood type and Rh factor. The donor of fresh sperm must undergo appropriate laboratory studies, which "may include, but are not limited to, venereal disease research laboratories, karyotyping, [gonococcus] culture, cytomegalo[virus], hepatitis, kem-zyme, Tay-Sachs, sickle-cell, ureaplasma, HTLV-III, and chlamydia."[117]

Although few statutory guidelines exist, physicians would face tort liability if they did not undertake proper screening of donors. Failure to do so could leave a physician liable for physical and emotional harm experienced by a recipient or her offspring as a result of the transmission of disease.

The U.S. Court of Appeals for the Sixth Circuit in 1992 considered the issue of screening in the surrogacy context.[118] The court held that the duty to protect the surrogate mother from harm may have been breached. The surrogate mother brought suit against the attorney arranging the surrogacy procedure, another attorney involved in establishing the surrogacy arrangement, and the physician for damages that arose when the child was born with severe birth defects.[119] The surrogate was artificially inseminated with the contracting man's semen. The surrogate, however, had engaged in sexual relations with her husband, and the child to whom she gave birth actually had been fathered by her husband. The child was born with a cytomegalovirus (CMV) infection that resulted in severe birth defects.[120] The child's parents alleged that the mother had contracted CMV infection from the semen of the donor, who was never tested for a sexually transmitted disease, nor was the semen sample tested.[121] In remanding the case for a jury trial, the court determined that "[I]t is for the jury to decide whether [the defendants] have provided the kind of care commensurate with the exercise of a high degree of diligence in protecting people from harm."[122]

In addition to the common law requirements, both the American Society for Reproductive Medicine (ASRM, formerly the AFS)[123] and the AATB[124] have developed extensive screening guidelines. These may be considered evidence of at least a minimal level of professional responsibility for screening. For example, the ASRM suggests excluding sperm donors who are at risk for having a sexually transmitted disease. They also suggest rescreening every 6 months and discontinuing the use of a donor if he has a new sexual partner or if there is a break in monogamy or abstinence.

The guidelines also recommend rejection of donors with a family history of certain enumerated genetic disorders as well as carriers of those disorders. The AATB Reproductive Council standards recommend selection of donors on the basis of a "personal, physical, and genetic examination and history" as well as in-depth semen analysis. The guidelines mandate rejection of a potential sperm donor if he is employed in a job that involves chemical or radiation exposure or if he is an alcohol or drug abuser.[125] Screening for infectious and genetic diseases should be conducted on egg or embryo donors as well.

Federal law requires assisted reproductive technology programs to report annually to the Secretary of Health and Human Services pregnancy success rates of the program with each reproductive technique. The report must also disclose the identity of each laboratory used by the program and whether such laboratory is certified.[126] As part of the certification standards, each laboratory shall follow a standard program for quality assurance and quality control.[127] The federal law grants the CDC authority to develop, inspect, and administer the certification program. The CDC has unofficially adopted the ASRM–College of American Pathologists (CAP) certification program.

RECORD-KEEPING AND CONFIDENTIALITY

Record-keeping

Confidential medical records should be kept that identify all the parties and include medical and genetic histories of donors and surrogates.[128] These histories should be available to the couples or individuals who use assisted reproduction and also to the children produced through these techniques. An Ohio law requires substantial but nonidentifying disclosures about sperm donors. The physician is required to provide to the recipient and her husband upon their request the medical and genetic history of the donor and people related to him, blood type, Rh factor, race, eye and hair color, age, height, weight, educational attainment and talents, religious background, and any other information that the donor has indicated may be disclosed.[129]

Efforts at record-keeping on providers of gametes have been minimal. Failure to keep adequate records presents the chance of harm to all parties. If a child is conceived with donated egg or sperm and has a medical problem due to a genetic disorder passed on through the donated gamete, without adequate records there is no way of identifying the donor to prevent using him or her for subsequent pregnancies. If the resulting child develops a medical problem that requires donation of genetically compatible organic material (such as bone marrow), if records are incomplete the child may be prevented from contacting a potential donor.

Reluctance by clinicians to keep records may stem from the fear that if donors could be identified, they might be held financially liable for the child. Physicians may argue that record-keeping is a burdensome task that diverts resources away from treating the patient[130]; however, physicians may be best suited for accepting this responsibility and ensuring confidentiality. Physicians' duty to keep records may be based on tort principles or professional codes of ethics.[131] A number of states require by statute that physicians keep records about donor insemination.[132] The Ohio law requires physicians to maintain a file for at least 5 years, separate from any regular medical chart, that includes the written consent form and information provided to the recipient.

Infertility programs must document whether they have in fact achieved a pregnancy and their pregnancy rates.[133] An analysis of such records provides the data to meet the requirements for informed consent.[134]

In addition to physicians' and clinics' keeping records about the participants in medically assisted reproduction (including donors and surrogates) and about resulting children, the state might have an interest in keeping information about the extent of use of alternative reproduction, the number of attempts, and rates of pregnancy, miscarriage, stillbirths, livebirths, and birth defects. Finally, state record-keeping could include maintaining a voluntary registry so that if both sides agree biologic children and their siblings or parents can be identified to each other.

Some states already have legislation that sets forth record-keeping requirements for specific procedures. For example, the artificial insemination statutes of 10 states require physicians to file with the appropriate state department the dates of all procedures they perform.[135] Three states require physicians to file information on the birth of children conceived through AID.[136]

Pennsylvania has such requirements for IVF but not for AID. Anyone conducting IVF is required to file quarterly reports with the department of health, including the names of everyone assisting in the procedure, the location in which the procedure is performed, names and addresses of sponsoring individuals or institutions (except the names of the donors or recipients of gametes), the number of ova fertilized, the number of embryos destroyed or discarded, and the number of women in whom the embryos are implanted.[137]

Confidentiality

State laws protect the physician-patient relationship by providing that the disclosure of confidential information is grounds for revocation of the physician's medical license or a basis for other disciplinary action. An ethical duty also exists, founded on the Hippocratic oath or the judicial ethics of the American Medical Association, that is paralleled by a legal duty set out in the disciplinary or testimonial privilege statutes in most states.

States that mandate filing a husband's consent to AID procedures also protect the confidentiality of such information and the privacy of the individuals. The information, generally confidential, may be opened by a court "for good cause shown." The extent and protection of confidentiality varies among jurisdictions. For example, the Ohio law provides that the physician maintaining a file on AID "shall not make this information available for inspections by any person" unless a court determines that inspection "is necessary for or helpful in the medical treatment of a child born as a result of artificial insemination."[138]

LEGAL AND BIOLOGIC PARENTAGE

Third-party involvement raises the potential for a distinction between legal and biologic parentage. In the context of AID, the courts recognized the consenting husband's legal parentage through a series of early cases that established the child's legal identity. Usually these cases arose out of a divorce proceeding. In one case the husband claimed he should not have to support the child because they were not genetically related.[139] In another, the wife tried to deny her husband visitation rights based on the same rationale.[140] Sometimes, in the earliest cases, the courts declared the child born as a result of artificial insemination to be illegitimate. It is well established, however, that the courts will protect the child financially and emotionally by finding the consenting husband to be the legal father with support responsibilities and visitation rights.

All of the 35 states that regulate AID clarify the paternity of a child by providing that the sperm recipient and her consenting husband are the legal parents.[141] The consenting husband is the legal father for legitimacy, inheritance, and support purposes.[142] Some statutes, such as those of Minnesota, Montana, Nevada, New Mexico, Virginia, Wisconsin, and Wyoming, require the husband's written consent to the procedure for him to be recognized as the legal parent.[143]

At least two of the states that regulate egg donation clarify parental responsibility. The laws state that a child born to a married woman as the result of egg donation is deemed to be the child of the marriage, and the egg donor has no parental rights or responsibilities.[144] The language and intent track sperm donation laws. A Florida law includes donated eggs and embryos in the marital presumption, as long as there is a written consent from the husband and wife.[145]

It appears that in cases involving surrogate gestational mothers, courts are adopting the position that the couple who provides the gametes are the legal parents. In *Smith v Jones*, a case involving a surrogate gestational mother who carried a couple's embryo, a district court recognized the genetic parents as the legal parents and granted them the right to have their names put on the birth certificate.[146] The gestational surrogate was not considered to be the mother, and the couple did not have to adopt the child.

In *Johnson v Calvert,* the California Supreme Court addressed the issue of parentage in a gestational surrogacy arrangement. It concluded that the genetic parents were the legal parents of the resulting child.[147] In making its determination, the court found that the parties' intent regarding parentage, as reflected by the contract, was the appropriate fact to consider.[148] An Ohio court was faced with the same issue of determining the parents of a child born through a gestational surrogacy arrangement.[149] The court determined that the spouses providing the genetic material were the legal and natural parents of the child.[150] Although the court reached the same decision as the court in *Johnson,* they were critical of the *Johnson* court's reliance on the parties' intent. The Ohio court found that two questions drive the determination of legal parentage: who provides the child's genes, and who will raise the child.[151] If the genetic parents have not relinquished their right to raise the child, then they must be deemed the legal and natural parents. The court held that "[t]he birth test becomes subordinate and secondary to genetics."[152]

The issue of determining the legal parents of the child can become even more complicated in the gestational surrogacy context when there is a conflict between the two gamete donors. Such a conflict was presented to the Court of Appeals of Arizona.[153] In that case, a couple entered into a gestational surrogacy arrangement with a woman who became pregnant with the couple's triplets. During the pregnancy, the couple filed for divorce. The wife requested shared custody of the unborn triplets with her divorcing husband. The husband tried to deny her request for custody, claiming that he was the biologic father of the triplets and the gestational surrogate was the legal mother of the children according to the Arizona surrogacy statute.[154] The trial court found that the statute was unconstitutional because the state had no compelling interest to justify denying the genetic mother the opportunity to prove her genetic link to the child (thus it was a violation of her due process rights). The court also found that the statute did not consider the importance of genetics in the legal recognition of parenthood. The appellate court agreed with the trial court. It held that the statute afforded the father an opportunity to rebut the presumption of paternity but did not afford the mother the same opportunity. Because the statute implicated a fundamental right, the right to bear a child, and it treated women differently from men, it violated the woman's equal protection right. Thus the court used strict scrutiny analysis and held that the Arizona statute violated both the state and federal constitutions.

A different result was reached by the New Jersey Supreme Court in the landmark *Baby M* decision, a case involving traditional rather than gestational surrogacy. Here the court held that the man providing the sperm was the legal father, and the woman providing the egg and gestating the embryo was the legal mother.

Another variation on determining parental rights was raised in *In re Marriage of Moschetta*.[155] *Moschetta,* like *Baby M* involved a traditional surrogacy arrangement. During the pregnancy, the contracting couple suffered marital problems, and at one point, the husband considered obtaining a divorce. The surrogate did not learn of the marital discord until the day before the baby was born. The surrogate responded to the news by refusing to place the child for adoption. She relented, though, and allowed the Moschettas to take the baby home once the couple told her that they would stay together. Within several months, Mr. Moschetta left the family home, taking the child. Mrs. Moschetta filed an action to establish a parental relationship with the child, and the surrogate sought to join the divorce action. The court, therefore, was confronted with determining the parental rights of Mrs. Moschetta and the surrogate and determined that the maternal rights to the child were vested in the surrogate mother.[156] The rationale for the decision rested on the fact that Mrs. Moschetta was not the biologic mother of the child—no genetic connection existed between her and the child.[157] It was clear that the surrogate not only gave birth but also was genetically related to the child.[158] The court acknowledged that the result was "disquieting" and expressed a need for "legislative guidance," however the existing state of the law compelled the decision that Mr. Moschetta and the surrogate were the legal parents of the child.[159]

A New York court did not rely on the genetic link to the child but rather the intention of the rearing parents to determine parental rights.[160] Mrs. McDonald gave birth to twins conceived by means of IVF with donated eggs and her husband's sperm. In a subsequent divorce action, the husband asserted that the children were illegitimate because they were not genetically related to the mother, and he should be granted sole custody. The court, relying on *Johnson v Calvert,*[161] relied on the couple's intent to establish a parental relationship and raise the twins. Thus the court found Mrs. McDonald was the natural mother and entitled to custody of the children.

The husband also requested access to all medical records concerning the IVF treatments, including information about the egg donor. The court denied the husband's motion because information about the egg donor was not relevant to the custody issue, and the egg donor was not a party to the action.

Arizona, Arkansas, the District of Columbia, Florida, Indiana, Kentucky, Louisiana, Michigan, Nebraska, Nevada, New Hampshire, New York, North Dakota, Utah, Virginia, and Washington specifically regulate surrogate motherhood arrangements.[162] Of these 16 states, only 7 specifically address paternity.[163] The Arkansas statute presumes that the legal mother of a child conceived by artificial insemination and born to an unmarried surrogate mother is the intended mother. In 12 states, statutes void paid surrogacy contracts,[164] and in 2 states, statutes ban surrogacy contracts.[165] Florida allows gestational surrogacy contracts to pay for reasonable living, legal, medical, psychologic, and psychiatric expenses.[166] If a dispute arose in states that have no surrogacy statute, the existing AID, adoption, and parentage statutes would provide a framework for determining paternity.

PAYMENT TO THIRD PARTIES

It is axiomatic in a market economy that providers of goods and services are compensated. Our society routinely compensates third parties for their time, effort, inconvenience, and availability in providing a service or product. The involvement of third parties in reproduction raises the question of compensating them for their efforts. A surrogate puts her own life at risk to give birth to a child for another couple. Should she be compensated, or does that commercialize the creation of life?

Sperm donors are routinely compensated for providing gametes. Payment to egg or embryo donors is often perceived to be different. One state explicitly forbids payment of egg donors in the context of IVF.[167] In addition, in at least six states the organ transplant laws are drafted so broadly that they could be used to ban payment to egg donors.[168] For example, a Virginia statute makes it "unlawful to sell, to offer to sell, to buy, to offer to buy or to procure through purchase" a human organ.[169] An organ is "any natural body part with the exception of hair, blood, or any other self-replacing body fluid."[170]

Some states regulate payment to a embryo donor rather than to an egg donor. Louisiana expressly prohibits payment to embryo donors.[171] Florida allows only reasonable compensation directly related to the donation of eggs, sperm, and embryos.[172] In addition, 11 statutes that prohibit a woman from selling a fetus for experimentation employ language potentially broad enough to forbid payment to a woman who undergoes in vivo fertilization by means of embryo transfer.[173]

Payment to surrogate mothers seems to have raised the most public discussion of reimbursement of third parties for their assistance in medically assisted reproduction. Nevada exempts paid surrogacy contracts from the prohibition against payment in connection with an adoption.[174] Laws in at least 23 states prohibit payment in connection with an adoption, which could be interpreted as restricting commercial surrogate motherhood.[175] Because the adoption laws were drafted with a different purpose, they may be differentiated from surrogate parenting and arguably may not restrict payment to a surrogate. Paying a surrogate a fee can be differentiated from paying an already pregnant woman for her child.

Courts have had to deal with payments to surrogates in the absence of legislative guidelines, and their reactions have been mixed. The New Jersey Supreme Court voided a surrogacy contract and held that statutes that ban payment in connection with an adoption prohibited payment to a surrogate.[176] This is similar to an earlier decision in which a Michigan court held that a statutory ban that prohibited payment in connection with an adoption also prohibited payment to a surrogate under a surrogate contract.[177] Other courts, specifically those in New York and Kentucky, have allowed compensation to the surrogate.[178] The Kentucky court concluded that contracts to pay surrogate mothers did not violate the statutory prohibition against payment in connection with an adoption.[179] A subsequently adopted Kentucky statute, however, voids paid surrogacy contracts.

Laws that restrict payment to third parties must be assessed in light of the individual's or couple's rights to privacy to make procreative decisions. People with particular infertility problems may be forced to remain childless if payment is not allowed, because it may not be possible to recruit donors or surrogate mothers without paying them. As with other statutory regulations that restrict alternative reproduction, laws that deny payment to third parties would be upheld only if they were to further a compelling state interest. For example, because the decision to use a surrogate is protected by the right to privacy, moral disapproval of payment as the commercialization of motherhood would be an insufficient reason to ban payment.

THE LAW, RESPONSIBILITY, AND NEW REPRODUCTIVE THERAPIES

The new reproductive therapies offer the hope of children to infertile couples, but with the promise comes additional responsibilities for all parties. Researchers who use the new opportunities for embryo and fetal research must comport with ethical standards. Clinicians' responsibilities include counseling and informing the participants in medically assisted reproduction and screening the third parties involved. An individual or a couple using the technologies will be faced with a host of new psychologic challenges. Society will be forced, in the course of questioning traditional notions of family, to decide how best to protect the fundamental rights of its citizenry. Finally, all those involved, from the researcher to society in general, must provide a safe, nurturing environment for the resulting children. The law will play a part in shaping the impact of the new reproductive technologies by protecting constitutional rights, setting the standards for research and practice, defining the rights and responsibilities of the parties and society, and contributing to the ethical considerations.

NOTES AND REFERENCES

1. *Skinner v Oklahoma,* 316 US 535 (1942)
2. *Skinner v Oklahoma,* 316 US 535, 541 (1942)
3. See, eg, *Griswold v Connecticut,* 381 US 479 (1965); *Eisenstadt v Baird,* 405 US 438 (1972); *Roe v Wade,* 410 US 113 (1973)
4. *Stanley v Illinois,* 405 US 645, 651 (1972)
5. *Eisentadt v Baird,* 405 US 438, 453 (1972)
6. *Roe v Wade,* 410 US 113, 155 (1973). In a subsequent case, the Supreme Court allowed a state to place some restrictions on a woman's access to abortion, but affirmed that state regulations must not place an undue burden on a woman's liberty right. The liberty right is composed of the "private sphere of the family" and the "bodily integrity of the pregnant woman." *Planned Parenthood of Southeastern Pennsylvania v Casey,* 112 SCt 2791, 60 USLW 4795, 4812 (1992)
7. Karst K: The freedom of intimate association. *Yale L J* 89:624, 1980
8. Andrews L, Hendricks: Legal and moral status of IVF/ET. In: Fredericks C, et al (eds), *Foundations of In Vitro Fertilization.* Washington, DC: Hemisphere 1987:312
9. Robertson J: Embryos, families, and procreative liberty: The legal structure of the new reproduction. *So Cal L Rev* 59:939, 1986
10. Andrews L: The legal status of the embryo. *Loyola L Rev* 32:357, 1986
11. *In re Baby M,* 217 NJ Super 313, 525 A2d 1128 (NJ 1987); 109 NJ 396, 537 A2d 1227 (1988)
12. Some states have prohibited payment for surrogate parenting arrangements in the hope of discouraging the practice, but they have not banned it outright.

13. Robertson J: Embryo research. *Univ W Ontario L Rev* 24:15, 1986
14. *Second International Dictionary of Medicine and Biology.* New York: Wiley, 1986
15. Clifford Grobstein introduced the notion that IVF opens a window to the embryo. Grobstein C: *From Chance to Purpose: An Appraisal of External Human Fertilization.* 1981: Reading, MA: Addison-Wesley
16. Robertson, Embryo research, 17
17. Ibid, 17
18. See, eg, Louisiana statute that prohibits the creation of embryos solely for research. La Rev Stat Ann §9:122 (West 1991)
19. Ariz Rev Stat Ann §36:2302 (1986); Ark Stat Ann §82-436 to 442 (Supp 1985); Cal Health & Safety Code §25956 (West 1984); Fla Stat Ann §§390.001(6), (7) (West 1986); 720 ILCS 510/6 (1994); Ind Code §35-1-58.5-6 (1986); Ky Rev Stat Ann §436-026 (Baldwin 1985); La Rev Stat Ann §9:122 (West 1991); Me Rev Stat Ann tit 22, §1593 (1980); Mass Ann Laws ch 112, §12J (Law, Co-op 1985); Mich Comp Laws Ann §§333-2685-.2692 (West 1980); Minn Stat Ann §§145.421-.422 (West Supp 1987); Mo Ann Stat §188.037 (Vernon 1983); Mont Code Ann §50-20-108(3) (1985); Neb Rev Stat §§28-342 to -346 (1985); NM Stat Ann 24-9A-1 (1981); ND Cent Code §14-02.02-1 to -02 (1981); Ohio Rev Code Ann §2919.14 (Baldwin 1982); Okla Stat Ann tit 63, §1-735 (West 1984); Pa Stat Ann tit 18, §3216 (Purdon 1983); RI Gen Laws §11-54-1 (1994); SD Codified Laws Ann §34-23A-17 (1986); Tenn Code Ann §39-4-208 (1982); Utah Code Ann §§76-7-310 to -311 (1978); Wyo Stat §35-6-115 (1977)
20. Only Utah does not have such a restriction.
21. Arizona, Indiana, Kentucky, Maine, Ohio, Wyoming. All these laws, except for that in Maine, apply only to research on aborted fetuses.
22. Arkansas, California, Florida, Missouri, Nebraska, Oklahoma, Pennsylvania, which apply only to live aborted fetuses. Illinois, Massachusetts, Montana, North Dakota, Rhode Island, which apply to live fetuses.
23. La Rev Stat Ann §9:122 (West 1991)
24. Arizona, Arkansas, California, Florida, Indiana, Kentucky, Missouri, Nebraska, Ohio, Oklahoma, Pennsylvania, Tennessee, Wyoming.
25. Robertson, Embryo research, 16.
26. Ibid, at 16
27. 45 CFR §46.203(c) (1986)
28. 58 *Federal Register* 7468 (Feb 5, 1993)
29. Gianelli D: Embryo research approved: With a catch. *Am Med News* 37:3, 1994
30. Ibid
31. Ibid
32. Marwick, C: Feds may fund study of existing embryos only. *JAMA* 273:97, 1995
33. Louisiana, Maine, Massachusetts, Michigan, North Dakota, Rhode Island, and Utah
34. NM Stat Ann §24-9A01(D) (1986)
35. 720 ILCS 510/6(7) (1994)
36. Bustillo M, Buster J, Cohen J, et al: Delivery of a healthy infant following nonsurgical ovum transfer. *JAMA* 251:889, 1984
37. Arizona, Arkansas, Indiana, Louisiana, Maine, Massachusetts, Michigan, Missouri, Montana, Nebraska, North Dakota, Ohio, Oklahoma, Pennsylvania, Rhode Island, Utah, Wyoming. This includes both statutes that specifically apply to embryos and those that neglect to define *fetus* or the term used to refer to the subject of research and might be interpreted to include, preimplantation embryos
38. Arizona, Arkansas, California, Florida, Indiana, Kentucky, Missouri, Nebraska, Ohio, Oklahoma, Tennessee, Wyoming
39. Illinois, Louisiana (applies to cryopreservation after IVF), Maine, Massachusetts, Michigan, North Dakota, Pennsylvania, Rhode Island, Utah
40. Robertson J, Embryos, families, and procreative liberty, 994–995
41. The American Fertility Society (AFS) considers it ethical to dispose of nontransferred embryos. Ethics Committee of the American Fertility Society: Ethical considerations of assisted reproductive technologies. *Fertil Steril* 62(Suppl 1):5, 1994
42. La Rev Stat Ann §9:121 (West 1991)
43. La Rev Stat Ann §9:122 (West 1991)
44. La Rev Stat Ann §9:129 (West 1991)
45. La Rev Stat Ann §9:127 (West 1991)
46. Ky Rev Stat Ann §311.715 (Michie 1990)
47. The Illinois statute, now repealed, granted custody to the physician of an in vitro fertilized egg. The physician was "deemed to have care and custody of a child" for purposes of an 1877 child abuse act. Ill Ann Stat ch 23, §2354 (Smith-Hurd 1968)
48. *Smith v Hartigan,* 556 FSupp 157 (ND Ill 1983)
49. ILCS 510/6(7) (1994)
50. *Del Zio v Manhattan's Columbia Presbyterian Medical Center,* No 74-3558 (SDNY November 14, 1978)
51. Arkansas, Florida, Illinois (specifically exempts IVF), Kentucky, Louisiana (only involves embryos created through IVF), Maine, Massachusetts, Michigan, Minnesota, Nebraska, New Mexico, North Dakota, Ohio, Oklahoma, Rhode Island, Utah.
52. Arkansas, Kentucky, Maine, Massachusetts, Michigan, Nebraska, North Dakota, Rhode Island, Wyoming.
53. Fla Stat Ann §873.05 (West Supp 1987); ILCS 510/6(7) (1994) (prohibits sale only); La Rev Stat Ann §9:122 (1991) (prohibits sale of IVF embryos)
54. *Lifchez v Hartigan,* 735 FSupp 1361 (ND Ill 1990)
55. Ibid
56. 794 F2d 994 (5th Cir 1986)
57. *Margaret S v Edwards,* 794 F2d 994 (5th Cir 1986)
58. Ibid, 999
59. Ibid
60. Ibid
61. La Rev Stat Ann §9:122 (West 1991)
62. La Rev Stat Ann §9:130 (West 1991)
63. La Rev Stat Ann §9:130 (West 1991)
64. La Rev Stat Ann §9:122 (West 1991)
65. Andrews L: Informed consent statutes and the decisionmaking process. *J Leg Med* 5:163, 1984
66. Andrews L: The rationale behind the informed consent doctrine. *J Med Pract* 1:59, 1985
67. Andrews L: Provision of genetic services: Informed consent and

other duties to disclose. In: Andrews L, *Medical Genetics: A Legal Frontier*. Chicago, American Bar Foundation, 1987:105–134

68. Andrews L: The rationale behind the informed consent doctrine, 60

69. *Natason v Kline,* 186 Kan 393, 350 P2d 1093 (1960), *reh'g denied* 187 Kan 186, 354 P2d 670 (1960). The case involved a woman who suffered extensive tissue and bone damage after a series of cobalt treatments for breast cancer. The court held that where there is a substantial risk of injury in administration of a treatment and no emergency exists, the physician has a duty to make a reasonable disclosure to the patient of the known risks and would be subject to liability for a failure to do so.

70. American Fertility Society, 87S–88S

71. Robertson, Embryos, families, and procreative liberty, 1036

72. 42 USCA §263a-1 et seq (West Supp 1994)

73. Andrews, The legal status of the embryo, 401

74. An international review found that by 1987 60 live births had resulted from pregnancies involving donated eggs. Andrews, *Medical Genetics,* 163

75. Andrews L, Hendricks, 315

76. *Davis v Davis,* 842 SW2d 588 (1992), *remanded on reh'g and reh'g denied in part,* No 34, 1992 Tenn Lexis 622 (Tenn Nov 23, 1992), *later proceeding sub nom Stowe v Davis,* 113 SCt 1042, *cert denied, Stowe v Davis,* 113 SCt 1259 (1993)

77. Ibid, 604

78. Ibid

79. La Rev Stat Ann §9:126 (West 1991)

80. *Kass v Kass,* 1995 WL 110368 (NY Sup Ct Nassau County, 1995)

81. Ibid

82. *Davis* involved a couple who were divorcing and had undergone IVF with several embryos still frozen at the time of their divorce. The parties disputed who should receive custody of the embryos. The judge awarded control over frozen embryos to the husband, who did not want the embryos implanted. After the court awarded custody to the husband, the embryos were allowed to expire.

83. *Kass v Kass,* 1995 WL 110368 (NY Sup Ct Nassau County 1995)

84. Andrews L, Hendricks, 315

85. Kritchevsky B: The unmarried woman's right to artificial insemination: A call for an expanded definition of family. *Harvard Women L J* 4:1, 1981

86. Ohio Rev Code Ann §3111.31 (Baldwin 1987); Or Rev Stat §677.365 (1977). The Ohio statute applies to artificial insemination for the purpose of impregnating a woman so that she can bear a child that she intends to raise as her child. The Oregon statute requires the consent of her husband "if she is married." Or Rev Stat §677.365 (1977)

87. As the US Supreme Court noted, "It is the right of the *individual,* married or single, to be free of unwarranted governmental intrusion in matters so fundamentally affecting a person as the decision whether to bear or beget a child." *Eisenstadt v Baird,* 405 US 438, 453 (1972) [emphasis in the original]

88. *Smedes v Wayne State University,* No 80-725.83 (ED Mich, filed July 16, 1980)

89. Similar issues are raised by an unmarried man's use of a surrogate mother. Recently, a 26-year-old single man who contracted with a surrogate mother was charged with homicide in connection with the infant's death. The infant died of a skull fracture and internal head injuries 6 weeks after he was relinquished to the father. S.L. Berry: Right to reproduce: Who decides? *Indianapolis News* January 26, 1995

90. McGuire M, Alexander NJ: Artificial insemination of single women. *Fertil Steril* 43:182–184, 1985

91. Raschke HJ, Raschke VJ: Family conflict and children's self concept: A comparison of intact and single parent families. *J Marriage Fam* 41:367, 1979. Weiss: Growing up a little faster. *J Soc Issues* 35:97, 1979

92. McGuire, and Alexander, 182

93. *Jhordan C v Mary K,* 179 Cal App 3d 386, 224 Cal Rptr 530, 537-8 (1986)

94. Ohio Rev Code Ann §3111.37(B) (Baldwin 1987). The statute does not define "woman" as a married woman.

95. *CM v CC,* 152 NJ Super 160, 377 A2d 821 (1977)

96. *CM v CC,* 152 NJ Super 160, 377 A2d 821, 824 (1977)

97. *CM v CC,* 152 NJ Super 160, 377 A2d 821, 824 (1977)

98. *CM v CC,* 152 NJ Super 160, 377 A2d 821, 824 (1977)

99. Fla Stat Ann §742.11(2) (West Supp 1995); ND Cent Code §14-18-04 (Supp 1995); Okla Stat Ann tit 10, §555 (West Supp 1995); Tex Fam Code Ann §12.03A (West Supp 1995); Va Code Ann §20—158 (1995)

100. Ibid

101. Alabama, Alaska, California, Colorado, Idaho, Illinois, Minnesota, Montana, Nevada, New Jersey, New Mexico, Ohio, Virginia, Washington, Wisconsin, Wyoming

102. Andrews L: Alternative modes of reproduction. In: Cohen S, Taub N (eds), *Reproductive Laws for the 1990's.* Clifton, NJ, Rutgers Press, 1989:377. Chapter relates that artificial insemination may be accomplished in the privacy of one's own home with instruments no more sophisticated than a turkey baster. The Ohio law seems to anticipate this: "[S]upervision requires the availability of a physician for consultation and direction, but does not necessarily require the personal presence of the physician who is providing the supervision." Ohio Rev Code Ann §3111.32 (Baldwin 1987)

103. Cal Civ Code §7005(a) (West 1983)

104. Andrews L: Alternative reproduction. In: Schatkin SB, Andrews MW, *Disputed Paternity Proceedings.* New York, Mathew Bender, 1986:30–1, 30–19

105. A national survey of physicians providing artificial insemination found that 10% of the procedures were performed for unmarried women. Curie-Cohen M, Luttrell M, and Shapiro S: Current practice of artificial insemination by donor in the United States: *N Engl J Med* 300:585–590, 1979. The findings are consistent with a later survey by the US Congressional Office of Technology Assessment: *Artificial insemination: Practice in the United States.* Washington, DC, US Govt Printing Office, 1988. One reason why most physicians, both those in private practice and those in hospitals, refuse to perform AID for unmarried women is that they erroneously fear the practice is illegal. A second reason is that some of the physicians believe that unmarried women and lesbians should not be mothers. Kritchevsky B: The unmarried woman's right to insemination, 68

106. *Jhordan C v Mary K,* 179 Cal App 3d 386, 224 Cal Rptr 530 (1986)
107. Cal Civ Code §7005(b) (West 1983)
108. *Jhordan C v Mary K,* 179 Cal App 3d 386, 224 Cal Rptr 530, 535 (1986)
109. Ibid
110. Andrews L: Yours, mine and theirs. *Psychol Today* 18:20, 1984
111. *Jhordan C v Mary K,* 179 Cal App 3d 386, 224 Cal Rptr 530, 535 (1986)
112. La Rev Stat Ann §9:128 (West 1991)
113. Andrews L: The aftermath of Baby M: Proposed state laws on surrogate motherhood. *Hastings Center Rep* 17:31, 1987
114. Idaho Code §39-5404 (Supp 1986); Or Rev Stat §677.370 (1981). See also a New York City ordinance that provides that carriers of genetic diseases or defects and men suffering from venereal disease or tuberculosis cannot be sperm donors. It also provides that the sperm donor and recipient must have compatible Rh factors. City of New York Health Code §§21.03, .05 (1973)
115. Idaho Code §39-5408 (Supp 1986)
116. Ohio Rev Code Ann §3111.33 (Baldwin 1987)
117. Ibid
118. Stiver v Parker, 975 F2d 261 (6th Cir 1992)
119. Ibid
120. Ibid, 263
121. Ibid, 266
122. Ibid, 272
123. American Fertility Society, 83S-86S
124. American Association of Tissue Banks: Addendum 2: Specific standards—reproductive council. *American Association of Tissue Banks Provisional Standards* 22, Sept 1984
125. For a complete description of the screening guidelines developed by The American Fertility Society and the American Association of Tissue Banks see Andrews L: *Medical Genetics,* 168–171
126. 42 USCA §263a-1, *et seq* (West Supp 1994)
127. 42 USCA §263a-2(d) (2) (West Supp 1994)
128. American Fertility Society: Guidelines for gamete donation. *Fertil Steril* 59(Suppl 1):2, 1993
129. Ohio Rev Code Ann §3111.35(2) (Baldwin 1987)
130. Office of Technology Assessment (see also ref. 105): In a survey, 83% of physicians offering artificial insemination by donor were opposed to the idea of a statutory requirement for keeping records on the child or the donors. Curie-Cohen M, Luttrell M, Shapiro S: Current practice of artificial insemination in the United States. *N Engl J Med* 300:585–590, 1979. See also Office of Technology Assessment, *Artificial Insemination,* 48, 70
131. Ontario Law Reform Commission: *Report on Human Artificial Reproduction and Related Matters.* 1985:184
132. See, eg, Cal Civ Code §7005 (West 1983); Ohio Rev Code Ann §3111.36 (Baldwin 1987)
133. 42 USCA §263a-1(a)-(b) (West Supp 1994)
134. Records should be available to the patients concerning embryo discard, storage, donation, research, and cost. Robertson, Embryos, families, and procreative liberty, 1039
135. Alabama, Colorado, Minnesota, Montana, Nevada, New Jersey, New Mexico, Washington, Wisconsin, Wyoming
136. Connecticut, Idaho, Oregon. Connecticut requires the information be filed with the probate court. Idaho and Oregon require the information be filed with the state registrar of vital statistics
137. 18 Pa Cons Stat Ann §3213(e) (Purdon Supp 1986)
138. Ohio Rev Code Ann §3111.36(C) (Baldwin)
139. *Anonymous v Anonymous,* 41 Misc 2d 886, 246 NYS2d 1835 (1964)
140. *NY v Dennett,* 15 Misc 2d 260, 184 NYS2d 178 (1958)
141. Similarly, laws of 16 of the 35 states explicitly provide that the man donating sperm to a woman who is not his wife is not the legal father of the child: Alabama, California, Colorado, Connecticut, Idaho, Illinois, Minnesota, Montana, Nevada, New Jersey (unless the woman and donor have entered into a contract to the contrary), New Mexico (unless the woman and donor have agreed in writing to the contrary), Oregon, Texas, Washington (unless the woman and donor have agreed in writing to the contrary), Wisconsin, Wyoming
142. Alabama, Alaska, Arkansas, California, Colorado, Connecticut, Florida, Georgia, Idaho, Illinois, Kansas, Louisiana, Maryland, Michigan, Minnesota, Missouri, Montana, Nevada, New Jersey, New Mexico, New York, North Carolina, Ohio, Oklahoma, Oregon, Tennessee, Texas, Virginia, Washington, Wisconsin, Wyoming
143. Minn Stat Ann §257.56(1) (West 1982); Mont Code Ann §40-6-106 (1985); Nev Rev Stat §126.061 (1986); NM Stat Ann §40-11-6(A) (1986); Va Code Ann §64.1-7.1 (1980); Wis Stat Ann §767.48(9) (West 1981); §891.40 (West Supp 1986); Wyo Stat §14-2-103 (1994)
144. 10 Okla Stat §554 (1995); Tex Fam Code §12.03B (1995)
145. Fla Stat Ann §742.11 (West Supp 1994)
146. *Smith v Jones,* No 85 532014 02 (Michigan Cir Ct, Wayne Co, March 14, 1986). There was a similar case, with the same result in California, *Smith v Jones,* No CF 025653 (Los Angeles Superior Ct, Los Angeles Co, June 9, 1987). A New York Court allowed the genetic parents' names to appear on the birth certificate. *Arredondo v Nodelman,* NY Supreme Court, Queens Co, (January 26, 1995)
147. *Johnson v Calvert,* 19 Cal Rptr 2d 494 (1993)
148. Ibid, 501
149. *Belsito v Clark,* 67 Ohio Misc 2d 54 (1994)
150. Ibid
151. Ibid, 64
152. Ibid
153. *Soos v Superior Court of the State,* 179 Ariz Adv Rep 22 (1994)
154. The Arizona surrogacy statute recognizes the birth mother as the legal mother of the child. Ariz Stat Ann §25-218 (1991)
155. 30 Cal Rptr 2d 893 (Cal Dist Ct App 1994)
156. Ibid, 903
157. Ibid, 897
158. Ibid
159. Ibid, 903
160. *McDonald v McDonald,* 1994 NY App Div Lexis 1463
161. *Johnson v Calvert,* 19 Cal Rptr 2d 494 (1993)
162. Ariz Stat Ann §25-218 (1991); Ark Stat Ann §9-10-201 (1991); DC Code §16-401 (1993); Fla Stat Ann §63.212 (West Supp

1991); Ind Code Ann §§31-8-1-1 to 31-8-2-3 (Burns 1988); Ky Rev Stat Ann §199.590 (Michie/Bobbs-Merrill 1988); La Rev Stat Ann §2713 (West 1991); Mich Comp Laws Ann §§722.851-.863 (West Supp 1988); Neb Rev Stat §25-21, 200 (1988); Nev Rev Ann §127.287 (Michie 1987); NH Rev Stat Ann §§168-B:1 to :31 (Supp 1991); ND Cent Code §§14-18-01 to 14-18-07 (1991); NY Dom Rel Law §123 (Consol 1993); Utah Code Ann §76-7-204 (Supp 1991); Va Code Ann §§20-156 to 20-165 (Supp 1991); Wash Rev Code Ann §§26.26.210-.260 (Supp 1991)

163. Arizona, Arkansas, Florida, New Hampshire, North Dakota, Utah, Virginia

164. Arizona, Florida, Indiana, Kentucky, Louisiana, Michigan, Nebraska, New York, North Dakota, Utah, Virginia, Washington

165. Arizona, District of Columbia

166. Fla Stat Ann §742.15(4) (West Supp 1994)

167. La Rev Stat Ann §9:122 (1991)

168. District of Columbia, Michigan, Maryland, Minnesota, Texas, Virginia

169. Va Code Ann §32.1-289.1 (1985)

170. Va Code Ann §32.1-289 (1985)

171. La Rev Stat Ann. §9:122 (1993). The Louisiana law applies to embryos created through in vitro fertilization

172. Fla Stat Ann §742.14 (West 1994)

173. Maine, Massachusetts, Michigan, Nebraska, North Dakota, Ohio, Oklahoma, Rhode Island, Tennessee, Utah, Wyoming. Nebraska, Ohio, Oklahoma, Wyoming cover only aborted embryos

174. Nev SB 272 to be codified at Nev Rev Stat ch 773, §6(5) (1987)

175. Alabama, Arizona, California, Colorado, Delaware, Florida, Georgia, Idaho, Illinois, Indiana, Iowa, Kentucky, Maryland, Massachusetts, Michigan, Nevada, New Jersey, New York, North Carolina, Ohio, South Dakota, Tennessee, Utah, Wisconsin. One court interpreted the statutory prohibition against payment in connection with an adoption to include prohibiting payment to a surrogate. *Doe v Kelley,* 106 Mich App 169, 307 NW2d 438 (Mich App Ct 1981), *cert denied,* 459 US 1138 (1983)

176. *In Re Baby M,* A-39-87, slip op (NJ Supreme Ct, February 3, 1988)

177. *Doe v Kelley,* 106 Mich App 169, 307 NW2d 438 (Mich App Ct 1981) *cert denied* 459 US 1138 (1983). In one court's analysis, "the net effect of the [Kelley] decision prohibits the use of surrogate mothers in the State of Michigan since few women other than perhaps a close family member would bear someone else's child without compensation." *In re Adoption of Baby Girl LJ,* 132 Misc 2d 972, 505 NYS2d 813, 816 (1986)

178. *In re Baby M,* 217 NJ Super 313, 525 A2d 1128 (NJ 1987); *In re Adoption of Baby Girl LJ,* 132 Misc 2d 972, 505 NYS2d 813 (1986); *Surrogate Parenting Associates Inc v Kentucky,* 704 SW2d 209 (Ky 1986)

179. *Surrogate Parenting Associates Inc v Kentucky,* 704 SW2d 209 (Ky 1986)

CHAPTER 48

Ethical Considerations in Infertility

MARY B. MAHOWALD

The paradigm	Consentual sexual intercourse between a man and woman married to each other
	Gestation and birth through the woman
	Expectation of competent parenting

Philosophical or Religious Considerations	Role Differences	General Considerations (Principles)	Particular Considerations (Variables)
Moral status of the preembryo, embryo, or fetus:	Practitioner	Respect for autonomy	Gender differences
Person	Researcher	Avoidance of harm	Marital status
Nonperson	Potential parent	Promotion of benefit	Cost, invasiveness, and probable success
Potential person	Third party	Fairness	Anticipated ability to parent

From philosophical and ethical perspectives, the following questions are relevant to infertility:

- What is it?
- Who is infertile?
- What should be done about it?

In response to the first question, we may consider whether infertility is (1) a disease, (2) a disability, or (3) a desideratum. To the second question, we may consider infertility as applicable to (1) men, (2) women, or (3) couples. Answers to the third question depend on three factors: whose role is being considered (the researcher's, the clinician's, the potential parents', the gamete providers'); the moral status, if any, attributed to the human fetus; and the possible interventions. The range of pos-

sible interventions includes not only medical but also social measures that affect individual men and women, couples, society, and potential children. All of these aspects are discussed in this chapter.

WHAT IS INFERTILITY?

Infertility is generally defined as "the inability of a couple to conceive after 1 year of sexual intercourse without using any type of contraception."[1] Those who have never had biologically related children in such circumstances experience primary infertility; those who already have had a child may experience secondary infertility. Both types of infertility differ from sterility mainly because sterility connotes a permanent condition, whereas infertility is changeable, at least sometimes. Depending on how the inability to have children is interpreted, neither infertility nor sterility is necessarily associated with childlessness or the absence of parenthood. Adoption and marriage to persons who already have children are means by which people become parents regardless of their biologic ability to procreate. Blended and extended families are further ways in which people fulfill a parental role toward children.

The word *have* in relation to children allows different interpretations.[2] In most cases, the ability to "have" a child refers to the biologic capability of a man or woman to provide the genetic material required for fertilization. It also refers to the woman's ability to gestate the fertilized ovum and give birth. But "having a child" may also mean that one functions in the capacity of parent to the child, as adoptive parents do. In anonymous gamete donation and in surrogate gestation, individuals never "have" a child in the sense of having a social parental relationship with him or her. To the extent that individuals are bound by their agreement to provide gametes or gestation for others, they forfeit their right to be social parents by "having" the children to whom they are biologically related through these roles. Similarly, if biologically related parents relinquish their child to adoptive parents after birth, or if children are removed from parental care because of alleged neglect or abuse, their biologic parents are no longer able to "have" them.

Infertility may be interpreted positively or negatively, depending on whether the ability to have children is desirable. For prepubertal children, for example, infertility is a normal, healthy state. For adults who prefer not to have children, infertility may be an advantage, relieving them in most cases of the need, inconvenience, and cost of contraceptive practice. For individuals who are no longer fertile or are sterile, such as menopausal women, infertility may also be viewed positively, that is, as a normal healthy state marked by freedom from concerns about menses. For many individuals and couples, however, infertility is not a desirable state, and for them, the inability to have children is experienced as a disease or disability deserving of medical attention.[3–7]

Health care is commonly and legitimately provided for treatment of disease and disability. It may be argued that infertility is not a disease because it does not affect the health status of the infertile person as such. In fact, infertility avoids the health risks that pregnancy entails for some women and the discomfort and inconvenience that it entails for virtually all pregnant women. Despite the risks and discomforts, however, pregnancy is a desired experience for many women, both fertile and infertile. Among the infertile, some women regret that they do not or cannot experience gestation and childbirth more than they regret the absence of a genetic tie to their offspring. In a study of 50 infertile women in England, most (28 women) said they would prefer to be birth mothers rather than genetic mothers if they could not be both.[8]

Even if infertility is not a disease, it is classifiable as a disability if the condition is present in an individual or couple who would ordinarily be able to have children through the usual route of sexual intercourse, in vivo fertilization, gestation, and birth. The "ordinary" time for having children is during one's reproductive years, which for women are the years between menarche and menopause. Inability to have children before menarche or after menopause is not classifiable as a disability unless menopause occurs early, as with some karyotypic abnormalities or autoimmune diseases.

It makes little ethical difference whether infertility is defined as a disease or a disability (or both) because either designation suggests that the individual is disadvantaged vis-à-vis peers who are healthy or able in the same regard.[3] The ethical value or principle that supports treatment of such patients is that of justice or equity, which may be articulated as a right of equal opportunity to reproduce. In this context, the goal of health care is to promote equality among human beings, or to reduce the inequalities that occur because of differences in health and abilities.

Although the obligation to treat those who are disadvantaged because of disease or disability seems straightforwardly compelling from a societal and a clinical perspective, treatment of those who are healthy and able is another matter. Nonetheless, medical treatment is increasingly sought by and provided to persons who already are equal, or at least relatively equal, to their peers. In such situations, the treatment may confer an advantage over other persons, increasing or maintaining inequity or injustice. Provision of growth hormone therapy to those who are not disabled by their shortness and cosmetic surgery to enhance appearance rather than correct deformities are examples in this regard. As health insurance companies recognize, such treatments are elective rather than medically necessary. They may appropriately be construed as health commodities or services to be bought rather than treatment that is required and deserved regardless of one's ability to pay. Physicians who supply such elective treatment are operating outside the traditional ethos of medicine as a profession.

One of the traditional marks of a profession as distinct from an occupation that is not a profession is that the former involves an altruistic component.[9] Providers of medical treatment for nonmedical reasons function more within the model of business ethics, in which, although standards of care must be observed, the profit motive is acknowledged as primary. No doubt, practitioners of elective treatment provide desired services, but satisfaction of others' desires is not the essential goal of health care as a profession. The essential goal of reproductive endocrinology as a profession is to assist individuals or couples in overcoming the infertility that they experience as a disadvantage or disability vis-à-vis their peers.

WHO IS INFERTILE?

Clinicians involved in infertility treatment commonly refer to their patients as couples. They may also refer to individual patients as infertile. The obvious rationale for "couple" terminology is the fact that human reproduction requires both male and female participation. Equally obvious, however, is the fact that the participation of men and women is disproportionately demanding in terms of time, risk, and discomfort.[10] Moreover, although the couple as a unit may be correctly described as fertile, either partner may be infertile as an individual and both partners may be fertile with another partner. It is misleading, therefore, to consider infertility solely as a couple problem.

Both men and women are examined and may be treated for infertility. In some cases, problems are remediable through separate treatment of the partner whose condition constitutes the impediment to conception. When techniques such as insemination, in vitro fertilization, gamete or zygote interfallopian tube transfer are used, however, it is women who undergo the rigors and risks of the procedure regardless of whether the infertility is caused by the man, the woman, or the couple as a unit. Ironically, this gender difference is consistent with the fact that women undergo risks and rigors not required of men in unassisted pregnancy and childbirth. Rightly or wrongly, it is also consistent with the fact that women tend to bear the main societal responsibility for rearing children.

Some feminists have challenged practices of assisted reproduction that involve treatment of women for conditions of their male partners.[11,12] The basis for this challenge is the inequity it suggests and possible pressures on women to undergo risks and discomforts for the sake of others. Although infertility involves psychologic burdens for men as well as women, studies have shown that women experience considerably more distress than men during the course of infertility treatment.[13] Reasons offered for the discrepancy include not only the fact that the woman's body is the object of treatment but also socialization influences by which women are more likely to define themselves and their worth through motherhood than men are through fatherhood.

Because of the impact of gender socialization, it may be difficult if not impossible to determine whether women fully exercise their autonomy when they consent to procedures intended to facilitate reproduction. This difficulty applies also to situations in which medical assistance is not needed for reproduction. Regardless of whether the man, woman, or couple is infertile, consent to treatment must come from the person to be treated, and clinicians are ethically bound to ensure as much as possible that such consent is fully informed and free. Despite possible pressures from others, it is surely possible for individual women to disagree with others, including their partners and clinicians, in their choices for or against specific procedures that may be used in medically assisted reproduction. For other women, however, autonomy may be manifestly compromised. The ethical challenge for the clinician is to maximize respect for the autonomy of the person most affected and to promote a balance of burdens and benefits among those affected by interventions or lack of intervention.

ROLE-BASED RESPONSIBILITIES

Ethically justified decisions in health care are often role dependent. In infertility treatment, for example, whether a clinician should offer or provide a specific procedure to a couple or individual depends on many factors that may be irrelevant to the decision making of the individual patient or couple. Some caregivers may be religiously or morally opposed to some methods of assisted reproduction; providing such assistance would then constitute a betrayal of their own moral values or beliefs. Some clinicians may have developed extraordinary expertise with one technique but only limited expertise with another; they may be obliged to refer an individual to another clinician if optimal treatment requires the other's expertise.

Although some individuals are both researchers and clinicians, the responsibilities of researchers as such are different from those of clinicians as such. Researchers are primarily committed to obtain knowledge that may be useful for future patients. In contrast, clinicians are primarily committed to the individual patients with whom they establish a relationship. It is not surprising, then, that infertility researchers have argued strongly for government support for research involving early embryos, whereas clinicians who are not researchers have been less vocal in this regard. Reproductive endocrinologists who are researchers as well as clinicians may occasionally face the conflict between the value of scientific knowledge, along with its potential benefit to future patients, and the needs or desires of particular clients or couples. In general, clinical obligations to current patients supersede the obligations of the researcher as such, reflecting a priority of health over knowledge and of immediate therapeutic impact over potential therapeutic effectiveness.

Those responsible for public policy have different ethical priorities to honor than do clinicians or researchers. If world health is the goal, infertility treatment of individuals or couples is probably not as important a need as detection and correction of environmental causes of infertility, which generally affect other areas of human health and well-being. Indeed, it may be argued that advances in reproductive technologies that facilitate and encourage an increase in the world's population, with little corresponding effort with regard to population control or restraint, are immoral because they impose on future generations a quality of life that is bound to be inferior to our own. Solely from a public health standard, therefore, it is questionable whether anything should be done about infertility as such.

In the United States, infertility treatment is commonly articulated as the right to have a biologically related child.[2] Because rights apply to individuals rather than groups, this right may be claimed by single persons as well as couples. But individual rights are rarely if ever absolute, and negative rights are generally more compelling than positive rights. An absolute right is one that demands respect in every case; most if not all rights are prima facie rather than absolute, which means that they are overridable in at least some cases. A positive right is one that implies responsibility on the part of another to do something; a negative right implies responsibility on the part of another to refrain from doing something.[2] Laws about child abuse and neglect show that the right to have a biologically related child may be limited by the state. The fact that an individual cannot have her or his own biologically related child without the participation of another, who has the right to refuse, also shows that this right is not absolute. Unless one's partner agrees, or unless clinicians agree in cases requiring medical assistance, no individual has an absolute right to have a biologically related child. If infertility treatment is elective rather than medically necessary, clinicians are not obliged to provide it either to couples or to individuals.

Although the right to have one's biologically related child may not be absolute or positive, it is surely a negative right, which as such entails responsibilities on the part of others not to interfere with its expression. Justifications for noninterference are often articulated as privacy claims, as are many practices involving sexuality and reproduction. In general, these claims are subsumable under the aegis of respect for autonomy: they have their limits, but they represent prima facie obligations for others.

Clearly, the different roles played by male and female partners in infertility treatment suggest different rights and responsibilities on the part of each. As with the legal right to abortion, to the extent that women's bodies are primarily affected by reproduction, women remain the primary decision makers regarding infertility treatment. As with medical treatment in general, however, men and women alike have the right to refuse any treatment that affects them directly, whether that treatment is likely to benefit themselves or others. The right to refuse bone marrow donation—even if one were the only match for a family member who urgently needed it—illustrates this in nonreproductive practice.

When infertility treatment involves the participation of third parties as providers of gametes or gestation, another role is added to the mix. Another right may then be asserted—the right to have a child for another or the right to give or sell one's genetic material to another. Here again, it seems clear that such asserted rights are negative and prima facie rather than positive or absolute. It also seems clear that such rights involve correlative responsibilities, such as the duty to disclose any known health risks that one's gametes or one's gestational role might entail for the potential offspring. Contractual agreements are used to ensure that both rights and duties are observed by all of the participants. For some, however, the use of contracts to determine the disposition of infants borne as a result of these arrangements is comparable to babyselling.[2]

MORAL STATUS OF THE DEVELOPING ORGANISM

The unique philosophical or religious question that must be addressed with regard to reproductive issues is the moral status of the developing human organism. Although this question has long been accompanied by sharp and emotionally charged debates in the United States as well as other countries, advances in reproductive technology have introduced new complexity into the discussion. Different views about the moral status of the preembryo or embryo, whether it exists in vitro or in vivo, suggest different degrees of permissiveness regarding infertility treatment and research.

Clinical texts define the embryonic period of human development as a period that starts with fertilization and ends when the basic organ systems are rudimentarily established, at about 6 weeks of gestation. Since the advent of in vitro fertilization, the term *preembryo* has been used to demarcate the earlier part of this development, that is, from fertilization until the onset of the primitive streak, which occurs about 14 days after fertilization.[14] At that point, implantation has been completed, individuation is established, and embryonic cells can be differentiated from those of the placenta and embryonic membranes. Although some consider the distinction between embryos and preembryos arbitrary, it has been endorsed by the American Fertility Society,[15] and increasingly adopted in medical and ethical discussions.

At least four factors must be considered in addressing the moral status of the embryo or preembryo. First, its immaturity; second, its presence within or its dependence on a woman's body for further development; third, its species membership; and fourth, its potential or capacity for personhood.[16]

On the first point, a mature human being is definable as one who has developed the ability to reproduce offspring. Children, fetuses, and embryos are immature by this standard. Embryos, preembryos, and most fetuses are also immature by a standard that measures the ability to survive outside of a woman's body, that is, viability. Because the probability of maturation associated with viability increases through the course of development, it is lowest immediately after fertilization, that is, in the case of very early embryos or preembryos. In fact, most of these early organisms are aborted spontaneously before pregnancy is physiologically detectable. Nature thus appears to favor loss over preservation of preembryos.

Although preembryos may exist for a time in vitro, they cannot continue their development without transfer to a woman's body. The ethical relevance of this point stems from the intuitively justifiable claim that the wishes and welfare of those most affected by the alternatives being considered should be weighed more heavily than the wishes or welfare of those who are less affected or unaffected. To the extent that transfer of the preembryos involves risk and discomfort to the (potentially) pregnant woman without directly affecting others, her wishes regarding the procedure are paramount. The potential father's wishes are next in importance because, after his partner, he is generally the one most affected by the disposition of the embryo. In custody disputes about frozen embryos, the argument for the potential father's right to determine the fate of the embryo is more compelling than it is when the embryo is developing in vivo. When women serve as egg donors, however, they experience greater health risk and discomfort than the potential father, and when they serve as gestators they experience greater health risk and discomfort than either of the potential parents. Apart from the moral or legal obligation to fulfill one's promises, such women have a stronger claim regarding interventions or lack of intervention than others do.

Regarding species membership, the embryo or preembryo that develops from human gametes is clearly human, as human as is the fetus or child that the embryo may eventually become, and as human as are the gametes themselves. Although some would differentiate radically between separate gametes and embryos by pointing to fertilization as the onset of a new human life (or lives), this view does not imply that the fertilized ovum is a person or has rights. Although the question whether human embryos are persons is debated by philosophers and theologians, their potential for personhood is accepted even by those who deny that they are persons.[17] The potential for personhood also distinguishes human embryos from other human tissue and organs.

The philosopher R. M. Hare maintains that human gametes are also potential persons, attributing that potential to separate cells existing in different bodies.[18] However, several important differences between gametes and embryos are undeniable. The human zygote is a single cell that may naturally develop toward birth and unquestionable personhood without intervention by others. Gametes cannot achieve this natural propensity unless individuals choose to establish it through sexual intercourse or assisted fertilization. Moreover, preembryos are diploid and embody the total genetic constitution of at least one new human individual. Gametes, in contrast, are haploid and embody only half of the genetic constitution of a new human being. Surely, these empirical differences between the two are morally relevant to decisions regarding their fate.

WHAT SHOULD BE DONE?

The question what should be done about infertility is answerable in three ways: as much as possible should be done, nothing should be done, or some things should be done. If the right to have a biologically related child were absolute and positive, then as much as possible should be done by those who are in a position to support this right. As we have seen, however, the right is neither absolute nor positive. Accordingly, clinicians are not obligated to provide infertility treatment to every individual or couple who seeks medical assistance for reproduction.

That nothing should be done to treat one for infertility is an even less defensible position. If the world's resources could not meet the basic needs of the population and no other means were available to constrain further growth, a total prohibition of infertility treatment would probably be justified. However, this is simply not the case. Hence, infertility treatment should not be denied to everyone.

This leaves us with the third answer to the question of what should be done about infertility: some things should be done. Just what those things are, and by whom they should be done, remains problematic not only with regard to the articulation of policies or laws but also with regard to the decisions of those involved in specific cases. Legal aspects of infertility treatment are considered elsewhere in this book. But laws as such do not adequately define the morality of individuals. If laws and institutional policies were totally permissive of interventions to promote fertility, individual men, women, couples, and practitioners would still face situations requiring them to decide for themselves whether to seek or provide such treatment. And if laws or institutional policies were totally restrictive of treatment of infertility, that fact would not suffice to provide ethical justification for the laws themselves or for the decisions of individuals addressing the issue.

Consideration of basic ethical principles or values as well as the unique factors of each case are essential to ensure that ethical judgments are justifiable in the clinical setting. Attention to both general and particular considerations is as necessary to moral decision making as it is to clinical decision making (see paradigm on page 823). The ethical principles of *respect for autonomy, avoidance of harms or risks, promotion of health benefits,* and *maximization of fairness* toward those who are unequally affected have all been discussed already, at least implicitly. The variables of specific cases include not only *gender differences,* including those related to the life cycle, such as menopause, but also factors such as *marital and economic status; cost, invasiveness, risk,* and *success rate* of different procedures; *involvement of third parties* as donors or gestators; and expectations regarding the *parental competence* of those seeking treatment. For each case, the variables need to be identified and the principles interpreted and applied in a manner that maximizes their observance for each of the moral agents involved.

perform TID, or is the very act a transgression to adultery? And what is the status of a TID offspring?

Experts agree that TID using the semen of a Jewish donor is forbidden. It is the severity of the prohibition that is debatable. The question is whether TID constitutes adultery, which is strictly forbidden by the Torah, or whether the injunction stems from the source—primarily the legal complications of the birth of a TID offspring—as most experts hold. Some rabbinic authorities permit TID if the donor is a non-Jew. This eliminates some of the legal complications related to the personal status of the offspring. If the donor is a gentile, the child is pagan (blemished); if the child is a girl, she is forbidden to marry a *Cohen* (priest).

Jewish law prohibits TID for a variety of reasons: incest, lack of genealogy, and problems related to inheritance. In addition, donors and the physicians who use the semen are violating the severe prohibition against masturbation.

Although some halakhic authorities prohibit a married woman who undergoes TID from continuing to live with her husband831 on the grounds that she has committed adultery, most rabbis believe that without intercourse being involved, the woman is not guilty of adultery and can remain with her husband. If the woman undergoes TID without her husband's knowledge and consent, she must accept a divorce and forfeit any rights to financial support, including her *Ketubah* and alimony.

A child conceived through TID is considered by many rabbinical scholars as having the status of *Mamzer,* bastard. The mark of bastardy severely limits the offspring's prospects of marriage and implies a severe functional handicap from a social point of view. Some rabbis believe the offspring to be legitimate, as Ben Sira was, whereas others consider it *safek mamzer.*

Various views exist regarding the legal relationship between the semen donor and the child born as a result of TID. Some rule that no relationship exists. Others rule that the child is considered the donor's with all the inherent legal complications, such as incest, inheritance, levirate marriage (marriage between a woman and her deceased husband's brother), and custody. The majority opinion is that the donor has not fulfilled the *mitzvah* of procreation when his sperm is used to produce a child.

Although it is difficult to view fertilization with donor sperm as an act of adultery, there may be a legal prohibition against IVF of an oocyte with donor sperm. This prohibition does not affect an unmarried woman as long as the possibility of bastardy is excluded. Scholars who oppose IVF, claiming that there is no parental relationship in IVF and embryo transfer (ET), may give an advantage to the offspring who results from the use of donor sperm and IVF. If no kinship exists, the offspring cannot be regarded as the product of unacceptable genetic union and is thus at least as good for society as the off-

spring of a non-Jew and can marry a Jewish man or woman. In this case, the paternity of the non-Jewish genetic father is not recognized, and the status of the offspring is that of an ordinary Jew almost without exception.

IVF and ET, especially their potential applications, create legal and religious issues that have special implications with regard to their implementation in different societies. This is especially true in Israel, because matters of personal status are governed by religious as well as civil authorities.

The various aspects of the "test tube baby" are of considerable interest. The basic fact that allows IVF-ET to be considered in the rabbinic literature at all is that the oocyte and the sperm originate from the wife and husband based on the commandment of procreation stated in the Bible.

What are some of the delineating factors that would nevertheless withhold Jewish law from allowing IVF-ET? Some individual rabbis take a strict position and suggest that legal and biologic ties are severed with the removal of the egg. The fact that the host environment is sustained by means of medical intervention, that is, culture media, could change the biologic and legal status of the child. The majority Jewish religious point of view, however, formulated by the chief rabbis of Israel, one of the Ashkenazi sector (European origin) and one of the Sephardic sector (Oriental origin), supports both IVF and ET. Jews living outside Israel are generally subjected to the laws of the country in which they live, except when they wish or are required to obey the Jewish traditional personal-status regulations. In such cases, rules applicable in the state of Israel are applied by local rabbinic authorities when such exist and are recognized.

In Israel, special legal problems have arisen because of the powers vested in rabbinic courts in matters of personal status. Although general laws are secularly legislated by the Knesset, matters concerning marriage, divorce, paternity, legitimacy, and bastardy are adjudicated by the rabbinic courts, which follow orthodox interpretation. Because the courts must recognize the legitimacy of the child's birth, they must determine the legal status of a child born through IVF-ET.

Jewish law places limits on semen collection, management of menstrual problems, and homologous and heterologous insemination. These factors are considered when IVF-ET is undertaken. As mentioned, the collection of semen can present problems because of the prohibition against masturbation and seed wasting. However, for fertility analysis, many rabbinic authorities permit the collection of semen by means of coitus interruptus or by the use of a condom with a perforation. If a condom is used, it must be of the type that will not damage sperm vitality. Using either natural cycles or induced cycles to prepare a woman for oocyte retrieval may interfere with the *Niddah* state. Despite these concerns, thousands of Jewish children have been born as a result of IVF procedures in Israel, many of them to very religious couples.

The main issue with regard to egg or embryo donation is whether the oocyte donor or the recipient should be considered the mother. Jewish law says that the religious status of the child is determined by the mother. Contrary to the Talmudic interpretation, the father of a child resulting from TID is the sperm donor. Thus there is a divisible partnership-ownership of the egg and the environment in which the embryo is conceived. The child is related to the one who finished its formation, the one who gave birth. A judgment in the Mishnah states that if a person starts an action but does not complete it and another person comes along and completes it, the one who completes the action is considered to have done it all.

Only the offspring of a Jewish mother is regarded as a Jew. For purposes of lineage, the recipient woman rather than the ovum donor is the mother, although the latter is certainly the genetic parent. If the recipient is Jewish, then the child is Jewish.

Cryopreservation of preembryos is routinely practiced in IVF programs. Because it stops the development and growth of the embryo, cryopreservation raises the basic question whether it cancels all rights of the preembryo's father. As far as the mother is concerned the problem is simple, since the embryo is transferred into her uterus later and will renew the mother-embryo relationship. As for the father, whose main function is to fertilize the oocyte to form the preembryo, the period of freezing may sever his relationship with the child. Freezing the sperm and preembryo is permitted in Judaism only when all measures are taken to ensure that the father's identity will not be lost.

When a woman with infertility due to uterine factors is unable to carry the embryo, her ovum is fertilized with the sperm of her husband, after which it is implanted in the uterus of another woman, who gives birth as a gestational carrier. Surrogacy occurs when a woman is inseminated with another woman's husband's sperm and donates her oocyte and leases her uterus. After the birth the child is given to the infertile couple for adoption.

The Jewish religion does not forbid gestational carriage or surrogacy. If surrogacy is practiced, the infant should be placed in the custody of the owner of the sperm. In the case of operational carriage after embryo donation, the question is not resolved, as with the case of ovum donation. From the religious point of view, the child belongs to the man who gave the sperm and the woman who gave birth.

The Legal Status of the Preembryo

The legal status of the preembryo is difficult to establish. If one suggests it is a person, or even potential person, it has no legal status according to the law in most countries. There is a suggestion that the embryo is property, but this definition offends ethical principles. All suggestions leave open the legal question of the right to use, to discard, to sell, and to purchase an embryo.

A preembryo or embryo seems not to be a human being for purposes of criminal law. Deliberately destroying one is not a criminal abortion act.

Legal protection for a preembryo may be difficult to achieve, except through specific legislation. The legal status of the preembryo is broadly discussed in the history of our civilization when the question of compensation for causing miscarriage is discussed. According to the Babylonian code, compensation for destruction of an embryo or fetus was paid according to the social status of the pregnant woman. According to old Hebrew law, the compensation was paid according to the severity of the damage. The Hittes code states that compensation should be paid according to the stage of gestation.

Modern assisted reproductive technologies, including preembryo research, are practiced by one of the following systems:

- Regulation
- Government regulation
- Regulation prepared by professional bodies
- Local hospital committees
- Personal standard

According to one survey, only 13 countries practice research on preembryos. In some countries, such as Germany, Ireland, Israel, Norway, and Switzerland, research on embryos is forbidden by law. Different countries have dealt with the issue of assisted reproductive technologies, including research on embryos. The most important reports are from the Walter Committee in Australia, the European Human Reproduction Society (ESHRE), the Society for Reproductive Medicine, and the European Parliament.

Preembryo Research

Benefits from human preembryo research can be achieved in the four main medical areas: infertility research, to improve clinical results; diagnosis of genetic aberrations and possible therapy; contraceptive research; and therapeutic use of embryonal tissue for transplantation in life-threatening conditions. The potential sources of preembryo for research are existing surplus from IVF; defective IVF preembryos; aborted preembryos or embryos obtained with flushing methods induced or spontaneous abortions; and those produced for research. Various ethical committees differ on this issue, but all agree that the following procedures should be forbidden: cloning, interspecies fertilization, genetic manipulation, and transfer of human embryo to another species.

Researchers should be allowed to induce in vitro preimplantation embryos for fertility research if a real chance exists that the sperm owner may benefit and have a child as a result. Jewish law forbids destruction and use of a preembryo as long as it has potential to be implanted. An in vitro blastocyst that hatched from its zona pellucida and lost its implantation potential may be used for research. However, a postimplantation preembryo cannot be so used unless the research is essential to save the embryo's life. The arbitrary limit of 14 days after fertilization for research on preembryos established by some ethics committees is not recognized by Jewish law.

With the new DNA amplification technology for IVF, it is possible to identify the X or Y gene in an embryo soon after it has been fertilized in vitro and to detect early genetic anomalies. Some genetic disorders are X or Y linked. Because the sex of the embryo can be detected before implantation, it is possible to choose embryos of a certain sex, guaranteeing that the embryo that develops is free of a sex-linked genetic disorder. Using specific gene probes, it is already possible to diagnose such disorders (as opposed to simply identifying the sex) at an early stage.

Although Halakha generally takes a conservative approach regarding abortion, many contemporary rabbinic decisions maintain that untransplanted embryos have no standing and may be discarded. Therefore screening for genetic diseases is permitted.

Abortion

A fetus is not considered a person (Hebrew *Nefesh,* "soul") until it is born. It is regarded as a part of the mother's body and not a separate being until it begins to egress from the womb during parturition. In fact, until 40 days after conception, the fertilized egg is considered mere fluid.

Abortion on demand is repulsive to the ethics of the Halakha; however, in many situations a pregnancy may be terminated. If the mother's life is in danger, each fetus is a *Rodef,* an aggressor who may (or must) be killed to save the individual in danger. Most rabbis permit and even mandate abortion when the health or life of the mother is threatened. Some authorities are stringent and require the mother's life to be in actual danger, however remote that danger, whereas others permit abortion for a serious threat to the mother's health. The procedure is prohibited for fetal or social indications.

Reduction on demand also goes against the ethics of Halakha. If the danger is to various fetuses as in the case of multiple pregnancy, and not the mother, each fetus is an aggressor and victim with equal status; it therefore might not be permissible to put aside one soul for the sake of another. If, however, it is absolutely certain that all fetuses would be lost whereas one might be viable, some authorities would allow fetal reduction.

The Jewish reform movement first considered questions of the new treatment of infertility in 1952. The early leadership agreed that all efforts should be made to help infertile couples, in part to meet the need to expand a declining population. Authorities in 1952 approved of TIH, but they split over TID, although all agreed that it did not involve any question of adultery. By the 1970s reform opinion had definitely accepted TID, and it therefore was not troubled by the concept of IVF or of surrogate motherhood. It also concluded that fetuses younger than 40 days were not in any way persons and could be used for experimentation, so there should be no problem with disposing of unimplanted zygotes in IVF.

Conservative Jewish opinion evolved over time. The Committee on Law and Standards in 1967 opposed TID for essentially the same reasons as the Orthodox leaders. However, even then, leading conservative figures were far from unanimous in that opposition. In more recent years, most leaders came to accept the legitimacy of TID with the consent of the husband as a final alternative when nothing else helped. This seems to be emerging as the attitude toward IVF as well. Finally, with similar reservations, the Law Committee in 1985 approved the practice of surrogate motherhood.

At present, because of political circumstances, rigid Orthodoxy is the only form of Judaism officially recognized in Israel, for example, in solemnizing marriages. But a large part of the population is remote from formal religion, and the modernist versions have difficulty making their message heard. On the other hand, Orthodoxy has enjoyed a remarkable resurgence after a long period of decline, and modernist groups are placing greater emphasis on tradition and ceremony.

ISLAM

Islam was founded about 1400 years ago by the Prophet Muhammad (c 570–632). He was born in Mecca and spent his early life as a merchant. In middle life an inner conviction dawned on him that he was the prophet chosen by Allah to convey eternal messages to the Arabs.

There are two broad subdivisions of Islam—Shi'ism and Sunnism. Shi'ism originally referred to the partisans (Shia) of Ali and over the centuries developed its own body of law. This differed in minor ways (inheritance and the status of women) from that of the majority of Sunnis.

Islamic law, Sharia, is the heart of Islamic religion. It defines the path in which God wishes humans to walk. It not only deals with matters of religious ritual but also regulates every aspect of political, social, and private life. The main roots from which it is derived are the Quran and the *Hadith,* the traditions of the Prophet Muhammad. The Sharia is binding primarily for Muslims, who are directly responsible for God, and it is not enforced by the state. According to orthodox Muslims, the law is founded in divine revelation, and since revelation ended with the death of Muhammad, the Sharia is immortal.

There are two sources of Sharia in Islam, primary and secondary. The following are primary sources of Sharia in chronologic order:

1. The holy Quran. The very word of God.
2. The Sunna (customs). Authentic tradition and sayings of the Prophet Muhammad, as collected by specialists in *Hadith* (tradition).
3. Ijma (consensus). The consensus of the community of believers, who, according to a saying of the Prophet, would not agree on any error.
4. Qiyas (analogy). The application of a decision of the past or the principles on which were based new questions, which is the intelligent reasoning with which to rule on events the Quran and Sunna do not mention by matching against similar or equivalent events ruled on.

A good Muslim resorts to secondary sources of Sharia in matters not dealt with in the primary sources.

The Sharia classifies all human actions without exception into one of five categories: obligatory, recommended, permitted, disapproved but not forbidden, and absolutely forbidden. Even if the action is forbidden, it may be undertaken if the alternative would cause harm. The Sharia is not rigid; it leaves room to adapt to emerging situations in different era and places. It can accommodate different honest opinions, as long as they do not conflict with the spirit of its primary sources and are directed to the benefit of humanity.

Muslim modernists, however, have proclaimed the right of every qualified person to examine the sources of the Sharia. The result is that in most Muslim countries today, the Sharia laws are restricted and dominate only personal affairs.

Even in personal matters, a great deal of attention is now given to ways of adapting Islamic law to modern life. The Muftis and Kadis adapt laws of personal status to the requirements of contemporary society. The progressive attitudes of some religious leaders are revealed not only in familiar law but also with respect to other matters, especially those having to do with medical developments in the field of reproduction.

Most pre-Islamic urban women lived in a male-dominated society in which their status was low and their rights negligible. They were continually under the thumb of either a male relative or a husband. Men's rights over their women were the same as their rights over any other property. Marriages were made by purchase or contract. The suitor paid a sum of money (the *mahr*) to the guardian of the bride-to-be (and possibly another sum, the *sadaq* to the woman herself), thereby purchasing her and making her his exclusive property. The marriage contract, in other words, was a contract between husband and guardian, with the bride the sales object. Furthermore, neither conventions nor laws existed to limit the number of wives that a man could have simultaneously, so the only restrictive considerations were economic ones.

The marriage laws enjoin women not only to strict monogamy but also to marriage with Muslims only. Muslim men, on the other hand are free to marry Jewish, Christian, and Sabian women, although not an idolater. Both the social status and the legal rights of Muslim women were improved through Quranic legislation. Among the laws that effected such improvement were the following:

1. Laws that put an end to the pre-Islamic custom of burying baby girls alive
2. Sanctions of marriage as a meritorious institution that invests it with importance and dignity
3. Laws that guarantee women the right to inherit and bequeath property
4. Laws that guarantee women the right to have full possession and control of their health, including the dower, while married and after divorce
5. The right of the wife to be properly fed and clothed at the husband's expense

The Quranic divorce laws that stipulated the obligatory *idda* (a waiting period of about 3 months after the final pronouncement of the divorce formula) also have to be mentioned, as they slightly ameliorate a woman's position. Whereas a pre-Islamic wife could be repudiated and turned out of her husband's home immediately, now an adequate time for reflection is mandated, and the woman must be treated fairly if the man ultimately resolves to divorce her. These laws, although they improve women's status, do not establish political, social, or economic equality of the sexes, since men are considered a degree above women.

The general attitude toward women reflected in the *Hadith* is positive. The *Hadith* elaborates on the Quran's teaching regarding the spiritual equality of women and men. The nature of women as reflected in the *Hadith* spans the whole spectrum from the saintly to the evil and unclean. The *Hadith* gives unquestionable evidence that the *Hijab,* which implies not only the face veil but also the sum of practices connected with the seclusion of women, was legislatively made obligatory for the wives of the Prophet. It also contains much evidence of women's visibility as well as full participation in communal matters in the early Islamic period. Later generations of pious scholars changed these patterns considerably; rather, they sanctioned such changes as occurred within Islam under foreign influence. Through the centuries, traditionalist commentators on the Quran emphasized restrictive norms with the distinct purpose of legitimizing the newly restricted status of women in Islam. The result was that restrictions increased with the progression of time.

Islam regulates sexual relations and outlines guidelines. Sexual practice is allowed only for married couples. All other forms of sex, both premarital and extramarital, are forbidden. The couple must avoid sexual intercourse during menstruation, puerperium, sickness, and disability. Homosexual relations for both men and women are forbidden.

The Quran also outlines a system for punishment of both men and women who commit adultery. It is worth mentioning that the method of punishment increased from detention at home, blame, and oral humiliation at the beginning of Islam, to whipping 100 times and even throwing stones at the guilty person later in Islam. The gradual increase in the severity of punishment shows the way Islam implemented its rules and instruction: adultery prevailed in the pre-Islamic era but was not tolerated later. To be lawful and modest makes humans truly happy and prosperous. Adultery is unnatural and mischievous, and its consequences are disastrous.

Islam links marital sex to procreation and family formation. The *Hadith Shareef* also emphasizes that link. The Quran restricts sexual intercourse to penis in vagina, because this is the route for procreation and continuation of humankind. A husband may enjoy his wife's body in any way except anal intercourse.

Celibacy is not acceptable. It is the duty of well-to-do Muslims to help a poor individual marry. This is the only way to save the person's immortal soul and enable him or her to lead a respectable life in society. The Quran says marriage is a person's natural right.

The literary genre in which ethics is discussed is the *Fatawa* (legal responses provided by religious scholars on request from laypersons or government authorities). This chapter concentrates on 20th century Egyptian *Fatawa.* Egypt is by no means a country governed by Islamic Sharia principles, yet its daily newspaper, its periodicals, and other news media contain increasing numbers of *Fatawa,* a large portion of which deal with medical issues. Muslims do not ask their religious scholars whether one form of treatment is medically more effective than another or when to use a drug and for how long. They usually want to know the attitude of the Sharia toward the treatment and whether the intake of that particular agent is permitted by Islamic law. They want to be assured that modern medicine as practiced is also acceptable by Sharia Islamic norms.

The following are the main characteristics of Islamic medical ethics based on Egyptian *Fatawa:*

1. There is a constant attempt to base modern medical treatment in the classic sources of Islamic law.
2. The problems raised are pertinent predominantly to Muslims or derive directly from the commandments and prohibitions of Islamic law.
3. When Islamic law and state law on certain medical ethics are contraindicatory, the *Fatawa* is issued to mediate.

4. Islamic medical ethics tend to be apologetic or show the superiority of the Islamic way of life over that of other societies, especially those in the West.
5. Islamic medical ethics are often inseparable from social and political issues.

Assisted Reproduction

Artificial reproduction was not mentioned in the primary sources of Sharia; however, these same sources affirmed the importance of marriage, family formation, and procreation. When procreation fails, Islam encourages treatment, especially because adoption is not an acceptable solution. Thus attempts to cure infertility not only are permissible but also are a duty. The Quran, as well as the Old Testament, states emphatically that to have progeny is a great blessing from God. The pursuit of a remedy for infertility is therefore legitimate and should not be considered rebellion against a fate decreed by God.

The duty of the physician is to help a barren couple achieve successful fertilization, conception, and delivery of a baby. The procedure of IVF-ET is acceptable, but it can be performed only if it involves only the husband and wife. The fusion of sperm and egg, a step beyond the sex act, should take place only within a legal marriage. Since marriage is a contract between wife and husband, during their marriage no third party can intrude into the marital functions of sex and procreation. A third party is not acceptable, whether providing egg, sperm, embryo, or uterus. If a marriage has come to an end through divorce or death of the husband, artificial reproduction cannot be performed on the woman even with sperm cells from her former husband.

The practice of TID is strictly condemned by Islamic law on the grounds that it is adulterous. It enhances the risk for inadvertent brother-sister marriage and violates the legal system of inheritance. The procedure also entails the lie of registering the offspring of a man who is not the real father and therefore leads to confusion of lines of genealogy, the purity of which is of prime importance in Islam. If a man's infertility is beyond cure, it should be accepted.

Ovum donation is similar to sperm donation in that it involves intervention of a third party other than the husband and wife and thus is not permitted. Donation of embryos also is prohibited.

Frozen preembryos are the property of the couple alone and may be transferred to the woman in a successive cycle. The preembryos may be used for research purposes with the free informed consent of the couple.

Micromanipulative insemination procedures that involve handling oocytes and sperm and are recommended for male-factor infertility should be considered by analogy a form of artificial reproduction and therefore are acceptable when indicated.

Genetic manipulation is desirable to avoid genetic defects. From the Islamic perspective human gene therapy should be restricted to therapeutic indications. Somatic cell gene therapy is encouraged because it remediates and alleviates human suffering. However, enhanced genetic engineering or eugenic genetic engineering involves changes in God's creation, which could lead to imbalance of the universe. Thus it should be prohibited. Gene therapy to manipulate hereditary traits such as intelligence, appearance, and the like is a serious offense, because it may create an imbalance.

Embryo Research

Research conducted on preembryos should be limited to therapeutic purposes. This should be applicable to research involving microsurgical techniques, sperm pronuclear extraction to correct polyspermy, and genetic diagnosis of a portion of the embryo, one blastomere, or its nucleus for a specific genetic defect.

Abortion

Attitudes toward abortion have changed over the centuries. In 1355 the Grand Mufti issued a dictum allowing contraception, but abortion was permissible only for reasons such as interruption of a lactating mother's milk, which would endanger the existing child. After quickening, abortion was prohibited in all circumstances.

A number of predominantly Islamic countries have since liberalized their laws. In 1964 the Grand Mufti of Jordan allowed abortion provided that the embryo had not achieved human shape, interpreted as occurring at 120 days' gestation. Other countries followed suit. Much depends on the relationship with the state. Some Muslim countries permit termination only to save the life of the mother.

CHRISTIANITY

Christianity is centered on Jesus Christ as the supreme revelation of God and as lord of his followers and is based on his teachings. Christianity comprises three principle divisions: the Roman Catholic church, Protestant churches, and Orthodox Catholic churches. It is particularly characterized by its universality and its attempts to extend this doctrine to all humanity by means of missionary activity. The most striking development in the evolution of Christianity from its Jewish origin was the transition from a national religion (of the Jewish nation) to a universal religion.

At the heart of Christianity are issues of sexuality, marriage, and parenthood. The intervention of the church in the field of reproduction is inspired by the love it feels for humans, helping them to recognize and respect their rights and duties. Advances in technology have now made it possible to procreate apart from sexual relations by means of IVF techniques.

The Old Testament and the New Testament form the scriptures that are sacred to Christians. The Old Testament emphasizes the idea of an agreement between God and his people and contains a record of Jewish history to show how faithfully this agreement was observed. The New Testament contains promises made by God to humanity, as shown in the teaching and experiences of Christ and his followers.

In the early times of Christianity, the church fathers in Rome articulated principles of the perspective on sexual intercourse. Their central concern was liberation of spirit from flesh and not reproduction and formation of a family. Although there was some room for the dignity of the human body and the propriety of reproduction, sexual intercourse was more often treated as a danger than as a positive act or a part of the divine plan.

Roman Catholic Church

Roman Catholics base their beliefs on both the Bible and the traditions of their church. The traditions come from the declarations of church councils and popes. They also come from short statements called creeds and from dogma. The Roman Catholic church recognizes in marriage and its indissoluble unity the only setting worth of truly responsible procreation. The church abides by principles used to guide believers. The first principle is related to the protection of the human being from its very beginning, which is conception; the right to life is fundamental. The second principle is that procreation is inseparable from the psychoemotional relationship of the parents. However, from the moral point of view, a child must be the fruit of the marriage. The fidelity of the spouses involves acknowledgment that they become a father and a mother only through each other; the child is a living image of the parents' love, the permanent sign of their conjugal union. Procreation is not performed by a physician; the physician may be in the position to help the parents achieve conception but is not the one who is the "baby maker." The third principle is related to the personal norm of human integrity and dignity, and it should be taken into consideration in medical decisions, especially in the field of infertility.

The Vatican statement on assisted reproduction is very clear: assisted reproduction is not accepted. In 1956, Pope Pius XII declared that attempts at artificial human fecundation in vitro must be rejected as immoral and absolutely unlawful. The church argues that IVF involves disregard for human life and separates human procreation from sexual intercourse.

The Vatican's instruction on respect for human life made an important contribution to discussion on the practice of new reproductive technologies. It was issued by the Congregation for the Doctrine of the Faith in February 1987, signed by Cardinal Joseph Ratzniger, and approved by Pope John Paul II. The document is a response to inquiries from episcopal conferences and individual bishops about the licity of interventions into human reproduction. The key value in the instructions is respect for the dignity of the human person. The criteria for evaluating these interventions are the respect, defense, and promotion of a human being and his or her primary and fundamental right to life and dignity as a person who is endowed with a spiritual soul and with moral responsibility.

Fertilization is licit when it is the result of a conjugal act, that is, sexual intercourse between husband and wife. From the moral point of view, procreation is deprived of its proper perfection when it is not desired as a result of the conjugal act, that is, the specific act of the spouses' union.

Assisted Reproduction

The instruction is quite clear in its judgment on reproductive technology. Although augmented by modern concepts of human dignity and moral rights, this position relies heavily on the traditional natural-law analysis that intercourse has inseparable procreative and unitive dimensions. There can be absolutely no separation of any dimension of any aspect of reproduction. Consequently, the instruction prohibits IVF, ET, surrogate motherhood, and cryopreservation of embryos.

The instruction rejects TIH and IVF on the grounds that they involve a separation between "the goods and meanings of marriage," that is, the unitive and the procreative. Separation of these two dimensions means that procreation thus achieved is "deprived of its proper perfection" and is therefore "not in conformity with the dignity of the person." A child must be conceived through an act of love and, indeed, of sexual intercourse.

Within marriage TIH cannot be accepted except for situations in which the procedure is not a substitute for the conjugal act but facilitates it so that the act attains its natural purpose. Gamete intrafallopian transfer (GIFT) is acceptable because sperm can be removed from the vagina after a normal sexual act and implanted into the fallopian tube, where fertilization occurs.

Heterologous artificial fertilization is contrary to the unity of marriage, to the dignity of the spouses, to the vocation proper to parents, and to a child's right to be conceived and brought into the world in and from marriage. As mentioned, this method of conception also violates the rights of the child, compromises his or her parental origins, and can interfere with the development of personal identity. This position eliminates any use of donor semen whether for artificial insemination or for IVF. Furthermore, artificial fertilization of a woman who is unmarried or a widow, whoever the donor may be, cannot be morally justified. The practice of ovum donation is prohibited on the same basis as sperm donation.

Embryo Research

From the first moment of its existence until birth, no moral distinction is considered among zygotes, preembryos, embryos or fetuses. The official teaching of the Roman Catholic church is that a new individual comes into existence at conception. The instruction has a strong bias against reproductive technology. It claims human embryo experiments are not acceptable. Research that results in the destruction of preembryo is unethical, because it kills a human person. Cryopreservation constitutes an offense against the respect of human beings by exposing them to great risk of death or horror.

Not all Roman Catholic ethicists and theologians support this official view. Some instead claim either that the individual is formed at a later time or that the formation of the zygote does not mark the beginning of a new individual.

Abortion

The traditional Roman Catholic view was that although a human embryo deserved respect from the moment of conception, it was not a human being, with the rights of a human being, until about the sixth week of gestation. It was then that the body of the embryo was sufficiently developed to allow the "infusion" of the soul that made it distinctively human. It was a sin to bring about the death or abortion of the embryo, but it was not a sin of murder or homicide. St. Augustine, St. Albertus Magnus, and St. Thomas Aquinas all held this view, and in effect rejected the notion that the embryo was a human being from the moment of fertilization.

A later stance was that we did not know, and could not know, when the human soul was infused into the embryo or fetus. It was therefore safer to presume that this occurred at the moment of conception and to treat the early embryo as though it were a human being in the full sense.

A more recent position that dates from a statement of Pope Pius XII in 1956 is that an embryo is a human being from the moment of conception. Therefore the abortion of an embryo or fetus, whatever its gestational stage, is equivalent to murder.

In 1995 Pope John Paul II, in an encyclical warning of the rise of a "culture of death" in modern society, used his strongest language to condemn abortion, which he claimed is "a crime which no human law can claim to legitimize." He called on Christians to resist laws that permit the "killing of an innocent human being whether a fetus or an embryo."

Eastern Orthodox Church

Eastern Orthodox beliefs are based on the Bible and on Holt tradition (doctrines established mostly during the early centuries of Christianity). The Eastern Orthodox church was formally formed in 1054 when a split between the eastern and western churches occurred.

The Eastern Orthodox religion consists of several independent and self-governing denominations and some that are not self-governing. The four principle self-governing denominations are Constantinople, Turkey; Alexandria, Egypt; Antioch (Damascus), Syria; and Jerusalem. Others in order of size are the churches of Russia, Rumania, Serbia, Greece, Bulgaria, Georgia, and Cyprus. Eastern Orthodox congregations also are located in western Europe, North America, Central Africa, and the Far East, but they are not fully self-governing.

The three main orders of clergy are bishops, priests, and deacons. The priesthood includes married and monastic clergy. Most married priests head parishes. Parochial clergy can marry before ordination, but only unmarried priests can become bishops. Marriage is one of the seven major sacraments. The church permits divorce and allows divorced persons to remarry, but the first marriage is the greatest in the eyes of God.

The Eastern Orthodox church supports medical and surgical treatment of infertility. However, IVF and other assisted reproductive technologies are absolutely rejected, and the church opposes gamete donation, especially TID, on the basis that it is an adulterous act.

Protestantism

Protestantism resulted chiefly from the Reformation, a religious and political movement that began in Europe in 1517. At its base was a protest against the bureaucracy and policies of the Roman Catholic church. The result was the formation of several Protestant denominations. Protestants disagree with other Christians about the relationship between humanity and God. As a result, certain of their beliefs differ from those of other Christians, specifically ones related to the nature of faith and grace and the authority of the Bible. Most Protestants believe that the Bible should be the only authority of their religion.

Protestantism is most widely practiced in Europe and North America. A Protestant religion is the state religion in a number of nations, including Denmark, Norway, and Sweden. Protestantism has strongly influenced the cultural, political, and social history of these and other countries. Protestant churches accept traditional treatment of infertility. For some, however, assisted reproductive techniques are acceptable only when the gametes are from the married couple and when the procedure avoids damage to the preembryo. Donation of sperm or oocytes is prohibited.

The Baptist, Methodist, Lutheran, Mormon, Presbyterian, Episcopal, United Church of Christ, Christian Science, Jehovah's Witness, and Mennonite religions have liberal attitudes toward infertility treatments. All denominations except Christian Science accept IVF with the spouse's gametes and no embryo wastage. Christian Science poses no objection to TIH but opposes IVF because of the use of drugs and surgical procedures. All of these religions oppose IVF with donated gametes and all oppose the practice of surrogacy.

Anglican Church

Before the Reformation the Church of England separated from the Roman Catholic church. Anglicanism became the state religion of England and spread as British colonists settled in North and South America, Africa, and Asia. It is the official faith of the United Kingdom.

Anglicans believe in the ancient faith of the Christian church as expressed in the Apostles and Nicene creeds. They base their religion on Scripture, tradition, and reason. They follow the Book of Common Prayer, which is the basis for doctrine and discipline as well as for worship, but they acknowledge the right of national churches to revise the Book according to their needs. Anglicans often view themselves as a bridge between Roman Catholics and Protestants.

Assisted reproductive technology was developed in Great Britain and Australia. The Anglican church is liberal on the use of IVF-ET and allows semen collection by means of masturbation for artificial insemination by the husband for IVF. However, it forbids the use of donor gametes, semen or oocytes, from a third party. Gamete donation is practiced by legislation in England and in some parts of Australia, Canada, and other countries where the Anglican church prevails.

Embryo Research

The Anglican church holds the view that human embryo experimentation beyond the stage of syngamy is unethical. The absolute protection given to the preembryo is consistent with the Roman Catholic view. Some Anglican theologians believe that it is not the formation of the zygote at fertilization that accords moral status of the preembryo. Moral status is important only when either individuality or personal identity is established. People who hold this view believe that carrying out these sorts of experiments is a human responsibility for elimination of genetic disease, gross malfunction, and human suffering.

HINDUISM

The beliefs, practices, and socioreligious institutions of the people known as Hindus, principally people of India and part of Pakistan, Bangladesh, Sri Lanka, Nepal, Sikkim but also of communities in other parts of the world, evolved from Vedism. Vedism was the religion of the ancient Indo-European peoples who settled in India during the second millennium BCE.

Hinduism has no single book that serves as the source of its doctrine, but it has many writings, all of which contribute to the fundamental beliefs of the religion. The most important of these writings are the Vedas, the Puranas, the Ramayana, the Mahabharata, the Bhagavad-Gita, and the Manu Smiriti. The Manu Smiriti (code of Manu) is a basic source of Hindu religious and social law. Part of it sets forth the basis of the caste system. Caste is India's strict system of social classes that began about 1500 BCE. It includes thousands of subcastes, each of which has its own rules of behavior. Through the years, the system has weakened, but it remains a strong influence in Indian life. Many support the notion that social and religious duties are differently determined according to birth and inherent ability. This is the underlying principle of Dharma, the religious and moral law that governs individual conduct.

Hinduism teaches that the soul never dies. When the body dies, the soul is reborn. The law of *karma* is closely related to reincarnation. It states that every action, no matter how small, influences how a person's soul will be born in the next incarnation until he or she achieves spiritual perfection. The soul then enters a new level of existence, called *moksha,* from which it never returns.

Hinduism exerts its influence from the power of its thought over society not by means of formal institutional authority. The Hindu attitude toward family is based on three concepts, as follows:

1. The pursue concept. Inheritance from the husband's bloodline.
2. The child concept. Creation of Suputra, meaning the birth of a child who is really wanted and because God has rewarded the parents.
3. The marriage concept. Considered religiously after an appropriate ceremony.

The important concepts related to the problem of infertility are that the soul is eternal and indestructible; the soul has no definite beginning or definite end, but is a continuous process; marriage is sacred and permanent; male-factor infertility is not a cause for divorce; reproduction is not just to have children but to have a male offspring; and it is a religious duty to provide a male offspring. Therefore the wife of a sterile man could be authorized to have intercourse with a brother-in-law or other member of the husband's family for the purpose of having a male child. This is allowed only after 8 years of infertility or 11 years of giving birth to all girls.

Assisted Reproduction

Indian society places a high premium on fertility and procreation, and couples sacrifice all they have to beget a child. Therefore, assisted reproductive techniques are acceptable. The most important condition is that the ovum and the spermatozoa are from the legally married couple. The Hindus practice sperm donation with the restriction that the donor has to be a close relative of the husband. In practice TID and oocyte and embryo donation are performed with an anonymous donor.

Abortion and Adoption

Hinduism shows a mild tendency to oppose abortion and to promote the continuity of the family, but there has been as much divergence between thought and practice in India as in the West. In any case, the classic principles and traditions of Hinduism do not seem to have generated a strong cultural basis for contemporary opposition to more permissive abortion laws. Adoption can be accepted by Hindus on the condition that the child comes from their extended family.

BUDDHISM

Buddhism was founded in India in about 500 BCE. At various times it has been a dominant religious, cultural, and social force in most of Asia, especially India, China, Japan, Korea, Vietnam, and Tibet. In each area, Buddhism has combined with elements of other religions such as Hinduism and Shintoism. Buddhism has never been organized around a central authority, so Buddhists of all types in the various countries are individualistic, and even their scriptures are not rigid. In the strictest sense, Buddhism is an experience rather than a doctrine or system of beliefs. The Buddha's teaching was an attempt to communicate the experience of awakening.

All Buddhists have faith in Buddha, his teaching, called the Dharma, and the religious community he founded, called the Sangha. Buddha preached that existence was a continuing cycle of death and rebirth. Each person's position and well-being in life was determined by his or her behavior in previous lives. *Sangha* sometimes refers to the ideal Buddhist community, which consists of those who have reached the higher stages of spiritual development.

The ritual or worship of early Buddhism is very simple. There are no priests or clergy. The Sramanas or Bhikshus (mendicants) are simply a religious order. To achieve the final, transcendent beatitude called *nirvana,* these monks have entered a course of greater sanctity and austerity than ordinary people; they have no sacraments to administer or rites to perform, for every Buddhist is his own priest.

Various Buddhist schools developed in India and in other Asian countries. The most influential of which include the Theravad, the Mahayana, the Mantrayana, and Zen. These schools have much in common, but they also differ in important ways. The principal centers of the Mantrayana school are in the Himalayan region, in Mongolia, and in Japan. This school emphasizes sexual symbolism and beliefs that sexual relations should be used for holy purposes. The Zen school is practiced chiefly in Japan.

In general, Buddhism asserts that distinctions of sex, age, social class, and vocation are irrelevant to life in religion. Rules govern the status of monks, and nuns are relegated to subordinate positions. Debate regarding the inferiority of women has been pursued, but sex is not considered relevant from a doctrinal perspective. Some early Buddhist literature portrays women as fully enlightened beings, as quick-witted teachers, compassionate friends, self-sacrificing saints, and courageous heroines.

Assisted Reproduction

Buddhists in different countries do not have an authorized view on new reproductive technologies. Buddhists believe three factors are necessary for the rebirth of a human being: the female ovum, the male sperm, and the *karma*. Marriage does not have the high priority that it does in monotheistic religions. In fact, it is considered the second best institution after monastic life. Traditionally, Buddhism imposes strict ethics on priests, whereas it takes a relatively lenient attitude toward laypeople. Thus the priests allow laypeople to do whatever they want as long as they do not harm others in concrete ways. Any technology used to achieve conception is morally acceptable, and treatment should be given to unmarried as well as to married women.

IVF has been practiced in Japan since 1982 and is also practiced in other countries with large Buddhist populations. Because the crucial factor in the formation of human beings is *karma* energy, it is not necessary for the sperm and the ovum to be in their natural environments, and therefore IVF is acceptable.

Donation of sperm is not prohibited, but it is suggested that Buddhists refrain from this procedure as much as possible for several reasons. First, parents may find it difficult to care for a child who does not have their genes, especially if the child has congenital malformation or disease. Second, there is a danger that donation of sperm or oocyte from a third party would involve commercialization and cause social problems. Third, donation of gametes could lead to eugenism.

Sperm donation is practiced in Japan, but ovum donation is prohibited. However, a child who is born after TID or ovum donation is accepted as the legitimate child of the father who gave consent to TID and of the mother who delivered it. The child also has the right to know his or her genetic father or mother when he or she reaches maturity.

Abortion

Buddhist scriptures are silent about infanticide and abortion. In the context of the philosophy, it is evident that there is total disapproval of abortion. Abortion is illegal in Myanmar (formerly Burma), and the Thai penal code stipulates that abortion is illegal unless it is performed to save the life or health of the woman or when pregnancy is the result of rape. Abortion is not permitted solely for socioeconomic reasons or because the child will be handicapped. Laws in Myanmar and Thailand are consistent with the religious doctrine that follows the Theravada school of Buddhist thought. It is suggested that the Mahayana school has the same attitude.

REFERENT LITERATURE

1. Code of Canon Law, 1061
2. Congregation for the Doctrine of the Faith: Instruction on respect for human life in its origin and on the dignity of procreation. Replies to certain questions of the day. Libreria Editrice Vaticanna. 1987
3. Pope John Paul II: AAS 72:1126, 1980
4. Pope John Paul II: AAS 74:96, 1982
5. Pope Pius XII: AAS 48:471, 1956
6. Richards C, Fallick M, Seibel MM: Gamete intrafallopian transfer and ultrasound guided transcervical fallopian tube canalization. In: Seibel MM, Kiessling AA, Bernstein J, Levin S (eds), *Technology and Infertility: Clinical, Psychosocial, Legal and Ethical Aspects.* New York, Springer-Verlag, 1993
7. Schenker JG: Genetic material donation: Sperm, oocyte, pre-embryo. *Int J Obstet Gynecol* 43, 1993
8. Schenker JG: The therapeutic approach to infertility in cases of ovarian failure. *Ann N Y Acad Sci* 626:414, 1991
9. Schenker JG: Ovum donation: Ethical and legal aspects. *J Assist Reprod Genet* 9:411, 1992
10. Schenker JG: Religious views regarding gamete donation. In: Seibel MM, Crockin SL (eds), *Family Building Through Egg and Sperm Donation: Medical, Legal and Ethical Issues.* Sudbury, MA, Jones & Bartlett, 1996:238–250

PART X

Adoption

10. Coon H, et al: Identifying children in the Colorado Adoption Project at risk for conduct disorder. *J Am Acad Child Adolesc Psychiatry* 31:503, 1992

11. Cadoret RJ, et al: Genetic and environmental factors in adoptee antisocial personality. *Eur Arch Psychiatry Neurol Sci* 239:231, 1990

12. Halman LJ, et al: Attitudes about infertility interventions among fertile and infertile couples. *Am J Pub Health* 82:191, 1992

13. Lobar SL, Phillips S: The couple choosing private infant adoption. *Pediatr Nurs* 20:141, 1994

14. Sachdev P: Achieving openness in adoption. *Am J Orthopsychiatry* 61:241, 1991

15. Berry M: Adoptive parents perceptions and comfort with open adoption. *Child Welfare* 72:231, 1993

16. Shireman J, Johnson PR: Single parent adoptions: A longitudinal study. *Child Youth Serv* 7:321, 1985

17. Jenista JA, Chapman D: Medical problems of foreign-born adopted children. *Am J Disabled Child* 141:298, 1987

18. Miller LC, et al: Developmental and nutritional status of international adopted children. *Arch Pediatr Adolesc Med* 149:40, 1995

19. Velhust FC, et al: Damaging backgrounds: Later adjustment of international adoptees. *J Am Acad Child Adolesc Psychiatry* 31:518, 1992

20. Kaspke JE, et al: Becoming parents: Feeling of adoptive mothers. *Pediatr Nurs* 17:333, 1991

21. Rosenthal JA, Groze VK: A longitudinal study of special-needs adoptive families. *Child Welfare* 73:689, 1994

22. Weshues A, Cohen JS: Preventing disruption of special needs adoptions. *Child Welfare* 69:141, 1990

PART XI

Patient Perspectives

CHAPTER 51

RESOLVE

Patient Support for the Infertility Experience

DIANE D. ARONSON

Founding of RESOLVE
Mission and Scope
Publications
Chapter Network
Helpline Support
Advocacy Program
National Infertility Awareness Week
News Media
Advisory Groups

RESOLVE Policies
Statements of Principle
  Access to medical treatment of
    infertility
  Assisted reproductive technologies
    and third-party arrangements
  Adoption
  Child-free living
  Research
Summary

Individuals or couples who learn about a diagnosis of infertility often experience a life crisis of considerable proportion. Depending on the prognosis, individuals may respond in a variety of ways—depression, feelings of isolation, anger, and sometimes determination to learn everything that they can about their particular diagnosis to accomplish their goal of parenting.

The grief experienced because of an infertility diagnosis can be overwhelming. People often plan life goals such as going to college, owning a car, getting a particular job, living in a specific area, or building a family. When faced with obstacles to a life goal, people often experience a tremendous feeling of defeat or a reaction to strive harder to achieve that goal, such as studying more to do better at school or working longer hours to earn enough for a down payment for a house. Obstacles are not often simply solved. Addressing infertility involves some complex considerations, including medical, psychosocial, legal, and ethical factors. It may also involve issues of equity, such as reaction by employers or access to health care coverage for treat-

ment. Patients undergoing treatment discover it is not just a matter of trying harder; dealing with the disease or condition of infertility is a daunting task for some. As treatment has advanced, there are a multitude of considerations for a couple to review. Sound information and support from others who are experiencing infertility can be of tremendous help during this personal crisis.

FOUNDING OF RESOLVE

RESOLVE was founded as a consumer and patient support organization in 1974 by Barbara Eck Menning, a registered nurse in Massachusetts who had received a bachelor's degree from the University of Wisconsin School of Nursing, a master's degree in maternal child health care from Boston University Graduate School of Nursing, a master's degree from Harvard School of Public Health and was experiencing her own infertility. In the process of exploring her options for parenting, Menning was asked to coordinate a workshop for the Open Door Society, an adoption organization. With few resources available for the topic she chose, the infertile couple, she developed a perspective for the presentation that integrated the concerns she had experienced in the infertility process. The response to the workshop was overwhelming. From this initiation, Menning coordinated the first support group for infertility.

From that day on, Menning began to receive referrals in her kitchen in Belmont, Massachusetts. She found that most of the calls were medically oriented. Barbara was amazed that a large number of calls she received regarding adoption information were from people in the middle of medical evaluations or who had received no medical evaluation at all. From these kitchen phone calls, a mission emerged.

MISSION AND SCOPE

Menning combined her professional background, her personal experience with infertility, and an intense dedication to produce an avenue of support for individuals who were struggling with infertility and striving to build a family. The mission of RESOLVE is to provide timely, compassionate support and information to people who are experiencing infertility and to increase awareness of infertility issues through advocacy and public education. RESOLVE has grown since 1974 to involve thousands of members and contacts nationwide and nearly 60 chapters across the United States. In addition, National RESOLVE has become a part of the international patient community by providing assistance to countless patient groups in countries around the world. RESOLVE is also a founding member of the International Federation of Patient Associations, a network of worldwide consumer groups who support individuals who are experiencing infertility.

RESOLVE is organized as a nonprofit national organization supported by membership dues, publication sales, and tax deductible contributions from concerned individuals, foundations, and corporations. Menning's legacy in founding RESOLVE laid the foundation for education, support, and advocacy to the thousands of individuals who contact RESOLVE each year. RESOLVE strongly believes in supporting individuals to become informed decision makers as they follow their paths to parenthood.

Membership in RESOLVE is open to all who inquire. In principle and in practice RESOLVE values and seeks a diverse membership. There is no barrier to full participation. Dues range from $45 for basic membership or up to $100 for professional dues (includes individuals who treat patients with infertility). There is also a $35 limited-income category and a scholarship membership program whereby free membership is provided to those in need. All dues are shared by fifty percent with local chapters.

PUBLICATIONS

RESOLVE provides a wide variety of resources and educational materials about the continuum of the infertility experience. The national newsletter, published quarterly, includes regular medical updates from physicians working in the field, articles on psychosocial issues, advocacy and chapter information, and letters to the editor.

RESOLVE has a variety of fact sheets, starter kits, and booklets. The booklets include "Donor Insemination: Facts and Decision-Making," an "Assisted Reproductive Technology Workbook," and "Infertility Insurance Advisor." Starter kits include an *Introduction to Infertility: The First Steps*, *Exploring Adoption*, and *Emotional Aspects of Infertility*. There are more than 60 fact sheets on issues ranging from coping and self-help, such as "How to Deal with Family and Friends" and "Coping with the Holidays," to medical information and family-building options such as surrogacy, adoption, and child-free living. Discounts on publications are available through membership.

RESOLVE also provides a variety of free services to the general public, including its published list of "Questions to Ask," which covers more than 15 topics, such as questions to ask when considering donor insemination, surrogacy, and medications.

In addition to consumer publications, RESOLVE has a variety of resources for its professional members, including a waiting room resource binder that contains background information on RESOLVE, the emotional aspects of infertility, a sample fact sheet, and a newsletter. In addition, RESOLVE has educational brochures available for waiting rooms on topics such as the myths and facts of infertility.

CHAPTER NETWORK

RESOLVE has chapters located nationwide to serve people struggling with their infertility. At the local level, chapters provide educational meetings, chapter newsletters, physician referrals, support groups, and a chapter HelpLine. The chapter network provides a vital link by connecting individuals who may be experiencing a similar situation as they strive to build a family. This connection with others provides support, encouragement, and avenues for resolution. Each chapter is coordinated by volunteers who receive periodic mailings from National RESOLVE to provide quality and unified programs. Chapters have a board of directors and a corps of volunteers committed to providing quality services on the local level.

HELPLINE SUPPORT

National RESOLVE runs a HelpLine (617-623-0744) that is staffed with professionals and volunteers who answer questions about infertility. The phone lines are open for information weekdays 9 am to 12 noon and 1 pm to 4 pm (eastern time) and are accessible to the general public and members. The national and chapter HelpLines provide information about the physician referral service, which is a screened list of approximately 800 infertility specialists located throughout the United States and Canada. There is also a comprehensive resource guide with information about other organizations and general resources about a variety of topics ranging from adoption and legal support to issues such as single parenting.

The national HelpLine provides member-only access to RESOLVE's medical call-in hours (staffed by a registered nurse) on Wednesday afternoons for medical questions that are beyond the scope of questions handled by HelpLine staff and volunteers. The HelpLine also provides access to RESOLVE's member-to-member contact system, which coordinates communication between people who have experienced a particular aspect of infertility, such as donor insemination and people who are considering the same option. Contact with someone who has been through a particular aspect of the infertility experience can be invaluable support.

ADVOCACY PROGRAM

The national office of RESOLVE coordinates a comprehensive program to advocate for concerns regarding aspects of family building. Issues of advocacy have included health care coverage for infertility, adoption concerns, and general education about family building for elected officials who often have misunderstandings about infertility and its treatment. RESOLVE holds national training programs on advocacy, conducts site visits to enhance chapter advocacy committees at the local level, and is involved in lobbying of elected officials by providing testimony at hearings, visits, and letter-writing campaigns.

NATIONAL INFERTILITY AWARENESS WEEK

National Infertility Awareness Week (NIAW), established in 1989, is held each October. The goal of NIAW is to educate and inform the general public about the medical and emotional issues and the options available for those experiencing infertility. This program provides the opportunity to focus on the concerns and advocacy goals of RESOLVE and highlights the supportive programs of RESOLVE. Each year the Barbara Eck Menning Founder's Award is presented to an individual or group who has demonstrated leadership in infertility concerns. A theme is coordinated each year and promoted through National RESOLVE and its chapter membership. Themes since 1989 have included a focus on infertility in the workplace, the involvement of the entertainment industry with the issue of infertility, and environmental effects on fertility.

NEWS MEDIA

National RESOLVE leadership is called on with great frequency by news media outlets such as the *New York Times*, the *Washington Post*, the *Boston Globe*, the *Today Show*, *Good Morning America*, local newspapers, local news outlets across the country, and major magazines. RESOLVE is asked to provide information about a variety of aspects of infertility, including the consumer perspective regarding medical, psychosocial, legal, ethical, and spiritual considerations. Representatives from RESOLVE have been featured on television talk shows and network news and in numerous national publications.

ADVISORY GROUPS

RESOLVE programs are enhanced and supported through its advisory groups. The physician advisory group was established to provide a resource for consultation about medical issues of concern. Physicians on the advisory group provide RESOLVE with up-to-date information, review criteria for the physician referral list and are available for consultation. The mental health advisory group includes experts in the field of infertility who provide support services for people striving to build families. The group members provide counsel and guidance to RESOLVE on psychosocial concerns.

RESOLVE POLICIES

The policies of RESOLVE have developed continually over the past 20 years. The programs and advocacy are supported by well-considered policies drawn from the expertise of professionals and other leaders in the field of infertility.

STATEMENTS OF PRINCIPLE

In an effort to seek diversity and inclusiveness in the organization, the philosophy of RESOLVE is to provide an open, accepting environment for decision making regarding appropriate medical treatment and other family-building options in which people from all ethical, political, and religious points of view who are experiencing infertility feel welcome to give and receive information, referral, and support. RESOLVE supports the right of individuals experiencing infertility to build their families through a variety of methods, including appropriate medical treatment, adoption, and the choice of child-free living. RESOLVE urges individuals to make informed choices in recognition of the long-term implications of their family-building decisions on their lives and the lives of others. RESOLVE believes that decisions regarding medical methods rest with individuals and their physicians.

Access to Medical Treatment of Infertility

RESOLVE supports the right of all individuals experiencing infertility to obtain access to medically appropriate treatment of their disease, including the right to comprehensive health insurance coverage equivalent to that provided for other illnesses.

Regulation of Medical Treatment for Infertility

RESOLVE supports uniform regulations, standards, and guidelines that protect the integrity of prospective parents and donors, their gametes, and any resulting children, but which do not limit access to medically appropriate treatment. Regulations and guidelines regarding treatment for infertility should strive to achieve quality assurance and minimization of risk, including provisions regarding licensing, certification, accreditation, informed consent, confidentiality, record keeping, and a national registry for uniform reporting. A system should be in place that assures safeguards, compliance, and an avenue of recourse for the patient/consumer.

Assisted Reproductive Technologies and Third-Party Arrangements

RESOLVE supports the right of all individuals experiencing infertility to build their families through assisted reproductive technologies, including appropriate arrangements with third-party participants such as gamete donors, gestational carriers, and traditional surrogates. RESOLVE views the decision to use these procedures and the exact methods used as a decision solely within the province of the individuals involved and their physicians. RESOLVE encourages all parties to seek advice from informed medical, mental health, and legal professionals and to obtain appropriate psychologic and legal counseling before entering into third-party and assisted reproduction arrangements. RESOLVE urges individuals experiencing infertility and choose these options to enter into arrangements that are humane and respectful of the rights and feelings of all involved and to keep as a foremost priority the legal status, security, and well-being of the child.

Gamete Donation

RESOLVE supports the right of individuals experiencing infertility to build their families through gamete donation. RESOLVE encourages medical professionals to adopt procedures and practices that ensure: (1) a professional donor screening process, including medical and genetic history of the donor; (2) the right to privacy of all the parties; (3) an agreement by both the donor and the recipients that the recipients have the sole obligations and rights as the parents of the child; and (4) centers using cryopreservation of donor gametes follow the guidelines of the American Society for Reproductive Medicine regarding screening of donors for communicable diseases. RESOLVE encourages individuals who use gamete donation to obtain adequate information to ensure that the donor has been appropriately screened.

RESOLVE recognizes that gamete donation may, at the election of the individuals involved, include varying degrees of privacy and disclosure. RESOLVE supports the rights of those involved to reach an informed, mutually acceptable decision on this issue.

RESOLVE supports the medically appropriate use of donor egg treatment of infertile women who are within the normal child-bearing years. The infrequent use of donor egg treatment of women beyond the normal child-bearing years involves considerations beyond those of infertility, and therefore RESOLVE takes no position on that issue.

Traditional Surrogacy and Gestational Carrier Arrangements

RESOLVE recognizes both traditional surrogacy and gestational carrier arrangements as options that should be available to individuals experiencing infertility. RESOLVE urges individuals who wish to enter into such arrangements to educate themselves thoroughly about all issues involved so that they can make informed decisions. RESOLVE believes that legal regulation is appropriate to ensure noncoercive and legally recognized agreements that reflect the intentions of the parties. RESOLVE opposes legislation that would prohibit or unduly restrict traditional surrogacy or gestational carrier arrangements. RESOLVE urges those experiencing infertility to keep informed about the status of laws and regulations in their own states.

Adoption

RESOLVE supports the right of individuals experiencing infertility to build their families through adoption, including agency adoption, private or independent adoption, and international adoption. RESOLVE encourages states and agencies to formulate nondiscriminatory policies and procedures that enable children to find permanent homes through adoption at the earliest possible time in their lives. RESOLVE also supports legislation that would require, at the earliest possible time, coverage of all medical expenses of a child who is to be adopted. Recognizing that adoption may involve varying degrees of privacy and disclosure, RESOLVE supports the right of adoptive and birth parents to reach a mutually accepted decision on this issue. RESOLVE urges those involved in the adoption process to keep as a foremost priority the legal status, security, and well-being of the child.

Child-free Living

RESOLVE supports the right of individuals to choose to live as a family without children as a positive resolution to infertility.

Research

RESOLVE supports socially and ethically responsible research that advances the understanding and treatment of infertility and other diseases of the reproductive system or any disorder that affects reproduction and that enhances the opportunity for individuals experiencing infertility to build families.

SUMMARY

When individuals move from a diagnosis of infertility toward a path to resolution, they are met with a variety of emotions, including despair, anger, grief, and hope. RESOLVE, as a resource, can be a tremendous support to help address many of the stages toward resolution that are beyond issues faced with medical treatment alone. Through its length of service (more than 20 years in operation), professional staff, and renowned national advisors, RESOLVE has grown to become an internationally respected organization supporting individuals who are experiencing infertility.

Referral to RESOLVE can often be of benefit to a medical practice because it can provide an outlet for feelings of disappointment and grief. The address is RESOLVE, 1310 Broadway, Somerville, MA 02144-1731. The telephone numbers are as follows:

Business line	617-623-1156
Fax	617-623-0252
HelpLine	617-623-0744

CHAPTER 52

Endometriosis and Infertility
The Patient Perspective

MARY LOU BALLWEG

Delayed Diagnosis
Pain and Disability of Endometriosis
Psychosocial Aspects of
    Endometriosis
Coping with Endometriosis
	Role of the Endometriosis
	    Association
	Dioxin, Infertility, and Endometriosis
	Summary

I was diagnosed 4 years ago with stage 3 endometriosis when I had an emergency laparoscopy after an endometrioma burst. I had only two weeks prior to this episode been thoroughly examined by both my gynecologist, who is a good, up-to-date doctor, as well as by my internist, who is also an excellent doctor, because I had felt "funny" and intuitively knew "something was growing inside me." Neither doctor, however, had detected anything. My problem was that out of ignorance, I did not know how to (1) note my symptoms when they occurred, and (2) take them seriously to think I should share this information with a doctor. It also was that I, like most women, did not take my intuition seriously, and was afraid of being labeled a "hypochondriac" by my doctors.

Lynne, Illinois

    Last year at age 29 and recently married, I really wanted to get an answer as to what the abdominal pains that had troubled me for four years were. The pains would begin about two weeks before my period (though latterly were a daily occurrence) and they were like strong menstrual cramps. In that time I went to five doctors, two nurse practitioners and three ob/gyns and either mentioned this in connection with my general health or very specifically as the frequency of pain increased, and I got the following answers:

- *Nothing to worry about, some women get this pain*
- *Nothing to worry about, some women get this pain—it would probably improve if you had a baby (not very useful advice if you are unmarried)*
- *Try the pill (it worked for a few months)*

- *Pain caused by over-production of prostaglandins so anti-prostaglandins were prescribed, but I had to take large quantities to have any effect*
- *Possibly endometriosis—try a stronger pill or get pregnant*
- *Colon problem*
- *Polycystic ovaries (after results of sonogram)*
  and lastly
- *Endometriosis (opinion of two ob/gyns after evaluation of sonogram results and my description of my symptoms)*

    During these same four years my life was undergoing considerable change. I had transferred to the USA with my job for two years, had moved back to my country (New Zealand) for a year, then returned to get married. When I received the two endometriosis diagnoses I had been married for six months, was settling back to life here, working a lot of overtime, looking for a new job, dealing with Immigration Dept. "red tape" to complete residency requirements and was taking a computer class.

    These two ob/gyns said that endometriosis would affect my fertility and if I was thinking of having a baby I should do so NOW. As I was recently married and rather emotionally and physically drained from dealing with the things mentioned above, I did not feel I was ready for pregnancy. I was shocked at how indifferent they were to me as a total person and took a very "hands off" attitude to any non-physical factors which were quite significant then. I got quite frustrated by the lack of information and statistics they could provide when I asked what effect it would have on my fertility if I waited one year to get pregnant.

TABLE 52–3. DELAY TO DIAGNOSIS IN AUSTRALIA

Type of Delay	Average Length of Delay (y)
Between onset of symptoms and diagnosis	6.1
Reporting symptoms to physician	1.6
Between first report to physician and diagnosis	4.3

Age at First Report (y)	Diagnosis Delay
15–19	8.3
30–34	1.3

Australian Endometriosis Association Survey of 748 women with confirmed endometriosis.

symptoms had longer delays to diagnosis than women who presented other symptoms. Interestingly, however, the symptoms that led to longer delays were among the most common symptoms of endometriosis—menstrual pain, heavy bleeding, back pain, and intestinal pain. Women who reported menstrual pain, for example, had a diagnostic delay of 5.2 years compared with 2.3 years for those who did not report period pain.[10] Yet severe dysmenorrhea has a 95% predictive value for endometriosis, according to a study by Naish et al.[11] These authors defined severe dysmenorrhea as pain severe enough to affect the ability to perform daily tasks. Patients who undergo long periods of anxiety and frustration before the diagnosis is confirmed experience much stress in addition to their presenting symptoms.

PAIN AND DISABILITY OF ENDOMETRIOSIS

Since 1989, I have been diagnosed as having severe endometriosis. Prior to that diagnosis, all my symptoms were associated with "irritable bowel syndrome" and "just bad PMS" and I, not knowing, just accepted it and took the "Xanax" that they prescribed saying "This will take the edge off of things." Believe it or not, this is a well known women's medical center here on Long Island. Besides making me go through a "barium enema," they never tested any further. As time went on, my symptoms became severe and finally another physician diagnosed the endometriosis. In turn, I was on Depo-Provera and Lupron and am now going on my fourth surgery. . . . My doctor is aware of my symptoms yet his goal right now is to deal with the infertility—and I too desire children.

My quality of life is so poor. I've been unable to work because of this and financially, the loss of my income has made matters worse for my husband and me. . . . I long to be employed again and I believe I have so much to offer.

Lisa, New York

As many of us I felt pain and discomfort from onset of menses at 11 or 12. My mother recalls all too well. I had bowel symptomatology and it worsened with time and/or age.

I was diagnosed with possible DES exposure at 19 years old. . . . At 27 I met a wonderful, gentle guy and got married. We were restoring an old home; I was traveling for an education team for a chain of hair salons. At age 29 the pain became constant. All the problems magnified.

Miracle of miracles, we tried once (I was in a lot of pain now), and I became pregnant. Weirdly within two to three weeks the pain elevated. By the third month I had enormous bowel problems. I now know everything was adhered together, bowel, uterus, bladder, and adhesions everywhere. Also an enormous endometrioma filled with blood. By month five I had horrid bladder spasms and frequency and infections. Month six was

trichimonas from where who knows, vaginal discharge and itching. Month seven toxemia and bed rest. I was induced after two weeks of being overdue. At last my baby was born after 24 hours of labor. I don't recommend it to anyone. . . .

I stayed home part time with my daughter and gave up a trip to Italy etc. Teaching my little one gardening was much more fun. She rewarded me for all that pain I endured and she was so healthy. I was still dealing with vaginal itching etc., but I was too happy to even walk into a doctor's office. I decided I would never go back until my next baby. It had been so easy to get pregnant and I was certainly fertile with all that discharge and mucus.

[Two years later], in July, I had very bad premenstrual cramps and was hit with horrid bladder spasms etc. . . . Shortly the pain became constant and on a scale of 1 to 10, it was 10 1/2. I was diagnosed in December with severe endometriosis—he said it was everywhere—no hope, can't possibly get it all—get pregnant. We were afraid. I now owned a business; I couldn't be any sicker—pregnancy was so good for me!?

[After several other treatments] all that was left was pregnancy (IVF) or hysterectomy (total of course). I could not bring myself to put more medications in my body which would be there at conception. After all I could be DES and this could have been second generation. I also share the conviction that as we educate ourselves we must make choices about passing this on. I fear for my four year old daughter.

Miriam, Iowa

In addition to the dysmenorrhea, data from the Endometriosis Association research registry of more than 3000 case histories indicate that women with endometriosis typically experience many symptoms[2] (Table 52–4). As is apparent, there is a wide range of symptoms and a great deal of potential for interference in a person's life. Eighty-three percent of patients reported pain throughout the menstrual cycle, not just at the time of the period, and the pain for the most part was in the moderate to severe range (Tables 52–5 and 52–6).

In addition, nearly 75% of the women said the disease kept them at times from their normal work and activities (Table 52–7).[2] Nearly 96% of the subjects in a small nursing study reported the disease had interfered in their lives. Descriptions of how endometriosis interfered in their lives included the following: interruptions in social and family life, moodiness, crying,

TABLE 52–4. SYMPTOMS OF ENDOMETRIOSIS AMONG 3020 PATIENTS

Symptom	No.	Percentage of Total
Dysmenorrhea or pain throughout the menstrual cycle	2904	96.2
Dyspareunia	1801	59.6
Infertility	1340	44.4
Heavy or irregular bleeding	1971	65.3
Nausea, stomach upset at time of menses	1744	57.7
Diarrhea, painful bowel movements, or other intestinal upsets with menses	2385	79.0
Dizziness, headaches with menses, or pain	1782	59.0
Fatigue, exhaustion, low energy	2478	82.1
Low-grade fever	889	29.4
Low resistance to infection	1182	39.1
No symptoms	80	2.6

Forty-five percent of respondents detailed other symptoms, including muscular aches and emotional fluctuations (10.2%).
From Endometriosis Association Data Registry.

TABLE 52–5. PAIN PROFILE RELATIVE TO MENSTRUAL CYCLE

Pain	No.	Percentage
No pain relative to menses	80	2.7
At time of menses only	384	12.9
At ovulation only	39	1.3
Throughout the menstrual cycle	2481	83.1
Total	**2984**	**100.0**
Missing data	36	1.2[a]

[a]Percentage based on total of 3020 patients.

TABLE 52–7. HAVE YOU EVER BEEN UNABLE TO CARRY OUT YOUR NORMAL WORK AND ACTIVITIES?

Answer	No.	Perfect
Yes	2241	74.8
No	755	25.2
Total	**2996**	**100.0**
Missing	24	0.8[a]

[a]Percentage based on total of 3020 patients.

pain all the time, severe monthly pain, painful intercourse, infertility, and multiple surgeries.[12]

The Roper Starch Worldwide survey[6] found that 22% of women with endometriosis typically miss 2 or 3 days of work each month, and 14% typically miss 4 or more days each month. Imagine what missing 2 or 3 days of work each month would do to one's practice and career. A U.S. Army study[13] of disability due to endometriosis found that among 6456 women with endometriosis, the mean number of inpatient sick days over 5 years was 8 for mild disease, 18 for moderate disease, and 30 for severe disease. The dollar cost for the lost time for the sample was calculated at $2.5 million (in early 1980s dollars). The authors added that their assessment did not account for outpatient visits, time lost waiting in clinics, or days that patients spent at bed rest or otherwise in their quarters. The authors concluded that if the disease is diagnosed at the earliest possible time, the days lost can be held to a minimum. They also noted that a history of endometriosis or examination findings consistent with endometriosis make women ineligible for entry into active duty according to present army regulations. The same is true for women with dysmenorrhea that results in hours away from routine activities.[13] A British Endometriosis Society survey[7] also found extensive disability among women with endometriosis—approximately one sixth of the women were unable to work for more than 24 days in the preceding

TABLE 52–6. PATIENTS' CHARACTERIZATION OF PAIN SEVERITY LEVELS

Pain	No.	Percentage
Mild	92	3.2
Mild to moderate	234	8.1
Moderate	310	10.7
Moderate to severe	1145	39.7
Severe	546	18.9
Varies, mild to severe	558	19.3
Total	**2885**	**100.0**
No pain	78	2.6[a]
No response	57	1.9[a]

[a]Percentage based on total of 3020 patients.

year because of endometriosis pain. Two thirds had been unable to work between 1 and 6 days over the preceding year.[7]

More damaging and harder to quantify is the phenomenon of women with endometriosis working part-time or in home businesses because of inability to work more and the inability to perform housework and child care. The British Endometriosis Society survey[7] found that more than half of those who worked outside the home felt the disease had a negative effect on their career prospects; as many as one in five had stopped work or lost a job because of the disease. Compared with 27% of the full-time workers, 57% of the part-time workers said their daily hours were limited by pain.[7]

There is preliminary evidence of other health problems and susceptibilities among women with endometriosis that may contribute to the morbidity of the disease. These include high rates of all types of atopic diseases, including allergies, food intolerances, asthma, eczema, and sometimes debilitating chemical sensitivities in the women and their families[14,15]; tendencies to infection[2]; history of mononucleosis[16]; problems with *Candida albicans*[15–17]; mitral valve prolapse[18,19]; fibromyalgia and chronic fatigue immune dysfunction syndrome[20,21]; greater risk for lupus[22]; and greater risk for Hashimoto's thyroiditis.[24]

The frequency of symptoms in infertility populations may vary. In the Institute for the Study and Treatment of Endometriosis study,[4] a lower rate of dysmenorrhea and a higher rate of infertility were found. A study of infertility patients with endometriosis in Milan also found differences: 26% of patients with stages 1 and 2 disease, and 39% with stages 3 and 4 disease versus 59% in our registry experienced dyspareunia.[23]

Attitudes are changing, but there is still a great deal of evidence that women and physicians do not always recognize the seriousness of symptoms of endometriosis early and wait until symptoms are unbearable or infertility is an issue before diagnosis. Beard wrote: "There is a definite gulf between the patient and the gynecologist. The patient actually goes to see the doctor because she has got something that is seriously interfering with her life, which is pain. The gynecologist, however, is more interested in what is causing the pain and not so much in the interference with her life. If he does not find what is causing the pain he tends to give up at that point, and that produces intense resentment on the patient's part . . ."[25] Given the preponderance of life-disrupting symptoms that occur for so many years, the message underlying delayed diagnosis can easily be that the girl or woman herself does not matter—only when she cannot become pregnant is any attention to the symptoms likely. In other words, the person's quality of life is less important than the potential life she may bear. What an ugly message.

The same message seems to underlie the belief that aggressive therapy such as excision of deep disease or intestinal disease, for instance, which offers the best hope of pain relief,[26–28] should be withheld if fertility is desired on the grounds that such therapy may increase the risk for adhesions and thereby increase the risk for infertility. Again, the well-being of the young woman herself, who is already here and ready to be a productive human being, is in danger of being sacrificed. If the disease is truly progressive[28–30] and may deteriorate without treatment, and one understands the potentially severe ramifications, one could argue that it is unethical to limit treatment. Moreover, it could be argued that removal of the disease and modification of the inflammatory and peritoneal factors that are part of the disease may improve fertility and quality of life, allowing the person to get on with her life, her schooling, building a work life, and building relationships that will be important if she decides to have a family.

The delay in diagnosis of early symptoms could contribute to the development of infertility. The relation between endometriosis and infertility is controversial, especially in mild disease, but it is generally agreed that the more severe the disease, the more likely is infertility to result. Evidence for the progression of the disease can be found in data such as the Army study noted earlier. The average age for mild and moderate endometriosis among the active-duty women was 26 years whereas the average age for severe endometriosis was 31 years. Among dependents of active and retired personnel, the average age for mild and moderate endometriosis was 28 years, whereas the average age for severe endometriosis was 35 years.[13]

Other investigators have shown that endometriosis progresses through a variety of color and appearance changes with age to the burned-out black powderburn and adhesive disease that may be most linked to infertility.[28,31] The incidence of ovarian disease apparently increases with age although it is possible there is greater difficulty in identifying early ovarian disease.[28,32] Perhaps if a 15-year-old patient with endometriosis and incapacitating pain received the correct diagnosis and treatment, she might not be infertile at 25 years of age.

Awareness and discussion of endometriosis have greatly increased in the last 15 years. The 1994 Roper Starch Worldwide survey[6] found, for instance, that 69% of U.S. women said they had heard of endometriosis, and 66% were able to correctly choose the definition from a list. In contrast, in 1980, when the Endometriosis Association was founded, most people had never heard of the disease. A 1982 Tampax Corporation survey found that most of Americans considered menstruation a topic unsuitable even for discussion. Because there is now much more awareness of the disease, *now* is the time to take the next step—faster diagnosis.

PSYCHOSOCIAL ASPECTS OF ENDOMETRIOSIS

My husband and I separated and I am now in the process of going to court. I am unable to work because of my illness . . . My ex-husband says that it's psychosomatic. . . . It took me 8 years to prove to the doctors that there was something wrong with me . . . My husband left me because he said that he can't live with a sick person anymore and that he would like to have children, and I can't give him that. I'm severely depressed and I feel like I can't cope anymore. I didn't think I would be going through all of this pain and heartache.

Teresa, Florida

After I was diagnosed I took Danocrine for 9 months of complete misery (not one good hour) with no benefit—only increasing pain. I found the thought of sex intolerable because of pain. I was doing everything I could think of to avoid it. Around this time my husband told me he believed I was seeing someone else because I avoided him. I never even considered it! Also, he continued to say the pain was in my head. All of this plus the pain of infertility. . . . Nothing altered his attitude until we visited Dr. E. together. Just hearing the doctor talk about the very same things I had been saying seemed to make the pain and distress real to my husband. He has been acting more like the loving, caring husband I used to have since . . . there are times when I wonder if the emotional pain of infertility will ever go away along with the feelings of anger and betrayal toward my husband for his lack of support during such a traumatic time. . . .

Mary, Michigan

Coping with endometriosis can stretch relationships to the limit; delay in diagnosis seems to add to the negative psychosocial ramifications of the disease (Table 52–8). In the Roper Starch survey, for instance, 39% of the survey respondents reported that their symptoms had a negative impact on their personal and family relationships before diagnosis. After diagnosis, only 17% reported their symptoms still had a negative impact on their relationships with loved ones. So having an explanation for symptoms helped women and their significant others. One can easily imagine how a symptom like pain with sex, for instance, which affects 59% of the women in the Endometriosis Association research registry, would negatively affect personal relationships and that an explanation would help. Husbands and partners might feel the woman does not love them or is avoiding intimacy, and the women themselves might not understand,

TABLE 52–8. IMPACT OF ENDOMETRIOSIS SYMPTOMS ON RELATIONSHIPS WITH FAMILY MEMBERS

Effect	Before Diagnosis (%)	After Diagnosis (%)
No effect	51	57
Negative effect	39	17
Positive effect	9	24

but with a diagnosis, they have an explanation for their sexual difficulties or avoidance.[6]

In the British survey of 2102 Endometriosis Society members,[7] 9% of respondents said that the disease had destroyed their relationship with their partner. Six percent said that their relationship had been devastated. Almost 25% said it had strengthened the relationship.

Delay in diagnosis also increases the emotional pain for the woman or girl because of lack of understanding and sympathy or adjustment for the symptoms. As noted in the Institute for the Study and Treatment of Endometriosis study,[4] most women were told that they were overreacting to the pain and that the symptoms were psychologic in origin. Women were told to learn to live with the pain. Families and friends were often not sympathetic when there was no explanation and sometimes when there was.

The number of emotional issues involved in this highly personal disease also contribute to its impact and can make it especially devastating (Table 52–9). Lack of information about the disease, the chronic nature of the disease, and the taboos and myths associated with symptoms of endometriosis (taboos surrounding menstruation, female sexuality, and infertility date back thousands of years) all combine to make endometriosis an emotionally painful disease.

Why the failure to recognize obvious symptoms of endometriosis? Why the willingness to let girls and women suffer for years without help? Why the easy sliding into "it's normal for women to experience pain with menstruation and sex"? This occurs for a number of reasons that have to do with the taboo nature of the symptoms of the disease and its all-female population. Women with the disease have been very much maligned—supposedly they are white, stressed-out, perfectionistic, upper socioeconomic level women who brought the disease on themselves by postponing childbearing (Table 52–10). Why is it that in the 20th century, post-World War II era in which there have been so many unprecedented changes, the first place physicians and society looked to lay blame for what seems to be a huge increase in the numbers of women with endometriosis is on the women themselves? Future generations of sociologists will study endometriosis as a touchstone for the sexism in our society.

One of the issues faced by women with endometriosis of

TABLE 52–9. EMOTIONAL ISSUES ASSOCIATED WITH ENDOMETRIOSIS

Fertility
Sexuality
Ability to work
Ability to care for a household
Ability to maintain personal relationships
Ability to enjoy life

TABLE 52–10. MYTHS ABOUT ENDOMETRIOSIS

Psychosomatic
Due to stress
Caused by delayed childbearing
Career woman's disease
White woman's disease
Disease primarily of women in their 30s and 40s not teens and 20s
Affects high-strung, thin, nervous perfectionist women
Affects well-educated women
Pregnancy cures it

special interest to infertility specialists is the frequent prescription of pregnancy as a treatment or even cure of endometriosis. The myth that pregnancy can cure the disease probably developed because the worst symptoms of endometriosis—the pain that occurs with the monthly period—cannot occur when one is pregnant and not having periods. However, to leap from that observation to the statement that pregnancy "cures" the disease is a leap of faith with no scientific evidence. In fact, what little scientific evidence on pregnancy and endometriosis there is leads in the other direction—that the disease process continues in pregnancy. The first physician statements on pregnancy and endometriosis date back to 1922, but the first rigorous study of what actually happens to endometrial implants during pregnancy was not conducted until 1967. The 1967 study found that for some patients symptoms increased during pregnancy; in others they decreased. In 12 of the 25 patients in the study, the implants grew larger during pregnancy. In an additional 6 patients they grew larger in the postpartum period. Some of the endometriomas grew and then receded during the pregnancies; others diminished in size initially and then began to grow again. The investigators concluded that the behavior of endometriosis during pregnancy is extremely variable and that "patients alleged to exhibit permanent regression following pregnancy are encountered much less frequently than patients with manifestly persistent disease."[33]

From the beginnings of the Endometriosis Association, women with endometriosis who had been pregnant, even several times, and still had the disease have been part of the group. Chatman[34] documented endometriosis in teenagers who had had babies before the age of 17 years.

Another frequently heard myth is that women with endometriosis feel great during pregnancy or have completely normal pregnancies, labor, and deliveries. In an important study conducted by Ansell and Gorchoff of the Yale School of Nursing Midwifery with the assistance of the Endometriosis Association, the actual pregnancy experiences of women with endometriosis were studied. The results on 187 pregnancies were astounding. The women experienced multiple discomforts during their pregnancies (73%, for example, experienced morning sickness); a high incidence of dysfunctional labor (26.7%); an extremely high rate of postpartum depression (54.6%, lasting an average of 8.75 weeks); return of symptoms with the return of periods (an average of 10 months after delivery—most in the study breastfed); and a faster return of symptoms among those who did not breastfeed. The study also reconfirmed past findings of high rates of miscarriage and ectopic pregnancy among women with endometriosis.[35]

It seems that the ethical issues are often overlooked in this myth about endometriosis. It is profoundly disrespectful of life—the woman's and the potential child's—to suggest to someone that she have a baby to "cure" a disease. To suggest to women, whether they be in their teens or older, single or coupled, heterosexual, homosexual, or celibate, in a relationship capable of sustaining a child or not, or even whether they want a child or not that they have a child because they have a disease is ludicrous even if it were to cure the disease. Women routinely report that they feel insulted by the prescription of pregnancy and see it as an intrusion into a highly personal life decision (they do, however, appreciate the warning that the disease can interfere with their fertility as well as nearly everything else in their lives).

Several studies, including one by the Endometriosis Association, have found that in the most severe cases of endometriosis, the risk that other family members will have the disease (and other health problems) is high. This awareness is not yet widespread, but it will present a devastating moral dilemma if physicians and others perpetuate the pregnancy-cure myth. That dilemma, to "cure" one's own disease by taking the risk of passing it and other problems on to a child is horrible. The already-complex childbearing decision for the woman with endometriosis and her partner has become even more difficult with the discovery that dioxin and other hormonally active immunotoxicants prevalent in the environment are linked to endometriosis and are passed along to children in utero and with breastfeeding, adding even more urgency to the need to reevaluate the pregnancy prescription practice.

Combined with the pain and difficulty imposed by the disease itself, endometriosis is an immensely challenging coping process for many patients because of the taboos and myths surrounding the symptoms of the disease, the misinformation about the disease, the delayed diagnosis, the problematic hit-and-miss treatments, and the fact that there is no cure for this painful, chronic, stubborn disease.

COPING WITH ENDOMETRIOSIS

Being an active partner in my health care has been my most effective means of coping. I've had eight operations and been through several drug therapies, as well as vitamins, chiropractic, diet changes, exercise, etc. . . . While I don't feel like an expert, I feel like an "informed consumer" with my doctors and a source of information and support to others in our local support group. . . .

Perhaps the most difficult aspect of endometriosis is the length of time one must cope with it. My mother has often advised me that "Life is a marathon—not a sprint race." While she had been referring to other aspects of my life, she might just as well have been speaking of endometriosis. I look back and see that I was treating endometriosis as a sprint—just one more hurdle to jump over—that somehow there would be an "end" to the "race." But as months became years and years became decades, it gets a lot harder to sprint. It has been difficult for me at times to maintain some balance of hope and a positive outlook against the knowledge that I've had this disease for a long time and will continue to have it for a long time. . . .

The length of time that endometriosis goes on is also hard on friends and family. No matter how supportive they are . . . the relationship suffers. It makes for another very difficult aspect of the disease to cope with: male bosses and co-workers unable to understand why I couldn't take a business trip or why I turned down a certain assignment because of a "women's problem" . . . women friends I've lost because I had to cancel too many social engagements, etc. After all, endometriosis is just bad cramps; they've had them and keep going, right? . . . Countering the myths: "You've had a baby—you should be cured [my child is 4 1/2 and I've had 2 operations since her birth]." "I thought you said the doctor got all the endometriosis—how could it come back?" "Could be worse—could be cancer." "Why not get it over with and have a hysterectomy?" My family is tired of me being sick. . . .

My fear is that my daughter will inherit my "legacy" (a very strong possibility given my family's history). It's tough enough coping with her reactions (and my feelings toward those reactions) right now.

Joyce, Kansas

There has been one well-designed study of coping mechanisms among women with endometriosis. Dr. Rona Silverton, a psychologist, found that 13 different coping strategies were used by women with endometriosis. The strategies clustered into two groups: passive-dependent coping, such as denial of the problems or passive resignation. The passive-dependent coping strategies led to failure to take the actions that could improve outcome. The other cluster of strategies used were active-independent coping strategies, such as what Silverton called reaffirmation of healthy functioning and seeking out social support (Table 52–11). The women who used active-independent coping strategies appeared to cope better, whereas passive-dependent strategies were associated with worse outcome. Silverton cautioned, however, not to simply categorize these strategies into positive or negative ways of coping. One strategy may be

TABLE 52–11. COPING MECHANISMS USED BY WOMEN WITH ENDOMETRIOSIS

Active-independent (Associated with healthy adjustment)	Passive-dependent (Associated with poor adjustment)
Problem solving	Avoidance
Seeking out social support	Helplessness or passive resignation
Tension release	Negativism
Optimism	Denial
Acceptance	Social withdrawal
Selective ignoring	
Reaffirmation of healthy functioning	
Reordering of priorities and goals	

helpful in one context and hurtful in another. For example, avoidance or social withdrawal can help a woman feel better when experiencing acute pain or sickness; however, these strategies can be detrimental if they lead to giving up and not seeking the necessary medical treatment or social support. Reaffirmation of healthy functioning was a "take charge" approach to dealing with endometriosis. These women were active despite pain and placed emphasis on actions that were health promoting, such as eating healthful foods, exercising, and reducing stress. These strategies helped the women build an internal image of being in control.[36]

A similar study conducted in Australia[37] found that symptoms and treatment and physician satisfaction were more significantly associated with the impact of endometriosis than the coping behaviors of the patient. This study also found, as did the Silverton study, that avoidance behaviors were maladaptive: those who used them reported more symptoms and more disruption in their lives.[37]

A vivid example of how avoidance behaviors can lead to more life disruption is the case, many years back, of one of the secretaries of the Endometriosis Association office. With classic symptoms of endometriosis, she was gently urged, on a number of occasions, to seek help and a possible diagnosis of endometriosis. She firmly refused, saying she was very afraid of ever having to have a hysterectomy and thus would not go to a gynecologist. Because the symptoms were severe, it is not difficult to see how the woman's avoidance behavior was greatly increasing the likelihood of worsening symptoms and, unfortunately, increasing her likelihood of eventually undergoing a hysterectomy. Someone who, in contrast, took charge of the situation, facing it head-on, might have been able to gain some control of the problem and lessen her chances for hysterectomy.

ROLE OF THE ENDOMETRIOSIS ASSOCIATION

I feel as if I am one of the "lucky" ones because of the Endometriosis Association. Because of the information from your group and my support group I have had the chance for some excellent treatment. My first doctor would have given me a hysterectomy by now.
Nina, Texas

When my son was born, I sat and looked at this wonderful little person. And I realized that his birth was really due to all the information and support I had received from the Association group in Vancouver, and what a difference that support group had made to my life. So I decided to organize a support group here. I thought, maybe the information and support will change these women's lives as much as it's changed mine.
Nanci, Yukon

Through the Association, I found other women who had similar experiences and frustrations. I was not alone. The Association through its newsletter has become more of a family that shares its joys and difficulties and most important, all of the new information and technology concerning this baffling disease. I enjoy hearing who has defied this dis-

ease by becoming pregnant and bearing a healthy child; a normal body process many take for granted.
Diane, Minnesota

I decided to become a Lifetime Member of the Endometriosis Association because of my experience with hundreds of couples with this condition. I am impressed by how much this medical problem can disrupt people's lives, and have felt fortunate to be able to assist in the health care of these patients. I only wish we could do more. I feel that education of all consumers is essential if we are to provide the highest quality of care to patients. Therefore, I strongly support the Endometriosis Association in its goals of education and psychological support, and of course, ongoing research to improve our understanding of endometriosis.
G. David Adamson, MD
Infertility Specialist, California

The studies of the best coping strategies for endometriosis may help explain why the Endometriosis Association has been such a vital force in the lives of women with the disease. Association programs give women the support and tools needed to implement a take-charge attitude toward the disease (Table 52–12). Health practitioners also rely on the help available from the Association. A 1993 survey of nurses found that 95% provide informational brochures to help patients cope with the disease. They also named books, educational videos, a toll-free hotline, and women's support networks as very helpful.[38] The Association provides all these resources.

The support program is especially important for women with endometriosis. It ends the feeling of being alone; reduces the stigma attached to menstrual symptoms; rebuilds lost self-

TABLE 52–12. ENDOMETRIOSIS ASSOCIATION

Support Program
Support groups and chapters
Crisis-call assistance
Individual help with endometriosis problems
Networking services (local contact lists; international correspondence networks)
Prescription drug savings program

Education Program
Accurate, informative literature
Newsletter with research news, coping help
Public education campaigns, including annual international Endometriosis Awareness Week last full week of March
Health practitioner educational program

Research Program
Established large data registry, 1980
Epidemiologic studies using registry, 1983–1988
Technical assistance for researchers, help locating subjects
Clearinghouse activities
Fundraising for research
Research linking endometriosis to dioxin, 1992-ongoing
Ongoing research program at Dartmouth Medical School

esteem; teaches coping skills; helps women come to grips with the denial process; debunks the myths of endometriosis; allows women to talk through difficult treatment decisions and helps in times of crisis; builds support for women within their families and communities; and increases the frequency of diagnosis by raising awareness of the disease in the community.

DIOXIN, INFERTILITY, AND ENDOMETRIOSIS

In 1991, a long-term U.S. Air Force study[39] showed that spontaneous endometriosis developed in monkeys exposed to radiation. "Endometriosis in our monkey colony was conclusively linked to whole-body-penetrating energies of ionizing radiation. Women receiving whole-body, or in particular, abdominal, exposure to penetrating doses of protons or x-rays should possibly be considered to be at higher risk of developing endometriosis than unexposed women," wrote the investigators.[39]

The production of spontaneous disease with any agent had not been possible in the many studies done up until that time. Endometrium had to be transplanted into the pelvic cavity, raising questions whether a true model of endometriosis was produced. (A recent study finding[40] lends support to the idea that transplanted endometrium is not a true disease.) The Air Force study reminded me of another study[41] in which spontaneous disease had developed reputedly in rhesus monkeys after exposure to polychlorinated biphenyls (PCBs), toxic pollutants. "The endometriosis in these rhesus monkeys was much more productive of inflammatory reaction than the otherwise similar process in humans," wrote the clinical investigator.[41]

Sixty of the PCB-treated monkeys achieved only 26 pregnancies with 9 stillbirths, 4 deaths 1 to 11 days after delivery, and 3 miscarriages. Sixteen control monkeys achieved 9 livebirths and 2 stillbirths. Removal of the ovaries was performed on some of the animals to control the disease but was not always successful[42] (lending further support to the studies that show removal of the ovaries in humans does not always cure the disease).

From Dr. Campbell I learned that two monkeys in a reproductive toxicology study of dioxin, a pollutant similar to PCB, had died of intestinal obstruction or kidney failure caused by ureteral obstruction due to extensive endometriosis. This study colony had also experienced markedly impaired reproduction. Unfortunately, the research team had long been disbanded, with the exception of the behavioral psychologist who studied behavioral changes in the offspring of the dioxin-exposed monkeys, and the colony was about to lose its funding.

The Endometriosis Association provided emergency funding for the colony and arranged for laparoscopy and immunologic studies to be conducted on the entire colony (low dose, high dose, and control group). Laparoscopic examinations

showed that 79% of the monkeys exposed to dioxin in the study had spontaneous endometriosis. Moreover, the disease increased in severity in proportion to the amount of dioxin exposure. Control monkeys tended to have minimal disease; exposed monkeys moderate or severe, depending on the amount of dioxin exposure (American Fertility Society and American Fertility Society-revised classifications).[43] Immune changes, particularly in levels of interleukin-6 and tumor necrosis factor, also were found. These findings are consistent with those of human studies that suggested immune mechanisms may contribute to the disease process.[44–47] The Association has maintained the monkey colony and invites researchers interested in conducting related studies to contact us: Endometriosis Association, International Headquarters, 8585 North 76th Place, Milwaukee, WI 53223. A study conducted in Germany[48] supported the link between pollutants and endometriosis. The investigators found that women with endometriosis and antithyroid antibodies have higher levels of PCBs in their blood.

Physicians have expressed surprise that women would be exposed to toxins such as dioxin and PCBs (Table 52–13). These chemicals are widely dispersed in our food, water, and environment. TCDD (2,3,7,8-tetrachlorodibenzo-p-dioxin) and PCBs are organochlorine pollutants that have been manufactured and distributed in this century (since 1929 for PCBs and the 1940s for TCDD) and are now found worldwide. TCDD, the most toxic of 75 dioxins, is known to cause immune suppression and to interfere with hormonal function. Dioxin is found in pesticides and herbicides, food, especially meat and animal products, byproducts of incineration, and pulp and paper manufacturing and products, including sanitary napkins and tampons.

PCBs were widely used as electrical insulators and were formerly used in carbonless paper, specialty inks, paints, and additives in plastics manufacturing. Allowable amounts occurred in dairy products, poultry, and eggs and other food products until they were banned in the United States (1979) and

TABLE 52–13. SOURCES OF DIOXIN AND POLYCHLORINATED BIPHENYLS (PCBs) IN THE ENVIRONMENT

Factors	Dioxin	PCBs
Sources	Pesticides, incineration, industrial byproducts	Electrical insulators
Pathway to animals and humans	Food, water	Water, soil, fish
	Accumulates in fatty tissue	
Life of compound in the human	14–22 years	Life
Transmission	Transmitted from mother to offspring in utero and by means of lactation	
Effects	Disrupts endocrine and immune systems	
	Functional deficits may not be apparent at birth and may not be fully manifested until adulthood	

Canada (1980). They are still widely prevalent in the environment, particularly in the Great Lakes basin, the most PCB-contaminated area of North America. Contaminated fish and drinking water and breast milk and in utero exposure are some of the sources of exposure. These chemicals can last hundreds of years and bioaccumulate in the fatty tissue of animals and humans. In addition, biomagnification occurs, that is, there is an increasing concentration of toxins as one moves up the food chain.

There are at least 23 chemical families of pollutants, such as dioxins and PCBs, that disrupt the endocrine system, according to a concensus statement issued by scientists gathered at a conference, Endocrine Disrupters in the Environment, in July 1991. The consensus statement read

Many wildlife populations are already affected by these compounds. The impacts include thyroid dysfunction in birds and fish; decreased fertility in birds, fish, shellfish, and mammals; decreased hatching success in birds, fish, and turtles; gross birth deformities in birds, fish, and turtles; metabolic abnormalities in birds, fish, and mammals; behavioral abnormalities in birds; demasculinization and feminization of male fish, birds, and mammals; defeminization and masculinization of female fish and birds; and compromised immune systems in birds and mammals. . . .

The mechanisms by which these compounds have their impact vary, but they share the general properties of (1) mimicking the effects of natural hormones by recognizing their binding sites; (2) antagonizing the effect of these hormones by blocking their interaction with their physiological binding sites; (3) reacting directly and indirectly with the hormone in question; (4) altering the natural pattern of synthesis of hormones; or (5) altering hormone receptor levels.[49]

The reproductive consequences of most of these endocrine-disrupting pollutants in human beings is unknown, although there have been many instances of increased frequencies of spontaneous abortion, impaired fertility, birth defects, and infant deaths in areas of known contamination. As demonstrated in a recent book for the general public on infertility, there are more than 60,000 chemicals in widespread commercial use today, most introduced since the second world war, but only three are regulated based on their documented effects on human reproduction. Most need much more reproductive study.[50]

Perhaps the most heartbreaking aspect of these pollutants is that they are transmitted from mother to infant both in utero and during breastfeeding. In the dioxin monkey colony, the mother monkeys dumped 20% of their body burden of dioxin into their infants—the infants received *more* dioxin per kilogram of weight than the mothers. Breastfeeding was the principal source of the dumping.[51] A similar phenomenon is very likely in humans. Dr. Arnold Schecter, a professor of preventive medicine at the State University of New York, Binghamton, was quoted as saying: "Our calculations show that with one year of breastfeeding, North American babies are exceeding the [dioxin intake] levels calculated by most governments as a do-not-exceed lifetime dose."[52] This is particularly worrisome because the embryo, fetus, and neonate are much more sensitive to the deleterious effects of these chemicals than adults. Because of this, the Michigan Medical Society, has advised that children and anyone, male or female, who ever plans to have children should eat no Great Lakes fish. According to another source,[53] pediatricians may recommend that women who have worked around pesticides should have their breast milk tested for dichlorodiphenyltrichloroethane (DDT) content. If the level is high, the pediatrician may recommend that mothers pump their breasts to remove as much toxin from their bodies as possible *but not to feed the milk to their babies*. Perhaps similar precautions should be taken with dioxin, PCBs, and other toxins.

Preventing exposure is especially important because effective methods of removing the toxins are not known. Because impaired fertility often can indicate toxic contamination, it behooves infertility specialists to become informed and involved. As Swain[54] has shown, it may take six generations before PCBs are cleared from our bodies even with no further exposure. This figure was calculated on the basis of the first mother in the six generations having the average level of PCBs in her breast milk currently found in Michigan mothers who consumed PCB-contaminated fish.[54]

SUMMARY

Hugely important social issues face us if endometriosis is a 20th century epidemic brought on by environmental toxins. One hopes infertility specialists will be at the forefront of alerting society about what may be serious threats to the fertility, reproduction, health, and survival of humans and other species. Endometriosis may be a paradigm in which these issues come together. As such, it behooves us all to look beyond the infertility aspect of the disease to the bigger picture.

REFERENCES

1. Muse K: Endometriosis and infertility. In: Wilson EA (ed), *Endometriosis*. New York, Alan R. Liss, 1987
2. Endometriosis Association Research Registry: *Endometriosis Assoc Newsletter* 10:2, 1989

3. Endometriosis Association, British Endometriosis Society, and Australian Endometriosis Association: In: Ballweg ML (ed), *Overcoming Endometriosis: New Help from the Endometriosis Association.* New York, Congdon & Weed, 1987:297

4. Halstead L, Pepping P, Haile L, Dmowski WP: Women's experiences with endometriosis: Delay and disbelief. In: Abstracts of the 3rd World Congress on Endometriosis, June 1992, Brussels, Belgium

5. Insight Canada Research: Canadian Women and Endometriosis. Survey for Syntex Laboratories, Canada, December 1990

6. Roper Starch Worldwide: Endometriosis and the American Woman. Survey for Zeneca Pharmaceuticals, January 1994

7. Endometriosis Society Survey: *Endometriosis Soc Newsletter* 2:70, 1994

8. Hysterectomies in the United States, 1965–84: Vital and Health Statistics, US Department of Health and Human Services, Public Health Service, Centers for Disease Control, National Center for Health Statistics, Series 13, no. 92, 1987

9. Lamb K, Breitkopf LJ, Hamilton K: Does hysterectomy and removal of the ovaries offer a cure for endometriosis? An exploratory study. In: Ballweg ML (ed), *The Endometriosis Sourcebook.* Chicago, Contemporary Books, 1995:130–143

10. Wood R: The pathway to diagnosis of women with endometriosis. In: Abstracts of the 3rd World Congress on Endometriosis, June 1992, Brussels, Belgium

11. Naish CE, Kennedy SH, Barlow DH: Correlation between pain symptoms and laparoscopic findings. In: Abstracts, 3rd World Congress on Endometriosis, June 1992, Brussels, Belgium

12. Christian A: The relationship between women's symptoms of endometriosis and self-esteem. *J Obstet Gynecol Neonat Nurs* 22:4, 1993

13. Boling RO, Abbasi R, Ackerman G, Schipul AH Jr, Chaney SA: Disability from endometriosis in the United States army. *J Reprod Med* 33:49, 1988

14. Nichols TR, Lamb K, Arkins JA: The association of atopic diseases with endometriosis. *Ann Allergy* 59:11, 1987

15. Ballweg ML: The endometriosis–candidiasis link. In: Ballweg ML (ed), *Overcoming Endometriosis: New Help from the Endometriosis Association.* New York, Congdon & Weed, 1987:198–219

16. Lamb K, Nichols TR: Endometriosis: A comparison of associated disease histories. *Am J Prev Med* 2:6, 1986

17. Ballweg ML: Research news: Candida–chronic fatigue link. *Endometriosis Assoc Newsletter* 10:4, 1989

18. Ballweg ML: A heart defect in endometriosis: Another clue to a bigger picture? In: Ballweg ML (ed), *Overcoming Endometriosis: New Help from the Endometriosis Association.* New York, Congdon & Weed, 1987:228–231

19. Fletcher N: Mitral valve prolapse. *Endometriosis Assoc Newsletter* 13:2, 1992

20. Ballweg ML: Fibromyalgia/endometriosis link? *Endometriosis Assoc Newsletter* 12:3, 1991

21. Thorson K: FMS and endometriosis. *Fibromyalgia Network Compendium* 2:18

22. Grimes DA, LeBolt SA, Grimes KRT, Wingo PA: Two-fold risk of endometriosis in hospitalized patients with lupus. *Am J Obstet Gynecol* 153:179, 1985

23. Parazzini F: Is pelvic pain more frequent in women with endometriosis? In: Crosignani PG, Vercellini P (eds), *Endometriosis and Pelvic Pain: Time of Review.* New York, Parthenon, 1994: 11–16

24. Brush MG: Increased incidence of thyroid autoimmune problems in women with endometriosis. In: Coventry Branch of the Endometriosis Society, *Endometriosis: A Collection of Papers Written by GPs, Researchers, Specialists and Sufferers about Endometriosis.* March, 1987

25. Kennedy S: What is important to the patient with endometriosis? Discussion. *Br J Clin Pract* 45(Suppl 72):11, 1991

26. Ripps BA, Martin DC: Focal pelvic tenderness, pelvic pain, and dysmenorrhea in endometriosis. *J Reprod Med* 36:470, 1991

27. Cornillie F, et al: Deeply infiltrating endometriosis: Histology and clinical significance. *Fertil Steril* 53:978, 1990

28. Koninckx PR, et al: Suggestive evidence that pelvic endometriosis is a progressive disease, whereas deeply infiltrating endometriosis is associated with pelvic pain. *Fertil Steril* 55:759, 1991

29. Telimaa S, Puolakka J, Ronnberg L, Kauppila A: Placebo-controlled comparison of danazol and high-dose medroxyprogesterone acetate in the treatment of endometriosis. *Gynecol Endocrinol* 1:13, 1987

30. Thomas EJ, Cooke ID: Impact of gestrinone on the course of asymptomatic endometriosis. *Br Med J* 294:272, 1987

31. Redwine DB: Age-related evolution in color appearance of endometriosis. *Fertil Steril* 48:1062, 1987

32. Redwine DB: The distribution of endometriosis in the pelvis by age groups and fertility. *Fertil Steril* 47:173, 1987

33. Gould SF, Shannon JM, Cunha GR: Nuclear estrogen binding sites seen in foci of endometriosis. *Fertil Steril* 39:4, 1983

34. Chatman DL: Endometriosis in the black woman. *Am J Obstet Gynecol* 125:7, 1976

35. Ballweg ML: Research review: Pregnancy, labor, and postpartum experiences of women with endometriosis. In: Ballweg ML (ed), *The Endometriosis Sourcebook.* Chicago, Contemporary Books, 1995:248–258

36. Schwebach LS: Coping strategies used by women with endometriosis. In: Ballweg ML (ed), *The Endometriosis Sourcebook.* Chicago, Contemporary Books, 1995:291–293

37. Research Report: coping behaviours in endometriosis. *Endometriosis Assoc (Victoria) Newsletter* April 1994

38. Roper Starch Worldwide: Endometriosis and the American Woman: Nurse Survey Data Tabulations. Survey for Zeneca Pharmaceuticals, August 1993

39. Fanton JW, Golden JG: Radiation-induced endometriosis in *Macaca mulatta. Radiat Res* 126:141, 1991

40. D'Hooghe TM, Bambra CS, Raeymaekers BM, De Jonge I, Hill JA, Koninckx PR: The effects of immunosuppression on development and progression of endometriosis in baboons (*Papio anubis*). *Fertil Steril* 64:1:172, 1995

41. Campbell JS, Wong J, Tryphonas L, et al: Is simian endometriosis an effect of immunotoxicity? Presented at the Ontario Association of Pathologists, October 1985, London, Ontario

42. Campbell J: Is reproductive wastage and failure related to environmental pollution? Considerations of human and data findings from a rhesus model. Presented at the Symposium on Toxicological Pathology: Quo Vadis? September, 1988, Ottawa, Ontario

43. Rier SE, Martin DC, Bowman RE, et al: Endometriosis in rhesus monkeys (*Macaca mulatta*) following chronic exposure to 2,3,7,8 tetrachlorodibenzo-p-dioxin. *Fundam Appl Toxicol* 21:4:433, 1993

44. Rier SE, Parsons AK, Becker JL: Altered interleukin-6 production by peritoneal leukocytes from patients with endometriosis. *Fertil Steril* 61:294, 1994

45. Rier SE, Zarmakoupis PN, Hu X, Becker J: Dysregulation of interleukin-6 responses in ectopic endometrial stromal cells: correlation with decreased soluble receptor levels in peritoneal fluid of women with endometriosis. *J Clin Endocrinol Metabol* 80:1431, 1995

46. Rier SE, Spangelo BL, Martin DC, Bowman RE, Becker JL: Production of interleukin-6 and tumor necrosis factor-alpha by peripheral blood mononuclear cells from rhesus monkeys with endometriosis. *J Immunol* 150:49A, 1992

47. Rier SE, Martin DC, Bowman RE, Becker JL: Immunoresponsiveness in endometriosis: Implications of estrogenic toxicants. *Environ Health Perspect* 103, 1995

48. Gerhard I, Runnebaum B: German der hormonsubstitution bei schadstoffbelastung und fertilitätsstörungen. *Zentralbl Gynakol* 114:593, 1992

49. Colborn T, Clement C (eds): *Advances in Modern Environmental Toxicology. Vol XXI. Chemically-Induced Alterations in Sexual and Functional Development: The Wildlife/Human Connection.* Princeton, Princeton Scientific, 1992

50. Berger GS, Goldstein M, Fuerst M: *The Couple's Guide to Fertility: How New Medical Advances Can Help You Have a Baby.* New York, Doubleday, 1989:61

51. Bowman RE, Schantz SL, Weerasinghe NCA, Gross ML, Barsotti DA: Chronic dietary intake of 2,3,7,8 tetrachlorodibenzo-p-dioxin (TCDD) at 5 or 25 parts per trillion in the monkey: TCDD kinetics and dose-effect estimate of reproductive toxicity. *Chemosphere* 18:243, 1989

52. McGuire R: Dioxin in mother's milk. *Med Trib* 27:34, 1986

53. Needleman HL, Landrigan PJ: *Raising Children Toxic Free: How to Keep Your Child Safe from Lead, Asbestos, Pesticides, and Other Environmental Hazards.* New York, Farrar, Straus & Giroux, 1994

54. Swain WR: Human health consequences of consumption of fish contaminated with organochlorine compounds. *Aquatic Toxicol* 11:357, 1988

PART XII

Statistics

CHAPTER 53

Statistical Analysis of Infertility Data

DAVID S. GUZICK

Special Features of Infertility Data
Measurements of outcome
Dependent versus independent
 variables
Dichotomous versus continuous
 variables
Impact of nonuniform follow-up
 after treatment

Statistical Techniques
Analysis when follow-up is not
 uniform
Analysis when follow-up is
 uniform
Computer software
Clinical Trials
Power analysis
 Example: intracervical versus
  intrauterine insemination
Summary

The word *statistics* originally meant the collection of population and economic information vital to the state. A statistic in this sense has come to mean an item of data. More generally, the subject area is now considered to encompass the entire science of decision making in the face of uncertainty. This covers enormous ground: Uncertainties are present when we experiment with a new drug, determine life insurance premiums, inspect manufactured products, rate the abilities of human beings, and make business decisions.

The practice of clinical medicine almost continuously involves making decisions in the face of uncertainty. In the case of infertility, clinical decisions often must be made in the absence of definitive information. Examples are how to treat mild or moderate endometriosis; whether to recommend in vitro fertilization (IVF) or fimbrioplasty to women with moderate to severe distal tubal disease; how many cycles of intrauterine insemination (IUI) to perform when the husband has severe oligospermia before recommending IVF or donor insemination;

and how optimally to induce ovulation in a particular anovulatory patient.

Statistical methods can help with these decisions because they allow one to make inferences about an entire population based on information gathered from a sample. For example, before investing in equipment needed for laparoscopic laser tubal surgery, one may want to know whether pregnancy rates after tuboplasties performed with the aid of a laser are higher than those performed with a microcautery. What one really wants to know is whether this is true in general, that is, for the entire population of women undergoing tuboplasty. Because there are only limited numbers of patients to study in a given geographic location, however, one collects information about a sample of patients undergoing one procedure or the other. The method of sampling is critical. The idea is that patients sampled from two surgical treatment groups should differ in no important respect other than the type of procedure performed. Underlying the sampling method is the assumption that the pregnancy rate

TABLE 53–1. CALCULATION OF CUMULATIVE PREGNANCY RATE BY MEANS OF THE LIFE-TABLE METHOD

Interval After Treatment (mos)	Last Report		Number Not Pregnant at Beginning of Interval	Number Exposed to Pregnancy	Probability of Pregnancy in Interval	Cumulative Pregnancy Rate
	Pregnant	Not Pregnant				
0–12	68	0	214	214.0	0.318	0.318
13–24	21	39	146	126.5	0.166	0.431
25–36	15	14	86	79.0	0.190	0.539
37–48	7	10	57	52.0	0.135	0.601
49–60	2	10	40	35.0	0.057	0.624
61–72	1	4	28	26.0	0.038	0.639

completed (O). Those who were either L or O are described as "censored." Fig 53–1B displays the same data after recording the time of entry into the study (that is, the time of treatment) as time zero. This is the starting point for the pregnancy life-table calculation.

The following life-table calculations are based on the original description by Berkson and Gage.[1] Table 53–1 is a life table constructed from data on 214 patients with endometriosis who were treated with conservative surgical management at the Johns Hopkins Hospital.[2] Each row represents data for a given interval of time after therapy. During the first 12 months after therapy, 68 patients conceived (column 2). None were censored (column 3), so all 214 patients who entered the study (column 4) were exposed to the possibility of pregnancy (column 5). The probability of pregnancy during this interval was equal to the

number of pregnancies (68) divided by the number of women exposed (214), or 31.8% (column 6).

Because 68 patients became pregnant during the first 12 months, 146 (214 minus 68) entered the second interval (column 4). Of these, 21 conceived (column 2). During this period, however, 39 patients were censored (column 3). We assume uniform dropout of these patients over the 12-month interval, that is, half of them, or 19.5, were exposed. Thus, a total of 146 − 19.5 = 126.5 patients were exposed (column 5), giving a probability of pregnancy for this interval of 21 ÷ 126.5 = 16.6% (column 6).

The cumulative probability of pregnancy was then obtained by successively applying the probabilities of pregnancy in each interval to a starting figure of 0% pregnant. Thus the probability of pregnancy during the first interval was 31.8%,

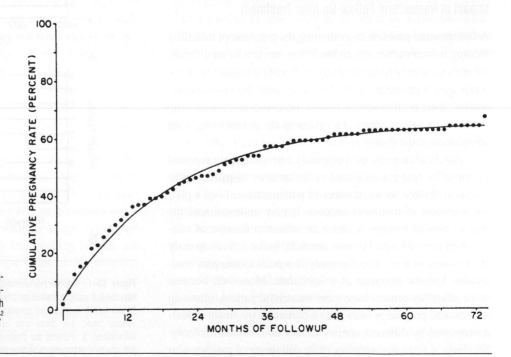

Figure 53–2. Comparison of the observed cumulative pregnancy curve (solid circles) after conservative surgical treatment of endometriosis with that predicted by the model of Guzick and Rock[2] (solid line).

and because none of the patients conceived before therapy, the cumulative pregnancy rate was also 31.8% (column 7). In the second interval, 16.6% of the remaining 68.2% of nonpregnant patients conceived, adding an estimated 11.3% patients (0.166 × 0.682) to the pregnancy rate. Thus in the second interval the cumulative pregnancy rate was 31.8% + 11.3% = 43.1%. This process continued for the remaining intervals.

The cumulative pregnancy curve can be plotted graphically (closed circles in Fig 53–2). One can infer certain features of the curve by examining the plot; that is, the curve seems to level off at a cumulative pregnancy rate of 60 to 65%, as compared with a crude pregnancy rate of 54% for these same data. To describe the curve more precisely, or to compare two or more such curves for different patient groups, however, a mathematical model is needed.

One model that has been advanced involves the assumption that the pregnancy rate per month (that is, the hazard rate) for all patients is constant over time.[3] Given a constant monthly pregnancy rate, the predicted cumulative pregnancy rate (CPR) can easily be calculated: assuming a 20% monthly pregnancy rate, CPR = 20% the first month. During the second month, 20% of the remaining 80% of patients conceive, or an additional 16%. Thus CPR = 36% after 2 months; similarly, it is 49% after 3 months, 59% after 4 months, and so on.

Applying such a model is straightforward. One simply calculates the average monthly pregnancy rate (or fecundability) by dividing the number of pregnancies by the total months of follow-up and then predicts CPR. Indeed, estimates of fecundability after treatment are now commonly reported in the infertility literature. Interpretation of such estimates is difficult, however, because the underlying assumption of a constant hazard rate is often incorrect. From the endometriosis data in Table 53–1, for example, it can be seen that the hazard rate declines rather markedly over time, as shown in Fig 53–3. It is not surprising, therefore, that the predicted cumulative pregnancy curve based on this model fits the observed data poorly (Fig 53–4). The CPR predicted by means of the model initially underestimates and then overestimates the observed CPR.

To develop a model of CPR that better approximates the observed data in a wide variety of infertility investigations, assume that the observed cumulative pregnancy curve is a weighted average of two cures, one for patients who will ultimately conceive (the "cured" group) and the other for those who will never conceive (the "uncured" group).[2] The curve for the uncured patients is a horizontal line at 0%. The proportion of patients in the uncured group increases as follow-up advances and pregnant patients in the cured group are progressively deleted from the sample, providing greater weight to the overall curve. This concept is shown graphically in Fig 53–5.

Mathematically, the model has been formalized as follows[2]:

$$P(t) = c[1 - exp(-\lambda t)]. \qquad (1)$$

That is, the cumulative pregnancy curve that gives the probability of pregnancy at any time t of follow-up, $P(t)$, can be expressed in terms of two parameters: the cure rate (c) and the hazard rate (or monthly probability of pregnancy) among those cured (λ). By "cure" we mean that a patient has the potential, after treatment, to conceive. This model can be estimated with nonlinear least squares[2] or a maximum-likelihood technique.[4,5] My associates and I have estimated the model for data sets on endometriosis,[2] polycystic ovary syndrome,[6] artificial insemination by donor,[7] tubal reanastomosis,[8,9] and IVF.[10] In these studies and in other examples in which the model has been used,[11,12] the fit has been uniformly excellent. For example, the results for the endometriosis data set are as follows:

$$P(t) = 0.645[1 - exp(0.056t)]. \qquad (2)$$

Thus it is estimated that 64.5% of patients were "cured" of their infertility problem, and among those the monthly probability of pregnancy was 5.6%. The estimated model fits the observed data quite well (see Fig 53–2). In Fig 53–5 it can be seen graphically that the predicated cumulative pregnancy curve for

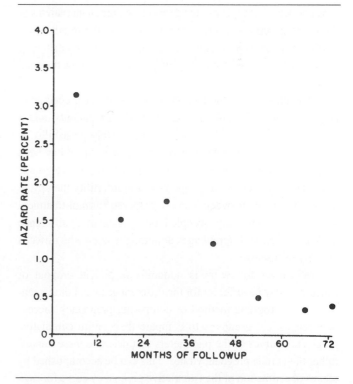

Figure 53–3. Hazard rate (i.e., probability of pregnancy) after conservative surgical treatment of endometriosis as a function of months of follow-up.

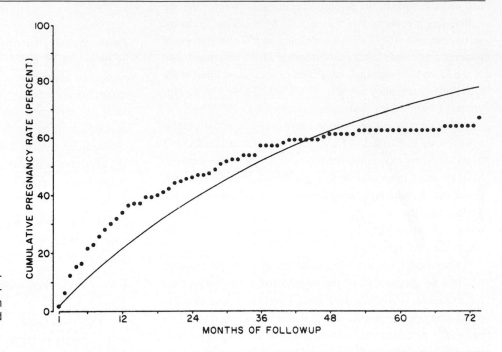

Figure 53–4. Comparison of the observed cumulative pregnancy curve (solid circles) after conservative surgical treatment of endometriosis with that predicted by the model of Cramer et al[3] (solid line).

the sample is the weighted average of two curves, one for the patients who ultimately conceive and one for those who will never conceive. As follow-up advances and pregnant patients in the cured group are deleted from the sample, the relative proportion of patients in the uncured group increases, contributing more weight to the probability of pregnancy among the total group.

The life-table method has been described as a procedure to adjust for nonuniformity in the follow-up of patients, and a method for estimating the cure rate and monthly probability of pregnancy represented by a given pregnancy curve has been presented. It is often of interest to compare two or more groups of patients with respect to pregnancy after infertility therapy. Is there a difference between a newly proposed form of treatment and the conventionally accepted one? Is there a difference among women of different ages or among women who differ in severity of disease?

Whenever follow-up is nonuniform, patient dropout or censoring may be different for the different groups. For this reason, the appropriate method of comparing pregnancy success between patient groups is to compare their entire cumulative pregnancy curves or the parameters that describe these curves, rather than crude pregnancy rates. This can be accomplished by means of estimation of the cumulative pregnancy curve for each patient group with the model described earlier, and then performing a statistical comparison of the estimated curves. My associates and I[4,5] have developed a likelihood-ratio method for

making such comparisons. Unfortunately, the sample size required for this type of estimation (a minimum of 30 to 40 subjects in each group) is often not available. Nonparametric methods of comparing life tables[13,14] are used in such instances.

Analysis When Follow-Up Is Uniform

If follow-up of patients is uniform, complete, and of sufficiently long duration, the crude pregnancy rate closely approximates the asymptotic pregnancy rate of the life table or the cure rate of the model. Under this circumstance, some simple and powerful statistical methods can be applied.

Suppose, for example, it is of interest to study factors associated with pregnancy success after tubal reanastomosis and that 60 patients with at least 2 years of follow-up are available. Potential factors that may be associated with pregnancy can be identified on the basis of a theoretic model or previous research findings. From these considerations, suppose that the particular factors hypothesized to be associated with pregnancy success are tubal length at the completion of the operation, type of tubal ligation performed, type of anastomosis (such as isthmic-isthmic), and patient age.

How can one assess the association between pregnancy success and each of these potentially prognostic variables? There are two broad categories of such independent or explanatory variables: categorical (type of tubal ligation, type of anastomosis) and continuous (age, tubal length). In the example, the

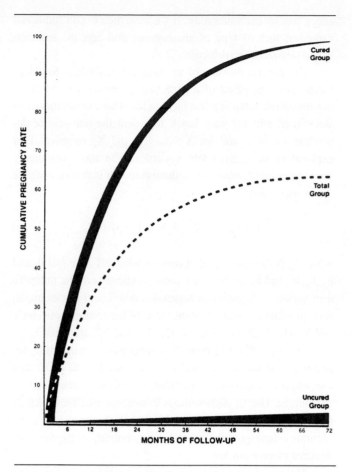

Figure 53–5. Schematic description of cumulative pregnancy model. Relative proportions of patients in the cured and uncured groups over time are represented by the thickness of the line.

dependent or outcome variable (pregnancy/no pregnancy) is categorical.

In general, to determine whether a relationship exists between one categorical variable and another, it is appropriate to perform a chi-square test. To determine whether a relationship exists between a dichotomous and a continuous variable, the appropriate test is a *t* test. Each of these tests allows one to make a decision about whether the observed relationship is greater than would have been expected by some predetermined chance level. That is, one can infer a statistically significant association between the variables.

Chi-Square Test

The data for a chi-square test of the relation between pregnancy outcome (pregnant/nonpregnant) after 2 years of follow-up and type of tubal ligation procedure performed are shown in Table 53–2. Each cell represents a frequency count of the number of patients who fall into a particular category (for example, five patients who underwent tubal cauterization conceived). Shown

TABLE 53–2. ILLUSTRATIVE CHI-SQUARE ANALYSIS FOR PREGNANCY VERSUS TYPE OF TUBAL LIGATION[a]

Clinical Pregnancy	Tubal Ligation Type			Totals
	Banding	*Cautery*	*Pomeroy*	
No	3	7	8	18
	(6)	(3.6)	(8.4)	
Yes	17	5	20	42
	(14)	(8.4)	(19.6)	
Totals	20	12	28	60

[a]Each cell contains the actual frequency observed and the expected frequency below it in parentheses.

in parentheses below these observed frequencies are the expected frequencies that would occur if the null hypothesis (no difference in pregnancy rate among types of tubal ligation) were true. These expected frequencies can be calculated from the row and column totals. For example, 70% of the patients conceived (42 of 60). If the null hypothesis were true and there were no differences in pregnancy rates among tubal ligation procedures, the proportion pregnant for each procedure type would also be 70%. For example, because 20 patients underwent tubal banding, it would be expected that 14 of these patients would have conceived.

After the observed (*o*) and expected (*e*) frequency counts in each cell have been tabulated, the chi-square statistic can be calculated as follows:

$$\chi^2 = \sum_{i=1}^{6} \frac{(o - e_i)^2}{e_i} = 6.76. \tag{3}$$

To determine whether this χ^2 value is statistically significant at the 5% level, one consults a χ^2 probability distribution to determine the value of χ^2 that represents a 5% probability of falsely rejecting the null hypothesis. Because the calculated χ^2 value of 6.76 exceeds this critical value of 4.6, we reject the null hypothesis of no association between tubal ligation and pregnancy success.

Student's t Test

One use for a *t* test is to examine the relation between a dichotomous and a continuous variable. Suppose one is interested in the relation between tubal length (continuous variable, in centimeters) and pregnancy success (dichotomous variable, yes/no). The Student's *t* test can be used to compare the mean tubal length of the pregnant group with that of the nonpregnant group.

The formula for the Student's *t* statistic is as follows:

$$t = \frac{\text{difference between means}}{\text{standard error of difference between means}} \tag{4}$$

Conceptually, the *t* statistic is the ratio of the difference between two samples and the variability between them. If the difference between the means of the two samples were high and variability low, the *t* statistic would be high, and it would be reasonable to conclude that the observed difference between the means reflects a true difference in tubal length between the populations of women who do and do not conceive. If the difference between the observed sample means were small and the standard error of the difference large, the *t* statistic would be low, and we could not reject the null hypothesis that there was no difference between the means; that is, the difference observed would probably be due to sampling variation.

In the example, the observed sample mean of tubal length among the pregnant group was 6.10, the sample mean of tubal length among the nonpregnant group was 4.83, and the standard error of difference between the means was 0.44. The *t* statistic is thus $(6.10 - 4.83)/0.44 = 2.88$. This value exceeds the critical value of 2.0 for a .05 level of significance (as determined from a table of critical points for Student's *t*). Thus we conclude that tubal length at completion of the operation was significantly higher among the pregnant group than among the nonpregnant group.

Multivariate Analysis and Logistic Regression

From the univariate analyses performed thus far, it appears that type of ligation and tube length are both directly associated with the likelihood of pregnancy after anastomosis. It is possible, however, that part of the reason higher pregnancy rates occur after anastomosis of a banded tube than a burned tube is that banding destroys less tissue, so that final tubal length is greater. If this were true, can we tease out the true independent contributions to the probability of pregnancy of tubal length and ligation type? The answer lies within the general framework of multivariate analysis.

The simplest type of multivariate analysis is cross-classification. Tubal length could be rounded to whole numbers in centimeters and a separate chi-square table of tubal ligation type (cautery, resection, banding) with pregnancy (yes, no) could be analyzed for each tube length. If a statistically significant relationship were found between ligation type and pregnancy at each tube length, we could conclude that ligation type has an effect on the probability of pregnancy even after controlling for tube length.

The cross-classification approach is simple but cumbersome. As the number of variables included in the analysis grows, so does the number of subjects required to address the question with meaning. Even with only the two explanatory variables in the example, one with three levels (tubal ligation type) and the other with six levels (tube length 3 to 8 cm), there are 18 subgroups. Given a sample size of 60, there are only about three subjects, on average, with whom to calculate a preg-

nancy rate for each subgroup. If we were then to add additional variables, such as type of anastomosis and age, the situation would be even more difficult.

The general purpose of multivariate analysis is to obtain estimates of the effect of a particular explanatory variable on outcome while statistically adjusting for other explanatory variables in an efficient way. Let Y represent the outcome or dependent variable, and let X_1, X_2 X_3, and X_4 represent four explanatory or independent variables. The most commonly used multivariate model in medical research is that of *multiple linear regression*:

$$Y = b_0 = b_1X_1 + b_2X_2 + b_3X_3 + b_4X_4 \qquad (5)$$

where b_0 is the intercept that obtains when all Xs equal 0, and b_1, b_2, b_3, and b_4 are the regression coefficients of the independent variables. A particular regression coefficient (for example, b_2) represents an estimate of the slope of the relation between Y and X_2 when "all other things" (X_1, X_3, and X_4) are equal.

The difficulty with using this linear model in infertility research is that it is based on the assumption that the dependent variable is continuous and normally distributed rather than dichotomous. Use of dichotomous dependent variables such as pregnancy (yes/no) in this model has been shown to lead to inaccurate estimates of the *b* when the probability of the outcome deviates much from 50%.

Multiple logistic regression[15] is a technique that was developed in the early 1960s to handle multivariate analysis with a dichotomous dependent variable. As applied to our example, in which the dependent variable is pregnancy (yes = 1; no = 0), the logistic model specifies that the likelihood of pregnancy *P* depends on the four explanatory variables X_1, X_2, X_3, and X_4 in the following way:

$$ln\,(P/Q) = b_0 + b_1X_1 + b_2X_2 + b_3X_3 + b_4X_4, \qquad (6)$$

where $Q = I - P$. The term $ln(PQ)$ is the log odds, or logit, of pregnancy. The parameters $b_i(b_0, b_1, b_2, b_3,$ and $b_4)$ are called *logistic regression coefficients*. It can be shown that for a dichotomous independent variable X_i, the antilog of b_i is equivalent to the *odds ratio* of pregnancy attributable to X_i, controlling for all other X's. The odds ratio for a given X_i is the odds of pregnancy if X_i were present ($X_i = 1$) divided by the odds of pregnancy if X_i were absent ($X_i = 0$). Equation 6 is called a *logit model*. Expressed in terms of logit, a unit change in the variable X_i changes the logit of pregnancy ($ln\,P/Q$) by the amount of b_i.

The set of explanatory variables X_i can be dichotomous, continuous, or both. When a categorical variable contains more than two levels, such as anastomosis type, we can use dichotomous variables. Thus we might use the variable isthmic-isthmic, or "ii" (yes = 1; no = 0). This variable would be entered into the logit model and its coefficients would be interpreted in relation to the other types of anastomoses (ampullary-ampullary and isthmic-ampullary) that were not entered. A coefficient of 1.01 for ii means that women who underwent isthmic-isthmic anastomosis have a logit of pregnancy after surgical treatment that is 1.01 units higher than that for women who had other types of anastomosis. Because the antilog of 1.01 is 2.75, we conclude that the odds of pregnancy among the ii group is 2.75 times higher than that among the non-ii groups.

Using the illustrative data set, estimation of the logistic model (by means of a method of estimation called *maximum likelihood* that is beyond the present scope) yields results that can be summarized as shown in Table 53–3. Age was not found to be related to pregnancy and thus was deleted from the logistic model. The *P* value shown below each coefficient estimate represents a test of whether the coefficient is significantly different from 0. The first equation in Table 53–3 is analogous to the univariate analysis. When cautery (yes or no) is entered as the only variable to explain pregnancy success (equation 1, Table 53–3) it has a highly significant negative coefficient. This means that it is associated with a *lower* probability of pregnancy after reversal than either banding or Pomeroy tubal ligation. When type of anastomosis (ii) is added (equation 2, Table 53–3), it can be seen that the probability of pregnancy is significantly higher for isthmic-isthmic anastomosis than for isthmic-ampullary or ampullary-ampullary, controlling for ligation type. But when tubal length is added to the model (equation 3, Table 53–3), ii loses its significance, whereas tubal length enters with a strongly positive coefficient. This implies that the apparent importance of isthmic-isthmic anastomosis was mainly due to its association with tube length; when tube length was controlled for, ii was no longer important. Tubal length appears to be highly important, however, even after controlling for type of ligation and type of anastomosis. Because ii was not found to be significant after tubal length was controlled for, a final model was estimated (equation 4, Table 53–3) that excluded ii.

TABLE 53–3. LOGISTIC REGRESSION RESULTS FOR ILLUSTRATIVE DATA ON TUBAL REANASTOMOSIS (DEPENDENT VARIABLE IS CLINICAL PREGNANCY)

Independent Variables (X_i)	Estimated Logistic Coefficients*			
	Eq. 1	*Eq. 2*	*Eq. 3*	*Eq. 4*
Intercept	0.43	1.98	−0.29	−0.31
Cautery (y = 1/n = 0)	−0.77	−0.69	−0.67	−0.78
	(.02)	(.06)	(.07)	(0.05)
Isthmic-isthmic (yes = 1/no = 0)		1.01	0.18	
		(.02)	(.53)	
Tube length (cm)			0.36	0.38
			(.02)	(0.02)

*P values are in parentheses below the estimated coefficients.

An additional benefit of logistic analysis is that it provides a method for estimating the probability of an outcome given particular combinations of prognostic factors.[15] In the example, one can calculate from equation 4 and Table 53–3 that a patient who underwent sterilization by means of tubal banding and who has 6 cm of tube after anastomosis would have a logit score (S) of $0.31 - 0.78(0) + 0.38(6) = 1.97$. The probability of pregnancy in this situation is estimated to be $exp(S)/[1 + exp(S)] = exp(1.97)[1 + exp(1.97)] = 7.17/8.17 = 0.878$. Similar calculations can be made for patients with other combinations of characteristics.

Computer Software

Fortunately, once the conceptual framework for the statistical techniques is understood, calculations by hand are unnecessary. All that one needs are the raw data organized in a format that is acceptable as input into preprogrammed statistical software. Consultation with a statistician is advisable before implementing a research design so that suitable statistical methods can be chosen and so that the data can be collected in a manner appropriate for the software available at a particular site.

CLINICAL TRIALS

The standard for experimental evaluation of infertility treatment is the randomized clinical trial. In randomized trials with sufficient statistical power, unambiguous evidence may be obtained concerning the efficacy of such treatment. Critical elements of a randomized clinical trial include a clear statement of a testable hypothesis, use of a control group, randomization of subjects between treatment and control groups, recruitment of an adequate number of subjects to test the hypothesis with sufficient power, and minimization of investigator bias in collecting and analyzing data. A discussion of these elements as applied to infertility studies can be found in a recent review.[16] For the present purposes, the important issue of statistical power, which is often not considered adequately in infertility studies, is reviewed herein. This concept is illustrated with clinical trials of intracervical versus intrauterine donor insemination.

Power Analysis

Much of the emphasis in statistical tests in the medical literature concerns the *P value* (Type I error or α), which reflects the probability of falsely concluding that treatment helps. To avoid such an error, most investigators set a low *P* value, typically .05. That is, if the difference in pregnancy rates between treatment and control groups is of such magnitude that there is less than a 5% probability that the observed difference is due to chance, the risk of a Type I error is considered low enough to reject the null hypothesis. Given the small sample size in most infertility studies, however, a much more common error (Type II error or β) is failure to reject the null hypothesis when a difference between groups does, in fact, exist. Because power is $1 - \beta$, such studies are said to lack statistical power.

Power analysis is one of the most important but commonly overlooked components of clinical trial design. A difference between study groups might be observed, but the investigator might conclude that there is no statistically significant difference because the power of the study is limited because of small sample size. For example, suppose four cycles of timed IUI were to be compared with four cycles of time intercourse as treatment of male-factor infertility. Suppose further that 50 patients were to be randomized to each group and that the pregnancy rates per patient are 20% and 10% for IUI and timed intercourse. If the investigator sets the P value at .05, the power of the study, or the probability that the null hypothesis will be rejected, is only 20%. That is, despite the fact that treatment leads to a doubling of pregnancy rate, the sample size available implies that there is an 80% chance that the investigator will conclude at the end of the study that there is "no difference." In fact, one would need 169 patients in each group to detect a twofold difference in pregnancy rates between timed intercourse and IUI.

In view of these considerations, it is important to conduct a power analysis *before* a clinical trial is initiated. With available data, the investigator estimates the likely result in the control group. The treatment group result that would represent a clinically important difference is then specified, along with desired levels for the P value and power. Typically, these are set at .05 and .80 (that is, Type II error = .20), implying a value judgment that a Type I error is four times more important to avoid than a Type II error. (Arguably, one might relax P and increase power if, for example, a drug is being tested that has no side effects and is inexpensive but may provide benefit against an illness with high morbidity and cost.) The sample size in each group needed to detect a clinically important difference at the 5% level of significance with 80% power could then be estimated from standard sources, or by use of computer programs such as POWER (Epicenter Software, Pasadena, CA). Such estimates can help an investigator decide whether a study is feasible given available resources, or, in a larger study with several planned groups, they can help the investigator focus on key hypotheses and groups.

Example: Intracervical Versus Intrauterine Insemination

Different routes of artificial insemination are being used. The two most common are intracervical insemination (ICI) and IUI. Theoretically, IUI may enhance pregnancy rates because of a higher density of spermatozoa placed closer to the ovulated egg. A literature search was performed to evaluate the randomized comparative trials of ICI versus IUI.[16] The results are shown in Table 53–4. Only studies with a randomized or alternating type of treatment allocation were included, which resulted in a total of four studies, all using frozen semen.[17–20] Of these, only the study by Peters et al,[20] which contained a nonrandomized, alternating treatment schedule, did not show a significant increase in pregnancy rates between IUI and ICI. The study by

TABLE 53–4. RANDOMIZED COMPARISON TRIALS OF INTRACERVICAL (ICI) VERSUS INTRAUTERINE (IUI) INSEMINATION

| Study | Randomization | Number of Subjects (Cycles) | | Length of Study (Cycles) | Pregnancy Rates per Cycle (%) | | Cumulative Pregnancy Rates (%) | | P Value | Power to Detect Increase Over Baseline | |
		IUI	ICI		IUI	ICI	IUI	ICI		50%	100%
Byrd et al[17]	Yes	77 (238)	77 (229)	6	9.7	3.9	70.6	38.2	< .05	0.11	0.36
							(12 months)				
Patton et al[19]	Yes	28 (82)	22 (79)	6	23.0	5.1	67.9	18.2	.02	0.05	0.15
							(6 months)				
Peters et al[20]	No	13 (40)	13 (41)	4	17.5	17.1	N/A	N/A	>.05	0.10	0.32
Hurd et al[18]	Yes	39 (60)	37 (52)	10	18.6	3.9	77.0	5.4	.023	0.03	0.36
							(4 months)				

N/A, not available.
Modified from Stovall DW, Guzick DA: Clinical trials: Uses, designs, limitations. Infertil Reproduc Med Clin North Am 5:337, 1994.

Byrd et al[17] was the largest of the four. It included 154 patients and 467 cycles and used a randomized, alternating treatment allocation. Given a low control (ICI) pregnancy rate of 3.9% per cycle, however, power was still low; the probability of detecting or doubling of the ICI pregnancy rate was only 36%. Among the sample in the study by Byrd et al,[17] a significant difference in pregnancy rates between IUI and ICI of frozen sperm was found (9.7% versus 3.9%) ($P < .05$). Taken as a whole, these data[17] support the hypothesis that IUI yields higher pregnancy rates than does ICI.

SUMMARY

Certain features of infertility investigations lend themselves to particular statistical techniques. Life-table methods are useful because follow-up after treatment is often nonuniform, and logistic regression (or a similar technique) is useful because of dichotomous outcome measures such as pregnancy/nonpregnancy. The importance of sound research design before data collection is worthy of reemphasis. Valid conclusions cannot be drawn with statistical tests unless the data are based on research design that is without intrinsic bias. In this context, the importance of randomized clinical trials cannot be overstated.

REFERENCES

1. Berkson I, Gage RP: Calculation of survival rates for cancer. *Mayo Clin Proc* 25:270, 1950
2. Guzick DS, Rock JA: Estimation of a model of cumulative pregnancy following infertility therapy. *Am J Obstet Gynecol* 140:573, 1981
3. Cramer DW, Walker AM, Schiff I: Statistical methods in evaluating the outcome in infertility therapy. *Fertil Steril* 32:80, 1979
4. Guzick DS, Bross DS, Rock JA: A parametric method for comparing cumulative pregnancy curves following infertility therapy. *Fertil Steril* 37:503, 1982
5. Guzick DS, Bross D: Convenient numerical procedures for estimating cumulative pregnancy curves. *Fertil Steril* 57:85, 1992
6. Adashi EY, Rock JA, Guzick DS, et al: Fertility following bilateral ovarian wedge resection: A critical analysis of 90 consecutive cases of the polycystic ovary syndrome. *Fertil Steril* 35:320, 1981
7. Bradshaw KD, Guzick DS, Gun B, Johnson N, Ackerman GA: Cumulative pregnancy rates for donor insemination according to ovulatory functions and tubal status. *Fertil Steril* 48:1051, 1987
8. Rock JA, Chang JS, Limpaphayon K, et al: Microsurgical tubal reanastomosis: A controlled trial in four Asian centers. *Microsurgery* 5:95, 1984
9. Rock JA, Guzick DS, Katz E, Zacur HA, King TM: Tubla anastomosis: Pregnancy success following reversal of Falope ring or monopolar cautery sterilization. *Fertil Steril* 48:13, 1987
10. Guzick DS, Hinkle C, Jones HW: Cumulative clinical pregnancy rates for in vitro fertilization and embryo transfer. *Fertil Steril* 46:663, 1986
11. Olive DL, Stohs GF, Metzger DA, Franklin RR: Expectant management and hydrotumations in the treatment of endometriosis-associated infertility. *Fertil Steril* 44:35, 1985
12. Olive DL, Martin DC: Treatment of endometriosis-associated infertility with CO_2 laser laparoscopy: The use of one- and two-parameter exponential models. *Fertil Steril* 48:18, 1987
13. Mantel N: Evaluation of survival data and two new rank order statistics arising in its consideration. *Cancer Chemother Rep* 50:163, 1966
14. Breslow N: A generalized Kreuskil-Willis test for comparing K samples subject to unequal patterns of censorship. *Biometrika* 57:579, 1974
15. Schiesselman JJ: *Case Control Studies.* Oxford, England, Oxford University Press, 1982
16. Stovall DW, Guzick DS: Clinical trials: Uses, designs, limitations. *Infertil Reprod Med Clin North Am* 5:337, 1994
17. Byrd W, Bradshaw K, Carr B, et al: A prospective randomized study of pregnancy rates following intrauterine and intracervical insemination using frozen donor sperm. *Fertil Steril* 53:521, 1990
18. Hurd WW, Randolph JF Jr, Ansbacher R, et al: Comparison of intracervical, intrauterine, and intratubal techniques for donor insemination. *Fertil Steril* 59:339, 1993
19. Patton PE, Burry KA, Thurmond A, et al: Intrauterine insemination outperforms intracervical insemination in a randomized, controlled study with frozen, donor semen. *Fertil Steril* 57:559, 1992
20. Peters AJ, Hecht B, Wentz AC, et al: Comparison of the methods of artificial insemination on the incidence of conception in single unmarried women. *Fertil Steril* 59:121, 1993

INDEX

Abortion
    rate, age and, 441
    religious aspects of, 834, 837, 838, 840, 841
    spontaneous, *see* Spontaneous abortion
ABP (androgen-binding protein), 230, 232
Acetylcholine, 36
Acetyl coenzyme A, metabolic pathways leading from, to cholesterol, 225*f*
Acquired immunodeficiency syndrome (AIDS), 264, 367
Acrosomal reaction, regulation of, 238
Acrosomic vesicle, 235
Activin, 379
Adenomyoma, 190
Adenomyosis, uterine, 160
Adhesiolysis, 616
Adhesions
    dense intrauterine, color plate facing 580
    hysteroscopy and, 582–583, 584–585
    pelvic, *see* Pelvic adhesions
    prevention of, in tubal surgery by laparotomy, 625–627
Adnexal adhesions, American Fertility Society classification of, 657*f*
Adoption, 845–849, 856–857
    conception after, 37
    concurrent pursuit of medical treatment and, 846–847
    cross-cultural, 848
    expansion of support services for, 847
    family building through, 849
    issues to resolve before, 846–848
    procedure for, 848–849
    risks of, 848
    stages of, 845
    traditional versus nontraditional, 847
Adrenal 21 hydroxylase deficiency, 124
Adrenal hyperplasia, congenital, 380
AFP (α-fetoprotein), 391–392
African Americans, genetic disorders related to, 394*t*
AFS, *see* American Fertility Society

Age
    abortion rate and, 441
    changes in length of menstrual cycle with, 12*t*
    effect of, on male fertility, 440–441
    endometriosis symptoms first presented, 861*t*
    female reproductive system and, 437–440
    fertility rates and, 436–437
    maternal, *see* Maternal age
    oocytes and, 681
    outcome of IVF and GIFT by, 730*t*
    ovarian reserve status and, 10
    paternal, conception rate and, 11*f*
    process of aging, 435
    reduction in fecundity and, 11
    reproduction and, 10–12, 435–441
    and risk for spontaneous abortion, 12*t*
Agglutination inhibition, 66, 67*f*
AID (artificial insemination by donor), physician involvement in, 813–814
AIDS (acquired immunodeficiency syndrome), 264, 367
Air bubbles giving appearance of fibroid, 20*f*
Alcoholic liver disease, 264
Alcohol use, chronic, 266
Allogenic leukocyte immunotherapy, for recurrent pregnancy loss, 428
Alloimmune factors in recurrent pregnancy loss, 423–424
α-fetoprotein (AFP), 391–392
Alzheimer's disease, Down syndrome and, 438
Amenorrhea, 114–117
    differential diagnosis of, 514*f*
    evaluating causes for, 63*f*
    evaluation of, 111
    hypothalamic, *see* Hypothalamic amenorrhea
    primary, 115–116
    secondary, 115, 116–117
    types of, 115*t*

American Fertility Society (AFS)
    classification of adnexal adhesions, 657*f*
    classification of endometriosis, 193, 194*f*
    pelvic adhesion scoring method, 658*f*
American Society for Reproductive Medicine (ASRM), *see* American Fertility Society
AMH (anti-müllerian hormone), 84
Amniocentesis, 393*t*
Amygdala, 403–404
Androgen-binding protein (ABP), 230, 232
Androgen biosynthesis, 224–227
Androgen deficiency, neurologic causes of, 401–402
Androgen insensitivity, 265
Androgenization, differential diagnosis of, 516*f*
Androgen receptor, 380
Androgens in epilepsy, 400–402
Androstenedione, 224
    polycystic ovary syndrome and, 127*f*
Aneuploidy, 382, 391
    fetal, 438
Angelman's syndrome, 377, 390
Angiotensin II, 157
Anglican aspects of reproduction, 839
Anorexia nervosa, 116
Anovulation, 117–118
    hyperprolactinemia and, 160–161
    ovulatory dysfunction and, 481–482
Anticardiolipin antibody, 423
Antiendometriotic medication, 195
Antimicrosomal antibodies, 174
Anti-müllerian hormone (AMH), 84
Antinuclear antibodies, 423
Antiphospholipid antibodies, recurrent pregnancy loss and, 426*t*
Antisperm antibodies, 344
    cervical mucus–penetrating ability and, 351–352
    infertility and, 345–353
    in women, 349
Antithyroid antibodies, miscarriage and, 184
Antithyroid peroxidase antibody, 175

Anxiety, 38

Appendiceal endometriosis, 210

Artificial insemination by donor (AID), physician involvement in, 813–814

ARTs, *see* Assisted reproductive treatments

Asherman's syndrome, 452

Ashkenazi Jews, genetic disorders related to, 394*t*

Aspirin, recurrent pregnancy loss and, 426–427

ASRM, *see* American Society for Reproductive Medicine

Assisted reproduction, 40–41

Assisted reproductive treatments (ARTs), 761

  of oligospermia, 297–306

   treatment and results, 304–305

   treatment selection, 303–304

Asthenospermia, 262

Asthenozoospermia, 49

Autoantibodies, 422–423

Autodisassociation enhancement lanthanide fluoroimmunoassay (DELFIA), 75

Autoimmune factors in recurrent pregnancy loss, 422–423

Autoimmune thyroid disease, 175, 182

Autoimmunity to sperm, 346

Automated immunoassay, 74–75

Autosomal dominant disorders, 389*t*

Autosomal Mendelian disorders, 388–389

Autosomal recessive disorders, 389*t*

Avidin-biotin interaction, 71

AxSYM system, 75

Azoospermia, 48

  evaluating endocrine linkage to, 64*f*

  obstructive, diagnosis and treatment of, 277–291

AZT (zidovudine), 264

Balbiani vitelline body, 86

Basal body temperature (BBT) chart, 19–20, 22*f*

Baseline ultrasonographic scan, 468–469

BBT (basal body temperature) chart, 19–20, 22*f*

B cells, 342

Benzodiazepine receptor, peripheral (PBR), 225–226

β blockers, 180

Bicornuate uterus, 8*f*, 9*f*

Bioassays, 59–61

Biologic parentage, 816–817

Bioluminescent assays, 73–74

Biopsy instruments, 596, 597*f*

Bipolar block, 623

Bipolar coagulation, 593

Bipolar coagulator and forceps, 613

Bladder endometriosis, 215–216

Blastocysts

  development of, 672–673

  hatching of, 673–674

Blastomere biopsy, 767

Blastomeres, multinucleate, 99*f*

Blended family, 849

Body fat, 409–412

Body weight, 409

  clomiphene citrate and, 414*f*

  ideal (IBW), 412–413

  reproduction and, 409–414

Braxton-Hicks contractions, 462

Breast budding, 112

Breast examination, prolactin and, 163*t*

Bromocriptine

  hyperprolactinemia and, 160

  pharmacology of, 559–562

  prolactin and, 558–559

  structural formula of, 558*f*

  in unexplained infertility, 331, 332*f*

Buddhist aspects of reproduction, 840–841

Buserelin

  chemical structure of, 197*t*

  high-density lipoprotein levels with, 196*f*

CA 125, 194

Cabergoline, 165, 557*t*, 563

  structural formula of, 562*f*

Calcitonin, prolactin and, 156

Calcium channel blockers, 663

Calmodulin, 539

cAMP (cyclic adenosine 3',5'-monophosphate), 223

Capillary tube mucus penetration test, 16

Cap phase of spermiogenesis, 235

Carbon dioxide

  fallopian tube insufflation with, 16

  in hysteroscopy, 576

Carbon dioxide lasers, 633–635, 660

Carbon disulfide, 266

Catecholamines, 35

Catechol compounds, structure of, 411*f*

CCCT (clomiphene citrate challenge test), 437

CCOF (chromosomally competent ovarian failure), 377

CD8+ lymphocytes, 419

CD56+ cells, 419, 423–424

Centromeres, 84

Cervical cannula, 596

Cervical factors

  iatrogenically induced, 515

  in infertility, 7

Cervical mucus, 343

  ferning pattern of, 14*f*

Cervical mucus-penetrating ability, antisperm antibodies and, 351–352

Cervical mucus penetration test, 16*f*

Cervix

  effect of age on, 440

  normal, 448

Cetrorelix, 709

Chemiluminescent assays, 72–74

Chiari–Frommel syndrome, 156

Chi-square test, 881

Chlamydial infection, 7

Chlamydia trachomatis, 363–364, 366

Chocolate cyst, 452, color plate facing 460

Cholesterol

  formation of pregnenolone from, 227*f*

  metabolic pathways leading from acetyl coenzyme A to, 225*f*

  polycystic ovary syndrome and, 128*f*

Chorionic gonadotropin, human, *see* hCG *entries*

Chorionic villus sampling, 393*t*

Christian aspects of reproduction, 837–839

Chromogranin-B, 158

Chromosomal abnormalities, 391–392

  by maternal age, 13*t*

Chromosomal analysis

  of preimplantation embryos, 721*t*

  recurrent pregnancy loss and, 418*t*, 420

Chromosomally competent ovarian failure (CCOF), 377

Chromosomally incompetent ovarian failure (CIOF), 374

Cigarette smoking, *see* Smoking

CIOF (chromosomally incompetent ovarian failure), 374

Circannual rhythm in sperm count, 23*f*

Circhoral secretion, 113

c-kit-KL ligand system, 86

Cleft lip and palate, 394

CLIA (Clinical Laboratory Improvement Act), 54–55

Clinical decisions about diagnostic tests, 327–330

Clinical Laboratory Improvement Act (CLIA), 54–55

Clinical trials, infertility data and, 883–885

Clomid, *see* Clomiphene citrate

Clomiphene citrate, 496, 564

  administration, 497–499

  adverse effects of, 500–502

  anovulatory response, 499*f*, 500*f*

  body weight and, 414*f*

  conception and, 499*t*

  conception failure and, 499–500

  conception rates with, 500

  contraindications for, 497

  developmental landmarks of, 496*f*

  dose effects of, 498*t*

  establishment of dosage for, 498–499

  hormonal monitoring of, 498*f*

indications for, 497
in vitro fertilization and, 706
in luteal-phase deficiency, 149
in male infertility, 271
monitoring, 497–498
multiple pregnancies and, 500
ovarian cancer and, 501–502
ovulation failure and, 499
ovulation initiation with, 495–502
ovulation rates with, 500
pharmacology, 496–497
polycystic ovary syndrome and, 130
stereochemical isomers of, 496*f*
structural formula of, 496*f*
treatment with, 63
in unexplained infertility, 332–333
Clomiphene citrate challenge test (CCCT), 437
CMV infection, 367
Co-culture systems, embryo, 720–721
COH, *see* Controlled ovarian hyperstimulation
Coherence, 629
Complement-fixation assay, 66, 67*f*
Complement system, 347–348
Conception
    after adoption, 37
    clomiphene citrate and, 499*t*
    cycles to, sperm motility and, 255*t*
    human menopausal gonadotropin and, 509*t*
Conception failure, clomiphene citrate and, 499–500
Conception rate
    intercourse frequency and, 12*f*
    paternal age and, 11*f*
Consent, informed, 811
Consent form for laparoscopy, 593*f*
Constitutional dimensions of reproduction, 807–808
Contact hysteroscope, 574, 575*f*
Continuous variables, 877
Controlled ovarian hyperstimulation (COH), 310, 471, 680, 689–690
    endometrial effects of, 680
Conversion factors for hormones, 62*t*
Cornual anastomosis, 617–619
Cornual occlusion
    bilateral, 21*f*
    pathologic, 616–617
Corpus luteum, 113, 136, color plate facing 460
Corpus luteum function, evaluation of, 137*f*
Cortical granules, 87
Corticotropin-releasing factor (CRF), 35
Counseling
    genetic, *see* Genetic counseling
    for intracytoplasmic single-sperm injection, 753
    long-term, 38
    in unexplained infertility, 334–335
CPAs (cryoprotective agents), 794

CRF (corticotropin-releasing factor), 35
Cross-cultural adoption, 848
Cryopreservation, 793–803
    in animal reproduction, 795–796
    concepts in, 794
    of embryos, 722–723, 799–801
    ethical issues in, 802–803
    historical overview of, 793–794
    legal considerations for, 811–812
    of spermatozoa, 796–799
    sperm function and, 796–797
Cryopreserved embryos, supernumerary, fate of, 801
Cryoprotective agents (CPAs), 794
Cryptorchidism, 263
Culdocentesis, 360, 648
Cumulus oocyte complexes, 89*f,* 91
Cumulus oophorus, 84, 463
CV205–502, 165
Cycle, *see* Menstrual cycle
Cyclic adenosine 3′,5′-monophosphate (cAMP), 223
Cyclin degradation, 94
Cyclosporine, 266
Cyproheptadine, 157
Cyproterone acetate, 131
Cytochalasin, 97–98
Cytochrome P450 enzyme group, 379
Cytogenetic abnormalities, 381
Cytoplasmic droplets, 52–53
Cytoplasmic vesicles, 86
Cytotrophoblasts, 673

Danazol, 195–196
    chemical structure of, 195*f*
    high-density lipoprotein levels with, 196*f*
    in unexplained infertility, 332
DBI (diazepam-binding inhibitor), 225–226
Decidua, 676
Decidua basalis, 676
Decidualization, structure of uterus and, 676–678
Dehydroepiandrosterone sulfate (DHEAS), 162
    normal ranges of, 62*t*
DELFIA (autodisassociation enhancement lanthanide fluoroimmunoassay), 75
Deoxyribonucleic acid, *see* DNA *entries*
Dependent variable, 877
DES, *see* Diethylstilbestrol
Determinants, 342
Dexon, 659
Dextran, 626, 663
Dextran-coated charcoal, 69
Dextrose 5% in water, 576
DHEAS, *see* Dehydroepiandrosterone sulfate
Diagnostic tests, clinical decisions about, 327–330

Diakinesis state of meiosis, 88
Dianette, 131
Diathermy, ovarian, 130–131
Diazepam-binding inhibitor (DBI), 225–226
Dibromochloropropane, 266
Dichotomous variables, 877
Dictuate or dictyotene stage of meiotic prophase, 84
Dietary history, 6
Diethylstilbestrol (DES), 451–452
    exposure, hysterosalpingogram of, 6*f*
Dieting, 412
Dimethylsulfoxide (DMSO), 95
Dioxin, endometriosis and, 868–869
Diplotene stage of meiotic prophase, 84
Distention media in hysteroscopy, 575–577
DMSO (dimethylsulfoxide), 95
DNA (deoxyribonucleic acid), 371–372
    recombinant, 373
DNA analysis, 372–374
DNA fingerprint, 373
DNA probes, 366–367
DNA replication, 372
Dominant disorders
    autosomal, 389*t*
    X-linked, 390
Donor insemination, pregnancy rates for, 11*f*
Dopamine, 35
    prolactin secretion and, 156
    structure of, 411*f*
Dopamine agonists
    hyperprolactinemia and, 557
    infertility treatment with, 557–565
    normoprolactinemic infertility and, 564–565
    polycystic ovary syndrome and, 565
Doppler velocimetry, 448, 475, 477–483
    of ovarian circulation, 480–483
    of uterine circulation, 477–480
Double decidual sac sign, 475, 476*f*
Down syndrome, 392, 441
    Alzheimer's disease and, 438
Doxycycline, 272
Dynamic instability, 96

Eastern Orthodox aspects of reproduction, 838–839
Ectopic pregnancy, 644–645, 678
    causes of, 645*t*
    clinical features, 645–649
    diagnosing by history and physical examination, 646*t*
    diagnosis and management of, 643–652
    etiology, 645
    hysterectomy and, 649
    laboratory studies, 646–647
    laparoscopy and, 648
    management of, 606–608

Ectopic pregnancy (*cont.*)
  methotrexate and, 651
  misdiagnoses of, 644*t*
  operations for, 610
  rate of, 644*f*
  salpingectomy and, 649
  salpingotomy for, 607–608
  second, management of, 650–651
  signs and symptoms, 645–646
  sites and incidence of, 644*f*
  surgical technique, 651–652
  tubal milking and, 649
  after tubal operations, 645*t*
  ultrasonography of, 647–648
EGF (epidermal growth factor), 94
Egg-penetration test, 350–351
Egg–sperm recognition, mechanisms of,
    239–240
EIAs (enzyme immunoassays), 70–71
Ejaculatory abstinence time, 46
Ejaculatory duct, obstruction of, 290
Ejaculatory dysfunction, 266–267
Electrocauterization, 660
Electromagnetic spectrum, 633*f*
ELISA (enzyme-linked immunosorbent
    assay), 70
Embryo biopsy, 734
Embryo co-culture systems, 720–721
Embryo culture
  culture environment for, 717
  culture medium for, 716–717
  in vitro fertilization and, 716–725
  oocyte collection and maturation in,
    717–718
  sperm preparation and insemination in,
    718–719
Embryo development, transfer, and freezing
    in intracytoplasmic single-sperm in-
    jection, 755–756
Embryo donation, legal considerations for,
    812
Embryo freezing, 794
Embryo implantation site, 146*f*
Embryonic aneuploidy, 382
Embryo quality, assessment of, 720
Embryos
  cryopreservation of, 722–723, 799–801
  cryopreserved, supernumerary, fate of, 801
  excess, 809–811
  moral status of, 826
  nidation of, 671
  parthenogenetic, 98
  preimplantation
    chromosomal analysis of, 721*t*
    lasers in micromanipulation of, 638–639
  uterine interactions with, during implanta-
    tion, 671–682

Embryotoxic factors, 427–428
Embryotoxicity assay, 424
Embryo transfers, 809
  guided by ultrasound, 474
  for in vitro fertilization, 723–725
  in ovum donation, 786
  pregnancy rate by number of, 731*t*
  transcervical, *see* In vitro fertilization
EMIT (enzyme multiple-immunoassay tech-
    nique), 71
Emotional aspects of infertility, 25, 29–41
  effects of, 34–37
  in evaluation, 30–31
  infertility therapy and, 32, 33
  for men, 31–32
  for women, 31
Emotions, fertility and, 30
Empty follicle syndrome, 467, 716
Empty sella syndrome, 161
Endocoagulator, 594, 595*f*
Endocrine testing in infertility, 59–75
  bioassays, 59–61
Endocrinology
  of female infertility, 81–184
  reproductive, 377–381
Endometrial biopsy, 20–21, 22*f*
  in luteal phase, 145–147
  recurrent pregnancy loss and, 421
  for unexplained infertility, 329
Endometrial cavity, hysteroscopic view of,
    color plate facing 580
Endometrial–cervical infertility of infectious
    causation, 364–365
Endometrial cysts, 192
Endometrial dating, 147*f*
Endometrial echo patterns, 714
Endometrial preparation, hormone require-
    ments for, 680–681
Endometrial receptivity
  clinical assessment of, 678–680
  evaluation of, 420–421
  uterine perfusion and, 479
Endometrial surface, 675
Endometrial thickness, 460
  as implantation predictor, 460–462
Endometriomas, 204
  management of, 207–208
  ovarian, 192
  resection of, 604*f*, 605*f*
Endometriosis, 189–216, 546, 704–705
  age and, 861*t*
  American Fertility Society classification
    of, 193, 194*f*
  appendiceal, 210
  bladder, 215–216
  chart of evaluation for, 203
  chart of management of, 189
  coping with, 866–867
  deep, 191*f*
  delayed diagnosis of, 860–862

  diagnosis of, 193–194
  dioxin and, 868–869
  emotional issues associated with, 865*t*
  factors in infertility in patients with, 206*t*
  flow chart of management of, 190*f*
  of genitourinary tract, 214–216
  GnRH agonists and, 197, 546
  hazard rate and, 879*f*
  hysterectomy for, 208–209
  impact of, 864*t*
  infertility and, 546
  infiltrative, laparoscopic management of,
    210–212
  interruption of pelvic nerves for pain relief
    in, 208
  intestinal, 209–214
  laparoscopic assessment of, 199
  laparoscopic laser cauterization with, 207*f*
  laparoscopic view of, 198, 205
  LH and, 192*f*
  mechanisms of infertility associated with,
    206*t*
  medical treatment, 194–197
    of infertility associated with, 197–200
  minimal, intrauterine insemination with,
    191*f*
  myths about, 865*t*
  operations for, 609–610
  ovarian, 191*f*
  ovarian dysfunction and, 192
  pain and disability of, 862–864
  pathophysiology of, 190–193
  patient perspective on, 859–869
  pelvic adhesions in, 192
  pelvic pain with, 204
  peritoneal, *see* Peritoneal endometriosis
  potential mechanisms of, 192–193
  presentation of, 204–206
  prevalence of, 190
  progestogens and, 195
  psychosocial aspects of, 864–866
  of small intestine, 212
  surgical treatment, 200, 203–216
  symptoms of, 862*t*
  techniques for management of,
    602–605
  tubal dysfunction and, 192–193
  ultrasound and, 452–455
  vaporization of, 636
Endometriosis Association, 867–868
Endometrium, 136–138, 676
  abnormal, 419
  menstrual cycle and, 458–460
  ultrasonography of, 421–422
Endoplasmic reticulum (ER), 86
Endorphins, 35
Enhancers, 372
Enzyme immunoassays (EIAs), 70–71
Enzyme-linked immunosorbent assay
    (ELISA), 70

Enzyme multiple-immunoassay technique (EMIT), 71
Epidermal growth factor (EGF), 94
Epididymal transit, 237
Epididymis
 freeing, 287*f*
 sperm maturation in, 237–238
 transection of, 281*f*
 vasectomy effects on, 280–282
 vasogram of, 286*f*
Epididymo-orchitis, 263
Epilepsy, 398
 androgens in, 400–402
 estradiol and, 402
 reproductive dysfunction and, 398–399
Epinephrine, 34
 structure of, 411*f*
Epitopes, 342
ER (endoplasmic reticulum), 86
Ergocornine, 558
Estradiol
 absolute level of, 712
 delivery, transdermal, 782–783
 epilepsy and, 402
 ethinyl, 131
 in menstrual cycle, 140*f*
 normal ranges of, 62*t*
Estradiol 17β, 93
Estrogen receptor, 380–381
Estrogens, 37
 assay of, 269
Ethical issues
 in cryopreservation, 802–803
 in infertility, 823–828
 in ovum donation, 789–790
 role-based responsibilities and, 825–826
Ethinyl estradiol, 131
Exercise history, 6
Explanted oocytes, 95

Fallopian tube infertility, 360–364
 antimicrobial therapy for, 362
 clinical follow-up care, 362–364
 Gainesville staging of, 361*t*
 microbiologic evaluation of, 365–367
 pathophysiology, 360–361
 therapeutic staging of, 361–362
Fallopian tubes
 effect of age on, 440
 function of, 16
 insufflation with carbon dioxide, 16
Family history taking, 394
Fat, body, 409–412
Fecundability rate, 436
Fecundity, reduction in, age and, 11
Female-factor infertility
 hyperthyroidism and, 177
 surgical treatment of, 573–666

Female infertility
 endocrinology of, 81–184
 hormonal treatment of, 495–565
 ultrasound and, 448–467
Female reproductive dysfunction, neurologic considerations of, 402–405
Female reproductive system, age and, 437–440
Females, *see* Women *entries*
Female subfertility, sperm count and, 258–259
Ferning pattern of cervical mucus, 14*f*
Fertility
 defined, 4
 emotions and, 30
 humoral immunity and, 193
 male, effect of age on, 440–441
 after vasoepididymostomy, 285–287
Fertility-preserving management, 650
Fertility rates, 436
 age and, 436–437
Fertilization, 673
 in vitro, *see* In vitro fertilization
 in in vitro fertilization, 719–720
Fertilization techniques, assisted, 751–756
Fetal aneuploidy, 438
Fetal ovarian development, 112
Fetal research, 808–809
Fetal tachycardia, 180
Fetal thyroid development, 171–172
Fetus, color plate facing 460
 moral status of, 826
FIA (fluorescence immunoassay), 72
Fibrinolytic agents, 663
Fibrioplasty, 621, 622*f*, 625
Fibroids
 air bubbles giving appearance of, 20*f*
 hysteroscopy and, 584, 585–586
 submucous, color plate facing 580
 uterine, *see* Uterine fibroids
 uterine cavity distorted by, 7*f*, 8*f*
Fibrous lattice, 86
Finasteride, 132
FISH (fluorescent in situ hybridization), 735–736, 769
Flow cytometry, 346
Flow velocity waveforms (FVWs), 475, 477
Flunitrazepan, 225
Fluorescence, 631
Fluorescence assay, 71–72
Fluorescence immunoassay (FIA), 72
Fluorescence-polarization immunoassay (FPIA), 72
Fluorescent in situ hybridization (FISH), 735–736, 769
Flutamide, 131
Folic acid, 392
Follicle-enclosed oocytes, in vitro growth of, 94–95

Follicles, resting, 85*f*
Follicle-stimulating hormone (FSH), 34, 508, 526
 clinical studies, 528–533
 in GnRH therapy, 197*f*
 with human chorionic gonadotropin as surrogate luteinizing hormone surge, 531–532
 microheterogeneity of, 510*t*
 normal ranges of, 62*t*
 ovulation induction with, 525–533
 ovulatory cycle after administration of low dose of, 530*f*
 physiology of, 527–528
 primary structure of, 526*t*
 production, 508
 recombinant (rFSH), 526, 710
 Sertoli cells and, 229–231
 structure and pharmacology, 526–527
 urinary, for in vitro fertilization, 532–533
Follicle stimulation protocols in gamete intrafallopian transfer, 690*t*
Follicular development, 512–514
 during gestation, 84–85
Follicular dominance, 514
Follicular growth
 induction of, 705–711
 ultrasound and, 469–470
Follicular phase of menstrual cycle, 113–114
 events in, 139–141
Follicular rescue, 512
Follicular selection, 513–514
Follicular volume, 464
Folliculogenesis, 81–85
FPIA (fluorescence-polarization immunoassay), 72
FSH, *see* Follicle-stimulating hormone
FVWs (flow velocity waveforms), 475, 477

GABA (γ-aminobutyric acid), 156
Gainesville staging of Fallopian tube infertility, 361*t*
Galactorrhea, 6
Galactosemia, 377
Galanin, 158
GalTase, 239
Gamete donation, 856
Gamete intrafallopian transfer (GIFT), 334, 587, 687–700, 751
 comparison of annual U.S. and Canadian procedure outcomes, 696*t*
 diagnoses among patients of, 689*t*
 follicle stimulation protocols in, 690*t*
 modifications of, 699–700
 oocyte retrieval for, 691–693
 outcome by age, 730*t*
 outcome in United States, 728*t*
 patient selection for, 688–689

Gamete intrafallopian transfer (GIFT) (*cont.*)
  results of, 696–699
    sperm collection and preparation for, 691
    transfer catheter loading for, 693–696
    ultrasound-guided, 474
Gametes, 391
  micromanipulation of, 730–734
  moral status of, 826
  preimplantation, lasers in micromanipulation of, 638–639
Gamete uterine transfer (GUT), 474, 696
Gametogenesis, 81–85
γ-aminobutyric acid (GABA), 156
γ-tubulin, 96
GAP (GnRH-associated peptide), 157, 377–378
Gap junctions, 85
Genes in reproduction, 374–377
Gene structure, 371–372
Genetic analysis, 734–736
Genetic aspects of in vitro fertilization, 721–722
Genetic counseling, 388
  principles of, 392–395
Genetic diagnosis, preimplantation, *see* Preimplantation genetic diagnosis
Genetic issues in reproduction, 387–395
Genetic risk, estimation of, 394–395
Genetics, medical, 387
Genital tract obstruction in male infertility, 266
Genitourinary tract, endometriosis of, 214–216
Germ cells, 233
  Sertoli cells and, interrelationships of, 231*f*, 232
Germinal aplasia, 263
Germinal cells, leukocytes and, 53
Germinal vesicle, 86
Gestation, follicular development during, 84–85
Gestational surrogacy, 788–789
Gestational transient thyrotoxicosis (GTT), 178, 179
Gestations, multiple, ultrasound and, 472
Gestrinone, 196–197
GH, *see* Growth hormone
GIFT, *see* Gamete intrafallopian transfer
Girls
  neonatal and prepubertal, 112
  pubertal events in, 112*t*
Glucocorticoids in male infertility, 271–272
Glycine, 577
GnRH (gonadotropin-releasing hormone), 377, 538
  agonists
    in assisted reproduction, 547–550

comparison between long and short protocols with, 548–549
  endometriosis and, 197, 546
  in in vitro fertilization, 708*t*
  miscarriage and, 550
  myoma and, 546–547
  ovarian hyperstimulation syndrome and, 549–550
  in ovulation induction, 707–708
  protocols for, 708–709
agonist stimulation test, 437–438
antagonists, 709–710
chemical structure of, 197*t*
deficiency, congenital, 271
in menstrual cycle, 540–543
ovulation induction with pulsatile, 537–551
pharmacology of, 539–540
physiology of, 538–543
prolactin and, 157
pump therapy, 543–546
secretion, limbic structures and, 401*f*
structural formula of, 539*f*
structure of decapeptide, 541*f*
test, 270
therapy, LH and FSH in, 197*f*
GnRH-associated peptide (GAP), 157, 377–378
GnRH/GAP gene, 377–378
Goldman perimetry, 165
Golgi apparatus, 86, 235
Golgi phase of spermiogenesis, 235
Gomel irrigator, 613
Gonadal mosaicism, 390
Gonadotropin
  human chorionic, *see* hCG *entries*
  human menopausal, *see* hMG *entries*
Gonadotropin assay, 269
Gonadotropin deficiency, 270–271
Gonadotropin genes, 378–379
Gonadotropin production, steps of, 511*t*
Gonadotropin-releasing hormone, *see* GnRH *entries*
Gonadotropin secretion, sleep-associated, 113*f*
Gonadotropin therapy
  monitoring of, 518
  selection of patients for, 514–516
Gonads, neural innervation of, 403
Gonocytes, 234
Gore-Tex surgical membrane, 664–665
Graafian follicles, 36, 113
Granins, 158
Graspers, 596, 597*f*
Graves' disease, 178–180, 181
Group therapy, 38
Growth hormone (GH)
  in vitro fertilization and, 710–711
  meiotic competence and, 90, 90*f*
GTT (gestational transient thyrotoxicosis), 178, 179

Guilt, 31, 32
GUT (gamete uterine transfer), 474, 696

Habitual abortion, *see* Recurrent pregnancy loss
Hamou microcolpohysteroscope, 574–575
Hashimoto's thyroiditis, 175, 181
Hatching
  assisted, 734
  of blastocysts, 673–674
Hazard rate, endometriosis and, 879*f*
hCG (human chorionic gonadotropin), 173, 508
  administration of
    optimum timing of, 549
    timing of, 470
  doubling times of, 647*t*
  with follicle-stimulating hormone as surrogate luteinizing hormone surge, 531–532
  maternal, during pregnancy, 173*f*
  monitoring of β titers, 648
hCG levels, male, 222–223
HDL, *see* High-density lipoprotein
Healing process, 656–657
Height and weight table for women, 412*t*
HelpLine, RESOLVE, 855
Hemorrhagic ovarian cyst, 190
Heparin, recurrent pregnancy loss and, 427
Herniorrhaphy, inguinal disruption of vas deferens after, 289
Heteroplasmy, 391
High-density lipoprotein levels, with buserelin and danazol, 196*f*
Hindu aspects of reproduction, 839–840
Hirsutism, 64
Histamine, 157
HIV (human immunodeficiency virus) infection, 264, 367
hMG (human menopausal gonadotropin), 333
  chemistry, clearance, and physiology, 510–512
  conception and, 509*t*
  congenital malformations with, 519–520
  historical perspectives, 508–509
  hyperstimulation, classification of, 519*t*
  in vitro fertilization and, 706–707
  long-term safety with, 520–521
  ovulation induction with, 507–521
  primary structure of, 526*t*
  results of treatment, 518–521
Homeobox genes, 382
Horizontal transmission, 389
Hormonal treatment of female infertility, 495–565
Hormone requirements for endometrial preparation, 680–681

Hormones, conversion factors for, 62*t*

Hormone testing, laboratory, indications for, 61–65

Hot flushes, 500

HSG, *see* Hysterosalpingography

Human chorionic gonadotropin, *see* hCG *entries*

Human Genome Project, 387, 761

Human immunodeficiency virus (HIV) infection, 264, 367

Human menopausal gonadotropin, *see* hMG *entries*

Humoral immunity, fertility and, 193

Hyaluronic acid, 664

HY antigen, 375

HyCoSy (hysterosalpingo-contrast-sonography), 458

Hydatidiform mole, 382–383

Hydergine, 557*t*, 564

Hydroflotation, 609

2-Hydroxyestrone, structure of, 411*f*

Hyperandrogenism
    hypothalamic-pituitary dysfunction associated with, 515–516
    polycystic ovary syndrome and, 131–132

Hyperemesis gravidarum, 179

Hyperprolactinemia, 124, 156
    anovulation and, 160–161
    bromocriptine and, 160
    diagnosis of, 162–164
    dopamine agonists and, 557
    evaluation for, 559
    functional, 161
    hypothyroidism and, 162
    in infertility, 160–162
    intermittent, 161–162
    management of, 164–165
    medical management of, 559
    natural history of, 165
    stress and, 35–36

Hyperspermia, 47

Hyperstimulated ovary, color plate

Hyperthyroidism, 177–180
    clinical features of, 178*t*
    female-factor infertility and, 177
    male-factor infertility and, 177
    neonatal, 180–181
    preconception planning with, 182
    pregnancy and, 178–180
    subclinical, 177

Hypoestrogenism, 412

Hypogonadism, 263, 401

Hypogonadotropic-hypogonadal syndrome, 61

Hypogonadotropic hypogonadism, 263–264

Hypogonadotropic hypopituitarism, 255

Hypoplastic uterine corpus, 425

Hypospermia, 47

Hypothalamic amenorrhea, 116*f*

follicle-stimulating hormone for ovulation induction in, 528–529

Hypothalamic-pituitary axis, 156–157

Hypothalamic-pituitary dysfunction associated with hyperandrogenism, 515–516

Hypothalamic-pituitary-gonadal axis, 61

Hypothalamic-pituitary insufficiency, 514

Hypothalamic-pituitary-ovarian feedback, 112

Hypothalamus, 397
    effect of age on, 439–440

Hypothyroidism, 173–177
    clinical features of, 173*t*
    diagnosis, 173–174
    hyperprolactinemia and, 162
    infertility and, 174–175
    maternal, 172
    neonatal, 180
    preconception planning with, 182
    pregnancy and, 175–177
    prepubertal, 174
    subclinical, 173
    TSH and, 174

Hypoxanthine, 92

Hyskon, 576, 663

Hysterectomy
    ectopic pregnancy and, 649
    for endometriosis, 208–209

Hysterosalpingo-contrast-sonography (HyCoSy), 458

Hysterosalpingogram of diethylstilbestrol exposure, 6*f*

Hysterosalpingography (HSG), 16–18, 450, 451
    hysteroscopy and, 580–581

Hysteroscopic myomectomy, 585–586

Hysteroscopy, 14, 573–587
    adhesions and, 582–583, 584–585
    ancillary instruments for, 577
    combined laparoscopy and, 581
    complications of, 578–580
    contraindications to, 578
    diagnostic, 580
    distention media in, 575–577
    fibroids and, 584, 585–586
    findings in, 581–583
    hysterosalpingography and, 580–581
    infertility and, 580
    instruments for, 574–577
    lasers and, 637–638
    operative, 584–587
    polyps and, 581–582, 584
    potential therapeutic applications of, 587
    recurrent pregnancy loss and, 580
    relevance of lesions detected at, 583–584
    technique for, 577–578
    uterine perforation by, 579
    uterine septa and, 584, 586–587

Hysterosonography, 18

Ice formation, intracellular, 722

ICI (intracervical insemination), intrauterine insemination versus, 884–885

ICSI, *see* Intracytoplasmic single-sperm injection

Ideal body weight (IBW), 412–413

Idiopathic infertility, 39–40

IEF (isoelectrofocusing), 527

IFMA (immunofluorometric assay), 72

IGF-1, *see* Insulin-like growth factor-1

Iliac vessels, laparoscopic view of, 449*f*

Immotile-cilia syndrome, 266

Immune complement, 347–348

Immune response, overview of, 342*f*

Immunities to spermatozoa, *see* Immunology

Immunoassays, 60–61
    automated, 74–75
    labeled-antibody, 68–69
    labeled-hormone, 68
    luminescent, 71–74
    nonlabeled, 66–68
    tag-labeled, 68

Immunobead binding, 346, 347*f*, 347*t*

Immunochemical reaction, 65–66

Immunofluorometric assay (IFMA), 72

Immunoglobulins, 342–345
    detection of, on sperm surface, 345
    present in reproductive tract, 343–344
    regulation of secretion of, in reproductive tract, 343
    structure of, 342*f*

Immunoinhibitory substance, 355

Immunology (immunities to spermatozoa), 341–355
    cause of, 353–355
        among women, 355
    evaluation of, 341
    experimental induction of infertility by, 344–345
    frequency of, 345*t*
    sperm production and, 353–355

Immunoradiometric assay (IRMA), 68

Immunotherapy for recurrent pregnancy loss, 426–428

Implantation, 764
    embryo–uterine interactions during, 671–682
    mechanisms of, 672
    stages of, 673–676

Implantation predictor, endometrial thickness as, 460–462

Imprinting, 390

Independent variables, 877

Infections, 359–368
    evaluation of, 359
    viral, reproduction and, 367

Infertile couple, 825
    approach to initial infertility investigation, 5–13
    basic tests for, 13–27

Infertile couple (*cont.*)
  choosing best treatment for, 18*t*
  concept of, as unit, 5
  diagnostic evaluation of, 3–25
    chart for, 3
  final steps in evaluation of, 23–25
  Jewish evaluation of, 829–830
  physical examination for, 13
  physicians and, 33–34
  proportion of, with unexplained infertility, 325*t*
  psychologic treatment of, 37–39
Infertility
  antisperm antibodies and, 345–353
  approach to initial investigation of, 5–13
  basic tests for, 13–27
  cervical factors in, 7
  crisis of, 32–33
  defined, 4, 823–824
  dopamine agonists and, 557–565
  duration of, pregnancy rate and, 331*f*
  emotional aspects of, *see* Emotional aspects of infertility
  endocrine testing in, *see* Endocrine testing in infertility
  endometrial–cervical, of infectious causation, 364–365
  endometriosis-associated, *see* Endometriosis
  ethical issues in, 823–828
  evaluation of, 3–75
    chart for, 3
  experimental induction of, by immunology, 344–345
  fallopian tube, *see* Fallopian tube infertility
  female, *see* Female infertility
  female-factor, *see* Female-factor infertility
  history of investigation of, 324
  hyperprolactinemia in, *see* Hyperprolactinemia
  hypothyroidism and, 174–175
  hysteroscopy and, 580
  idiopathic, 39–40
  incidence of, 4
  legal aspects of, 807–818
  male, *see* Male infertility
  male-factor, *see* Male-factor infertility
  molecular genetics and, 371–383
  neurologic considerations in, 397–405
  ovulatory factors in, 6
  pelvic adhesions and, *see* Pelvic adhesions
  peritoneal factors in, 6–7
  polycystic ovary syndrome and, 130–131
  prevalence of, 4
  psychogenic, 37
  psychoneuroendocrinology of, 34–36

reaction to, 33
specific categories of, 323–441
stress effects in, 40
ultrasound in, 447–485
unexplained, *see* Unexplained infertility
uterine factors in, 7
uterine perfusion and, 478–480
Infertility care, general principles of, 4–5
Infertility data
  clinical trials and, 883–885
  special features of, 876–877
  statistical analysis of, 875–885
Infertility therapy
  emotional aspects of infertility and, 32, 33
  length of, 30
  persistence in, 25
Informed consent, 811
Inheritance
  Mendelian patterns of, 388–390
  mitochondrial, 391
  multifactorial, 392
  patterns of, 388–392
  Y-linked, 390
Inhibin, 231–232, 379
  in menstrual cycle, 140*f*
Insemination, therapeutic
  by donor, *see* Therapeutic insemination by donor
  with husband's sperm, *see* Therapeutic insemination with husband's sperm
Insufflator, 592–593, 594*f*
Insulin, hypersecretion of, 126–128
Insulin concentration, menstrual cycles and, 127*f*
Insulin-like growth factor-1 (IGF-1), 94, 232
  system, 513
Integrins, 422, 675
Integrin $\alpha v\beta 3$, 138
Interceed, 664–665
Intercourse frequency, conception rate and, 12*f*
Intermenstrual intervals, 114
Intestinal adhesions, lysis of, 209
Intestinal endometriosis, 209–214
Intestine, small, endometriosis of, 212
Intracellular ice formation, 722
Intracervical insemination (ICI), intrauterine insemination versus, 884–885
Intracytoplasmic single-sperm injection (ICSI), 733–734, 752
  clinical evaluation of, 752–756
  embryo development, transfer, and freezing in, 755–756
  obstetric outcome, prenatal diagnosis, and follow-up study with children of, 756
  oocyte damage after, 755
  oocyte handling for, 753–754
  ovarian stimulation for, 753–754
  patient selection and counseling for, 753

  procedure for, 754–755
  semen evaluation and preparation for, 754
Intradecidual sign, 475, 476*f*
Intrafallopian transfer
  gamete, *see* Gamete intrafallopian transfer
  zygote, *see* Zygote intrafallopian transfer
Intratubal insemination, 699–700
Intrauterine contraceptive device (IUD), ultrasound and, 452
Intrauterine insemination (IUI), 191, 304
  infectious complications of, 367
  intracervical insemination versus, 884–885
  with minimal endometriosis, 191*f*
  unexplained infertility and, 333–334
Intrauterine polyp, 10*f*
Intrauterine synechiae, 6*f*
Intravenous immunoglobulin (IVIg) therapy, 424, 427, 428–429
Intrinsic aging, 435
In vitro fertilization (IVF), 40–41, 298, 304–305, 703–736, 751, 774, 808
  clinical pregnancy and delivery rates, 729*t*
  clomiphene citrate and, 706
  embryo culture and, 716–725
  embryo transfer in, 723–725
  fertilization in, 719–720
  genetic aspects of, 721–722
  GnRH agonists for ovarian stimulation in, 547–550, 708*t*
  growth hormone and, 710–711
  human menopausal gonadotropin and, 706–707
  legal considerations for, 811
  lessons from, 680
  luteal phase, 725–727
  oocyte retrieval for, 715–716
  outcome by age, 730*t*
  outcome in United States, 728*t*
  patient selection for, 704–705
  progesterone levels and, 713
  quality assurance in, 814–815
  record-keeping and confidentiality in, 815–816
  results and outcome, 727–730
  unexplained infertility and, 334
  urinary follicle-stimulating hormone for, 532–533
In vitro maturation of oocytes, 723
In vitro sperm migration tests, 15–16
Iodide during pregnancy, 173
Ionization, 632
IRMA (immunoradiometric assay), 68
Islamic aspects of reproduction, 834–837
Iso-B-prolactin, 162
Isoelectrofocusing (IEF), 527
Isojima test, 348
Isolation, 32
IUD, *see* Intrauterine contraceptive device
IUI, *see* Intrauterine insemination

---

t indicates table; *f* indicates figure

IVF, *see* In vitro fertilization
IVIg (intravenous immunoglobulin) therapy, 424, 427, 428–429

Jewish aspects of reproduction, 829–834
Jewish evaluation of infertile couple, 829–830
Juxtacrine concept, 158

Kallikreins, 271
Kallmann's syndrome, 271, 377–378
Karyotypic abnormalities, 381
Kinetochore, 96
Kirschner retractor, 612*f*
Kleppinger bipolar forceps, 594*f*
Klinefelter's syndrome, 262
KL ligand, 82–83
KTP laser, 635

Labeled-antibody immunoassay, 68–69
Labeled complex, separation of, 69–70
Labeled-hormone immunoassay, 68
Laboratory hormone testing, indications for, 61–65
Lack of penetrance, 388
Lactotrophs, prolactin and, 158
Laparoscopic laser cauterization with endometriosis, 207*f*
Laparoscopic management of infiltrative endometriosis, 210–212
Laparoscopic myomectomy, 605–606
Laparoscopic tubal anastomosis, 620–621
Laparoscopic tubal transfer, *see* Zygote intrafallopian transfer
Laparoscopy, 24–25, 591–610
  adjunctive agents, 608–609
  combined hysteroscopy and, 581
  consent form for, 593*f*
  ectopic pregnancy and, 648
  general considerations, 598–599
  instrumentation for, 592–598
  laser, 635–637
  operating team, 592
  operative procedures, 599–608
  patient preparation, 592
  second-look (SLL), 665
  surgical results, 609–610
  for unexplained infertility, 329–330
Laparotomy, tubal surgery by means of, *see* Tubal surgery by laparotomy
Laser drilling, 637
Laser energy, 595
Laser laparoscopy, 635–637
Laser light, 629–630

Laser physics in reproductive medicine, 629–640
Lasers
  delivery systems for, 633–635
  effects and technical details of, 634*t*
  hysteroscopy and, 637–638
  in micromanipulation of preimplantation embryos and gametes, 638–639
  in pelvic reconstruction, 632–633
  physical principles of, 629–630
Laser safety, 632
Laser–tissue interactions, 630–632
Laser zona drilling, 639
Latranculin, 97–98
LCAH (congenital lipoid adrenal hyperplasia), 226
Legal aspects of infertility, 807–818
Legal parentage, 816–817
Leptin, 128–129
Leptin level, 117
Leptotene stage of meiotic prophase, 84
Leukocyte antibody detection test, 424
Leukocytes, germinal cells and, 53
Leuprolide, chemical structure of, 197*t*
Leuprolide acetate, 783–784
Leydig cells, 221–224
  peritubular cells and, 233
  Sertoli cells and, 228–229, 232–233
LH, *see* Luteinizing hormone
Life-table method, pregnancy rate by, 878*t*
Limbic structures, GnRH secretion and, 401*f*
Linear regression, 882
Lipoid adrenal hyperplasia, congenital (LCAH), 226
Lisuride, 557*t*, 564
Liver disease, chronic, 264
Logistic regression, multiple, 882
Logistic regression coefficients, 882
Long-term counseling, 38
Loupes, 615
LPD, *see* Luteal-phase deficiency
Luciferin and luciferase, 73
LUF (luteinized unruptured follicle) syndrome, 192, 466, 482
Luminescence, 71
Luminescent immunoassay, 71–74
Luteal activity, progesterone and, 145
Luteal conversion, 481
Luteal dysfunction, physiologic, 139
Luteal function
  confirmation of, 144
  tests of, 144–145
  variability in, 139*t*
Luteal phase, *see* Luteal phase of menstrual cycle
Luteal-phase deficiency (LPD), 138–144, 679
  clomiphene citrate in, 149
  management of, 147–150
  progesterone and, 142*f*

progesterone supplementation therapy in, 150
progesterone vaginal suppositories in, 149–150
treatment protocols, 149–150
Luteal-phase events, 141–143
Luteal-phase inadequacy, 135–151
  evaluation of, 135
Luteal phase of menstrual cycle, 114, 136
  abnormal, definition of, 147
  endometrial biopsy in, 145–147
  evaluation of, in clinical setting, 144–147
  in vitro fertilization, 725–727
  relaxin in, 145
Luteal-phase physiology, 136–138
Luteal rescue, 136, 143–144
Luteinization, 136
  premature, 515
  prolactin and, 159
Luteinized unruptured follicle (LUF) syndrome, 192, 466, 482
Luteinizing hormone (LH), 34, 508
  endometriosis and, 192*f*
  in GnRH therapy, 197*f*
  hypersecretion of, 128–129
  normal ranges of, 62*t*
  polycystic ovary syndrome and, 127*f*
  premature surges in, 681
  primary structure of, 526*t*
  secretion, male, 222–223
  secretory pattern in puberty, 410*f*
  surge
    day of, 776*f*
    premature, inhibition of, 545
    surrogate, human chorionic gonadotropin with follicle-stimulating hormone as, 531–532
  testosterone and, 228
Luteinizing hormone-to-follicle-stimulating hormone (LH/FSH) ratio, 497
Lutrelin, chemical structure of, 197*t*
Lymphocytes, 344
Lymphocytic hypophysitis, 181
Lymphocytic thyroiditis, 181

Macroadenoma, pituitary, 164*f*
Macrophages, testicular, 233
Macroprolactinomas, 164
Magnetic resonance imaging (MRI), 451, 454
Male-factor infertility, 12–13, 705
  abnormal semen values and, 253–359
  criteria for, 691*t*
  evaluating, 65
  hyperthyroidism and, 177
  relative severity of, 303
  ultrasound and, 483–485
Male fertility, effect of age on, 440–441

Male infertility, 221–318
  approach for couple with, 297
  clinical evaluation of, 268–270
  clomiphene citrate in, 271
  evaluation of, 261
  functional endocrine tests for, 269–270
  genital tract obstruction in, 266
  glucocorticoids in, 271–272
  laboratory evaluation for, 269
  medical management of, 270–272
  pathologic conditions in, 262–268
  prednisolone in, 271–272
  questionnaire for, 268t
  radiologic investigation of, 270
  surgical management of, 277–294
  tamoxifen in, 271
Male reproductive dysfunction, neurologic
    considerations of, 400–402
Males
  emotional aspects of infertility for, 31–32
  reproductive physiology of, 221–241
  stress and, 31–32
MAPK (microtubule-associated protein
    kinase), 91
MAR (mixed agglutination reaction),
    345–346
Maternal age
  chromosomal abnormality by, 13t
  recurrent pregnancy loss and, 418
Maternal hypothyroidism, 172
Maternal thyroid status, 172
Matrix metalloproteinases (MMP), 676
Maturation-promoting factor (MPF), 91, 96f
Maximum likelihood method of estimation,
    883
MCR (metabolic clearance rate), 511
Mechlorethamine, 265
Medial temporal lobe structures, 398
Medical genetics, 387
Mediterraneans, genetic disorders related to,
    394t
MEIA (microparticle enzyme immunoassay),
    75
Meiosis, 84, 233, 234, 763
Meiotic competence, 88–91
  failure of, 91
  GH and, 90, 90f
Meiotic completion, 96–98
  failure of, 98–101
Meiotic maturation, control of, 88–94
Meiotic oocytes, 82
Meiotic resumption, regulation of, 91–94
Melatonin, 34–35
Membranum granulosum, 84
Men, see Male entries
Menarche, 112
Mendelian patterns of inheritance, 388–390

Mendelian single-gene disorders, 388–389
Mendelian single-gene inheritance, 388
Menopausal gonadotropin, human, see hMG
    entries
Menopause, 112
Menotropins, 564
Menotropin therapy, 150
Menstrual cycle, 113–114
  changes in length of, with age, 12t
  endometrium and, 458–460
  estradiol in, 140f
  gonadotropin-releasing hormone in,
    540–543
  inhibin in, 140f
  insulin concentration and, 127f
  ovarian changes during, 462–464
  ovarian circulation during, 480–481
  pain profile relative to, 863t
  pathophysiology of, 114–118
  progesterone in, 140f
Menstrual dysfunction, causes of, 118t
MESA (microsurgical epididymal sperm
    aspiration), 301–302
Mesothelium, 190
Mesterolone, 271
Mesulergine, 557t
Metabolic clearance rate (MCR), 511
Metaphase II stage, 88
Metergoline, 564
Methotrexate, ectopic pregnancy and, 651
d-Methyl-p-tyrosine, 34
Metrodin HP, 508–509, 526
Metroplasty, 425
Microadenoma, pituitary, 163f
Microcephalic sperm, 51
Microfilaments, 97–98
Microhysteroflator, 578f
Micromanipulation of gametes, 730–734
Microparticle enzyme immunoassay
    (MEIA), 75
Microsatellite repeat loci, 373
Microtubule-associated protein kinase
    (MAPK), 91
Microtubule-associated proteins, 96
Microtubule configurations, 100f
Microtubule-organizing center, 97
Midtubal anastomosis, 619–620
Minilaparotomy, segmental resection
    through, 214
Miscarriage
  antithyroid antibodies and, 184
  autoimmune thyroid disease and, 182
  gonadotropin-releasing hormone agonists
    and, 550
Mitochondria, 86, 391
Mitochondrial inheritance, 391
Mitosis, 83
Mitotic divisions, beginning of, 96–98
Mixed agglutination reaction (MAR),
    345–346

MMP (matrix metalloproteinases), 676
Molecular diagnosis, 767–769
Molecular genetics, 371–374
  infertility and, 371–383
Monoclonal antibodies, 65
Monopolar coagulator and microelectrode,
    612–613
Monopolar electrosurgical technique,
    594–595
Monosomy, 391
Moral status of developing organism,
    826–827
Morcellator, 598
Mosaicism, 390
Mouse breast bioassay, 61
MPF (maturation-promoting factor), 91, 96f
MRI (magnetic resonance imaging), 451,
    454
Müllerian duct anomalies, 425
Multicystic ovaries, 121–122
Multifactorial inheritance, 392
Multinucleate blastomeres, 99f
Multiple logistic regression, 882
Multivariate analysis, 882
Mutations, unstable, 390
Mycobacterium tuberculosis, 365–366
Mycoplasma hominis, 365
Myoma, gonadotropin-releasing hormone
    agonists and, 546–547
Myomectomy, 547
  hysteroscopic, 585–586
  laparoscopic, 605–606
  laser, 637
Myometrial contractions, subendometrial,
    462

Nabothian cysts, 448, 449f
Nafarelin, chemical structure of, 197t
Nal–Glu, 709
Naloxone, 35
National Infertility Awareness Week
    (NIAW), 855
Nd:YAG laser, 635
Necrozoospermia, 49
Needle holders, 596, 597f
Neonatal and prepubertal girls, 112
Neural innervation of gonads, 403
Neural tube defects, 394
Neurologic considerations
  of female reproductive dysfunction,
    402–405
  in infertility, 397–405
  of male reproductive dysfunction,
    400–402
Neurotensin, 157
NIAW (National Infertility Awareness
    Week), 855
Nicotine, see Smoking

Nidation of embryo, 671
Nitabuch's layer, 677
Nonseparating assay, 72
Norepinephrine, 34, 36
    structure of, 411f
Normoprolactinemic infertility, dopamine
        agonists and, 564–565
Northern blots, 373
Northern European Caucasians, genetic dis-
        orders related to, 394t
Novak curette, 146
Null hypothesis, 876

Obstetric outcome, prenatal diagnosis, and
        follow-up study with children of in-
        tracytoplasmic single-sperm injec-
        tion, 756
Obstructed ureter, 215
Obstructive azoospermia, diagnosis and
        treatment of, 277–291
OCCC (oocyte–corona–cumulus complex),
        718f
Odds ratio, 882
Office visits, stamps used for, 24f
Ofloxacin, 272
OHSS, see Ovarian hyperstimulation syn-
        drome
Okadaic acid, 91
Oligospermia, 262
    assisted reproductive treatments of,
        297–306
    idiopathic, 271
    pregnancy rate and, 256t
    severe, evaluating endocrine linkage to,
        64f
Oligoteratoasthenozoospermia, 705
Oligozoospermia, 48
Olympus halogen light source, 594f
Omentectomy, 616f, 625
Omentopexy, 616f, 625
OMI (oocyte maturation inhibitor), 92
Oocyte collection and maturation in embryo
        culture, 717–718
Oocyte–corona–cumulus complex (OCCC),
        718f
Oocyte damage after intracytoplasmic single-
        sperm injection, 755
Oocyte depletion, 438
Oocyte development, 81–101
Oocyte freezing, 794, 801–802
Oocyte handling for intracytoplasmic single-
        sperm injection, 753–754
Oocyte maturation, stages of, 764f
Oocyte maturation inhibitor (OMI), 92
Oocyte proteins, 88
Oocyte retrieval
    for gamete intrafallopian transfer,
        691–693

guided with ultrasound, 472–474
for in vitro fertilization, 715–716
for ovum donation, 784
transvaginal, 473–474
Oocytes, 81, 763
    age and, 681
    explanted, 95
    follicle-enclosed, in vitro growth of,
        94–95
    growing, 85–88
    in vitro maturation of, 723
    meiotic, 82
    primary, 84
    secondary, 88
Oogonia, 83
Oolemma, 86–87
Ophthalmic scalpel, 615f
Opiate abuse, 266
Optical trapping, sperm manipulation with,
        638–639
Osteopontin, 422
Ovarian autoimmune involvement, 117
Ovarian blood flow during ovulation induc-
        tion therapy, 482–483
Ovarian cancer, clomiphene citrate and,
        501–502
Ovarian changes during menstrual cycle,
        462–464
Ovarian circulation
    Doppler velocimetry of, 480–483
    during menstrual cycle, 480–481
Ovarian cysts
    draining, 599
    hemorrhagic, 190
Ovarian development, fetal, 112
Ovarian diathermy, 130–131
Ovarian dysfunction, endometriosis and,
        192
Ovarian endometrioma, 192
Ovarian endometriosis, 191f
Ovarian function
    decline in, 437–439
    prolactin and, 158–159
Ovarian hyperstimulation, controlled, see
        Controlled ovarian hyperstimulation
Ovarian hyperstimulation syndrome (OHSS),
        123, 470–471
    avoidance of, 545
    GnRH agonists and, 549–550
Ovarian irregularity, 64
Ovarian reserve, diminished, 776–777
Ovarian reserve status, age and, 10
Ovarian stimulation for intracytoplasmic
        single-sperm injection, 753–754
Ovarian volume, measurements of, 125f
Ovariectomy, 403
Ovaries
    effect of age on, 437–439
    hyperstimulated, color plate facing 460
    multicystic, 121–122

normal, 448
polycystic, see Polycystic ovaries
    with polycystic appearance, 126f
    ultrasound monitoring of, 469–470
Overweight women, treatment of, 413–
        414
Oviductins, 87
Ovulation, 113
Ovulation failure, clomiphene citrate and,
        499
Ovulation induction
    clinical monitoring of, 711–715
    with clomiphene citrate, 495–502
    complications of, 470–472
    with follicle-stimulating hormone,
        525–533
    gonadotropin-releasing hormone agonists
        in, 707–708
    principles of, 516–517
    with pulsatile gonadotropin-releasing hor-
        mone, 537–551
    ultrasound and, 467–468
Ovulation induction therapy, ovarian blood
        flow during, 482–483
Ovulatory cycle
    after administration of low dose of FSH,
        530f
    natural, 477–478
Ovulatory dysfunction, anovulation and,
        481–482
Ovulatory factor, 19–22
Ovulatory factors in infertility, 6
Ovum, formation of, 90t
Ovum donation, 773–790
    donor and recipient synchronization for,
        784–786
    donor stimulation and oocyte retrieval for,
        784
    embryo transfer and posttransfer care in,
        786
    ethical issues in, 789–790
    evaluation and screening of donors for,
        779–780
    evaluation for, 773
    evaluation of potential recipients for,
        778–779
    gestational surrogacy and, 788–789
    historical perspective on, 774–775
    indications for, 777t
    as in vivo model for early reproductive
        processes, 787–788
    milestones of, 774f
    outcome of, 786–787
    patient selection and indications for,
        775–778
    for patients without ovarian function,
        781–783
    for patients with ovarian function,
        783–784
    preparation of recipient for, 780–784

Pain profile relative to menstrual cycle, 863*t*

Pain relief in endometriosis, interruption of pelvic nerves for, 208

Panoramic hysteroscope, 574

Papanicolaou stains for semen smears, 50

PAPP-A (pregnancy-associated plasma protein-A), 649

Paracrine regulation of spermatogenesis, 232

Parentage, legal and biologic, 816–817

Parenthood, single, 812–813

Parenting, shared, 846

Parlodel, 557*t*, 558

Parlodel LAR, 165

Parlodel SRO, 164

Parthenogenetic embryos, 98

Partial zonal dissection (PZD), 731, 752

Paternal age, conception rate and, 11*f*

Patient perspectives
    endometriosis and infertility, 859–869
    RESOLVE, 853–857

Payment to third parties, 817–818

PBR (peripheral benzodiazepine receptor), 225–226

PCBs (polychlorinated biphenyls), 868–865

PCC (premature chromosome condensation), 98

PCO, *see* Polycystic ovary syndrome

PCR (polymerase chain reaction), 373–374, 735, 767–769

PdG (pregnanediol glucuronide), 145

PDT (photodynamic therapy), 639–640

Pelvic adhesions, 655
    adjuvants for reduction of, 661–665
    American Fertility Society scoring method, 658*f*
    diagnosis, 656
    in endometriosis, 192
    infertility and, 655–666
    pathophysiologic process of formation of, 656–658
    prevention of, 659–661
    recommendations for prevention of, 659*t*

Pelvic inflammatory disease (PID), 7
    in ultrasound, 455–456

Pelvic nerves, interruption of, for pain relief in endometriosis, 208

Pelvic pain with endometriosis, 204

Pelvic reconstruction, lasers in, 632–633

Pelvi-Trainer, 592*f*

Pentoxifylline, 271

Percoll gradient, 300, 718–719

Pergolide, 557*t*, 563
    structural formula of, 562*f*

Pergolide mesylate, 165

Perimenopause, 114

Peritoneal endometriosis, 190
    terminology used for, 191*t*
    vaporized or excised, 207

Peritoneal factors
    in infertility, 6–7
    in ultrasound, 455–457

Peritoneal fluid, 193

Peritoneal lesions, nonendometriotic, 193*t*

Peritoneal platforms, 625, 626*f*

Peritubular cells
    Leydig cells and, 233
    Sertoli cells and, 232

PESA (percutaneous epididymal sperm aspiration), 302

P450c21 (21-hydroxylase), 379–380

PGCs (primordial germ cells), 82–83

PGD, *see* Preimplantation genetic diagnosis

Phenothiazine, 34

pH of semen, 48

Phosphorescence, 72

Photoablation, 631

Photochemistry, 631

Photodynamic therapy (PDT), 639–640

Photosensitization, 639–640

Physical examination for infertile couple, 13

Physicians
    and artificial insemination by donor, 813–814
    infertile couple and, 33–34

PI, *see* Pulsatility index

PID, *see* Pelvic inflammatory disease

Pigments, 631

Pineal gland, 34

Pinopode formation, 137, 138*f*

Pinopodes, 675

Pipelle catheter, 146

Pituitary gland, 508

Pituitary–Leydig cell axis, 228–229

Pituitary macroadenoma, 164*f*

Pituitary microadenoma, 163*f*

Pituitary necrosis, postpartum, 181

Pituitary–seminiferous tubule axis, 229–233

Pituitary–testicular axis of spermatogenic regulation, 221–229

Placentation, 676

Plasma formation, 632

Pluriglandular endocrine gland failure, autoimmune, 117

Polar body, 88, 98

Polar-body biopsy, 765, 766

Poloxamer 407, 664

Polyadenylated (poly[A]) RNA, 87

Polychlorinated biphenyls (PCBs), 868–869

Polyclonal antibodies, 65

Polycystic ovaries, 121, 122–123
    characteristics of women with, 125*t*
    ultrasound scan of, 125*f*

Polycystic ovary (PCO) syndrome, 64, 121–132
    androstenedione and, 127*f*
    cholesterol and, 128*f*
    clinical features of, 123–129, 126*t*
    clomiphene citrate and, 130
    definitions in, 121–122
    dopamine agonists and, 565
    endocrine findings in, 123–124
    etiology of, 129–130
    follicle-stimulating hormone for ovulation induction in, 529–533
    heterogeneity of, 124–126
    hormonal imbalance observed in, 528*f*
    hyperandrogenism and, 131–132
    infertility and, 130–131
    LH and, 127*f*
    management of, 130–132
    neuroendocrine disturbances in, 129*t*
    testosterone and, 127*f*
    ultrasound and, 464–466

Polydioxanone, 659

Polygenic disorders, 392

Polymerase chain reaction (PCR), 373–374, 735, 767–769

Polyploidy, 391

Polyps
    hysteroscopy and, 581–582, 584
    intrauterine, 10*f*

Polyspermy, silent, 99

Polyzoospermia, 49

Population parameter, 876

Postcoital test, 328
    poor, evaluation of, 349–350
    Sims–Huhner, 14–16

Postpartum thyroid disease, 181, 182

Power analysis, 883–884

Power density, lasers, 630

Prader–Willi syndrome, 377, 390

Precipitin assay, 66–67

Precision in testing, 60

Prednisolone in male infertility, 271–272

Prednisone, recurrent pregnancy loss and, 427

Preeclampsia, 678

Preembryo, 763
    legal status of, 833
    moral status of, 826
    term, 764

Preembryo biopsy, 765, 766–767

Preembryo research, religious aspects of, 833–834, 837, 838, 839

Pregnancy
    baseline risks of abnormal outcome of, 388*t*
    ectopic, *see* Ectopic pregnancy
    hyperthyroidism and, 178–180
    hypothyroidism and, 175–177
    iodide during, 173

---

t indicates table; *f* indicates figure

maternal TSH and hCG during, 173*f*
multiple, clomiphene citrate and, 500
thyroid physiology in, 172–173
tubal, *see* Tubal pregnancy
ultrasound monitoring, 474–475
Pregnancy-associated plasma protein-A
    (PAPP-A), 649
Pregnancy loss
    clinical versus preclinical, 419
    recurrent, *see* Recurrent pregnancy loss
Pregnancy rate, 4–5
    according to cycle rank, 730*t*
    cumulative and life-table, 257*f*
    for donor insemination, 11*f*
    duration of infertility and, 331*f*
    by life-table method, 878*t*
    by number of embryo transfers, 731*t*
    oligospermia and, 256*t*
    semen morphology and, 257–258
    sperm counts and, 256–257
    with therapeutic insemination by donor,
        258, 317–318
Pregnancy-specific β-1 glycoprotein (SP1),
    649
Pregnancy tests, 59–60
    limits of detection of blood and urine,
        647*f*
Pregnanediol glucuronide (PdG), 145
Pregnenolone
    formation of, from cholesterol, 227*f*
    metabolic pathways from, to testosterone,
        224*f*
Preimplantation embryos, chromosomal
    analysis of, 721*t*
Preimplantation genetic diagnosis (PGD),
    734–736, 761–770
    polar-body biopsy, 765, 766
    preembryo biopsy, 765, 766–767
Premature chromosome condensation (PCC),
    98
Premature ovarian failure, 64
Prenatal diagnostic tests, 393*t*
Preprolactin, 158
Prepubertal hypothyroidism, 174
Primary follicle, 84
Primary oocytes, 84
Primordial follicles, 84–85, 463
    recruitment, growth, and degeneration of,
        512*f*
Primordial germ cells (PGCs), 82–83
PRL, *see* Prolactin
Probability distribution, 876
Procreation, *see* Reproduction
Progesterone, 37
    luteal activity and, 145
    luteal-phase deficiency and, 142*f*
    in menstrual cycle, 140*f*
    normal ranges of, 62*t*
Progesterone deficiency in recurrent preg-
    nancy loss, 426

Progesterone levels, 21–22
    in vitro fertilization and, 713
    premature elevation of, 681
    salivary, 145
Progesterone supplementation therapy in
    luteal-phase deficiency, 150
Progesterone vaginal suppositories in luteal-
    phase deficiency, 149–150
Progestogens, endometriosis and, 195
Prolactin, 94, 156
    assay of, 269
    breast examination and, 163*t*
    bromocriptine and, 558–559
    calcitonin and, 156
    GnRH and, 157
    lactotrophs and, 158
    luteinization and, 159
    normal ranges of, 62*t*
    ovarian function and, 158–159
    physiology and pathophysiology, 558
    steroidogenesis and, 159
    testicular function and, 159–160
Prolactin disorders, 155–166
    evaluation of, 155
Prolactinemia, 62
Prolactin inhibitor, 156
Prolactinomas, 160–161
Prolactin secretion
    autoregulation and paracrine control of,
        157–158
    dopamine and, 156
    physiology of, 156–160
Promethazine, 661–662
Pronuclear stage transfer (PROST), 698–
    699
Pronuclear status after intracytoplasmic
    single-sperm injection, 755
Pronuclei, 751
Prophase of meiosis, 84
Propylthiouracil (PTU), 179, 180
PROST (pronuclear stage transfer), 698–
    699
Prostatitis, chronic, 272
Protein hormones, 61
Protestant aspects of reproduction, 839
Pseudoautosomal region, 375
Psychogenic infertility, 37
Psychologic treatment of infertile couple,
    37–39
Psychoneuroendocrinology of infertility,
    34–36
PTU (propylthiouracil), 179, 180
Pubertal events in girls, 112*t*
Puberty, 112–113
    LH secretory pattern in, 410*f*
Pulsatility index (PI), 475, 477, 714
    threshold value of, 478–479
Pulsed-wave Doppler system, 477
P value, 883–884
PZD (partial zonal dissection), 731, 752

Quality assurance in in vitro fertilization,
    814–815
Quality laboratory for semen analysis,
    54–55
Quinagolide, 557*t,* 563–564
    structural formula of, 562*f*

Radioimmunoassay (RIA), 68
Radiometric labeling, type of, 69
Random variable, 876
Recessive disorders
    autosomal, 389*t*
    X-linked, 389–390
Recombinant DNA, 373
Recombinant follicle-stimulating hormone
    (rFSH), 710
Record-keeping and confidentiality in in
    vitro fertilization, 815–816
Recurrent pregnancy loss, 417–429
    allogenic leukocyte immunotherapy for,
        428
    alloimmune factors in, 423–424
    antiphospholipid antibodies and, 426*t*
    aspirin and, 426–427
    autoimmune factors in, 422–423
    chromosomal analysis and, 418*t*, 420
    diagnosis, 420–424
    endometrial biopsy and, 421
    evaluation of, 417, 420*t*
    genetic aspects of, 381–383
    heparin and, 427
    hysteroscopy and, 580
    immunotherapy for, 426–428
    maternal age and, 418
    prednisone and, 427
    prevalence of diagnosis among couples
        with, 425*t*
    progesterone deficiency in, 426
    proposed mechanisms of, 418–419
    treatment of, 424–428
Reduction division, 763
Reinke crystals, 222
Relaxin in luteal phase, 145
Renal failure, chronic, 264
Reproduction
    age and, 10–12, 435–441
    assisted, 40–41
        gonadotropin-releasing hormone ago-
            nists in, 547–550
    body weight and, 409–414
    constitutional dimensions of, 807–
        808
    genes in, 374–377
    genetic issues in, 387–395
    religious aspects of, 829–841
    role of, 4
    smoking and, 7–10
    viral infections and, 367

Reproductive dysfunction
   epilepsy and, 398–399
   female, neurologic considerations of,
      402–405
   male, neurologic considerations of,
      400–402
Reproductive endocrinology, 377–381
Reproductive function, drugs and toxins
      affecting, 265t
Reproductive medicine, laser physics in,
      629–640
Reproductive physiology of men, 221–
      241
Reproductive processes, early, ovum dona-
      tion as in vivo model for, 787–
      788
Reproductive system, female, see Female
      reproductive system
Reproductive technology, 671–841
Reproductive tract
   autonomic control of, 36–37
   immunoglobulins present in, 343–344
   regulation of secretion of immunoglobu-
      lins in, 343
Reproductive treatments, assisted, see
      Assisted reproductive treatments
Research
   fetal, 808–809
   preembryo, religious aspects of, 833–834,
      837, 838, 839
Reserpine, 34
RESOLVE, 853–857
   founding of, 853–854
   mission and scope, 854
   statements of principle, 855–857
Resting follicles, 85f
Resting primordial follicles, 84
Restriction enzymes, 372–373
Restriction fragment length polymorphisms
      (RFLPs), 373
Retroverted uterus, 17f
RFLPs (restriction fragment length polymor-
      phisms), 373
rFSH (recombinant follicle-stimulating hor-
      mone), 526, 710
RIA (radioimmunoassay), 68
Ribosome number, 86
Risk, genetic, estimation of, 394–395
RNA
   polyadenylated (poly[A]), 87
   synthesized, 87–88
Role-based responsibilities and ethical
      issues, 825–826
Roman Catholic aspects of reproduction,
      837–838
RU-486, 677

Safety, laser, 632
Salivary progesterone levels, 145
Salpingectomy
   complete, 609f
   ectopic pregnancy and, 649
   partial, 608f
Salpingitis, see Fallopian tube infertility
Salpingo-ovariolysis, 599–600
Salpingostomy, 601, 602f, 622–623,
      624f
   linear, 649–650
   terminal, 636
Salpingotomy for ectopic pregnancy,
      607–608
Sample statistic, 876
Sandwich-labeled assay, 69
SAP (steroidogenesis activator polypeptide),
      225
SC (secretory component), 343
SCPs (sterol carrier protein), 224–225
SCSGF (Sertoli cell-secreted growth factor),
      232
Seatbelt region, 526
Secondary follicle, 84
Secondary oocytes, 88
Second choice or second best, terms, 846
Secretogranin-2, 158
Secretory component (SC), 343
Segmental resection
   complete, with transanal or transvaginal
      prolapse, 213–214
   through minilaparotomy, 214
Semen
   color of, 47
   consistency of, 47–48
   liquefaction of, 46–47
   pH of, 48
   volume of, 47
Semen analysis, 22–23, 45–56, 254–256,
      269
   components of, 46t
   limitations of, 55–56
   macroscopic, 46–48
   microscopic, 48–54
   normal, 240–241
   quality laboratory for, 54–55
Semen autopreservation, 797–798
Semen evaluation and preparation for intra-
      cytoplasmic single-sperm injection,
      754
Semen morphology, pregnancy rate and,
      257–258
Semen preparation for therapeutic insemina-
      tion with husband's sperm, 311–
      313
Semen smears, preparation of, 50
Semen specimen collection, 45–46
Semen values, abnormal
   evaluation for men with, 253
   male-factor infertility and, 253–259

Seminal plasma, separating spermatozoon
      from, 300–301
Seminiferous epithelium, organization of,
      236
Seminiferous growth factor (SGF), 232
Seminiferous tubule failure, 270
Sensitivity in testing, 60
Serophene, see Clomiphene citrate
Serotonin, 35
Sertoli-cell-only syndrome, 263
Sertoli cells, 233
   FSH and, 229–231
   germ cells and, interrelationships of, 231f,
      232
   Leydig cells and, 228–229, 232–233
   peritubular cells and, 232
Sertoli cell-secreted growth factor (SCSGF),
      232
Sex determination, 374–377
   scheme for, 375f
Sex selection, therapeutic insemination with
      husband's sperm for, 315
SF-1 (steroidogenic factor-1), 374
SGF (seminiferous growth factor), 232
Shared parenting, 846
Sheehan's syndrome, 181
SHIFT (synchronized hysteroscopic insemi-
      nation of fallopian tube), 587
Silent polyspermy, 99
Silicone mat, 612f
Sims–Huhner postcoital test, 14–16
Single-gene disorders, Mendelian, 388–389
Single-gene inheritance, Mendelian, 388
Single parenthood, 812–813
Sleep-associated gonadotropin secretion,
      113f
SLL (second-look laparoscopy), 665
Smoking, 266
   reproduction and, 7–10
Sorbitol, 577
Southeast Asians and Chinese, genetic disor-
      ders related to, 394t
Southern blots, 373
SP1 (pregnancy-specific β-1 glycoprotein),
      649
SPA, see Sperm penetration assay
Specificity in testing, 60
Sperm
   autoimmunity to, 346
   immotile, 266
   interaction with zona, 352–353
   microcephalic, 51
Sperm antibodies, 267
Sperm antibody testing, 16
Sperm aspiration
   microsurgical epididymal (MESA),
      301–302
   percutaneous epididymal (PESA), 302
Spermatocytes, secondary, 234
Spermatocytogenesis, 233–234

Spermatogenesis
    arrangement of, 285*f*
    duration of, 236–237
    histologic aspects of, 233–237
    paracrine regulation of, 232
    stages of, 283*f*
Spermatogenic cycle, stages of, 236*f*
Spermatogenic regulation, pituitary-testicular
        axis of, 221–229
Spermatogonial forms, 234
Spermatozoon, 235–236
    cryopreservation of, 796–799
    immunities to, *see* Immunology
    separating, from seminal plasma, 300–301
Sperm capacitation, 238
Sperm classification, 51–53
Sperm collection for gamete intrafallopian
        transfer, 691
Sperm concentration, 48–49
Sperm counts, 240
    circannual rhythm in, 23*f*
    female subfertility and, 258–259
    frequency distribution of, 254*t*, 255*t*
    literature review on, 254–256
    pregnancy rate and, 256–257
Sperm-directed antibody test, 328–329
Sperm-egg recognition, mechanisms of,
        239–240
Sperm extraction, testicular (TESE), 302
Sperm freezing, 793–794
Sperm function, cryopreservation and,
        796–797
Sperm granuloma, 280*f*
Sperm harvesting, methods of, 301–302
Sperm heads
    degenerated, 281*f*
    shapes of, 241*t*
Spermiogenesis, 233, 234–235
Sperm manipulation with optical trapping,
        638–639
Sperm maturation in epididymis, 237–238
Sperm migration tests, in vitro, 15–16
Sperm morphology, 23, 50–51
Sperm motility, 49–50
    assessing, 240–241
    changes in, 238
    cycles to conception and, 255*t*
    frequency distribution of, 254*t*, 255*t*
Sperm-panning test, 346
Sperm penetration assay (SPA), 298–300
    clinical indications for, 301*f*
Sperm penetration test, 15
Sperm polypeptide p95, 239–240
Sperm preparation and insemination in
        embryo culture, 718–719
Sperm production, immunology and,
        353–355
Sperm protein Sp56, 239
Sperm surface, detection of immunoglobu-
        lins on, 345

Sperm transport system failure, 484–485
Spinnbarkeit, 14, 15
Spironolactone, 131
Spontaneous abortion, 418
    age and risk for, 12*t*
    recurrent, *see* Recurrent pregnancy loss
Stamps used for office visits, 24*f*
Stangel retrograde lavage cannula, 613
StAR (steroidogenic acute regulatory pro-
        tein), 226–227
Statistical analysis
    of infertility data, 875–885
    when follow-up is not uniform, 877–880
    when follow-up is uniform, 880–883
Statistical significance, 876
Statistical techniques, 877–883
Stein–Leventhal syndrome, 123
Sterility, defined, 4
Steroid hormones, 379–381
Steroidogenesis, prolactin and, 159
Steroidogenesis activator polypeptide (SAP),
        225
Steroidogenic acute regulatory protein
        (StAR), 226–227
Steroidogenic factor-1 (SF-1), 374
Steroids, 37
Sterol carrier protein (SCP2), 224–225
Stress, 5
    effects in infertility, 40
    hyperprolactinemia and, 35–36
    men and, 31–32
Student's *t* test, 881–882
Subendometrial myometrial contractions,
        462
Subfertility
    female, sperm count and, 258–259
    history of, 418–419
Substance P, 157
Subzonal sperm insertion (SUZI), 732–733,
        752
Suction irrigator, 595
Sulfasalazine, 266
Supercooling, 794
Supernumerary cryopreserved embryos, fate
        of, 801
Surgicel, 664
Surrogacy, gestational, 788–789
SUZI (subzonal sperm insertion), 732–733,
        752
Synapsis, 763
Synchronized hysteroscopic insemination of
        fallopian tube (SHIFT), 587
Syncytiotrophoblasts, 673
Synechiae, intrauterine, 6*f*

T$_3$ (triiodothyronine), 172
T$_4$ (tetraiodothyronine), 172
Tachycardia, fetal, 180

Tag-labeled immunoassay, 68
Tamoxifen in male infertility, 271
Tanner staging, 112
TAS (transabdominal ultrasonography), 448
TBG (thyroid hormone binding globulin),
        172
T cells, 342
TeBG (testosterone–estradiol-binding globu-
        lin), 227–228
Technology, reproductive, 671–841
Teflon-coated dissecting rods, 614*f*
Temporal lobe epilepsy (TLE), 398–399
Teratospermia, 262
Terguride, 557*t*, 564
Tertiary follicle, 84
TESE (testicular sperm extraction), 302
Testes, *see* Testis
Testicle, undescended, microsurgery for,
        291–294
Testicular autotransplantation, rationale for,
        291–293
Testicular biopsy, 270
    quantitative interpretation of findings at,
        282–283
Testicular dysfunction, systemic illness asso-
        ciated with, 264–265
Testicular failure
    primary, 262–264
    ultrasound and, 483–484
Testicular feminization, 265
Testicular function
    drugs and toxins affecting, 265–266
    prolactin and, 159–160
Testicular macrophages, 233
Testicular sperm extraction (TESE), 302
Testicular torsion, 263
Testicular trauma and inflammation, 263
Testis, 221
    changes in, 222
    effects of temperature on, 267–268
    measurement of, 268
    vasectomy effects on, 280–282
    volume of, 13
Testolactone, 271
Testosterone, 222
    assay of, 269
    chemical structure of, 195*f*
    LH and, 228
    metabolic pathways from pregnenolone to,
        224*f*
    normal ranges of, 62*t*
    polycystic ovary syndrome and, 127*f*
Testosterone biosynthesis, 224
Testosterone–estradiol-binding globulin
        (TeBG), 227–228
Testosterone transport and metabolism,
        227–228
Tetrads, 84
Tetraiodothyronine (T$_4$), 172
TGF-β_1 (transforming growth factor β_1), 82

Therapeutic insemination by donor (TID), 256, 393, 831–832
  donor selection and screening for, 315–317
  evaluation for, 310
  guidelines for, 316*t*
  history of, 310–311
  indications for, 315
  legal aspects of, 318
  pregnancy rate with, 258, 317–318
  timing of, 317
  use of frozen donor semen in, 798–799
Therapeutic insemination with husband's sperm (TIH), 309–318, 831
  complications of, 313–314
  evaluation for, 309, 311
  indications for, 311
  semen preparation for, 311–313
  for sex selection, 315
  success rates with, 314–315
  techniques for, 313
  timing of, 311
Thioridazine, 40
Threshold PI value, 478–479
Thyroglobulin, 173
Thyroid antibodies, 423
Thyroid development, fetal, 171–172
Thyroid disease
  autoimmune, 175, 182
  postpartum, 181, 182
Thyroid disorders, 171–184
  treatment of patient with infertility with, 182–184
  TSH and, 183*f*
Thyroid dysfunction, neonatal, 180–181
Thyroid hormone binding globulin (TBG), 172
Thyroid nodules and cancer, 181
Thyroid physiology in pregnancy, 172–173
Thyroid status, maternal, 172
Thyroid-stimulating hormone (TSH), 171–172
  hypothyroidism and, 174
  maternal, during pregnancy, 173*f*
  normal ranges of, 62*t*
  thyroid disorders and, 183*f*
Thyroid storm, 180
Thyrotoxicosis, 177
  gestational transient (GTT), 178, 179
Thyrotropin-releasing hormone (TRH), 156–157
Thyroxine, free, normal ranges of, 62*t*
TID, *see* Therapeutic insemination by donor
TIH, *see* Therapeutic insemination with husband's sperm
Tissue–laser interactions, 630–632
Tissue retrieval bags, 598

TLE (temporal lobe epilepsy), 398–399
TLX (trophoblast/lymphocyte cross-reactive) antigen, 364
Toxic multinodular goiter, 179
Transabdominal ultrasonography (TAS), 448
Transanal or transvaginal prolapse, complete segmental resection with, 213–214
Transanal or transvaginal resection, partial, 213
Transcervical embryo transfer, *see* In vitro fertilization
Transdermal estradiol delivery, 782–783
Transfer catheter loading for gamete intrafallopian transfer, 693–696
Transforming growth factor β_1 (TGF–β_1), 82
Translocations, 391
Transvaginal oocyte retrieval, 473–474
Transvaginal ultrasonography (TVS), 447–448
TRH (thyrotropin-releasing hormone), 156–157
Triiodothyronine (T_3), 172
Triple 7 regimen, 497–498
Trisomy, 391
Trisomy 21, 392
Trophoblastic cells, 419
Trophoblastic disease, 179
Trophoblast invasion, 675–676
  unrestricted, 678
Trophoblast/lymphocyte cross-reactive (TLX) antigen, 364
Trophoblasts, 673
Trophoectoderm biopsy, 767
TSH, *see* Thyroid-stimulating hormone
T-shaped uterus, 451–452
Tubal anastomosis, laparoscopic, 620–621
Tubal catheterization guided by ultrasound, 458
Tubal disease, 704
Tubal dysfunction, endometriosis and, 192–193
Tubal factors in ultrasound, 455–457
Tubal milking, ectopic pregnancy and, 649
Tubal mobility, effect of age on, 440
Tubal occlusion, 362
Tubal operations, ectopic pregnancy after, 645*t*
Tubal ostium, cannulation of, color plate facing 580
Tubal patency, demonstration of, 457–458
Tubal pregnancy, management of, 636–637
Tubal surgery by laparotomy, 611–627
  adhesion prevention in, 625–627
  instruments for, 612–615
  operative procedures, 616–623
  results of, 624–625
Tubal transfer, laparoscopic, *see* Zygote intrafallopian transfer
Tubo-ovarian abscess, 456, 457*f*

Tubo-ovarian complex, 362
  ruptured, 362
Turner's syndrome, 115, 374
TVS (transvaginal ultrasonography), 447–448
Tyrosine autophosphorylation, 126

Ultrasonographic scan, baseline, 468–469
Ultrasound, 447
  embryo transfer guided by, 474
  endometriosis and, 452–455
  female infertility and, 448–467
  follicular growth and, 469–470
  gamete intrafallopian transfer guided by, 474
  in infertility, 447–485
  intrauterine contraceptive device and, 452
  male-factor infertility and, 483–485
  monitoring of ovaries, 469–470
  monitoring pregnancy, 474–475
  monitoring therapy with, 467–470
  multiple gestations and, 472
  oocyte retrieval guided with, 472–474
  ovulation induction and, 467–468
  pelvic inflammatory disease in, 455–456
  polycystic ovary syndrome and, 464–466
  procedures guided by, 472–474
  testicular failure and, 483–484
  tubal and peritoneal factors in, 455–457
  tubal catheterization guided by, 458
  uterine anomalies and, 451–452
  uterine fibroids and, 448–451
Underweight women, treatment of, 412–413
Undescended testicle, microsurgery for, 291–294
Unexplained infertility, 323–335, 705
  baseline prognosis without treatment, 330–331
  bromocriptine in, 331, 332*f*
  clomiphene citrate in, 332–333
  contributing factors, 324–325
  counseling in, 334–335
  danazol in, 332
  diagnostic tests having normal results in, 327*t*
  duration of infertility with, 326*f*
  epidemiology of, 324–325
  evaluation of, 323
  intrauterine insemination and, 333–334
  in vitro fertilization and, 334
  judging effectiveness of treatment, 331
  management of, 330–334
  prevalence of, 324
  problems defining, 326–327
  proportion of couples with, 325*t*
Unicornuate uterus, 8*f*
Unstable mutations, 390
Ureaplasma urealyticum, 365

Ureter, obstructed, 215
Uterine adenomyosis, 160
Uterine anomalies, ultrasound and, 451–452
Uterine cavity distorted by fibroid, 7f, 8f
Uterine circulation, Doppler velocimetry of, 477–480
Uterine corpus, hypoplastic, 425
Uterine factors in infertility, 7
Uterine fibroids, ultrasound and, 448–451
Uterine perforation by hysteroscopy, 579
Uterine perfusion
    endometrial receptivity and, 479
    infertility and, 478–480
Uterine septa, hysteroscopy and, 584, 586–587
Uterine suspension, 625
Uterine synechiae, 452, 453f, 579
Uterosacral ligament, ablation of, 636
Uterus
    bicornuate, 8f, 9f
    effect of age on, 439
    embryo interactions with, during implantation, 671–682
    examination of, 420
    normal, 448
    retroverted, 17f
    structure of, decidualization and, 676–678
    three-dimensional ultrasound scan of, color plate facing 460
    unicornuate, 8f

Vaginal fluid, 343
Vaginal suppositories, progesterone, in luteal-phase deficiency, 149–150
Varicoceles, 267, 484
Vas deferens
    congenital absence of, 290–291

inguinal disruption of, after herniorrhaphy, 289
Vasectomy
    effects on testis and epididymis, 280–282
    evaluation of obstruction not caused by, 287–289
Vasectomy reversal, see Vasovasostomy
Vasoactive intestinal polypeptide (VIP), 157
Vasoepididymostomy
    crossover, 289, 290f
    fertility after, 285–287
    microsurgical, 283–285
    specific tubule technique for, 287f
Vasogram
    of epididymis, 286f
    performing, 288
Vasovasostomy, 255–256, 277
    microsurgical approach, 277–279
    results of, 279–280
Vertical transmission, 389
Vickers–Owens needle carriers, 614f
Vicryl, 659
VIP (vasoactive intestinal polypeptide), 157
Viral infections, reproduction and, 367
Vitrification method, 722

Weathering, 435
Weight, body, see Body weight
Weight and height table for women, 412t
Weight loss, 410
Western blots, 373
Women, see also Female entries
    antisperm antibodies in, 349
    cause of immunology among, 355
    emotional aspects of infertility for, 31
    height and weight table for, 412t

overweight, treatment of, 413–414
underweight, treatment of, 412–413

X-chromosome aneuploidy, 382
X chromosomes, 374
X-linked dominant disorders, 390
X-linked recessive disorders, 389–390
47,XYY, 262

Y chromosomes, 375
    map of, 376f
Y-linked inheritance, 390
Yolk sac, 475

Zidovudine (AZT), 264
ZIFT (zygote intrafallopian transfer), 298, 305, 689, 751
Zinc finger proteins, 375
Zoladex, chemical structure of, 197t
Zona-free hamster egg penetration test, 350–351
Zona interaction with sperm, 352–353
Zona-opening procedures, 730–732
Zona pellucida, 87
Zona pellucida drilling, 731
    laser, 639
Zona reaction, 87
Zondek pregnancy test, 60
ZP3 glycoprotein, 239
Zygote, 391
Zygote intrafallopian transfer (ZIFT), 298, 305, 689, 751
Zygotene stage of meiotic prophase, 84